Paramedic Care: Principles & Practice

Fifth Edition

Volume 3

Medical Emergencies

BRYAN E. BLEDSOE, DO, FACEP, FAAEM, EMT-P
Professor of Emergency Medicine
University of Nevada, Las Vegas School of Medicine
University of Nevada, Reno School of Medicine
Attending Emergency Physician
University Medical Center of Southern Nevada
Medical Director, MedicWest Ambulance
Las Vegas, Nevada

RICHARD A. CHERRY, MS, EMT-P
Training Consultant
Northern Onondaga Volunteer Ambulance
Liverpool, New York

LEGACY AUTHOR

ROBERT S. PORTER

Pearson

330 Hudson Street, NY, NY 10013

Publisher: Julie Levin Alexander
Publisher's Assistant: Sarah Henrich
Editor: Sladjana Repic Bruno
Editorial Assistant: Lisa Narine
Development Editor: Sandra Breuer
Copyeditor: Deborah Wenger
Director, Publishing Operations: Paul DeLuca
Team Lead, Program Management: Melissa Bashe
Team Lead, Project Management: Cynthia Zonneveld
Manufacturing Buyer: Maura Zaldivar-Garcia
Art Director: Mary Siener
Cover and Interior Designer: Mary Siener
Managing Photography Editor: Michal Heron
Vice President of Sales & Marketing: David Gesell
Vice President, Director of Marketing: Margaret Waples
Senior Field Marketing Manager: Brian Hoehl
Marketing Assistant: Amy Pfund
Senior Producer: Amy Peltier
Media Producer and Project Manager: Lisa Rinaldi
Full-Service Project Manager: Amy Kopperude/ iEnergizer Aptara®, Ltd.
Composition: iEnergizer Aptara®, Ltd.
Printer/Binder: LSC Communications
Cover Printer: LSC Communications
Cover Image: ollo/Getty Images, Rudi Von Briel/ Getty Images

Notice
The author and the publisher of this book have taken care to make certain that the information given is correct and compatible with the standards generally accepted at the time of publication. Nevertheless, as new information becomes available, changes in treatment and in the use of equipment and procedures become necessary. The reader is advised to carefully consult the instruction and information material included in each piece of equipment or device before administration. Students are warned that the use of any techniques must be authorized by their medical advisor, where appropriate, in accordance with local laws and regulations. The publisher disclaims any liability, loss, injury, or damage incurred as a consequence, directly or indirectly, of the use and application of any of the contents of this book.

Library of Congress Cataloging-in-Publication Data

Names: Bledsoe, Bryan E., author. | Cherry, Richard A., author. | Porter, Robert S., author.
Title: Paramedic care : principles & practice | Bryan E. Bledsoe, Richard A. Cherry, Robert S. Porter.
Description: Fifth edition. | Boston : Pearson Education, Inc., 2016- | Includes bibliographical references and index.
Identifiers: LCCN 2016009904 | ISBN 9780134538730 (pbk. : alk. paper) | ISBN 0134538730 (pbk. : alk. paper)
Subjects: | MESH: Emergencies | Emergency Medical Services | Emergency Medical Technicians
Classification: LCC RC86.7 | NLM WB 105 | DDC 616.02/5—dc23 LC record available at http://lccn.loc.gov/2016009904

Pearson

ISBN 10: 0-13-453873-0
ISBN 13: 978-0-13-453873-0

23 2022

This text is respectfully dedicated to all EMS personnel
who have made the ultimate sacrifice. Their memory
and good deeds will forever be in our thoughts and prayers.

BEB, RAC

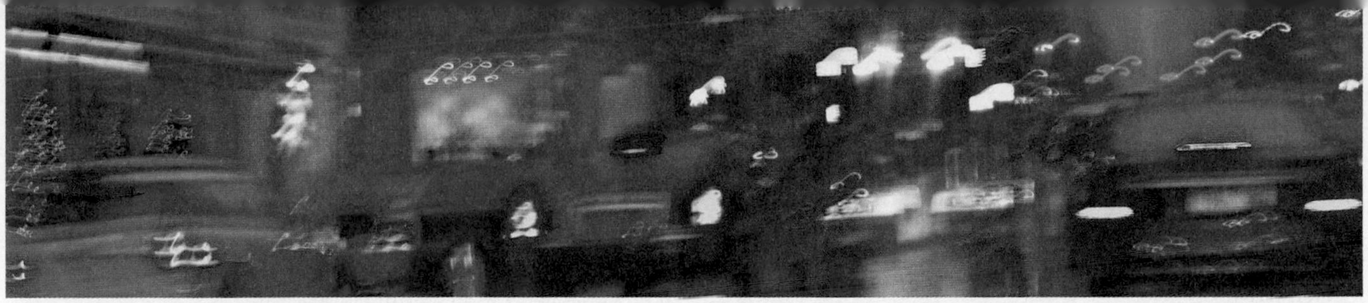

Contents

Preface to Volume 3 xi
Acknowledgments xiii
About the Authors xvii

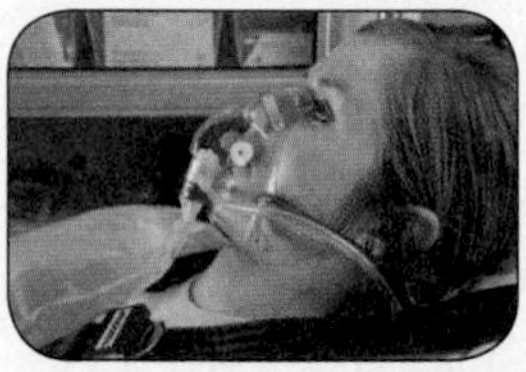

1 Pulmonology 1

Introduction 3
Review of Respiratory Anatomy and Physiology 3
- Upper Airway Anatomy 3
- Lower Airway Anatomy 5
- Physiologic Processes 7

Pathophysiology 12
- Disruption in Ventilation 13
- Disruption in Diffusion 14
- Disruption in Perfusion 14

Assessment of the Respiratory System 14
- Scene Size-Up 14
- Primary Assessment 15
- Secondary Assessment 16

Management of Respiratory Disorders 24
- Management Principles 24

Specific Respiratory Diseases 25
- Upper Airway Obstruction 25
- Noncardiogenic Pulmonary Edema/Acute Respiratory Distress Syndrome 26
- Obstructive Lung Disease 27
- Emphysema 30
- Chronic Bronchitis 31
- Asthma 32
- Upper Respiratory Infection 36
- Pneumonia 37
- Severe Acute Respiratory Syndrome (SARS) 39
- Middle East Respiratory Syndrome (MERS) 39
- Lung Cancer 40
- Toxic Inhalation 41
- Carbon Monoxide Inhalation 41
- Pulmonary Embolism 43
- Spontaneous Pneumothorax 44
- Hyperventilation Syndrome 44
- Central Nervous System Dysfunction 45
- Dysfunction of the Spinal Cord, Nerves, or Respiratory Muscles 45

2 Cardiology 49

Introduction 52
Cardiovascular Anatomy 53
- Anatomy of the Heart 53
- Anatomy of the Peripheral Circulation 57

Cardiac Physiology 57
- The Cardiac Cycle 57
- Nervous Control of the Heart 61
- The Heart as an Endocrine Organ 62
- Role of Electrolytes 62
- Electrophysiology 62

Electrocardiographic Monitoring 65
- The Electrocardiogram 66
- Relationship of the ECG to Electrical Events in the Heart 68
- Interpretation of Rhythm Strips 74

Arrhythmias 75
- Mechanism of Impulse Formation 75
- Classification of Arrhythmias 76
- Arrhythmias Originating in the SA Node 76
- Arrhythmias Originating in the Atria 82
- Arrhythmias Originating within the AV Junction (AV Blocks) 88
- Arrhythmias Sustained or Originating in the AV Junction 93
- Arrhythmias Originating in the Ventricles 96
- Artificial Pacemaker Rhythm 105
- Pulseless Electrical Activity 108
- Arrhythmias Resulting from Disorders of Conduction 108
- ECG Changes from Electrolyte Abnormalities and Hypothermia 109

Assessment of the Cardiovascular Patient 111
- Scene Size-up and Primary Assessment 111
- History 111
- Physical Examination 114

Management of Cardiovascular Emergencies 117
- Basic Life Support 117
- Advanced Life Support 117

Monitoring ECG in the Field 117
Vagal Maneuvers 119
Precordial Thump 119
Pharmacological Management 120
Defibrillation 122
Emergency Synchronized Cardioversion 125
Transcutaneous Cardiac Pacing 125
Carotid Sinus Massage 128
Support and Communication 130
Managing Specific Cardiovascular Emergencies 130
Acute Coronary Syndrome 131
Angina Pectoris 131
Myocardial Infarction 133
Heart Failure 139
Cardiac Tamponade 143
Hypertensive Emergencies 145
Cardiogenic Shock 147
Cardiac Arrest 149
Peripheral Vascular and Other Cardiovascular Emergencies 154
Reviewing the Cardiac Conductive System 157
ECG Recording 157
ECG Leads 158
Bipolar Limb Leads 158
Unipolar or Augmented Limb Leads 159
Precordial Leads 161
Mean QRS Axis Determination 162
Axis Deviation 162
The Normal 12-Lead ECG 164
Disease Findings 164
Evolution of Acute Coronary Syndrome 166
Localization of Acute Myocardial Infarction 167
Early Repolarization Versus STEMI 177
Conduction Abnormalities 177
AV Blocks 177
Bundle Branch Blocks 178
Chamber Enlargement 182
Prehospital ECG Monitoring 187
Prehospital 12-Lead ECG Monitoring 187

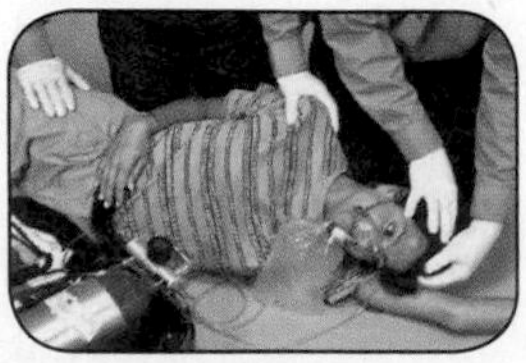

3 Neurology 195
Introduction 197
Anatomy and Physiology 197
The Central Nervous System 198
The Peripheral Nervous System 203
Pathophysiology 205
Alteration in Cognitive Systems 205
Central Nervous System Disorders 206
Cerebral Homeostasis 206
Peripheral Nervous System Disorders 206
Autonomic Nervous System Disorders 207
General Assessment Findings 207
Scene Size-Up and Primary Assessment 207
Secondary Assessment 208
Ongoing Assessment 213
Management of Specific Nervous System Emergencies 213
Altered Mental Status 213
Stroke and Intracranial Hemorrhage 214
Seizures and Epilepsy 220
Syncope 223
Headache 223
Cranial Nerve Disorders 225
"Weak and Dizzy" 226
Neoplasms 226
Brain Abscess 228
Degenerative Neurologic Disorders and Dementia 228
Back Pain and Nontraumatic Spinal Disorders 231

4 Endocrinology 237
Introduction 239
Anatomy and Physiology 239
Hypothalamus 240
Pituitary Gland 243
Thyroid Gland 244
Parathyroid Glands 244
Thymus Gland 244
Pancreas 244
Adrenal Glands 245
Gonads 246
Pineal Gland 246
Other Organs with Endocrine Activity 246
Endocrine Disorders and Emergencies 247
Disorders of the Pancreas 247
Disorders of the Thyroid Gland 255
Disorders of the Adrenal Glands 257

5 Immunology 261
Introduction 263
Pathophysiology 263
The Immune System 263
Allergies 264
Anaphylaxis 266
Assessment Findings in Anaphylaxis 266
Management of Anaphylaxis 268
Protect the Airway 270
Administer Medications 270
Offer Psychological Support 271

Assessment Findings in Allergic Reaction 271
Management of Allergic Reactions 271
Patient Education 272

6 Gastroenterology 275
Introduction 277
General Pathophysiology, Assessment, and Treatment 277
General Pathophysiology 277
General Assessment 278
General Treatment 280
Specific Illnesses 280
Upper Gastrointestinal Diseases 281
Lower Gastrointestinal Diseases 287
Accessory Organ Diseases 293

7 Urology and Nephrology 300
Introduction 302
Anatomy and Physiology 303
Kidneys 303
Ureters 306
Urinary Bladder 306
Urethra 306
Testes 307
Epididymis and Vas Deferens 307
Prostate Gland 307
Penis 307
General Mechanisms of Nontraumatic Tissue Problems 308
General Pathophysiology, Assessment, and Management 308
Pathophysiologic Basis of Pain 308
Causes of Pain 308
Types of Pain 308
Assessment and Management 308
Renal and Urologic Emergencies 311
Acute Kidney Injury 311
Chronic Kidney Disease 314
Renal Calculi 318
Priapism 320
Testicular Torsion 320
Urinary Tract Infection 320

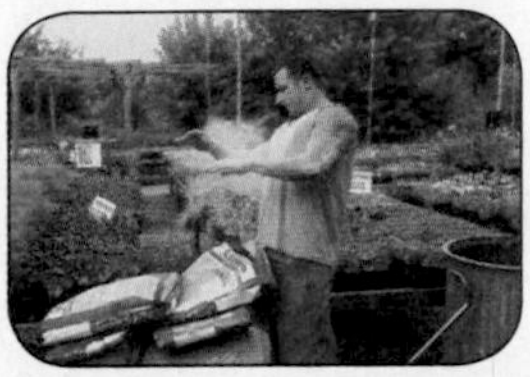

8 Toxicology and Substance Abuse 325
Introduction 326
Epidemiology 327
Poison Control Centers 327
Routes of Toxic Exposure 327
Ingestion 328
Inhalation 328
Surface Absorption 328
Injection 328
General Principles of Toxicologic Assessment and Management 329
Scene Size-Up 329
Primary Assessment 329
Secondary Assessment 329
Treatment 329
Ingested Toxins 331
Assessment 331
Inhaled Toxins 332
Surface-Absorbed Toxins 333
Specific Ingested, Inhaled, and Absorbed Toxins 333
Carbon Monoxide 333
Cyanide 341
Cardiac Medications 343
Caustic Substances 344
Hydrofluoric Acid 345
Alcohol 345
Hydrocarbons 345
Tricyclic Antidepressants 346
MAO Inhibitors 346
Newer Antidepressants 347
Lithium 348
Salicylates 348
Acetaminophen 349
Other Nonprescription Pain Medications 349
Theophylline 350
Metals 350
Lead and Mercury 351
Contaminated Food 351
Poisonous Plants and Mushrooms 352
Injected Toxins 352
General Principles of Management 352
Bites and Stings 353
Snakebites 356
Substance Abuse and Overdose 359
Alcohol Abuse 362
Physiologic Effects 362
General Alcoholic Profile 363
Consequences of Chronic Alcohol Ingestion 363

9 Hematology 368
Introduction 369
Anatomy, Physiology, and Pathophysiology 370
Components of Blood 370
Hemostasis 376
Blood Products and Blood Typing 377
Transfusion Reactions 379

General Assessment and Management 379
- Scene Size-Up 379
- Primary Assessment 379
- Secondary Assessment 380
- General Management of Hematopoietic Emergencies 382

Managing Specific Hematopoietic Disorders 383
- Diseases of the Red Blood Cells 383
- Diseases of the White Blood Cells 385
- Diseases of the Platelets/Blood Clotting Abnormalities 386
- Other Hematopoietic Disorders 388

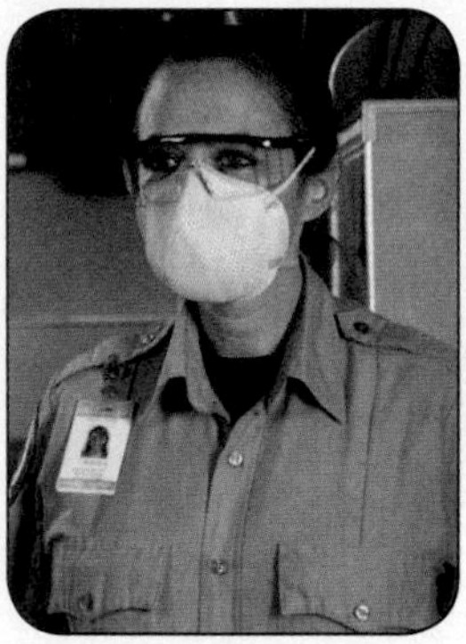

10 Infectious Diseases and Sepsis 391

Introduction 393

Public Health Principles 394

Public Health Agencies 394

Microorganisms 395
- Bacteria 395
- Viruses 396
- Other Microorganisms 396

Contraction, Transmission, and Stages of Disease 397
- Phases of the Infectious Process 399

The Body's Defenses Against Disease 399
- The Immune System 399
- The Complement System 400
- The Lymphatic System 400
- Individual Host Immunity 401

Infection Control in Prehospital Care 401
- Preparation for Response 401
- Response 402
- Patient Contact 403
- Recovery 406
- Infectious Disease Exposures 408

Assessment of the Patient with Infectious Disease 408
- Past Medical History 409
- The Physical Examination 409

Specific Infectious Diseases 410
- Diseases of Immediate Concern to EMS Providers 410
- Other Infectious Conditions of the Respiratory System 427
- GI System Infections 428
- Nervous System Infections 429
- Sexually Transmitted Diseases 433
- Diseases of the Skin 436
- Bedbugs 437
- Nosocomial Infections 438

Patient Education 438

Preventing Disease Transmission 438

Sepsis/Systemic Inflammatory Response Syndrome (SIRS) 439

11 Psychiatric and Behavioral Disorders 444

Introduction 446

Behavioral Emergencies 446

Pathophysiology of Psychiatric Disorders 446
- Biological 446
- Psychosocial 447
- Sociocultural 447

Assessment of Behavioral Emergency Patients 447
- Scene Size-Up 447
- Primary Assessment 448
- Secondary Assessment 448
- Mental Status Examination 449
- Psychiatric Medications 449

Specific Psychiatric Disorders 449
- Cognitive Disorders 450
- Schizophrenia 450
- Anxiety and Related Disorders 451
- Mood Disorders 452
- Substance-Related Disorders 453
- Somatoform Disorders 454
- Factitious Disorders 454
- Dissociative Disorders 454
- Eating Disorders 455
- Personality Disorders 455
- Personality Disorder Clusters 455
- Impulse Control Disorders 456
- Suicide 456
- Age-Related Conditions 457
- Excited Delirium Syndrome 457

Management of Behavioral Emergencies 458
- TASERed Patients 458
- Medical Care 459
- Psychological Care 459

Violent Patients and Restraint 460
- Methods of Restraint 460

12 Diseases of the Eyes, Ears, Nose, and Throat 465

Introduction 466

Eyes 467
- Anatomy of the Eye 467
- Medical Conditions of the Eye 468

Ears 472
Anatomy of the Ear 472
Medical Conditions of the Ear 473
Nose 475
Anatomy and Physiology of the Nose 475
Medical Conditions of the Nose 476
Throat 478
Anatomy and Physiology of the Mouth and Throat 478
Medical Conditions of the Mouth and Throat 480

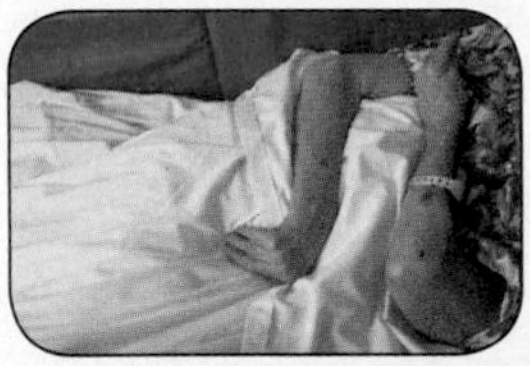

13 Nontraumatic Musculoskeletal Disorders 485

Introduction 486
Anatomy and Physiology Review 487
Skeletal System 487
Muscular System 490
Assessment and Findings 491
Nontraumatic Musculoskeletal Conditions 491
Overuse/Repetitive-Motion Disorders 491
Degenerative Conditions 493
Inflammatory Conditions 494
Infectious Conditions 496
Neoplastic Processes 498
Chronic Pain Syndrome 498
Pediatric Conditions 499

Precautions on Bloodborne Pathogens and Infectious Diseases 503
Suggested Responses to "You Make the Call" 505
Answers to Review Questions 510
Glossary 512
Index 527

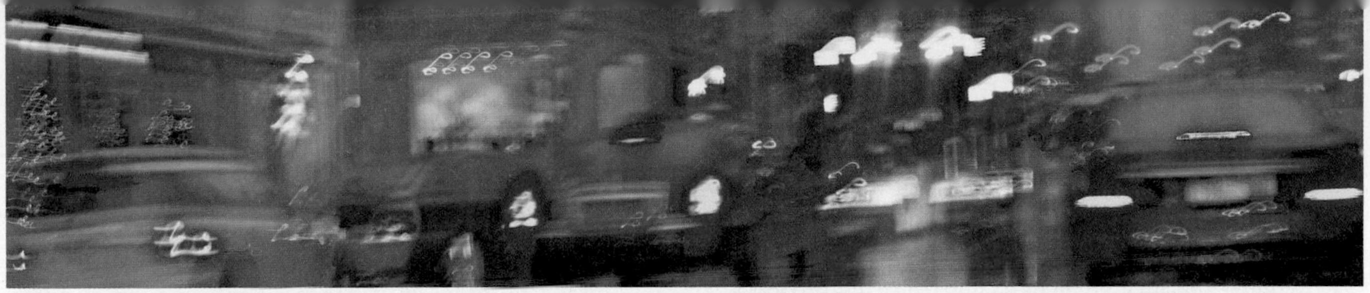

Preface to Volume 3

Advanced life support (ALS) and paramedic care were initially developed to treat cardiac problems in the field, specifically sudden death. Many people were suffering acute coronary events and dying before reaching the hospital. Physicians with foresight believed that rapid prehospital intervention could mean the difference between life and death for many people. The earliest origins of EMS were this initial emphasis on prehospital cardiac care, which developed simultaneously with the early advances in trauma care. Over the years, EMS proved effective in treating different types of cardiac emergencies. As EMS evolved, prehospital care was expanded to many other types of medical emergencies, including diabetic emergencies and respiratory emergencies.

Under the current *National EMS Education Standards* and the accompanying *Paramedic Instructional Guidelines*, paramedics are responsible for a much more detailed understanding of medical emergencies. Those Standards and Instructional Guidelines, on which this book is based, address in detail the various types of medical emergencies. Cardiac emergencies still represent the most common reason EMS is summoned, and the discussion of cardiac emergencies remains the most comprehensive in the text and is consistent with the *2015 American Heart Association Guidelines for Cardiopulmonary Resuscitation and Emergency Cardiovascular Care*.

Paramedics are also expected to have a high level of understanding of emergencies involving other body systems. In this volume, we briefly review important anatomy and physiology as it applies to each emergency, followed by a discussion of the relevant pathophysiology. Finally, we present focused prehospital assessment and treatment for each type of medical emergency. *Paramedic Care: Principles & Practice*, Volume 3, *Medical Emergencies*, provides a detailed discussion of virtually all types of medical emergencies likely to be encountered in the prehospital setting.

This volume follows a systems approach that also parallels the various subspecialties of internal medicine.

Overview of the Chapters . . . and What's New in the 5th Edition?

CHAPTER 1 Pulmonology introduces the paramedic student to commonly encountered respiratory system emergencies. Emphasis is on the recognition and treatment of reactive airway diseases such as asthma.

New in the 5th Edition: Emphasis on administering just enough oxygen to achieve **normoxia** if hypoxia is determined. (Dangers of hyperoxia are stressed.) There is a new section on **Middle Eastern Respiratory Syndrome (MERS)**.

CHAPTER 2 Cardiology presents the material crucial to advanced prehospital cardiac care. The first part of the chapter reviews essential anatomy and physiology and introduces electrophysiology. The second part of the chapter deals with cardiac emergencies and peripheral vascular system emergencies. The third part addresses 12-lead ECG interpretation and prehospital application of 12-lead ECG diagnostics and monitoring.

New in the 5th Edition: A detailed new section on **cardiac arrest in pregnancy** has been added. This chapter (and all chapters in all five volumes) updated as needed for consistency with the 2015 AHA guidelines.

CHAPTER 3 Neurology reviews the anatomy and physiology of the central and peripheral nervous systems. This is followed by a detailed discussion of neurologic emergencies.

CHAPTER 4 Endocrinology is a detailed discussion of the endocrine system, which, along with the nervous system, is an alternative control system for the body. Emphasis is placed on diabetic emergencies, as they are by far the most common endocrine emergency encountered by paramedics.

CHAPTER 5 Immunology reviews the immune system, with particular emphasis on hypersensitivity reactions (allergic reactions). The chapter emphasizes prehospital recognition and treatment of allergic reactions, particularly the severe reactions known as anaphylaxis.

CHAPTER 6 Gastroenterology is a detailed discussion of emergencies arising within the gastrointestinal system. The chapter initially reviews the relevant anatomy and physiology and follows this with a discussion of assessment and treatment of gastroenterologic emergencies.

New in the 5th Edition: A new section on **cyclical vomiting syndrome (CVS)** and a new section on **irritable bowel disease (IBS)** have been added.

CHAPTER 7 Urology and Nephrology presents an overview of emergencies that arise from the genitourinary system and the male reproductive system. This includes a discussion of infectious emergencies, renal failure, and other problems.

CHAPTER 8 Toxicology and Substance Abuse provides a detailed description of basic toxicology as it applies to prehospital care. The chapter reviews both common and uncommon causes of poisoning. In addition to accidental poisoning, there is a detailed discussion of the various drugs of abuse that are frequently seen in prehospital care.

New in the 5th Edition: Tables listing **toxic syndromes** and **drugs of abuse** have been updated.

CHAPTER 9 Hematology is a comprehensive chapter covering the blood and the reticuloendothelial system. The beginning of the chapter provides a detailed discussion of the blood and blood-forming organs. This is followed by a discussion of hematologic emergencies seen in emergency care.

CHAPTER 10 Infectious Diseases and Sepsis addresses an important but often overlooked aspect of prehospital care. Infectious diseases pose a risk to both the paramedic and the patient. This chapter reviews the basics of infectious disease, including disease transmission. This is followed by a discussion of infectious diseases likely to be encountered in prehospital care.

New in the 5th Edition: The following have been added to update this chapter's information on infectious diseases: New information on the **brain-eating amoeba** (*Naegleria fowler*); a new section on **Middle East respiratory syndrome (MERS)**; a new section on **Ebola virus disease**; a new section on **Zika virus disease**; a new section on **Chikungunya virus disease**; an extensive new section on the **Centers for Disease Control and Prevention Enhanced Precautions** to protect EMS personnel at risk of exposure to Ebola or other highly contagious disease; information on **antiviral drugs to treat hepatitis C**; information on the **increase in the occurrence of measles related to "anti-vaccine" movement** among some parents.

CHAPTER 11 Psychiatric and Behavioral Disorders provides an overview of psychiatric and behavioral problems. Paramedics are often the first health care professionals encountered by a patient with a psychiatric disorder. Because of this, paramedics must be ready to recognize and manage these emergencies appropriately.

New in the 5th Edition: Information added regarding increasing use of **ketamine as a chemical restraint** in the prehospital management of excited delirium.

CHAPTER 12 Diseases of the Eyes, Ears, Nose, and Throat presents an overview of the relevant anatomy and physiology and specific medical conditions that may affect each element that makes up this category of disease–the eyes, the ears, the nose, and the throat.

CHAPTER 13 Nontraumatic Musculoskeletal Disorders begins with a review of the anatomy and physiology of the skeletal system and the muscular system, then discusses relevant assessment and findings and details specific nontraumatic (medical) disorders that may affect these systems.

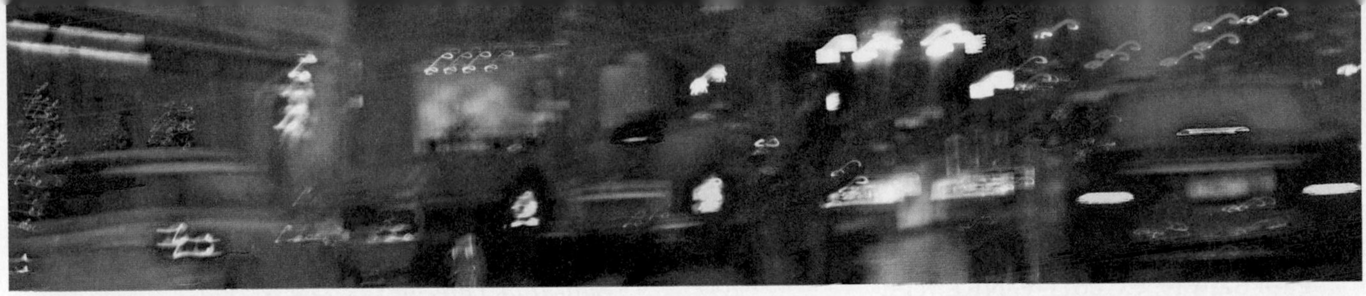

Acknowledgments

Chapter Contributors

We wish to acknowledge the remarkable talents of the following people who contributed to this five volume series. Individually, they worked with extraordinary commitment. Together, they form a team of highly dedicated professionals who have upheld the highest standards of EMS instruction.

Paul Ganss, MS, NRP (Volume 1, Chapter 2)
Michael F. O'Keefe (Volume 1, Chapter 5)
Wes Ogilvie, MPA, JD, LP (Volume 1, Chapter 7)
Kevin McGinnis, MPS, EMT-P (Volume 1, Chapter 9)
Jeff Brosious, EMT-P (Volume 1, Chapter 10)
W.E. Gandy, JD, NREMT-P (Volume 1, Chapter 15)
Darren Braude, MD, MPH, FACEP (Volume 1, Chapter 15)
Joseph R. Lauro, MD, EMT-P (Volume 2, Chapter 6)
Brad Buck, NRP, CCEMT-P (Volume 3, Chapter 10)
Andrew Schmidt, DO, MPH (Volume 4, Chapter 10)
Justin Sempsrott, MD (Volume 4, Chapter 10)
David Nelson, MD, FAAP, FAAEM (Volume 5, Chapter 4)
Mike Abernethy, MD, FAAEM (Volume 5, Chapter 10)
Ryan J. Wubben, MD, FAAEM (Volume 5, Chapter 10)
Louis Molino, NREMT-I (Volume 5, Chapter 11)
Dale M. Carrison, DO, FACEP, FACOEP (Volume 5, Chapter 14)
Dan Limmer, AS, NRP (Volume 5, Chapter 14)
Deborah J. McCoy-Freeman, BS, RN, NREMTP (Volume 5, Chapter 15)

BEB, RAC

Instructor Reviewers

The reviewers of this edition of *Paramedic Care: Principles & Practice* have provided many excellent suggestions and ideas for improving the text. The quality of the reviews has been outstanding, and the reviews have been a major aid in the preparation and revision of the manuscript. The assistance provided by these EMS experts is deeply appreciated.

Fifth Edition

Michael Smith, MS, Educator, Kilgore College, Longview, TX

Edward Lee, A.A.S., BS, Ed.S., NRP, CCEMT-P, EMT Paramedic Program Coordinator, Trident Technical College, Summerville, SC

Ryan Batenhorst, BA, NRP, EMS-I, Program Director, Paramedic Program, Southeast Community College, Milford, NE

Brett Peine, BS, NRP, Director, Southern State University, Joplin, MO

Fourth Edition

Ronald R. Audette, NREMT-P
Vice President
Educational Resource Group LLC
East Providence, RI

Troy Breitag, BS, NREMT-P, Fire Lt.
Department Supervisor – Med/Fire Rescue
Lake Area Technical Institute
Watertown, SD

Joshua Chan, BA, NREMT-P
EMS Educator
Cuyuna Regional Medical Center
Crosby, MN

Thomas E. Ezell, III, NREMT-P, CCEMT-P, CHpT
Fire/Rescue Captain (Ret.)
James City County Fire Department
Williamsburg, VA

Sean P. Haaverson, AA, NR/CCEMT-P
EMS Faculty
Central New Mexico Community College
Albuquerque, NM

L. Kelly Kirk, III, AAS, BS, EMT-P
Director of Distance Education
Randolph Community College
Asheboro, NC

Paul Salway, CCEMT-P, NREMT-P
Firefighter/EMT-P
South Portland Fire Department
South Portland, ME

R. Thomy Windham, BS
Director
Pee Dee Regional Community Training Center
Florence, SC

We also wish to express appreciation to the following EMS professionals who reviewed the third edition of Paramedic Care: Principles & Practice. *Their suggestions and perspectives helped to make this program a successful teaching tool.*

Mike Dymes, NREMT-P
EMS Program Director
Durham Technical Community College
Durham, NC

Wes Hamilton, RN, BSN, CCRN, CFRN, CTRN, NREMT-P, FP-C
Clinical Educator
Clinical Care Services Division
Air-Evac Lifeteam
West Plains, MO

Sean Kivlehan, EMT-P
St. Vincent's Hospital, Manhattan
New York, NY

Darren P. Lacroix, AAS, EMT-P
Del Mar College
Emergency Medical Service Professions
Corpus Christi, TX

Mike McEvoy, PhD, REMT-P, RN, CCRN
EMS Coordinator
Saratoga County, NY

Greg Mullen, MS, NREMT-P
National EMS Academy
Lafayette, LA

Deborah L. Petty, BS, EMT-P I/C
Training Officer
St. Charles County Ambulance District
St. Peter's, MO

B. Jeanine Riner, MHSA, BS, RRT, NREMT-P
GA Office of EMS and Trauma
Atlanta, GA

Michael D. Smith, LP
Kilgore College
Longview, TX

Allen Walls
Department of Fire & EMS
Colerain Township, OH

Brian J. Wilson, BA, NREMT-P
Education Director
Texas Tech School of Medicine
El Paso, TX

Photo Acknowledgments

All photographs not credited adjacent to the photograph or in the photo credit section below were photographed on assignment for Brady/Prentice Hall/Pearson Education.

Organizations

We wish to thank the following organizations for their assistance in creating the photo program for this project:

Michael J. Grant, President & CEO
Ambitrans Medical Transport, Inc.,
Punta Gorda, FL

Alan J. Skavroneck, Vice-President & COO
Ambitrans Medical Transport, Inc.

Debbie Harrington, BS, NREMT, Director
Community Relations, Ambitrans Medical Transport, Inc.

Companies

The following companies assisted in our photo program by donating EMS products to use in our photo shoots:

Persys Medical. NIO and BIG interosseous

Pyng Medical. FAST interosseous

Teleflex Corp. LMAs

Photo Coordinators/ Technical Advisors

Thanks to the following for valuable assistance directing the medical accuracy of the shoots and coordinating models, props, and locations for our photos:

Skippi Farley, EMT-P

Rodney VanOrsdol, FF/EMT-P

Photographers who have contributed to this project

Michael Gallitelli, Michal Heron, Kevin Link and Richard Logan

Photographer for the Fifth edition

Maria Lyle/Maria Lyle Photography
Sarasota, Florida

Models

Thanks to the following people from the Flower Mound Fire Department, Flower Mound, Texas, and from Winter Park Fire-Rescue, Winter Park, Florida, who provided locations and/or portrayed patients and EMS providers in our photographs.

FAO/Paramedic Wade Woody

FF/Paramedic Tim Mackling

FF/Paramedic Matthew Daniel

FF/Paramedic Jon Rea

FF/Paramedic Waylon Palmer

FF/EMT Jesse Palmer

Captain/EMT Billy McWhorter

Linda Kirk, Director, Winter Park Towers, Winter Park, FL

Andrew Isaacs

Richard Rodriguez

Tod Meadors

Jeff Spinelli

Mark Vaughn

Victoria Devereaux

Teresa George

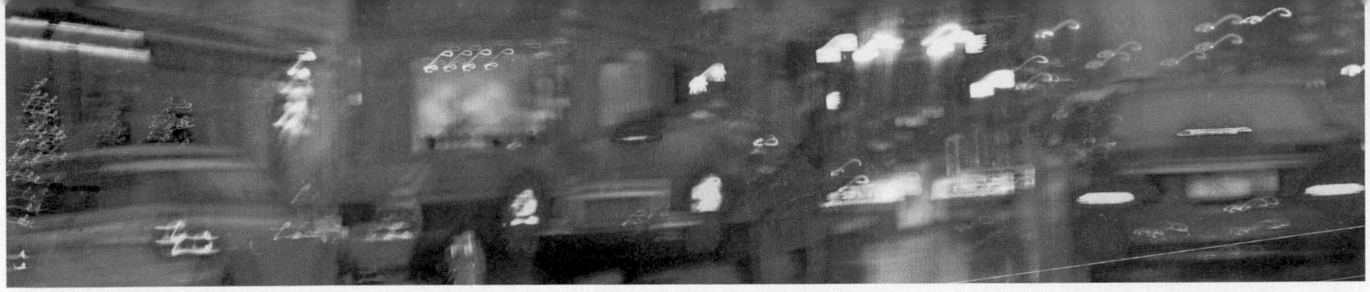

About the Authors

BRYAN E. BLEDSOE, DO, FACEP, FAAEM, EMT-P

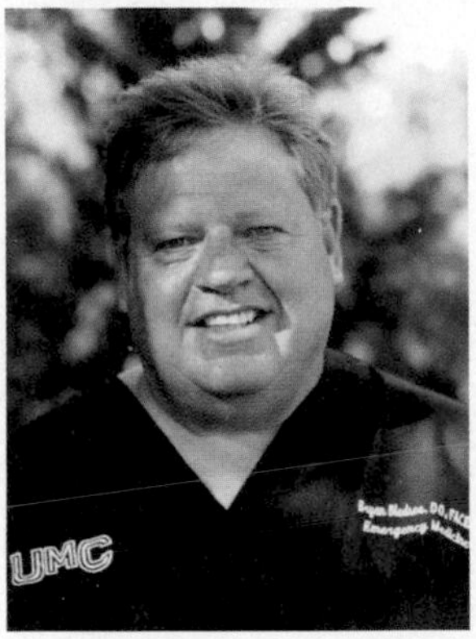

Dr. Bryan Bledsoe is an emergency physician, researcher, and EMS author. Presently he is Professor of Emergency Medicine at the University of Nevada School of Medicine and an Attending Emergency Physician at the University Medical Center of Southern Nevada in Las Vegas. He is board-certified in emergency medicine and emergency medical services. Prior to attending medical school, Dr. Bledsoe worked as an EMT, a paramedic, and a paramedic instructor. He completed EMT training in 1974 and paramedic training in 1976 and worked for six years as a field paramedic in Fort Worth, Texas. In 1979, he joined the faculty of the University of North Texas Health Sciences Center and served as coordinator of EMT and paramedic education programs at the university.

Dr. Bledsoe is active in emergency medicine and EMS research. He is a popular speaker at state, national, and international seminars and writes regularly for numerous EMS journals. He is active in educational endeavors with the United States Special Operations Command (USSOCOM) and the University of Nevada at Las Vegas. Dr. Bledsoe is the author of numerous EMS textbooks and has in excess of 1 million books in print. Dr. Bledsoe was named a "Hero of Emergency Medicine" in 2008 by the American College of Emergency Physicians as a part of their 40th anniversary celebration and was named a "Hero of Health and Fitness" by *Men's Health* magazine as part of their 20th anniversary edition in November of 2008. He is frequently interviewed in the national media. Dr. Bledsoe is married and divides his time between his residences in Midlothian, TX, and Las Vegas, NV.

RICHARD A. CHERRY, MS, EMT-P

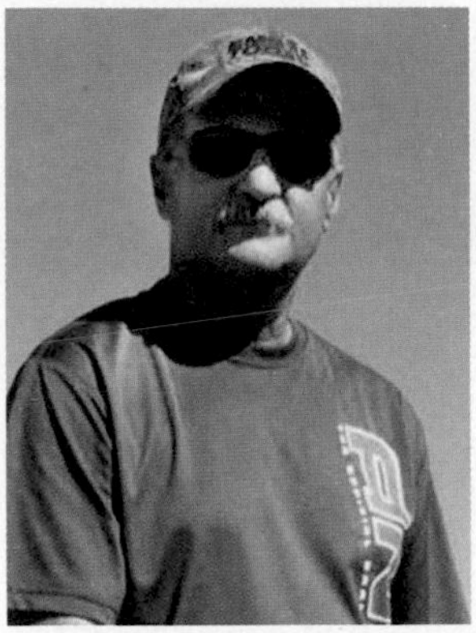

Richard Cherry is a Training Consultant for Northern Onondaga Volunteer Ambulance (NOVA) in Liverpool, New York, a suburb of Syracuse. He is also a program reviewer for The Continuing Education Coordinating Board for Emergency Medical Services (CECBEMS). He formerly held positions in the Department of Emergency Medicine at Upstate Medical University as Director of Paramedic Training, Assistant Emergency Medicine Residency Director, Clinical Assistant Professor of Emergency Medicine, and Technical Director for Medical Simulation. His experience includes years of classroom teaching and emergency fieldwork. A native of Buffalo, Mr. Cherry earned his bachelor's degree at nearby St. Bonaventure University in 1972. He taught high school for the next ten years while he earned his master's degree in education from Oswego State University in 1977. He holds a permanent teaching license in New York State.

Mr. Cherry entered the emergency medical services field in 1974 with the DeWitt Volunteer Fire Department, where he served his community as a firefighter and EMS provider for more than 15 years. He took his first EMT course in 1977 and became an ALS provider two years later. He earned his paramedic certificate in 1985 as a member of the area's first paramedic class. He then worked both as a paid and volunteer paramedic for the next 15 years.

Mr. Cherry has authored several books for Brady. Most notable are *Paramedic Care: Principles & Practice, Essentials of Paramedic Care, Intermediate Emergency Care: Principles & Practice,* and *EMT Teaching: A Common Sense Approach.* He has made presentations at many state, national, and international EMS conferences on a variety of EMS clinical and teaching topics. He and his wife, Sue, reside in Sun City West, Arizona. In addition to riding horses, hiking, and playing softball, they volunteer their time at Banner Del Webb Medical Center. Mr. Cherry also plays lead guitar in a Christian band.

A GUIDE TO KEY FEATURES

Emphasizing Principles

LEARNING OBJECTIVES

Terminal Performance Objectives and a separate set of Enabling Objectives are provided for each chapter.

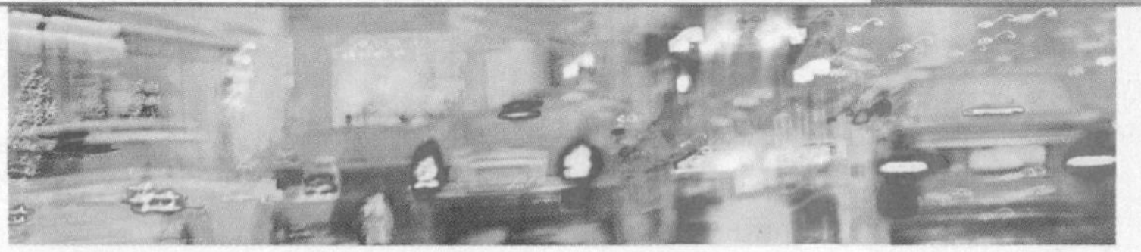

Chapter 1

Introduction to Paramedicine

Bryan Bledsoe, DO, FACEP, FAAEM

STANDARD

Preparatory (EMS Systems)

COMPETENCY

Integrates comprehensive knowledge of EMS systems, the safety and well-being of the paramedic, and medical–legal and ethical issues, which is intended to improve the health of EMS personnel, patients, and the community.

Learning Objectives

Terminal Performance Objective: After reading this chapter your should be able to discuss the characteristics of the profession of paramedicine.

Enabling Objectives: To accomplish the terminal performance objective, you should be able to:

1. Define key terms introduced in this chapter.
2. Compare and contrast the four nationally recognized levels of EMS providers in the United States.
3. Describe the requirements that must be met for EMS professionals to function at the paramedic level.
4. Discuss the traditional and emerging roles of the paramedic in health care, public health, and public safety.
5. List and describe the various health care settings paramedics may practice in with an expanded scope of practice.

KEY TERMS

Advanced Emergency Medical Technician (AEMT), p. 3
community paramedicine, p. 4
critical care transport, p. 7
Emergency Medical Responder (EMR), p. 3
Emergency Medical Services (EMS) system, p. 2
Emergency Medical Technician (EMT), p. 3
mobile integrated health care, p. 4
National Emergency Medical Services Education Standards: Paramedic Instructional Guidelines, p. 5
Paramedic, p. 3
paramedicine, p. 4

1

KEY TERMS

Page numbers identify where each key term first appears, boldfaced, in the chapter.

more rapid are the pulse and respiratory rates.

3.0 and 3.5 kg. Because of the excretion of extracellular

As newborns make the transition from fetal to pulmonary circulation in the first few days of life, several important

Table 11-1 Normal Vital Signs

	Pulse (Beats per Minute)	Respiration (Breaths per Minute)	Blood Pressure (Average mmHg)	Temperature	
Infancy:					
At birth:	100–180	30–60	60–90 systolic	98–100°F	36.7–37.8°C
At 1 year:	100–160	30–60	87–105 systolic	98–100°F	36.7–37.8°C
Toddler (12 to 36 months)	80–110	24–40	95–105 systolic	96.8–99.6°F	36.0–37.5°C
Preschool age (3 to 5 years)	70–110	22–34	95–110 systolic	96.8–99.6°F	36.0–37.5°C
School-age (6 to 12 years)	65–110	18–30	97–112 systolic	98.6°F	37°C
Adolescence (13 to 18 years)	60–90	12–26	112–128 systolic	98.6°F	37°C
Early adulthood (19 to 40 years)	60–100	12–20	120/80	98.6°F	37°C
Middle adulthood (41 to 60 years)	60–100	12–20	120/80	98.6°F	37°C
Late adulthood (61 years and older)	*	*	*	98.6°F	37°C

*Depends on the individual's physical health status.

TABLES

A wealth of tables offers the opportunity to highlight, summarize, and compare information.

components of the rule of threes. Whenever BVM ventilation is difficult, however, the rule of threes should be employed.

CONTENT REVIEW

- The Rule of Threes for Optimal BVM Ventilation
  - Three providers
  - Three inches
  - Three fingers
  - Three airways
  - Three PSI
  - Three PEEP

- ***Three providers.*** One provider on the mask, one on the bag, and one for cricoid pressure.
- ***Three inches.*** A reminder to place the patient in the sniffing position (elevate the head three inches) if not contraindicated.
- ***Three fingers.*** Three fingers on the cricoid cartilage to perform cricoid pressure.
- ***Three airways.*** In a worst-case scenario, the airway can be maintained, if necessary, with an orophrayngeal airway and two nasopharyngeal airways (one in each nostril).

CONTENT REVIEW

Content review boxes set off from the text are interspersed throughout the chapter. They summarize key points and serve as a helpful study guide—in an easy format for quick review.

PHOTOS AND ILLUSTRATIONS

Carefully selected photos and a unique art program reinforce content coverage and add to text explanations.

index, and middle finger of one hand. If a lesser-trained provider is performing the maneuver, you should confirm that they are in the correct position (Figure 15-47).

Use caution not to apply so much pressure as to deform and possibly obstruct the trachea; this is a particular danger in infants. The necessary pressure has been estimated as the amount of force that will compress a capped 50-mL syringe from 50 mL to the 30 mL marking. In the event that the patient actively vomits, it is imperative to release the pressure to avoid esophageal rupture. Similarly, if cricoid pressure is being performed during intubation, reduce or release the pressure if the intubator is having difficulty visualizing the vocal cords.

Optimal BVM Ventilation Using the Rule of Threes

The *rule of threes* was developed to help providers recall the components of optimal BVM ventilation. Many patients can be easily oxygenated and ventilated without using all

- ***Three PSI.*** A gentle reminder to use the lowest pressure necessary to see the chest rise.
- ***Three seconds.*** A reminder to ventilate slowly and allow time for adequate exhalation.
- ***Three PEEP.*** Or up to 15 cm/H_2O positive-end expiratory pressure (PEEP) as needed to improve oxygen saturations.

Bag-Valve Ventilation of the Pediatric Patient

The differences in the pediatric patient's anatomy require some variation in ventilation technique. First, the child's relatively flat nasal bridge makes achieving a mask seal more difficult. Pressing the mask against the child's face to improve the seal can actually obstruct the airway, which is more compressible than an adult's. You can best achieve the mask seal with the two-person BVM technique, using a jaw-thrust to maintain an open airway.

For BVM ventilation, the bag size depends on the child's age. Full-term neonates and infants will require a pediatric BVM with a capacity of at least 450 mL. For children up to 8 years of age, the pediatric BVM is preferred, although for patients in the upper portion of that age range you can use an adult BVM with a capacity of 1,500 mL if you do not maximally inflate it. Children older than 8 years require an adult BVM to achieve adequate tidal volumes. Additionally, be

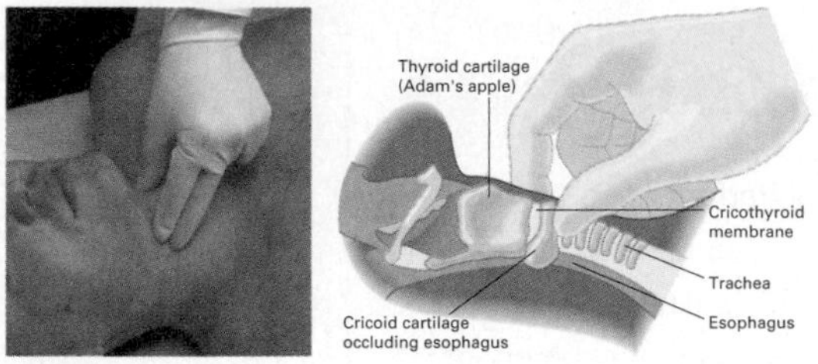

FIGURE 15-47 Cricoid pressure.

Summary

The scene size-up is the initial step in the patient care process. Sizing up the scene and situation begins at your initial dispatch and does not end until you are clear of the call. As the call unfolds, you should be making constant observations and adjustments to your plan of action. Remember that your safety and the safety of your partner are paramount—it is hard to effectively treat both yourself and others.

Scene size-up should be practiced so much that it becomes second nature to you. It is like noticing veins on people in public after you begin starting IVs. (You have all done it—looked across the room at the back of someone's hand and noticed what nice veins they had.) Sizing up a scene is no different. After a while, you begin to notice mechanisms of injury and other important details almost subconsciously. But be careful and do not get complacent! Always make it a point to pause for just a few seconds and consciously look around the scene before proceeding into any situation.

Scene size-up is not a step-by-step process, but a series of decisions you make when confronted with a variety of circumstances that are often beyond your control. It is a way to make order out of chaos, keep yourself and your crew safe, and ensure that all necessary resources are focused on patient care and outcomes. With time and experience, you will learn to perform a scene size-up quickly and focus on important issues. Your careful size-up lays the foundation for an organized and timely approach toward patient care and scene management. And always remember that scene size-up is not a one-time occurrence. It is an ongoing process.

SUMMARY

This end-of-chapter feature provides a concise review of chapter information.

YOU MAKE THE CALL

A scenario at the end of each chapter promotes critical thinking by requiring students to apply principles to actual practice.

airway management in every patient, you should learn and use advanced skills such as intubation, RSI, and cricothyrotomy. You must maintain proficiency in all airway skills, especially the more advanced techniques, through ongoing continuing education, physician medical direction, and testing with each EMS service. If you cannot do this, it is in the patient's best interest to focus on less sophisticated airway skills. If you anticipate that every airway will be complicated, apply basic airway skills before using advanced procedures, and perform frequent reassessments, you will give the patient his best chance for meaningful survival.

You Make the Call

You and your paramedic partner, Preston Connelly, are assigned to District 4, a quiet suburban neighborhood, on a warm Saturday in June. At 2:00 P.M., you are dispatched to care for a choking child at the Happy Hotdog Restaurant on Main Street. On your way to the location, the dispatcher advises you that they are currently giving prearrival choking instructions to the bystanders at the scene. On arrival, you find a frantic mother who tells you that her 6-year-old son was eating a hot dog and drinking a soda when he started coughing and gasping for air. She keeps yelling for you to do something. Bystanders surround the child and are attempting to perform the Heimlich maneuver without success. On your primary assessment, you find a 6-year-old boy lying on the floor, unconscious and apneic, with a pulse rate of 130. There is cyanosis surrounding his lips and fingernail beds, with a moderate amount of secretions coming from his mouth. There are no signs of trauma. You and Preston immediately start management of this child.

1. What is your primary assessment and management of this child?
2. What are your first actions?
3. What are your options for managing the airway after the obstruction is relieved?
4. What are the major anatomic differences between pediatric and adult patients in terms of airway management?

See Suggested Responses at the back of this book.

REVIEW QUESTIONS

These questions ask students to review and recall key information they have just learned.

Review Questions

1. When you couple the physical assessment findings with the patient's medical history, you are able to derive a list of ____________
   a. clinical diagnostics.
   b. field prognoses
   c. chief complaints
   d. differential field diagnoses.
2. The pain, discomfort, or dysfunction that caused your patient to request help is known as the ____________
   a. primary problem.
   b. nature of the illness.
   c. differential diagnosis.
   d. chief complaint.
3. You are assessing a patient who complains of cardiac-type chest pain that is felt in the jaw and down the left arm. This pattern of pain is known as ____________
   a. sympathetic pain.
   b. tenderness.
   c. referred pain.
   d. associated pain.
4. Your patient has smoked 2 packs of cigarettes each day for the past 35 years. He is a ____________ pack/year smoker.
   a. 35 c. 730
   b. 70 d. 25,550
5. The CAGE questionnaire is used as an evaluation tool to assess a patient with what type of history?
   a. Alcoholism c. Allergies
   b. Lung disease d. Pregnancy
6. What interviewing mnemonic should be used for each presenting problem a patient has?
   a. SAMPLE
   b. DCAP–BTLS
   c. OPQRST–ASPN
   d. AEIOU–TIPS
7. The mnemonic GPAL is used to evaluate a patient's ____________
   a. alcoholism.
   b. allergies.
   c. pregnancy history.
   d. endocrine dysfunction.

Match the following elements of the present illness of the patient with a chief complaint of chest pain with their respective examples:

1.	O	a. Pain is 6 on a scale of 1–10
2.	P	b. Patient also complains of shortness of breath and nausea
3.	Q	c. Pain had a sudden onset
4.	R	d. Pain began 2 hours ago
5.	S	e. Pain worsens while lying down
6.	T	f. Patient denies dizziness
7.	AS	g. Pain goes through to the back
8.	PN	h. Pain is heavy and vise-like

See Answers to Review Questions at the back of this book.

6. Which radio frequencies may be used by cities and municipalities for their ability to better transmit through concrete and steel?
   a. UHF c. 800-mHz
   b. VHF d. none of the above
7. Which frequency band is typically used by county and suburban agencies due to its ability to transmit over various terrains and longer distances?
   a. UHF c. 800-mHz
   b. VHF d. none of the above
8. What is the name of the basic communications system that uses the same frequency to both transmit and receive?
   a. Multiplex c. Simplex
   b. Duplex d. Complex
9. A communications system that uses a different transmit and receive frequency allowing for simultaneous communications between two parties is called ____________
   a. multiplex.
   b. duplex.
   c. simplex.
   d. complex.
10. ____________ communications systems are capable of transmitting both voice and electronic patient data simultaneously.
    a. Multiplex c. Simplex
    b. Duplex d. Complex

See answers to Review Questions at the back of this book.

References

1. Department of Homeland Security. SAFECOM. (Available at http://www.dhs.gov/safecom/)
2. National EMS Information System (NEMSIS). The NEMSIS Technical Assistance Center (TAC). (Available at http://www.nemsis.org//.)
3. American College of Emergency Physicians (ACEP). "Automatic Crash Notification and Intelligent Transportation Systems." *Ann Emerg Med* 55 (2010): 397.
4. National Emergency Number Association (NENA). National Emergency Number Association. (Available at: http://www.nena.org)
5. Association of Public-Safety Communications Officials (APCO). [Available at: http://www.apco911.org/]
6. Department of Transportation, Research and Innovative Technology Administration. Next Generation 911. (Available at: http://www.its.dot.gov/ng911/.)
7. Centers for Disease Control and Prevention. Recommendations from the Expert Panel: Advanced Automatic Collision Notification and Triage of the Injured Patient. (See NHTSA summary at http://www.nhtsa.gov/Research/Biomechanics+&+Trauma/Advanced+Automatic+Collision+Notification+-+AACN)
8. Wilson, S., M. Cooke, R. Morrell et al. "A Systematic Review of the Evidence Supporting the Use of Priority Dispatch of Emergency Ambulances." *Prehosp Emerg Care* 6 (2002): 42–29.
9. Billittier, A. J., 4th, E. B. Lerner, W. Tucker, and J. Lee. "The Lay Public's Expectations of Prearrival Instructions When Dialing 911." *Prehosp Emerg Care* 4 (2000): 234–237.
10. Munk, M. D., S. D. White, M. L. Perry, et al. "Physician Medical Direction and Clinical Performance at an Established Emergency Medical Services System." *Prehosp Emerg Care* 13 (2009): 185–192.
11. Cheung, D. S., J. J. Kelly, C. Beach, et al. "Improving Handoffs in the Emergency Department." *Ann Emerg Med* 55 (2010): 171–180.
12. Chan, T. C., J. Killeen, W. Griswold, and L. Lenert. "Information Technology and Emergency Medical Care during Disasters." *Acad Emerg Med* 11 (2004): 1229–1236.
13. DREAMS Ambulance Project. (See article at: https://www.ems1.com/ems-products/technology/articles/1183110-DREAMS-revolutionizes-communication-between-ER-and-ambulance/.)
14. Haskins, P. A., D. G. Ellis, and J. Mayrose. "Predicted Utilization of Emergency Medical Services Telemedicine in Decreasing Ambulance Transports." *Prehosp Emerg Care* 6 (2002): 445–448.

Further Reading

Bass, R., J. Potter, K. McGinnis, and T. Miyahara. "Surveying Emerging Trends in Emergency-related Information Delivery for the EMS Profession." *Topics in Emergency Medicine* 26 (April–June 2004): 2, 93–102.

Fitch, J. "Benchmarking Your Comm Center." *JEMS* 2006: 98–112.

McGinnis, K. K. "The Future of Emergency Medical Services Communications Systems: Time for a Change." *N C Med J* 68 (2007): 283–285.

McGinnis, K. K. *Future EMS Technologies: Predicting Communications Implications*. National Public Safety Telecommunications Council, National Association of State EMS Officials, National Association of EMS Physicians, June, 2010.

McGinnis, K. K. "The Future Is Now: Emergency Medical Services (EMS) Communications Advances Can Be as Important as Medical Treatment Advances When It Comes to Saving Lives." *Interoperability Today* (SafeCom, U.S. Department of Homeland Security), Volume 3, 2005.

McGinnis, K. K. *Rural and Frontier Emergency Medical Services Agenda for the Future*. National Rural Health Association Press: October 2004.

REFERENCES

This listing is a compilation of source material providing the basis of updated data and research used in the preparation of each chapter.

FURTHER READING

This list features recommendations for books and journal articles that go beyond chapter coverage.

cleaning, p. 70
Code Green Campaign, p. 78
disinfection, p. 70
exposure, p. 70
isotonic exercise, p. 61
pathogens, p. 65
personal protective equipment (PPE), p. 66
sterilization, p. 70
stress, p. 74
stressor, p. 74
Tema Conter Memorial Trust, p. 78

CASE STUDY

This feature at the start of each chapter draws students into the reading and creates a link between text content and real-life situations.

Case Study

Howard is a 15-year veteran of a high-volume, inner-city EMS service. When he first started his career, Howard thought he knew what he was getting into, but the years have taught him differently.

Right now, Howard is in the spotlight for saving the life of a police officer who was shot in a hostage situation. "That call forced me to reflect on a few important things," he says. "Two years ago, I had a minor heart problem, and it was a good wake-up call. Since then I've been lifting weights and running, so I was able to get to the officer with enough strength to carry him to safety.

"Another thing is that I always use personal protective equipment. I never go to work without steel-toed boots and I never leave the ambulance without a pair of disposable gloves. Can you believe there are still paramedics who knock the concept of infection control? If any one of my partners sticks a needle into the squad bench in my ambulance, they know I'll speak up."

Howard, a mild-mannered, nondescript man, doesn't realize that his young colleagues regard him as a role model. They've seen him handle himself at chaotic scenes as well as when a situation demands sensitivity, patience, and gentleness. "Howard is the man I'd want to tell bad news to my mother," one of his partners says. "He can handle people involved in just about any circumstance—death situations, panicked parents, lonely elderly people, and even hostile drunks. I've never seen anyone treat others with such dignity and respect. He's the best partner anyone could want, especially when we have to manage patients who are thrashing around. But that was not always so, was it, Howard?"

"No, it wasn't," Howard replies. "There was a time when no one wanted to work with me. I was a rebel, and I figured there was only one way to do things: my way. But an incident that occurred a few years ago changed all that. It's a long story. But the upshot is that when I recovered from the stress, my outlook had been altered. I realized that though I couldn't save the world, I could save myself. That's when I learned how to deal with the effects of a stressful job. I started eating right, lost a lot of weight, and adopted a new attitude. Anyway, if I can maintain my own well-being, I can do a lot more to help others. Right? Isn't that what we're about?"

Introduction

The safety and well-being of the workforce is a fundamental aspect of top-notch performance in EMS.[1] As a paramedic, it includes your physical well-being as well as your mental and emotional well-being. If your body is fed well and kept fit, if you use the principles of safe lifting, observe safe driving practices, and avoid potentially addictive and and insidious infections. If you let your spirit appreciate the fear and sadness on other faces, you will find ways to combat your prejudices and treat people with dignity and respect. By doing all these things, you will also be able to promote the benefits of well-being to your EMS colleagues.

Death, dying, stress, injury, infection, fear—all these threaten your wellness and conspire to interfere with your good intentions. However, you can do something about

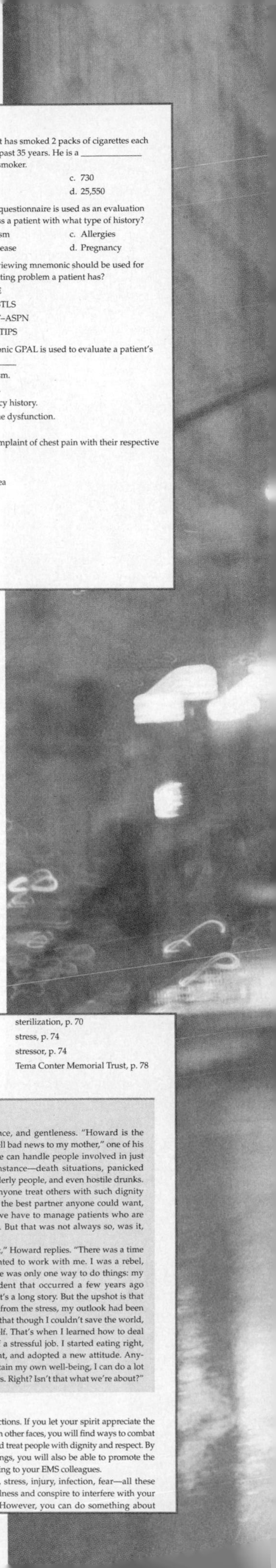

PROCEDURE SCANS

Visual skill summaries provide step-by-step support in skill instruction.

Procedure 7-4 Reassessment

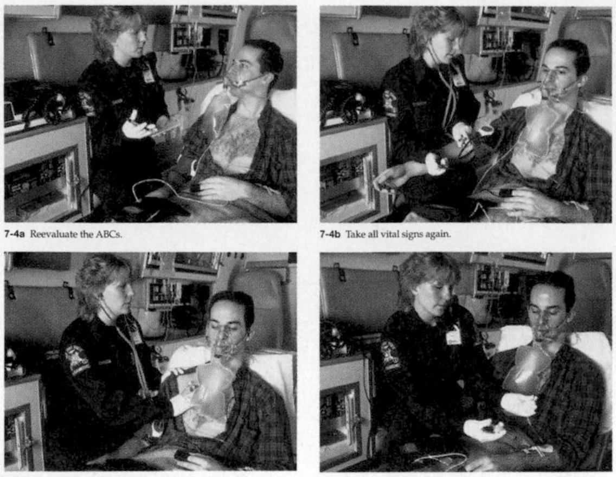

7-4a Reevaluate the ABCs.

7-4b Take all vital signs again.

7-4c Perform your focused assessment again.

7-4d Evaluate your interventions' effects.

laryngospasm may be occurring. Airway and breathing management requires constant reevaluation.

oxygenation. Lip cyanosis indicates central hypoxia (overall oxygen status), whereas peripheral cyanosis indicates decreased oxygen to the tissues. Pallor and coolness sug-

Special Features

the present illness. Common sense and clinical experience will determine how much of the following history to use.

Preliminary Data

For documentation, always record the date and time of the physical exam. Determine your patient's age, sex, race, birthplace, and occupation. This provides a starting point for the interview and establishes you as the interviewer. Who is the source of the information you receive about your patient? Is it the competent patient himself, his spouse, a friend, or a bystander? Are you receiving a report from a first responder, the police, or another health care worker? Do you have the medical record from a transferring facility?

After you have gathered the information, you should establish its reliability, which will vary according to the source's knowledge, memory, trust, and motivation. Again, reconfirm the information with the patient, if possible. This is a judgment call based on your experience. For example, if the patient information you received from a particular EMT first responder has been accurate in the past, you probably will trust it again. On the other hand, if the nurse at a physician's office has repeatedly provided you with erroneous information, you probably will doubt its accuracy.

scious patient, the chief complaint becomes what someone else identifies or what you observe as the primary problem. In some trauma situations, for instance, the chief complaint might be the mechanism of injury, such as "a penetrating wound to the chest" or "a fall from 25 feet."

Patho Pearls

The renowned Canadian physician Sir William Osler said, "Listen to the patient, and he will tell you what is wrong." This advice is as true today as it was 100 years ago. A great deal of information can be determined from a skillful history taking. As you listen to a patient's medical history, try to understand the underlying pathophysiologic processes that might cause the symptoms the patient describes. This will help you to fully comprehend the disease process or processes affecting the patient.

For example, consider the following case. Mrs. J. Franklin is a 72-year-old pensioner, twice widowed, who lives in an older section of town. She summons EMS with what initially seem like vague complaints. She reports to the dispatcher, when queried, that she is "just sick." You arrive and begin an assessment, starting with a pertinent history. The patient reports that her symptoms began about two weeks ago after several family members came to her house with dinner, which included a baked ham. Since that time, she has developed some fatigue, progressive dyspnea, and occasional chest pain. She now reports that she often wakes up at 3:00 A.M. with breathing trouble that resolves when she walks around the room or

PATHO PEARLS

Offer a snapshot of pathological considerations students will encounter in the field.

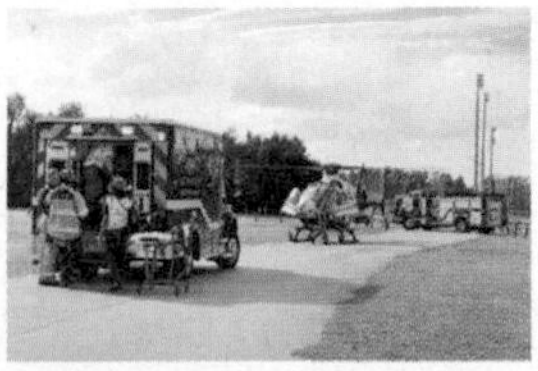

FIGURE 2-11 Patients may be transported by ground or air. Medical helicopter transport was introduced in the 1950s during the Korean War. *(© Ed Effron)*

Vietnam, and success of military evacuation procedures led to their use in civilian ambulance systems. In 1970, the Military Assistance to Safety and Traffic (MAST) program was established. This demonstration project set up 35 helicopter transportation programs nationwide to test the feasibility of using military helicopters and paramedics in

Legal Considerations

Emergency Department Closures. Numerous factors have resulted in emergency department closures and ambulance diversions. This can have a significant impact on the EMS system. All systems must address this situation so that patient care does not suffer.

In 1974, in response to a request from the DOT, the General Services Administration (GSA) developed the "KKK-A-1822 Federal Specifications for Ambulances." This was the first attempt at standardizing ambulance design to permit intensive life support for patients en route to a definitive care facility. The act defined the following basic types of ambulance:

- *Type I (Figure 2-13).* This is a conventional cab and chassis on which a module ambulance body is mounted, with no passageway between the driver's and patient's compartments.
- *Type II (Figure 2-14).* A standard van, body, and cab form an integral unit. Most have a raised roof.

LEGAL CONSIDERATIONS

Offer a snapshot of pathological considerations students will encounter in the field.

An important part of patient assessment is gathering information that is accurate, complete, and relevant to the present emergency. To begin, you must identify the patient's chief complaint. Although dispatch probably will have given you an idea of what the emergency is about, it is

Cultural Considerations

Eye contact is a major form of nonverbal communication. Short eye contact is often seen as friendly, whereas prolonged eye contact may be interpreted as threatening. Thus, timing is an important factor in how a person interprets eye contact.

One's culture also influences how eye contact is interpreted. Eye contact can mean respect in one culture and disrespect in another. Often, Asians will avoid eye contact even when they have nothing to hide. Eye contact between people of different sexes is problematic in Muslim cultures, in which a prolonged look in the face of a member of the opposite sex might be misinterpreted. Because of this, people in Middle Eastern countries might look a person of the same sex in the eye and not look into the eyes of a person of the opposite sex.

If you work in a culturally diverse community, you should learn the customs of eye contact and other forms of nonverbal communication of those you might encounter during the course of your work.

unexpected but important facts. For example, instead of asking your patient with abdominal pain, "Did you have breakfast today?" which can be answered with either a "yes" or a "no," ask: "What have you eaten today?"

- ***Use direct questions when necessary.*** Direct questions, or **closed questions**, ask for specific information. ("Did you take your pills today?" or "Does the abdominal pain come and go like a cramp, or is it constant?") These questions are good for three reasons: They fill in information generated by open-ended questions. They help to answer crucial questions when time is limited. And they can help to control overly talkative patients, who might want to tell you about their gallbladder surgery in 1969 when their chief complaint is a sprained ankle.
- ***Ask only one question at a time, and allow the patient to complete his answers.*** If you ask more than one question, the patient may not know which one to answer and may leave out portions of information or become confused. Equally important is having one person do the interview. Don't force your patient to discern questions from multiple interviewers.
- ***Listen to the patient's complete response before asking the next question.*** By doing so, you might find that

CULTURAL CONSIDERATIONS

Provide an awareness of beliefs that might affect patient care.

ASSESSMENT PEARLS

Offer tips, guidance, and information to aid in patient assessment.

Provocation/Palliation

What provokes the symptom (makes it worse)? Does anything palliate the symptom (make it better)? In many

Assessment Pearls

Chest pain is a common reason that people summon EMS. However, the causes of chest pain are numerous. In emergency medicine or EMS, we often look to exclude the most serious causes before determining whether chest pain is of a benign origin. Internal organs do not have as many pain fibers as do such structures as the skin and other areas. Pain arising from an internal organ tends to be dull and vague. This is because nerves from various spinal levels innervate the organ in question. The heart, for example, is innervated by several thoracic spinal nerve segments. Thus, cardiac pain tends to be dull and is sometimes described as pressure. It also tends to cause referred pain (i.e., pain in an area somewhat distant to the organ), such as pain in the left arm and jaw. Dull pain that is hard to localize (or to reproduce with palpation) may be due to cardiac disease. One sign often seen with patients suffering cardiac disease is Levine's sign. With Levine's sign, the patient will subconsciously clench his fist when describing the chest pain. Levine's sign is associated with pain of a cardiac origin (e.g., angina or acute coronary syndrome).

Ask about any activity, medication, or other circumstance that either alleviates or aggravates the chief complaint.

Quality

How does your patient perceive the pain or discomfort? Ask him to explain how the symptom feels, and listen carefully to his answer. Does your patient call his pain crushing, tearing, oppressive, gnawing, crampy, sharp, dull, or otherwise? Quote his exact descriptors in your report.

Region/Radiation

Where is the symptom? Does it move anywhere else? Identify the exact location and area of pain, discomfort, or dysfunction. Does your patient complain of pain "here," while holding a clenched fist over the sternum, or does he grasp the entire abdomen with both hands and moan? If your patient has not done so, ask him to point to the painful area. Identify the specific location, or the boundary of the pain if it is regional.

Determine whether the pain is truly pain (occurring independently) or **tenderness** (pain on palpation). Also determine whether the pain moves or radiates. Localized pain occurs in one specific area, whereas radiating pain

PEDIATRIC PEARLS

Offer tips, guidance, and information on how to deal with pediatric patients encountered in the field.

the result of a head injury, hypothermia, severe hypoxia, or drug overdose. Bradycardia is a common finding in the well-conditioned athlete, but it may be found in almost anyone. Treat bradycardia only if it compromises your patient's cardiac output and general circulatory status.

Tachycardia usually indicates an increase in sympathetic nervous system stimulation as the body compensates for another problem, such as blood loss, fear, pain, fever, drug overdose, or hypoxia. It is an early indicator of shock and may indicate ventricular tachycardia, a life-threatening cardiac dysrhythmia.

The pulse's quality can be weak, strong, or bounding. Weak, thready pulses indicate a decreased circulatory status, such as shock. Strong, bounding pulses may indicate high blood pressure, heat stroke, or increasing intracranial pressure. The pulse location may be another indicator of your patient's clinical status. The presence of a carotid pulse generally means that his systolic blood pressure is at least 60 mmHg. The presence of peripheral pulses indicates a higher blood pressure; their absence suggests circulatory collapse. Practice locating each of the pulse locations (Figure 5-12). As with other vital signs, take your patient's pulse frequently in the emergency setting and note any trends.

To take the pulse of a conscious adult or large child, the most accessible and commonly used location is the radial artery. With the pads of your first two or three

Pediatric Pearls

In infants and small children, use the brachial artery or auscultate for an apical pulse. Remember that auscultating an apical pulse does not provide information about your patient's hemodynamic status. To locate the brachial artery, feel just medial to the biceps tendon. Auscultate the apical pulse just below the left nipple.

fingers, compress the radial artery onto the radius, just below the wrist on the thumb side (Procedure 5-1b). In the unconscious patient, begin by checking his carotid pulse. To locate the carotid pulse, palpate medial to and just below the angle of the jaw. Locate the thyroid cartilage (Adam's apple) and slide your fingers laterally until they are between the thyroid cartilage and the large muscle in the neck (sternocleidomastoid).

First, note your patient's pulse rate by counting the number of beats in 1 minute. If his pulse is regular, you can count the beats in 15 seconds and multiply that number by 4. If his pulse is irregular, you must count it for a full minute to obtain an accurate total. Also note the pulse's rhythm and quality.

Blood Pressure

Blood pressure is the force of blood against the arteries' walls as the heart contracts and relaxes. It is equal to cardiac output times the systemic vascular resistance. Any

CUSTOMER SERVICE MINUTE

Shows how extending extra kindness and compassion can make an important difference to patients and families coping with an emergency.

Customer Service Minute

Following Up. Last week, a man took his dog to the vet for an upper respiratory infection. The dog was pretty sick, but the vet assured the owner that she was not critical, and with antibiotics she would be better in a few days, so he brought her home. The next day, the veterinarian called to find out how the dog was doing. She called every day until the dog was back to normal. Needless to say, the man was delighted in the service he received from that vet.

Physicians' offices, dentists' offices, and veterinary offices often call their patients a few days following a visit to see how things are going. Why don't we? Before you leave your patient and the family, why not ask them for permission to call the next day or in a few days to see how they're doing? If they say no or are hesitant to give permission, drop it. If they give permission, call them and see if there is anything you can do for them.

The follow-up has many benefits. You get to reconnect with the people in your community. It is great for public relations. It is educational because you can see whether your diagnosis was accurate. It's a winner from every angle. When they hang up, they'll be thinking, "Wow!"

Introduction

Patient assessment means conducting a problem-oriented evaluation of your patient and establishing priorities of your patient en route to the hospital to detect changes in patient condition.

Your proficiency in performing a systematic patient assessment will determine your ability to deliver the highest quality of prehospital **advanced life support** (ALS) to sick and injured people. Paramedic patient assessment is a straightforward skill, similar to the assessment you might have performed as an EMT. It differs, however, in depth and in the kind of care you will provide as a result.

Your assessment must be thorough, because many ALS procedures are potentially dangerous. Safely and appropriately performing advanced procedures such as administration of drugs, defibrillation, synchronized cardioversion, needle decompression of the chest, or endotracheal intubation will depend on your assessment and correct field diagnosis. If your assessment does not reveal your patient's true problem, the consequences can be devastating.

As always, common sense dictates how you proceed in the field. When you assess the responsive medical patient, the history reveals the most important diagnostic information and takes priority over the physical exam. For the trauma patient and the unresponsive medical patient, the reverse is true. However, trauma may cause a medical emergency, and, conversely, a medical emergency may cause trauma. Only by performing a thorough patient assessment can you discover the true cause of your patient's problems. This chapter provides problem-oriented patient assessment examples based on the information and techniques presented in the previous six chapters.

IN THE FIELD

Provides extra tips that can help ensure success in real-life emergency situations.

In the Field

The Tools of Your Trade: *The Ophthalmoscope*

An **ophthalmoscope** (Figure 5-27) is a medical instrument used to examine the internal eye structures, especially the retina, located at the back of the eye. Although it is most often used to diagnose eye conditions, you can discover information that may be relevant to other medical and traumatic events.

The ophthalmoscope is basically a light source with lenses and mirrors. It has a handle, which houses the batteries, and a head, which includes a window through which you visualize the internal eye; an aperture dial, which changes the width of the light beam; a lens dial to bring the eye into focus; and a lens indicator, which identifies the lens magnification number (i.e., 0 to +40 or 0 to −20). You examine the eye by looking through a monocular eyepiece into the eye of your patient. You can view different depths of the eye at different magnifications by rotating a disk of varying lenses within the instrument itself.

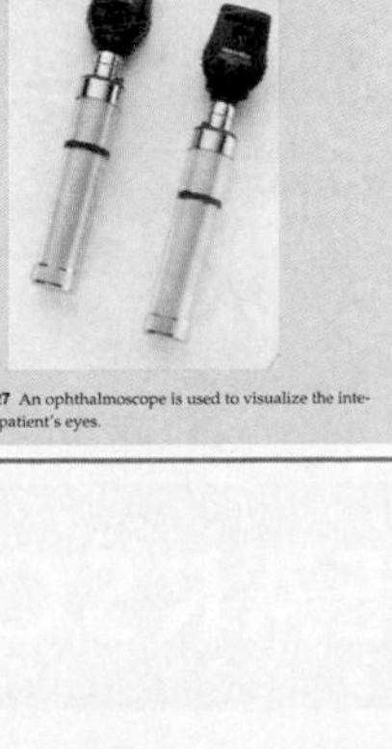

FIGURE 5-27 An ophthalmoscope is used to visualize the interior of your patient's eyes.

eye while the patient continues to fix his gaze on an object in the distance. Adjust the lens disk as needed to focus on the retina. Farsighted patients will require more "plus" diopters (black or green numbers), whereas nearsighted patients will require more "minus" diopters (red numbers) to keep the retina in focus.

Try to keep both your eyes open and relaxed. The optic disk should come into view when you are about 1.5 to 2 inches from the eye while you are still aiming your light 15 to 25 degrees nasally. If you are having difficulty finding the disk, look for a branching (bifurcation) in a retinal blood vessel. Usually the bifurcation will point toward the disk.

Follow the vessel in the direction of the bifurcation and you should arrive at the optic disk. The disk should appear as a yellowish-orange to pink round structure. Within the center of the disk there should be a central physiologic cup, which normally appears as a smaller, paler circle. The cup should be less than half the diameter of the disk. An enlarged cup may indicate chronic open-angle glaucoma. Indistinct borders or elevation of the optic disk may indicate papilledema, which is a marker of increased intracranial pressure.

Next, look at the arteries and veins of the retina. The arteries are usually brighter and smaller than the veins. Spontaneous venous pulsations are normal. Abnormalities of the retina such as hemorrhages, arteriovenous (AV) nicking, and cotton wool spots may indicate local or systemic disease such as retinal vein occlusion, hypertension, or many other conditions.

Finally, look at the fovea and surrounding macula. This area is where vision is most acute. It is located about two disk diameters temporal to the optic disk. You may also find the macula by asking the patient to look directly into the light of your ophthalmoscope. Prepare for a fleeting glimpse as this area is very sensitive to light and may be uncomfortable for your patient to maintain. A "cherry red" macula with surrounding pallor of tissue in the setting of acute painless monocular visual loss indicates a central retinal artery occlusion. Irreversible damage occurs

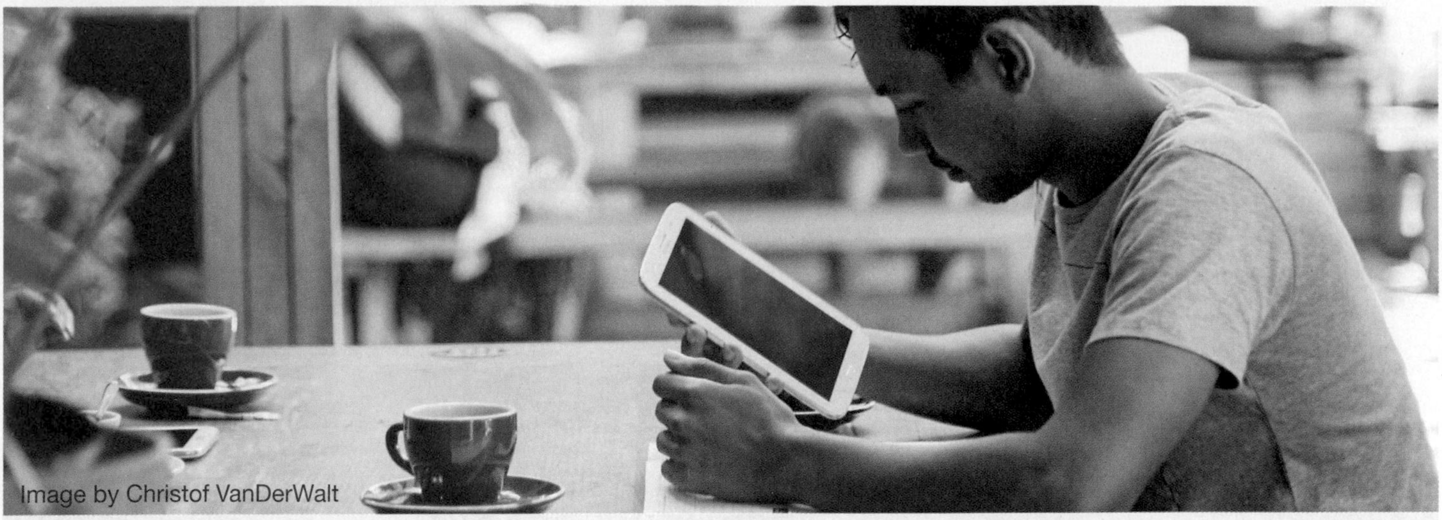
Image by Christof VanDerWalt

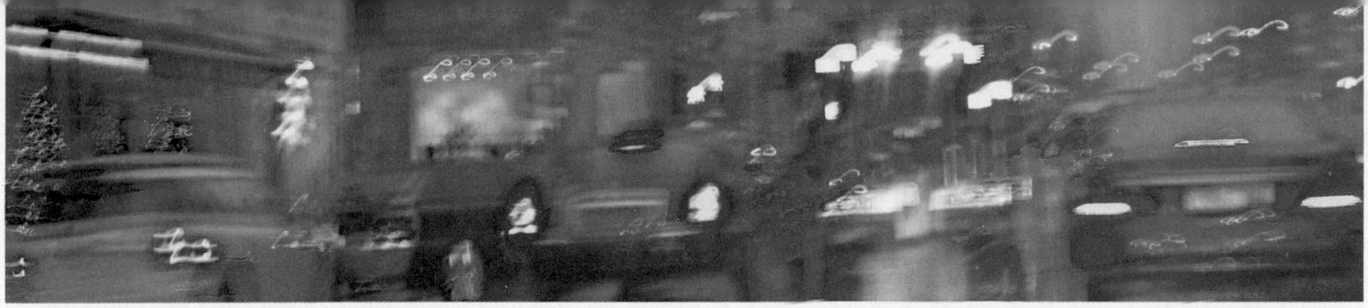

Chapter 1
Pulmonology

Bryan Bledsoe, DO, FACEP, FAAEM, EMT-P

STANDARD
Medicine (Respiratory)

COMPETENCY
Integrates assessment findings with principles of epidemiology and pathophysiology to formulate a field impression and implement a comprehensive treatment/disposition plan for a patient with a medical complaint.

Learning Objectives

Terminal Performance Objective: After reading this chapter, you should be able to integrate patient assessment findings, patient history, and knowledge of anatomy, physiology, pathophysiology, and basic and advanced life support interventions to recognize and manage patients with pulmonary disorders.

Enabling Objectives: To accomplish the terminal performance objective, you should be able to:

1. Define key terms introduced in this chapter.
2. Identify risk factors that increase the likelihood of developing a respiratory disease.
3. Review the anatomy and physiology of the pulmonary system.
4. Describe pathophysiological changes that lead to disruption of ventilation, diffusion, and perfusion as they relate to the pulmonary system.
5. Integrate the scene size-up, primary assessment, patient history, secondary assessment, and use of monitoring technology to arrive at field impressions and differentials for pulmonary patients.
6. Recognize signs and symptoms of airway compromise, respiratory distress, and respiratory failure.
7. Explain the pathophysiology of respiratory disorders commonly seen in the prehospital environment by the paramedic.
8. Use a process of clinical reasoning to guide and interpret the patient assessment findings and develop a management plan for patients with pulmonary disorders in the prehospital environment.
9. Given a variety of scenarios, discuss the integration of assessment and management guidelines as they relate to pulmonary emergencies.

KEY TERMS

acute respiratory distress syndrome (ARDS), p. 26
apnea, p. 13
asphyxia, p. 16
bradypnea, p. 20
carbaminohemoglobin, p. 12
carboxyhemoglobin, p. 42
carina, p. 5
chronic obstructive pulmonary disease (COPD), p. 3
cor pulmonale, p. 30
crepitus, p. 18
cyanosis, p. 15
deoxyhemoglobin, p. 11
diaphoresis, p. 15
diffusion, p. 11
dyspnea, p. 16
flail chest, p. 13
free radicals, p. 25
hemoglobin, p. 11
hemoptysis, p. 16
hemothorax, p. 13
hyperoxia, p. 25
hypoxia, p. 25
nasal flaring, p. 16
normoxia, p. 25
orthopnea, p. 16
oxidative stress, p. 25
oxyhemoglobin, p. 11
pallor, p. 15
paroxysmal nocturnal dyspnea, p. 16
perfusion, p. 11
pH, p. 10
pleuritic, p. 38
pneumothorax, p. 13
polycythemia, p. 30
positive end-expiratory pressure (PEEP), p. 27
reactive oxygen species (ROS), p. 25
respiration, p. 12
spontaneous pneumothorax, p. 44
subcutaneous emphysema, p. 18
surfactant, p. 6
tachycardia, p. 16
tachypnea, p. 20
tactile fremitus, p. 18
tracheal deviation, p. 18
tracheal tugging, p. 16
ventilation, p. 7

Case Study

Paramedics Tony Alvarez and Lee Smith are just finishing their barbecue lunch when they are toned out for a "medical emergency." They quickly go to the ambulance for the rest of the dispatch information. The emergency communications center dispatches them to 423 Black Champ Road, where a male patient is reportedly having difficulty breathing. The dispatcher also informs the crew that first responders from the Maypearl Fire Department are already en route. The paramedics are familiar with this area. It is a rural part of the county with mainly cotton farms. The response time is approximately 12 minutes. Upon arrival at the farmhouse, Alice Swenson, an emergency medical responder from the Maypearl Volunteer Fire Department, meets the paramedics. Alice reports that they have a 55-year-old white male who is having difficulty breathing. She further states that oxygen is already being administered.

The paramedics grab the drug box, monitor/defibrillator, airway kit, and stretcher. They then enter the small farmhouse. A quick scene size-up reveals no immediate dangers. Tony and Lee find the patient seated at the kitchen table, obviously short of breath. They quickly perform a primary assessment. The airway is clear, the patient is moving little air, and he has a strong pulse. Tony replaces the nasal cannula placed by the first responders with a nonrebreather mask. Lee and Tony then complete a focused history and physical exam. The patient has diminished breath sounds and occasional rhonchi, and is using the accessory muscles of respiration. There is a hint of cyanosis around his mouth.

The team learns that, several years ago, doctors at the Veterans Administration (VA) hospital diagnosed the patient as having emphysema. Over the past 24 hours, he has had progressive dyspnea and didn't sleep at all the previous night. His wife reports that he paced the floor and repeatedly opened and closed windows. Vital signs reveal a blood pressure of 140/78 mmHg, a pulse of 96 beats per minute, and a respiratory rate of 28 breaths per minute. The monitor shows a sinus rhythm. Pulse oximetry reveals an oxygen saturation of 90 percent while receiving supplemental oxygen. The patient is mentally alert but slightly anxious. His current medications include an albuterol (Ventolin) metered-dose inhaler, montelukast (Singulair), and azithromycin (Zithromax). He still smokes a pack and a half of cigarettes per day and has done so for 40 years, accumulating a 60-pack/year history.

The patient wants to be transported to the VA hospital. Lee contacts medical direction and provides a brief patient report. Medical direction approves transport to the VA hospital, as it is only 5 miles farther away than the nearest hospital. The transport time will be approximately 40 minutes. The paramedics place a saline lock. In addition, medical direction orders a nebulizer treatment with levalbuterol (Xopenex). Because of the long transport time, medical direction also orders the administration of 125 milligrams of methylprednisolone (Solu-Medrol) by IV push.

Halfway through the nebulizer treatment, the patient shows marked improvement. His respiratory rate slows to 20 breaths per minute, and his oxygen saturation reading increases to 94 percent. Transport to the VA hospital is uneventful. He remains at the VA hospital for two days and is discharged.

Introduction

The respiratory system is a vital body system responsible for providing oxygen to the tissues, while at the same time removing the metabolic waste product, carbon dioxide. Oxygen is required for the conversion of essential nutrients into energy and must be constantly available to all body tissues.

Respiratory emergencies are among the most common emergencies EMS personnel are called on to treat. You will encounter many patients in respiratory distress during your career. As a paramedic, you must promptly recognize and appropriately treat respiratory problems in order to reduce mortality and morbidity.

Several risk factors increase the likelihood of developing respiratory disease. *Intrinsic risk factors* are those that are influenced by or are from within the patient. The most important intrinsic risk factor is genetic predisposition. The likelihood of developing respiratory disease, such as bronchial asthma, **chronic obstructive pulmonary disease (COPD)**, and lung carcinoma (cancer), is increased in patients who have family members with these diseases.

Certain respiratory conditions are increased in patients who have underlying cardiac or circulatory problems. For example, patients with cardiac conditions that result in ineffective pumping of blood are prone to the development of pulmonary edema. In addition, both cardiac and circulatory disease may allow blood to pool in the large veins of the pelvis and lower extremities, leading to the development of pulmonary emboli. Both pulmonary edema and pulmonary emboli often present with a respiratory complaint as the primary complaint. Finally, the patient's level of stress may increase the severity of any respiratory complaint. Remember that stress can actually precipitate acute episodes of asthma or COPD.

CONTENT REVIEW

- Factors in Respiratory Disorder Development
  - Most important *intrinsic factor:* genetic predisposition
  - Most important *extrensic factor:* smoking

Extrinsic risk factors, those that are external to the patient, are also important in increasing the likelihood of developing respiratory disease. The most important of these is cigarette smoking. There is a strong link between cigarette smoking and the development of pulmonary diseases such as lung carcinoma and COPD. Additionally, diseases such as pneumonia and pulmonary emboli are more likely in patients who smoke. Finally, cigarette smoking has been implicated as a risk factor in the development of cardiac disease that may lead to the development of pulmonary edema. In any case, underlying lung damage caused by cigarette smoke causes virtually all lung disorders to be worse in smokers.

Another important extrinsic risk factor is environmental pollutants. Patients who live in highly industrialized areas, particularly where there is little movement of air, are at particular risk for respiratory problems. The prevalence of patients with COPD is markedly increased in areas with high environmental pollutants. The number and severity of acute attacks of both asthma and COPD are also worse under these conditions.

This chapter will help you to develop an understanding of the pathophysiology of respiratory disease, then integrate this knowledge with your assessment findings to develop a field impression and manage the patient with respiratory problems. (Before continuing with this chapter, you may want to review the chapter "Airway Management and Ventilation.")

Review of Respiratory Anatomy and Physiology

As you may recall, the airway is divided anatomically into the upper airway and the lower airway (Figure 1-1).

Upper Airway Anatomy

The upper airway (Figure 1-2) is responsible for warming and humidifying incoming air. It is also very effective in air purification. Each day, approximately 10,000 liters of air are filtered, warmed, humidified, and exchanged by the adult respiratory system.

CONTENT REVIEW

- The Upper Airway
  - Nasal cavity
  - Pharynx
  - Larynx

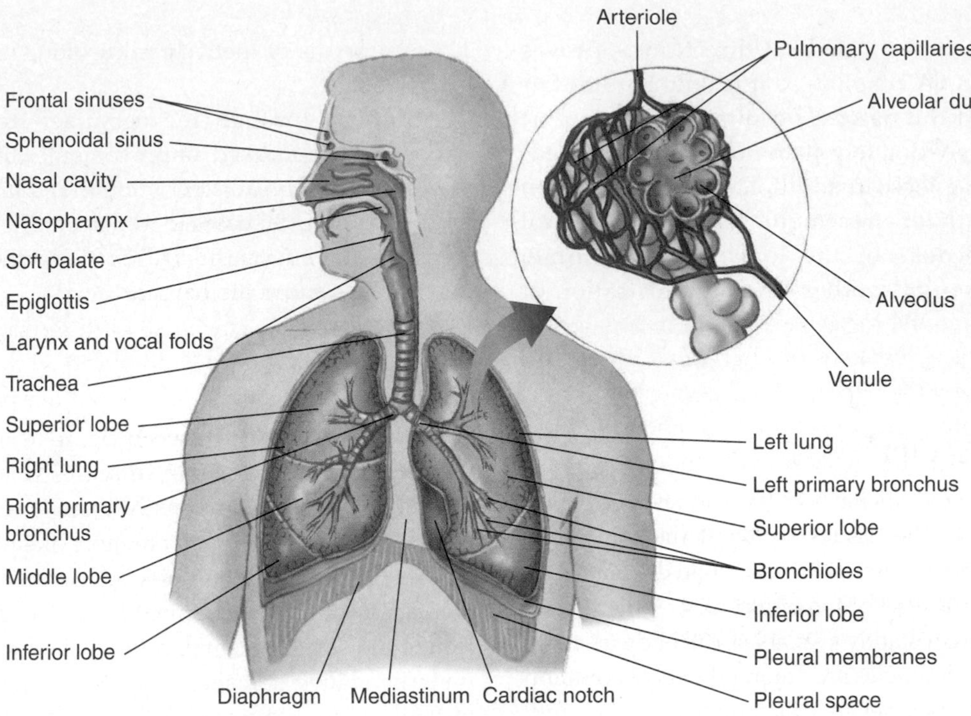

FIGURE 1-1 Overview of the upper and lower airways.

Nasal Cavity

Air enters the upper airway through the nose. It initially passes through the external nares, or nostrils, and enters the nasal cavity. The nasal cavity is divided into two chambers (right and left) by the nasal septum. In the anterior portion of the nose are many hair follicles that help trap large dust particles. The lateral wall of the nasal cavity is marked by three bony prominences called the *turbinates.* Between each set of turbinates is a passageway, or *meatus,* that leads to the *paranasal sinuses* (Figure 1-3). The turbinates cause turbulence in the incoming airflow. This facilitates the entrapment and removal of any inhaled foreign particles, such as dust.

As air passes posteriorly, the thin layer of mucus that lines the nose traps any small inhaled particles not filtered by the hair follicles. This mucus is constantly produced by goblet cells found in the mucous membrane. Some of the

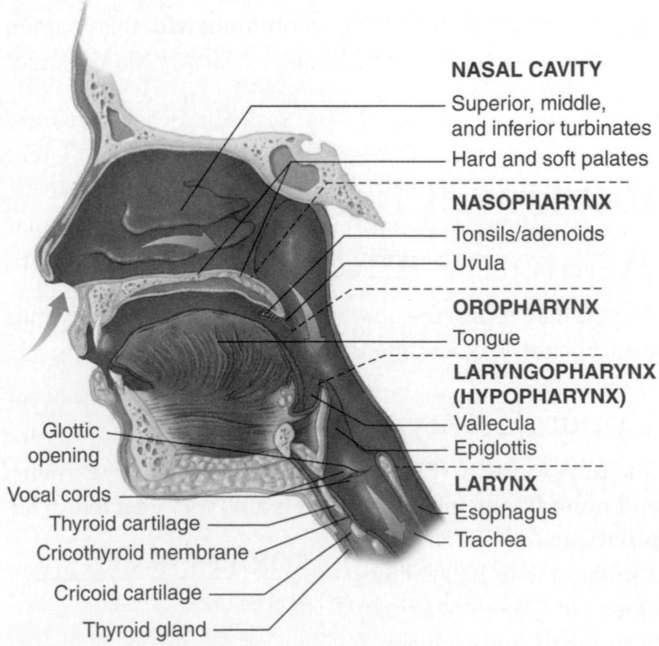

FIGURE 1-2 Anatomy of the upper airway.

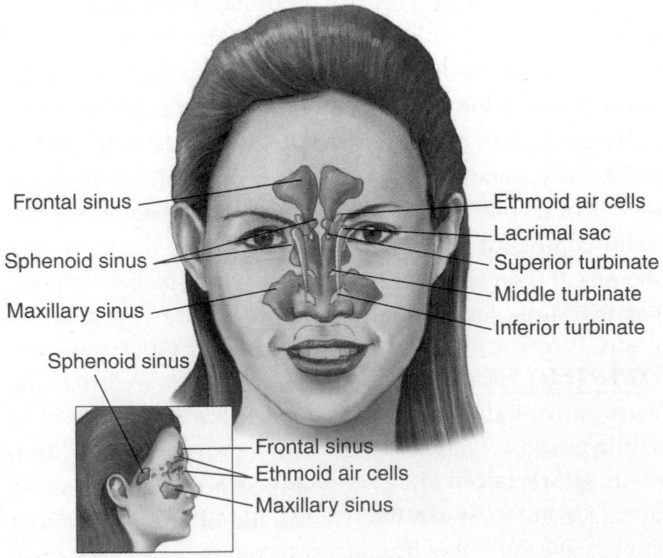

FIGURE 1-3 Paranasal sinuses.

cells lining the respiratory tract have *cilia.* Cilia are thin, fingerlike projections that have the ability to contract in a single direction. In the nose, the cilia move in a manner that produces a steady posterior flow of mucus, at the same time removing any entrapped particles. Once the mucus and any entrapped particles reach the posterior part of the nasopharynx, they are swallowed and removed from the body via the digestive tract.

There is a rich supply of blood vessels, referred to as *Kiesselbach's plexus,* in the lower nasal septum that warms the inspired air. These functions of filtering and warming are also supported by the paranasal sinuses, which are air cavities in the frontal, ethmoid, sphenoid, and maxillary portions of the skull. All are connected to the nasal cavity. The superior portion of the nose contains nerve fibers that are important to our sense of smell (olfactory sense). These fibers, derived from the first cranial nerve (CN-I, the olfactory nerve), pass through the thin cribriform plate that separates the nasal cavity from the cranial cavity.

Pharynx

The *pharynx* is a funnel-shaped structure that connects the nose and mouth to the larynx. It has three divisions: the nasopharynx, the oropharynx, and the laryngopharynx. The *nasopharynx* is the portion of the pharynx that is posterior to the nose and is the most superior aspect of the pharynx. Filtering, humidification, and warming of inspired air continue in the nasopharynx. Both food and air are conducted through the lower divisions of the pharynx, the *oropharynx* and the *laryngopharynx.* The tonsils are nodules of lymphoid tissue that are located in the posterior pharynx. There are three types of tonsils. The pharyngeal tonsils, also called the adenoids, are found in the nasopharynx. The palatine tonsils and lingual tonsils are located in the oropharynx.

Larynx

In addition to its role in speech, the larynx serves as a filtering device for the digestive and respiratory tracts. Externally, you can locate the larynx by feeling the thyroid cartilage, or Adam's apple. The larynx is composed of three pairs of cartilage (arytenoid, corniculate, and cuneiform), the thyroid cartilage, the cricoid cartilage, and the epiglottis. The larynx also possesses two pairs of folds that are derived from the internal lining of the larynx. The upper lining forms a pair of folds called the *vestibule,* or false vocal cords. The lower pair forms the true vocal cords. The vocal cords and the space in between them are referred to as the *glottic opening.* During inspiration, the three paired cartilages remain widely separated, and the epiglottis sits upright so that air can freely enter the trachea. With swallowing, the epiglottis tips backward and the cartilage pairs close, diverting food to the esophagus.

Lower Airway Anatomy

CONTENT REVIEW

- The Lower Airway
  - Trachea
  - Bronchi
  - Alveoli
  - Lungs

Trachea

During inspiration, air exits the upper airway and passes through the larynx into the *trachea* (Figure 1-4). The trachea is approximately 11 cm in length and is composed of a series of C-shaped cartilaginous rings. It is lined with the same kind of cells that line the nares. Mucus produced by these cells continues to trap air contaminants, and the cilia propel the mucus toward the pharynx. Additionally, stimulation of the trachea by food or other ingested products triggers a coughing response that helps keep the airway free of foreign material. Cigarette smoking ultimately leads to destruction of the cilia, leaving the cough reflex as the only protective mechanism.

Bronchi

At the **carina**, the trachea divides into the right and the left mainstem bronchi. The carina has many nerve endings and stimulation of this area produces violent coughing. The right mainstem bronchus is almost a straight continuation of the trachea, whereas the left mainstem bronchus angles more acutely to the left. This anatomic difference between the two mainstem bronchi helps to explain why gastric contents or other aspirated material tend to pass down the right mainstem bronchus into the lungs. It also explains why pneumonia that results from aspiration occurs more commonly in the right lung. Additionally, this is why, in most instances, an endotracheal tube advanced too far into the trachea will pass into the right mainstem bronchus.

The mainstem bronchi divide into the secondary (lobar) bronchi. These secondary bronchi divide into tertiary (segmental) bronchi, which ultimately divide into the bronchioles, or the small airways. The bronchioles are approximately 1 mm thick and contain smooth muscle that can contract, thus reducing the diameter of the airway.

The conduit system, from the trachea to the terminal bronchioles, must be intact for air to enter the lungs. Both the upper airway and lower airway must be patent so that air may pass through the bronchial system into the alveoli. The upper airway is the gateway to the body's respiratory system, and occlusion by the patient's tongue or a foreign body prevents air from reaching the alveoli. Lower airway disease such as bronchial asthma can have the same result. You can see, therefore, how important it is to maintain a patent airway as you attempt to resuscitate a patient.

After approximately 22 divisions, the bronchioles become terminal bronchioles. The terminal bronchioles divide into the respiratory bronchioles, and it is at this point that the airway shifts from being a conduit for air to

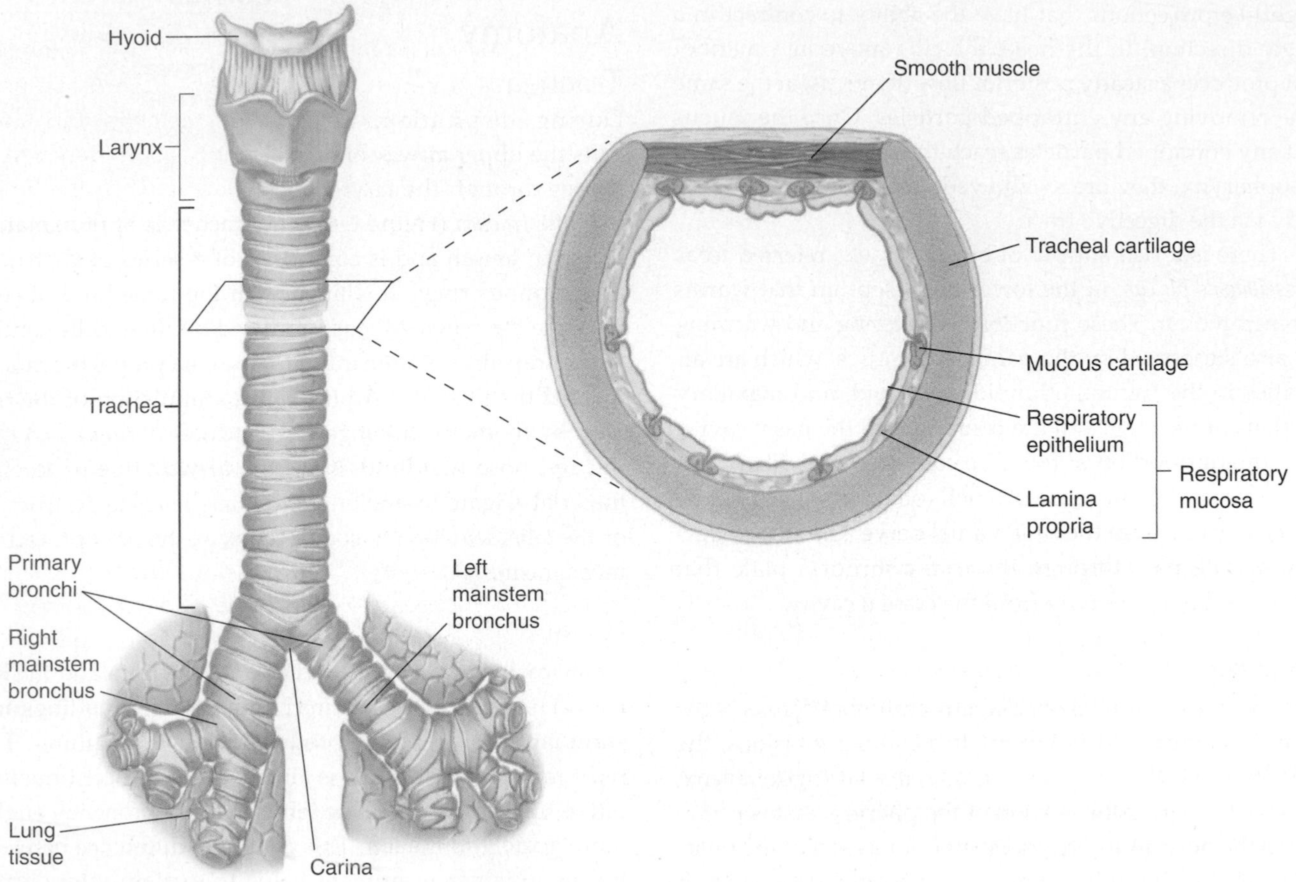

FIGURE 1-4 Anatomy of the lower airway.

an organ of gas exchange. The respiratory bronchioles contain mostly smooth muscle and have limited gas exchange ability.

Alveoli

The respiratory bronchioles divide into the alveolar ducts. These terminate in the alveolar sacs, or alveoli. It is estimated that there may be 300 million alveoli in the lungs. Most of the gas exchange (exchange of oxygen and carbon dioxide) takes place in the alveoli (Figure 1-5), although limited gas exchange may occur in the alveolar ducts and respiratory bronchioles.

The alveolar wall consists of a thin layer of cells (type I cells) that lines the surface of the lung. In close proximity to the alveoli are the pulmonary capillaries. These capillaries carry carbon dioxide-rich blood from the heart into the lungs and oxygen-rich blood away from the lungs for return to the heart. A small amount of supportive tissue contained in the interstitial space separates the capillaries from the alveolar surface (Figure 1-6).

The alveolar lining, supportive tissue, and capillaries make up the *respiratory membrane.* This gas exchange surface measures approximately 70 m^2. Diseases such as emphysema destroy the walls between the alveoli and reduce the total surface area available for gas exchange. When this surface area is reduced by more than two-thirds, oxygen diffusion will be unable to meet the needs of the resting patient.

The alveoli are moistened and kept open because of the presence of an important chemical called **surfactant**

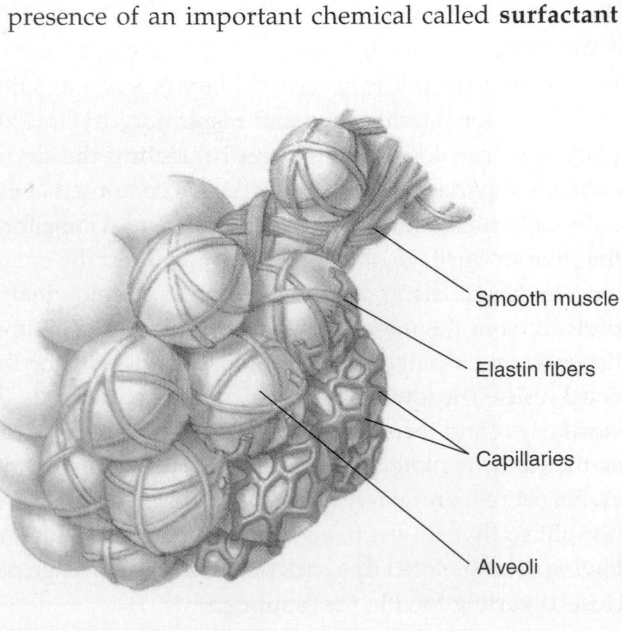

FIGURE 1-5 The alveoli and the pulmonary capillaries.

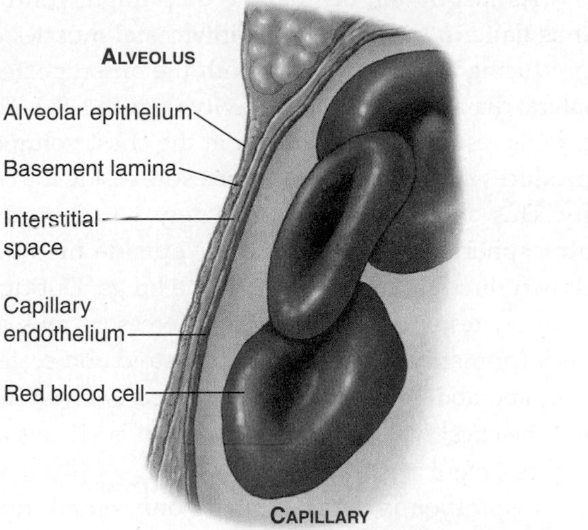

FIGURE 1-6 Supportive tissue contained in the interstitial space that separates capillaries from the alveolar surface.

that is secreted by type II cells found on the alveolar surface. Surfactant tends to decrease the surface tension of the alveoli, thus keeping them open for gas exchange. The alveolar macrophages are another type of cell found within the alveoli. These cells are part of the body's immune system and function to digest particles, bacteria, and other foreign material.

Remember that, in a normal patient, not all of the alveoli remain patent during gas exchange. This means that a small percentage of blood will pass through the alveoli without exchanging oxygen and carbon dioxide. This is referred to as *physiologic shunt* and affects approximately 2 percent of the total blood flow to the lungs.

Lungs

The lungs are the main organs of respiration. The right lung contains three main divisions, or *lobes*, whereas the left lung has only two lobes. The lungs are covered by connective tissue called *pleura*. Unattached to the lung, except at the *hilum* (the point at which the bronchi and blood vessels enter the lungs), the pleura consists of two layers, visceral and parietal. The *visceral pleura* covers the lungs and does not contain nerve fibers. In contrast, the *parietal pleura* lines the thoracic cavity and contains nerve fibers. A small amount of pleural fluid is usually found in the pleural space, a potential space between the two layers of pleura. This fluid serves as a lubricant for lung movement during respiration. The surface tension maintains the contact between the lungs and chest wall (similar to the attractive force that is generated when you place water between two glass slides).

Pulmonary and Bronchial Vessels

Blood is supplied to the lungs through two systems: the pulmonary vessels and the bronchial vessels. The pulmonary arteries transport deoxygenated, carbon dioxide-rich blood from the heart and present it to the lungs for oxygenation. The pulmonary veins then transport the oxygenated blood from the lungs back to the heart. The lung tissue itself receives little of its blood supply from the pulmonary arteries and veins. Instead, bronchial arteries that branch from the aorta provide most of the blood supply to the lungs. Bronchial veins return blood from the lungs to the superior vena cava.

Physiologic Processes

The major function of the respiratory system is to exchange gases with the environment. Oxygen is taken in while carbon dioxide is eliminated, a process known as gas exchange.

Oxygen is vital to our bodies, allowing us to generate the energy that drives our many body functions. Oxygen from the atmosphere diffuses into the bloodstream through the lungs. Oxygen is then available for use in cellular metabolism by the body's 100 trillion cells. Waste products, including carbon dioxide, produced by cellular metabolism must be eliminated from the body. In the lungs, carbon dioxide is exchanged for oxygen, and the carbon dioxide is excreted from the lungs.

Three important processes allow gas exchange to occur:

- Ventilation
- Diffusion
- Perfusion

Ventilation

Ventilation is the mechanical process of moving air in and out of the lungs. For ventilation to occur, several body structures must be intact, including the chest wall, nerve pathways, diaphragm, pleural cavity, and brainstem.

The chest wall consists of a series of ribs that are supported posteriorly by the thoracic spine and anteriorly by the sternum and costal cartilages. Each set of ribs is connected by a thick array of muscles called the *intercostal muscles*. A paired artery and vein, the intercostal vessels, nourish these muscles, which receive their nerve supply from the intercostal nerve. The nerve and blood vessels lie along the lower edge of each rib in a groove on the posterior surface (Figure 1-7). The chest wall is an important component of ventilation and also serves to protect the heart, lungs, and other organs of the thorax.

The *diaphragm*, a dome-shaped muscle, separates the thorax and abdomen. Nerve impulses from the phrenic nerve, which begins in the region of the cervical portion of the spinal cord

CONTENT REVIEW

➤ Processes of Gas Exchange
- Ventilation
- Diffusion
- Perfusion

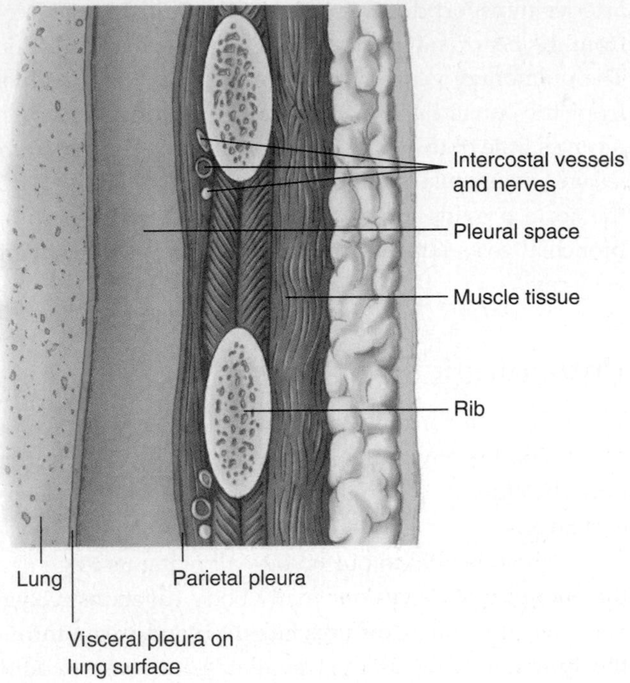

FIGURE 1-7 The intercostal vessels and nerves are located at the inferior borders of the ribs.

and travels through the chest cavity, stimulate the diaphragm to contract. Several traumatic, infectious, and even neoplastic conditions (cancer, tumors) can interrupt the nerve supply to the diaphragm.

INSPIRATION AND EXPIRATION Ventilation is divided into two phases: inspiration and expiration. During inspiration, air is drawn into the lungs. During expiration, air leaves the lungs. These phases of ventilation depend on changes in the volume of the thoracic cavity.

As inspiration begins, the diaphragm contracts and thus flattens. In addition, the intercostal muscles contract, producing an expansion in both the anteroposterior and lateral diameter of the chest cavity (Figure 1-8a). These two actions result in an expansion in the chest volume, which produces a decrease in the air pressure inside the chest cavity. This decrease to approximately 1 to 2 mmHg *below* atmospheric pressure causes air outside the body to be drawn through the trachea into the lungs. During periods of heavy respiratory demand, the accessory muscles of the neck (primarily the sternocleidomastoid and scalene muscles) and abdominal wall are recruited to assist in increasing the chest wall volume. Inspiration is always an active process, requiring energy.

Inspiration is dependent not only on an intact chest wall, but also on an intact pleural cavity. The pleural space has a pressure between 4 and 8 mmHg less than atmospheric pressure. This pressure difference between the lung and pleural space, as well as the surface tension of the pleural fluid, ensures that the lungs will move in concert with the chest wall. You can see how an opening into the pleural cavity from a knife or gunshot wound would severely disrupt the normal ventilatory mechanism. A wound opening would eliminate the negative pressure that exists in the pleural space that causes the lungs to expand with the chest wall.

During expiration, both the chest wall and diaphragm recoil to their normal resting state, which increases the pressure inside the chest to approximately 1 to 2 mmHg *above* atmospheric pressure (Figure 1-8b). This drives air out of the lungs. Expiration is generally a passive process that does not require energy. In some disease states, such as emphysema, however, the normal elasticity of the lungs is

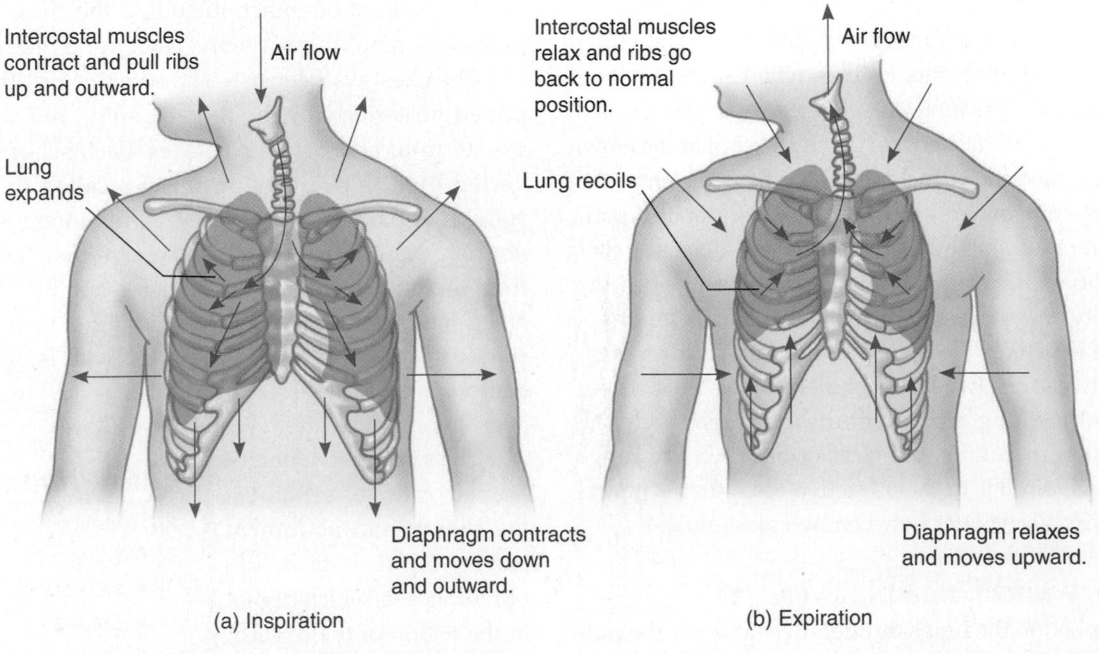

FIGURE 1-8 The phases of respiration: (a) inspiration; (b) expiration.

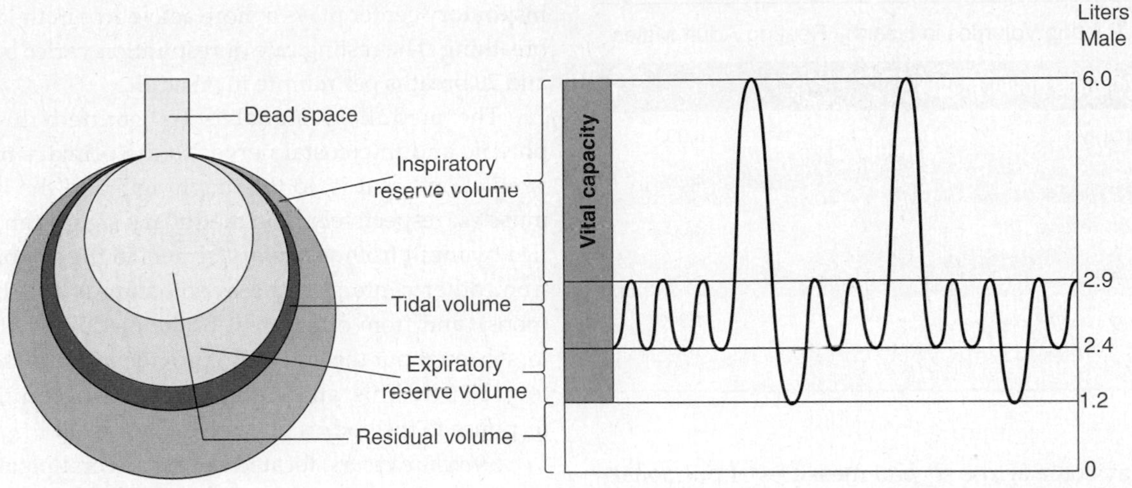

FIGURE 1-9 The lung volumes.

lost. Additionally, during heavy exercise, use of expiratory muscles (such as the rectus muscle and some of the intercostal muscles) is required to generate a larger expiratory effort. In either of these situations, expiration of air becomes an active process, requiring energy.

AIRWAY RESISTANCE AND LUNG COMPLIANCE

The amount of airflow into the lungs (ventilation) is dependent not only on the difference between the pressure in the atmosphere and that inside the chest cavity, but also on two additional factors: airway resistance and lung compliance.

The more *airway resistance* (or drag to the flow of air) exists, the less air flows into the chest cavity. Of the passages that conduct air into the alveoli, the medium-sized bronchi offer the greatest resistance to airflow. In patients who have asthma, the smooth muscle within these structures is stimulated by environmental allergens, cold weather, infection, and other factors. This stimulation leads to *bronchospasm* (widespread constriction of the bronchial smooth muscle) and increased resistance to airflow. This makes breathing more strenuous for the patient. The bronchi contain smooth muscle that is also very sensitive to input from the sympathetic nervous system. This is why sympathetic stimulants such as epinephrine, or parasympathetic blocking agents such as atropine or ipratropium bromide (Atrovent), are useful in the treatment of asthma.

Another factor that influences airflow into the lungs is *lung compliance*. Simply stated, compliance refers to the ease with which the chest expands. More specifically, it is defined as the change in volume of the chest cavity that results from a specific change in pressure within the chest cavity. The more the chest wall expands as the result of a change in pressure, the greater the lung compliance. One natural change that occurs with aging is a decrease in lung compliance. This is caused by a loss of elasticity in the muscles, ribs, and cartilage that form the chest wall, which results in a shrinking of the chest wall. The reverse is true with emphysema patients. Because elastic tissue is destroyed in these patients, their lung compliance is abnormally high, so that small changes in pressure result in large expansion of lung volume.

LUNG VOLUMES The volume of air entering the lungs varies based on the metabolic needs of the patient. Several important lung volumes can be measured (Figure 1-9). Factors such as age, sex, physical conditioning, and medical illness will alter these volumes. During quiet respiration, approximately 500 mL of air move in and out of the lungs of a 70-kg adult. This is referred to as the *tidal volume*. The lungs are capable of drawing in an additional volume of air beyond the volume inspired during quiet respiration. This is referred to as the *inspiratory reserve volume*. In an adult male, this volume is approximately 3,000 mL. Similarly, the amount of air that can be forcibly expired out of the lung after a normal breath is referred to as the *expiratory reserve volume* and measures approximately 1,200 mL. An additional 1,200 mL of air remains in the lungs at all times and is important in maintaining the patency of the alveoli. This is called the *residual volume*.

Several calculated volumes can be derived from these volumes that we have already discussed. Such derived volumes are referred to as *lung capacities*. The *inspiratory capacity* is the sum of the tidal volume and inspiratory reserve volume. This is approximately 3,500 mL in adult males. The sum of the expiratory reserve volume and the residual volume is the *functional residual capacity*, which measures approximately 2,400 mL. The *vital capacity* is the amount of air that is measured from a full inspiration to a full expiration. This is the sum of the inspiratory reserve volume, tidal volume, and expiratory reserve volume and measures 4,800 mL. The total volume of air in the lungs, called the *total lung capacity*, measures approximately 6,000 mL in an adult male (Table 1-1).

Table 1-1 Lung Volumes in Healthy Resting Adult Males

Capacity/Volumes (male, in mL)	
Total lung capacity	6,000
Vital capacity	4,800
Inspiratory reserve	3,000
Tidal volume	500
Expiratory volume	1,200
Residual volume	1,200

You may come across several measures of pulmonary function when caring for patients with respiratory disorders. These measurements reflect the dynamic nature of air movement in and out of the lungs. The *minute respiratory volume* is the amount of air moved in and out of the lungs during 1 minute. It is calculated by multiplying the tidal volume and the respiratory rate. For an adult male, the typical minute respiratory volume is approximately 6,000 mL (or 500 mL × 12 breaths per minute). Similarly, the *minute alveolar volume* is the volume of air moving through the alveoli in 1 minute. It is calculated by subtracting the dead space (approximately 150 mL; explanation follows) from the tidal volume and multiplying by the respiratory rate.

The *forced expiratory volume (FEV)* is the volume of air exhaled over a measured period of time. Most commonly, the FEV_1 measures the volume of air expelled during the first second of a forced expiration. Similarly, a *peak flow* measures the maximum rate of airflow during a forced expiration. This is measured in liters of air expiration per minute. Both these measurements are commonly used in the assessment of patients with lung diseases, such as asthma or COPD, in which the expiration of gases may be impaired.

Remember that when a patient breathes in a tidal volume of 500 mL, some of that air rests in the trachea, mainstem bronchi, and bronchioles and is unavailable for gas exchange. This is called the *anatomical dead space* and is approximately 150 mL. You should also remember that under certain conditions, some alveoli might be unavailable for gas exchange (because they are collapsed or are filled with fluid). This is referred to as *alveolar dead space*. This volume varies depending on the degree of alveolar collapse.

REGULATION OF VENTILATION The lower portions of the brainstem, specifically the *medulla*, control ventilation. This area of the brain sends a constant, repetitive signal to the lungs to initiate inspiration. The medulla contains both an inspiratory and an expiratory center. However, because expiration is generally a passive process, the inspiratory center plays a more active role in the rhythm of breathing. The resting rate of respiration varies between 12 and 20 breaths per minute in an adult.

The medullary signal is transmitted through the phrenic and intercostal nerves to the primary muscles of ventilation—that is, to the diaphragm and the intercostal muscles, respectively. The medullary signal can be modified by input from voluntary centers in the cerebral cortex, from other centers in the hypothalamus and brainstem (pons), and from other areas of the medulla. Other receptors throughout the body also provide input to the respiratory center. This allows tight control of ventilation in response to the body's physiologic needs.

Stretch receptors, located on the visceral pleura and on the walls of the bronchi and bronchioles, are important body structures that provide input to the medulla's respiratory center. As the patient continues to inhale, signals from these receptors become stronger until they completely inhibit impulses transmitted from the medulla. As the lungs begin to recoil, the signals become less intense, allowing the medulla to begin another inspiratory phase. This mechanism prevents overinflation of the lungs and is called the *Hering-Breuer reflex*. The medulla also receives input to increase the ventilatory rate from receptors that are stimulated by irritants in the lung and bronchial tree and, additionally, from receptors that detect increased activity in muscles and joints.

The most important determinant of the ventilatory rate is the arterial PCO_2. An increase in the patient's arterial PCO_2 results in a decrease in the **pH** of the blood. An increase in carbon dioxide in the blood also results in an increase in carbon dioxide in *cerebrospinal fluid* (the fluid that bathes the brain and spinal cord). Carbon dioxide and water combine to produce an acid, resulting in a lowering of the pH (increasing the concentration of hydrogen ions) in the cerebrospinal fluid. Chemical receptors in the area of the medulla detect this decrease in the pH, which produces an increase in the ventilatory rate, which helps the body eliminate excess CO_2 and return the pH to a normal level. There are also chemical receptors in the carotid artery and aorta that are directly sensitive to the arterial PCO_2. Stimulation of these receptors by an increase in arterial PCO_2 will also stimulate respiration. Remember that there is instantaneous feedback through these chemical receptors to the medulla so that, once changes in cerebrospinal fluid pH and arterial PCO_2 are corrected, the stimulus to increase respiration ceases.

Unfortunately, regulation of ventilation in patients with COPD does not take place as described. In patients with this disorder, the body becomes less responsive to changes in arterial PCO_2. Instead, the major stimulus to breathing comes from the level of oxygen detected in arterial blood by receptors in the aortic arch. As a result, patients with COPD will achieve a delicate balance in the

PO_2, with the level being low enough to continually stimulate the medulla's respiratory center while having enough oxygen to maintain normal body functions. Measured PO_2 levels of between 50 and 60 mmHg are not uncommon in this patient population.

Diffusion

Diffusion is the process by which gases move between the alveoli and the pulmonary capillaries. Remember that gases tend to flow from areas in which there is a high concentration of gas into an area of low concentration. The normal concentration of oxygen in the alveoli is 104 mmHg, as opposed to a concentration of 40 mmHg in the pulmonary arterial circulation. Therefore, oxygen will move from the oxygen-rich alveoli into the oxygen-poor capillaries in response to the gradient that exists in the concentration of gases. As the red blood cells move through the pulmonary capillaries, they become enriched with oxygen. Less oxygen will pass into the bloodstream as the gradient between alveolar and capillary oxygen concentration decreases.

Similarly, carbon dioxide passes out of the blood in response to a gradient that exists between the concentration of carbon dioxide in the blood in the pulmonary capillaries (45 mmHg) and in the alveoli (40 mmHg). By the time blood leaves the pulmonary capillaries, it has a dissolved concentration of oxygen of 104 mmHg and a carbon dioxide concentration of 40 mmHg.

The respiratory membrane, which normally measures 0.5 to 1.0 micrometer in thickness, must remain intact for gas exchange to occur. Any disorder that damages the alveoli or allows them to collapse will impede oxygen from entering the body and will reduce carbon dioxide elimination. Changes in the respiratory membrane or any increase in the interstitial space will also impede the process of diffusion. For example, fluid accumulation in the interstitial space as the result of pulmonary edema or pneumonia will prevent proper diffusion of gases. Finally, the endothelial lining of the capillaries must be intact for exchange of oxygen and carbon dioxide to occur. Diseases that produce thickening of the endothelial lining will also interfere with the process of diffusion.

There are certain measures you can take to address problems with lung diffusion. Providing the patient with high concentrations of oxygen is one simple step that can be used. Remember that the concentration gradient provides the driving force in moving oxygen into the capillaries. Therefore, the larger the difference between the concentration of oxygen in the alveoli and the capillaries, the greater the diffusion of oxygen into the bloodstream. Similarly, when fluid accumulation or inflammation is the underlying cause of the thickening of the interstitial space within the alveoli, medications such as diuretic agents or anti-inflammatory drugs (corticosteroids) are given to reduce fluid and inflammation.

Perfusion

One additional process that occurs in the lungs is **perfusion**. Lung perfusion is the circulation of blood through the lungs or, more specifically, the pulmonary capillaries. Lung perfusion is dependent on three conditions:

- Adequate blood volume
- Intact pulmonary capillaries
- Efficient pumping of blood by the heart

For perfusion to proceed effectively, there must be an adequate volume of blood in the bloodstream. Equally important is the concentration of **hemoglobin**, which is the transport protein that carries oxygen in the blood. Remember that oxygen is transported in the bloodstream in one of two ways: bound to hemoglobin or dissolved in the plasma. Under normal conditions, less than 2 percent of all oxygen is transported dissolved in plasma (as measured by the PO_2), whereas more than 98 percent is carried by hemoglobin. Hemoglobin with oxygen bound is referred to as **oxyhemoglobin**. Hemoglobin without oxygen is called **deoxyhemoglobin**.

Hemoglobin has some unique properties. It is made up of four iron-containing heme molecules and a protein-containing globin portion. Oxygen molecules bind to the heme portion of the hemoglobin molecule. As oxygen binds to hemoglobin, its structure changes so that it more readily binds additional oxygen molecules. Similarly, as fully oxygen-bound hemoglobin begins to release oxygen, it more readily sheds additional oxygen. The relationship is described by the *oxygen dissociation curve* (Figure 1-10). You can see that, between 10 and 50 mmHg, there is a marked increase in the saturation of hemoglobin. However, as the PO_2 increases above 70 mmHg, there is only a small change in the saturation of hemoglobin, which is already near 100 percent.

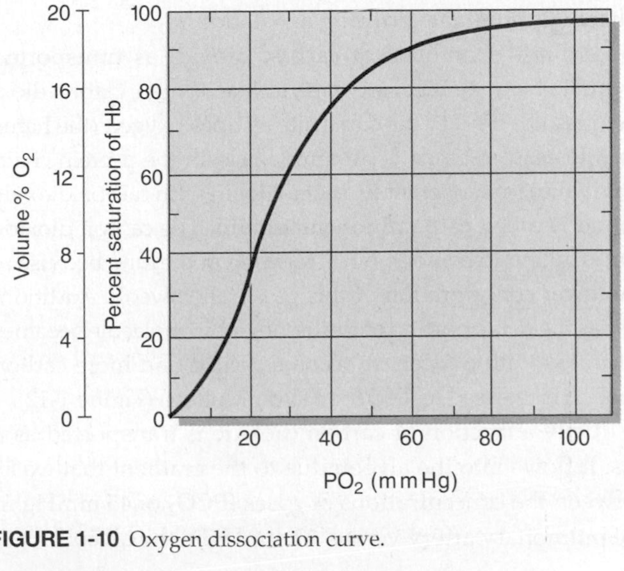

FIGURE 1-10 Oxygen dissociation curve.

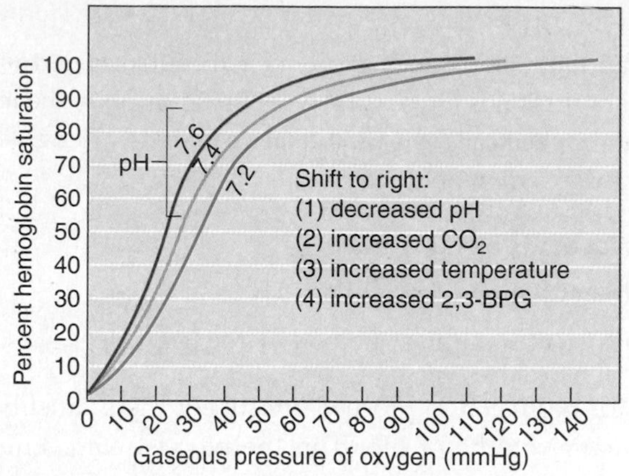

FIGURE 1-11 The Bohr effect.

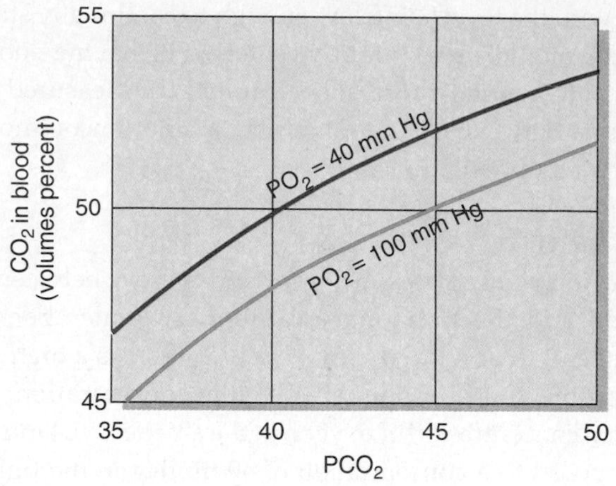

FIGURE 1-12 The Haldane effect.

Changes in the body temperature, the blood pH, and the PCO_2 can alter the oxygen dissociation curve. Within the tissues, as hemoglobin becomes bound with carbon dioxide, it loses its affinity for oxygen. As a result, more oxygen is released and is thus available to cells for metabolism (called the Bohr effect) (Figure 1-11).

Carbon dioxide is transported from the cells to the lungs in one of three ways:

- As bicarbonate ion (70 percent)
- Bound to the globin portion of the hemoglobin molecule (23 percent)
- Dissolved in plasma (measured as PCO_2) (7 percent)

As just noted, the vast majority of carbon dioxide is transported in the form of bicarbonate ion. As the CO_2 is released into the capillaries, it enters the red blood cell where an enzyme (carbonic anhydrase) combines carbon dioxide with water to form two ions, hydrogen (H^+) and bicarbonate (HCO_3^-). Bicarbonate is then released from the red blood cell and transported in plasma. In the lungs, the reverse process takes place, producing water and carbon dioxide. The carbon dioxide then diffuses into the alveoli, where it is eliminated during exhalation.

A limited amount of carbon dioxide is transported bound to hemoglobin. However, unlike oxygen, carbon dioxide does not bind to the same site as does oxygen (the heme site). Instead, it binds to an amino acid in the protein chain that makes up hemoglobin. Hemoglobin with carbon dioxide bound is called **carbaminohemoglobin**. The carbon dioxide that is bound to hemoglobin is released in the lung because of the lower concentration of this gas in the alveoli. Additionally, as the heme portion of the hemoglobin molecule becomes saturated with oxygen, it becomes acidic and more carbon dioxide is released (called the Haldane effect) (Figure 1-12).

Only a fraction of carbon dioxide is transported as a gas. It flows into the alveoli due to the gradient that exists between the concentrations of gases (PCO_2 of 45 mmHg in the pulmonary artery versus 40 mmHg in the alveoli).

For perfusion to take place, in addition to having adequate blood volume, the pulmonary capillaries must be able to transport blood through all portions of the lung tissue. These vessels must be open and not occluded, or blocked. For example, a pulmonary embolism will occlude the pulmonary artery in which it lodges, making that artery unavailable for perfusion of the portion of the lung it usually supplies with blood. Finally, the heart must pump efficiently to push blood effectively through the pulmonary capillaries to perfuse the lung tissues.

To maintain perfusion, you must ensure that the patient has an adequate circulating blood volume. In addition, take the necessary steps to improve the pumping action of the heart. For example, in patients with acute pulmonary edema, the use of diuretic agents reduces the blood return (preload) to an ineffectively pumping heart and improves cardiac efficiency.

The entire system we have just discussed provides for **respiration**, which is the exchange of gases between a living organism and its environment. Pulmonary respiration occurs in the lungs when the respiratory gases are exchanged between the alveoli and the red blood cells in the pulmonary capillaries through the respiratory membranes. Cellular respiration, on the other hand, occurs in the peripheral capillaries. It involves the exchange of the respiratory gases between the red blood cells and the various tissues. Many of the principles of gas exchange that occur in the lungs are reversed in the tissues, with oxygen being released to the cells and carbon dioxide accumulating in the plasma and red blood cells.

Pathophysiology

Remember that many disease states affect the pulmonary system and interfere with its ability to acquire the oxygen required for normal cellular metabolism. Additionally, respiratory diseases limit the body's ability to get rid of waste products such as carbon dioxide. Your understanding of normal anatomy and physiology—ventilation, diffusion, and perfusion—will aid in understanding the mechanism of each disease process and will direct you toward the appropriate corrective actions. Ultimately, any disease process that impairs the pulmonary system will result in a derangement in ventilation, diffusion, perfusion, or a combination of these processes.

Disruption in Ventilation

Diseases that affect ventilation will result in obstruction of the normal conducting pathways of the upper or lower respiratory tract, impairment of the normal function of the chest wall, or abnormalities involving the nervous system's control of ventilation.

Upper and Lower Respiratory Tracts

Disease states that affect the upper respiratory tract will result in obstruction of airflow to the lower structures. Upper airway trauma, for example, produces both significant hemorrhage and swelling. Infections of the upper airway structures, including epiglottitis, soft tissue infections of the neck, tonsillitis, and abscess formation within the pharynx (peritonsillar abscess and retropharyngeal abscess), can obstruct airflow. A common condition, obstructive sleep apnea, occurs when the tongue (or adjoining tissues) blocks the airway during deep sleep. This results in periods of apnea that usually awaken the patient. Similarly, lower airway obstruction may be produced by trauma, foreign body aspiration, mucus accumulation (as in asthmatics), smooth muscle constriction (in asthma and COPD), and airway edema produced by infection or burns.

Chest Wall and Diaphragm

As you read earlier, the chest wall and diaphragm are mechanical components that are essential for normal ventilation. Traumatic injuries to these areas will disrupt the normal mechanics, causing loss of negative pressure within the pleural space. This occurs in patients with **pneumothorax**, including open pneumothorax, tension pneumothorax, or **hemothorax**. Infectious processes such as empyema (pus accumulation in the pleural space) or inflammatory conditions produce similar effects. Chest wall injuries, including rib fractures or **flail chest** and diaphragmatic rupture, limit the patient's ability to expand the thoracic cavity. Certain neuromuscular diseases, such as muscular dystrophy, multiple sclerosis, or amyotrophic lateral sclerosis (ALS or Lou Gehrig's disease), impair muscular function so as to limit the ability to generate a negative pressure within the chest cavity.

Nervous System

Any disease process that impairs the nervous system's regulation of breathing may also alter ventilation. Central nervous system depressants, such as alcohol, benzodiazepines, or barbiturates, alone or in combination, can alter the brain's response to important signals such as rising PCO_2. Similarly, stroke, diseases, or injuries that involve the respiratory centers within the central nervous system can change the normal ventilatory pattern. In fact, certain abnormal respiratory patterns are produced by specific brain injury (Figure 1-13):

- *Cheyne-Stokes respirations* are a ventilatory pattern with progressively increasing tidal volume, followed by a declining volume, separated by periods of **apnea** at the end of expiration. This pattern is typically seen in older patients with terminal illness or brain injury.
- *Kussmaul's respirations* are deep, rapid breaths that result as a corrective measure against conditions such as diabetic ketoacidosis that produce metabolic acidosis.

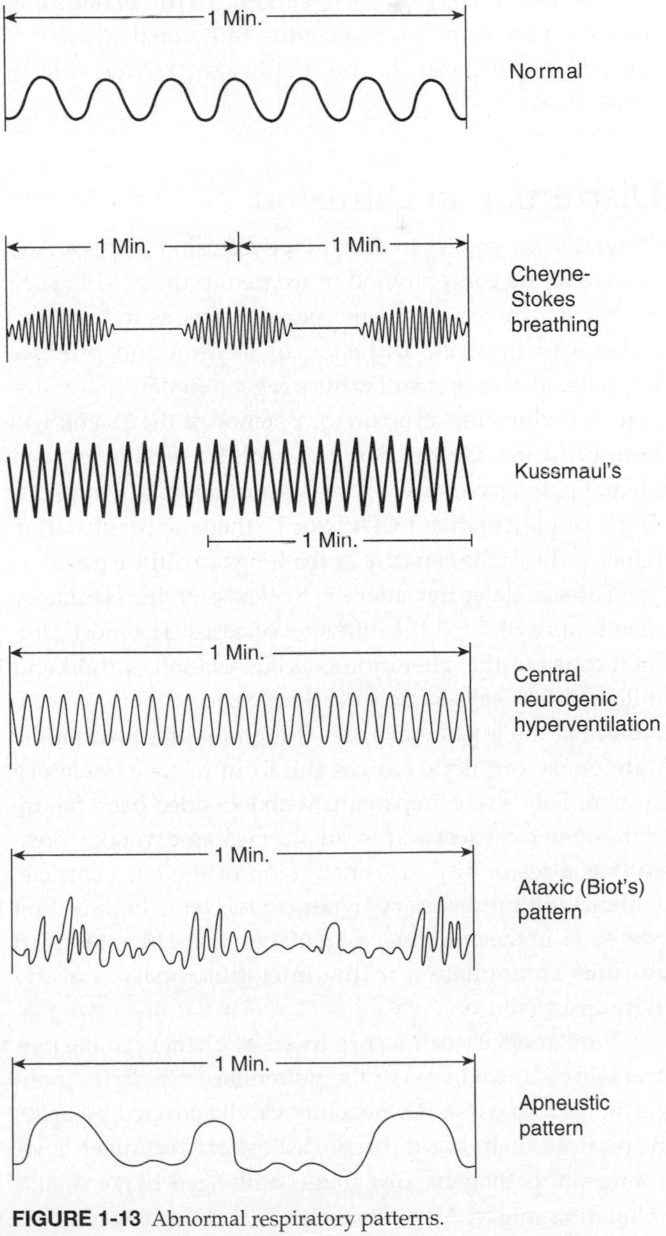

FIGURE 1-13 Abnormal respiratory patterns.

- *Central neurogenic hyperventilation* also produces deep, rapid respirations that are caused by strokes or injury to the brainstem. In this case, there is loss of normal regulation of ventilatory controls and respiratory alkalosis is often seen.
- *Ataxic (Biot's) respirations* are characterized by repeated episodes of gasping ventilations separated by periods of apnea. This pattern is seen in patients with increased intracranial pressure.
- *Apneustic respiration* is characterized by long, deep breaths that are stopped during the inspiratory phase and separated by periods of apnea. This pattern is a result of stroke or severe central nervous system disease.

Also remember that damage to the major peripheral nerves that supply the diaphragm and intercostal muscles, the phrenic nerve, and intercostal nerves will also affect normal ventilatory mechanics. Traumatic disruption of the phrenic nerve during chest surgery, with penetrating trauma, or by neoplastic (cancerous, tumorous) invasion of the nerve can paralyze the diaphragm on the side of involvement.

Disruption in Diffusion

Other disease states can disrupt the diffusion of gases. Any change in the concentration of oxygen in the alveoli, such as that which occurs when a person ascends to high altitudes, can limit the diffusion of oxygen and produce **hypoxia**, a state of insufficient oxygen. Similarly, any disease that alters the structure or patency of the alveoli will limit diffusion. Destruction of alveoli by certain environmental pathogens, such as asbestos or coal (black lung disease), in patients with COPD or in those with inhalation injury reduces the capacity of the lungs to diffuse gases.

Disease states that alter the thickness of the respiratory membrane will limit the diffusion of gases. The most common cause of this alteration is accumulation of fluid and inflammatory cells in the interstitial space. Fluid can accumulate in the interstitial space if high pressure within the pulmonary capillaries forces fluid out of the circulatory system. This is seen in patients with left-sided heart failure (cardiogenic causes) and is due to increased venous pressure as a result of poor functioning of the left ventricle. Patients with pulmonary hypertension have high resting pressures in the pulmonary circulation that ultimately lead to fluid accumulation in the interstitial space, causing right-heart failure.

Similar effects can be produced by changes in the permeability (or leakiness) of the pulmonary capillaries (noncardiogenic causes). Permeability can be affected by acute respiratory distress syndrome, asbestosis and other environmental pathogens, drowning, prolonged hypoxia, and inhalation injury. Also remember that disease states that alter the pulmonary capillary endothelial lining, such as advanced atherosclerosis or vascular inflammatory states, can affect diffusion.

Disruption in Perfusion

As detailed earlier, any alteration in appropriate blood flow through the pulmonary capillaries will limit normal gas exchange in the lungs. Any disease state that reduces the normal circulating blood volume—such as trauma, hemorrhage, dehydration, shock, or other causes of hypovolemia—will limit normal perfusion of the lungs. Remember that hemoglobin is the major transport protein for oxygen and plays a significant role in the elimination of carbon dioxide. Therefore, any reduction in the normal circulating hemoglobin will also affect perfusion. All causes of anemia, a condition in which the number of red blood cells or amount of hemoglobin in them is below normal, must be considered. Such causes include acute blood loss, iron or vitamin deficiency, malnutrition, and anemia from chronic disease states.

Remember that blood must be available to all the lung segments for maximum gas exchange to occur. When an area of lung tissue is appropriately ventilated but no capillary perfusion occurs, available oxygen is not moved into the circulatory system. This is referred to as a *pulmonary shunting*. In patients with pulmonary embolism, a blockage of a division of the pulmonary artery by a clot prevents perfusion of the lung segments supplied by that branch of the artery. As a result, there may be significant shunt with return of deoxygenated blood to the pulmonary venous circulation.

Assessment of the Respiratory System

Assessment of the respiratory system is a vital aspect of prehospital care. You must quickly assess the airway and ventilation status during the primary assessment. If the patient's complaints suggest that the respiratory system is involved in the patient's problem, the focused history and physical examination should be directed to this aspect of the assessment.

Scene Size-Up

When you approach the scene, consider two major questions: (1) Is the scene safe to approach the patient? (2) Are there visual clues that might provide information regarding the patient's medical complaint?

Remember that several hazards may result in respiratory complaints by the patient that are also potentially dangerous for emergency care providers. Certain gases and toxic products that are causing respiratory complaints from the patient may also present a significant risk to you. Dust particles are also a risk. Some rescuers involved in the World Trade Center attacks in 2001 and the Oklahoma City bombing in 1995 developed both acute and chronic respiratory problems following dust exposure. Carbon monoxide, for example, is a colorless and odorless gas that may be present in quantities large enough to overcome unsuspecting emergency care personnel. Other toxins from incomplete combustion produced in fires or industrial processes pose a similar risk. Past incidents involving chemical agents such as sarin gas or biologic agents such as anthrax highlight the need for emergency care providers to be aware of hazards to themselves as well as to their patient.

You should also be aware that in certain rescue environments, the concentration of available oxygen is significantly reduced. This would include areas such as grain silos, enclosed storage containers, or any enclosed space in which there is an active fire. You must take the appropriate precautions before entering such environments, including the use of your own supplemental oxygen supply.

In any situation in which you believe there is a hazard to you as a care provider, make sure that the scene is appropriately secured before you enter. If specific protective items such as hazardous materials suits, self-contained breathing apparatus (SCBA), or supplemental oxygen are needed, make sure they are available before you attempt to care for your patient. Similarly, if other personnel such as fire suppression units or hazmat teams are required, contact dispatch and have them available on scene before putting yourself at risk.

Once it is safe to enter the scene, look for clues that will provide information regarding the patient's complaints. Do you see evidence of cigarette packs or ashtrays to suggest that the patient or family members are smokers? Look for any home nebulizer machines or supplemental oxygen tanks that may suggest a patient with underlying COPD or asthma. Look for possible sources of carbon monoxide exposure. If the patient is a small child, look for small items lying around the house that could suggest potential ingested foreign bodies. Using your eyes, ears, and nose can lead you to several important clues that are useful as you begin your assessment of the patient.

Primary Assessment

General Impression

Take the following considerations and steps to help form your initial impression of the patient's respiratory status:

- ***Position.*** Consider the patient's position. Patients with respiratory diseases tend to tolerate an upright posture better than lying flat. Indications of severe respiratory distress include a patient who is sitting upright with feet dangling over the side of the bed. In the most severe cases, the patient will assume the "tripod" position in which he leans forward and supports his weight with the arms extended (Figure 1-14).

CONTENT REVIEW

➤ General Impression of Respiratory Status
- Position
- Color
- Mental status
- Ability to speak
- Respiratory effort

- ***Color.*** Patients with severe respiratory distress display **pallor** and **diaphoresis**. **Cyanosis** is a late finding and may be absent even with significant hypoxia. Peripheral cyanosis (bluish discoloration involving only the distal extremities) is not a specific finding and is also found in patients with poor circulation. Peripheral cyanosis reflects the slowing of blood flow and increased extraction of oxygen from red blood cells. Central cyanosis (involving the lips, tongue, and truncal skin) is a more ominous finding seen in hypoxia.
- ***Mental status.*** Briefly assess the patient's mental status. The hypoxic patient will become restless and agitated. Confusion is seen with both hypoxia (deficiency of oxygen) and hypercarbia (excess of carbon dioxide). When respiratory failure is imminent, the patient will appear severely lethargic and somnolent. The eyelids will begin to droop and the head will bob with each respiratory effort.
- ***Ability to speak.*** Assess the patient's ability to speak in full, coherent sentences. Determine the ease with

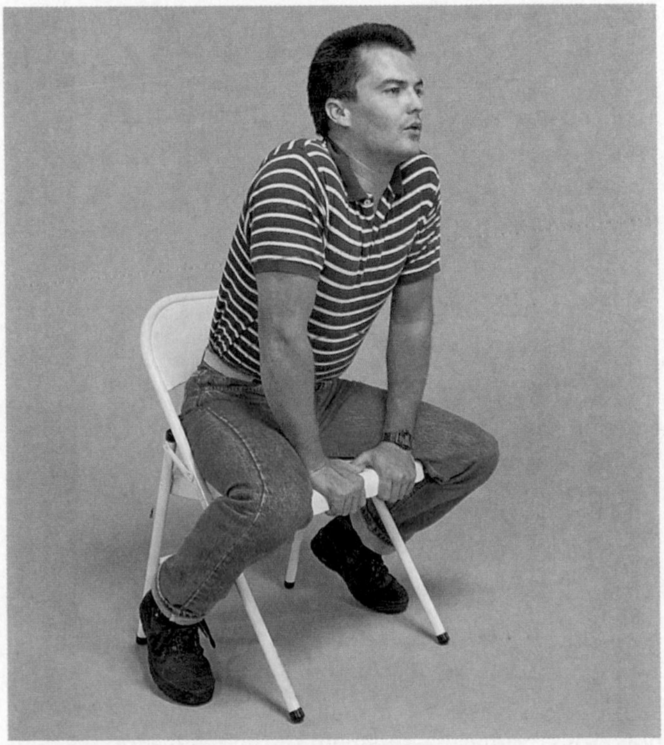

FIGURE 1-14 Tripod position.

which the patient can discuss symptoms. Patients with respiratory distress will be able to speak only one to two words before they need to pause to catch their breath. Rambling, incoherent speech indicates fear, anxiety, or hypoxia.

- ***Respiratory effort.*** As described, normal ventilation is an active process. However, the use of accessory muscles in the neck (scalenes and sternocleidomastoids) and visible contractions of the intercostal muscles indicate significant breathing effort.

As you form your general impression, also make specific note of any of the following signs of respiratory distress:

- **Nasal flaring**
- Intercostal muscle retraction
- Use of the accessory respiratory muscles
- Cyanosis
- Pursed lips
- **Tracheal tugging**

Your primary assessment of the patient is directed at identification of any life-threatening conditions resulting from compromise of airway, breathing, or circulation (the ABCs). Remember that in presumed cardiac arrest, circulation comes before airway and breathing. Because this chapter concerns the respiratory system, we focus here on assessment of airway and breathing.

Airway

Remember that oxygen is one of the most basic necessities for life, and the respiratory system is responsible for supplying it to the body tissues. As a result, any significant abnormality in the respiratory tract must be viewed as potentially life threatening.

After quickly forming your general impression, immediately focus on the patient's airway. When assessing the airway, keep these principles in mind:

- Noisy breathing nearly always means partial airway obstruction.
- Obstructed breathing is not always noisy.
- The brain can survive only a few minutes in **asphyxia**.
- Artificial respiration is useless if the airway is blocked.
- A patent airway is useless if the patient is apneic.
- If you note airway obstruction, do not waste time looking for help or equipment. Act immediately.

If the airway is compromised, quickly institute basic airway management techniques. Once you have secured a patent airway, ensure that the patient has adequate ventilation. Your primary assessment of the respiratory system should be brief and directed. A more detailed examination should be conducted once you have been able to establish that an immediate threat to life does not exist.

Breathing

The following signs should suggest a possible life-threatening respiratory problem in adults. They are listed in order from most ominous to least severe.

- Alterations in mental status
- Severe central cyanosis
- Absent breath sounds
- Audible stridor
- One-to-two-word **dyspnea** (need to breathe after every word or two)
- **Tachycardia** ≥ 130 beats per minute
- Pallor and diaphoresis
- Presence of intercostal and sternocleidomastoid retractions
- Use of accessory muscles

If any of these signs are present, direct your efforts toward immediate resuscitation and transport of the patient to a medical facility.

Secondary Assessment

History

The history and physical exam should be directed at problem areas as determined by the patient's chief complaint or primary problem. Patients with respiratory diseases will often present with a complaint of "shortness of breath" (dyspnea). Obtain a SAMPLE history. If the chief complaint suggests respiratory disease, ask the OPQRST questions, including the following questions about the current symptoms. The answers to these or similar questions will provide you with a pertinent patient history.

- How long has the dyspnea been present?
- Was the onset gradual or abrupt?
- Is the dyspnea better or worse by position? Is there associated **orthopnea** or **paroxysmal nocturnal dyspnea**?
- Has the patient been coughing?
- If so, is the cough productive?
- What is the character and color of the sputum?
- Is there any **hemoptysis** (coughing up of blood)?
- Is there any chest pain associated with the dyspnea?
- If so, what is the location of the pain?
- Was the onset of pain sudden or slow?
- What was the duration of the pain?
- Does the pain radiate to any area?

- Does the pain increase with respiration?
- Are there associated symptoms of fever or chills?
- What is the patient's past medical history?
- Does the patient have obstructive sleep apnea?
- Has the patient experienced wheezing?
- Is the patient or close family member a smoker?

It is also important to ask the patient whether he has ever experienced similar symptoms in the past. Patients with chronic medical conditions such as COPD or asthma can usually relate the severity of their current presenting complaints to other episodes that they have experienced. Question the patient or family about prior hospitalizations for respiratory disease. In particular, you should try to determine whether the patient required care in the intensive care unit (ICU) for breathing problems. Ask whether the patient has ever required endotracheal intubation and ventilatory support. Consider patients who have been previously intubated to be potentially seriously ill and approach them with great caution.

Similarly, it is important to ask the patient whether he already has a known respiratory disease. The most common reason for a call to emergency care personnel is a worsening of an already present respiratory disease. This is typical for patients with COPD, asthma, or lung cancer. If you are not familiar with the patient's diagnosis (for example, alpha-1 antitrypsin deficiency), try to determine whether the disease is affecting the process of ventilation, diffusion, or perfusion.

Continue history taking by determining:

- What current medications is the patient taking? (Pay particular attention to oxygen therapy, oral bronchodilators, corticosteroids, and antibiotics.)
- Does the patient have any allergies?

A good history of medication use is essential and may provide useful clues to the diagnosis. If time permits, gather the patient's current medications and transport them with the patient. This is a great benefit to the emergency department personnel who will be evaluating the patient. Pay particular attention to any medications that suggest pulmonary disease. These would include inhaled or oral sympathomimetics such as albuterol and related agents that are used to treat diseases such as COPD or asthma. Also ask about steroid preparations, which are used in these conditions. Other common medications used by patients with COPD or asthma include cromolyn sodium, methylxanthines (e.g., theophylline), and antibiotic agents.

Ask if the patient has a home nebulizer unit and how frequently it is used. Inquire about the use of a continuous positive airway pressure (CPAP) device (or similar device) for obstructive sleep apnea.

Also ask about drugs used for cardiac conditions, as cardiac patients often present with dyspnea. Patients with cardiac disease commonly use nitrates, calcium channel blockers, diuretic agents, digoxin, and certain antiarrhythmic agents.

CONTENT REVIEW

- ➤ Physical Exam of the Respiratory System
  - Head
  - Neck
  - Chest
    - Inspection
    - Palpation
    - Percussion
    - Auscultation
  - Extremities

Finally, inquire about medication allergies. This information is important because it helps to avoid administering agents to which the patient is allergic. It is also possible that a specific medication may be the cause of an allergic reaction that has resulted in upper airway edema and respiratory complaints.

Physical Examination

First address the patient's head and neck. Look at the lips. Pursed lips indicate significant respiratory distress. This is the patient's way of maintaining positive pressure during expiration and preventing alveolar collapse. Also examine the nose, mouth, and throat for any signs of swelling or infection that might be causing upper airway obstruction.

Occasionally, the patient may produce sputum, which can suggest an underlying cause of the patient's complaints. An increase in the amount of sputum produced suggests infection of the lungs or bronchial passages (bronchitis). Thick green or brown sputum is characteristic of these infections. On the other hand, thin yellow or pale gray sputum is more typical of inflammation or an allergic cause. Pink, frothy sputum is a sign of severe pulmonary edema. Truly bloody sputum (hemoptysis) may be seen with cancer, tuberculosis, and bronchial infection.

Assess the neck for signs of swelling or infection. Remember to look at the jugular veins for evidence of distention (Figure 1-15). This occurs when the right side of

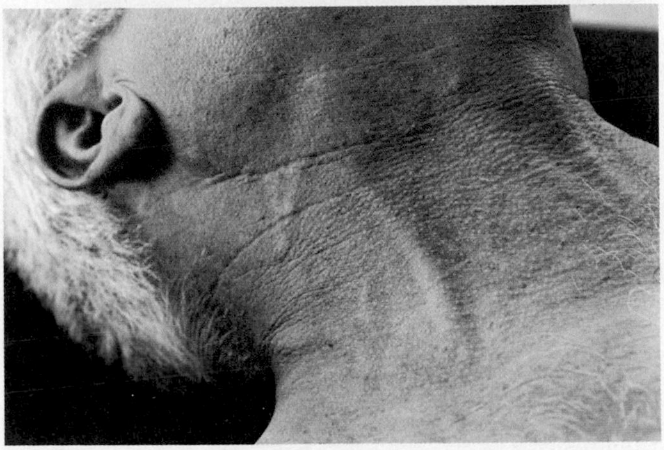

FIGURE 1-15 Jugular vein distention.

the heart is not pumping blood effectively, causing a "backup" in the venous circulation. Such findings are often accompanied by left-sided heart failure and pulmonary edema.

Physical examination of the respiratory system should follow the standard steps of patient assessment: inspection, palpation, percussion, and auscultation.

- ***Inspection.*** Inspection should include an examination of the anterior–posterior dimensions and general shape of the chest (Figure 1-16). An increased anterior–posterior diameter is suggestive of COPD. Inspect the chest for symmetrical movement. Any asymmetry may be suggestive of trauma. A paradoxical movement (moving in a fashion opposite to that expected) is suggestive of flail chest. Note any chest scars, lesions, wounds, or deformities.
- ***Palpation.*** Palpate the chest, both front and back, for abnormalities (Figure 1-17). Note any tenderness, **crepitus**, or **subcutaneous emphysema**. Palpate the anterior chest first, then the posterior. Inspect your gloved hands for blood each time you remove them from behind the patient's chest. In some instances, it may be appropriate to evaluate **tactile fremitus**, the vibration felt in the chest during speaking. When evaluating tactile fremitus, compare one side of the chest with the other. Simultaneously, palpate the trachea for **tracheal deviation**, which is suggestive of a tension pneumothorax.

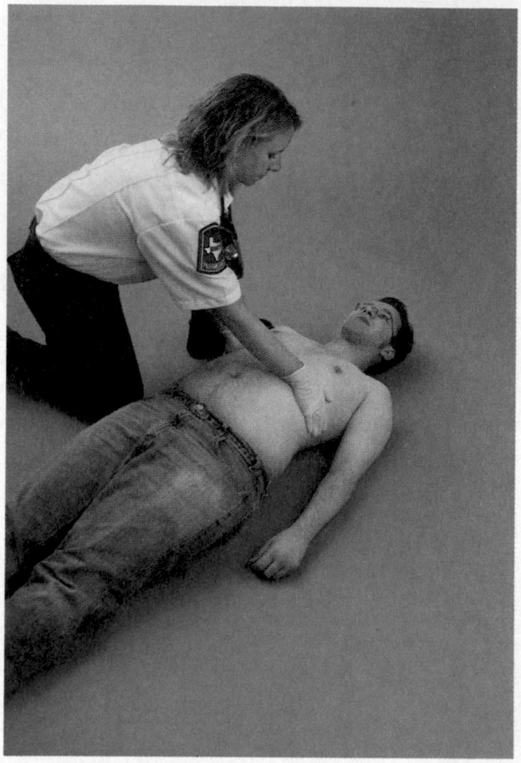

FIGURE 1-17 The chest should be palpated.

- ***Percussion.*** If indicated, quickly percuss the chest (Figure 1-18). Limit percussion to suspected cases of pneumothorax and pulmonary edema. A hollow sound on percussion is often indicative of pneumothorax or

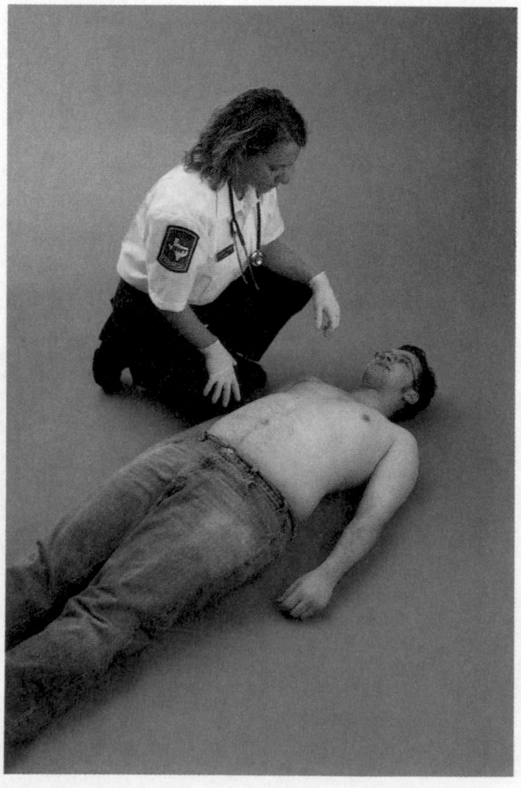

FIGURE 1-16 Inspection of the chest.

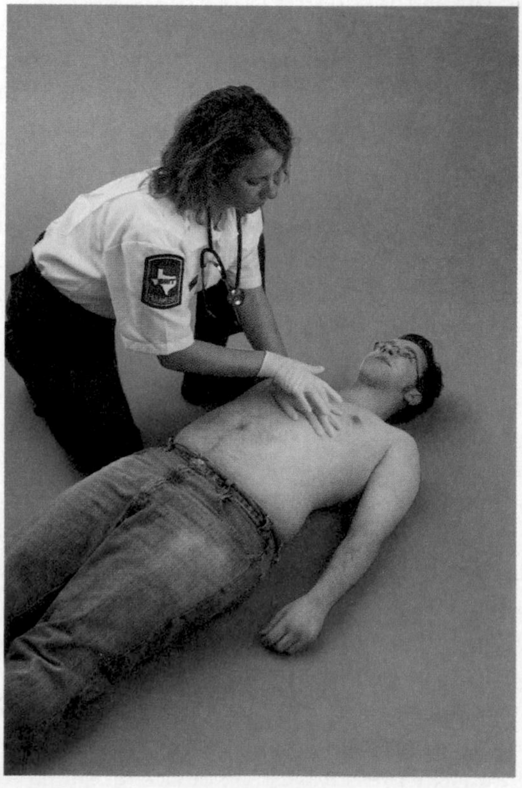

FIGURE 1-18 If indicated, the chest should be percussed.

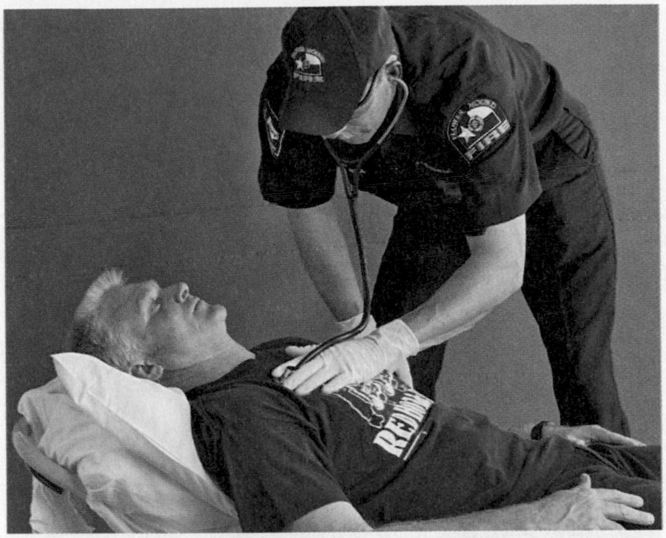

FIGURE 1-19 The chest should be auscultated.

emphysema. In contrast, a dull sound is indicative of pulmonary edema, hemothorax, or pneumonia. Remember, however, that percussion may be of little value in the noisy environment typical of most emergency scenes.

- ***Auscultation.*** Auscultate the chest. Begin by listening to the patient without a stethoscope and from a distance. Note any loud stridor, wheezing, or cough. If possible, the patient should be in the sitting position and the chest auscultated in a symmetrical pattern. When the patient cannot sit up, auscultate the anterior and lateral parts of the chest (Figure 1-19). Each area should be auscultated for one respiratory cycle.

Normal breath sounds heard during auscultation can be characterized according to the following descriptions.

Normal Breath Sounds

- Bronchial (or tubular)
  - Loud, high-pitched breath sounds heard over the trachea
  - Expiratory phase lasts longer than inspiratory phase
- Bronchovesicular
  - Softer, medium-pitched breath sounds heard over the mainstem bronchi (below clavicles or between scapulae)
  - Expiratory phase and inspiratory phase equal
- Vesicular
  - Soft, low-pitched breath sounds heard in the lung periphery

While the patient breathes in and out deeply with the mouth open, note any abnormal breath sounds and their location. Many terms are used to describe abnormal breath sounds. The following list includes some of the more common terms.

Abnormal Breath Sounds

- ***Snoring.*** Occurs when the upper airway is partially obstructed, usually by the tongue.
- ***Stridor.*** Harsh, high-pitched sound heard on inspiration and characteristic of an upper airway obstruction such as croup.
- ***Wheezing.*** Whistling sound due to narrowing of the airways by edema, bronchoconstriction, or foreign materials.
- ***Rhonchi.*** Rattling sounds in the larger airways associated with excessive mucus or other material.
- ***Crackles*** (also called rales). Fine, moist crackling sounds associated with fluid in the smaller airways.
- ***Pleural friction rub.*** Sounds like dried pieces of leather rubbing together; occurs when the pleura become inflamed, as in pleurisy.

Also examine the extremities. Look for peripheral cyanosis, which may indicate hypoxia. Examine the extremities for swelling, redness, and a hard, firm cord indicating a venous clot. This may suggest a possible cause for pulmonary embolism. Look for clubbing of the fingers (Figure 1-20), suggesting long-standing hypoxemia. This is typical of patients with COPD or cyanotic heart disease. Finally, the patient may demonstrate *carpopedal spasm*, in which the fingers and toes are contracted in flexion. This is found in patients with hyperventilation and is caused by transient shifts in the blood calcium concentration due to changes in the serum CO_2 and pH levels.

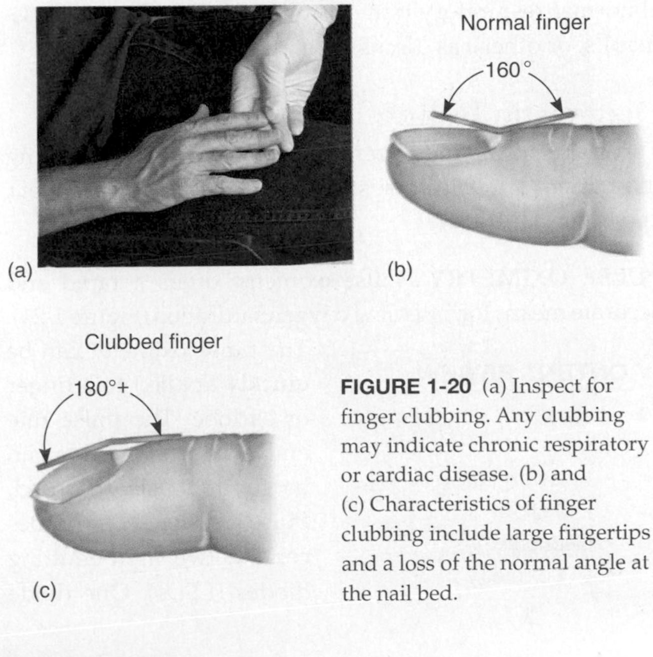

FIGURE 1-20 (a) Inspect for finger clubbing. Any clubbing may indicate chronic respiratory or cardiac disease. (b) and (c) Characteristics of finger clubbing include large fingertips and a loss of the normal angle at the nail bed.

Vital Signs

The patient's vital signs may also provide information regarding the severity of the respiratory complaints. In general, tachycardia (rapid heart rate) is a very nonspecific finding, seen with fear, anxiety, and fever. In patients with respiratory complaints, however, tachycardia may also indicate hypoxia. Remember that the patient may have recently used sympathomimetic drugs such as albuterol, which will accelerate the heart rate. These same drugs will elevate the patient's blood pressure as well. During your assessment of the blood pressure, a patient will occasionally exhibit *pulsus paradoxus,* a drop in the systolic blood pressure of 10 mmHg or more with each respiratory cycle. *Pulsus paradoxus* is associated with COPD and cardiac tamponade. As a rule, however, you should not take the time to look for *pulsus paradoxus.*

A change in a patient's respiratory rate may be one of the earliest indicators of respiratory disease. The patient's respiratory rate can be influenced by several factors, including respiratory difficulty, fear, anxiety, fever, and underlying metabolic disease. Assume that an elevated respiratory rate in a patient with dyspnea is caused by hypoxia. Although fluctuations in the respiratory rate are common, a persistently *slow* rate indicates impending respiratory arrest.

Continually reassess the patient's respiratory rate during the time that you are caring for the patient. Trends in the respiratory rate (for example, an increasing rate) can give you an overall assessment of the effectiveness of any intervention you have made. Also assess the patient's respiratory pattern. The normal respiratory pattern (eupnea) is steady, even breaths occurring 12 to 20 times per minute with an expiratory phase that lasts between 3 to 4 times as long as the inspiratory phase. **Tachypnea** describes a respiratory pattern with a rate that exceeds 20 breaths per minute. **Bradypnea** describes a respiratory pattern with a rate slower than 12 breaths per minute. Look also for any abnormal respiratory patterns (e.g., Cheyne-Stokes, Kussmaul's, or other), as discussed earlier in the chapter.

Diagnostic Testing

Three diagnostic measurements are of value in assessing the patient's respiratory status: *pulse oximetry, peak flow,* and *capnography.*

PULSE OXIMETRY Pulse oximetry offers a rapid and accurate means for assessing oxygen saturation (Figure 1-21). The pulse oximeter can be quickly applied to a finger or earlobe. The pulse rate and oxygen saturation can be continuously recorded. Pulse oximeter probes contain two light-emitting diodes (LEDs). One diode emits light in the red range (660 nm) and the other emits light in the infrared (940 nm) range. Photodetectors on the opposite side of the probe detect the two wavelengths of light that penetrate the tissues. Deoxyhemoglobin absorbs more red light than does oxyhemoglobin. Oxyhemoglobin absorbs more infrared light than red light. The ratio of the two types of absorbed light is calculated by the oximeter and compared against standardized values. The concentration of oxyhemoglobin (and thus oxygen saturation) is displayed as a percentage called the *hemoglobin oxygen saturation*. The oxygen saturation measurement obtained through pulse oximetry is abbreviated as SpO_2. Oxygen saturations obtained through blood gas analysis in hospitals are abbreviated SaO_2. Normally, the SpO_2 and SaO_2 are the same.

CONTENT REVIEW

- Prehospital Diagnostic Tests
  - Pulse oximetry
  - Peak flow
  - Capnometry
  - CO-oximetry

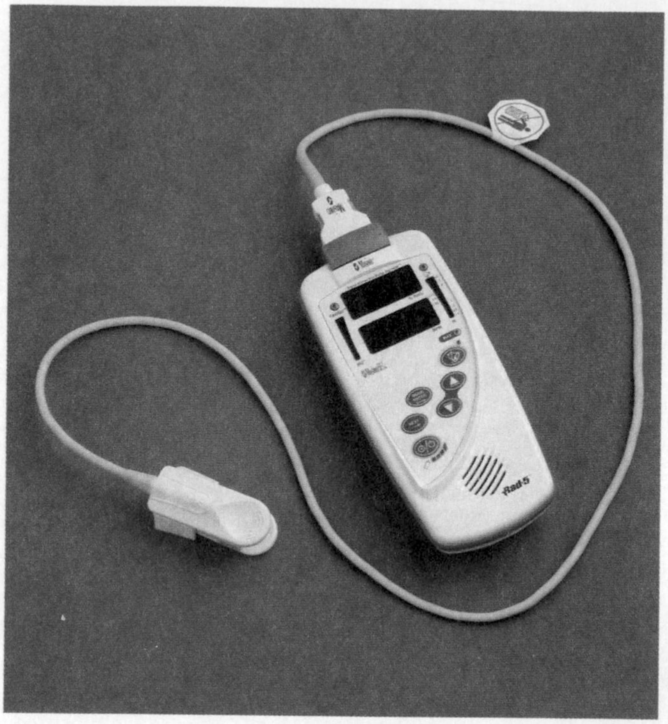

FIGURE 1-21 Sensing unit for pulse oximetry. This device transmits light through a vascular bed, such as in the finger, and can determine the oxygen saturation of red blood cells. To use the pulse oximeter, it is only necessary to turn the device on and attach the sensor to a finger. The desired graphic mode on the oximeter should be selected. The oxygen saturation and pulse rate can be continuously monitored.

Older pulse oximeters were prone to give abnormal or inconsistent readings in patients with peripheral vasoconstriction (as in sepsis or hypothermia) or low-flow states. They also tended to be inaccurate under conditions in which an abnormal substance such as carbon monoxide was bound to hemoglobin, as the instrument measures the saturation of hemoglobin without indicating which substance has saturated it. Fortunately, second-generation pulse oximeters have technology (filters, signal processors) that minimizes these effects, making them much more accurate and much less sensitive to extraneous factors.

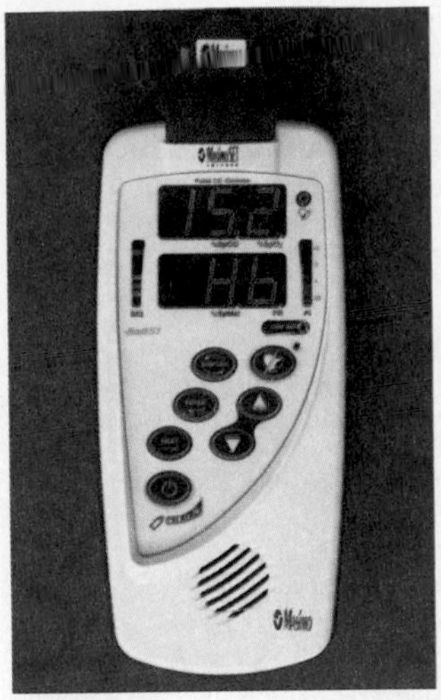

FIGURE 1-22 The ability to noninvasively determine the amount of hemoglobin present (SpHb) is available on certain monitoring technologies.

(© Dr. Bryan E. Bledsoe)

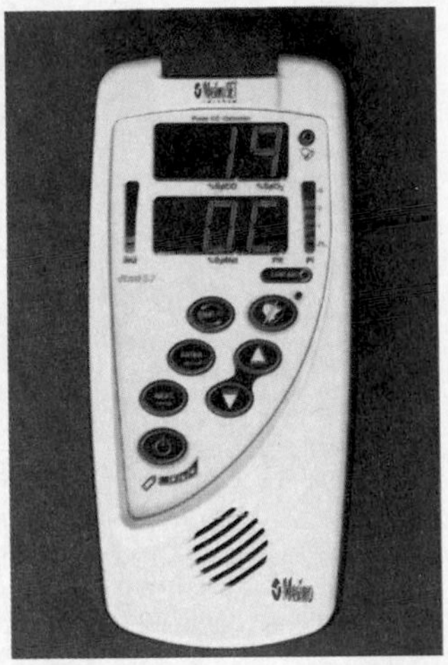

FIGURE 1-23 Combining the oxygen saturation (SpO_2) with the total hemoglobin (SpHb) allows for the calculation of the oxygen content of arterial blood (SpOC).

(© Dr. Bryan E. Bledsoe)

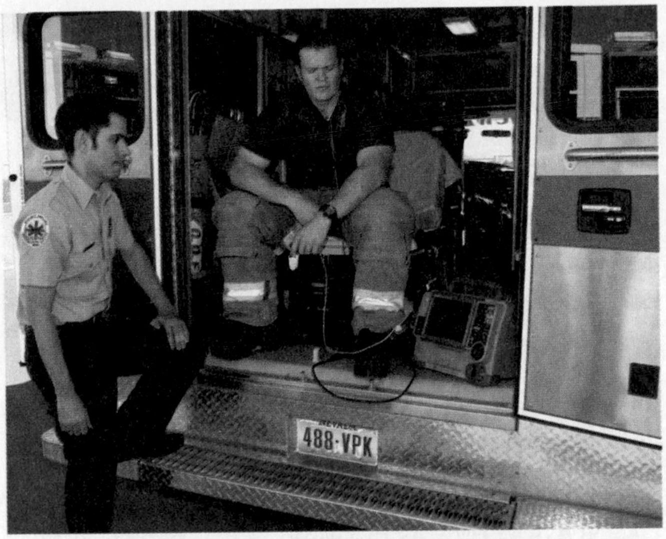

FIGURE 1-24 Modern prehospital patient monitors now allow for continuous monitoring of multiple physiologic parameters.

(© Dr. Bryan E. Bledsoe)

It is important to note that the SpO_2 reflects the oxygen saturation of available hemoglobin. Most pulse oximeters cannot discern between normal and abnormal levels of hemoglobin. For example, in a patient with anemia or who has suffered significant hemorrhage, the total amount of hemoglobin available to transport oxygen is reduced. However, most pulse oximeters will reflect a normal SpO_2 despite the fact that tissue delivery of oxygen may be impaired because of inadequate hemoglobin. Some of the newer pulse oximeters have the capability of noninvasively measuring total hemoglobin (SpHb) in addition to SpO_2 and other parameters (Figure 1-22).[1] This provides more accurate information about the total amount of oxygen being transported. This value is referred to as the *oxygen content* and, when being measured noninvasively, is referred to as the SpOC (Figure 1-23).

Use of the pulse oximeter, if available, is encouraged for any patient complaining of dyspnea or respiratory problems (Figure 1-24). It is important to remember that the pulse oximeter is designed to supplement the physical examination and not replace it. However, oxygen saturation readings can help you guide care. Table 1-2 details how to interpret oxygen saturation readings and suggested interventions.

PEAK FLOW Handheld devices are available for use in determining the patient's peak expiratory flow rate (PEFR). The normal expected peak flow rate is based on the patient's sex, age, and height. Remember that the measurement of the peak expiratory flow rate is somewhat effort dependent; you must have a cooperative patient who understands the use of the device to get an accurate reading.

Table 1-2 Treatment Strategies Based on Pulse Oximetry Readings

SpO_2	Interpretation	Suggested Intervention
95–100%	Normal	Increase or decrease the FiO_2 to maintain a normal SpO_2
91–94%	Mild hypoxemia	Increase FiO_2 to increase oxygen saturation
85–90%	Moderate hypoxemia	Increase FiO_2 to increase oxygen saturation Assess and increase ventilation as indicated
<85%	Severe hypoxemia	Increase FiO_2 to increase oxygen saturation Increase ventilation

The PEFR is obtained using a Wright spirometer (Figure 1-25), which is inexpensive and easy to use. Place the disposable mouthpiece into the meter. First have the patient take in the deepest possible inspiration. Then encourage the patient to seal his lips around the device and

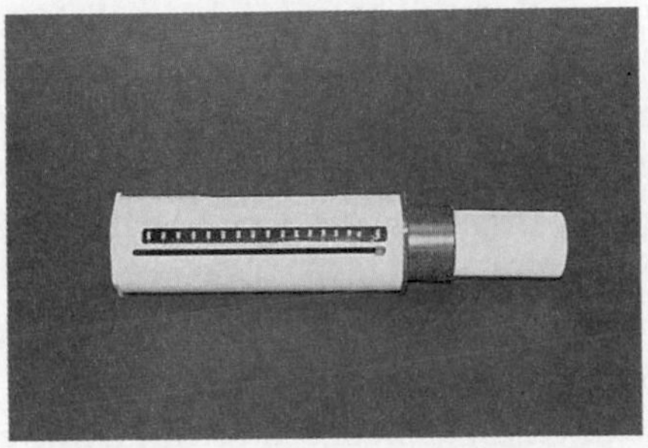

FIGURE 1-25 Wright spirometer for determining peak expiratory flow rate (PEFR).

Table 1-3 Spirometry and Peak Flow Values for Adults

Severity	FEV_1 (liters)	FVC (%)	Peak Flow (liters/min)
Normal	4.0–6.0	80–90	550–650 (Male) 400–500 (Female)
Mild	3.0	70	300–400
Moderate	1.6	50	200–300
Severe	0.6	40	100

forcibly exhale. The peak rate of exhaled gas is recorded in liters per minute. This should be repeated twice, with the highest reading recorded as the patient's PEFR (Table 1-3).

CAPNOGRAPHY As discussed in the chapter "Airway Management and Ventilation," capnography has become a commonly used diagnostic tool for prehospital care. Capnography is a noninvasive method of measuring the levels of carbon dioxide (CO_2) in the exhaled breath.

The following terms have been applied to capnography:

- ***Capnometry:*** the measurement of expired CO_2. (It typically provides a numeric display of the partial pressure of CO_2 [in torr or mmHg] or the percentage of CO_2 present.)
- ***Capnography:*** a graphic recording or display of the capnometry reading over time
- ***Capnograph:*** a device that measures expired CO_2 levels
- ***Capnogram:*** the visual representation of the expired CO_2 waveform
- ***End-tidal CO_2 ($ETCO_2$):*** the measurement of the CO_2 concentration at the end of expiration (maximum CO_2)
- ***$PETCO_2$:*** the partial pressure of end-tidal CO_2 in a mixed gas solution
- ***$PaCO_2$:*** the partial pressure of CO_2 in the arterial blood

CO_2 is a normal end product of metabolism and is transported by the venous system to the right side of the heart. It is then pumped from the right ventricle to the pulmonary artery and eventually enters the pulmonary capillaries. There, it diffuses into the alveoli and is removed from the body through exhalation. When circulation is normal, CO_2 levels change with ventilation and are a reliable estimate of the partial pressure of carbon dioxide in the arterial system ($PaCO_2$). Normal $ETCO_2$ is 1 to 2 mm less than the partial pressure of carbon dioxide ($PaCO_2$), or approximately 5 percent. A normal partial pressure of end-tidal CO_2 ($PETCO_2$) is approximately 38 mmHg (0.05×760 mmHg = 38 mmHg). ($ETCO_2$ is normally expressed as a percentage, whereas $PETCO_2$, a partial pressure, is expressed in mmHg.) When perfusion decreases, as in shock or cardiac arrest, $ETCO_2$ levels reflect pulmonary blood flow and cardiac output, not ventilation.

Table 1-4 Basic Rules of Capnography

Symptom	Possible Cause
Sudden drop of $ETCO_2$ to zero	• Esophageal intubation • Ventilator disconnection or defect in ventilator • Defect in CO_2 analyzer
Sudden decrease of $ETCO_2$ (not to zero)	• Leak in ventilator system; obstruction • Partial disconnect in ventilator circuit • Partial airway obstruction (secretions)
Exponential decrease of $ETCO_2$	• Pulmonary embolism • Cardiac arrest • Hypotension (sudden) • Severe hyperventilation
Change in CO_2 baseline	• Calibration error • Water droplet in analyzer • Mechanical failure (ventilator)
Sudden increase in $ETCO_2$	• Accessing an area of lung previously obstructed • Release of tourniquet • Sudden increase in blood pressure
Gradual lowering of $ETCO_2$	• Hypovolemia • Decreasing cardiac output • Decreasing body temperature; hypothermia; drop in metabolism
Gradual increase in $ETCO_2$	• Rising body temperature • Hypoventilation • CO_2 absorption • Partial airway obstruction (foreign body); reactive airway disease

Decreased CO_2 levels can be found in shock, cardiac arrest, pulmonary embolism, bronchospasm, and with incomplete airway obstruction (such as mucus plugging). Increased CO_2 levels are found with hypoventilation, respiratory depression, and hyperthermia (Table 1-4).

Capnometry provides a noninvasive measure of CO_2 levels, thus providing medical personnel with information about the status of systemic metabolism, circulation, and ventilation. It can be used to detect certain conditions by examining the waveform in the context of the physical examination. The use of capnography has become commonplace in the operating room, emergency department, and prehospital setting.

When first introduced into prehospital care, CO_2 monitoring was used exclusively to verify proper endotracheal tube placement in the trachea, and it is still used for this purpose. The presence of adequate CO_2 levels following intubation confirms that the tube is in the trachea through the presence of exhaled CO_2. CO_2 is detected by using either a colorimetric or an infrared device.

Colorimetric Devices The colorimetric device is a disposable CO_2 detector that contains pH-sensitive, chemically impregnated paper encased within a plastic chamber (Figure 1-26). It is placed in the airway circuit between the patient and the ventilation device. When the paper is

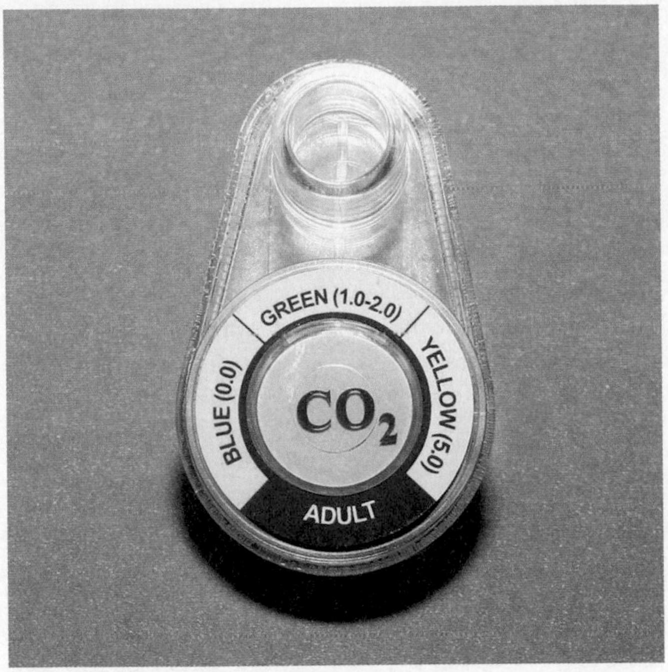

FIGURE 1-26 Colorimetric end-tidal CO_2 detector.
(© Dr. Bryan E. Bledsoe)

exposed to CO_2, hydrogen ions (H^+) are generated, causing a color change in the paper. The color change is reversible and changes from breath to breath. A color scale on the device estimates the CO_2 level. Colorimetric devices cannot detect hypercarbia or hypocarbia (increased or decreased CO_2 levels). If gastric contents or acidic drugs (e.g., endotracheal epinephrine) contact the paper in the device, subsequent readings may be unreliable.

Electronic Devices Electronic capnography detectors use an infrared technique to detect CO_2 in the exhaled breath (Figure 1-27). A heated element in the sensor generates infrared radiation. The CO_2 molecules absorb infrared light at a very specific wavelength and can thus be measured. Electronic $ETCO_2$ detectors may be either qualitative (i.e., they simply detect the presence of CO_2) or quantitative (i.e., they determine how much CO_2 is present). Quantitative devices are now routinely used in prehospital care. Most can provide a digital waveform (capnogram) that reflects the entire respiratory cycle (Figure 1-28).

Capnogram The capnogram reflects CO_2 concentrations over time. It is typically divided into four phases (Figure 1-29).

- *Phase I* (AB in Figure 1-29) is the respiratory baseline. It is flat when no CO_2 is present and corresponds to the late phase of inspiration and the early part of expiration (in which dead-space gases without CO_2 are released).
- *Phase II* (BC in Figure 1-29) is the respiratory upstroke. This reflects the appearance of CO_2 in the alveoli.

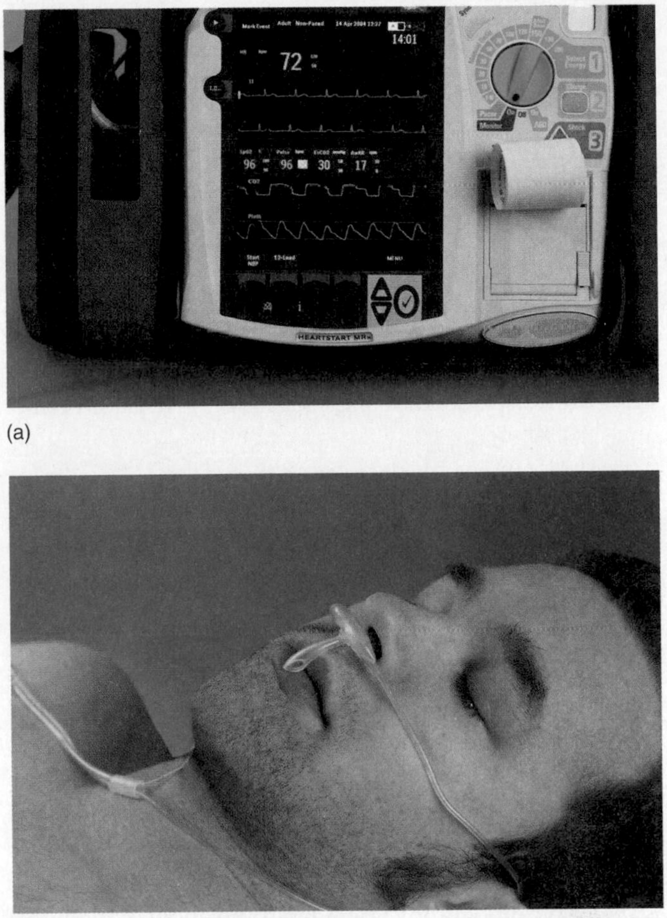

FIGURE 1-27 (a) Electronic capnography. (b) Electronic capnography sensor on a patient.

- *Phase III* (CD in Figure 1-29) is the respiratory plateau. It reflects the airflow through uniformly ventilated alveoli with a nearly constant CO_2 level. The highest level of the plateau (point D in Figure 1-29) is called the $ETCO_2$ and is recorded as such by the capnometer.

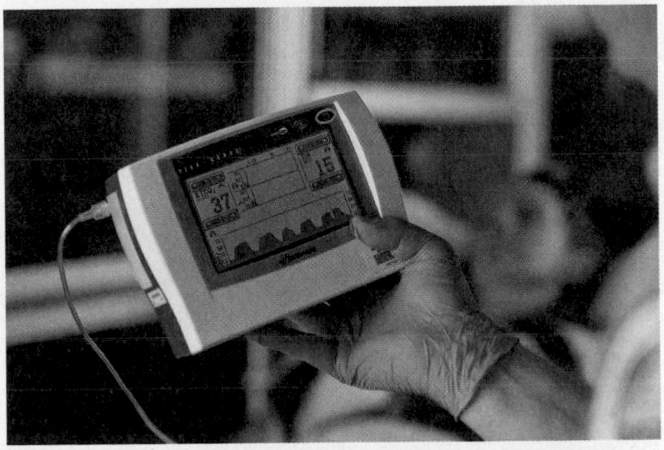

FIGURE 1-28 Capnography devices provide a digital waveform (capnogram) that reflects the entire respiratory cycle.

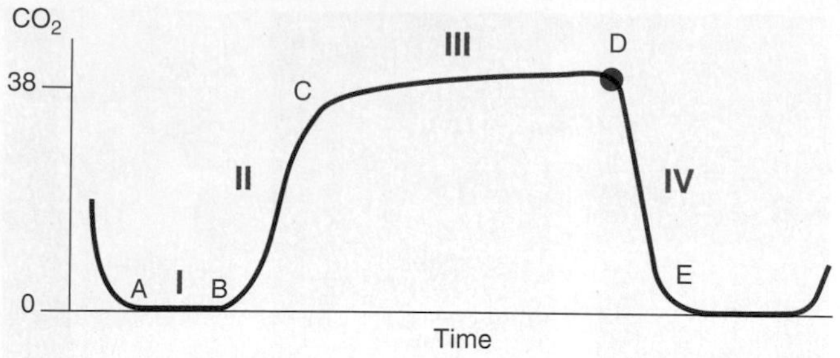

FIGURE 1-29 Normal capnogram. AB = *Phase I:* late inspiration, early expiration (no CO_2). BC 5 *Phase II:* appearance of CO_2 in exhaled gas. CD = *Phase III:* plateau (constant CO_2). D = highest point ($ETCO_2$). DE = *Phase IV:* rapid descent during inspiration. EA = respiratory pause.

- ***Phase IV*** (DE in Figure 1-29) is the inspiratory phase. It is a sudden downstroke and ultimately returns to the baseline during inspiration. The respiratory pause restarts the cycle (EA in Figure 1-29).

Clinical Applications Initially, as noted earlier, CO_2 detection was used only to determine proper endotracheal tube placement. Typically, a qualitative $ETCO_2$ device was applied to the airway circuit following intubation. If CO_2 levels were detected, then proper tube placement was verified. However, it is difficult to continuously monitor the airway with a quantitative device. Now, continuous waveform capnography is available and allows continuous monitoring of airway placement and ventilation for intubated patients. Continuous waveform capnography also has utility in monitoring nonintubated patients. By following trends in the capnogram, prehospital personnel can continuously monitor the patient's condition, detect trends, and document the response to medications.

CO_2 detection is also useful in CPR. During cardiac arrest, CO_2 levels fall abruptly following the onset of cardiac arrest. They begin to rise with the onset of effective CPR and return to near-normal levels with a return of spontaneous circulation. During effective CPR, CO_2 levels have been found to correlate well with cardiac output, coronary perfusion pressure, and even with the effectiveness of CPR compressions.

Continuous waveform capnography is rapidly becoming a standard of care in EMS (Figure 1-30). Misplaced endotracheal tubes represent a significant area of liability in EMS, and the documentation provided by this technology can provide irrefutable evidence of proper endotracheal tube placement.

Management of Respiratory Disorders

The following sections address the pathophysiology, assessment, and management of the more common respiratory disorders encountered in prehospital care. The discussion begins with a look at general principles that can and should be applied to all respiratory emergencies.

Management Principles

In cases of acute respiratory insufficiency, the following principles should guide your actions in the prehospital setting:

- The airway always has first priority. In trauma victims who may have associated cervical spine injuries,

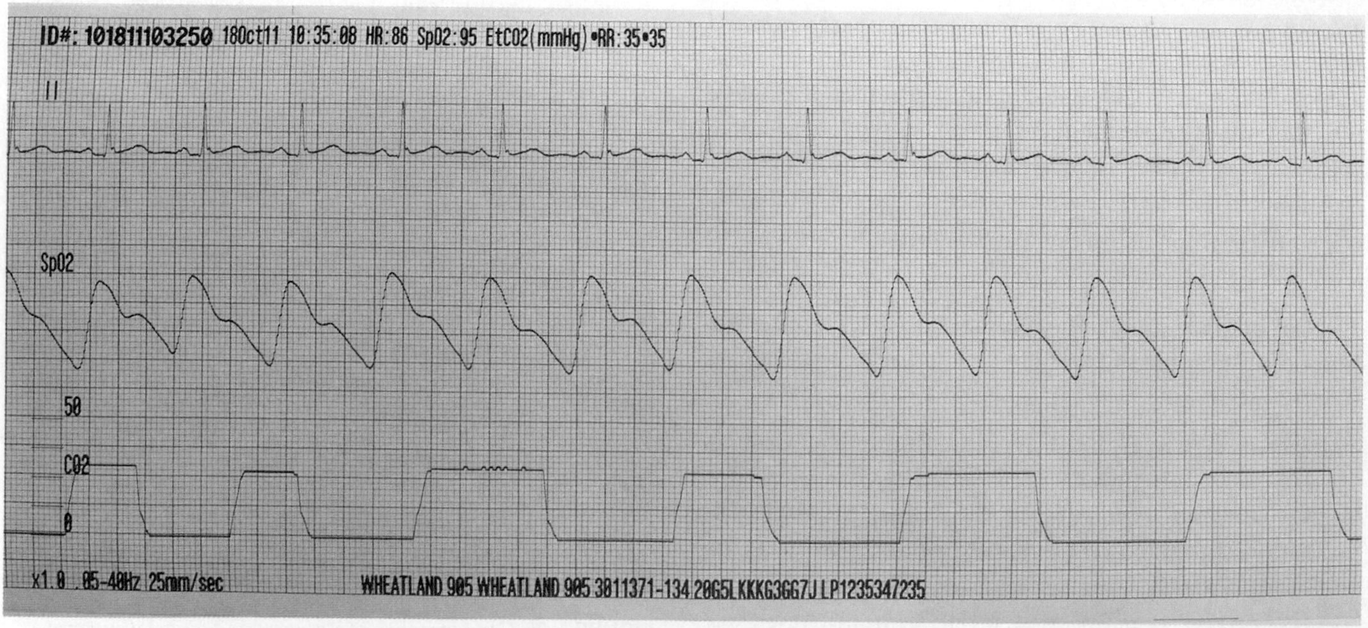

FIGURE 1-30 Continuous waveform (bottom tracing).

protect and maintain the airway without extending the neck.

- Any patient with hypoxia should receive oxygen.
- Any patient whose illness or injury suggests the possibility of hypoxia should receive oxygen until pulse oximetry is available.
- If there is a question whether oxygen should be given, as in COPD, administer enough oxygen to maintain an adequate SpO_2 level (typically ≥96 percent). This state of normal, adequate oxygen is known as **normoxia**. You should strive for normoxia in your patient and avoid both hypoxia and **hyperoxia** (too little or too much oxygen), if possible.

Oxygenation

Supplemental oxygen administration has always been the mainstay of respiratory emergency management. Although supplemental oxygen is an essential and important therapy in prehospital care, several recent studies have demonstrated that administering too much oxygen can actually worsen patient outcomes.[2,3,4] **Hypoxia**, a state of excess oxygen, can result in the formation of toxic chemicals called **free radicals**. These chemicals, also called **reactive oxygen species (ROS)**, can damage body cells and tissues—a process called **oxidative stress**. Because of this, the goal of oxygen therapy is to provide just enough oxygen to treat hypoxia (as guided by pulse oximetry) without causing hyperoxia. Oxygen should be treated like any other drug in the formulary. It should be used when needed, but judiciously. As already emphasized, the goal is normoxia (Figure 1-31).

Keep these precautions in mind as you read through the descriptions of pathophysiology, assessment, and management of respiratory disorders frequently encountered in the field.

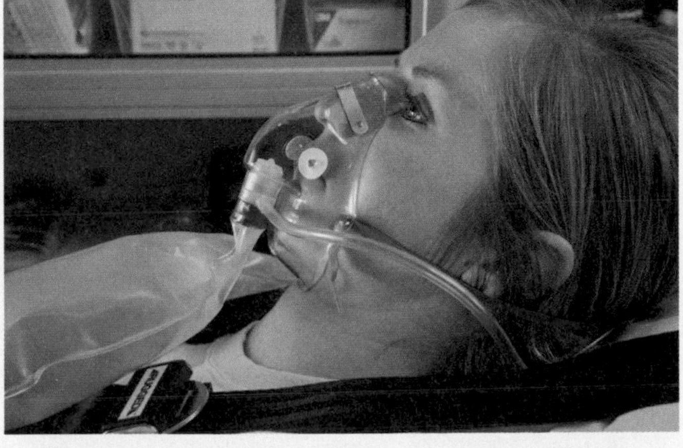

FIGURE 1-31 Excess amounts of oxygen (hyperoxia) have been associated with worsened outcomes in critically ill patients. Always provide enough oxygen to treat hypoxia but avoid hyperoxia.

Specific Respiratory Diseases

Upper Airway Obstruction

The most common cause of upper airway obstruction is the relaxed tongue. In an unconscious patient in the supine position, the tongue can fall into the back of the throat and obstruct the upper airway. Additionally, such common materials as food, dentures, or other foreign bodies can obstruct the upper airway. A typical example of upper airway obstruction is the "café coronary," which tends to occur in middle-aged or elderly patients who wear dentures. These people often are unable to sense how well they have chewed their food. Thus, they accidentally inhale a large piece of food (often meat) that obstructs their airway. Concurrent alcohol consumption is often implicated in the café coronary. Furthermore, obstruction of the upper airway can be the result of facial or neck trauma, upper airway burns, or allergic reactions. In addition, the upper airway can become blocked by an infection that causes swelling of the epiglottis (epiglottitis) or subglottic area (croup).

Foreign bodies may cause either a mild or a severe airway obstruction. Intervention is usually required only if there is a severe airway obstruction. Signs of a severe airway obstruction include a silent cough, cyanosis, and the inability to speak or breathe. If the patient is conscious, ask, "Are you choking?" If the victim indicates yes (by nodding the head) without speaking, you should assume that the obstruction is severe.

Assessment

Assessment of the patient with an upper airway obstruction varies, depending on the cause of the obstruction and the history of the event. The unresponsive patient should be evaluated for snoring respirations, possibly indicating tongue or denture obstruction. If confronted by a patient suffering a café coronary, determine whether the victim can speak. Speech indicates that, at present, the obstruction is incomplete. If the victim is unresponsive and has been eating, strongly suspect a food bolus lodged in the trachea. If a burn is present or suspected, assume laryngeal edema until proven otherwise.

CONTENT REVIEW

➤ Common Causes of Airway Obstruction
- Tongue
- Foreign matter
- Trauma
- Burns
- Allergic reaction
- Infection

Patients who may be having an allergic reaction to food or medications will often report an itching sensation in the palate followed by a "lump" in the throat. The situation may progress to hoarseness, inspiratory stridor, and complete obstruction. Pay particular attention to the presence of urticaria (hives). Intercostal muscle retraction and use of the strap muscles of the neck for breathing suggest attempts to ventilate against a partially closed airway.

Capnography can be useful in identifying upper airway obstruction. Generally, depending on the degree of upper airway obstruction, you will see a steady increase in CO_2 levels.

Management

Management of the obstructed airway is based on the nature of the obstruction. Blockage by the tongue can be corrected by opening the airway, using either the head-tilt, chin-lift, jaw-thrust, or jaw-thrust without head extension maneuver. The airway can be maintained by employing either a nasopharyngeal or oropharyngeal airway. If possible, remove obstructing foreign bodies using the following basic airway maneuvers for an adult.[5] (For management of a foreign body airway obstruction in an infant or child, see the chapter "Pediatrics.")

CONSCIOUS ADULT In an adult patient (or child >1 year of age) who is conscious:

1. Determine whether there is a complete obstruction or poor air exchange. Ask the patient: "Are you choking?" "Can you speak?" If the patient can speak, he should be asked to produce a forceful cough to expel the foreign body.
2. If the patient has a severe obstruction or poor air exchange, provide rapid abdominal thrusts in rapid sequence until the obstruction is relieved. If abdominal thrusts are ineffective (or if the patient is obese), attempt chest thrusts instead. If the patient is pregnant, omit the abdominal thrusts and proceed straight to chest thrusts. Often, more than one technique is required. These should be applied in rapid sequence until the obstruction is relieved.

UNCONSCIOUS ADULT If the patient is unconscious or loses consciousness:

1. Use the head-tilt, chin-lift, jaw-thrust, or jaw-thrust without head extension maneuver in an attempt to open the airway.
2. Begin CPR.
3. Each time you open the airway during CPR, look for an object in the victim's mouth and remove it.
4. If the obstruction persists and ventilation cannot be provided, visualize the airway with the laryngoscope. If you can see the foreign body, grasp it with the Magill forceps and remove. Once the obstruction has been removed, begin ventilation and administer supplemental oxygen (if hypoxia is detected or suspected).

In cases of airway obstruction caused by laryngeal edema (e.g., anaphylactic reactions, angioedema), establish the airway by the head-tilt, chin-lift, jaw-thrust, or jaw-thrust without head extension maneuver. Then administer supplemental oxygen if hypoxia has been determined by pulse oximetry. Attempt bag-valve-mask ventilation. Often, air can be forced past the obstruction and the patient adequately ventilated using this technique. Next, start an IV with a crystalloid solution and administer intravenous or intramuscular epinephrine. Then administer diphenhydramine (Benadryl). Transtracheal ventilation may be required if the patient does not respond to the treatments described. (See the "Pediatrics" chapter for pediatric techniques.)

Noncardiogenic Pulmonary Edema/ Acute Respiratory Distress Syndrome

Acute respiratory distress syndrome (ARDS) is a life-threatening condition that adversely affects gas exchange in the lungs. It is a form of pulmonary edema that is caused by fluid accumulation in the interstitial space within the lungs. Patients with *cardiogenic* pulmonary edema have a poorly functioning left ventricle. This leads to increases in hydrostatic pressure and fluid accumulation in the interstitial space. In patients with ARDS, however, fluid accumulation occurs as the result of increased vascular permeability and decreased fluid removal from the lung tissue. This occurs in response to a wide variety of lung insults including:

- Sepsis, particularly with Gram-negative organisms
- Aspiration
- Pneumonia or other respiratory infections
- Pulmonary injury
- Burns
- Inhalation injury
- Oxygen toxicity
- Drugs such as aspirin or opiates
- High altitude
- Hypothermia
- Near-drowning
- Head injury
- Emboli from blood clot, fat, or amniotic fluid
- Tumor destruction
- Pancreatitis
- Procedures such as cardiopulmonary bypass or hemodialysis
- Other insults such as hypoxia, hypotension, or cardiac arrest

The mortality in patients who develop ARDS is quite high, approaching 70 percent. Although many patients die as the result of respiratory failure, many succumb to failure of several organ systems, including the liver and kidneys.

Pathophysiology

ARDS is a disorder of lung diffusion that results from increased fluid in the interstitial space. Each of the underlying conditions cited previously results in the inability to maintain a proper fluid balance in the interstitial space. Severe hypotension, significant hypoxemia as the result of cardiac arrest, drowning, seizure activity or hypoventilation, high-altitude exposure, environmental toxins, and endotoxins released in septic shock all can cause disruption of the alveolar–capillary membrane. Increases in pulmonary capillary permeability, destruction of the capillary lining, and increases in osmotic forces act to draw fluid into the interstitial space and contribute to interstitial edema. This increases the thickness of the respiratory membrane and limits diffusion of oxygen. In advanced cases, fluid also accumulates in the alveoli, causing loss of surfactant, collapse of the alveolar sacs, and impaired gas exchange. This results in a significant amount of pulmonary shunting with deoxygenated blood returning to the circulation. The result is significant hypoxia (Figure 1-32).[6]

Assessment

Specific clinical symptoms are related to the underlying cause of ARDS. For example, patients who develop ARDS as the result of sepsis will have symptoms related to their underlying infection. Determine whether there is a history of prolonged hypoxia, head or chest trauma, inhalation of gases, or ascent to a high altitude without prior acclimation, all of which can suggest an underlying cause for the respiratory complaints.

Patients with ARDS experience a gradual decline in their respiratory status. In rare cases, a seemingly healthy patient has a sudden onset of respiratory failure and hypoxia. Such a presentation is characteristic of patients with high-altitude pulmonary edema (HAPE).

Dyspnea, confusion, and agitation are often found in patients with noncardiogenic pulmonary edema. Patients may also report fatigue and reduced exercise ability. Symptoms such as orthopnea, paroxysmal nocturnal dyspnea, or sputum production are not commonly reported but may be seen.

The prominent physical findings are generally those associated with the underlying lung insult. Tachypnea and tachycardia are often found in association with ARDS. Crackles (rales) are audible in both lungs. Wheezing may also be heard if there is any element of bronchospasm. Severe tachypnea, central cyanosis, and signs of imminent respiratory failure are seen in severe cases. Pulse oximetry will demonstrate low oxygen saturations in patients with advanced disease. In patients requiring ventilatory support, decreased lung compliance will be noted. (It will require more operator force to deliver an adequate lung volume.)

Management

Specific management of the patient's underlying medical condition is the hallmark of treatment for this disorder. Treatment of Gram-negative sepsis with appropriate antibiotics, removal of the patient from any inciting toxin, or rapid descent to a lower altitude in patients with HAPE are the most important therapies for this condition. The patient will usually tolerate an upright position with the legs dangling off the cart.

Because the hypoxia seen in ARDS is the result of diffusion defects, supplementation is often essential for all patients with this condition. Establish intravenous access, but provide fluids only if hypovolemia exists. Establish cardiac monitoring. Suctioning of lung secretions is often required to maintain airway patency.

Use positive pressure ventilation to support any ARDS patient who demonstrates signs of respiratory failure. Use bag-valve-mask ventilation for initial respiratory support while preparing a continuous positive airway pressure (CPAP) device. Use of CPAP can often avoid the need for endotracheal intubation and mechanical ventilation. **Positive end-expiratory pressure (PEEP)**, via CPAP, will help to maintain patency of the alveoli and adequate oxygenation. Diuretics and nitrates, which are used in patients with cardiogenic pulmonary edema, are usually not helpful in patients with ARDS. Your medical director may occasionally order corticosteroids for patients with ARDS/noncardiogenic pulmonary edema. Corticosteroids are thought to stabilize the alveolar–capillary membrane, although clinical studies have not demonstrated any benefit to their use.

Maintain cardiac monitoring and pulse oximetry throughout transport of the patient. Transport patients to a facility capable of advanced hemodynamic monitoring (including via Swan-Ganz catheter) and mechanical ventilation support.

Obstructive Lung Disease

Obstructive lung disease is widespread in our society. The most common obstructive lung diseases encountered in prehospital care are asthma, emphysema, and chronic bronchitis (the last two are often discussed together as chronic obstructive pulmonary disease, or COPD). Asthma afflicts 4 to 5 percent of the U.S. population and COPD is found in 25 percent of all adults. Chronic bronchitis alone

CONTENT REVIEW

➤ Obstructive Lung Diseases
- Emphysema
- Chronic bronchitis
- Asthma

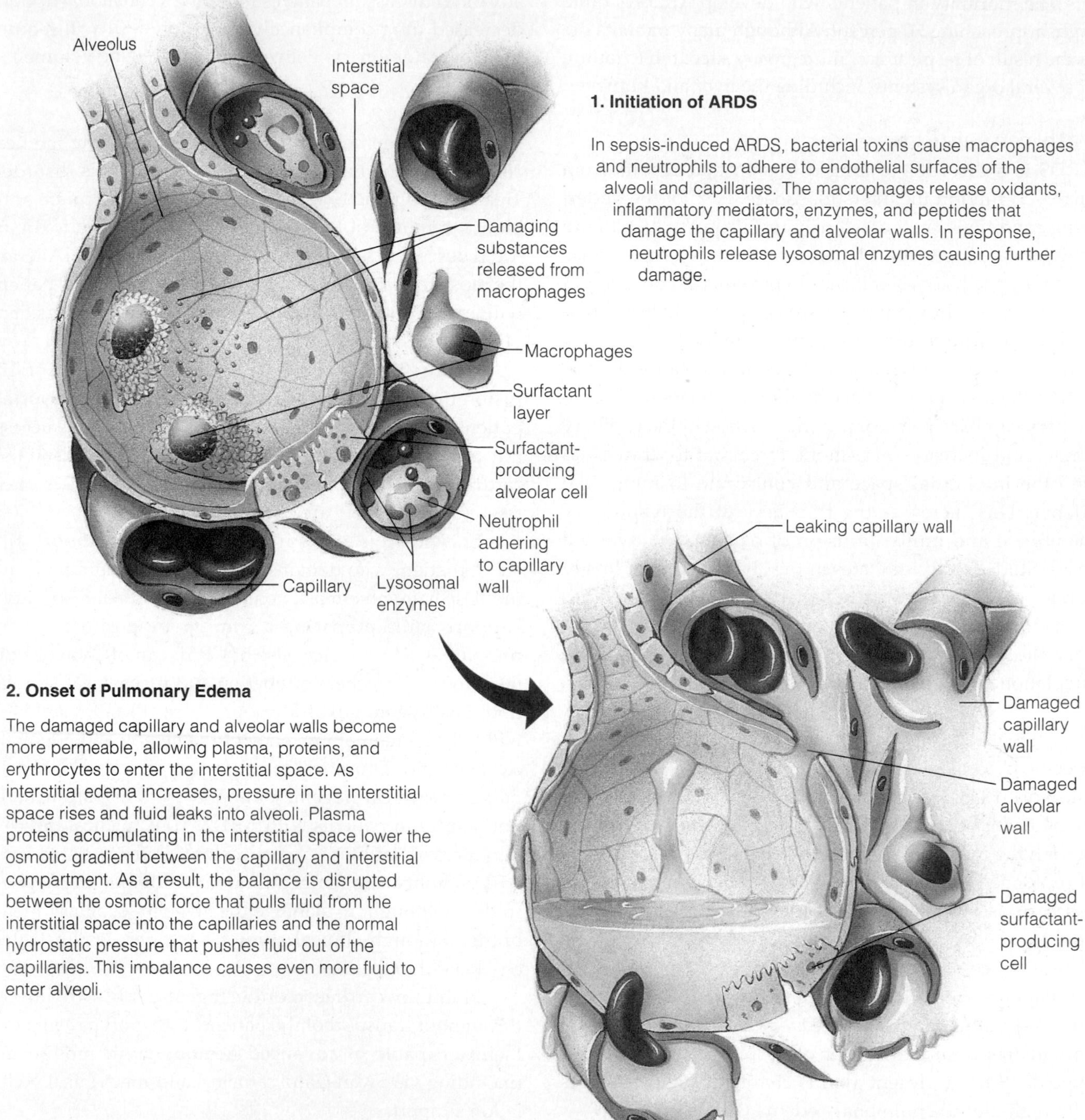

FIGURE 1-32

1. ***Initiation of ARDS*** In septic ARDS, bacterial toxins cause inflammation that damages the alveolar and capillary walls.
2. ***Onset of Pulmonary Edema*** The damaged alveolar and capillary walls become more permeable, allowing plasma and other substances to enter the interstitial space, thus causing fluid entry into the alveoli.
3. ***End-Stage ARDS*** Fibrin and cell debris form hyaline membranes that reduce alveolar compliance and adversely affect diffusion.
4. ***Alveolar Collapse*** Protein-rich fluid accumulates in the alveoli and damages the cells that manufacture surfactant, causing stiffening of the alveoli and atelectasis.

affects one in five adult males. Patients with COPD have a 50 percent mortality within 10 years of the diagnosis.

Although asthma may have a genetic predisposition, COPD is known to be directly caused by cigarette smoking and environmental toxins. Other factors have been shown to precipitate symptoms in patients who already have obstructive airway disease. Intrinsic factors include stress, upper respiratory infections, and

3. Alveolar Collapse

Protein-rich fluid accumulates in the alveoli, inactivating surfactant and damaging type II alveolar cells that produce surfactant. (Surfactant is important in maintaining alveolar compliance—the ability of tissue to stretch or distend.) As active surfactant is lost, the alveoli stiffen and collapse, leading to atelectasis, which increases breathing effort.

Decreased alveolar compliance, atelectasis, and fluid-filled alveoli interfere with gas exchange across the alveolar-capillary membrane. Blood oxygen (PaO_2) levels fall. Because carbon dioxide diffuses more readily than oxygen, however, blood carbon dioxide ($PaCO_2$) levels also fall initially as tachypnea causes more CO_2 to be expired.

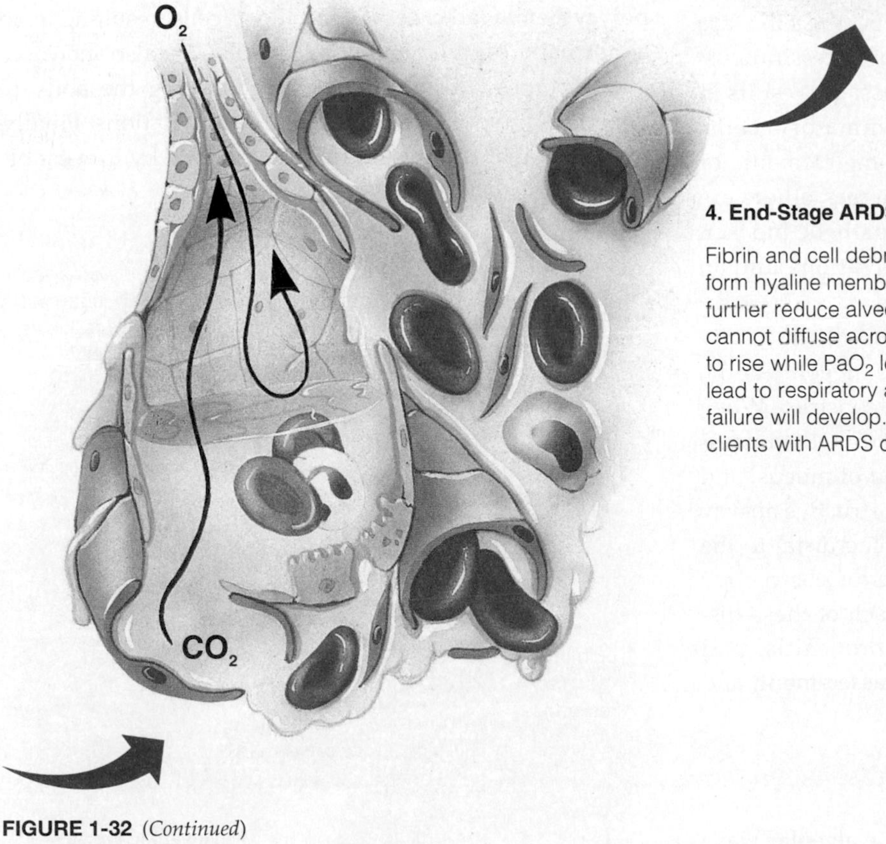

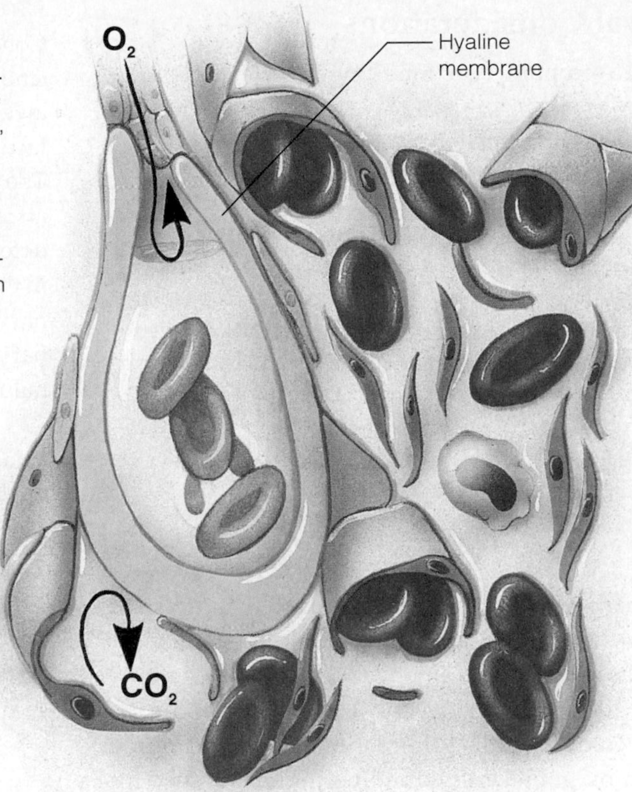

4. End-Stage ARDS

Fibrin and cell debris from necrotic cells combine to form hyaline membranes, which line the interior of the alveoli and further reduce alveolar compliance and gas exchange. Because CO_2 cannot diffuse across hyaline membranes, $PaCO_2$ levels now begin to rise while PaO_2 levels continue to fall. Rising $PaCO_2$ levels can lead to respiratory acidosis. Without respiratory support, respiratory failure will develop. Even with aggressive treatment, almost 50% of clients with ARDS die.

FIGURE 1-32 *(Continued)*

exercise. Extrinsic factors include tobacco smoke, drugs, occupational hazards (chemical fumes, dust, and others), and allergens such as foods, animal danders, dusts, and molds.

Obstructive lung diseases all have abnormal ventilation as a common feature. This abnormal ventilation is a result of obstruction that occurs primarily in the bronchioles. Several changes occur within these air conduits.

Cultural Considerations

Cultural Acceptance of Smoking. Cigarette smoking has clearly been demonstrated to be a contributing factor in the development of respiratory disease—especially chronic obstructive pulmonary disease and bronchogenic cancers. Although the use of tobacco products in the United States has declined overall, it is still more acceptable in some areas of the country than in others. For example, in some southern and eastern states where tobacco is the cash crop, there is a higher incidence of tobacco use. Smoking also is more acceptable and better tolerated in some cultures than in others, and tobacco products are more readily available where these cultures prevail. Thus, over time, one would expect the incidence of chronic obstructive pulmonary diseases and bronchogenic cancers to be higher in these groups.

Bronchospasm (sustained smooth muscle contraction) occurs, which may be reversed by beta-adrenergic receptor stimulation. Agents such as albuterol (Ventolin, Proventil), levalbuterol (Xopenex), and epinephrine are used to accomplish this stimulation. Increased mucus production by goblet cells that line the respiratory tree also contributes to obstruction. This effect may be worsened by the fact that in many patients, the cilia are destroyed, resulting in poor clearance of excess mucus. Finally, inflammation of the bronchial passages results in the accumulation of fluid and inflammatory cells. Depending on the underlying cause, some elements of bronchial obstruction are reversible, whereas others are not. Ipratropium (Atrovent), a parasympathetic blocker, may aid in the drying of bronchial secretions and in reversing bronchospasm.

During inspiration, the bronchioles will naturally dilate, allowing air to be drawn into the alveoli. As the patient begins to exhale, the bronchioles constrict. When this natural constriction occurs—in addition to the underlying bronchospasm, increased production of mucus, and inflammation that exist in patients with obstructive airway disease—the result is significant air trapping distal to the obstruction. This is one of the hallmarks of obstructive lung disease. The next sections discuss each of these disease processes—emphysema, chronic bronchitis, and asthma—detailing the pathophysiology, assessment, and treatment of each.

Emphysema

Emphysema results from destruction of the alveolar walls distal to the terminal bronchioles. It is more common in men than in women. The major factor contributing to emphysema in our society is cigarette smoking. Significant exposure to environmental toxins is another contributing factor.

Pathophysiology

Continued exposure to noxious substances, such as cigarette smoke, results in the gradual destruction of the walls of the alveoli. This process decreases the alveolar membrane surface area, thus lessening the area available for gas exchange. The progressive loss of the respiratory membrane results in an increased ratio of air to lung tissue. The result is diffusion defects. Additionally, the number of pulmonary capillaries in the lung is decreased, thus increasing resistance to pulmonary blood flow. This condition ultimately causes pulmonary hypertension, which in turn may lead to right-heart failure, **cor pulmonale**, and death (Figure 1-33).

Emphysema also causes weakening of the walls of the small bronchioles. When the walls of the alveoli and small bronchioles are destroyed, the lungs lose their capacity to recoil and air becomes trapped in the lungs. Thus, residual volume increases while vital capacity remains relatively normal. The destroyed lung tissue (called *blebs*) results in alveolar collapse. To counteract this effect, patients tend to breathe through pursed lips. This creates continued positive pressure similar to PEEP (positive end-expiratory pressure) and prevents alveolar collapse.

As the disease progresses, the PaO_2 further decreases, which may lead to increased red blood cell production and **polycythemia** (an excess of red blood cells, resulting in an abnormally high hematocrit). The $PaCO_2$ also increases and becomes chronically elevated, forcing the body to depend on hypoxic drive to control respirations. Finally, remember that emphysema is characterized by irreversible airway obstruction.

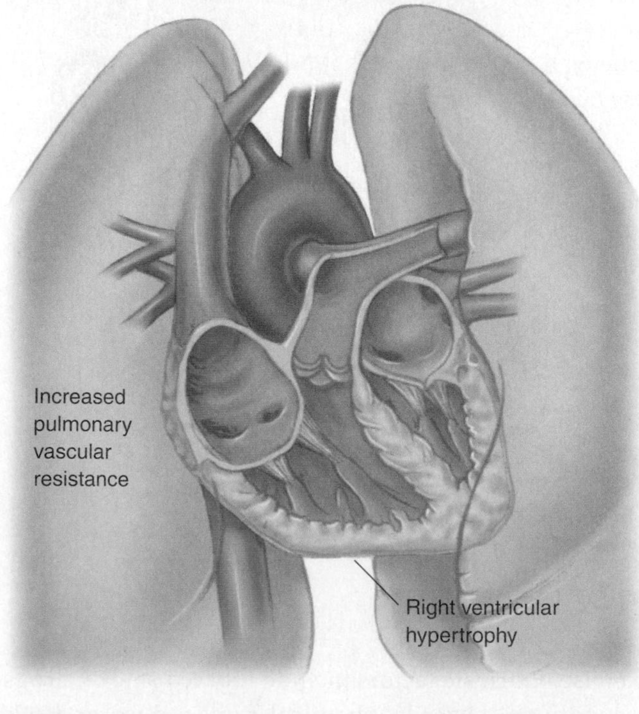

FIGURE 1-33 Chronic obstructive pulmonary disease of long duration can cause pulmonary hypertension, which in turn may lead to cor pulmonale.

Patients with emphysema are more susceptible to acute respiratory infections, such as pneumonia, and to cardiac arrhythmias. Chronic emphysema patients ultimately become dependent on bronchodilators, corticosteroids, and, in the final stages, supplemental oxygen.

Assessment

The patient with emphysema may report a history of recent weight loss, increased dyspnea on exertion, and progressive limitation of physical activity. Unlike chronic bronchitis, discussed in subsequent sections, emphysema is rarely associated with a cough, except in the morning. Question the patient about cigarette and tobacco usage. This is generally reported in pack/years. Ask the number of cigarette packs (20 cigarettes/pack) smoked per day and the number of years the patient has smoked. Multiply the number of packs smoked per day by the number of years. For example, a man who has smoked 2 packs per day for 15 years would have a 30-pack/year smoking history. Medical problems related to smoking, such as emphysema, chronic bronchitis, and lung cancer, usually begin after a patient surpasses a 20-pack/year history, although this can vary significantly.

Physical exam of the emphysema patient usually reveals a barrel chest, evidenced by an increase in the anterior/posterior chest diameter. You may also note decreased chest excursion with a prolonged expiratory phase and a rapid resting respiratory rate. Patients with emphysema are often thin because they must use a significant amount of their caloric intake for respiration. They tend to be pink in color due to polycythemia (excess of red blood cells) and are often referred to as "pink puffers." Emphysema patients often have hypertrophy of the accessory respiratory muscles (Figure 1-34).

The patient will often involuntarily purse his lips to create continuous positive airway pressure. Clubbing of the fingers is common. Breath sounds are usually diminished. Wheezes and rhonchi may or may not be present, depending on the amount of obstruction to airflow. The patient may exhibit signs of right-heart failure, as evidenced by jugular vein distention, peripheral edema, and hepatic congestion. Signs of severe respiratory impairment in all patients with obstructive lung disease include confusion, agitation, somnolence, one-to-two-word dyspnea, and use of accessory muscles to assist ventilation.

CONTENT REVIEW

➤ Emphysema and Chronic Bronchitis: Management Goals
- Relieve hypoxia.
- Reverse bronchoconstriction.

Management

Although emphysema differs in the disease process from chronic bronchitis, the two respiratory disorders share several of the same symptoms and pathophysiology. As a result, you will treat the two disorders in a similar manner. The discussion of management of emphysema will be taken up with chronic bronchitis in the following section.

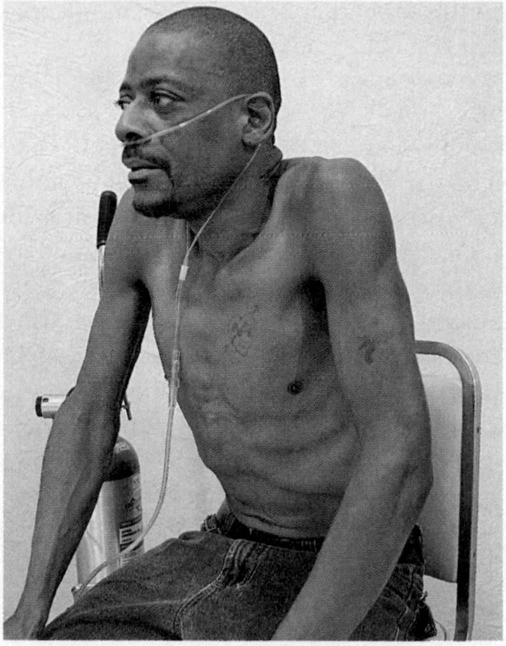

FIGURE 1-34 Typical appearance of patient with emphysema. There are well-developed accessory muscles and suprasternal retraction.

(© Ray Kemp/Science Source)

Chronic Bronchitis

Chronic bronchitis results from an increase in the number of the goblet (mucus-secreting) cells in the respiratory tree (Figure 1-35). It is characterized by the production of a

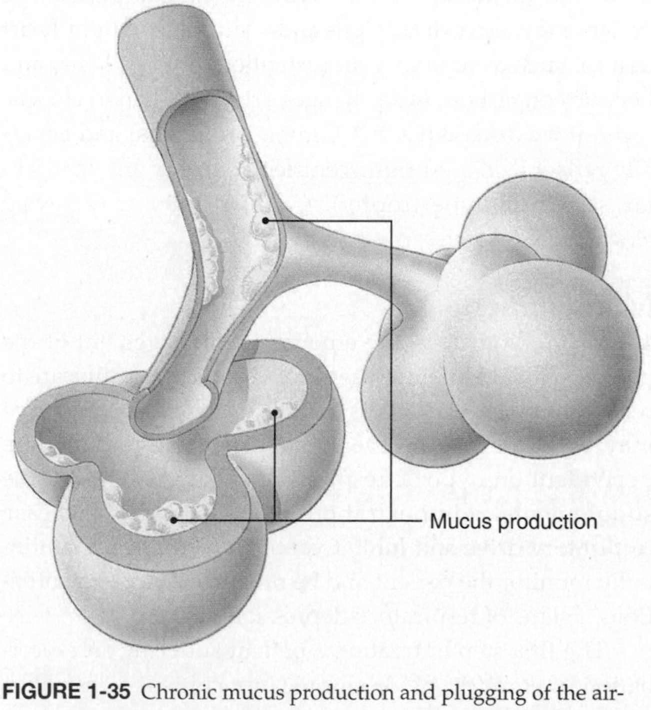

FIGURE 1-35 Chronic mucus production and plugging of the airways occur in chronic bronchitis.

large quantity of sputum. This often occurs after prolonged exposure to cigarette smoke.

Pathophysiology

Unlike emphysema, in chronic bronchitis the alveoli are not severely affected and diffusion remains normal. Gas exchange is decreased because of the lowered alveolar ventilation, which ultimately results in hypoxia and hypercarbia. Hypoxia may increase red blood cell production, which, in turn, leads to polycythemia (as occurs in emphysema). Increased $PaCO_2$ levels may lead to irritability, somnolence, decreased intellectual abilities, headaches, and personality changes. Physiologically, an increased $PaCO_2$ causes pulmonary vasoconstriction, resulting in pulmonary hypertension and, eventually, cor pulmonale. Unlike emphysema, the vital capacity is decreased, whereas the residual volume is normal or decreased.

Assessment

The patient with chronic bronchitis often will have a history of heavy cigarette smoking, but the disease may also occur in nonsmokers. There may also be a history of frequent respiratory infections. In addition, these patients usually produce considerable quantities of sputum daily. Clinically, the patient is described as having a productive cough for at least three months per year for two or more consecutive years.

Patients with chronic bronchitis tend to be overweight and can be cyanotic. Because of this, they are often referred to as "blue bloaters." This can be contrasted with the "pink puffer" image of emphysema patients just described. Auscultation of the thorax often will reveal rhonchi due to occlusion of the larger airways with mucus plugs. The patient may also exhibit signs and symptoms of right-heart failure, such as jugular vein distention, ankle edema, and hepatic congestion. ECG changes are often seen in chronic respiratory disease (COPD, chronic bronchitis) and generally reflect increased right ventricular size (right ventricular strain or hypertrophy). Capnography may reveal elevated CO_2 levels.[7]

Management

The primary goals in the emergency management of the patient with either emphysema or chronic bronchitis are to relieve hypoxia and reverse any bronchoconstriction that may be present. However, many of these patients are dependent on hypoxic respiratory drive. As a result, the supplemental administration of oxygen may decrease respiratory drive and inhibit ventilation. You must continually monitor the patient and be prepared to assist ventilations if signs of respiratory depression develop.

The first step in treating a patient suffering an exacerbation of emphysema or chronic bronchitis is to establish an airway. Then place the patient in a seated or semi-seated position to assist the accessory respiratory muscles. Apply a pulse oximeter and determine the blood oxygen saturation (SpO_2). Administer supplemental oxygen at a low flow rate while maintaining an oxygen saturation greater than 90 to 95 percent. A nasal cannula can often be used, but you must constantly monitor the respiratory rate and depth as well as oxygen saturation. If hypoxia or respiratory failure is evident, then increase the concentration of delivered oxygen. Be prepared to support the ventilation with bag-valve-mask assistance. CPAP may prove beneficial in COPD and can, in some instances, prevent the need for endotracheal intubation. It is best to keep PEEP pressures 10 cm/H_2O to prevent possible barotraumas. Regardless, intubation may be required if CPAP fails and respiratory failure is imminent.

Place a saline lock in case medication or fluid administration is required. Fluid administration is suggested if there are signs of dehydration present. This may also aid in loosening thick mucus secretions. Then, if ordered by medical direction, administer a bronchodilator medication such as albuterol, levalbuterol, or metaproterenol through a small-volume nebulizer. Consider the addition of ipratropium bromide (Atrovent) during the initial nebulizer treatment. Corticosteroids are also commonly used in the early management of patients with COPD.

Asthma

Asthma is a common respiratory illness that affects many people. Although deaths from other respiratory diseases are steadily declining, deaths from asthma have significantly increased during the last decade. Most of the increased asthma deaths have occurred in patients aged 45 years or older. In addition, the death rate for black asthmatics has been twice as high as for their white counterparts. Approximately 50 percent of patients who die from asthma do so before reaching the hospital. Thus, EMS personnel are frequently called on to treat patients suffering an asthma attack. Prompt recognition followed by appropriate treatment can significantly improve the patient's condition and enhance his chance of survival.

Pathophysiology

Asthma is a chronic inflammatory disorder of the airways. In susceptible individuals, this inflammation causes symptoms usually associated with widespread but variable airflow obstruction. In addition to airflow obstruction, the airway becomes hyperresponsive. The airflow obstruction and hyperresponsiveness are often reversible with treatment. These conditions may also reverse spontaneously.

Asthma may be induced by one of many different factors. These factors, commonly referred to as "triggers" or "inducers," vary from one individual to the next. In allergic individuals, environmental allergens are a major cause

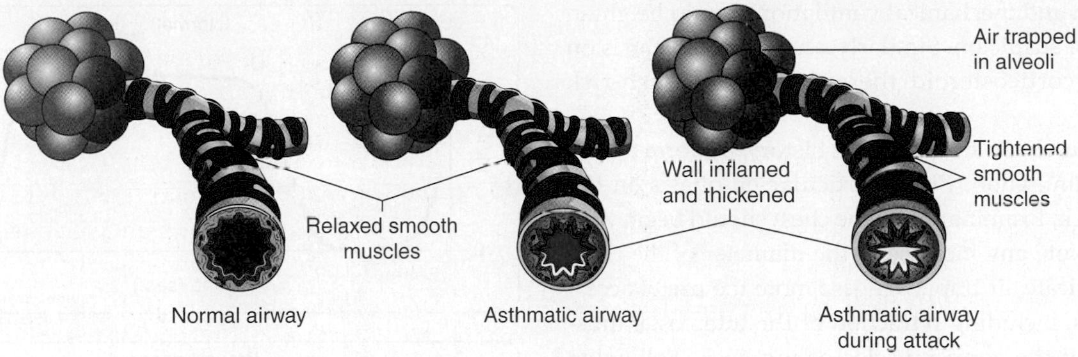

FIGURE 1-36 (a) Normal airway, (b) asthmatic airway, and (c) asthmatic airway during an attack.

of inflammation. These may occur both indoors and outdoors. In addition to allergens, cold air, exercise, foods, irritants, stress, and certain medications may trigger asthma. Often, a specific trigger cannot be identified. Extrinsic triggers tend predominantly to affect children, whereas intrinsic factors trigger asthma in adults.

Within minutes of exposure to the offending trigger, a two-phase reaction occurs. The first phase of the reaction is characterized by the release of chemical mediators such as histamine. These mediators cause contraction of the bronchial smooth muscle and leakage of fluid from peribronchial capillaries. This results in both bronchoconstriction and bronchial edema. These two factors can significantly decrease expiratory airflow, causing the typical "asthma attack" (Figure 1-36).

Often, the asthma attack will resolve spontaneously in 1 to 2 hours or may be aborted by the use of inhaled bronchodilator medications such as albuterol. However, within 6 to 8 hours after exposure to the trigger, a second reaction occurs. This late phase is characterized by inflammation of the bronchioles as cells of the immune system (eosinophils, neutrophils, and lymphocytes) invade the mucosa of the respiratory tract. This leads to additional edema and swelling of the bronchioles and a further decrease in expiratory airflow.

The second phase reaction will not typically respond to inhaled beta-agonist drugs such as metaproterenol or albuterol. Instead, anti-inflammatory agents such as corticosteroids are often required. It is important to point out that the severe inflammatory changes seen in an acute asthma attack do not develop over a few hours or even a few days. The inflammation will often begin several days or several weeks before the onset of the actual asthma attack.

Assessment

Begin the primary prehospital assessment of the asthmatic by considering immediate threats to the airway, breathing, or circulation. Then turn your attention to the focused history and physical examination.

The most common presenting symptoms of asthma are dyspnea, wheezing, and cough. Wheezing results from turbulent airflow through the inflamed and narrowed bronchioles. Many asthmatics will have a persistent cough. This is primarily due to hyperresponsiveness of the airway. It is important to point out that some asthmatics do not wheeze. Instead, their initial presentation may be a frequent and persistent cough. As asthma severity increases, the patient may exhibit hyperinflation of the chest due to trapping of air in the alveoli. In addition, tachypnea (rapid respiration) will occur. The patient may start to use accessory muscles to aid respiration.

Symptoms of a severe asthma attack include one-to-two-word dyspnea (the inability to complete a phrase or sentence without having to stop to breathe), *pulsus paradoxus* (a drop of systolic blood pressure of 10 mmHg or more with inspiration), tachycardia, and decreased oxygen saturation on pulse oximetry. As hypoxia develops, the patient may become agitated and anxious.

When conducting the focused history and physical examination, start by obtaining a brief patient history. Most asthmatics will report that they suffer from asthma. In addition, the patient's home medications may help confirm a history of asthma. Common asthma medications include inhaled beta-agonists (albuterol, levalbuterol, metaproterenol), inhaled corticosteroids (betamethasone, beclomethasone), inhaled cromolyn sodium, and inhaled anticholinergics (ipratropium bromide). Often the patient will be taking oral bronchodilators, such as theophylline, or may be taking oral corticosteroids (prednisone).

Determine when symptoms started and what the patient has taken in an attempt to abort the attack. Also, find out whether the patient is allergic to any medications. Question the patient about hospitalizations for asthma. If the patient has been hospitalized, ask whether the patient has ever required intubation and mechanical ventilation. A prior history

CONTENT REVIEW

➤ Asthma: Common Presenting Signs
- Dyspnea
- Wheezing
- Cough

of intubation and mechanical ventilation should heighten your index of suspicion. Similarly, an asthmatic who is on continuous corticosteroid therapy is also a high-risk patient.

After you obtain the pertinent history, perform a brief physical examination. Place particular emphasis on the chest and neck. Examination of the chest should begin with inspection. Note any increase in the diameter of the chest that may indicate air trapping. Also, note the use of accessory muscles, including retraction of the intercostal muscles or use of the strap muscles of the neck. Following inspection, palpate the chest, noting any deformity, crepitus, or asymmetry. Next, auscultate the posterior chest. Note any abnormal breath sounds such as wheezing or rhonchi. Listen to the symmetry of breath sounds. Unilateral wheezing may indicate an aspirated foreign body or a pneumothorax.

Obtain accurate vital signs. One of the most important vital signs is the respiratory rate. An increase in the respiratory rate is one of the earliest symptoms of a respiratory problem. Many EMS personnel inaccurately measure the respiratory rate. The easiest method is to simply place your fingers on the patient's radial artery as if you were measuring the pulse rate. This will make the patient think you are obtaining the pulse rate, and he will not alter his breathing pattern. Measure the respiratory rate for at least 30 seconds. At the same time, note any alterations in the respiratory pattern. Pulse oximetry is an excellent adjunct to respiratory assessment. It will provide you with data regarding the oxygen saturation status (SpO_2) as well as an audible measure of the pulse rate.

EMS systems should be able to measure the peak expiratory flow rate (PEFR). (Review Figure 1-28 and Table 1-3.) The PEFR is a reliable indicator of airflow. If possible, measure peak flow rates to determine the severity of an asthma attack and the degree of response to treatment. The more severe the asthma attack, the lower will be the PEFR.

Continuous waveform capnography can assist in identifying asthma (and other types of lung disease) and can also help determine the severity of airflow obstruction. Patients with an acute asthma exacerbation will often exhibit a "shark fin" configuration on their capnogram (Figure 1-37). This results from slower emptying of the alveoli, which causes a decrease in the slope of the ascending phase and the alveolar plateau. During an acute asthma exacerbation, patients tend to hyperventilate to maintain adequate oxygenation. This causes a fall in the $ETCO_2$ level (usually <35 mmHg). As the exacerbation progresses untreated, the patient will begin to tire and the $ETCO_2$ will rise back to the normal range (35–45 mmHg). If effective treatment is not provided or the patient fails to respond to treatment, the $ETCO_2$ levels will continue to rise to dangerous levels (>50 mmHg) (Table 1-5). Thus, considering both the "shark fin" configuration and the $ETCO_2$ level, it is possible to detect asthma and estimate the severity of an asthma patient's exacerbation.

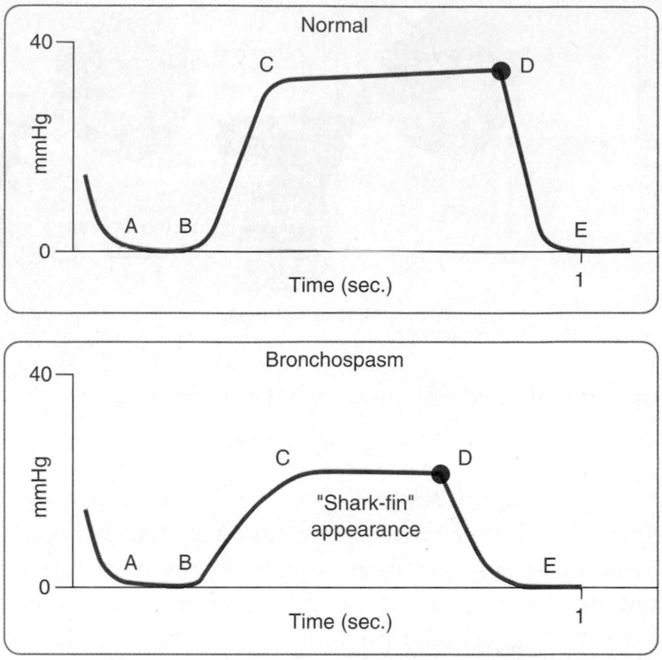

FIGURE 1-37 Comparison of normal and asthmatic capnogram waveforms.

Table 1-5 Phases of Acute Asthma Exacerbation

Phase	Clinical Assessment	$ETCO_2$ Levels (mmHg)
Mild	Hyperventilating	<35
Moderate	Tiring	35–50
Severe	Tired	>50

Management

Treatment of asthma is designed to correct hypoxia, reverse any bronchospasm, and treat the inflammatory changes associated with the disease.[8] Administer supplemental oxygen to correct hypoxia. Establish intravenous access and place the patient on an ECG monitor. Direct initial treatment at reversing any bronchospasm present. The most commonly used drugs are the inhaled beta-agonist preparations such as albuterol (Ventolin, Proventil) or levalbuterol (Xopenex) in conjunction with ipratropium bromide (Atrovent). These can be easily administered with a small-volume oxygen-powered nebulizer (Procedure 1-1).

The goal of the beta-agonist preparations is to reverse any bronchospasm. In advanced and prolonged asthma attacks,

CONTENT REVIEW

- Asthma: Management Goals
  - Correct hypoxia.
  - Reverse bronchospasm.
  - Reduce inflammation.

Procedure 1-1 Administration of Nebulized Medications

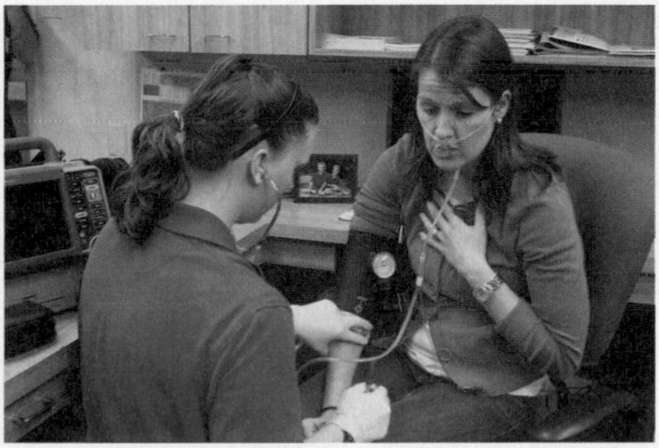

1-1A Complete the primary assessment.

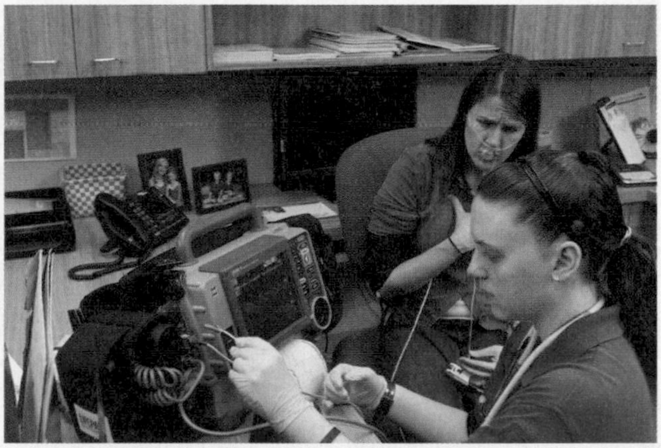

1-1B Place the patient on appropriate monitors.

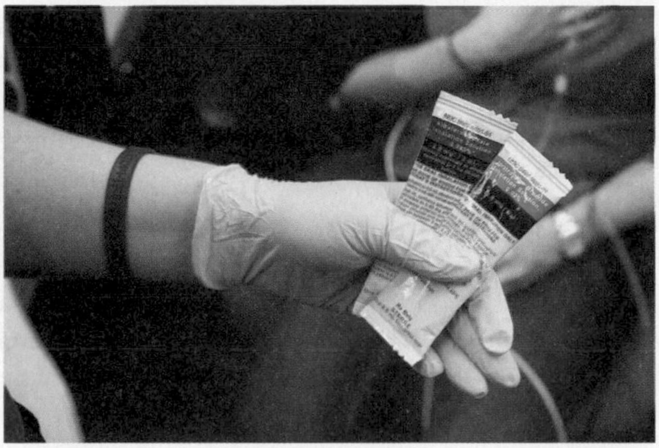

1-1C Select the desired medication(s).

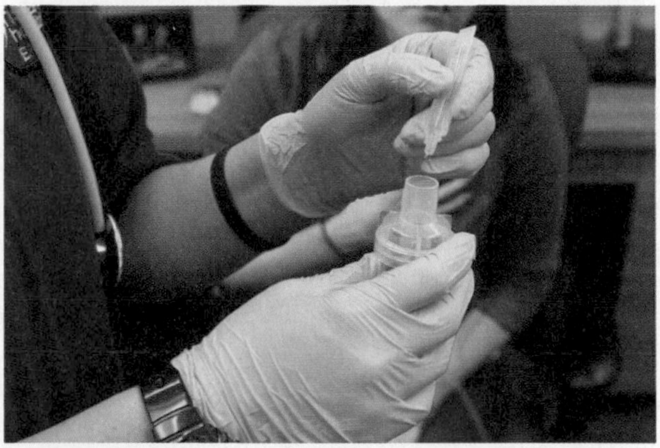

1-1D Add medication to the nebulizer.

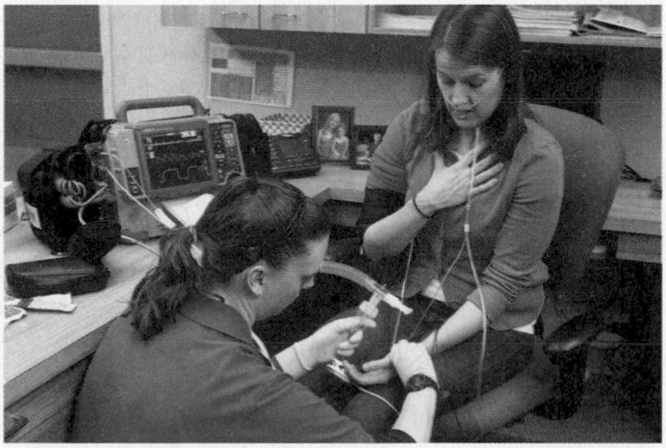

1-1E Assemble the nebulizer and determine pretreatment pulse rate.

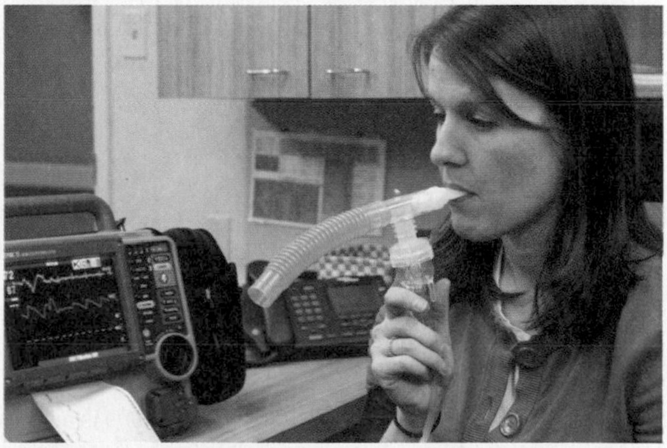

1-1F Administer the medication.

(*Continue*)

Procedure 1-1 *Continued*

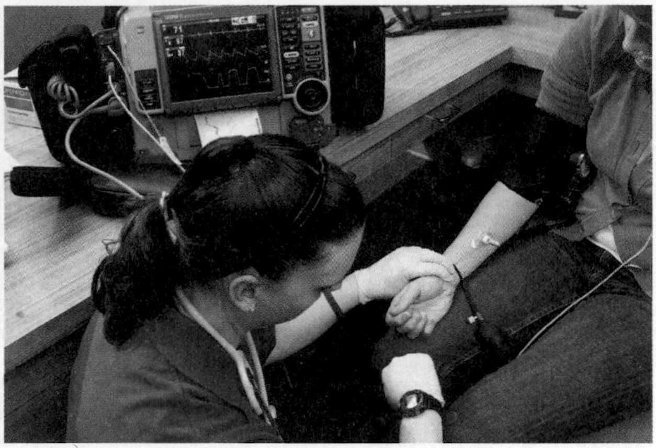

1-1G Determine posttreatment pulse rate.

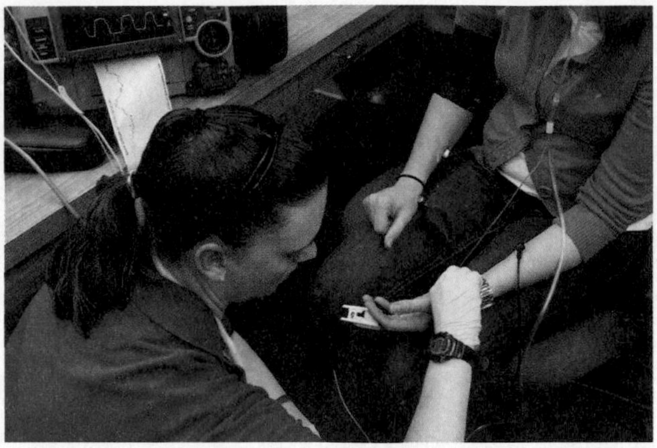

1-1H Reassess the patient.

inflammation is just as significant a problem. This is typically treated with corticosteroids and similar medications. The role of these agents in prehospital care varies from region to region. Certainly, EMS services with a long transport time should consider the use of corticosteroids and similar medications for patients with refractory asthma. Magnesium sulfate can sometimes be beneficial in refractory cases. Monitor the patient's response to these medications by noting improvement in PEFR, capnography, and pulse oximetry readings.

Many asthmatic patients will wait before summoning EMS. The longer the time interval from the onset of the asthma attack until treatment, the less likely it will be that bronchodilator medications will work. Often, after a prolonged asthma attack, the patient may become fatigued. A fatigued patient can quickly develop respiratory failure and subsequently require intubation and mechanical ventilation. Always be prepared to provide airway and respiratory support for the asthmatic.

Special Cases

Although most cases of asthma conform to the preceding descriptions, you may run into several special cases in the field. Asthma conditions that require special concern include status asthmaticus and asthmatic attacks in children.

STATUS ASTHMATICUS *Status asthmaticus* is a severe, prolonged asthma attack that cannot be broken by repeated doses of bronchodilators. It is a serious medical emergency that requires prompt recognition, treatment, and transport. The patient suffering status asthmaticus frequently will have a greatly distended chest from continued air trapping. Breath sounds, and often wheezing, may be absent. The patient is usually exhausted, severely acidotic, and dehydrated. The management of status asthmaticus is basically the same as for asthma. *Recognize that respiratory arrest is imminent and be prepared for endotracheal intubation.* Transport immediately and continue aggressive treatment en route.

ASTHMA IN CHILDREN Asthma in children is common. The pathophysiology and treatment are essentially the same as in adults, with altered medication dosages. Several additional medications are used in the treatment of childhood asthma. (Asthma in children is discussed in greater detail in the "Pediatrics" chapter.)

Upper Respiratory Infection

Infections involving the upper airway and respiratory tract are among the most common infections for which patients seek medical attention. Although these conditions are rarely life threatening, upper respiratory infections (URIs) can make many existing pulmonary diseases worse or lead to direct pulmonary infection. The best defenses against the spread of URIs are common practices such as good hand washing and covering the mouth during coughing and sneezing. Attention to such details is important when caring for patients with underlying pulmonary disease or those who are immunosuppressed (HIV infection, cancer) because URIs are more severe in these populations. Because of the prevalence of such infections, complete protection is impossible.

Pathophysiology

Remember that the upper airway begins at the nose and mouth, passes through the pharynx, and ends at the larynx. Other related structures are the paranasal sinuses and the eustachian tubes that connect the pharynx and the middle ear. In addition, several collections of lymphoid tissue found in the pharynx (palatine, pharyngeal, and lingual tonsils) produce antibodies and provide immune protection.

Viruses cause the vast majority of URIs. A variety of bacteria may also produce infection of the upper respiratory tract. The most significant is group A streptococcus, which is the causative organism in "strep throat" and accounts for up to 30 percent of URIs. These bacteria are also implicated in sinusitis and middle ear infections. Up to 50 percent of patients who have pharyngitis (inflammation of the pharynx) are not found to have a viral or bacterial cause. Fortunately, most URIs are self-limiting illnesses that resolve after several days of symptoms.

Assessment

The major symptoms of URI are determined by the portion of the upper respiratory tract that is predominantly affected (Table 1-6). Patients with URIs will often have accompanying symptoms such as fever, chills, myalgias (muscle pains), and fatigue.

Remember that any child with suspected epiglottitis (see the "Pediatrics" chapter) should be supported in a position of comfort. Do not attempt examination of the throat because this may produce severe laryngospasm. Adults occasionally also develop epiglottitis, but this is generally a more benign condition.

Management

In most cases, the diagnosis and treatment of upper respiratory conditions is based on the history and physical findings. Patients with pharyngitis are often diagnosed by obtaining a throat culture that confirms the presence of a bacterial cause of symptoms. A rapid test is also available. In patients with sinusitis and otitis media, treatment is based on a presumed bacterial cause.

As with other medical conditions, focus your attention on the patient's airway and ventilation. Generally, no intervention is required except in children with epiglottitis and in some complicated upper respiratory infections in which a collection of pus may occlude the airway. Give oxygen supplementation to any patient who has underlying pulmonary disease to treat hypoxia (avoid hyperoxia).

Most upper respiratory infections are treated symptomatically. Acetaminophen or ibuprofen is prescribed for fever, headache, and myalgias. Encourage patients to drink plenty of fluids. Saltwater gargles may be used for throat discomfort. Decongestants and antihistamines may be used to reduce mucus secretion. Encourage patients being treated with antibiotics for bacterial causes of URI to continue these agents.

In some patients with asthma or COPD, a URI may produce a worsening of their underlying medical condition. Use inhaled bronchodilators and corticosteroid agents according to local protocols or on advice of medical direction. Transport patients with underlying medical conditions to a health care facility capable of continued evaluation and management of the underlying condition. Continue appropriate monitoring with pulse oximetry and ECG during transport.

Pneumonia

Pneumonia is an infection of the lungs and is a common medical problem, especially in the aged and those infected with the human immunodeficiency virus (HIV). In fact, pneumonia is one of the leading causes of death in both groups of patients and is the fifth leading overall cause of death in the United States.

Patients with HIV infection and those on immune-suppressive therapy (cancer patients) are at high risk of developing pneumonia. In addition, the very young and very old are at higher risk of acquiring pneumonia because of ineffective protective mechanisms. Other risk factors include a history of alcoholism, cigarette smoking, and exposure to cold temperatures.

Table 1-6 Locations and Signs and Symptoms of Upper Respiratory Infections

Structure	Infection	Symptoms	Signs
Nose	Rhinitis	Runny nose, congestion, sneezing	Rhinorrhea
Pharynx	Pharyngitis	Sore throat, pain on swallowing	Erythematous pharynx, tonsil enlargement, pus on tonsils, cervical lymph node enlargement
Middle ear	Otitis media	Ear pain, decreased hearing	Red, bulging eardrum, pus behind eardrum, lymph node enlargement in front of or behind ear
Larynx	Laryngitis	Sore throat, hoarseness, pain on speaking	Red pharynx, hoarse quality to voice, cervical lymph node enlargement
Epiglottis	Epiglottitis	Sore throat, drooling, ill appearing	Upright position, drooling, ill appearing
Sinuses	Sinusitis	Headache, congestion	Tenderness over the sinuses, worsening of pain with leaning forward, yellow nasal discharge

Pathophysiology

Pneumonia is a collection of related respiratory diseases caused when any of a variety of infectious agents invades the lungs. Earlier in this chapter, you learned about the roles of mucus production and the action of respiratory tract cilia in protecting the body against bacterial invasion. When considering which patients are at risk, the unifying concept is that there is a defect in mucus production, ciliary action, or both.

Bacterial and viral pneumonias are the most frequent, although fungal and other forms of pneumonia exist. More unusual forms of pneumonia are seen in those patients who are currently or recently have been hospitalized, where they are exposed to a more unusual variety of microorganisms. This is referred to as *hospital-acquired pneumonia*. (Cases that develop in the out-of-hospital setting are described as *community-acquired pneumonia*.)

The infection begins in one part of the lung and often spreads to nearby alveoli. The infection may ultimately involve the entire lung. As the disease progresses, fluid and inflammatory cells collect in the alveoli, and alveolar collapse may occur (Figure 1-38). Pneumonia is primarily a ventilation disorder. Occasionally, the infection will extend beyond the lungs into the bloodstream and to more distant sites in the body. This systemic spread may lead to septic shock.

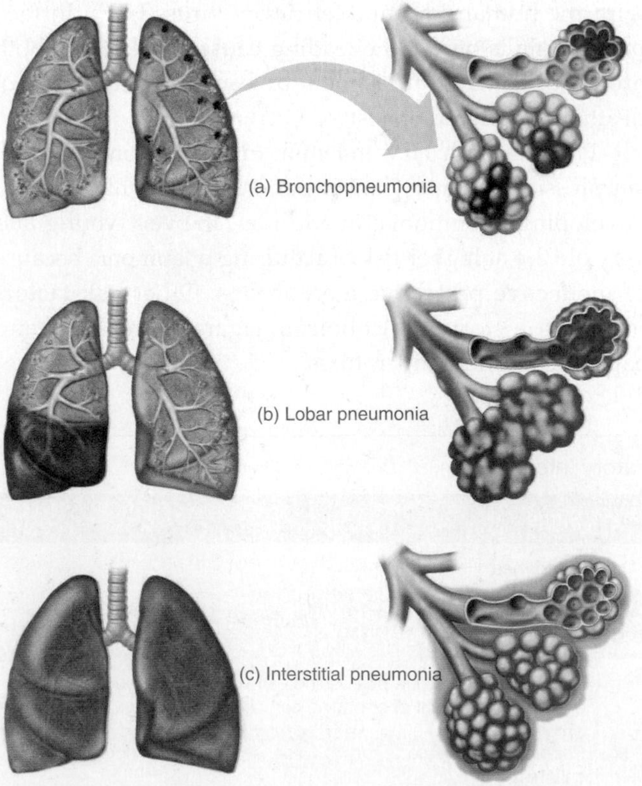

FIGURE 1-38 Types of pneumonia: (a) Bronchopneumonia with localized pattern. (b) Lobar pneumonia with diffuse pattern within the lung lobe. (c) Interstitial pneumonia is typically diffuse and bilateral.

Assessment

A patient with pneumonia will generally appear ill. He may report a recent history of fever and chills. These chills are commonly described as "bed shaking." There is usually a generalized weakness and malaise. The patient will tend to complain of a deep, productive cough and may expel yellow to brown sputum, often streaked with blood. Many cases involve associated **pleuritic** chest pain. Therefore, pneumonia should be considered in any patient who presents complaining of chest pain, especially if accompanied by fever and/or chills. In pneumonia involving the lower lobes of the lungs, a patient may complain of nothing more than upper abdominal pain.

Physical examination will commonly reveal fever, tachypnea, tachycardia, and a cough. Respiratory distress may be present. Auscultation of the chest usually demonstrates crackles (rales) in the involved lung segment, although wheezes or rhonchi may be heard. There usually is decreased air movement in the areas filled with infection. Percussion of the chest may reveal dullness over these areas. *Egophony* (a change in the spoken "E" sound to an "A" sound on auscultation) may also be noted.

In the forms of pneumonia involving viral, fungal, and rare bacterial causes, the typical symptoms as described are not seen. Instead, these patients may report a nonproductive cough with less prominent lung findings. Systemic symptoms such as headache, malaise, fatigue, muscle aches, sore throat, and abdominal complaints including nausea, vomiting, and diarrhea are more prominent. Fever and chills are not as impressive as in bacterial pneumonia.

Management

Pneumonia is generally diagnosed on the basis of physical examination, X-ray findings, and laboratory cultures. Therefore, diagnosis in the field is unlikely. The primary treatment is antibiotics to which the causative organism is susceptible. In the field, however, antibiotics are not indicated and treatment is purely supportive.

Place the patient in a comfortable position and administer supplemental oxygen to correct hypoxia. Use pulse oximetry to assess the patient's oxygen requirements. In severe cases, ventilatory assistance is needed and endotracheal intubation may be required. Establish intravenous access and base fluid resuscitation on the patient's hydration status. Administering fluids for dehydration is appropriate, but overhydration can also worsen the respiratory condition. Medical direction may sometimes order a breathing treatment with a beta-agonist, particularly if wheezing is present. Because patients with pneumonia often have some bronchospasm, these drugs will afford the patient some symptomatic relief. Give antipyretic agents such as acetaminophen or ibuprofen to reduce a high fever. A cool, moistened washcloth may soothe the patient.

Remember to be extremely careful when caring for patients over age 65 with suspected pneumonia. These patients have high mortality and complication rates. Transport them to a facility capable of handling the significant complications associated with the disease for this population.

Severe Acute Respiratory Syndrome (SARS)

Severe acute respiratory syndrome (SARS) is a viral respiratory illness that first appeared in southern China in November 2002. It became a global threat in March 2003 by spreading internationally via Hong Kong. Ultimately, 8,098 people worldwide were affected with SARS during that outbreak. Of these, 774 died. SARS entered Canada and several other countries and spread rapidly. Toronto was particularly affected. In fact, SARS placed a significant stress on the Toronto EMS system. Four paramedics contracted the disease, and more than 400 paramedics were placed on "working quarantine." The four paramedics who contracted SARS reportedly did so before mandatory PPE measures were undertaken. SARS appears to be an ongoing threat because of the highly infectious nature of the illness.

Pathophysiology

The virus that causes SARS, which was previously unrecognized, is called SARS-associated coronavirus (SARS-CoV). Coronaviruses play a major role in upper respiratory infections and the common cold. Preliminary studies indicated that SARS-CoV might survive in the environment for several days. Other infectious agents may play a role in SARS as well.

SARS is spread by close person-to-person contact. Respiratory droplets produced when an infected person coughs or sneezes transmit SARS-CoV. Disease transmission occurs when these droplets are deposited on the mucous membranes of the mouth, nose, and eyes of persons who are nearby. People touching a surface or object contaminated by infectious droplets can also transmit SARS-CoV.

The incubation period (time from exposure until onset of symptoms) is generally 2 to 7 days, although some cases have had an incubation period of as long as 10 to 14 days. A person with SARS is considered to be contagious as long as he has symptoms. Furthermore, there have been no reported cases of disease transmission before the source patient develops symptoms. Persons with documented SARS should be quarantined to their home for at least 10 days after the fever has abated and symptoms have cleared.

Assessment

If a SARS outbreak has been identified, all personnel should use appropriate PPE on every call or as directed by local health authorities. If, in a non-SARS epidemic area, a case is encountered that has SARS-like symptoms, all involved should immediately don appropriate PPE.

As for any patient with a respiratory illness, first address signs of severe respiratory distress. Look for altered mental status, one-to-two-word speech dyspnea, cough, cyanosis, and hypoxia as documented by pulse oximetry. Patients with underlying respiratory disease (asthma, emphysema, chronic bronchitis) and those with chronic illnesses are at increased risk of SARS-related problems.

Signs and symptoms that have been associated with SARS include sore throat, rhinorrhea (runny nose), chills or rigors (sudden paroxysmal chills), myalgias (muscle aches), headache, and diarrhea. This can progress to cough, sputum production, respiratory distress, and eventual respiratory failure.

Management

From a management standpoint, any patient suspected of SARS should be treated as any patient with suspected pneumonia or other respiratory illness. Place the patient in a comfortable position and administer supplemental oxygen to correct hypoxia. Use pulse oximetry to assess the patient's oxygenation requirements. In severe cases, ventilatory assistance may be needed and endotracheal intubation may be required. Establish intravenous access, and base fluid administration on the patient's hydration status. If the patient is wheezing, consider the administration of a nebulized bronchodilator. If SARS is suspected, notify the receiving hospital of your suspicions so that it can take appropriate measures for isolation of the patient and protection of health care workers.

Middle East Respiratory Syndrome (MERS)

Middle East respiratory syndrome (MERS) is a viral respiratory infection that is new to humans. First reported in Jordan and Saudi Arabia in 2012, it has spread to several other countries, including the United States. It is caused by the Middle East respiratory syndrome coronavirus (MERS-CoV). MERS is a dangerous infection, causing death in 3 to 4 of every 10 patients infected. It appears to be spread from person to person through close contact, including caring or living with a person who has the infection. It tends to affect all age groups. The incubation period appears to be 5 to 6 days, but can range from 2 days to 2 weeks. The primary signs and symptoms of MERS are:

- Fever
- Cough
- Shortness of breath

Some MERS patients will develop nausea, vomiting, and diarrhea. People with coexisting illnesses (e.g., diabetes, cancer, chronic lung disease, heart disease, kidney disease) are more severely affected and can develop pneumonia and renal failure. Currently there is no vaccine for MERS and there is no specific treatment. Standard respiratory illness protection measures are recommended (similar to those employed for SARS).

Lung Cancer

Lung cancer (neoplasm) is the leading cause of cancer-related death in the United States in both men and women. Most patients with lung cancer are between the ages of 55 and 65 years. There is a high mortality rate for patients with lung cancer after only 1 year with the disease.

There are currently four major types of lung cancer based on the predominant cell type. Twenty percent of cases involve only the lung tissue. Another 35 percent involve spread to the lymphatic system, and 45 percent have distant metastases (cancer cells spreading to other tissues). In cases in which there is lung tissue invasion, the primary problem is disruption of diffusion. In some larger cancers, there may also be alterations in ventilation by obstruction of the conducting bronchioles.

Cigarette smoking has long been known to be a risk factor for development of lung cancer. Environmental exposures to asbestos, hydrocarbons, radiation, and fumes from metal production have also been identified as risk factors. Finally, home exposure to radon has been implicated in the development of lung cancer. Preventive strategies include educating teenagers about the dangers of cigarette smoking and encouraging current smokers to quit. Implementing environmental safety standards that reduce the risk of exposure to such substances as asbestos will also reduce the risk of lung cancer. Finally, cancer screening of populations at risk is encouraged.

Pathophysiology

Although cancers that start elsewhere in the body can spread to the lungs, the vast majority of lung cancers are caused by carcinogens (cancer-producing substances) from cigarette smoking. A small portion of lung cancers are caused by inhalation of occupational agents such as asbestos and arsenic. These substances irritate and adversely affect the various tissues of the lung, ultimately leading to the development of abnormal (cancerous) cells.

There are four major types of lung cancers, depending on the type of lung tissue involved. The most common type of lung cancer is referred to as *adenocarcinoma.* This cancer arises from glandular-type (i.e., mucus-producing) cells found in the lungs and bronchioles. The next most frequently encountered type of lung cancer is *small cell carcinoma* (also called "oat cell" carcinoma). Small cell carcinoma arises from bronchial tissues. The third type of lung cancer is referred to as *epidermoid carcinoma.* Finally, *large cell carcinoma* is the fourth major type of lung cancer. Like small cell carcinoma, epidermoid and large cell carcinomas typically arise from the bronchial tissues. Lung cancers generally have a poor prognosis, with most patients dying within a year of the diagnosis (Figure 1-39).

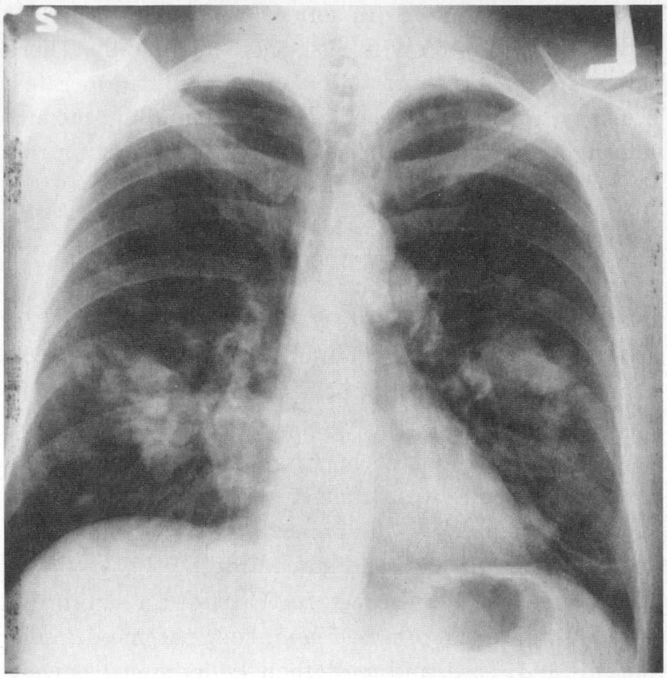

FIGURE 1-39 Chest X-ray showing lung cancer.
(© National Cancer Institute)

Assessment

As with other respiratory diseases, your first priority is to address signs of severe respiratory distress. Look for altered mental status, one-to-two-word dyspnea, cyanosis, hemoptysis, and hypoxia as documented by pulse oximeter. Severe uncontrolled hemoptysis can be a particularly life-threatening presentation.

Patients with lung cancer will present with a variety of complaints, depending on whether they are related to direct lung involvement, invasion of local structures, or metastatic spread. Patients with localized disease will present with cough, dyspnea, hoarseness, vague chest pain, and hemoptysis. Fever, chills, and pleuritic chest pain are seen in patients who develop pneumonia. Symptoms related to local invasion include pain on swallowing (dysphagia), weakness or numbness in the arm, and shoulder pain. Metastatic symptoms are related to the area of spread and include headache, seizures, bone pain, abdominal pain, nausea, and malaise.

Physical findings are nonspecific. Patients with advanced disease have profound weight loss and cachexia

CONTENT REVIEW

- Lung Cancer: Management Goals
  - Administer oxygen (if patient is hypoxic).
  - Support ventilation.
  - Be aware of any DNR order.
  - Provide emotional support to the patient and family.

(general physical wasting and malnutrition). Crackles (rales), rhonchi, wheezes, and diminished breath sounds may be heard in the affected lung. Venous distention in the arms and neck may be present if there is occlusion of the superior vena cava (called *superior vena cava syndrome*).

Management

Administer supplemental oxygen as needed based on the clinical status and pulse oximetry measurement. Support the patient's ventilation as needed and intubate as necessary. Be attentive, however, for any Do Not Resuscitate order or other advance directive, such as a living will, and follow your local protocol regarding these legal instruments. Consult medical direction if questions arise.

Initiate an IV of 0.9 percent normal saline and provide fluids if signs of dehydration are present. Follow your local protocol regarding the access of permanent indwelling catheters that many cancer patients have in place.

Prehospital drug therapy consists of bronchodilator agents and corticosteroids when signs of obstructive lung disease are present. Continue any prescribed antibiotics. Transport the patient and monitor mental status, vital signs, and oxygen status, as appropriate. Be prepared to provide emotional support for both the patient and family during transport.

Toxic Inhalation

Inhalation of toxic substances into the respiratory tract can cause pain, inflammation, or destruction of pulmonary tissues. Significant inhalations can affect the ability of the alveoli to exchange oxygen, thus resulting in hypoxemia.

Pathophysiology

The possibility of inhalation of products toxic to the respiratory system should be considered in any dyspneic patient. Causes of toxic inhalation include superheated air, toxic products of combustion, chemical irritants, and inhalation of steam. Each of these agents can result in upper airway obstruction due to edema and laryngospasm. In such cases, bronchospasm and lower airway edema may also appear. In severe inhalations, disruption of the alveolar–capillary membranes may result in life-threatening pulmonary edema.

Assessment

When assessing the patient with possible toxic inhalation exposure, determine the nature of the inhalant or the combusted material. Several products can result in the formation of corrosive acids or alkalis that irritate and damage the airway. These include:

- Ammonia (ammonium hydroxide)
- Nitrogen oxide (nitric acid)
- Sulfur dioxide (sulfurous acid)
- Sulfur trioxide (sulfuric acid)
- Chlorine (hydrochloric acid)

It is also crucial to determine the duration of the exposure, whether the patient was in an enclosed area at the time of the exposure, or if he experienced a loss of consciousness. Loss of consciousness may cause the airway to become vulnerable as a result of the loss of airway protective mechanisms.

During physical examination, pay particular attention to the face, mouth, and throat. Note any burns or particulate matter. Next, auscultate the chest for the presence of any wheezes or crackles (rales). Wheezing may indicate bronchospasm, whereas crackles may suggest pulmonary edema.

Management

After ensuring the safety of rescue personnel, remove the patient from the hazardous environment. Next, establish and maintain an open airway. Remember that the airway is often irritable and attempts at endotracheal intubation may result in laryngospasm, completely obstructing the airway. Laryngeal edema, as evidenced by hoarseness, brassy cough, and stridor, is ominous and may require prompt endotracheal intubation. Administer humidified oxygen to correct hypoxia. As a precaution, place a saline lock for venous access. Transport promptly.

Carbon Monoxide Inhalation

Carbon monoxide is an odorless, tasteless, colorless gas produced from the incomplete burning of fossil fuels and other carbon-containing compounds. It is the number-one cause of poisoning in industrialized countries. Carbon monoxide can be encountered in industrial sites, such as mines and factories. It is present in the environment in various concentrations primarily because of automotive exhaust emissions. Most poisonings occur from automobile emissions and home heating devices used in poorly ventilated areas.

CONTENT REVIEW

- Toxic Inhalation: Management Sequence
  - Ensure the safety of rescue personnel.
  - Remove the patient from the toxic environment.
  - Maintain an open airway.
  - Provide humidified high-concentration oxygen.

Carbon monoxide is often used in suicide attempts. In addition, it is a particular hazard for firefighters and rescue personnel.

Pathophysiology

Carbon monoxide exposure is potentially life threatening because it easily binds to the hemoglobin molecule. It has an affinity for hemoglobin 200 to 250 times that of oxygen. Once bound, receptor sites on the hemoglobin can no longer transport oxygen to the peripheral tissues. Hemoglobin with carbon monoxide bound is referred to as **carboxyhemoglobin**. The result is hypoxia at the cellular level and, ultimately, metabolic acidosis. Additionally, carbon monoxide binds to iron-containing enzymes and proteins (myoglobin) within the cells, leading to worsening cellular acidosis.[9]

Assessment

When confronted by a patient suffering possible carbon monoxide poisoning, determine the source of exposure, its length, and the location. Less time is required to develop a significant exposure in a closed space compared with one in an area that is fairly well ventilated.

Signs and symptoms of carbon monoxide poisoning include headache, nausea and vomiting, confusion, agitation, loss of coordination, chest pain, loss of consciousness, and even seizures. On physical examination, the skin may be cyanotic or it may be bright cherry red (a very late finding). There may be other signs of hypoxia, such as peripheral cyanosis or confusion.

Carboxyhemoglobin levels can now be measured noninvasively in the prehospital setting through CO-oximetry (Figure 1-40). A CO-oximeter is similar to a pulse oximeter, but uses eight wavelengths of light instead of two. It can detect carboxyhemoglobin, methemoglobin (on certain models), oxyhemoglobin, and deoxyhemogobin. Carboxyhemoglobin levels (SpCO) are reported as percentage of carboxyhemoglobin present. Normally, carboxyhemoglobin levels are less than 1 percent in nonsmokers and 3 percent in smokers. Table 1-7 lists CO severity by CO level and by signs and symptoms. SpCO levels may not always correlate with symptoms.

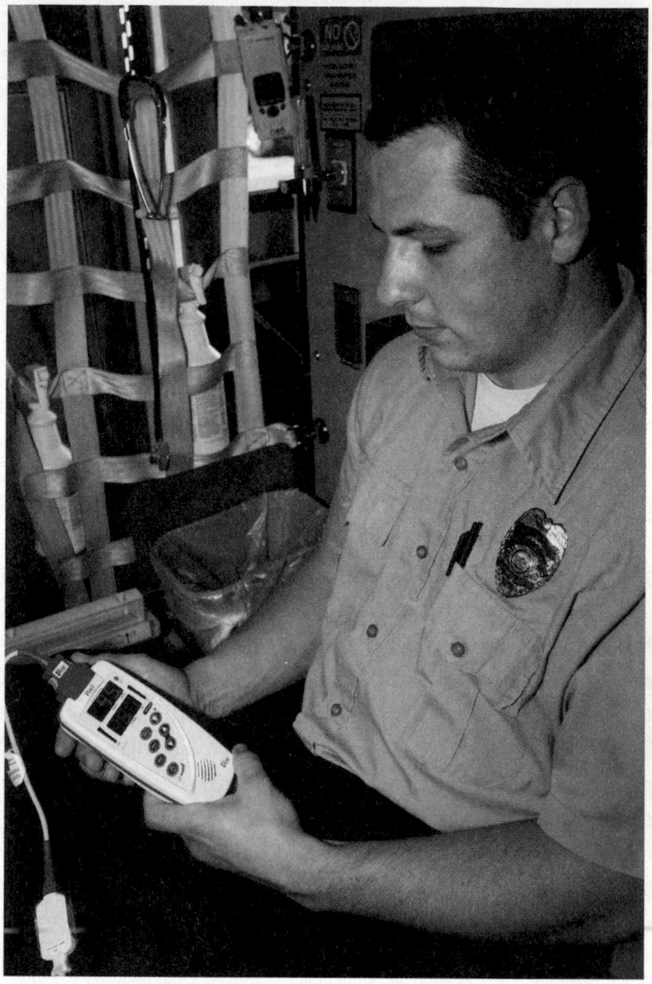

FIGURE 1-40 The CO-oximeter can rapidly and noninvasively determine and monitor carboxyhemoglobin levels in the prehospital setting.

(© Dr. Bryan E. Bledsoe)

CONTENT REVIEW

- Carbon Monoxide Inhalation: Management Sequence
  - Ensure the safety of rescue personnel.
  - Remove the patient from the exposure site.
  - Maintain an open airway.
  - Provide high-flow, high-concentration oxygen.

Management

Upon detection of carbon monoxide poisoning, first ensure the safety of rescue personnel, and then remove the patient from the site of exposure. Ensure and maintain the airway. Administer supplemental oxygen at the highest possible concentration. If the patient is breathing spontaneously, apply a *tight-fitting* nonrebreather mask. Consider the use of CPAP for moderate to severe exposures. If respiratory depression is noted, assist respirations. If shock is present, treat it. Prompt transport is essential.

Hyperbaric oxygen (HBO) therapy may be used in the treatment of severe carbon monoxide poisoning, although the effectiveness of this treatment is questionable. Many

Table 1-7 Severity of Carbon Monoxide Poisoning

CO-Hb	Severity	Signs and Symptoms
<15–20%	Mild	Headache, nausea, vomiting, dizziness, blurred vision
21–40%	Moderate	Confusion, syncope, chest pain, dyspnea, tachycardia, tachypnea, weakness
41–60%	Severe	Arrhythmias, hypotension, cardiac ischemia, palpitations, respiratory arrest, pulmonary edema, seizures, coma, cardiac arrest
>60%	Fatal	Death

EMS systems have protocols established whereby patients suffering from carbon monoxide poisoning are transported to hospitals with HBO therapy facilities. Hyperbaric oxygen increases the PaO_2, thus promoting increased oxygen uptake and displacement of the carbon monoxide from the hemoglobin. As mentioned earlier, however, the effectiveness of hyperbaric oxygen therapy in carbon monoxide poisoning remains unclear.[10]

Pulmonary Embolism

A pulmonary embolism is a blood clot (thrombus) or some other particle that lodges in a pulmonary artery, effectively blocking blood flow through that vessel. This condition is potentially life threatening because it can significantly decrease pulmonary blood flow, thus leading to hypoxemia (inadequate levels of oxygen in the blood). Pulmonary thromboembolism accounts for 50,000 deaths annually in the United States. In fact, one in five cases of sudden death are caused by pulmonary emboli. The great majority of patients with pulmonary emboli survive; only one in ten cases of documented pulmonary emboli results in death.

The incidence of pulmonary emboli is increased in certain populations. Any condition that results in immobility of the extremities can increase the risk of thromboembolism. Such conditions include recent surgery, long bone fractures (with immobilization in casts or splints), bedridden condition, or prolonged immobilization, as with long-distance travel. Venous pooling that occurs during pregnancy can also lead to pulmonary emboli. Certain disease states increase the likelihood of blood clot formation. These include cancer, infections, thrombophlebitis, atrial fibrillation, and sickle cell anemia. The incidence of thromboembolic disease is increased in patients taking oral birth control pills, particularly among smokers.

Pathophysiology

Sources of pulmonary emboli include air embolism, such as can occur during the placement of a central line; fat embolism, which can occur following a fracture; amniotic fluid embolism; and blood clots. It is also possible for a foreign body (such as part of a venous catheter) to become dislodged in the venous circulation. The vast majority of cases, however, are caused by blood clots that develop in the deep venous system of the lower extremities.

As a rule, a significant amount of blood passes through the veins of the lower extremity. During normal use of our legs, muscular contractions propel the blood through the venous system with the aid of valves that are present in the lower extremity veins. This action prevents blood from flowing backward through the venous system. When there is infection, venous injury, or any other condition that leads to pooling of blood in the deep veins of the lower extremity, clot formation occurs. If a portion of the clot becomes dislodged, it will pass through the right side of the heart and become lodged in the pulmonary vasculature.

When a pulmonary embolism occurs, the blockage of blood flow through the affected artery causes the right heart to pump against increased resistance. This results in an increase in pulmonary capillary pressure. The area of the lung supplied by the occluded pulmonary vessel can no longer effectively function in gas exchange because it receives no effective blood supply. The major derangement in patients with pulmonary emboli is a perfusion disorder. The involved lung segment is still ventilated, producing a ventilation–perfusion mismatch.[11]

Assessment

Signs and symptoms of a patient suffering a pulmonary embolism will vary, depending on the size and location of the obstruction. The patient suffering acute pulmonary embolism may report a sudden onset of severe unexplained dyspnea, which may or may not be associated with pleuritic chest pain. The patient may also report a cough that is usually not productive but may occasionally produce blood (hemoptysis). There may be a recent history of immobilization, such as hip fracture, surgery, or debilitating illness.

The physical examination may reveal labored breathing, tachypnea, and tachycardia. In massive pulmonary emboli, there may be signs of right-heart failure, such as jugular venous distention and, in some cases, falling blood pressure. In many cases, auscultation of the chest may reveal no significant lung findings, although rare crackles and wheezing may be noted. Occasionally, a pleural friction rub (dry, leathery sound with inspiration—like two pieces of leather rubbing together) may be heard.

Always examine the extremities. In up to 50 percent of cases, findings suggestive of deep venous thrombosis will be evident. These include a warm, swollen extremity with a thick cord palpated along the medial thigh and pain on palpation or when extending the calf.

In extreme cases, the patient may present with extreme confusion as the result of hypoxia, severe cyanosis, profound hypotension, and even cardiac arrest. Physical examination may reveal petechiae (small hemorrhagic spots) on the arms and chest wall in these cases.

Management

As with all respiratory conditions, your first priorities are the airway, breathing, and circulation. Remember that a large pulmonary embolism may lead to cardiac arrest. Perform CPR if needed.

If you suspect a patient is suffering a pulmonary embolism, establish and maintain an airway. Assist ventilations as required. Administer supplemental oxygen at the highest possible concentration. Endotracheal intubation may be required.

Place a saline lock. The diagnosis of pulmonary embolism is often difficult and requires a high index of suspicion. Remember that patients with suspected pulmonary embolism may require a significant amount of care. This disorder has a high complication rate and significant mortality. Carefully monitor the patient's vital signs and cardiac rhythm. Quickly transport the patient to a facility with the capabilities to care for the critical needs of the patient. Treatment in the hospital setting may include the use of various medications such as fibrinolytic agents and blood thinners like heparin.

Spontaneous Pneumothorax

A **spontaneous pneumothorax** is defined as a pneumothorax that occurs in the absence of blunt or penetrating trauma. Spontaneous pneumothorax is a common clinical condition, with 18 cases occurring for every 100,000 population. There is also a high recurrence rate. Fifty percent of patients will have a recurrent episode within 2 years.

There is a 5:1 ratio of male to female patients with spontaneous pneumothorax. Other risk factors include a tall, thin stature and a history of cigarette smoking. This disorder tends to develop in patients between the ages of 20 and 40 years. Patients with COPD have a higher incidence of spontaneous pneumothorax, presumably because of the presence of thinned lung tissue (blebs) that may rupture.

Pathophysiology

The primary derangement is one of ventilation, as the negative pressure that normally exists in the pleural space is lost. This prevents proper expansion of the lung in concert with the chest wall. A pneumothorax occupying 15 to 20 percent of the chest cavity is generally well tolerated by the patient unless there is significant underlying lung disease.

Assessment

The patient with a spontaneous pneumothorax presents with a sudden onset of sharp, pleuritic chest or shoulder pain. Often, coughing or lifting precipitates the symptoms. Dyspnea is commonly reported. The degree of symptoms is not strictly related to the size of the pneumothorax.

The physical examination is usually not impressive. Decreased breath sounds on the involved side may be difficult to note. They may be best heard at the lung apex. Even subtler is hyperresonance to percussion of the chest. Occasionally, the patient may have subcutaneous emphysema, which may be palpated as a crackling under the skin overlying the chest. Tachypnea, diaphoresis, and pallor are also seen. Cyanosis is rarely found.

Management

Use the patient's symptoms and pulse oximetry readings as guides to therapy. For most cases of spontaneous pneumothorax, supplemental oxygen is all that is required. Ventilatory support and endotracheal intubation are rarely required.

Be careful when managing patients with a spontaneous pneumothorax who require positive pressure ventilation by mask or endotracheal tube. They are at risk for the development of a *tension pneumothorax*. You may note that the patient will become physically difficult to ventilate. Hypoxia, cyanosis, and hypotension may also develop. In addition to the usual signs of a pneumothorax, the patient will develop jugular vein distention and deviation of the trachea away from the pneumothorax. Needle decompression of a tension pneumothorax may be required.

Other management measures should include placing the patient in a position of comfort. Reserve intravenous access and electrocardiographic monitoring for patients with significant symptoms or severe underlying respiratory disease. Carefully monitor such patients during transport.

Hyperventilation Syndrome

Rapid breathing, chest pains, numbness, and other symptoms usually associated with anxiety or situational stress characterize hyperventilation syndrome. However, as shown in Table 1-8, anxiety and stress are not the only possible causes of hyperventilation syndrome. Many serious medical problems can cause hyperventilation. To avoid improper treatment, consider hyperventilation an indication of a serious medical problem until proven otherwise.

Pathophysiology

Hyperventilation syndrome frequently occurs in anxious patients. The patient often senses that he cannot "catch his breath." The patient will then begin to breathe rapidly.

Table 1-8 Causes of Hyperventilation Syndrome

Acidosis	Interstitial pneumonitis, fibrosis, edema
Beta-adrenergic agonists	Metabolic disorders
Bronchial asthma	Methylxanthine derivatives
Cardiovascular disorders	Neurologic disorders
Central nervous system infection or tumors	Pain
Congestive heart failure	Pneumonia
Drugs	Pregnancy
Fever, sepsis	Progesterone
Hepatic failure	Psychogenic or anxiety hypertension
High altitude	Pulmonary disease
Hypotension	Pulmonary emboli, vascular disease
Hypoxia	Salicylate

Hyperventilation in a purely anxious patient results in the excess elimination of CO_2, causing a respiratory alkalosis. This increases the amount of bound calcium, producing a relative hypocalcemia. This results in cramping of the muscles of the feet and hands, which is called *carpopedal spasm*.

Assessment

With a hyperventilating patient, you may elicit a history of fatigue, nervousness, dizziness, dyspnea, chest pain, and numbness and tingling around the mouth, hands, and feet. The physical examination will reveal an anxious patient with tachypnea and tachycardia. As noted, spasm of the fingers and feet may also be present. If the patient has a history of seizure disorder, the hyperventilation episode may precipitate a seizure. Other symptoms are related to the underlying cause of the hyperventilation syndrome.

Management

The primary treatment for hyperventilation syndrome is reassurance. Instruct the patient to voluntarily reduce his respiratory rate and depth of breathing. Mechanisms that will assist in increasing the PCO_2, such as breath holding or breathing into a paper bag, are discouraged in prehospital care. Check the oxygen saturation by applying a pulse oximeter. Hyperventilating patients may require oxygen if their SpO_2 levels are $\leq 96\%$. Allowing them to rebreathe into a paper bag can be deadly. Many EMS systems permit paramedics to use rebreathing techniques only on physician order. It is important to exclude other medical causes before determining that a patient is hyperventilating.

The hyperventilating patient can often present a dilemma for prehospital personnel. Although anxiety is the most common cause of hyperventilation, other, more serious, diseases can present in exactly the same manner. For example, pulmonary embolism or acute myocardial infarction can exhibit symptoms similar to hyperventilation syndrome.

Central Nervous System Dysfunction

Central nervous system dysfunction, with the exception of drug overdose and massive stroke, is a relatively rare cause of respiratory emergencies. However, always consider the possibility of central nervous system dysfunction in any dyspneic patient.

Pathophysiology

Central nervous system dysfunction can be a causative factor in respiratory depression and arrest. Causes include head trauma, stroke, brain tumors, and various drugs. Several medications, such as narcotics and barbiturates, make the respiratory centers in the brain less responsive to increases in $PaCO_2$. These agents also depress areas of the brain responsible for initiating respirations.

Assessment

The assessment of patients with central nervous system dysfunction should follow the same approach as for any respiratory emergency. However, you should be alert for nonrespiratory system problems, such as CNS trauma or drug ingestion. Be careful to note any variation in the respiratory pattern, which can be an indication of central nervous system dysfunction.

Management

If central nervous system dysfunction is suspected, establish and maintain an open airway. If respiratory depression is noted or if respirations are absent, initiate mechanical ventilation. Administer supplemental oxygen if hypoxia is detected by pulse oximetry and establish a saline lock for venous access. Direct specific therapy at the underlying problem, if it is known.

Dysfunction of the Spinal Cord, Nerves, or Respiratory Muscles

Several disease processes can affect the spinal cord, nerves, and/or respiratory muscles. Dysfunction of these structures can lead to hypoventilation and progressive hypoxemia.

Pathophysiology

Numerous disorders can interfere with respiratory function. These include spinal cord trauma, polio, amyotrophic lateral sclerosis (ALS or Lou Gehrig's disease), and myasthenia gravis. Viral infections, in certain cases, can cause dysfunction of the nervous system. An example of this is *Guillain-Barré syndrome (GBS)*. In GBS, the myelin covering of the nerve is damaged, resulting in relative loss of nerve impulse conduction. This affects virtually every peripheral nerve. Approximately 30 percent of patients with GBS will require ventilatory assistance, as the nerves that stimulate respiration are impaired.

Certain tumors can impinge on the spinal cord, depressing respiratory function. These disorders result in an inability of the respiratory muscles to contract normally, thus causing hypoventilation. Tidal volume and minute volume are decreased. You should also be aware that patients with these disorders do not have the ability to generate an adequate cough reflex and as a result are at risk of developing pneumonia.

Assessment

Patients with possible dysfunction of the spinal cord, nerves, or respiratory muscles may have a history of trauma that is not readily apparent. Always question the patient about injuries or falls. If there is any doubt about a possible injury, act accordingly and immobilize the cervical spine. Also, inquire about signs or symptoms that may suggest a problem with the peripheral nerves. These include such findings as numbness, pain, or sensory dysfunction. The assessment of patients with possible dysfunction of the spinal cord, nerves, or respiratory muscles should follow the same approach as for any respiratory emergency. However, be alert for subtle findings that may indicate a problem with the peripheral nervous system. Always be ready to protect the airway and support ventilation if the patient has symptoms of possible airway obstruction or respiratory failure.

Management

Management of spinal cord and respiratory muscle dysfunction is purely supportive. Establish an airway and provide ventilatory support. If myasthenia gravis is present and if transport time is long, the physician may request the administration of one of several agents effective in treating such patients.

Summary

Respiratory emergencies are commonly encountered in prehospital care. It is important to recognize that all respiratory disorders may produce derangements in ventilation, perfusion, or diffusion. Recognition and treatment must be prompt. Understanding the underlying cause of the respiratory disorder can guide therapy. The primary treatment is to correct hypoxia. Necessary steps include establishing and maintaining the airway, assisting ventilations as required, and administering supplemental oxygen. Appropriate pharmacological agents may be subsequently ordered by local protocols.

Whether you are dealing with a suspected pulmonary embolus, exacerbation of asthma, foreign body airway obstruction, or ARDS, your primary responsibility never changes: Make sure your patient has an open airway and is breathing well enough to maintain normoxia. Whenever the airway and breathing are affected, the astute paramedic will treat abnormalities as they are found. Oxygen is the primary medication of choice, but remember to use it sparingly. Your goal is normoxia, not hyperoxia. Remember, hyperoxia and hypoxia both have dangerous effects on the patient.

Paramedics today have a number of diagnostic tools available to help determine respiratory status and even its causes. Tools such as capnography, end-tidal CO_2, pulse oximetry, and even carbon monoxide detectors are readily available for determining a respiratory patient's status. Don't overlook these valuable tools. Use them to help you make an informed decision regarding your care plan for the patient. Once again, do not become lulled by the technology nor allow the technology to replace good old-fashioned assessment and common sense. When combined with a thorough physical assessment and proper judgment, these tools can be invaluable in guiding patient care and progress.

You Make the Call

You and your partner respond to the scene of a 69-year-old male patient who is reported to have difficulty breathing. Once you are sure the scene is safe, you enter and find a very dyspneic patient breathing 56 times per minute. His pulse is strong and rapid, at 140 beats per minute. He is using accessory muscles and has cyanosis about the lips and fingers. The patient is confused. His wife states that he has both COPD and lung cancer and reports that he had been a very heavy smoker up until the last few months. He has also had an increasing cough and fever over the past few days. The patient's initial pulse oximetry reading is 82 percent.

1. What pathophysiologic abnormality of the respiratory system do you suspect?
2. How would you initially manage this patient?
3. Why is the finding of cough and fever significant in this patient?

See Suggested Responses at the back of this book.

Review Questions

1. What type of risk factors are those that are influenced by or are from within the patient?
   a. Intrinsic
   b. Inherent
   c. Extrinsic
   d. Generic

2. The anatomic difference between the two mainstem bronchi helps to explain why ________
   a. aspirated gastric contents tend to pass into the right lung.
   b. the left lung is smaller and thus does not require as much airflow.
   c. endotracheal tubes advanced too far into the trachea will pass into the right mainstem bronchus.
   d. all of the above.

3. What is secreted by type II pneumocytes found on the alveolar surface that helps to decrease the surface tension of the alveoli?
   a. Tryptosin
   b. Histamine
   c. Surfactant
   d. Macrophage

4. Stimulatory impulses that travel from the spinal cord to the diaphragm do so down which nerve?
   a. Vagal
   b. Cranial
   c. Phrenic
   d. Hypoglossal

5. What term is used to describe the overall volume of air in the lungs after a full, complete inhalation?
   a. Total lung capacity
   b. Minute alveolar volume
   c. Minute respiratory volume
   d. Forced expiratory volume

6. The most important determinant of the ventilatory rate is the arterial ____________
   a. PO_2.
   b. pH.
   c. PCO_2.
   d. Hg.

7. The oxygen dissociation curve can be altered by changes in the ____________
   a. PCO_2.
   b. blood pH.
   c. body temperature.
   d. PCO_2, blood pH, and body temperature.

8. Cellular respiration occurs in the peripheral ____________
   a. veins.
   b. arteries.
   c. capillaries.
   d. arterioles.

9. What type of abnormal breathing pattern is characterized by long, deep breaths that are stopped during the inspiratory phase (i.e., breath holding) and separated by periods of apnea?
   a. Kussmaul's respirations
   b. Apneustic respirations
   c. Ataxic (Biot's) respirations
   d. Central neurogenic hyperventilation

10. Medications commonly used by patients with COPD include all of the following *except* ____________
    a. prednisone.
    b. albuterol.
    c. ipratropium.
    d. methacholine.

11. A whistling or musical sound due to narrowing of the airways by edema, bronchoconstriction, or foreign materials describes what abnormal breath sound?
    a. Stridor
    b. Snoring
    c. Rhonchi
    d. Wheezing

12. What is the preferred abbreviation to describe oxygen saturation measurement?
    a. O_2
    b. SpO_2
    c. PaO_2
    d. SaO_2

13. Which term is used to describe a graphic recording or display of the capnometry reading over time?
    a. Capnogram
    b. Capnoscreen
    c. Capnography
    d. Capnowave

14. What is the term for an excess of red blood cells, resulting in an abnormally high hematocrit?
    a. Anemia
    b. Hypoxemia
    c. Polycythemia
    d. Thrombocytopenia

15. Which medical assessment tool should the paramedic use when determining the severity of an asthma attack and/or the degree of response to treatment?
    a. CO_2
    b. PCO_2
    c. PEFR
    d. $ETCO_2$

16. What drug class is used for patients who have bronchoconstriction from asthma but are still able to maintain an acceptable minute ventilation?
    a. Corticosteroids
    b. Bronchodilators
    c. Antibiotics
    d. Methylxanthines

17. A CO-oximeter reading of 25 percent indicates what degree of CO poisoning?
    a. Mild
    b. Moderate
    c. Severe
    d. Fatal

18. Most patients with neuromuscular disorders that affect the patient's ability to ventilate will end up with which medical device?
    a. AED
    b. Insulin pump
    c. Home ventilator
    d. CPAP or BiPAP machine

See Answers to Review Questions at the back of this book.

References

1. Macknet, M. R., M. Allard, R. L. Applegate, and J. Rook. "The Accuracy of Noninvasive and Continuous Total Hemoglobin Measurement by Pulse CO-Oximetry in Human Subjects Undergoing Hemodilution." *Anesth Analg* 111 (2010): 1424–1426.
2. Austin, M. A., K. E. Wills, L. Blizzard, E. H. Walters, and R. Wood-Baker. "Effect of High Flow Oxygen on Mortality in Chronic Obstructive Pulmonary Disease Patients in Prehospital Setting: Randomised Controlled Trial." *BMJ* 341 (2010): c5462.
3. Kilgannon, J. H., A. E. Jones, N. I. Shapiro, et al. "Association between Arterial Hyperoxia Following Resuscitation from Cardiac Arrest and In-Hospital Mortality." *JAMA* 303 (2010): 2165–2171.
4. Moradkhan, R. and L. I. Sinoway. "Revisiting the Role of Oxygen Therapy in Cardiac Patients." *J Am Coll Cardiol* 56 (2010): 1013–1016.
5. Berg, R. A., R. Hemphill, B. S. Abella, et al. "Part 5: Adult Basic Life Support 2010 American Heart Association Guidelines for Cardiopulmonary Resuscitation and Emergency Cardiac Care." *Circulation* 122 (suppl 3) (2010): S685–S705.
6. Tsushima, K., L. S. King, N. R. Aggarwal, A. De Gorordo, F. R. D'Alessio, and K. Kubo. "Acute Lung Injury Review." *Intern Med* 48 (2009): 621–630.
7. Bailey, C. D., R. Wagland, R. Dabbour, A. Caress, J. Smith, and A. Molassiotis. "An Integrative Review of Systematic Reviews Related to the Management of Breathlessness in Respiratory Illnesses." *BMC Pulm Med* 10 (2010): 63.
8. Lazarus, S. C. "Clinical Practice. Emergency Treatment of Asthma." *N Engl J Med* 363 (2010): 755–764.
9. Thom, S. R., V. M. Bhopale, S. T. Han, J. M. Clark, and K. R. Hardy. "Intravascular Neutrophil Activation Due to Carbon Monoxide Poisoning." *Am J Respir Crit Care Med* 174 (2006): 1239–1248.
10. Buckley, N. A., D. N. Juurlink, G. Isbister, M. H. Bennett, and E. J. Lavonas. "Hyperbaric Oxygen for Carbon Monoxide Poisoning." *Cochrane Database Syst Rev* 4 (2011): CD002041.
11. Heit, J. A. "The Epidemiology of Venous Thromboembolism in the Community: Implications for Prevention and Management." *J Thromb Thrombolysis* 21 (2006): 23–29.

Further Reading

Dalton, A. L., D. Limmer, J. J. Mistovich, and H. A. Werman. *EMPACT.* Upper Saddle River, NJ: Pearson/Prentice Hall, 2012.

Marieb, E. N., ed. "The Respiratory System," in *Human Anatomy and Physiology*. 10th ed. San Francisco: Pearson, 2015.

Martini, R. H., E. F. Bartholomew, and B. E. Bledsoe. *Anatomy and Physiology for Emergency Care.* 2nd ed. Upper Saddle River, NJ: Pearson/Prentice Hall, 2008.

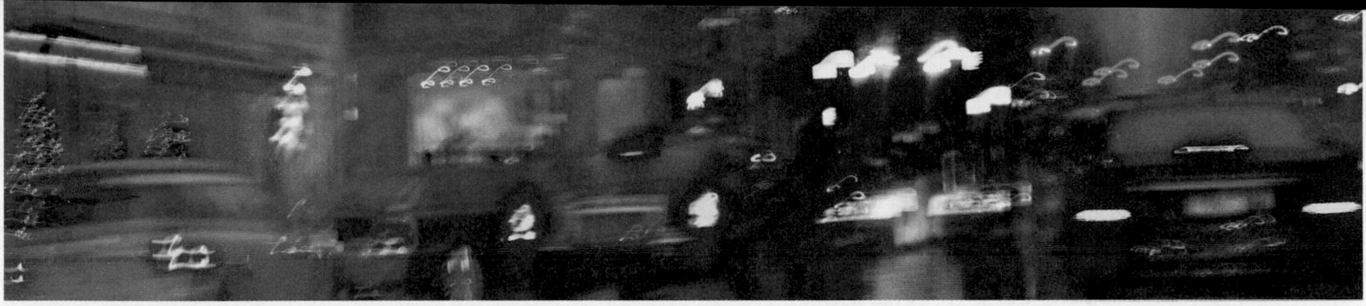

Chapter 2
Cardiology

Bryan Bledsoe, DO, FACEP, FAAEM, EMT-P

STANDARD
Medicine (Cardiovascular)

COMPETENCY
Integrates assessment findings with principles of epidemiology and pathophysiology to formulate a field impression and implement a comprehensive treatment/disposition plan for a patient with a medical complaint.

Learning Objectives

Terminal Performance Objective: After reading this chapter, you should be able to integrate patient assessment findings, patient history, and knowledge of anatomy, physiology, pathophysiology, and basic and advanced life support interventions to recognize and manage patients with cardiac disorders.

Enabling Objectives: To accomplish the terminal performance objective, you should be able to:

1. Define key terms introduced in this chapter.
2. Describe the epidemiology and other demographic findings for cardiovascular disease in the United States.
3. Identify risk factors for cardiovascular disease and public health initiatives aimed at lowering these risks and disease incidence.
4. Review the anatomy and physiology of the cardiovascular system, to include cardiac cycle physiology, electrophysiology, and ECG rhythm generation.
5. Explain electrocardiographic monitoring as it relates to rhythm acquisition, types of leads, and ECG graph paper.
6. Relate the normal waves and intervals of an ECG tracing to the electrical and mechanical events in the heart.
7. Explain the basic process for interpreting ECG rhythms when they deviate from normal.
8. Explain a systematic analysis of ECG rhythms, apply knowledge of abnormal cardiac rhythms, interpret ECG arrhythmias, and identify potential causes of these arrhythmias.
9. Given multiple ECG tracings and clinical presentation, describe the treatments generally indicated in the prehospital environment.

10. Adapt the scene size-up, primary assessment, history, secondary assessment, and use of monitoring technology to arrive at a field impression and differentials for cardiovascular emergencies.
11. Explain general BLS and ALS management principles for cardiovascular emergencies.
12. Describe the pathophysiology of cardiovascular disorders commonly seen in the prehospital environment by the paramedic.
13. Use a process of clinical reasoning to guide and interpret the patient assessment findings and develop a management plan for patients with cardiovascular disorders in the prehospital environment.
14. Describe the roles of diagnostic procedures in the evaluation of myocardial infarction, including 12-lead ECGs and laboratory tests.
15. Describe the roles of fibrinolytic therapy, percutaneous coronary interventions, coronary artery bypass grafts, and pharmacological treatments in the management of myocardial infarction.
16. List and describe the phases leading to biological death in cardiac arrest, and relate the appropriate prehospital treatment for each phase.
17. Explain management principles for arrested patients who achieve ROSC prehospitally.
18. Describe considerations in withholding resuscitation in cardiac arrest and in terminating resuscitative efforts in the field.
19. Describe the process and purpose of 12-lead ECG interpretation.
20. Given a variety of scenarios, discuss the integration of assessment and management guidelines as they relate to cardiovascular emergencies.

KEY TERMS

aberrant conduction, p. 108
abdominal aortic aneurysm, p. 154
absolute refractory period, p. 72
action potential, p. 63
acute arterial occlusion, p. 155
acute coronary syndrome (ACS), p. 131
acute pulmonary embolism, p. 155
afterload, p. 58
anastomosis, p. 56
aneurysm, p. 154
angina pectoris, p. 131
arrhythmia, p. 75
arteriosclerosis, p. 154
artifact, p. 67
atherosclerosis, p. 154
augmented leads, p. 68
automaticity, p. 64
bipolar leads, p. 67
bradycardia, p. 74
bruit, p. 85
bundle branch block, p. 108
bundle of Kent, p. 109
cardiac arrest, p. 149
cardiac cycle, p. 57
cardiac output, p. 58
cardiac tamponade, p. 143
cardiogenic shock, p. 147
cardiovascular disease (CVD), p. 52
cardiovascular system, p. 53
chronotropy, p. 61
claudication, p. 154
compensatory pause, p. 94
conductivity, p. 64
congestive heart failure (CHF), p. 140
contractility, p. 64
coronary artery disease (CAD), p. 52
corrected QT (QTc), p. 72
coupling interval, p. 100
current of injury (injury current), p. 164
cystic medial necrosis, p. 154
deep venous thrombosis, p. 155
defibrillation, p. 122
denervated, p. 62
depolarization, p. 63
diastole, p. 57
dissecting aortic aneurysm, p. 154
downtime, p. 152
dromotropy, p. 61
dysrhythmia, p. 75
early repolarization, p. 177
ectopic beat, p. 75
ectopic focus, p. 75
Einthoven's triangle, p. 67
ejection fraction, p. 58
electrocardiogram (ECG), p. 66
excitability, p. 64
heart failure, p. 139
hypertensive emergency, p. 145

hypertensive encephalopathy, p. 145
hypertrophy, p. 182
indeterminate axis, p. 162
induced therapeutic hypothermia (ITH), p. 152
injury current, p. 164
inotropy, p. 61
intercalated disks, p. 62
interpolated beat, p. 99
left axis deviation, p. 162
limb leads, p. 67
myocardial infarction (MI), p. 133
myocardial injury, p. 164
myocardial ischemia, p. 164
myoglobin, p. 149
noncompensatory pause, p. 83
non–ST-segment elevation myocardial infarction (NSTEMI), p. 134
normal sinus rhythm, p. 75
paroxysmal nocturnal dyspnea (PND), p. 141
peripheral arterial atherosclerotic disease, p. 155
Poiseuille's law, p. 57
precordial (chest) leads, p. 67
preload, p. 58
Prinzmetal's angina, p. 132
prolonged QT interval, p. 72
pulmonary embolism (PE), p. 140
QRS axis, p. 162
QT interval, p. 71
reciprocal, p. 171
refractory period, p. 72
relative refractory period, p. 72
repolarization, p. 63
resting potential, p. 63
resuscitation, p. 152
return of spontaneous circulation (ROSC), p. 152
rhythm strip, p. 66
right axis deviation, p. 162
Starling's law of the heart, p. 58
stroke volume, p. 58
ST-segment elevation myocardial infarction (STEMI), p. 134
subendocardial infarction, p. 134
sudden death, p. 149
survival, p. 152
synchronized cardioversion, p. 125
syncytium, p. 62
systole, p. 57
tachycardia, p. 74
total downtime, p. 152
transmural infarction, p. 134
unipolar leads, p. 68
varicose veins, p. 155
vasculitis, p. 155
vector, p. 162

Case Study

As soon as they complete the morning equipment check, Paramedic Unit 4 is dispatched to a difficulty-breathing call in a suburb of the city they serve. The response time is approximately 5 minutes. They arrive on scene at the same time as BLS first responders from the Pine Hill Fire Protection District. The house is a typical suburban residence; a woman is on the front porch waving at the rescuers. Paramedics Chris Clark and Kim Jones grab the equipment and head for the residence. First responders from the fire department get the stretcher from the ambulance and go to assist.

The crew enters the comfortable living room and sees a man in his 60s in obvious distress. He is sitting stark upright, pale, and breathing at 34 times a minute. The crew learns that he is Hubert Williams, a 69-year-old man who awakened early this morning extremely short of breath. He placed a call to his doctor but has not had a response. When he appeared to be getting worse, his wife called 911. His wife says he has a history of congestive heart failure and high blood pressure and had prostate surgery 8 weeks earlier.

The paramedics begin a primary assessment. The patient is in severe distress. He denies any pain, including chest pain. He is very anxious and able to communicate only in brief one-word sentences. Crackles (rales) are heard without a stethoscope. Oxygen is immediately administered at 100 percent via a nonrebreather mask. Despite that, the SpO_2 remains at 83 percent. The remainder of the physical examination reveals moderate jugular venous distention and loud crackles through all lung fields. A prominent S3 is heard, and there is mild pitting pretibial edema. Vital signs are blood pressure 140/98 mmHg, pulse 130 per minute, and respirations 32 per minute. A 12-lead ECG reveals atrial fibrillation with a rapid ventricular response.

The paramedics immediately apply the continuous positive airway pressure (CPAP) device and continue 100 percent oxygen administration—now with a PEEP of 10 cm H_2O. They apply 1 inch of nitroglycerin paste to his chest. Kim starts a saline lock in the left forearm.

Mr. Williams's wife brings in a shoebox full of medications. The paramedics note that Mr. Williams takes an aspirin a day, digoxin (Lanoxin), furosemide (Lasix), enalopril (Vasotec), nitroglycerin (Isordil), and acebutolol (Sectral). There is a prescription for acetaminophen with codeine (Tylenol #3) that she states he is not taking. He also takes several herbal supplements and vitamins. He has had no recent medication changes. He is not allergic to any medications.

Following application of the CPAP and nitroglycerin, Mr. Williams appears markedly better. However, he is still tachypneic, with a respiratory rate of 26 breaths per minute and a SpO_2 of 90 percent. According to their protocols, the paramedics administer 25 milligrams of captopril (Capoten) sublingually.

The paramedics ready the intubation equipment. However, Mr. Williams is much improved, and they don't think it will be needed. He is moved to the ambulance and reassessed. His respiratory rate is down to 20 breaths per minute and his heart rate is down to 100 beats per minute. He is able to speak in phrases and his SpO_2 is now 94 percent with the CPAP.

Mr. Williams is transported to Rockport Community Hospital, where he is diagnosed with flash pulmonary edema. The medical staff continues the CPAP and Mr. Williams improves to such a degree that he is admitted to the intermediate unit instead of the intensive care unit (ICU). He quickly responds to treatment and his medication regimen is adjusted. He is discharged home 48 hours later and is doing well. No obvious cause for the acute decompensation could be determined.

Introduction

According to current estimates, more than 60 million Americans have some form of **cardiovascular disease (CVD)**. **Coronary artery disease (CAD)**, a type of CVD, is the single largest killer of Americans (approximately 370,000 people annually). Each year, on average, 610,000 people die of heart disease (1 in every 4 deaths). Approximately 225,000 of them, a little more than half, die before ever reaching the hospital.[1] Another way of looking at the impact of CVD is this: An American will suffer a nonfatal heart attack every 29 seconds. About once every minute, an American will die from CAD. These deaths are usually sudden and often due to lethal cardiac rhythm disturbances that result in cardiac arrest.

Sudden death from CAD is often preventable. To decrease the chances of sudden death, the patient must recognize the signs and symptoms early and seek health care. Then, the health care system must provide definitive care promptly, usually within the first hour after the onset of symptoms.

Cultural Considerations

Culture and Cardiovascular Disease. Cardiovascular disease remains the number-one cause of death in the United States and Canada. The incidence of cardiovascular disease increased steadily during the 20th century, although it has stabilized somewhat over the past decade or so.

Cardiovascular deaths have increased for multiple reasons. For example, in the 1800s and the earlier part of the 1900s, many people died of infectious diseases. As a result, the average life span was much shorter than it is today. Thus, cardiovascular disease may not have been a significant factor because people did not live long enough to suffer the effects of the disease. However, with the advent of antibiotics in the mid-1900s, the average life span increased and people began to die from cardiovascular disease, cancers, and other causes that generally take longer to develop.

In addition, in the mid- to late 1900s, significant changes occurred in diet. Previously, foods were usually home grown and prepared (agrarian). Meat products and processed foods were not commonplace. Much of today's diet is fast food and processed foods. With that, we have seen a general decline in the intake of fiber and an increase in the intake of fats. And, unlike some Scandinavian and Asian countries, the U.S. diet does not include significant amounts of cold-water fish, which contain oils that decrease cholesterol. Thus, it could be said that a significant reason for the increase in cardiovascular disease is cultural dietary changes.

Public education about CVD has focused on two strategies. The first is to educate the public about the risk factors for the development of CVD. This program encourages patients to modify their lifestyle to minimize these risk factors. The following factors have been *proven* to increase the risk of cardiovascular disease:

- Smoking
- Older age
- Family history of CVD
- Hypertension (high blood pressure)
- Hypercholesterolemia (excessive cholesterol in the blood)
- Carbohydrate intolerance (diabetes mellitus)
- Substance abuse
- Male gender
- Lack of exercise

Factors that are *thought* to increase the risk of CVD include:

- Diet
- Obesity
- Oral contraceptives (birth control pills)
- Type A personality (competitive, aggressive, hostile)
- Psychosocial tensions (stress)

The second component of public education is to teach recognition of the signs and symptoms of heart attack. Patients can benefit from medical intervention only if they recognize the signs and symptoms and promptly access the health care system. Patients are encouraged to access the EMS system early. As a paramedic, you will treat patients who already have developed the manifestations of CVD. This will be an opportunity for you to further serve your patients by teaching preventive strategies, including early recognition of symptoms, education, and alteration of lifestyle.

This chapter discusses the advanced prehospital care of cardiovascular emergencies. First, we will review the pertinent anatomy and physiology, and then we will use that knowledge to discuss assessing, recognizing, and treating cardiovascular disorders.

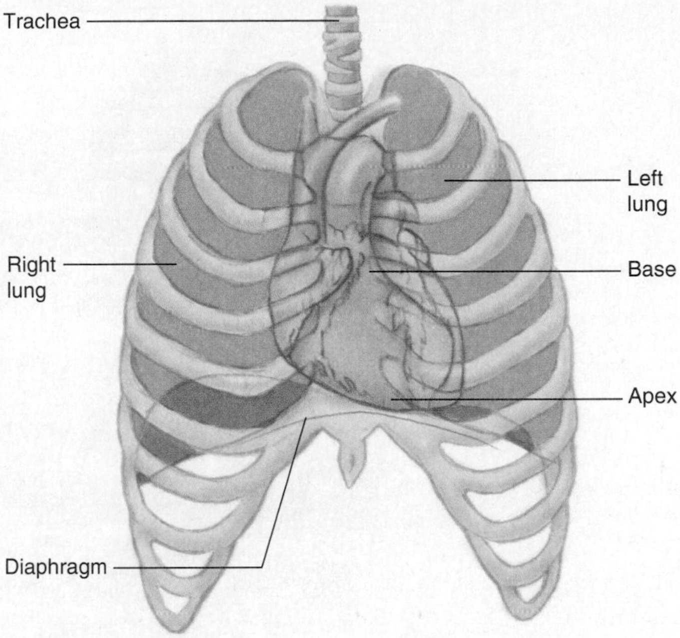

FIGURE 2-1 Location of the heart within the chest.

PART 1: Cardiovascular Anatomy and Physiology, ECG Monitoring, and Arrhythmia Analysis

Cardiovascular Anatomy

The two major components of the **cardiovascular system** are the heart and the peripheral blood vessels. Prehospital care of cardiovascular patients requires a sound knowledge of the anatomy and physiology of the cardiovascular system. Accurately assessing your patient, making a correct field diagnosis, and providing the best management possible will depend on your understanding of the heart and the peripheral blood vessels and how they work.

Anatomy of the Heart

The *heart* is a muscular organ, approximately the size of the patient's closed fist. It is in the center of the chest in the mediastinum, anterior to the spine and posterior to the sternum (Figure 2-1). Approximately two-thirds of the heart's mass is to the left of the midline, with the remainder to the right. The bottom of the heart, or *apex,* is just above the diaphragm, left of the midline. The top of the heart, or *base,* lies at approximately the level of the second rib. The great vessels connect to the heart through the base.

TISSUE LAYERS The heart consists of three tissue layers: endocardium, myocardium, and pericardium (Figure 2-2). The *endocardium* is the innermost layer. It lines the heart's chambers and is bathed in blood. The *myocardium* is the thick middle layer of the heart. Its cells are unique in that they physically resemble skeletal muscle but have electrical properties similar to those of smooth muscle. These cells also contain specialized structures that help to rapidly conduct electrical impulses from one muscle cell to another, enabling the heart to contract. The *pericardium* is a protective sac surrounding the heart. It consists of two layers, visceral and parietal. The *visceral pericardium,* also called the *epicardium,* is the inner layer, in contact with the heart muscle itself. The *parietal pericardium* is the outer, fibrous layer. In the pericardial cavity, between these two layers, is about 25 mL of pericardial fluid, a straw-colored lubricant that reduces friction as the heart beats and changes position. Certain disease processes and injuries can increase the amount of fluid in this sac, compressing the heart and decreasing cardiac output.

CHAMBERS The heart contains four chambers (Figure 2-3). The *atria,* the two superior chambers, receive incoming blood. The *ventricles,* the two larger, inferior chambers, pump blood out of the heart. The right and left atria are separated by the *interatrial septum.* The ventricles are separated by the *interventricular septum.* Both septa contain fibrous connective tissue as well as contractile muscle. The walls of the atria are much thinner than those of the ventricles and do not contribute significantly to the heart's pumping action.

VALVES The heart contains two pairs of valves, the *atrioventricular valves* and the *semilunar valves,* made of endocardial and connective tissue (Figure 2-4). The atrioventricular valves control blood flow between the atria and the ventricles. The right atrioventricular valve is called the *tricuspid valve* because it has three leaflets, or cusps. The left atrioventricular valve, called the *mitral valve,* has two leaflets. These valves are connected to specialized *papillary*

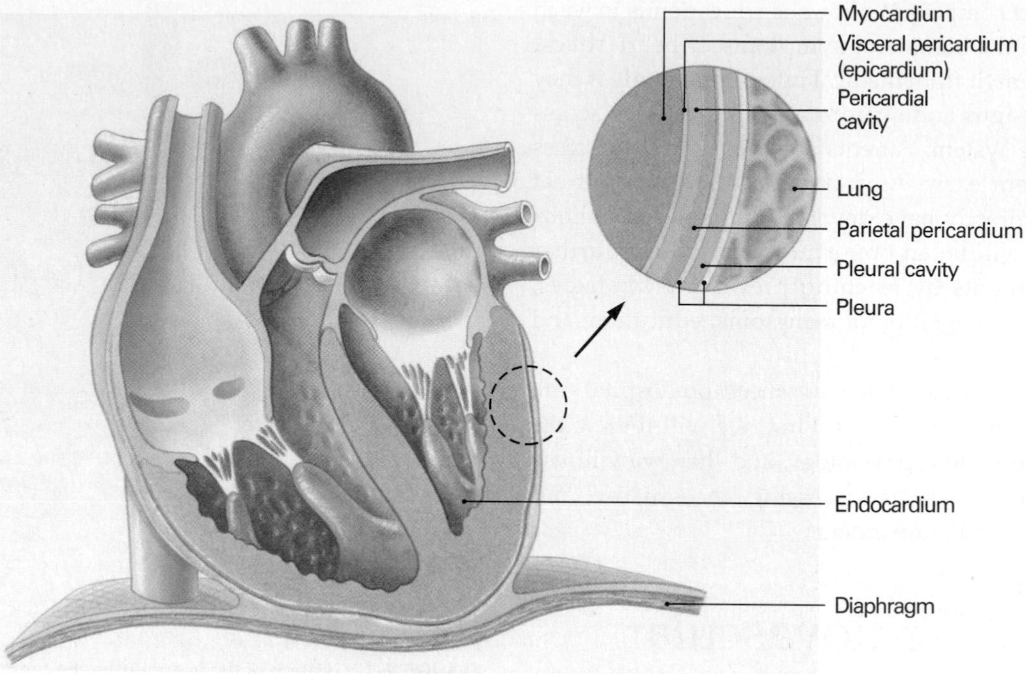

FIGURE 2-2 Layers of the heart.

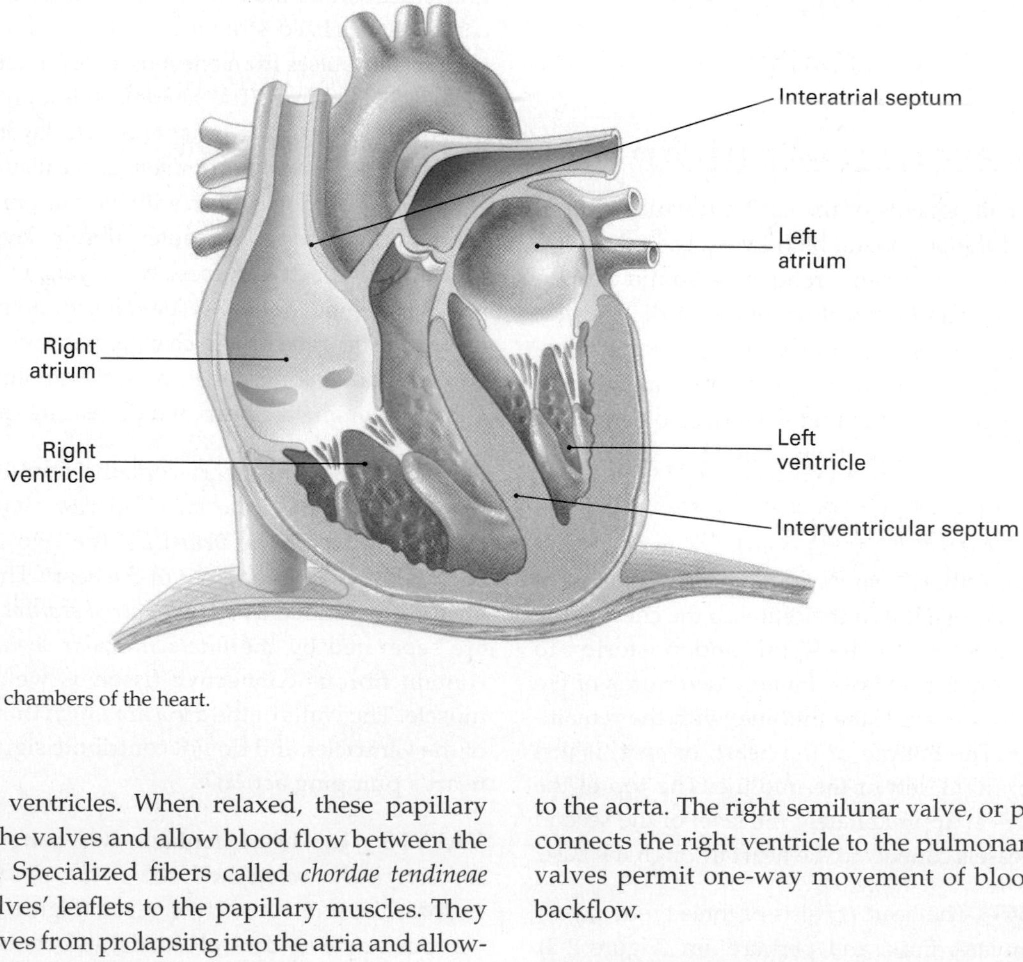

FIGURE 2-3 The chambers of the heart.

muscles in the ventricles. When relaxed, these papillary muscles open the valves and allow blood flow between the two chambers. Specialized fibers called *chordae tendineae* connect the valves' leaflets to the papillary muscles. They prevent the valves from prolapsing into the atria and allowing backflow during ventricular contraction.

The semilunar valves regulate blood flow between the ventricles and the arteries into which they empty. The left semilunar valve, or aortic valve, connects the left ventricle to the aorta. The right semilunar valve, or pulmonic valve, connects the right ventricle to the pulmonary artery. These valves permit one-way movement of blood and prevent backflow.

BLOOD FLOW The right atrium receives deoxygenated blood from the body via the superior and inferior venae cavae (Figure 2-5). The *superior vena cava* receives deoxygenated blood from the head and upper extremities, the *inferior*

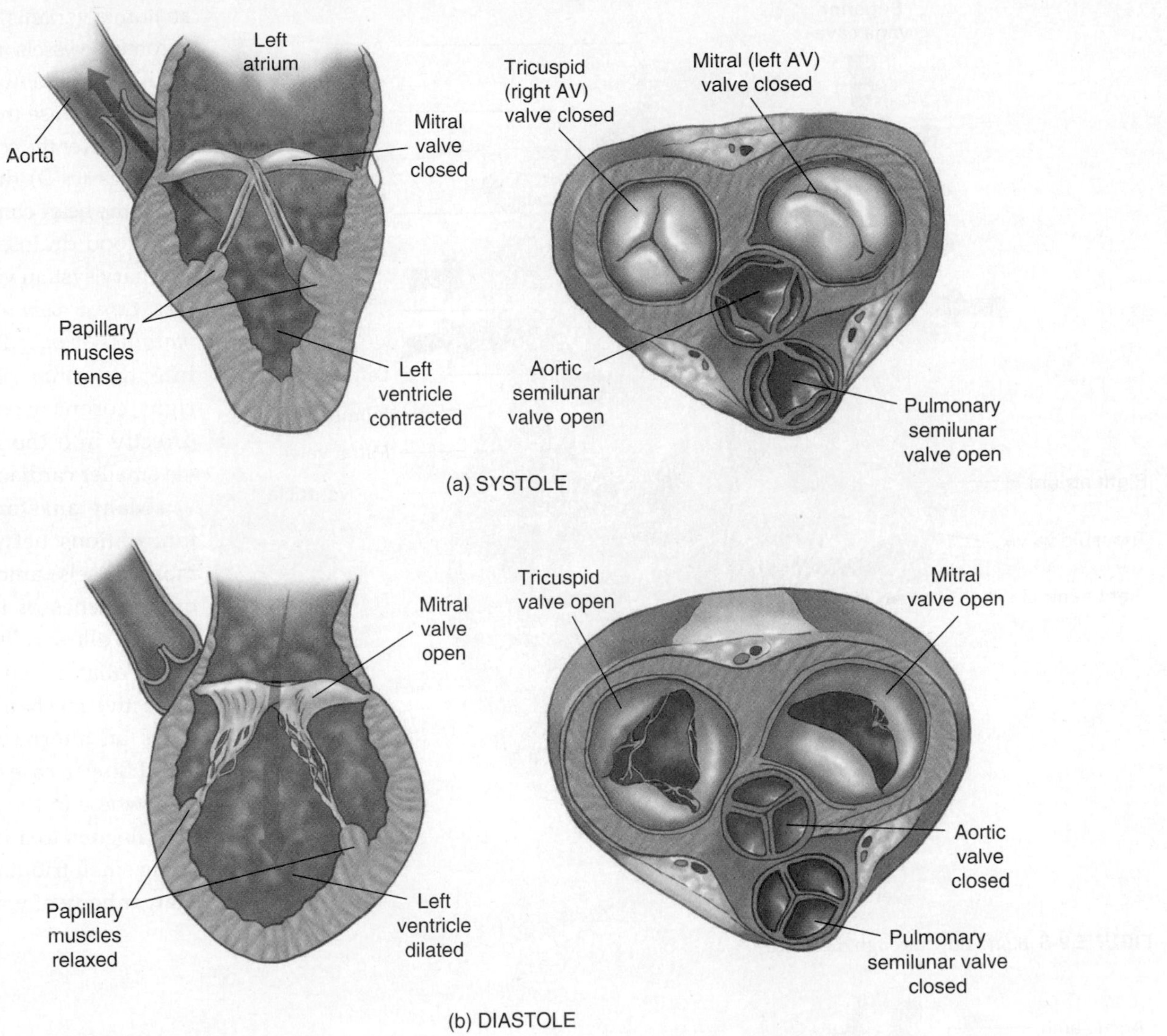

FIGURE 2-4 The valves of the heart.

vena cava from the areas below the heart. The right atrium pumps this blood through the tricuspid valve and into the right ventricle. The right ventricle then pumps the deoxygenated blood through the pulmonic valve to the *pulmonary artery* and on to the lungs. (The pulmonary artery is the only artery in the body that carries deoxygenated blood.)

After the blood circulates through the lungs and becomes oxygenated, it returns to the left atrium via the *pulmonary veins.* (The pulmonary veins are the only veins in the body that carry oxygenated blood.) The left atrium sends this oxygenated blood through the mitral valve and into the left ventricle. Finally, the left ventricle pumps the blood through the aortic valve to the aorta, which feeds the oxygenated blood to the rest of the body. Intracardiac pressures are higher on the left than on the right because the lungs offer less resistance to blood flow than the systemic circulation. Thus, the left myocardium is thicker than the right.

The major vessels of the body all branch off the aorta, which has three main parts. The *ascending aorta* comes directly from the heart. The *thoracic aorta* curves inferiorly and goes through the chest (or thorax). The *abdominal aorta* goes through the diaphragm and enters the abdomen.

CORONARY CIRCULATION Although the endocardium is bathed in blood, the heart does not receive its nutrients from the blood within its chambers but from the *coronary arteries* (Figure 2-6). The coronary arteries originate in the aorta, just above the leaflets of the aortic valve. The main coronary arteries lie on the surface of the heart, and small penetrating arterioles supply the myocardial muscle. The *left coronary artery* supplies the left ventricle, the interventricular septum, part of the right ventricle, and the heart's conduction system. Its two major branches are the *anterior descending artery* and the *circumflex artery.* The *right coronary artery* supplies a portion of the right atrium and right ventricle and part of the conduction system. Its two major branches are the *posterior descending artery* and the *marginal artery.* (Although the blood supply to most people's hearts follows this pattern,

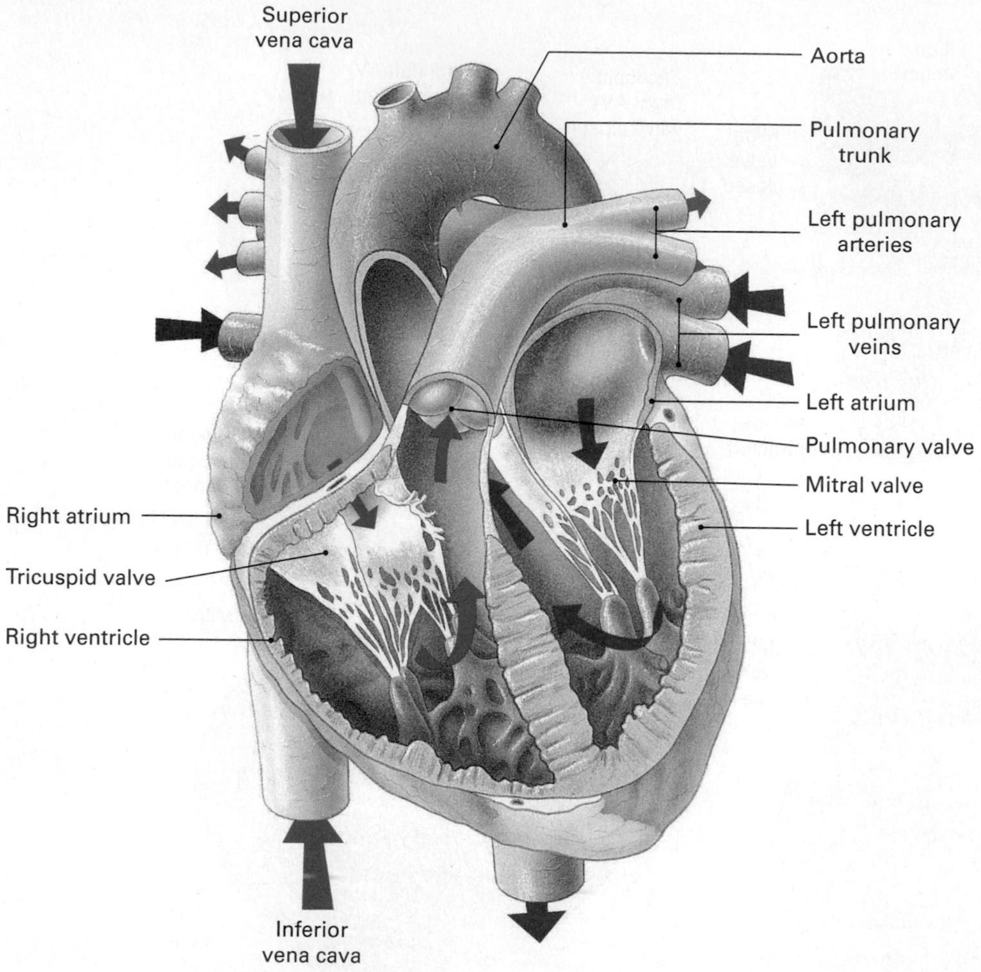

FIGURE 2-5 Blood flow through the heart.

anatomic variants do exist.) The coronary vessels receive blood during diastole, when the heart relaxes, because the aortic valve leaflets cover the coronary artery openings (*ostia*) during systole, when the heart contracts.

Blood drains from the left coronary system via the *anterior great cardiac vein* and the *lateral marginal veins.* These empty into the *coronary sinus.* The right coronary vein empties directly into the right atrium via smaller cardiac veins.

Many **anastomoses** (communications between two or more vessels) among the various branches of the coronary arteries allow *collateral circulation.* Collateral circulation is a protective mechanism that provides an alternative path for blood flow in case of a blockage somewhere in the system. This is analogous to a river's developing small tributaries to reach a larger body of water.

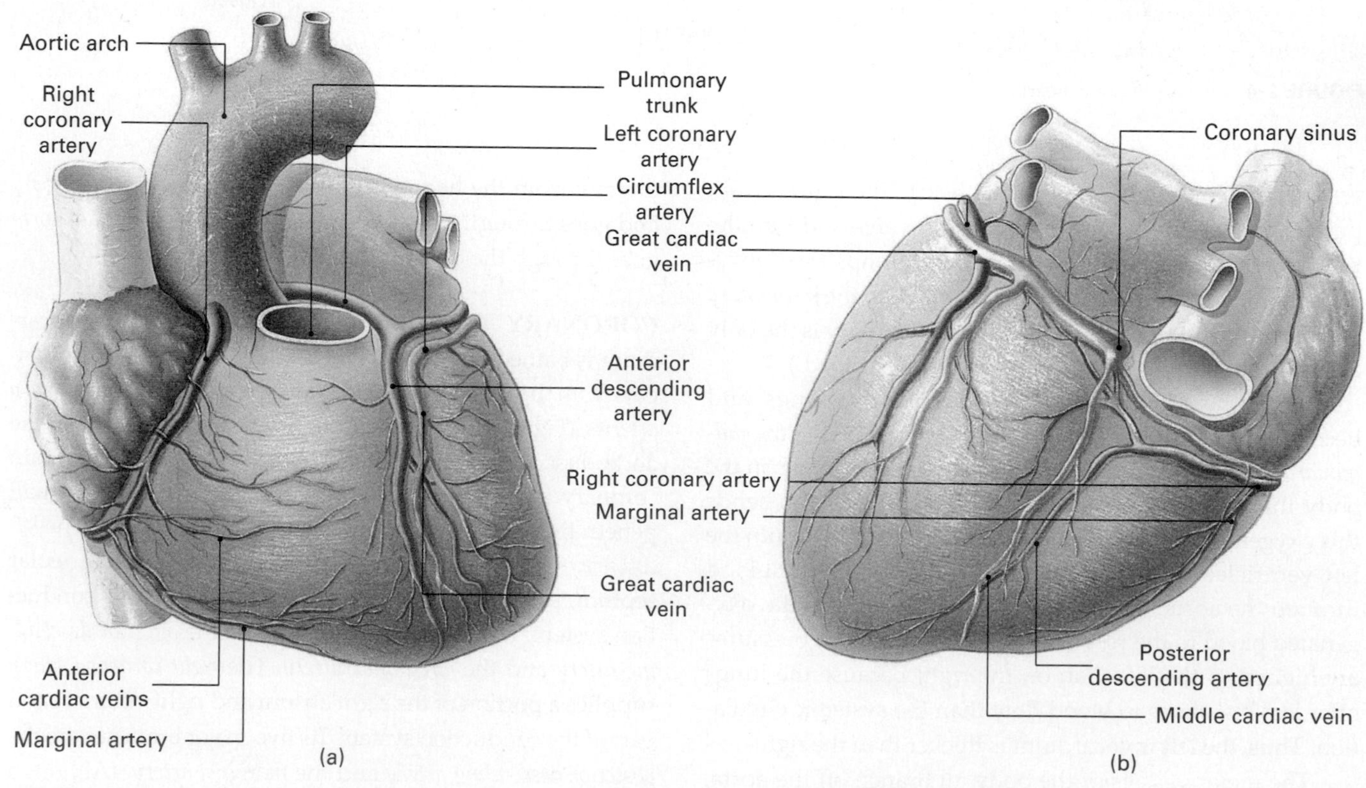

FIGURE 2-6 The coronary circulation: (a) anterior and (b) posterior.

Anatomy of the Peripheral Circulation

The peripheral circulation transports oxygenated blood from the heart to the tissues and subsequently transports deoxygenated blood back to the heart. Oxygenated blood leaves the heart via the arterial system, whereas deoxygenated blood returns via the venous system. (As noted earlier, the exceptions to this rule are the pulmonary artery and the pulmonary veins.)

A capillary wall consists of a single layer of cells. The walls of arteries and veins, however, are composed of several layers (Figure 2-7). The arteries' and veins' innermost lining, the *tunica intima,* is a single cell layer thick. The middle layer, the *tunica media,* consists of elastic fibers and muscle. It gives blood vessels their strength and recoil, which results from the difference in pressure inside and outside the vessel. The tunica media is much thicker in arteries than in veins. The outermost lining is the *tunica adventitia,* a fibrous tissue covering. It gives the vessel strength to withstand the pressures generated by the heart's contractions. The cavity inside a vessel is the *lumen.*

The vessels' diameters vary significantly and are directly related to the amount of blood they can transport. The larger the diameter, the greater the blood flow. In fact, according to **Poiseuille's law**, the blood flow through a vessel is directly proportional to the fourth power of the vessel's radius. For example, a vessel with a relative radius of 1 would transport 1 mL per minute of blood at a pressure difference of 100 mmHg. If the vessel's radius were increased to 4, keeping the pressure difference constant, the flow would increase to 256 mL (4^4) per minute.

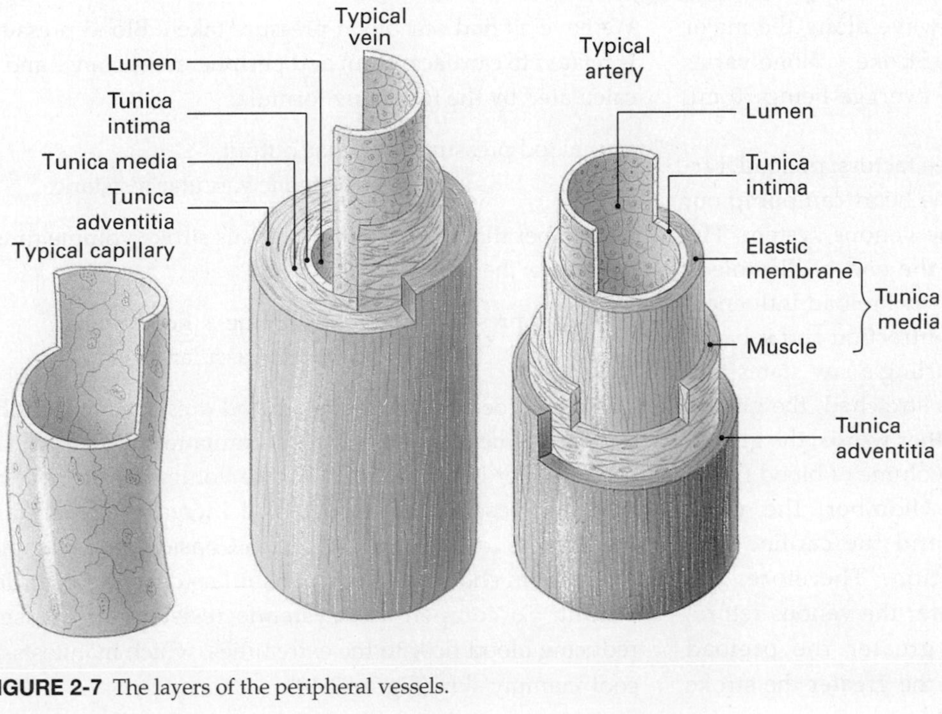

FIGURE 2-7 The layers of the peripheral vessels.

ARTERIAL SYSTEM The *arterial system,* which carries oxygenated blood from the heart, functions under high pressure. The larger arterial vessels are the *arteries.* The arteries branch into smaller structures called *arterioles,* which control blood flow to various organs by their degree of resistance. The arterioles continue to divide until they become *capillaries,* which are the connection points between the arterial and venous systems. The vascular system and the tissues are able to exchange gases, fluids, and nutrients through the very thin capillary walls.

VENOUS SYSTEM The *venous system* transports blood from the peripheral tissues back to the heart. It functions under low pressure with the aid of surrounding muscles and one-way valves within the veins. Blood enters the venous system through the capillaries, which drain into the *venules.* The venules, in turn, drain into the *veins,* the veins into the venae cavae, and the venae cavae into the right atrium.

Cardiac Physiology

The Cardiac Cycle

Although the heart's right and left sides perform different functions, they act as a unit. The right and left atria contract at the same time, filling both ventricles to their maximum capacities. Both ventricles then contract at the same time, ejecting blood into the pulmonary and systemic circulations. The pressure of the contraction closes the tricuspid and mitral valves and opens the aortic and pulmonic valves at the same time.

The **cardiac cycle** is the sequence of events that occurs between the end of one heart contraction and the end of the next. To evaluate heart sounds and read electrocardiographs, you must thoroughly understand the pumping action of the cardiac cycle (Figure 2-8). **Diastole**, the first phase of the cardiac cycle, is the *relaxation phase.* This is when ventricular filling begins. Blood enters the ventricles through the mitral and tricuspid valves. The pulmonic and aortic valves are closed. During the second phase, **systole**, the heart

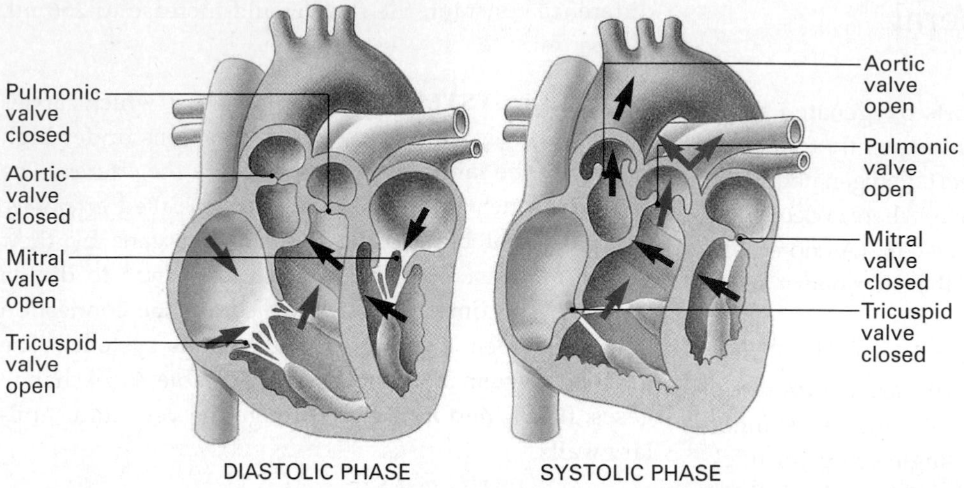

FIGURE 2-8 Relation of blood flow to cardiac contraction.

contracts. The atria contract first, to finish emptying their blood into the ventricles. Atrial systole is relatively quick and occurs just before ventricular contraction; in healthy hearts, this atrial "kick" boosts cardiac output. The pressure in the ventricles now increases until it exceeds the pressure in the aorta and pulmonary artery. At this point blood flows out of the ventricles through the pulmonic and aortic valves and into the arteries. The pressure also closes the mitral and tricuspid valves and, if working properly, prevents backflow of blood into the atria. When pressures in the aorta exceed the pressures in the ventricles, the valves close and diastole begins again.

The normal ventricle ejects about two-thirds of the blood it contains at the end of systole. This ratio is the **ejection fraction**. The amount of blood ejected is the **stroke volume**. Each time the ventricle pumps blood into the aorta, it generates a pressure wave along the major arteries, which we feel as a pulse. Stroke volume varies between 60 and 100 mL, with the average being 70 mL (Figure 2-9).

Stroke volume depends on three factors: preload, cardiac contractility, and afterload. The heart can pump out only the blood it receives from the venous system. The pressure in the filled ventricle at the end of diastole is called **preload**, or *end-diastolic volume.* Preload influences the force and amount of the next contraction and is based on **Starling's law of the heart**. Starling's law states that the more the myocardial muscle is stretched, the greater its force of contraction will be. In other words, the greater the volume of blood filling the chamber, the more forceful the cardiac contraction. Therefore, the greater the venous return, the greater the preload and the greater the stroke volume. Myocardial muscle, however, has its limits. If stretched too far, it will not contract properly and will weaken. Think of blowing up a tire. The tension in the walls increases as you put more air in the tire. If you were to put too much air in the tire, the tire would break or bulge from the side. If either of these happened, the tension in the wall would decrease, and if you filled the tire again it would not perform as well as before. **Afterload** is the resistance against which the ventricle must contract. An increase in peripheral vascular resistance will decrease stroke volume, and conversely, a decrease in peripheral vascular resistance will allow stroke volume to increase.

CONTENT REVIEW

➤ Factors Affecting Stroke Volume
- Preload
- Cardiac contractility
- Afterload

Cardiac output is the volume of blood that the heart pumps in 1 minute. It is a function of stroke volume and heart rate, as the following formula states:

$$\text{stroke volume (mL)} \times \text{heart rate (bpm)} = \text{cardiac output (mL/min)}$$

The normal heart rate is 60 to 100 beats per minute, and the average stroke volume is 70 mL. Thus an average cardiac output is about 5 L/min (5,000 mL/min), calculated as follows:

$$\text{stroke volume} \times \text{heart rate} = \text{cardiac output } 70 \text{ mL} \times 70 \text{ bpm} = 4{,}900 \text{ mL/min}$$

We have all had our blood pressure taken. Blood pressure is related to cardiac output and peripheral resistance and is calculated by the following formula:

$$\text{blood pressure} = \text{cardiac output} \times \text{systemic vascular resistance}$$

Remember that cardiac output equals stroke volume times heart rate; therefore,

$$\text{blood pressure} = (\text{stroke volume} \times \text{heart rate}) \times \text{systemic vascular resistance}$$

The body does its best to keep blood pressure constant by regulating the elements of this formula to compensate for changes. For instance, when stroke volume decreases, the systemic vascular resistance will increase to maintain blood pressure at a constant value. Consider, for example, a patient in shock. A shock patient has decreased cardiac output. To compensate, systemic resistance increases, reducing blood flow to the extremities, which manifests as cool, clammy skin (Figure 2-10).

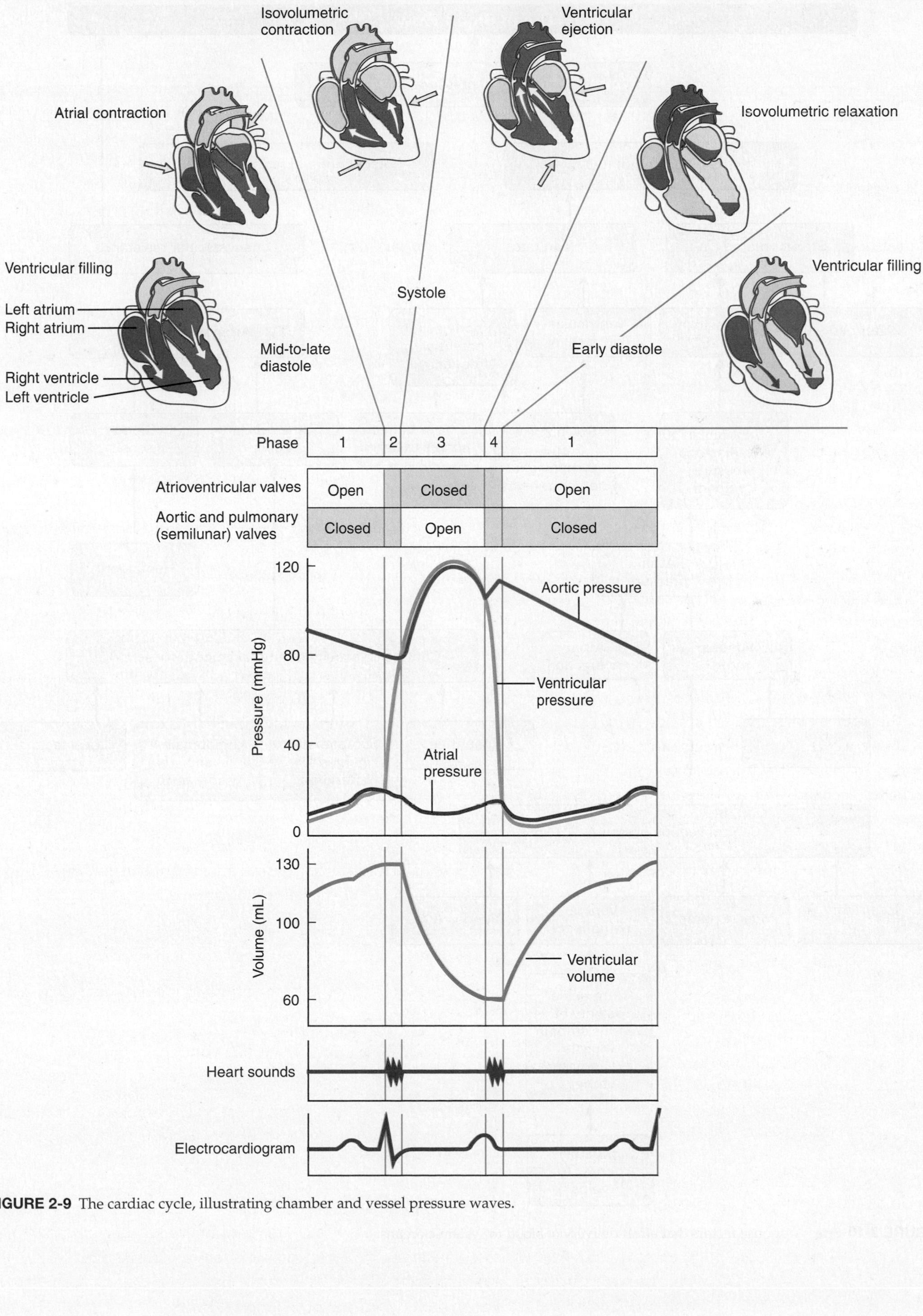

FIGURE 2-9 The cardiac cycle, illustrating chamber and vessel pressure waves.

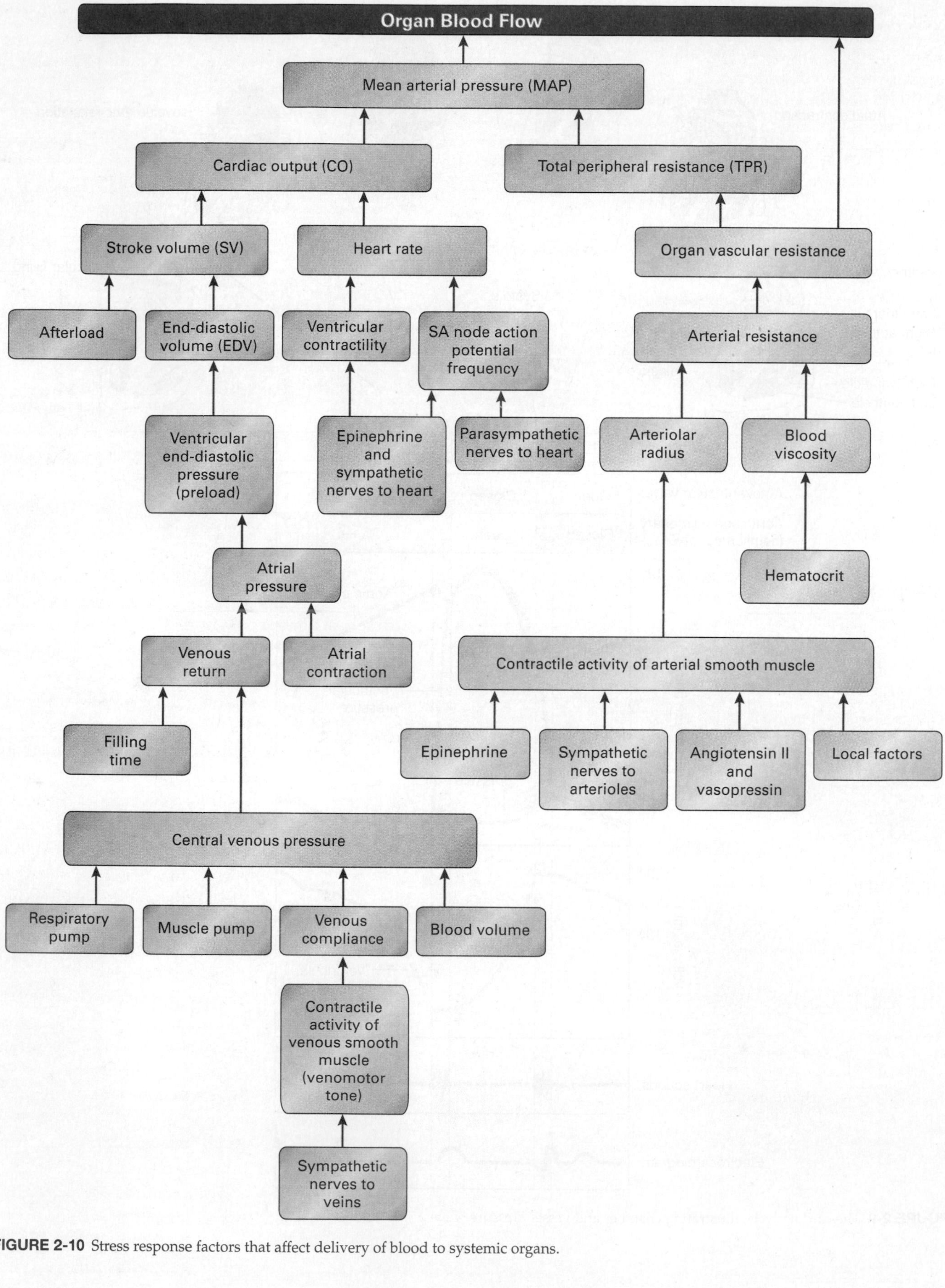

FIGURE 2-10 Stress response factors that affect delivery of blood to systemic organs.

Nervous Control of the Heart

The sympathetic and parasympathetic components of the autonomic nervous system work in direct opposition to one another to regulate the heart. In the heart's normal state, the two systems balance. In stressful situations, however, the sympathetic system becomes dominant, whereas during sleep the parasympathetic system dominates. The sympathetic nervous system innervates the heart through the *cardiac plexus,* a network of nerves at the base of the heart (Figure 2-11). The sympathetic nerves arise from the thoracic and lumbar regions of the spinal cord, then leave the spinal cord and form the sympathetic chain, which runs along the spinal column. The cardiac plexus arises, in turn, from ganglia in the sympathetic chain and innervates both the atria and ventricles. The chemical *neurotransmitter* for the sympathetic nervous system, and thus for the cardiac plexus, is *norepinephrine.* Its release increases heart rate and cardiac contractile force, primarily through its actions on beta-receptors.

The sympathetic nervous system has two principal types of receptors, alpha and beta. *Alpha-receptors* are located in the peripheral blood vessels and are responsible for vasoconstriction. *Beta$_1$ receptors,* primarily located in the heart, increase the heart rate and contractility. *Belu$_2$ receptors,* principally located in the lungs and peripheral blood vessels, cause bronchodilation and peripheral vasodilation. Medications specific to these various receptors cause different physiologic effects. For instance, beta-blockers slow the heart rate and lower blood pressure by blocking the beta$_1$ receptors, whose job is to increase heart rate and contractility.

Parasympathetic control of the heart occurs through the *vagus nerve* (the tenth cranial nerve). The vagus nerve descends from the brain to innervate the heart and other organs. Vagal nerve fibers primarily innervate the atria, although some innervate the upper ventricles. The neurotransmitter for the parasympathetic nervous system, and thus the vagus nerve, is *acetylcholine.* Its release slows both the heart rate and atrioventricular conduction. Several maneuvers can stimulate the vagus nerve, including the Valsalva maneuver (forced expiration against a closed glottis, which can occur when lifting heavy objects), pressure on the carotid sinus (carotid sinus massage), and distention of the urinary bladder.

The terms *chronotropy, inotropy,* and *dromotropy* describe autonomic control of the heart. **Chronotropy** refers to heart rate. A *positive chronotropic agent* increases the heart rate. Conversely, a *negative chronotropic agent* decreases the heart rate. **Inotropy** refers to the strength of a cardiac muscular contraction. A *positive inotropic agent* strengthens the cardiac contraction, while a *negative inotropic agent* weakens it. **Dromotropy** refers to the rate of nervous impulse

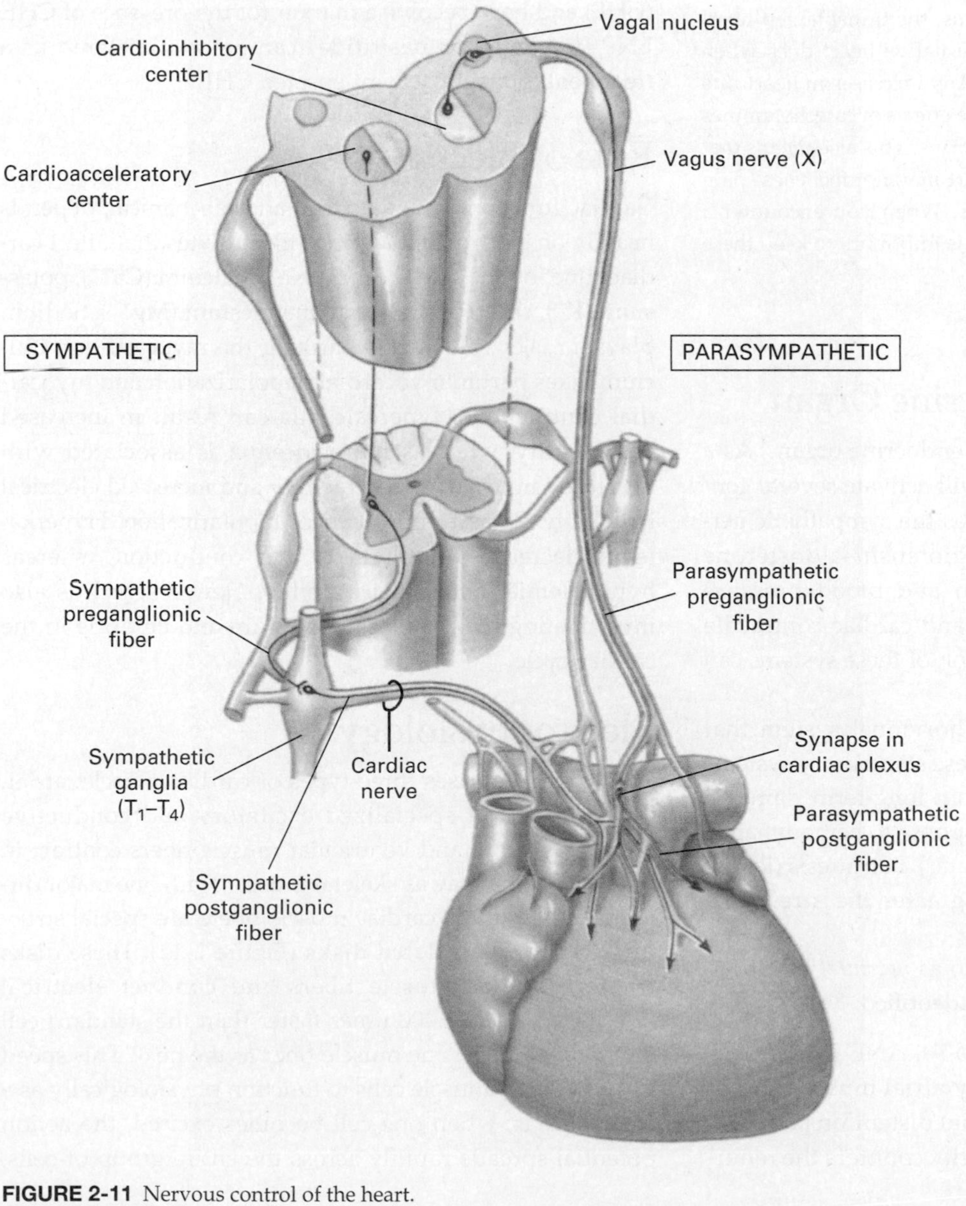

FIGURE 2-11 Nervous control of the heart.

conduction. A positive dromotropic agent speeds impulse conduction, whereas a negative dromotropic agent slows conduction.

Patho Pearls

One of the greatest innovations of 20th century medicine was the development of organ transplantation. The first heart transplant occurred in 1967 in Cape Town, South Africa. Now, numerous centers throughout the world routinely transplant hearts. The development of antirejection drugs has made organ transplantation a viable option for people with numerous end-stage diseases. As a paramedic, you are likely eventually to encounter a patient who has had a heart transplant. Generally, heart transplant patients are not treated any differently from any other patient with a cardiac-related complaint. However, it is important to recognize that the transplanted heart is **denervated**. This means that the transplanted heart does not have the nervous system connections that were present in the original native heart (these are cut during the transplant operation). Because of this, the transplanted heart does not respond as quickly as the native heart does when increases in heart rate are needed. Any increases in heart rate in a transplanted heart are due to the effects of catecholamines such as epinephrine and norepinephrine. This also means that the patient with a transplanted heart may not feel chest pain if coronary artery disease develops. When you encounter a patient with a transplanted heart, it is important to keep these considerations in mind.

The Heart as an Endocrine Organ

The heart is both a pump and an endocrine organ.[2] As a rule, left ventricular dysfunction will activate several control systems. These systems, such as the sympathetic nervous system and the renin–angiotensin–aldosterone system, help maintain perfusion and blood pressure through an increase in heart rate and cardiac contractile force. However, prolonged activation of these systems can be harmful to the heart.

Fortunately, the heart has a hormonal system that tends to counteract the effects of these stimulatory systems and provides some protection from long-term damage. These hormones are secreted in response to hemodynamic stress and cause diuresis (loss of water), natriuresis (loss of sodium), and vasodilation. The greater the stress, the greater the subsequent secretion.

These hormones are referred to as *natriuretic peptides*. Thus far, three peptides have been identified:

- ***Atrial natriuretic peptide (ANP).*** ANP is manufactured, stored, and released by atrial muscle cells in response to such things as atrial distention and sympathetic stimulation. It primarily counters the renin–angiotensin–aldosterone system and causes a reduction in blood volume resulting in decreased central venous pressure (CVP), cardiac output, and blood pressure.
- ***Brain natriuretic peptide (BNP).*** BNP was initially discovered in the brain. However, it is secreted principally by the ventricles of the heart in response to excessive stretching of myocytes. It also serves to counter the renin–angiotensin–aldosterone system and causes a reduction in blood volume, resulting in decreased CVP, cardiac output, and blood pressure. The half-life of BNP is twice as long as that of ANP.
- ***C-type natriuretic peptide (CNP).*** A third type of natriuretic peptide has been identified. Unlike ANP and BNP, this peptide appears to be secreted from the endothelium of blood vessels and appears to have a vasodilatory effect.

BNP levels are elevated in congestive heart failure (CHF) and have become a marker for the presence of CHF. BNP (marketed as nesiritide) can be administered as a treatment for acute decompensated CHF.

Role of Electrolytes

Cardiac function, both electrical and mechanical, depends heavily on electrolyte balances. Electrolytes that affect cardiac function include sodium (Na^+), calcium (Ca^{++}), potassium (K^+), chloride (Cl^-), and magnesium (Mg^{++}). Sodium plays a major role in depolarizing the myocardium. Calcium takes part in myocardial depolarization and myocardial contraction. Hypercalcemia can result in increased contractility, whereas hypocalcemia is associated with decreased myocardial contractility and increased electrical irritability. Potassium influences repolarization. Hyperkalemia decreases automaticity and conduction, whereas hypokalemia increases irritability. New research is also investigating the roles of magnesium and chloride in the cardiac cycle.

Electrophysiology

The heart comprises three types of cardiac muscle: atrial, ventricular, and specialized excitatory and conductive fibers. The atrial and ventricular muscle fibers contract in much the same way as skeletal muscle, with one major difference. Within the cardiac muscle fibers are special structures called **intercalated disks** (Figure 2-12). These disks connect cardiac muscle fibers and conduct electrical impulses quickly—400 times faster than the standard cell membrane—from one muscle fiber to the next. This speed allows cardiac muscle cells to function physiologically as a unit. That is, when one cell becomes excited, the action potential spreads rapidly across the entire group of cells,

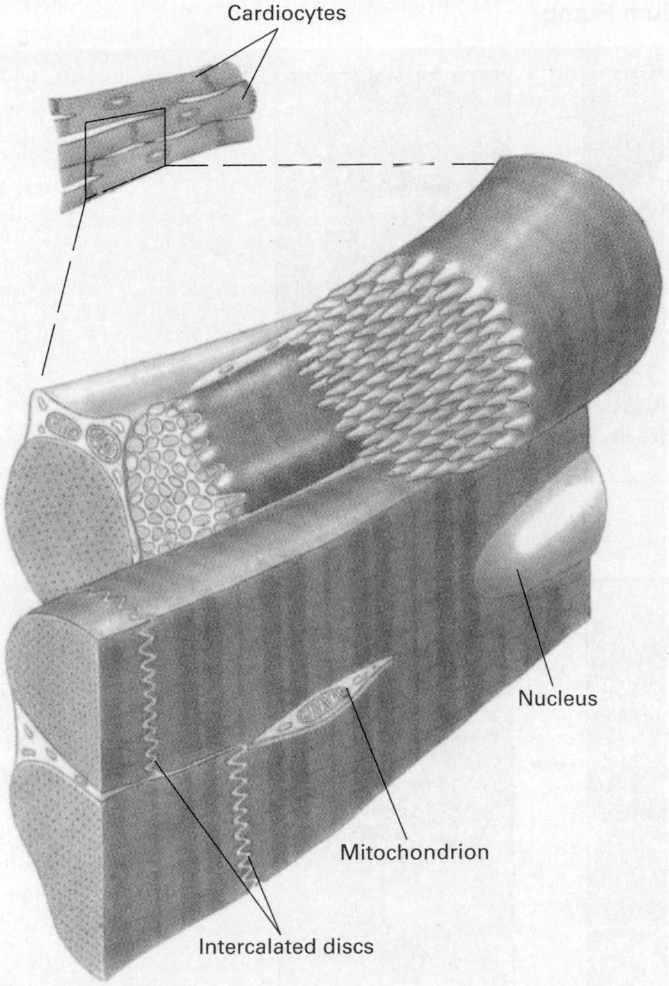

FIGURE 2-12 Microscopic appearance of cardiac muscle. The intercalated disks speed transmission of the electrical potential quickly from one cell to the next.

resulting in a coordinated contraction. This functional unit is a **syncytium**.

The heart has two syncytia—the *atrial syncytium* and the *ventricular syncytium.* The atrial syncytium contracts from superior to inferior, so the atria express blood to the ventricles. The ventricular syncytium, on the other hand, contracts from inferior to superior, expelling blood from the ventricles into the aorta and pulmonary arteries. The syncytia are separated from one another by the fibrous structure that supports the valves and physically separates the atria from the ventricles. The only way an impulse can be conducted from the atria to the ventricles is through the *atrioventricular (AV) bundle.* Cardiac muscle functions according to an "all-or-none" principle. That is, if a single muscle fiber becomes *depolarized,* the action potential will spread through the whole syncytium. Stimulating a single atrial fiber will thus completely depolarize the atria, and stimulating a single ventricular fiber will completely depolarize the ventricles.

Cardiac Depolarization

Understanding cardiac **depolarization** is essential to interpreting electrocardiograms (ECGs). Normally, an ionic difference exists on the two sides of a cell membrane. The cell's sodium–potassium pump expels sodium (Na^+) from the cell. However, the sodium–potassium pump moves three sodium ions to the outside and only two potassium ions to the inside (Figure 2-13). This leaves more negatively charged anions inside the cell than positively charged cations. Thus, the inside of the cell is more negatively charged than the outside. This difference, called the **resting potential**, can be measured experimentally by placing one probe inside the cell and another outside the cell and determining the difference, in millivolts. The resting potential in a myocardial cell is approximately –70 mV (Figure 2-14).

When the myocardial cell is stimulated, the membrane surrounding the cell changes instantaneously to allow sodium ions to rush into the cell, bringing with them their positive charge. This charge is so strong that it gives the inside of the cell a positive charge approximately +30 mV greater than the outside. This influx of sodium and change of membrane polarity is the **action potential**. After the influx of sodium, a slower influx of calcium ions (Ca^{++}) through the calcium channels increases the positive charge inside the cell. Once *depolarization* occurs in a muscle fiber, it is transmitted throughout the entire syncytium, via the intercalated disks, until the entire muscle mass is depolarized. Contraction of the muscle follows depolarization (Figure 2-15).

The cell membrane remains permeable to sodium for only a fraction of a second. Thereafter, sodium influx stops and potassium escapes from inside the cell. This returns the charge inside the cell to normal (negative). In addition, sodium is actively pumped outside the cell, allowing **repolarization** of the cell and return to its normal resting state. See Table 2-1 for details.

Cardiac Conductive System

The cardiac conductive system stimulates the ventricles to depolarize in the proper direction. As mentioned earlier, the atria contract from superior to inferior, and the ventricles from inferior to superior. If the depolarization impulse originated in the atria and spread passively to the ventricles, then the ventricles would depolarize from superior to inferior and would be ineffective. The cardiac conduction system, therefore, must initiate an impulse, spread it through the atria, transmit it quickly to the apex of the heart, and thence stimulate the ventricles to depolarize from inferior to superior. To do this, the conduction system relies on specialized conductive fibers comprising muscle cells that transmit the depolarization potential through the heart much faster than can regular myocardial cells.

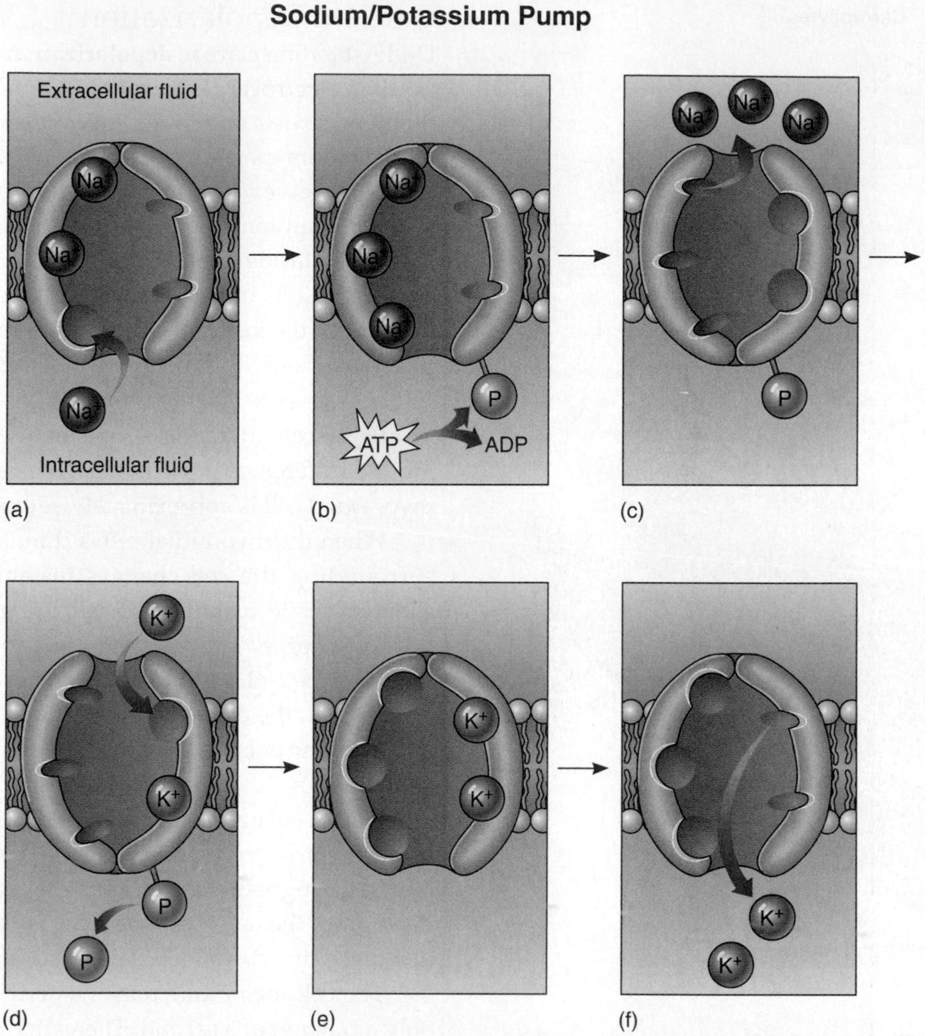

FIGURE 2-13 The sodium–potassium pump. The pump contains three sodium and two potassium binding sites and uses ATP to transport sodium out of the cell, at the same time transporting potassium into the cell. (a) Intracellular Na^+ ions bind to the pump protein. (b) The binding of three Na^+ ions triggers phosphorylation of the pump by ATP. (c) Phosphorylation induces a conformational change in the protein that allows the release of Na^+ into the extracellular fluid. (d) Extracellular K+ ions bind to the pump protein and trigger release of the phosphate group. (e) Loss of the phosphate group allows the protein to return to its original conformation. (f) K^+ ions are released into the cytosol and the Na^+ sites become available for binding again.

To accomplish their task, the cells of the cardiac conductive system have the important properties of excitability, conductivity, automaticity, and contractility.

- **Excitability**. The cells can respond to an electrical stimulus, like all other myocardial cells.
- **Conductivity**. The cells can propagate the electrical impulse from one cell to another.
- **Automaticity**. The individual cells of the conductive system can depolarize without any impulse from an outside source. This property is also called *self-excitation*. Generally, the cell in the cardiac conductive system with the fastest rate of discharge, or automaticity, becomes the heart's pacemaker. As a rule, the highest cell in the conductive system has the fastest rate of automaticity. Normally, this cell is in the *sinoatrial (SA) node,* high in the right atrium; however, if one pacemaker cell fails to discharge and depolarize, then the cell with the next fastest rate becomes the pacemaker.
- **Contractility**. Because the cells of the cardiac conductive system are specialized cardiac muscle cells, they retain the ability to contract.

Internodal atrial pathways connect the SA node to the AV node (Figure 2-16). These internodal pathways conduct the depolarization impulse to the atrial muscle mass and through the atria to the AV junction. The AV junction (the "gatekeeper") slows the impulse and allows the ventricles time to fill. Then, the impulse passes through the AV junction into the AV node and on to the AV fibers, which conduct the impulse from the atria to the ventricles. In the ventricles, the AV fibers form the *bundle of His.*

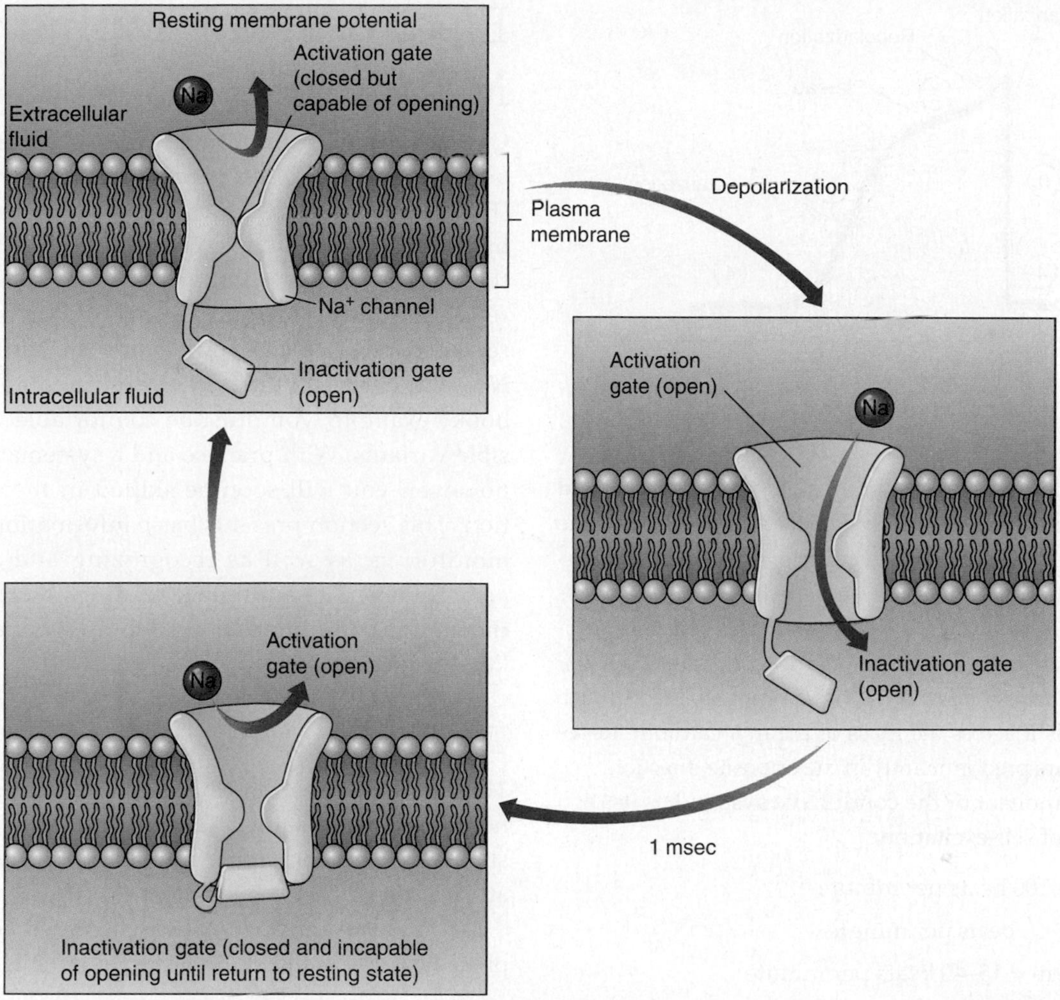

FIGURE 2-14 The sodium channels. The sodium channels are shown here with two gates. At rest, the sodium inactivation gate is open and the activation gate is closed (but can open in response to a depolarization stimulus). After a depolarizing stimulus, both the activation and deactivation gates are open, allowing sodium to move through the channel. Approximately 1 millisecond after the depolarizing stimulus, the inactivation gate closes and remains closed until the cell has repolarized to its resting state.

Table 2-1 Cardiac Polarization

	Resting	Depolarization	Repolarization	After Hyperpolarization
Membrane potential	–70 mV	+70 mV to +30 mV	+30 mV to 270 mV	–70 mV to –85 mV
Voltage-gated sodium channel	Closed	Open	Closed	Closed
Activation gate	Closed	Open	Open	Closed
Inactivation gate	Open	Open	Closed	Open
Sodium flow	Low inward, through leak channels	High inward, through voltage-gated channels	Low inward, through leak channels	Low inward, through leak channels
Voltage-gated potassium channel	Closed	Closed	Open	Closed
Potassium flow	Low outward, through leak channels	Low outward, through leak channels	High outward, through voltage-gated channels	High outward, through voltage-gated channels, but decreasing*

*Even though, at any given time, ions move through both voltage-gated channels and leak channels, the conductance through the leak channel is negligible compared to that through voltage-gated channels.

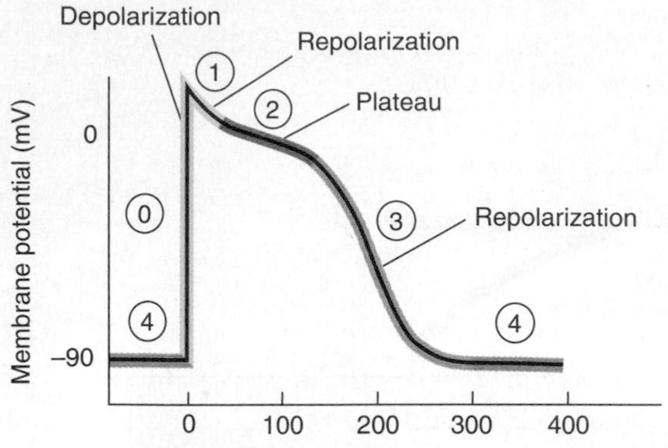

FIGURE 2-15 The cardiac action potential.

The bundle of His subsequently divides into the right and left bundle branches. The *right bundle branch* delivers the impulse to the apex of the right ventricle. From there, the *Purkinje system* spreads it across the myocardium. The *left bundle branch* divides into *anterior* and *posterior fascicles* that also ultimately terminate in the Purkinje system. At the same time that the impulse is transmitted to the right ventricle, the Purkinje system spreads it across the mass of the myocardium. Repolarization occurs predominantly in the opposite direction.

Each component of the conductive system has its own intrinsic rate of self-excitation:

SA node = 60–100 beats per minute

AV node = 40–60 beats per minute

Purkinje system = 15–40 beats per minute

Electrocardiographic Monitoring

One of your most important skills as a paramedic will be obtaining and interpreting electrocardiographic (ECG) **rhythm strips**. Your patient's subsequent treatment will be based on rapid, accurate interpretation of these strips. At first, rhythm strips may seem difficult to read, for only through classroom instruction and repeated practice can you master their interpretation. Nor will every rhythm strip you encounter be a "textbook" example; you must be comfortable with all possible variants. With practice and a systematic approach, however, you will soon be skilled in their interpretation. This section presents basic information about ECG monitoring, as well as recognizing and interpreting arrhythmias. The additional readings recommended at the end of the chapter will help you expand this knowledge.

The Electrocardiogram

The **electrocardiogram (ECG)** is a graphic record of the heart's electrical activity. However, it tells you nothing about the heart's pumping ability, which you must evaluate by pulse and blood pressure.

The electrocardiogram was invented by the Dutch physiologist Dr. Willem Einthoven in 1903. The device was

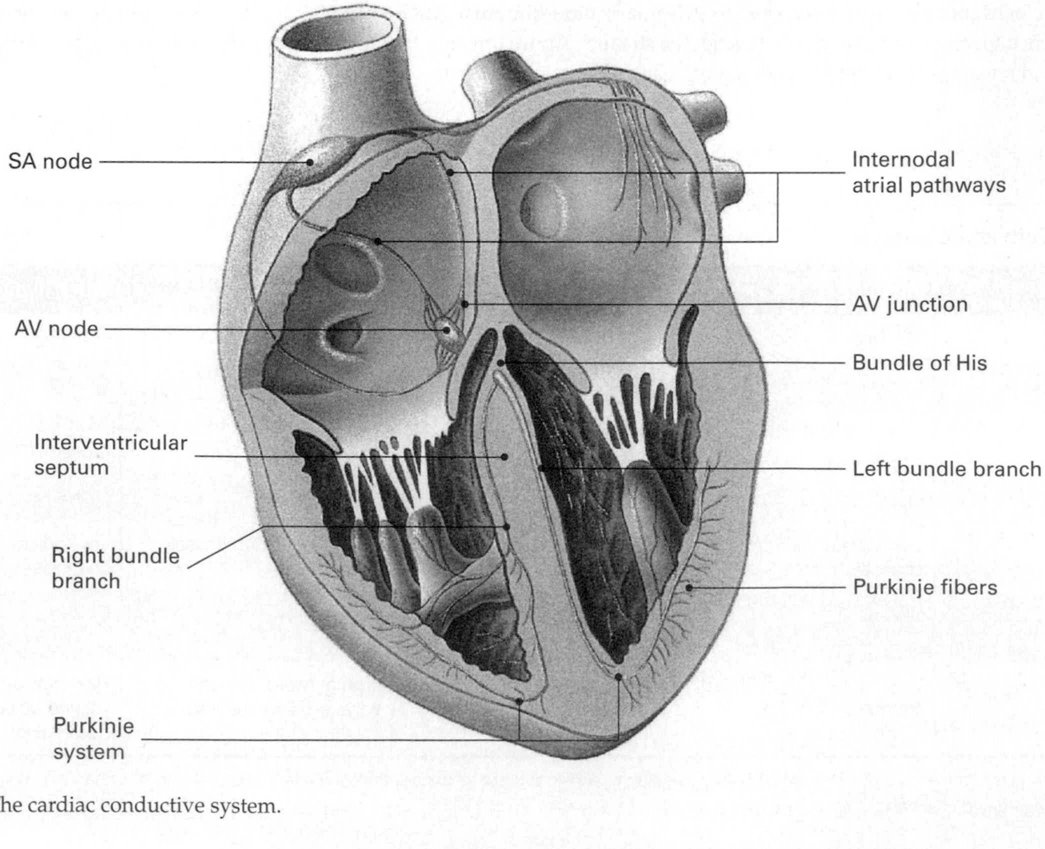

FIGURE 2-16 The cardiac conductive system.

first described in Dutch and referred to as an *elektrokardiograaf*, and thus the abbreviation *EKG* was applied. The abbreviation *EKG* is often interchanged with the English abbreviation *ECG*. Interestingly, Einthoven chose the letters *P, Q, R, S,* and *T* to describe points along the ECG waveform simply because they were in the middle of the alphabet and would not be confused with mathematic variables and similar commonly used letters.[3]

The body acts as a giant conductor of electricity, and the heart is its largest generator of electrical energy. Electrodes on the skin can detect the total electrical activity within the heart at any given time. The electrical impulses on the surface of the skin have a very low voltage. The ECG machine amplifies these impulses and records them over time on ECG graph paper or a monitor. *Positive impulses* appear as *upward* deflections on the paper, *negative impulses* as *downward* deflections. The absence of any electrical impulse produces an *isoelectric line,* which is flat.

Artifacts are deflections on the ECG produced by factors other than the heart's electrical activity. Common causes of artifacts include:

- Muscle tremors
- Shivering
- Patient movement
- Loose electrodes
- 60-hertz interference
- Machine malfunction

It is important for ECGs to be free of artifacts. When an artifact is present, you must first try to eliminate it before recording the ECG. Loose electrodes should be replaced. Occasionally, patients may be quite diaphoretic, thus preventing the electrodes from adhering well to the skin. In these cases, you may need to wipe the skin and apply tincture of benzoin before applying the electrode.

ECG Leads

You can obtain many views of the heart's electrical activity by monitoring the voltage change through *electrodes* placed at various places on the body surface. Each pair of electrodes is a *lead.* In the hospital, 12 leads are normally used. As a rule, most EMS systems use only 3 leads in the field. In fact, a single lead is adequate for detecting life-threatening arrhythmias. With the advent of fibrinolytic therapy and computer interpretation, however, 12-lead ECGs are becoming more common in the field, especially in rural EMS systems. (Part 3 of this chapter presents an introductory discussion of the 12-lead ECG.)

CONTENT REVIEW

- ➤ ECG Leads
  - Bipolar (limb)
  - Augmented (unipolar)
  - Precordial

The three types of ECG leads are bipolar, augmented, and precordial. **Bipolar leads**, the kind most frequently used, have one positive electrode and one negative electrode. Any electrical impulse moving toward the positive electrode will cause a positive (upward) deflection on the ECG paper. Any electrical impulse moving toward the negative electrode will cause a negative (downward) deflection. The absence of a positive or negative deflection means either that there is no electrical impulse or that the impulse is moving perpendicular to the lead. Leads I, II, and III, commonly called **limb leads**, are bipolar. They are the most frequently used leads in the field. Table 2-2 lists their placement sites.

Table 2-2 Bipolar Lead Placement Sites

Lead	Positive Electrode	Negative Electrode
I	Left arm	Right arm
II	Left leg	Right arm
III	Left leg	Left arm

These three bipolar leads form **Einthoven's triangle**, named after the inventor of the ECG machine (Figure 2-17). The direction from the negative to the positive electrode is the

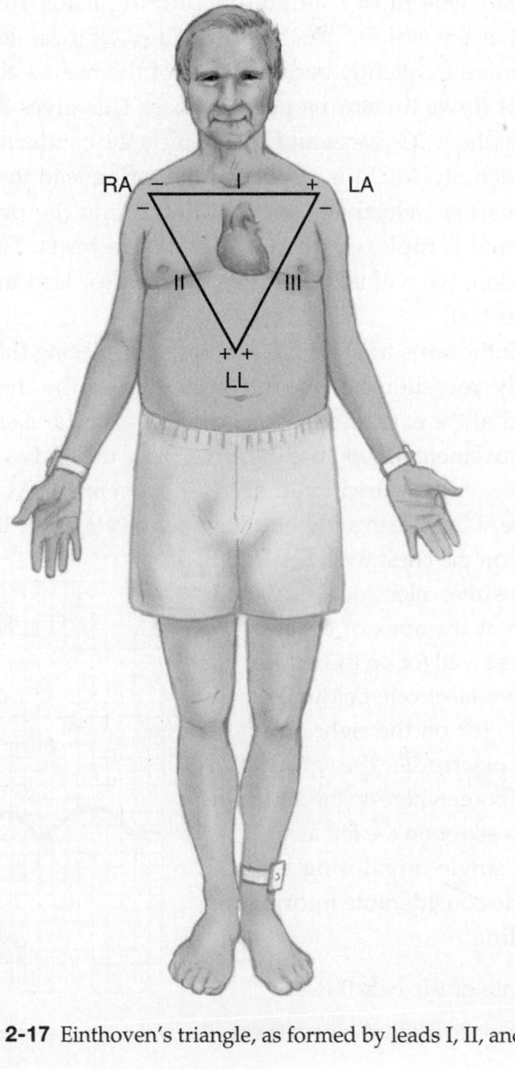

FIGURE 2-17 Einthoven's triangle, as formed by leads I, II, and III.

lead's *axis*. Each lead shows a different axis of the heart. Lead I, at the top of Einthoven's triangle, has an axis of 0°. Lead II forms the right side of the triangle and has an axis of 60°. Lead III forms the left side of the triangle and has an axis of 120°.

The bipolar leads provide only three views of the heart. **Augmented**, or **unipolar, leads** provide additional views that are sometimes useful. Although these leads evaluate different axes than the bipolar leads, they use the same electrodes. They do this by electronically combining the negative electrodes of two of the bipolar leads to obtain an axis. These augmented leads are designated aVR, aVL, and aVF. The letter *a* indicates that the lead is augmented. The letter *V* identifies it as a unipolar lead. The *R, L,* and *F* identify the extremity on which the lead is placed (R =right arm, L = left arm, and F = left foot).

In addition, six **precordial leads** can be placed across the surface of the chest to measure electrical cardiac activity on a horizontal axis. These leads help in viewing the left ventricle and septum. They are designated V_1 through V_6, with the letter *V* identifying them as unipolar leads.

Routine ECG Monitoring

Whether in the ambulance, emergency department, or coronary care unit, routine ECG monitoring generally uses only one lead. The most common monitoring leads are either lead II or the *modified chest lead 1* (MCL_1). Of these, lead II is used more frequently because most of the heart's electrical current flows toward its positive axis. This gives the best view of the ECG waves and best depicts the conduction system's activity. MCL_1 is a special monitoring lead that some systems use selectively to help determine the origin of abnormal complexes, such as premature beats. To avoid confusion, we will use lead II as the monitor lead throughout this text.

Einthoven's triangle offers a basis for placing the leads. Usually you should place the electrodes on the chest wall instead of the extremities. This helps to reduce artifacts from arm movement. (If you use the arms, place the lead as high as possible on the extremity to decrease movement.) Make certain the skin is clean and free of hair before you place the electrodes on the chest wall. For lead II, the positive electrode is usually placed at the apex of the heart on the chest wall (or on the left leg), the negative electrode below the right clavicle (or on the right arm). The third electrode, the ground, is placed somewhere on the left, upper chest wall (or on the left arm).

A single monitoring lead can provide considerable information, including:

- Rate of the heartbeat
- Regularity of the heartbeat
- Time it takes to conduct the impulse through the various parts of the heart

A single lead cannot provide the following information:

- Presence or location of an infarct
- Axis deviation or chamber enlargement
- Right-to-left differences in conduction or impulse formation
- Quality or presence of pumping action

ECG Graph Paper

ECG graph paper is standardized to allow comparative analysis of ECG patterns. The paper moves across the stylus at a standard speed of 25 mm/second (Figure 2-18). The *amplitude* of the ECG *deflection* is also standardized. When properly calibrated, the ECG stylus should deflect two large boxes when 1 mV is present. Most machines have calibration buttons, and a calibration curve should be placed at the beginning of the first ECG strip. Many machines do this automatically when they are first turned on.

The ECG graph is divided into a grid of light and heavy lines. The light lines are 1 mm apart, and the heavy lines are 5 mm apart. The heavy lines thus enclose large squares, each containing 25 of the smaller squares formed by the lighter lines (Figure 2-19). The following relationships apply to the horizontal axis:

1 small box = 0.04 sec

1 large box = 0.20 sec (0.04 sec $\times$ 5 = 0.20 sec)

These increments measure the duration of the ECG complexes and time intervals. The vertical axis reflects the voltage amplitude in millivolts (mV). Two large boxes equal 1 mV.

In addition to the grid, ECG paper has time interval markings at the top. These marks are placed at 3-second intervals. Each 3-second interval contains 15 large boxes (0.2 sec × 15 boxes = 3.0 sec). The time markings measure heart rate.

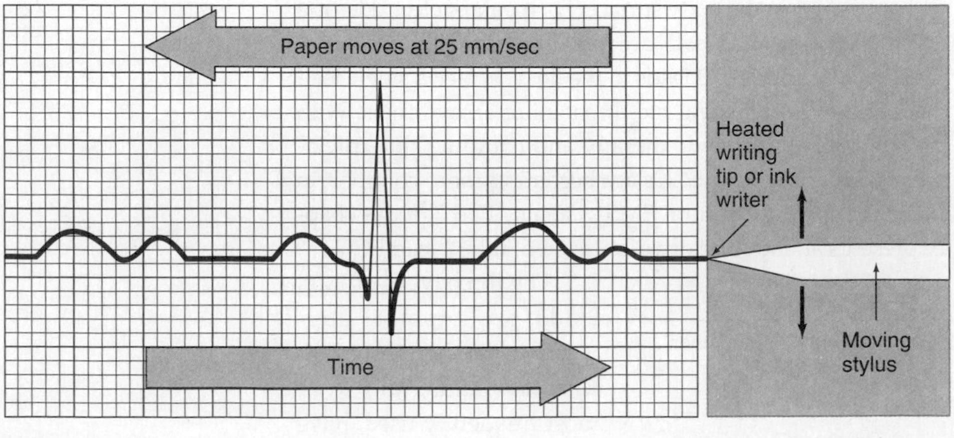

FIGURE 2-18 Recording of the ECG.

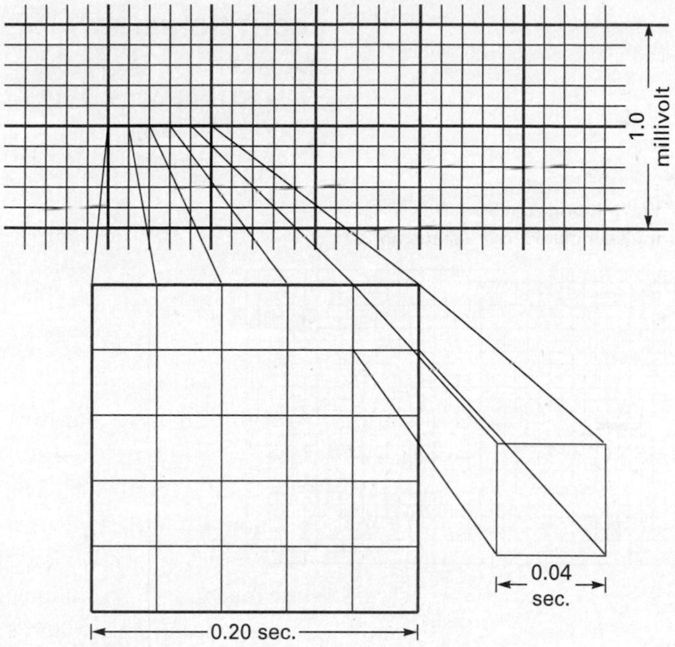

FIGURE 2-19 The ECG paper and markings.

Relationship of the ECG to Electrical Events in the Heart

The ECG tracing's components reflect electrical changes in the heart (Figure 2-20).

- ***P wave.*** The first component of the ECG, the P wave corresponds to atrial depolarization. On lead II, it is a positive, rounded wave before the QRS complex (Figures 2-21 to 2-25).
- ***QRS complex.*** The QRS complex reflects ventricular depolarization. The *Q wave* is the first negative deflection after the P wave; the *R wave* is the first positive deflection after the P wave; and the *S wave* is the first negative deflection after the R wave. Not all three waves are always present, and the shape of the QRS complex can vary among individuals (Figure 2-26).
- ***T wave.*** The T wave reflects repolarization of the ventricles. Normally positive in lead II, it is rounded and

CONTENT REVIEW

➤ ECG Components
- P wave
- QRS complex
- T wave
- U wave

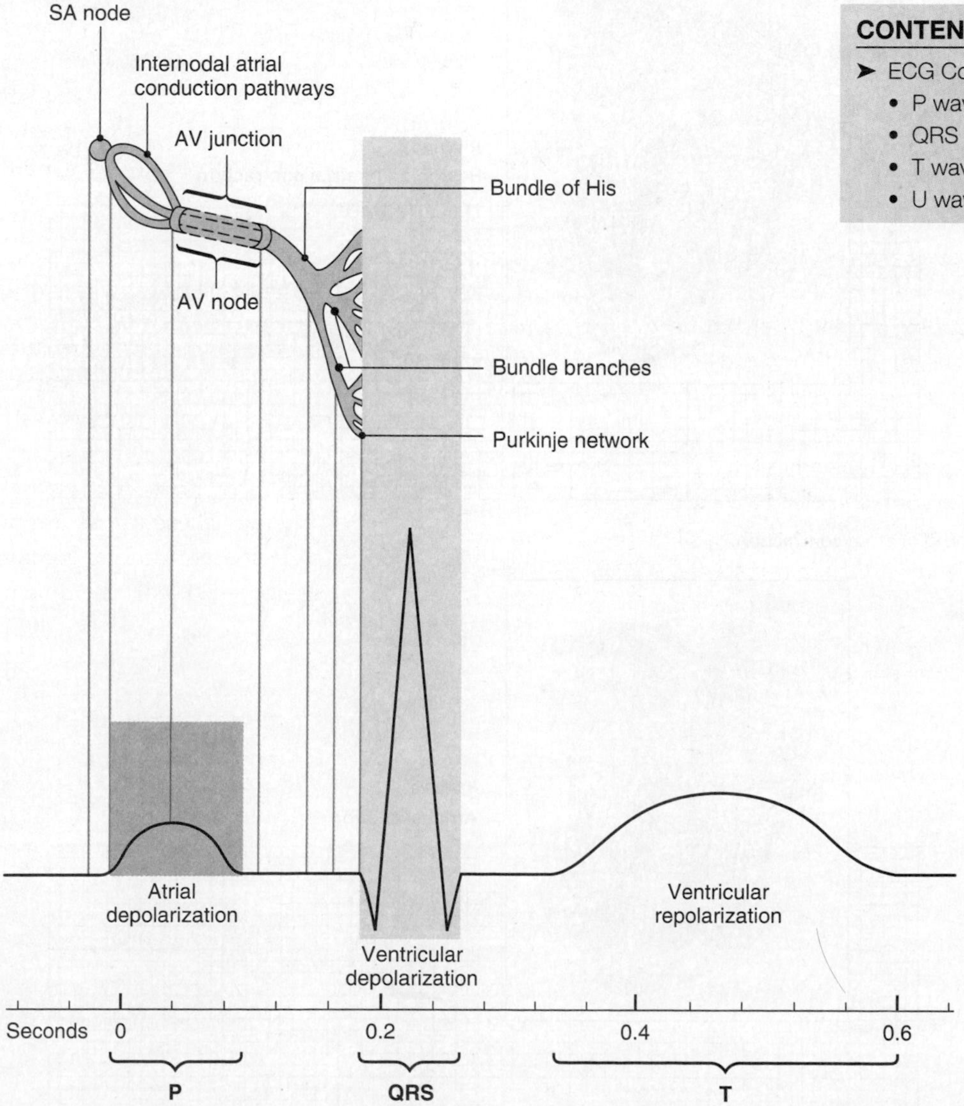

FIGURE 2-20 Relationship of the ECG to electrical activities in the heart.

CONTENT REVIEW

➤ ECG Time Intervals
- PR interval
- QRS interval
- ST segment

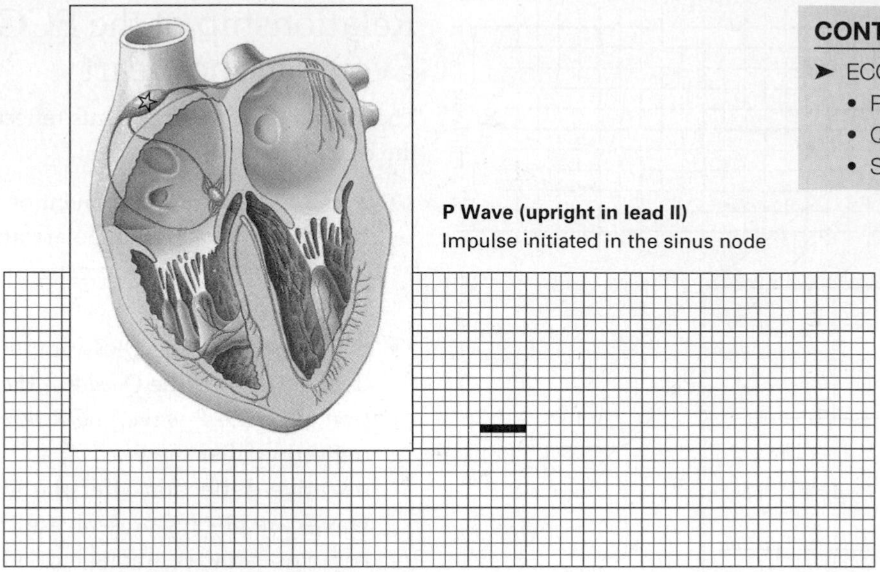

FIGURE 2-21 Impulse initiation in the SA node.

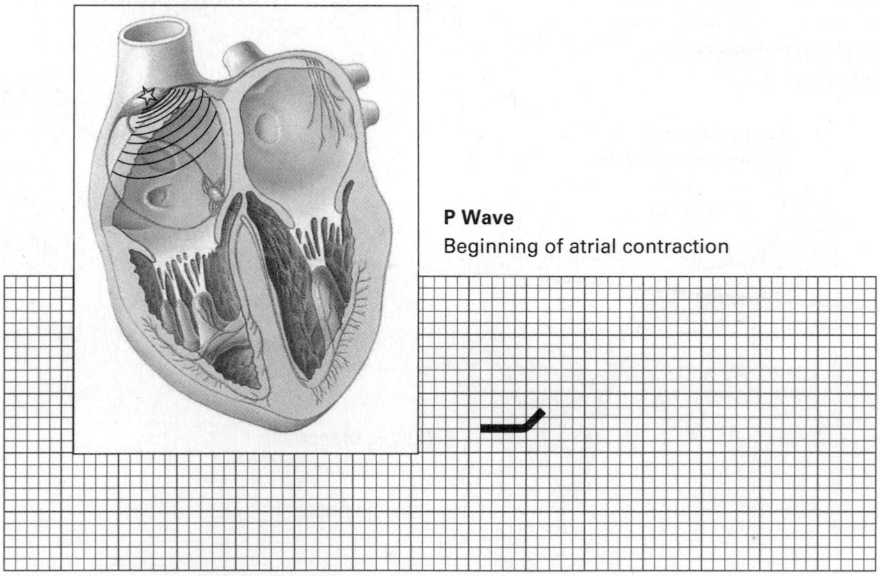

FIGURE 2-22 Beginning of atrial contraction.

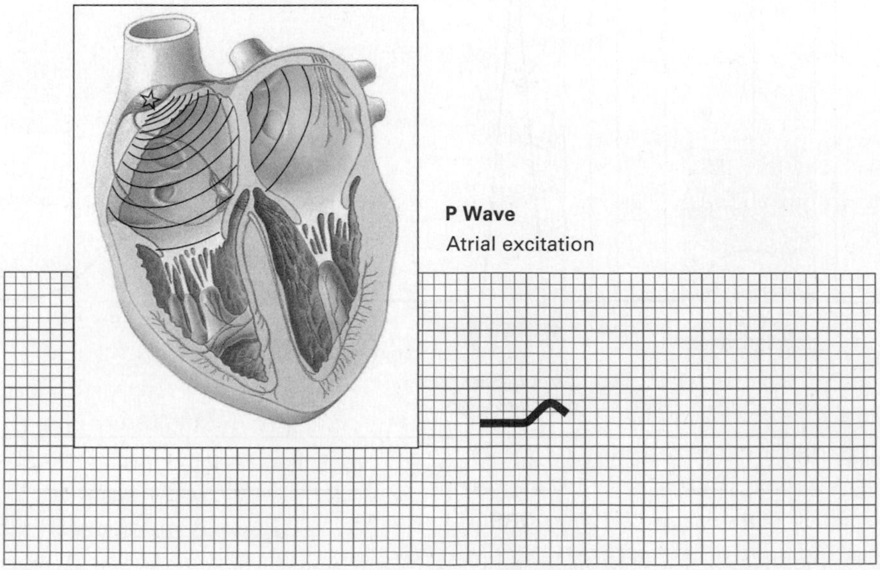

FIGURE 2-23 Atrial excitation.

> **CONTENT REVIEW**
> ➤ Normal Interval Durations
> - PR 0.12–0.20 sec
> - QRS 0.04–0.12 sec
> - QT 0.33–0.42 sec

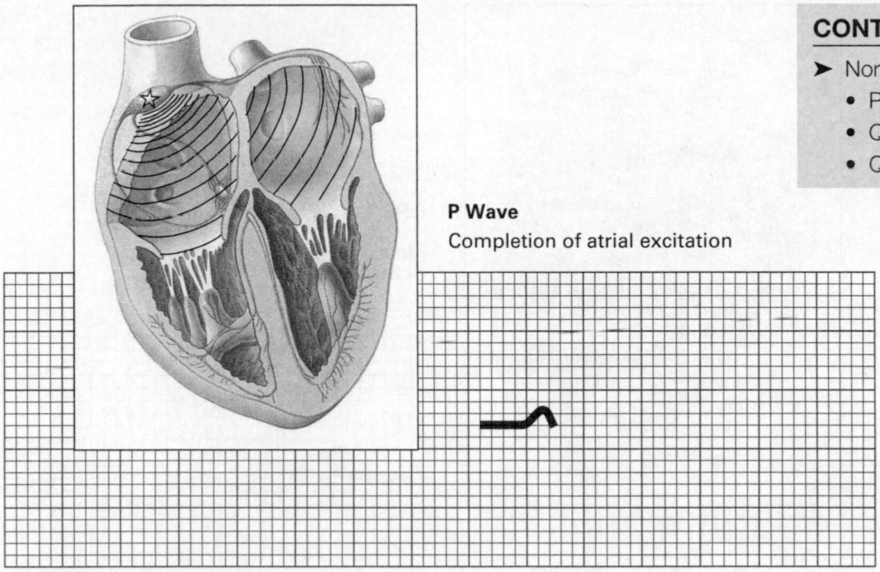

FIGURE 2-24 Completion of atrial excitation.

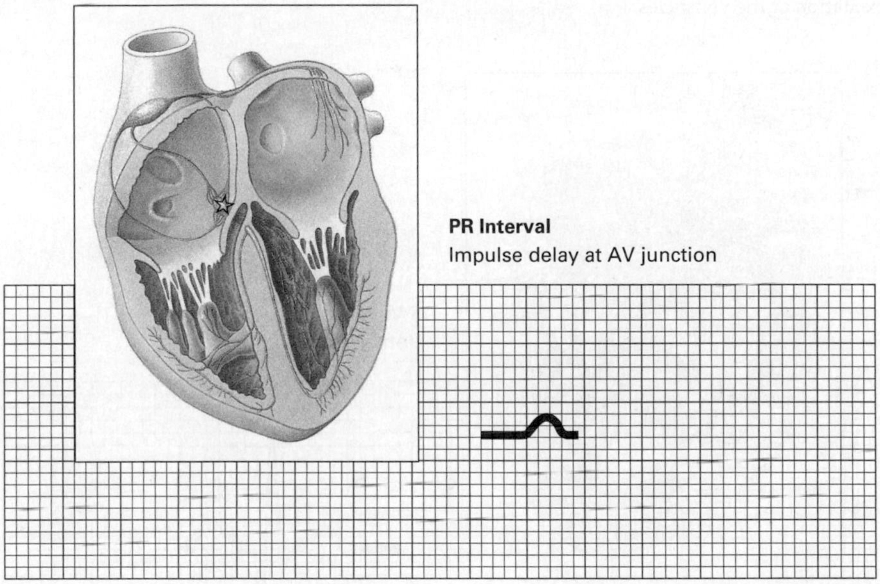

FIGURE 2-25 Impulse delay at the AV junction.

usually moves in the same direction as the QRS complex (Figure 2-27).

- ***U wave.*** Occasionally, a U wave appears. U waves follow T waves and are usually positive. U waves may be associated with electrolyte abnormalities, or they may be a normal finding.

In addition to the waveforms described, the ECG tracing reflects these important time intervals (Figure 2-28):

- ***PR interval (PRI) or P-Q interval (PQI).*** The PR interval is the distance from the beginning of the P wave to the beginning of the QRS complex. It represents the time the impulse takes to travel from the atria to the ventricles. Occasionally, the R wave is absent, in which case this interval is called the P-Q interval. The terms "PR interval" and "P-Q interval" may be used interchangeably.
- ***QRS interval.*** The QRS interval is the distance from the first deflection of the QRS complex to the last. It represents the time necessary for ventricular depolarization.
- ***ST segment.*** The ST segment is the distance from the S wave to the beginning of the T wave. Usually it is an isoelectric line; however, it may be elevated or depressed in certain disease states such as ischemia.

A normal PR interval is 0.12 to 0.20 second. A short PRI lasts less than 0.12 second; a prolonged PRI lasts longer than 0.20 second. A prolonged PRI indicates a delay in the AV node. A normal QRS complex lasts between 0.04 and 0.12 second. A value of less than 0.12 second means that the ventricles depolarized in a normal length of time.

The **QT interval** represents the total duration of ventricular depolarization. A normal QT interval is 0.33 to 0.42 second. QT intervals and heart rate have an inverse relationship:

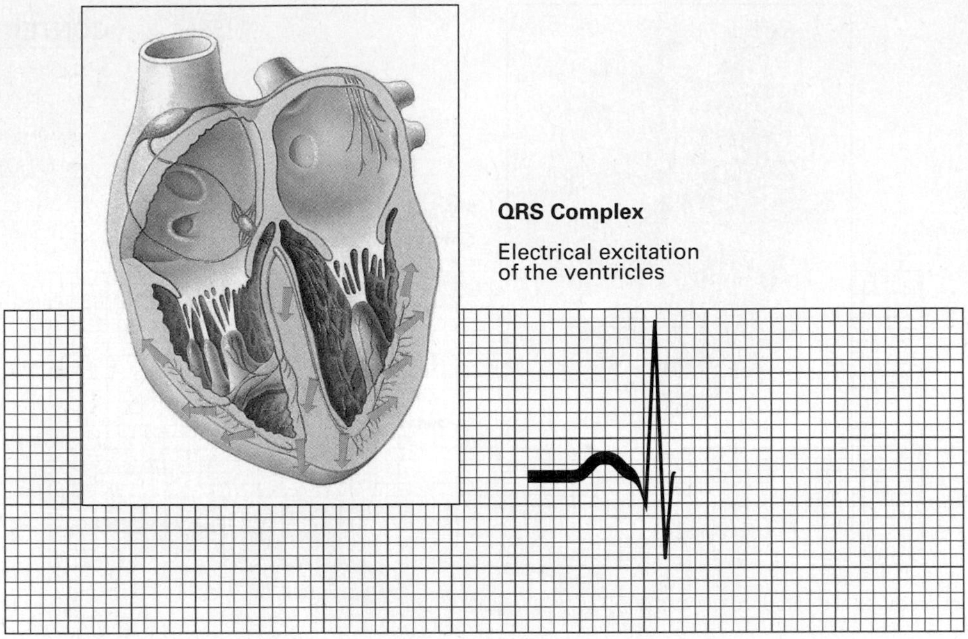

FIGURE 2-26 Electrical excitation of the ventricles.

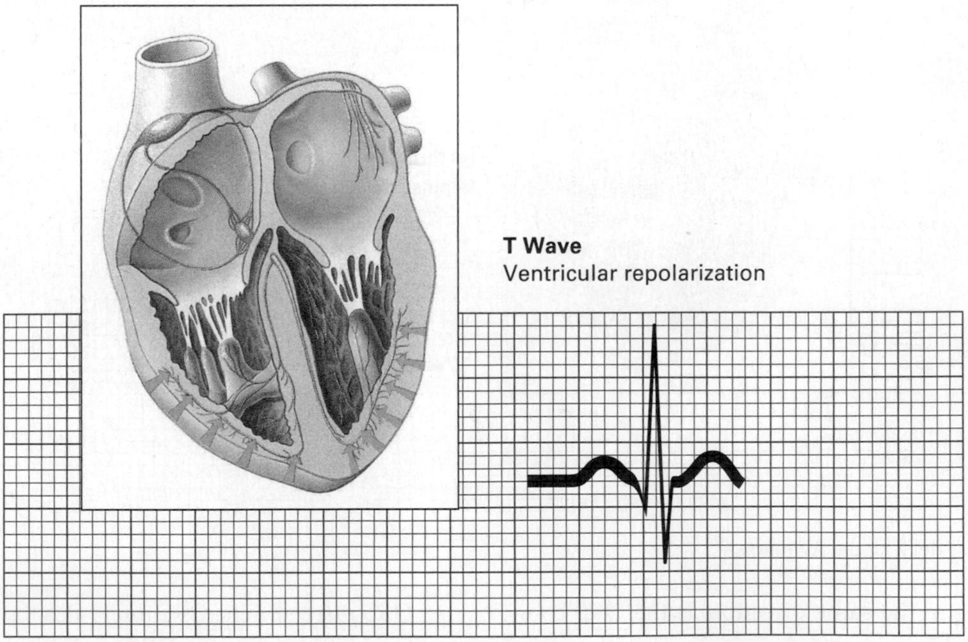

FIGURE 2-27 Ventricular repolarization.

Increases in heart rate usually decrease the QT interval, whereas decreases in heart rate usually prolong it. Generally, the QT interval is expressed as a **corrected QT (QTc)** by taking the QT interval and dividing it by the square root of the RR interval (interval between ventricular depolarizations):

$$QTc = \frac{QT}{\sqrt{RR}}$$

This allows an assessment of the QT interval that is independent of heart rate. Normal corrected QTc intervals are less than 0.44 second. A **prolonged QT interval** is thought to be related to an increased risk of certain ventricular arrhythmias and sudden death. Numerous medications, particularly some of the antipsychotic medications, have been associated with prolongation of the QT interval.

The all-or-none nature of myocardial depolarization results in an interval when the heart cannot be restimulated to depolarize. From our earlier discussion, you will recall that during this time, the myocardial cells have not yet repolarized and cannot be stimulated again (Figure 2-29). This **refractory period** has two parts: an **absolute refractory period** and a **relative refractory period**. During the

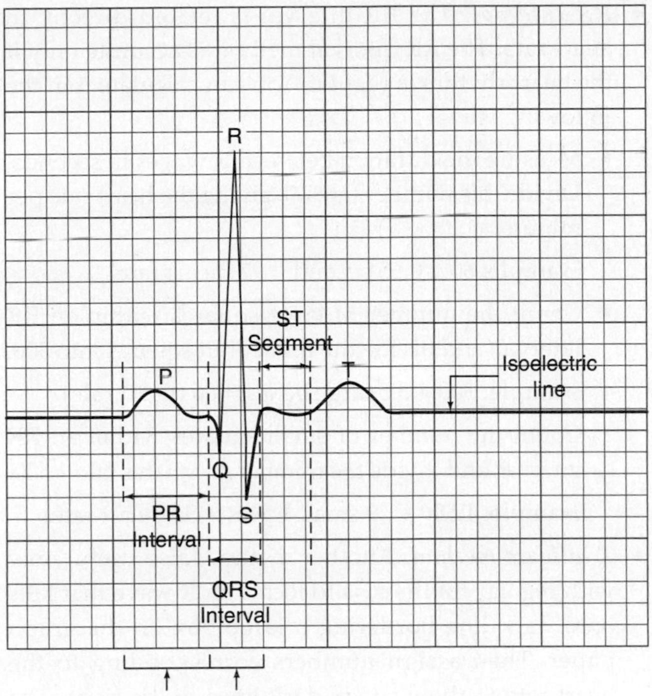

FIGURE 2-28 The ECG.

absolute refractory period, stimulation produces no depolarization whatsoever. This usually lasts from the beginning of the QRS complex to the apex of the T wave. During the relative refractory period, a sufficiently strong stimulus may produce depolarization. This usually corresponds to the T wave's downslope.

ST SEGMENT CHANGES The ST segment is usually an isoelectric line. Myocardial infarctions, which are caused by lack of blood flow to a part of the heart, produce changes in this line. The affected area is then electrically dead and cannot conduct electrical impulses. Myocardial infarctions usually follow this sequence:

1. Ischemia (lack of oxygen)
2. Injury
3. Necrosis (cell death, infarction)

Each of these stages results in distinct ST segment changes. Ischemia causes ST segment depression or an inverted T wave. The inversion is usually symmetrical.

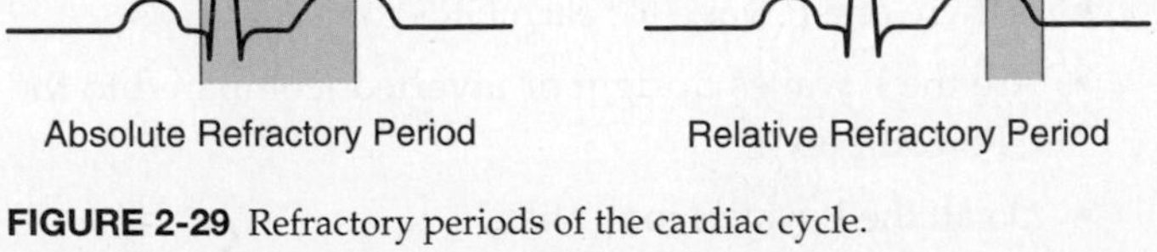

FIGURE 2-29 Refractory periods of the cardiac cycle.

Injury elevates the ST segment, most often in the early phases of a myocardial infarction. As the tissue dies, a significant Q wave appears. As we noted earlier, small, insignificant Q waves may show up in normal ECG tracings. A significant Q wave is at least one small square wide, lasting 0.04 second, or is more than one-third the height of the QRS complex. Q waves may also indicate extensive transient ischemia.

LEAD SYSTEMS AND HEART SURFACES Using the various ECG leads is comparable to waiting for a train at a railroad crossing. You will want to know how long you have to wait (in other words, how long is the train), but you can see only the front of the train. If you had cameras at other viewpoints, you could see how long the train actually was. Similarly, by combining the different ECG leads, you can view different parts of the heart.

Leads V_1–V_4 view the anterior surface of the heart. Leads I and aVL view the lateral surface of the heart. The inferior surface of the heart can be visualized in leads II, III, and aVF. These leads can show ischemia, injury, and necrotic changes and can provide information about the corresponding heart surface (Table 2-3). For example, significant ST elevation in V_1–V_4 may indicate anterior involvement, whereas elevation in leads II, III, and aVF may indicate inferior involvement. Part 3 of this chapter, on 12-lead ECG analysis, discusses these leads in more detail.

Medical procedures (percutaneous coronary intervention) and drugs (fibrinolytics) can treat acute myocardial infarction. The earlier they are initiated, the better the patient's potential outcome. Earlier identification in the field of patients with acute myocardial infarction (AMI) will allow for earlier interventions, but the 12-lead ECG's role in out-of-hospital care remains unresolved. Its use may not be appropriate in many EMS settings. Individual EMS medical directors will determine the application and use of the 12-lead ECG in their specific EMS settings.

Table 2-3 Overview of ECG Lead Groupings

Leads	Portion of the Heart Examined
I and aVL	Left side of the heart in a vertical plane
II, III, and aVF	Inferior (diaphragmatic) side of the heart
aVR	Right side of the heart in a vertical plane
V_1 and V_2	Right ventricle
V_3 and V_4	Interventricular septum and the anterior wall of the left ventricle
V_5 and V_6	Anterior and lateral walls of the left ventricle

Interpretation of Rhythm Strips

CONTENT REVIEW

➤ Normal Sinus Rhythm
- Rate: 60–100
- Rhythm: regular
- P waves: normal, upright, only before each QRS complex
- PR interval: 0.12–0.20 sec
- QRS complex
- Morphology: normal
- Duration: <0.12 sec

The key to interpreting rhythm strips is to approach each strip logically and systematically. Attempts to nonanalytically "eyeball" the strip often lead to incorrect interpretations. Your approach to rhythm strip interpretation should include the following basic criteria:

- Always be consistent and analytical.
- Memorize the rules for each arrhythmia.
- Analyze a given rhythm strip according to a specific format.
- Compare your analysis to the rules for each arrhythmia.
- Identify the arrhythmia by its similarity to established rules.

The health care profession uses several standard formats for ECG analysis. We will use the following five-step procedure. Analyze the:

1. Rate
2. Rhythm
3. P waves
4. PR interval
5. QRS complex

ANALYZING RATE The first step in ECG strip interpretation is to analyze the heart rate. Usually this means the ventricular rate; however, if the atrial and ventricular rates differ, you must calculate both. The normal heart rate is 60 to 100 beats per minute. A heart rate greater than 100 beats per minute is a **tachycardia**. A heart rate less than 60 beats per minute is a **bradycardia**. You can use any of the following methods to calculate the rate:

- ***Six-second method.*** Count the number of complexes in a 6-second interval. Mark off a 6-second interval by noting two 3-second marks at the top of the ECG paper. Then multiply the number of complexes within the 6-second strip by 10.
- ***Heart rate calculator rulers.*** Commercially available heart rate calculator rulers allow you to determine heart rates rapidly. Always use them according to the accompanying directions, as variations occur among different manufacturers. Also learn a manual method so you can still calculate rates if you forget your ruler.
- ***RR interval.*** The RR interval is related directly to heart rate. The RR interval method is accurate only if the heart rhythm is regular. You can calculate it in the following ways:
  - Measure the duration between R waves in seconds. Divide this number into 60, giving the heart rate per minute.

    Example: 60 ÷ 0.65 second = 92 (heart rate)
  - Count the number of large squares within an RR interval, and divide the number of squares into 300.

    Example: 300 ÷ 3.5 large boxes = 86 (heart rate)
  - Count the number of small squares within an RR interval, and divide the number of squares into 1,500.

    Example: 1,500 ÷ 29 small **boxes** = 52 (heart rate)
- ***Triplicate method.*** Another method, also useful only with regular rhythms, is to locate an R wave that falls on a dark line bordering a large box on the graph paper. Then assign numbers corresponding to the heart rate to the next six dark lines to the right. The order is: 300, 150, 100, 75, 60, and 50. The number corresponding to the dark line closest to the peak of the next R wave is a rough estimate of the heart rate.

Pick one of these methods and become comfortable with it. Use it to determine the rate on all strips that you analyze.

ANALYZING RHYTHM The next step is to analyze the rhythm. First, measure the RR interval across the strip. Normally, the RR rhythm is fairly regular. Some minimal variation, associated with respirations, should be expected. If the rhythm is irregular, note whether it fits one of the following patterns:

- Occasionally irregular (only one or two RR intervals on the strip are irregular)
- Regularly irregular (patterned irregularity or group beating)
- Irregularly irregular (no relationship among RR intervals)

ANALYZING P WAVES The P waves reflect atrial depolarization. Normally, the atria depolarize away from the SA node and toward the ventricles. In lead II, this appears as a positive, rounded P wave. When analyzing the P waves, ask yourself the following questions:

- Are P waves present?
- Are the P waves regular?
- Is there one P wave for each QRS complex?
- Are the P waves upright or inverted (compared to the QRS complex)?
- Do all the P waves look alike?

ANALYZING THE PR INTERVAL The PR interval represents the time needed for atrial depolarization and conduction of the impulse up to the AV node. Remember, the normal PR interval is 0.12 to 0.20 second (three to five small boxes). Any deviation is an abnormal finding. The PR interval should be consistent across the strip.

ANALYZING THE QRS COMPLEX The QRS complex represents ventricular depolarization. When evaluating the QRS complex, ask yourself the following questions:

- Do all of the QRS complexes look alike?
- What is the QRS duration?

Remember, the QRS duration is usually 0.04 to 0.12 second. Anything longer than 0.12 second (three small boxes) is abnormal.

Arrhythmias

On a normal ECG, the heart rate is between 60 and 100 beats per minute. The rhythm is regular (both P-P and RR). The P waves are normal in shape, upright, and appear only before each QRS complex. The PR interval lasts 0.12–0.20 second and is constant. The QRS complex has a normal morphology, and its duration is less than 0.12 second. All of these factors indicate a **normal sinus rhythm** (Figure 2-30). Any deviation from the heart's normal electrical rhythm is called an **arrhythmia**. (Literally, arrhythmia means the absence of cardiac electrical activity. A related term, **dysrhythmia**, means abnormal rhythm. Dysrhythmia is a better descriptor of a rhythm that varies from the normal, but arrhythmia is more commonly used to describe heart rhythm abnormalities. For this reason *arrhythmia* is the term we use in this text.)

The causes of arrhythmias include:

- Myocardial ischemia, necrosis, or infarction
- Autonomic nervous system imbalance
- Distention of the chambers of the heart (especially in the atria, secondary to congestive heart failure)
- Blood gas abnormalities, including hypoxia and abnormal pH
- Electrolyte imbalances (Ca^{++}, K^{+}, Mg^{++})
- Trauma to the myocardium (cardiac contusion)
- Drug effects and drug toxicity
- Electrocution
- Hypothermia
- CNS damage
- Idiopathic events
- Normal occurrences

Arrhythmias in the healthy heart are of little significance. No matter what the etiology or type of arrhythmia, treat the patient and his symptoms, not the arrhythmia. You will hear this repeated over and over: Treat the patient, not the monitor.

Mechanism of Impulse Formation

Several physiologic mechanisms can cause cardiac arrhythmias. The depolarization impulse is normally transmitted forward (*antegrade*) through the conductive system and the myocardium. In certain arrhythmias, however, the depolarization impulse is conducted backward (*retrograde*).

ECTOPIC FOCI One cause of arrhythmias is *enhanced automaticity*. This condition results when **ectopic foci** (heart cells other than the pacemaker cells) automatically depolarize, producing **ectopic (abnormal) beats**. Premature ventricular contractions and premature atrial contractions are examples of ectopic beats. Ectopic beats can be intermittent or sustained.

REENTRY Reentry may cause isolated premature beats, or *tachyarrhythmias*. It occurs when ischemia or another disease process alters two branches of a conduction pathway, slowing conduction in one branch and causing a unidirectional block in the other. An antegrade depolarization wave travels slowly through the branch with

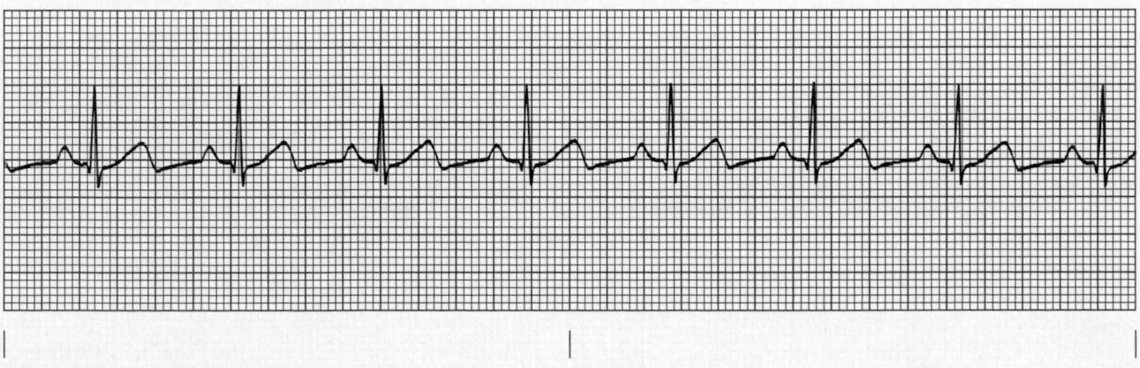

FIGURE 2-30 Normal sinus rhythm.

ischemia and is blocked in the branch with a unidirectional block. After the depolarization wave goes through the slowed branch, it enters the branch with the unidirectional block and is conducted retrograde back to the branch's origin. By now, the tissue is no longer refractory, and stimulation occurs again. This can result in rapid rhythms such as paroxysmal supraventricular tachycardia or atrial fibrillation.

Classification of Arrhythmias

Arrhythmias can be classified in any number of ways. Some of the classification methods include:

- Nature of origin (changes in automaticity versus disturbances in conduction)
- Magnitude (major versus minor)
- Severity (life threatening versus non-life threatening)
- Site of origin

Classifying arrhythmias by site of origin is closely related to basic physiology and, thus, is easy to understand. This approach divides arrhythmias into the following categories:

- Originating in the SA node
- Originating in the atria
- Originating within the AV junction
- Sustained in or originating in the AV junction
- Originating in the ventricles
- Resulting from disorders of conduction

Arrhythmias Originating in the SA Node

Arrhythmias originating in the SA node most often result from changes in autonomic tone. However, disease can exist in the SA node itself. Arrhythmias that originate in the SA node include:

- Sinus bradycardia
- Sinus tachycardia
- Sinus arrhythmia
- Sinus arrest
- Sinus block
- Sinus pause
- Sick sinus syndrome

Sinus Bradycardia

Description *Sinus bradycardia* results from slowing of the SA node.

Etiology Sinus bradycardia may result from any of the following conditions:

- Increased parasympathetic (vagal) tone
- Intrinsic disease of the SA node
- Drug effects (digitalis, beta-blockers, calcium channel blockers)
- Normal finding in healthy, well-conditioned persons

Rules of interpretation/lead II monitoring (Figure 2-31):

Rate—less than 60

Rhythm—regular

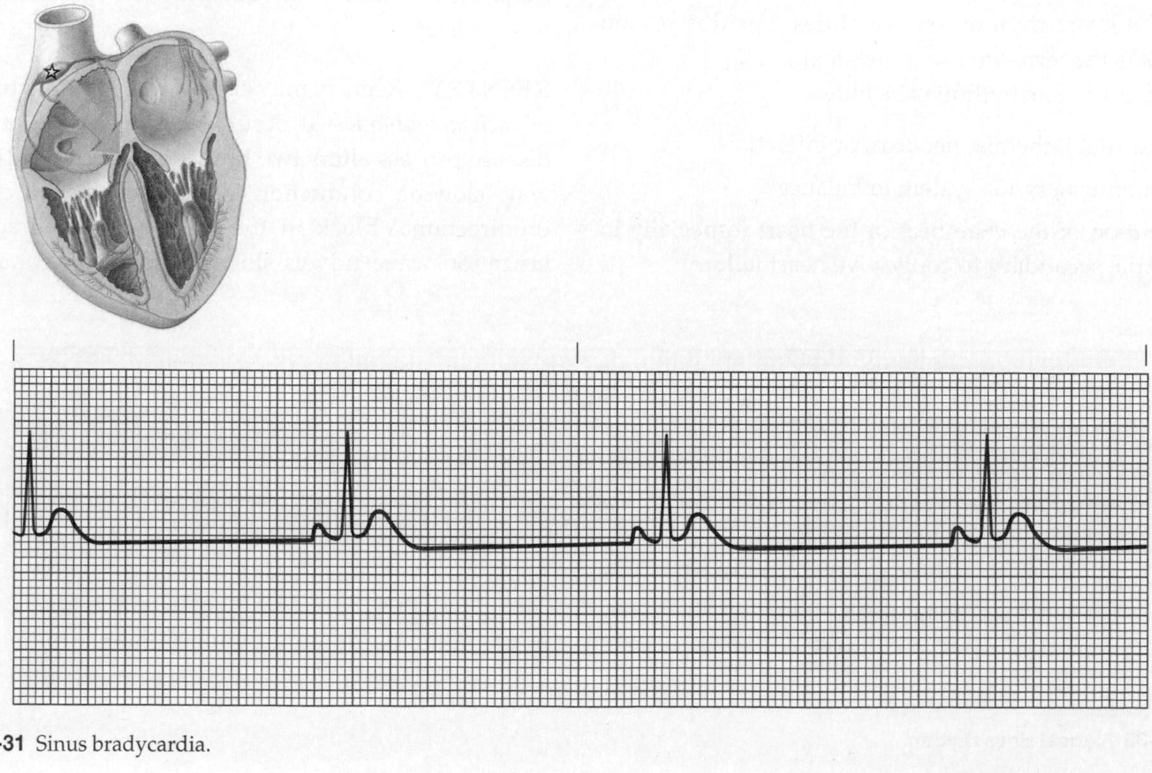

FIGURE 2-31 Sinus bradycardia.

Pacemaker site—SA node

P waves—upright and normal in morphology

PR interval—normal (0.12–0.20 second and constant)

QRS complex—normal (0.04–0.12 second)

Clinical significance The decreased heart rate can cause decreased cardiac output, hypotension, angina, or CNS symptoms. This is especially true for rates slower than 50 beats per minute. The slow heart rate may also lead to atrial ectopic or ventricular ectopic rhythms. In a healthy athlete, sinus bradycardia may be normal and have no clinical significance.

Treatment Treatment is generally unnecessary unless signs of poor perfusion (e.g., acute altered mental status, ongoing chest pain, hypotension or other signs of shock) are present. If there are signs of poor perfusion, prepare for transcutaneous pacing. Consider administering a 0.5-mg bolus of atropine sulfate. Repeat every 3 to 5 minutes until you have obtained a satisfactory rate or have given 3.0 mg of the drug. If atropine fails, consider transcutaneous cardiac pacing (TCP) or a catecholamine infusion.

Sinus Tachycardia

Description *Sinus tachycardia* results from an increased rate of SA node discharge.

Etiology Sinus tachycardia may result from any of the following:

- Exercise
- Fever
- Anxiety
- Hypovolemia
- Anemia
- Pump failure
- Increased sympathetic tone
- Hypoxia
- Hyperthyroidism

Rules of interpretation/lead II monitoring (Figure 2-32):

Rate—greater than 100

Rhythm—regular

Pacemaker site—SA node

P waves—upright and normal in morphology

PR interval—normal

QRS complex—normal

Clinical significance Sinus tachycardia is often benign. In some cases, it is a compensatory mechanism for decreased stroke volume. If the rate is greater than 140 beats per minute, cardiac output may fall because ventricular filling time is inadequate. Very rapid heart rates increase myocardial oxygen demand and can precipitate

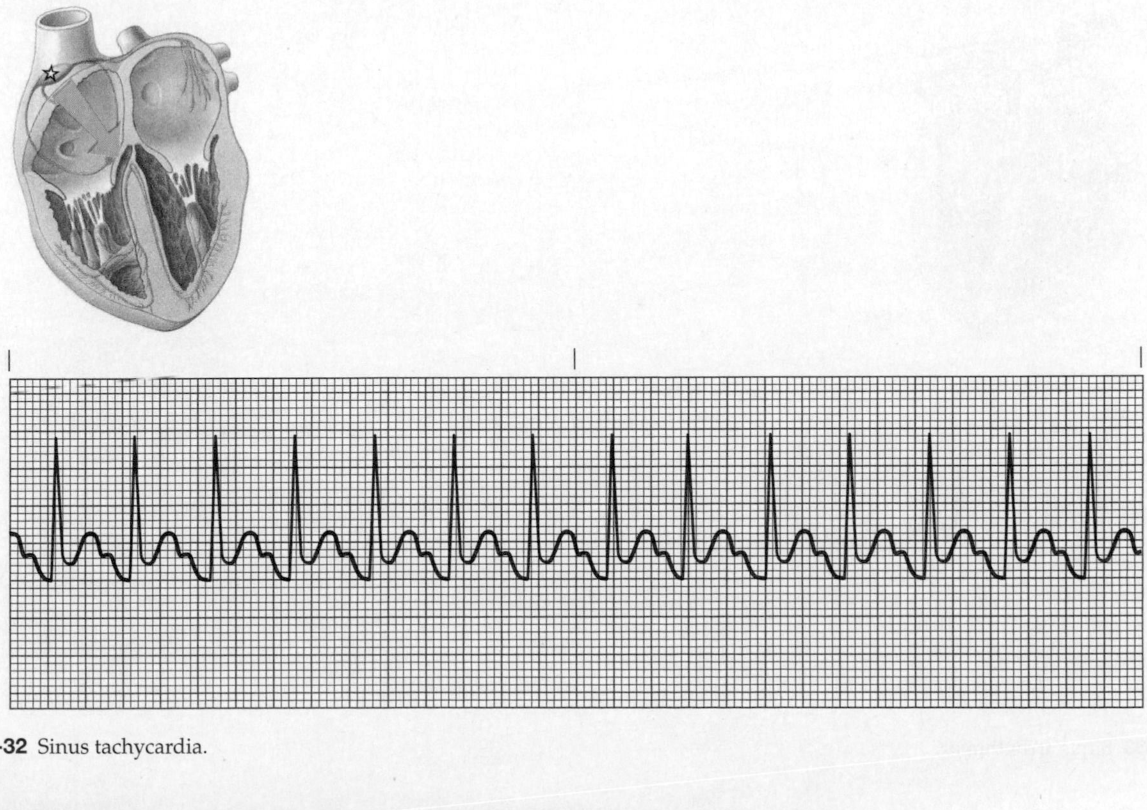

FIGURE 2-32 Sinus tachycardia.

ischemia or infarct in diseased hearts. Prolonged sinus tachycardia accompanying acute myocardial infarction (AMI) is often an ominous finding, suggesting cardiogenic shock.

Treatment Treatment is directed at the underlying cause. Hypovolemia, fever, hypoxia, or other causes should be corrected.

Sinus Arrhythmia

Description *Sinus arrhythmia* often results from a variation of the RR interval.

Etiology Sinus arrhythmia is often a normal finding and is sometimes related to the respiratory cycle and changes in intrathoracic pressure. It is quite common in children. Pathologically, sinus arrhythmia can be caused by enhanced vagal tone.

Rules of interpretation/lead II monitoring (Figure 2-33):

Rate—60–100 (varies with respirations)

Rhythm—irregular

Pacemaker site—SA node

P waves—upright and normal in morphology

PR interval—normal

QRS complex—normal

Clinical significance Sinus arrhythmia is a normal variant, particularly in the young and the aged.

Treatment Typically, none required.

Sinus Arrest

Description *Sinus arrest* occurs when the sinus node fails to discharge for a brief period, resulting in short periods of cardiac standstill. One or more of the subsequent PQRST complexes will be missing. This standstill can persist until pacemaker cells lower in the conductive system discharge (escape beats) or until the sinus node resumes discharge. Because the node fails to fire, the RR interval following the dropped beat will vary (e.g., the pause will NOT be a multiple of the previous RR interval).

Etiology Sinus arrest can result from any of the following conditions:

- Ischemia of the SA node
- Digitalis toxicity
- Excessive vagal tone
- Degenerative fibrotic disease

Rules of interpretation/lead II monitoring (Figure 2-34):

Rate—normal to slow, depending on the frequency and duration of the arrest

Rhythm—irregular

Pacemaker site—SA node

P waves—upright and normal in morphology

PR interval—normal

QRS complex—normal

Clinical significance Frequent or prolonged episodes may compromise cardiac output, resulting in syncope

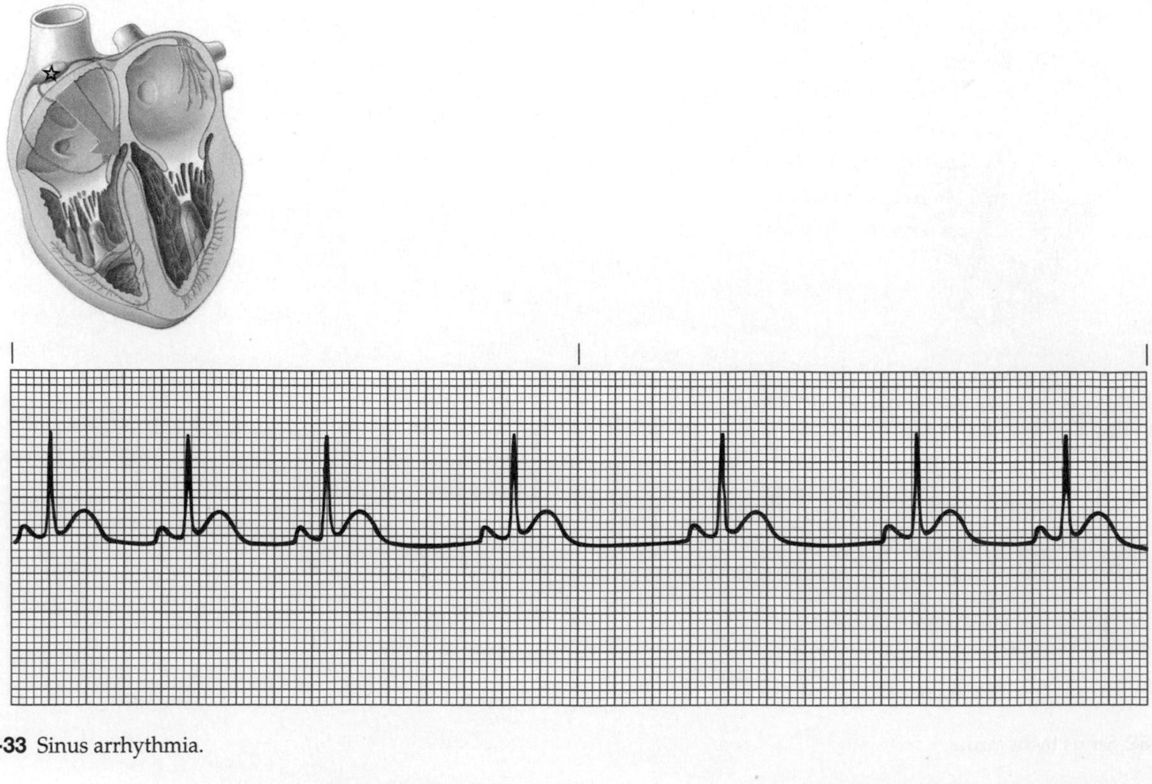

FIGURE 2-33 Sinus arrhythmia.

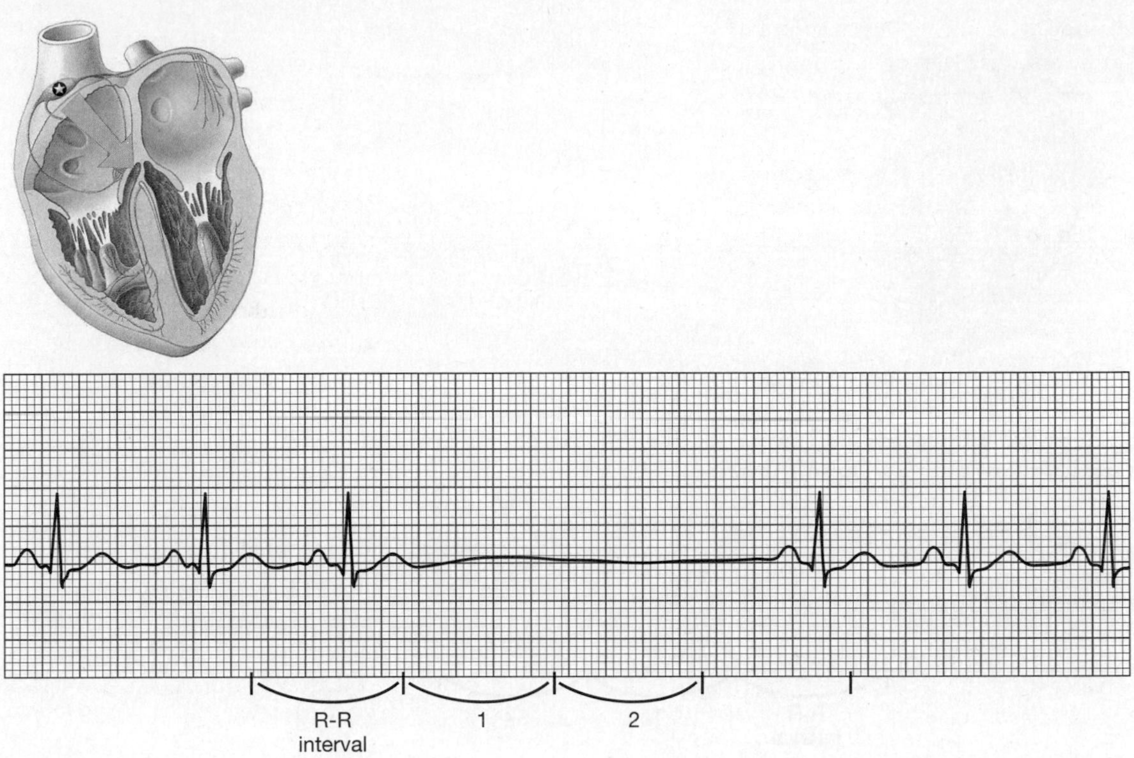

FIGURE 2-34 Sinus arrest.

(fainting) and other problems. There is always the danger of complete cessation of SA node activity. Usually, an escape rhythm develops; however, cardiac standstill occasionally can result.

Treatment If the patient is asymptomatic, observation is all that is required unless there are signs of poor perfusion (e.g., acute altered mental status, ongoing chest pain, hypotension or other signs of shock). If there are signs of poor perfusion, prepare for transcutaneous pacing. Consider administering a 0.5-mg bolus of atropine sulfate. Repeat every 3 to 5 minutes until you have obtained a satisfactory rate or have given 3.0 mg of the drug. If atropine fails, consider transcutaneous cardiac pacing (TCP) or a catecholamine infusion.

Sinus Block

Description *Sinus block*, also called *sinus exit block*, occurs when the sinus node fires on time but the impulse is blocked before it exits the sinus node. This results in a pause that varies in length depending on how many sinus beats are blocked. Because the SA node fires, the RR intervals after the last beat will be constant (e.g., the pause will be a multiple of the previous RR interval).

Etiology Sinus block can result from any of the following conditions:

- Ischemia of the SA node
- Digitalis toxicity
- Excessive vagal tone
- Degenerative fibrotic disease

Rules of interpretation/lead II monitoring (Figure 2-35):

Rate—normal to slow, depending on the frequency and duration of the arrest

Rhythm—regular

Pacemaker site—SA node

P waves—upright and normal in morphology

PR interval—normal

***QRS** complex*—normal

Clinical significance Frequent or prolonged episodes may compromise cardiac output, resulting in syncope (fainting) and other problems. There is always the danger of complete cessation of SA node activity. Usually, an escape rhythm develops; however, cardiac standstill occasionally can result.

Treatment If the patient is asymptomatic, observation is all that is required unless there are signs of poor perfusion (e.g., acute altered mental status, ongoing chest pain, hypotension or other signs of shock). If there are signs of poor perfusion, prepare for transcutaneous pacing. Consider administering a 0.5-mg bolus of atropine sulfate. Repeat every 3 to 5 minutes until you have obtained a satisfactory rate or have given 3.0 mg of the drug. If atropine fails, consider transcutaneous cardiac pacing (TCP) or a catecholamine infusion.

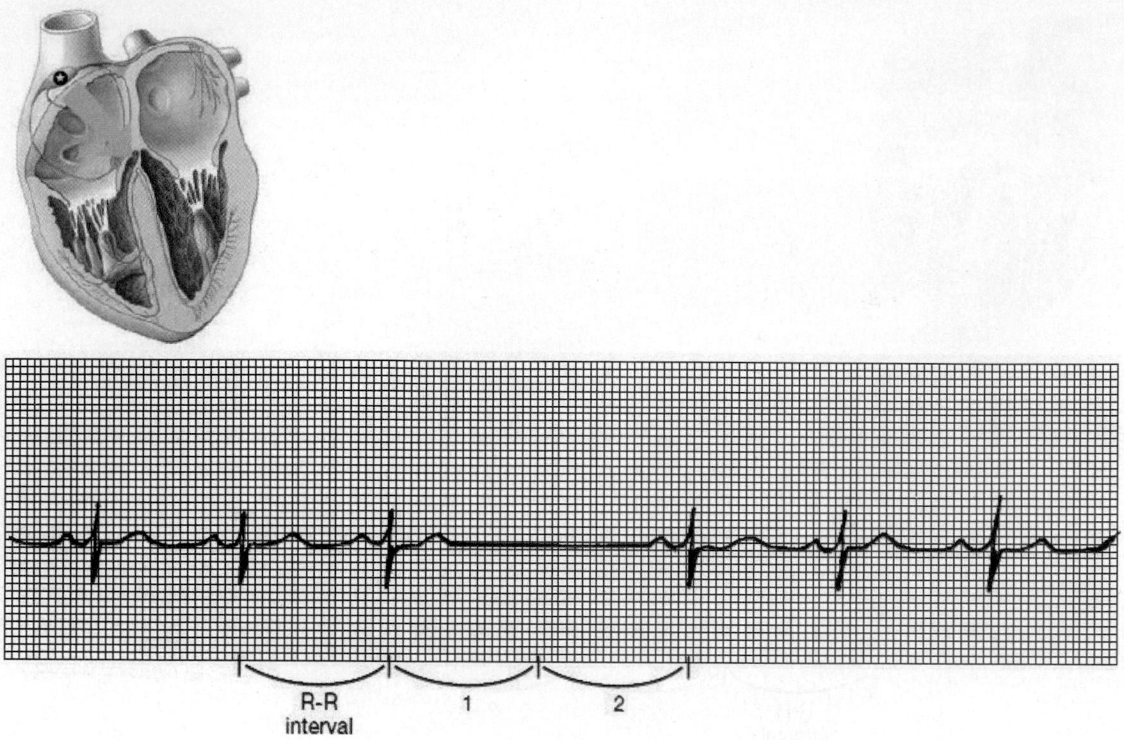

FIGURE 2-35 Sinus block.

Sinus Pause

Description A *sinus pause* occurs when the sinus node fails to discharge for a brief period, resulting in missing a single PQRST complex. A sinus pause differs from sinus arrest in that only a single beat is missed with a sinus pause, whereas multiple beats may be missed with a sinus arrest. Because the node fails to fire, the RR interval following the dropped beat will vary (e.g., the pause will NOT be a multiple of the previous RR interval).

Etiology Sinus pause can result from any of the following conditions:

- Ischemia of the SA node
- Digitalis toxicity
- Excessive vagal tone
- Degenerative fibrotic disease

Rules of interpretation/lead II monitoring (Figure 2-36):

Rate—normal to slow, depending on the frequency and duration of the arrest

Rhythm—irregular

Pacemaker site—SA node

P waves—upright and normal in morphology

PR interval—normal

QRS complex—normal

Clinical significance Frequent or prolonged episodes may compromise cardiac output, resulting in syncope (fainting) and other problems. There is always the danger of complete cessation of SA node activity. Usually, an escape rhythm develops; however, cardiac standstill occasionally can result.

Treatment If the patient is asymptomatic, observation is all that is required unless there are signs of poor perfusion (e.g., acute altered mental status, ongoing chest pain, hypotension or other signs of shock). If there are signs of poor perfusion, prepare for transcutaneous pacing. Consider administering a 0.5-mg bolus of atropine sulfate. Repeat every 3 to 5 minutes until you have obtained a satisfactory rate or have given 3.0 mg of the drug. If atropine fails, consider transcutaneous cardiac pacing (TCP) or a catecholamine infusion.

Sick Sinus Syndrome

Description Technically, *sick sinus syndrome* is not an arrhythmia per se, but a combination of arrhythmias. Sick sinus syndrome occurs when the sinus node is diseased or ischemic. It is characterized by wild swings in the heart rate—often moving rapidly from a profound bradycardia to a severe tachycardia and back. Sinus blocks are also commonly seen with sick sinus syndrome. The sinus node fails to discharge for a brief period, resulting in missing a single PQRST complex.

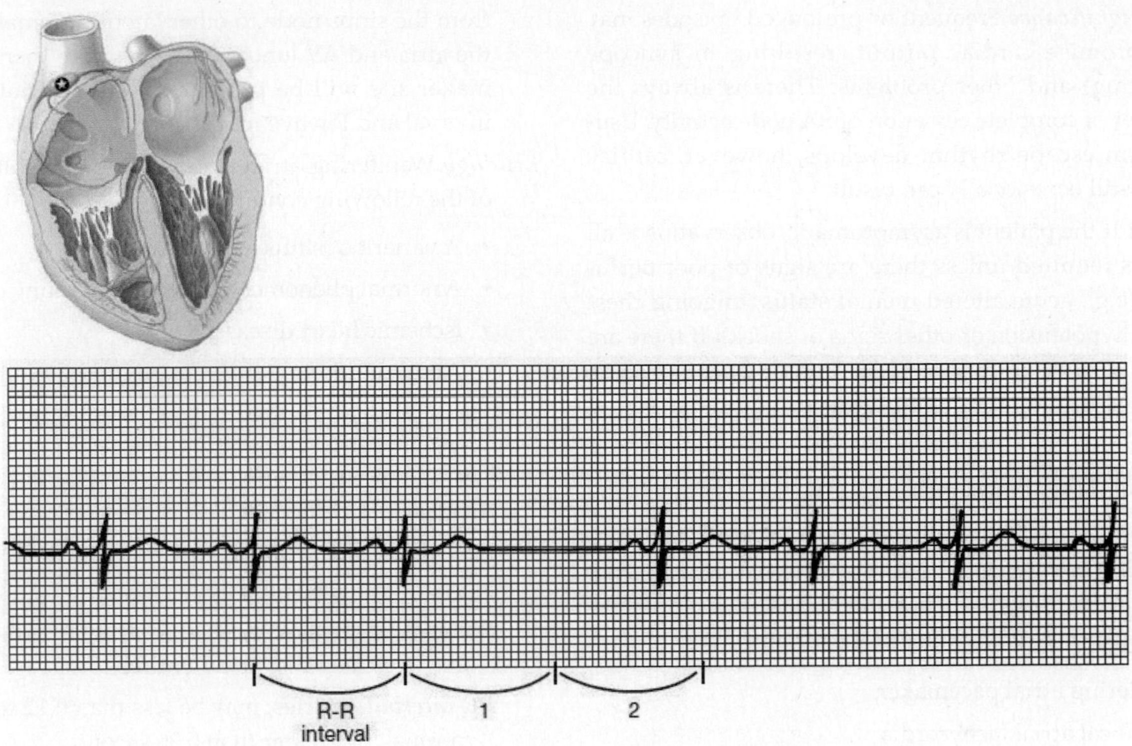

FIGURE 2-36 Sinus pause.

Because the node fails to fire, the RR interval following the dropped beat will vary (e.g., the pause will NOT be a multiple of the previous RR interval).

Etiology Sick sinus syndrome can result from any of the following conditions:

- Ischemia of the SA node
- Digitalis toxicity
- Degenerative fibrotic disease

Rules of interpretation/lead II monitoring (Figure 2-37):

Rate—extremely variable

Rhythm—irregular

Pacemaker site—SA node

P waves—upright and normal in morphology

PR interval—normal

QRS complex—normal

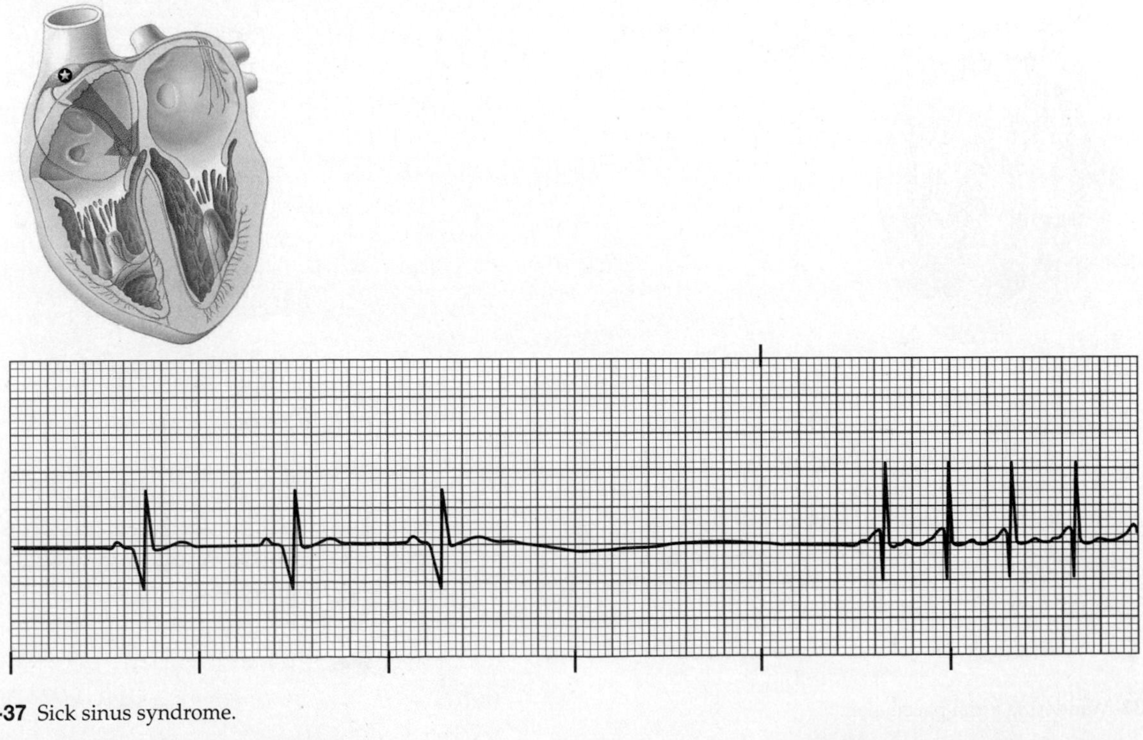

FIGURE 2-37 Sick sinus syndrome.

Clinical significance Frequent or prolonged episodes may compromise cardiac output, resulting in syncope (fainting) and other problems. There is always the danger of complete cessation of SA node activity. Usually, an escape rhythm develops; however, cardiac standstill occasionally can result.

Treatment If the patient is asymptomatic, observation is all that is required unless there are signs of poor perfusion (e.g., acute altered mental status, ongoing chest pain, hypotension or other signs of shock). If there are signs of poor perfusion, begin transcutaneous pacing or consider a catecholamine infusion.

Arrhythmias Originating in the Atria

Arrhythmias can originate outside the SA node in the atrial tissue or in the internodal pathways. Ischemia, hypoxia, atrial dilation, and other factors can cause atrial arrhythmias. Arrhythmias originating in the atria include:

- Wandering atrial pacemaker
- Multifocal atrial tachycardia
- Premature atrial contractions
- Paroxysmal supraventricular tachycardia
- Supraventricular tachycardia
- Atrial flutter
- Atrial fibrillation

Wandering Atrial Pacemaker

Description *Wandering atrial pacemaker* (also called *ectopic tachycardia*) is the passive transfer of pacemaker sites from the sinus node to other latent pacemaker sites in the atria and AV junction. Often, more than one pacemaker site will be present, causing variation in RR interval and P wave morphology.

Etiology Wandering atrial pacemaker can result from any of the following conditions:

- A variant of sinus arrhythmia
- A normal phenomenon in the very young or the aged
- Ischemic heart disease
- Atrial dilation

Rules of interpretation/lead II monitoring (Figure 2-38):

Rate—usually normal

Rhythm—slightly irregular

Pacemaker site—varies among the SA node, atrial tissue, and the AV junction

P waves—morphology changes from beat to beat; P waves may disappear entirely

PR interval—varies; may be less than 0.12 second, normal, or greater than 0.20 second

QRS complex—normal

Clinical significance Wandering atrial pacemaker usually has no detrimental effects. Occasionally, it can be a precursor of other atrial arrhythmias, such as atrial fibrillation. It sometimes indicates digitalis toxicity.

Treatment If the patient is asymptomatic, observation is all that is required. If the patient is symptomatic, consider adenosine.

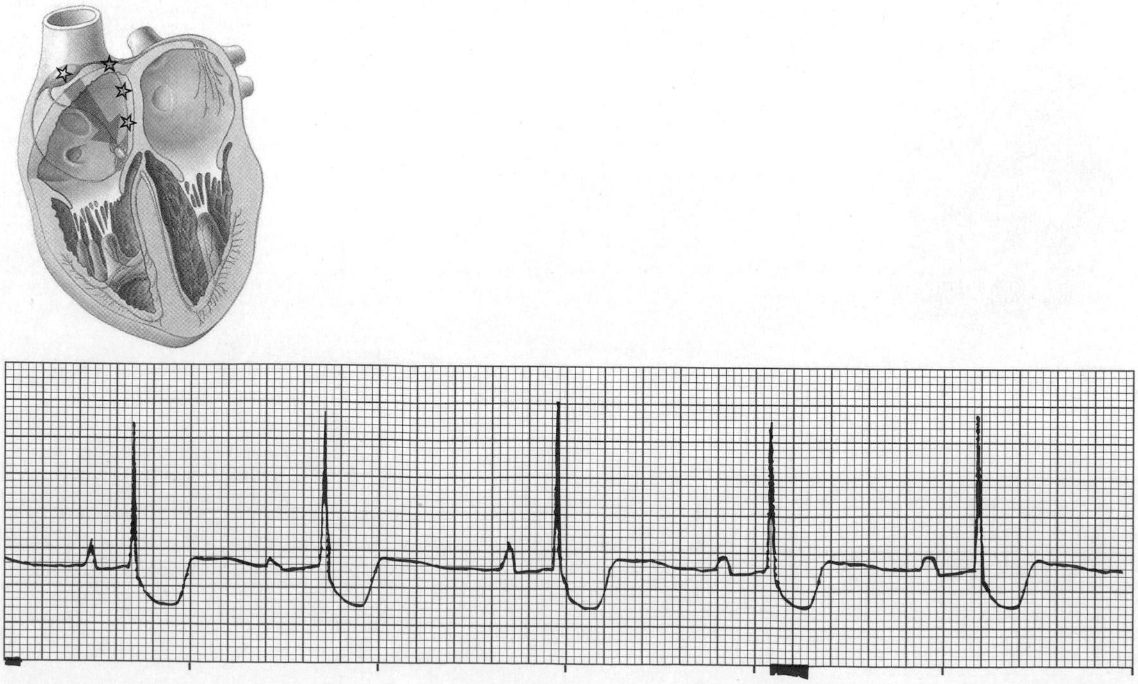

FIGURE 2-38 Wandering atrial pacemaker.

Multifocal Atrial Tachycardia

Description *Multifocal atrial tachycardia (MAT)* is usually seen in acutely ill patients. Basically, MAT is a wandering pacemaker rhythm with a rate greater than 100. Significant pulmonary disease is seen in about 60 percent of these patients. Certain medications used to treat lung disease (such as the beta-agonists and theophylline) may worsen the arrhythmia. Three different P waves are noted, indicating various ectopic foci.

Etiology Multifocal atrial tachycardia can result from any of the following conditions:

- Pulmonary disease
- Metabolic disorders (hypokalemia)
- Ischemic heart disease
- Recent surgery

Rules of interpretation/lead II monitoring (Figure 2-39):

Rate—more than 100

Rhythm—irregular

Pacemaker site—ectopic sites in atria

P waves—organized, discrete nonsinus P waves with at least three different forms

PR interval—varies

QRS complex—may be less than 0.12 second, normal, or greater than 0.20 second, depending on the AV node's refractory status when the impulse reaches it

Clinical significance Frequently, these patients are acutely ill; this arrhythmia may indicate a serious underlying medical illness.

Treatment Treatment of the underlying medical disease usually resolves the arrhythmia. Specific antiarrhythmic therapy is not frequently required.

Premature Atrial Contractions

Description *Premature atrial contractions (PACs)* result from a single electrical impulse originating in the atria outside the SA node, which, in turn, causes a premature depolarization of the heart before the next expected sinus beat. Because it depolarizes the atrial syncytium, this impulse also depolarizes the SA node, interrupting the normal cadence. This creates a **noncompensatory pause** in the underlying rhythm.

Etiology A premature atrial contraction can result from any of the following conditions:

- Use of caffeine, nicotine, or alcohol
- Sympathomimetic drugs
- Ischemic heart disease
- Hypoxia
- Digitalis toxicity
- No apparent cause (idiopathic)

Rules of interpretation/lead II monitoring (Figure 2-40):

Rate—depends on the underlying rhythm

Rhythm—depends on the underlying rhythm; usually regular except for the PAC

Pacemaker site—ectopic focus in the atrium

P waves—the P wave of the PAC differs from the P wave of the underlying rhythm. It occurs earlier than the next expected P wave and may be hidden in the preceding T wave.

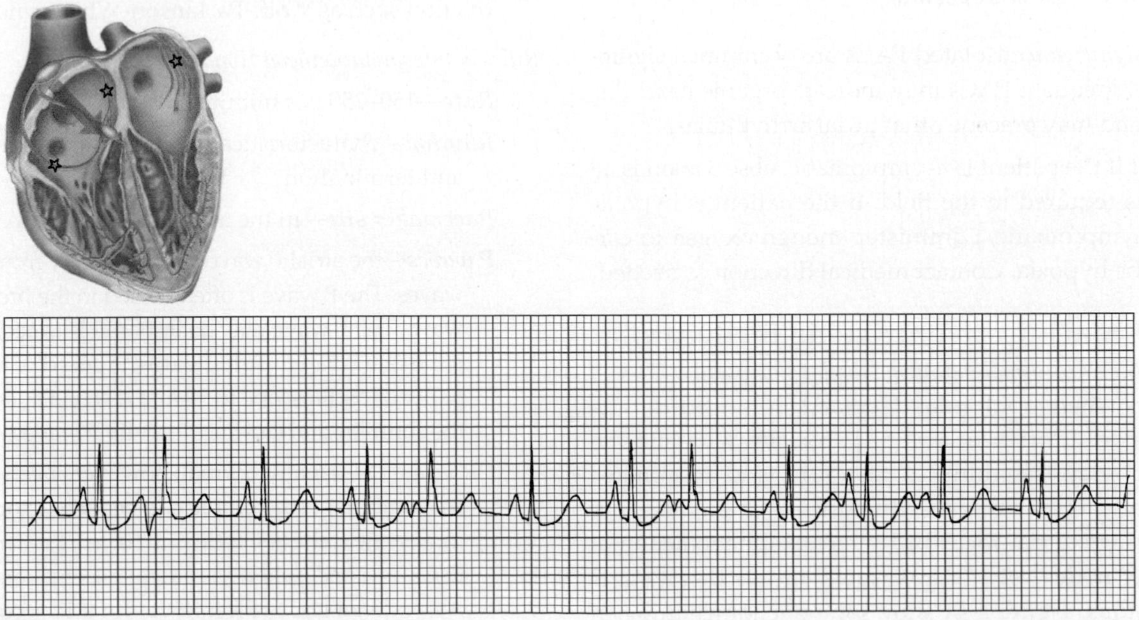

FIGURE 2-39 Multifocal atrial tachycardia.

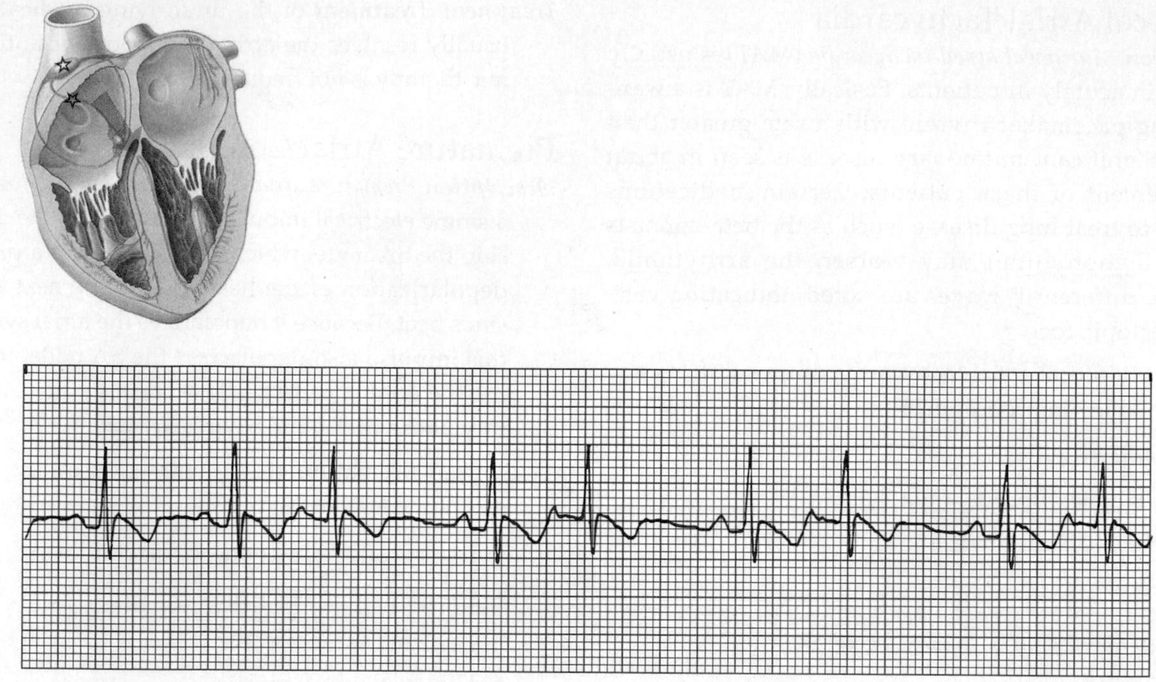

FIGURE 2-40 Premature atrial contractions.

PR interval—usually normal; can vary with the location of the ectopic focus. Ectopic foci near the SA node will have a PR interval of 0.12 second or greater, whereas ectopic foci near the AV node will have a PR interval of 0.12 second or less.

QRS complex—usually normal; may be greater than 0.12 second if the PAC is abnormally conducted through partially refractory ventricles. In some cases, the ventricles are refractory and will not depolarize in response to the PAC. In these cases, the QRS complex is absent.

Clinical significance Isolated PACs are of minimal significance. Frequent PACs may indicate organic heart disease and may precede other atrial arrhythmias.

Treatment If the patient is asymptomatic, observation is all that is required in the field. If the patient is hypoxic and symptomatic, administer enough oxygen to correct the hypoxia. Contact medical direction as needed.

Paroxysmal Supraventricular Tachycardia

Description *Paroxysmal supraventricular tachycardia (PSVT)* occurs when rapid atrial depolarization overrides the SA node. It often occurs in paroxysm with sudden onset, may last minutes to hours, and terminates abruptly. It may be caused by increased automaticity of a single atrial focus or by reentry phenomenon at the AV node. *Note:* "Paroxysmal" means that it starts and stops. Figure 2-41 shows the phenomenon when the paroxysm is active. Often, the paroxysms would *not* be seen on a rhythm strip. To diagnose PSVT, the paroxysms must be seen.

Etiology Paroxysmal supraventricular tachycardia may occur at any age and often is not associated with underlying heart disease. It may be precipitated by stress, overexertion, smoking, or ingestion of caffeine. It is, however, sometimes associated with underlying atherosclerotic cardiovascular disease and rheumatic heart disease. PSVT is rare in patients with myocardial infarction. It can occur with accessory pathway conduction such as Wolff-Parkinson-White syndrome.

Rules of interpretation/lead II monitoring:

Rate—150–250 per minute

Rhythm—characteristically regular, except at onset and termination

Pacemaker site—in the atria, outside the SA node

P waves—the atrial P waves differ slightly from sinus P waves. The P wave is often buried in the preceding T wave. The P wave may be impossible to see, especially if the rate is rapid. Turning up the speed of the graph paper or oscilloscope to 50 mm/second spreads out the complex and can help identify P waves.

PR interval—usually normal; however, it can vary with the location of the ectopic pacemaker. Ectopic pacemakers near the SA node will have PR intervals close to 0.12 second, whereas ectopic pacemakers near the AV node will have PR intervals of 0.12 second or less.

QRS complex—normal

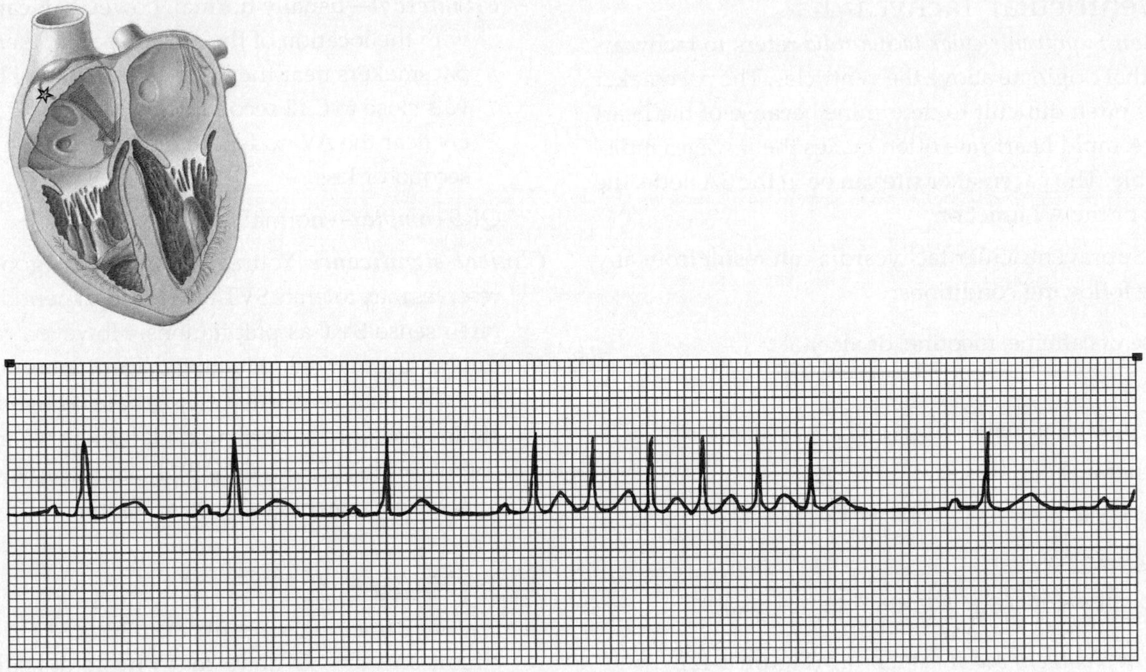

FIGURE 2-41 Paroxysmal atrial (supraventricular) tachycardia.

Clinical significance Young patients with good cardiac reserves may tolerate PSVT well for short periods. Patients often sense PSVT as palpitations. However, rapid rates can cause a marked reduction in cardiac output because of inadequate ventricular filling time. The reduced diastolic phase of the cardiac cycle can also compromise coronary artery perfusion. PSVT can precipitate angina, hypotension, or congestive heart failure.

Treatment If the patient is stable, obtain a 12-lead ECG, establish IV access, and do the following:

1. ***Vagal maneuvers.*** Ask the patient to perform a Valsalva maneuver. This is a forced expiration against a closed glottis, or the act of "bearing down" as if to move the bowels. This results in vagal stimulation, which may slow the heart. If this is unsuccessful, attempt carotid artery massage, if the patient is eligible. Do not attempt carotid artery massage in patients with carotid **bruits** or known cerebrovascular or carotid artery disease.
2. ***Pharmacological therapy.*** Adenosine (Adenocard) is safe and highly effective in terminating PSVT, especially if its etiology is reentry. Administer 6 mg of adenosine by rapid IV bolus over 1 to 3 seconds through the medication port closest to the patient's heart or central circulation. (Adenosine has a very short half-life, and you must immediately follow administration with a bolus of normal saline to allow the medication to reach its site of action while it is still effective.) If the patient does not convert after 1 to 2 minutes, administer a second bolus of 12 mg over 1 to 3 seconds in the medication port closest to the patient's heart or central circulation. If this fails and the patient has a normal blood pressure, then look again at the width of the cardiac QRS. Discerning narrow-complex tachycardia from wide-complex tachycardia can be difficult. It is sometimes helpful to look at lead V_1 (or MCL_1) to determine whether the arrhythmia is actually a narrow- or wide-complex tachycardia. In many instances, a narrow-complex tachycardia will be complicated by a bundle branch block, which can be more apparent in these leads. This determination is important, as the treatments are considerably different for the two arrhythmias. If the patient has a narrow-complex tachycardia and is stable, provide supportive care. If the patient becomes unstable, it is prudent to proceed with synchronized cardioversion.

If the patient is unstable (e.g., altered mental status, ongoing chest pain, hypotension, or other signs of shock), do the following:

1. ***Electrical therapy.*** Use synchronized cardioversion (described later in the chapter) if the rate is greater than 150 beats per minute. If time allows, sedate the patient and apply synchronized DC countershock of 50 to 100 joules (or biphasic equivalent). If this is unsuccessful, repeat the countershock at increased energy (200 joules monophasic, 120 joules biphasic) as ordered by medical direction. DC countershock is contraindicated if you suspect digitalis toxicity as the PSVT's cause.

Supraventricular Tachycardia

Description *Supraventricular tachycardia* refers to tachycardias that originate above the ventricles. The pacemaker site is often difficult to determine because of the heart rate. A rapid heart rate often makes the P waves indiscernible. The pacemaker site can be in the SA node, the atria, or the AV junction.

Etiology Supraventricular tachycardia can result from any of the following conditions:

- Use of caffeine, nicotine, or alcohol
- Cocaine
- Sympathomimetic drugs
- Ischemic heart disease
- Hypoxia
- Digitalis toxicity
- No apparent cause (idiopathic)

Rules of interpretation/lead II monitoring (Figure 2-42):

Rate—150–250 per minute

Rhythm—characteristically regular, except at onset and termination

Pacemaker site—in the atria, outside the SA node

P waves—The P wave may be impossible to see, especially if the rate is rapid. Turning up the speed of the graph paper or oscilloscope to 50 mm/second spreads out the complex and can help identify P waves.

PR interval—usually normal; however, it can vary with the location of the ectopic pacemaker. Ectopic pacemakers near the SA node will have PR intervals close to 0.12 second, whereas ectopic pacemakers near the AV node will have PR intervals of 0.12 second or less.

QRS complex—normal

Clinical significance Young patients with good cardiac reserves may tolerate SVT well for short periods. Patients often sense SVT as palpitations. However, rapid rates can cause a marked reduction in cardiac output because of inadequate ventricular filling time. The reduced diastolic phase of the cardiac cycle can also compromise coronary artery perfusion. SVT can precipitate angina, hypotension, or congestive heart failure.

Atrial Flutter

Description *Atrial flutter* results from a rapid atrial reentry circuit and an AV node that physiologically cannot conduct all impulses through to the ventricles. The AV junction may allow impulses in a 1:1 (rare), 2:1, 3:1, or 4:1 ratio or greater, resulting in a discrepancy between atrial and ventricular rates. The AV block may be consistent or variable.

Etiology Atrial flutter may occur in normal hearts, but it is usually associated with organic disease. It rarely occurs as the direct result of an MI. Atrial dilation, which occurs with congestive heart failure, is a cause of atrial flutter.

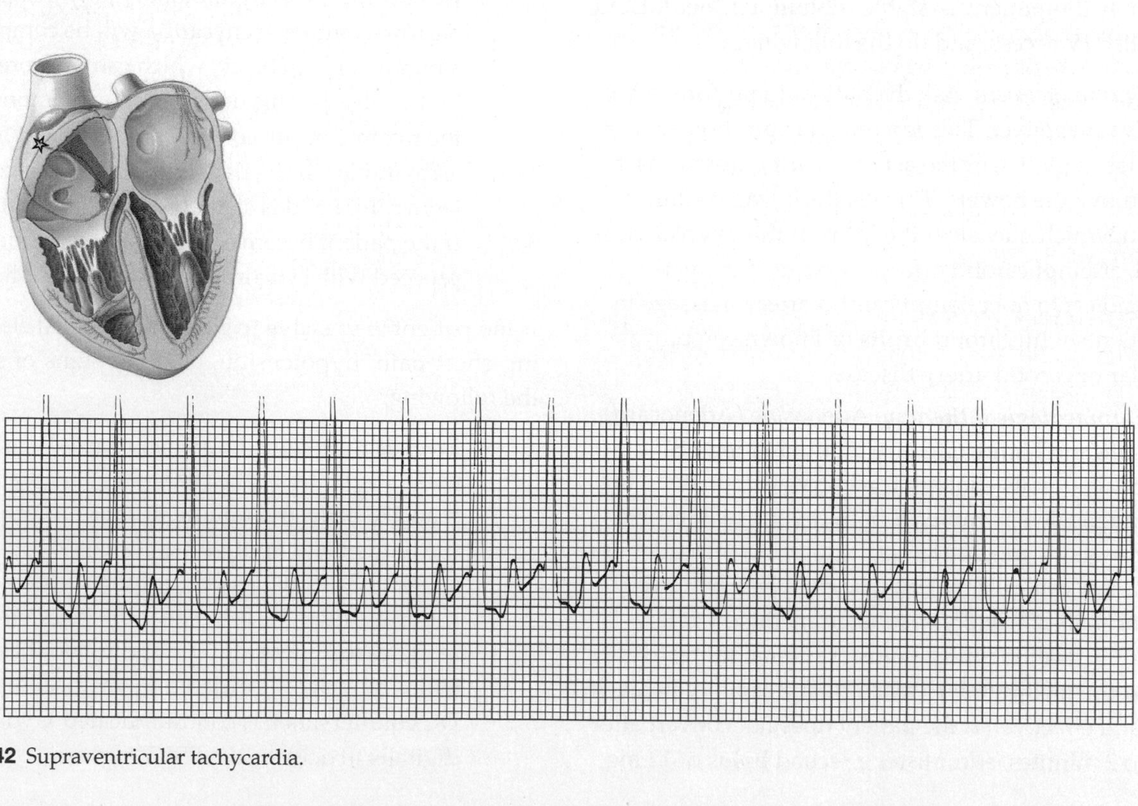

FIGURE 2-42 Supraventricular tachycardia.

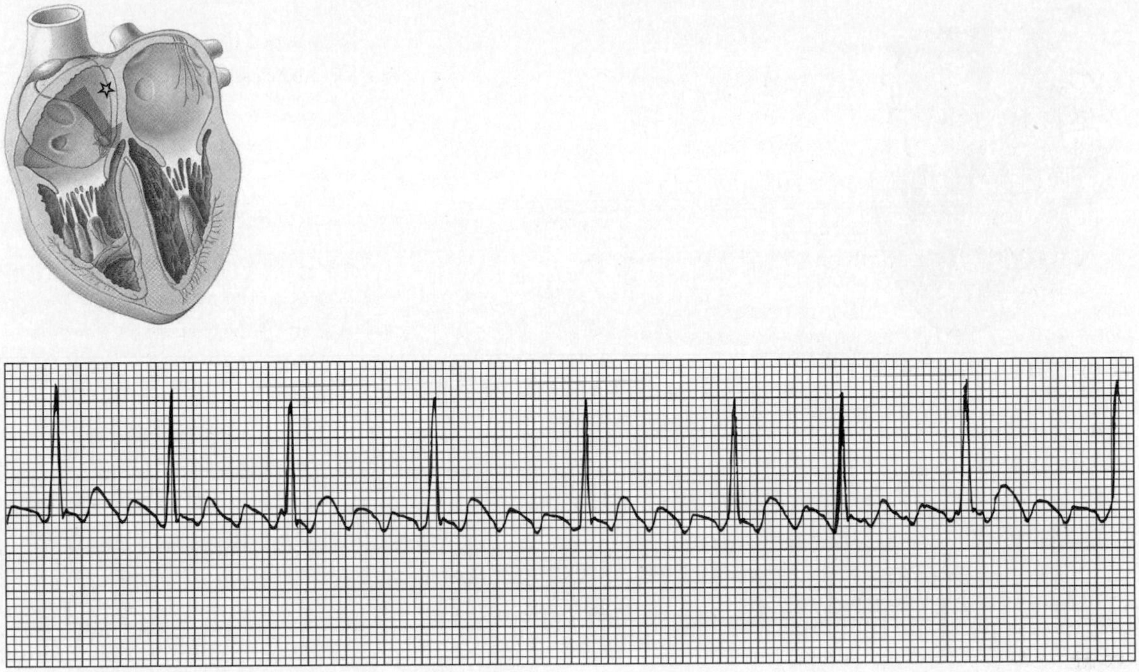

FIGURE 2-43 Atrial flutter.

Rules of interpretation/lead II monitoring (Figure 2-43):

Rate—atrial rate is 250–350 per minute. Ventricular rate varies with the ratio of AV conduction.

Rhythm—atrial rhythm is regular; ventricular rhythm is usually regular, but can be irregular if the block is variable.

Pacemaker site—sites in the atria outside the SA node

P waves—flutter (F) waves are present, resembling a sawtooth or picket-fence pattern. This pattern is often difficult to identify in a 2:1 flutter. However, if the ventricular rate is approximately 150, suspect 2:1 flutter.

PR interval—usually constant but may vary

QRS complex—normal

Clinical significance Atrial flutter with normal ventricular rates is generally well tolerated. Rapid ventricular rates may compromise cardiac output and result in symptoms. Atrial flutter often occurs in conjunction with atrial fibrillation and is referred to as "atrial fib-flutter."

Treatment If the patient is stable, obtain a 12-lead ECG, establish IV access, and do the following:

Pharmacological therapy—Consider rate control with diltiazem or beta-blockers if the patient is unstable (e.g., altered mental status, ongoing chest pain, hypotension or other signs of shock).

Electrical therapy—Use synchronized cardioversion (described later in the chapter) if the rate is greater than 150 beats per minute. If time allows, sedate the patient and apply synchronized DC countershock of 50 to 100 joules (or biphasic equivalent).

Atrial Fibrillation

Description *Atrial fibrillation* results from multiple areas of reentry within the atria or from multiple ectopic foci bombarding an AV node that physiologically cannot handle all the incoming impulses. AV conduction is random and highly variable. It is the most common sustained cardiac arrhythmia.

Etiology Atrial fibrillation may be chronic and is often associated with underlying heart disease such as rheumatic heart disease, atherosclerotic heart disease, or congestive heart failure. Atrial dilation occurs with congestive heart failure and often causes atrial fibrillation. Atrial fibrillation is often classified as follows:

- *First detected episode.* The patient has no known history of atrial fibrillation prior to the current episode.
- *Recurrent arrhythmia.* The patient has a known history of atrial fibrillation prior to the current episode.
- *Paroxysmal.* The arrhythmia is self-terminating.
- *Persistent.* Continues until medical treatment is provided.
- *Permanent.* Continues for more than a year despite medical treatment.

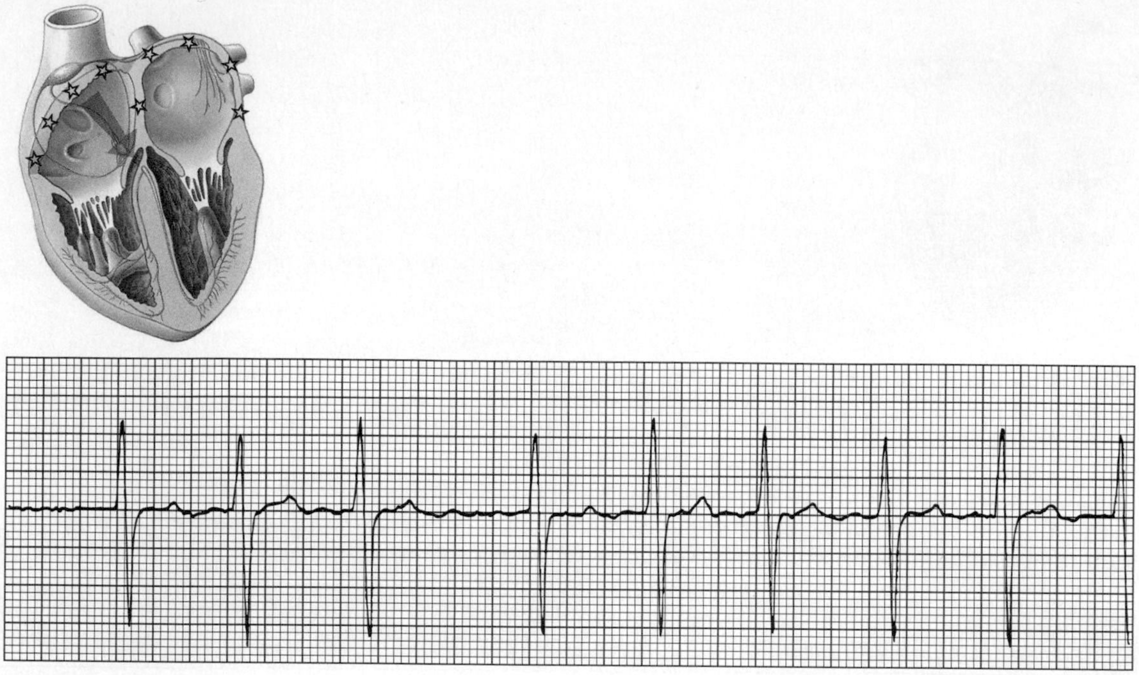

FIGURE 2-44 Atrial fibrillation.

Rules of interpretation/lead II monitoring (Figure 2-44):

Rate—atrial rate is 350–750 per minute (cannot be counted); ventricular rate varies greatly, depending on conduction through the AV node.

Rhythm—irregularly irregular

Pacemaker site—numerous ectopic foci in the atria

P waves—none discernible. Fibrillation (f) waves are present, indicating chaotic atrial activity.

PR interval—none

QRS complex—normal

Clinical significance In atrial fibrillation, the atria fail to contract and the so-called atrial kick is lost, thus reducing cardiac output by 20 to 25 percent. There is frequently a *pulse deficit* (a difference between the apical and peripheral pulse rates). If the rate of ventricular response is normal, as often occurs in patients on digitalis, the rhythm is usually well tolerated. If the ventricular rate is less than 60, cardiac output can fall. Suspect digitalis toxicity in patients taking digitalis with atrial fibrillation and a ventricular rate less than 60. If the ventricular response is rapid, coupled with the loss of atrial kick, cardiovascular decompensation may occur, resulting in hypotension, angina, infarct, congestive heart failure, or shock. Atrial fibrillation is often characterized by the associated ventricular rate (e.g., atrial fibrillation with a rapid ventricular response).

Treatment If the patient is stable, obtain a 12-lead ECG, establish IV access, and do the following:

Pharmacological therapy—Consider rate control with diltiazem or beta-blockers.

If the patient is unstable (e.g., altered mental status, ongoing chest pain, hypotension, or other signs of shock), do the following:

Electrical therapy—Use synchronized cardioversion (described later in the chapter) if the rate is greater than 150 beats per minute. If time allows, sedate the patient and apply synchronized DC countershock of 50 to 100 joules (or biphasic equivalent).

Arrhythmias Originating within the AV Junction (AV Blocks)

Two potential problems in the AV junction (or AV node) may result in arrhythmias. One is an atrioventricular (AV) block, in which the electrical impulse is slowed or blocked as it passes through the AV node. The other is arrhythmias due to a malfunction of AV junctional cells themselves.

The AV junction is an important part of the conductive system, serving two important physiologic purposes (Figure 2-45). First, it effectively slows the impulse between the atria and the ventricles to allow for atrial emptying and ventricular filling. Second, it serves as a backup pacemaker if the SA node or cells higher in the conductive system fail to fire. Parts of the AV tissues function as a pacemaker node and other parts serve as the junction between the atria and the ventricles.

The internodal fibers that blend to form the AV junction are called *transitional fibers*. These small fibers slow the impulse. The transitional fibers then blend into the AV junction. The lower portion of the AV node penetrates the fibrous tissue that separates the atria from the ventricles.

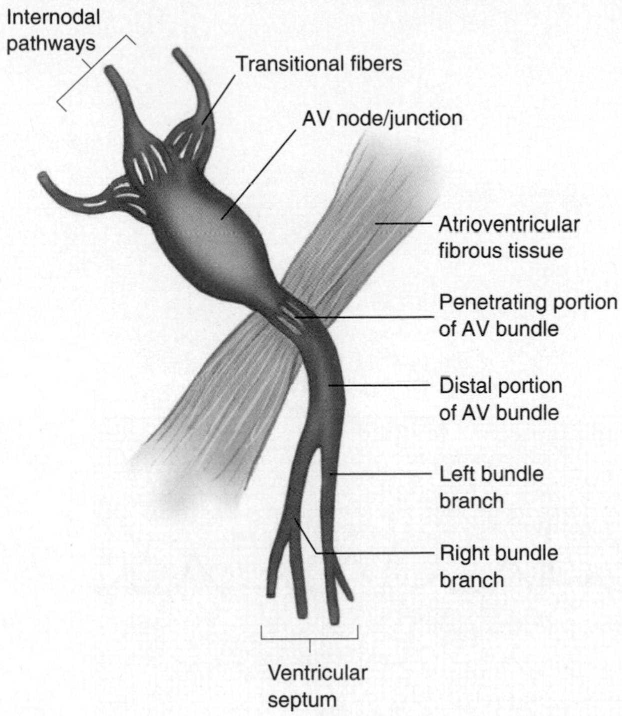

FIGURE 2-45 Organization of the AV node.

This part of the node also slows impulse conduction. After penetrating the fibrous band, the AV node then becomes the AV bundle, which is also called the bundle of His. The bundle of His subsequently divides into the left and right bundle branches.

Atrioventricular Blocks

An *AV block* delays or interrupts impulses between the atria and the ventricles. These arrhythmias can be caused by pathology of the AV junctional tissue or by a physiologic block, such as occurs with atrial fibrillation or flutter. Their causes include AV junctional ischemia, AV junctional necrosis, degenerative disease of the conductive system, and drug toxicity (particularly from digitalis).

AV blocks can be classified according to the site or the degree of the block. Blocks may occur at the following sites:

- At the AV node
- At the bundle of His
- Below the bifurcation of the bundle of His

Our discussion classifies AV blocks by the following degrees (traditional classification):

- First-degree AV block
- Type I second-degree AV block (Mobitz I, or Wenckebach)
- Type II second-degree AV block (Mobitz II, or infranodal)
- 2:1 AV block
- Third-degree AV block

First-Degree AV Block

Description A *first-degree AV block* is a delay in conduction at the level of the AV node rather than an actual block. First-degree AV block is not a rhythm in itself, but a condition superimposed on another rhythm. The underlying rhythm must also be identified (for example, sinus bradycardia with first-degree AV block).

Etiology AV block can occur in the healthy heart. However, ischemia at the AV junction is the most common cause.

Rules of interpretation/lead II monitoring (Figure 2-46):

Rate—depends on underlying rhythm

Rhythm—usually regular; can be slightly irregular

Pacemaker site—SA node or atria

P waves—normal

PR interval—greater than 0.20 second (diagnostic)

QRS complex—usually less than 0.12 second; may be bizarre in shape if conductive system disease exists in the ventricles

Clinical significance First-degree block is usually no danger in itself. However, a newly developed first-degree block may precede a more advanced block.

Treatment Generally, no treatment is required except observation, unless the heart rate drops significantly. If possible, avoid drugs that slow AV conduction, such as lidocaine and procainamide.

Type I Second-Degree AV Block

Description A *type I second-degree AV block* (also called *second-degree Mobitz I*, or *Wenckebach*) is an intermittent block at the level of the AV node. It produces a characteristic cyclic pattern in which the PR intervals become progressively longer until an impulse is blocked (not conducted). The cycle is repetitive, and the P-P interval remains constant. The ratio of conduction (P waves to QRS complexes) is commonly 5:4, 4:3, 3:2, or 2:1. The pattern may be constant or variable.

Etiology Low-grade AV blocks (first-degree and second-degree Mobitz I) can occur in the healthy heart. However, ischemia at the AV junction is the most common cause. Increased parasympathetic tone and drugs are also common etiologies.

Rules of interpretation/lead II monitoring (Figure 2-47):

Rate—atrial rate is unaffected; the ventricular rate may be normal or slowed.

Rhythm—atrial rhythm is typically regular; ventricular rhythm is irregular because of the nonconducted beat

Pacemaker site—SA node or atria

P waves—normal; some P waves are not followed by QRS complexes.

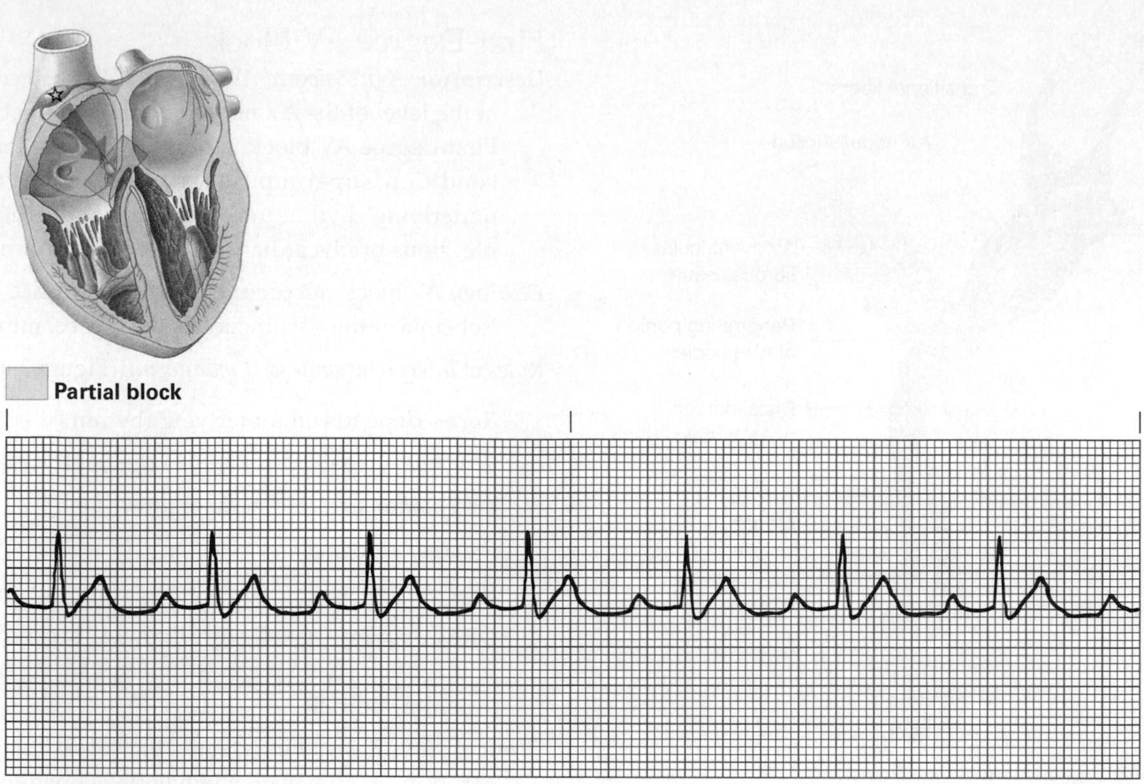

FIGURE 2-46 First-degree AV block.

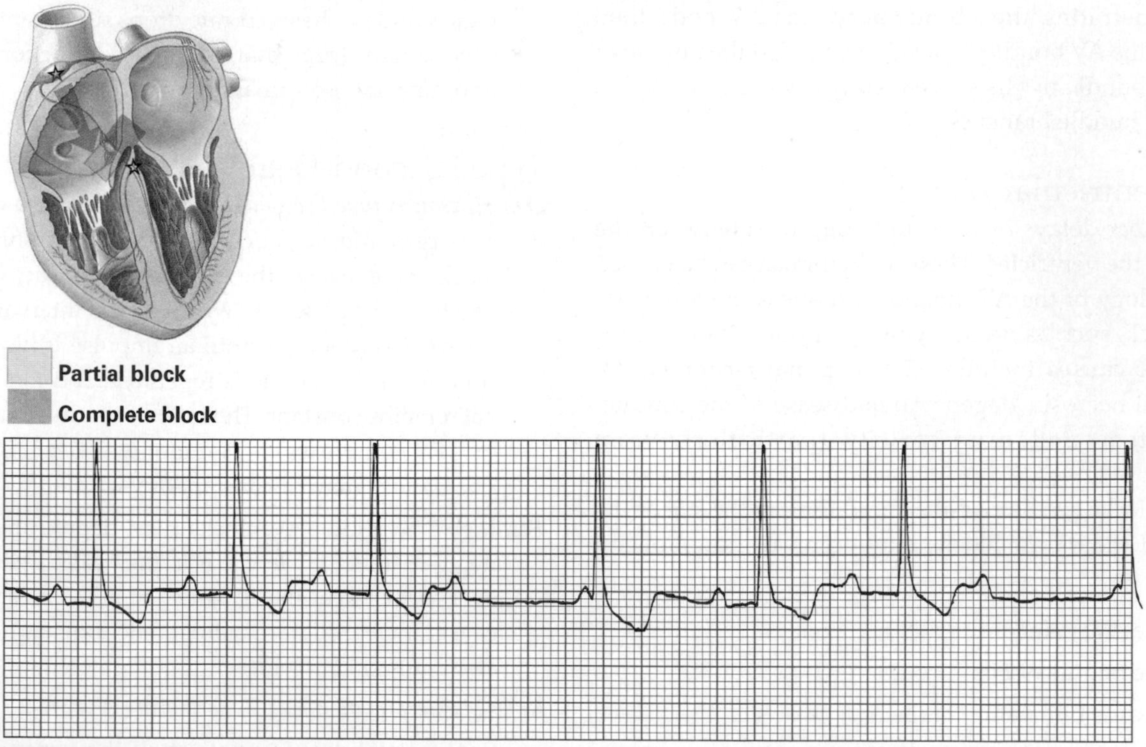

FIGURE 2-47 Type I second-degree AV block.

PR interval—becomes progressively longer until the QRS complex is dropped; the cycle then repeats.

QRS complex—usually less than 0.12 second; may be bizarre in shape if conductive system disease exists in the ventricles

Clinical significance If beats are frequently dropped, second-degree block can compromise cardiac output by causing problems such as syncope and angina. This block is often a transient phenomenon that occurs immediately after an inferior wall myocardial infarction.

Treatment Generally, no treatment other than observation is required. If possible, avoid drugs that slow AV conduction, such as lidocaine and procainamide. If the heart rate falls and the patient becomes symptomatic, administer 0.5 mg of atropine IV. Repeat every 3 to 5 minutes until you have obtained a satisfactory rate or have given 3.0 mg of the drug. If atropine fails, consider transcutaneous cardiac pacing (TCP) or catecholamine infusion.

Type II Second-Degree AV Block

Description A *type II second-degree AV block* (also called *second-degree Mobitz II,* or *infranodal*) is an intermittent block characterized by P waves that are not conducted to the ventricles, but without associated lengthening of the PR interval before the dropped beats. The ratio of conduction (P waves to QRS complexes) is commonly 4:1, 3:1, or 2:1. The ratio may be constant or may vary. A 2:1 Mobitz II block is often indistinguishable from a 2:1 Mobitz I block.

Etiology Second-degree AV block, Mobitz II, is usually associated with acute myocardial infarction and septal necrosis.

Rules of interpretation/lead II monitoring (Figure 2-48):

Rate—atrial rate is unaffected; ventricular rate is usually bradycardic

Rhythm—regular or irregular, depending on whether the conduction ratio is constant or varied

Pacemaker site—SA node or atria

P waves—normal; some P waves are not followed by QRS complexes.

PR interval—constant for conducted beats; may be greater than 0.20 second.

QRS complex—may be normal; however, it is often greater than 0.12 second because of abnormal ventricular depolarization sequence.

Clinical significance A Mobitz II block can compromise cardiac output, causing problems such as syncope and angina if beats are frequently dropped. Because this block is often associated with cell necrosis resulting from myocardial infarction, it is considered much more serious than Mobitz I. Many Mobitz II blocks develop into full AV blocks.

Treatment Treatment is generally unnecessary unless signs of poor perfusion (e.g., acute altered mental status, ongoing chest pain, hypotension or other signs of shock) are present. If there are signs of poor perfusion, prepare for transcutaneous pacing. Consider administering a 0.5-mg bolus of atropine sulfate. Repeat every 3 to 5 minutes until you have obtained a satisfactory rate or have given 3.0 mg of the drug. If atropine fails, consider transcutaneous cardiac pacing (TCP) or catecholamine infusion.

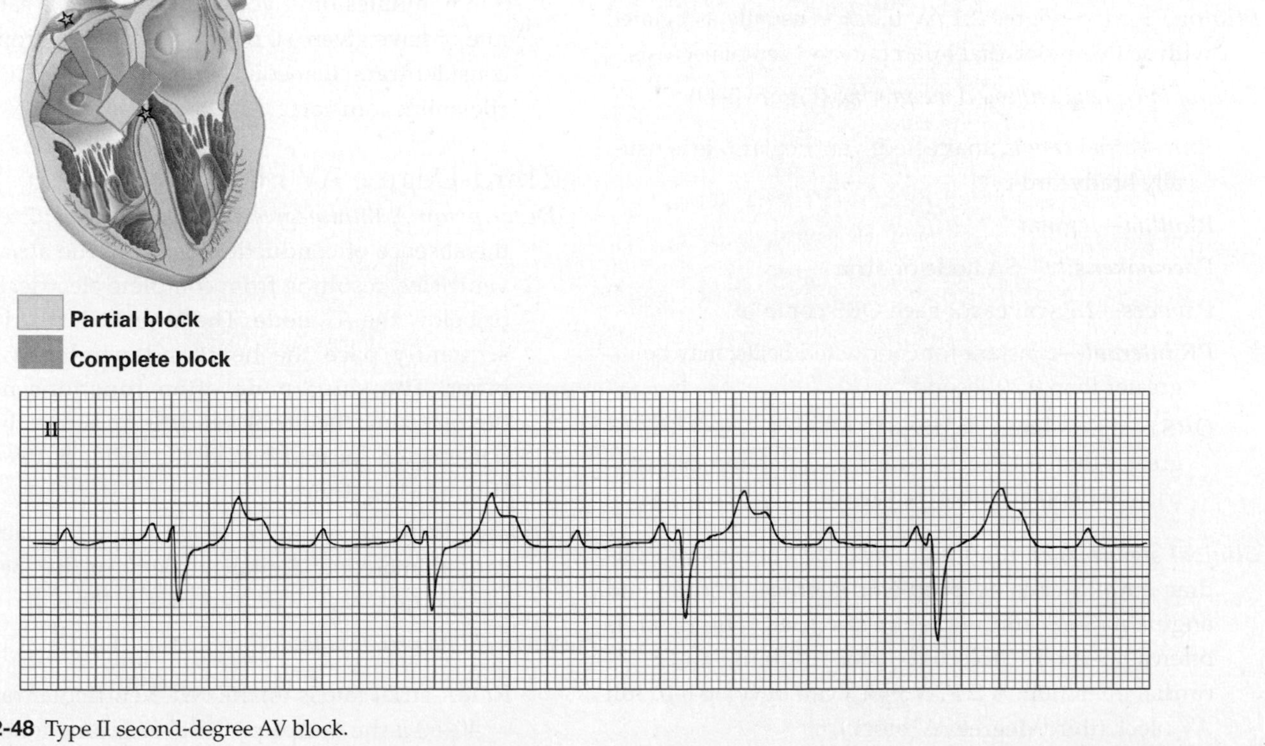

FIGURE 2-48 Type II second-degree AV block.

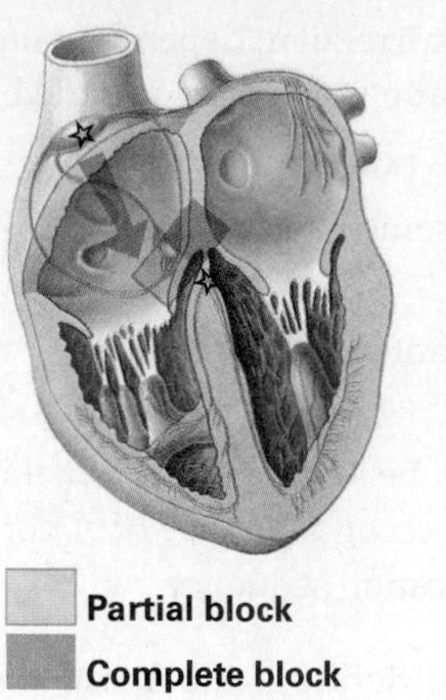

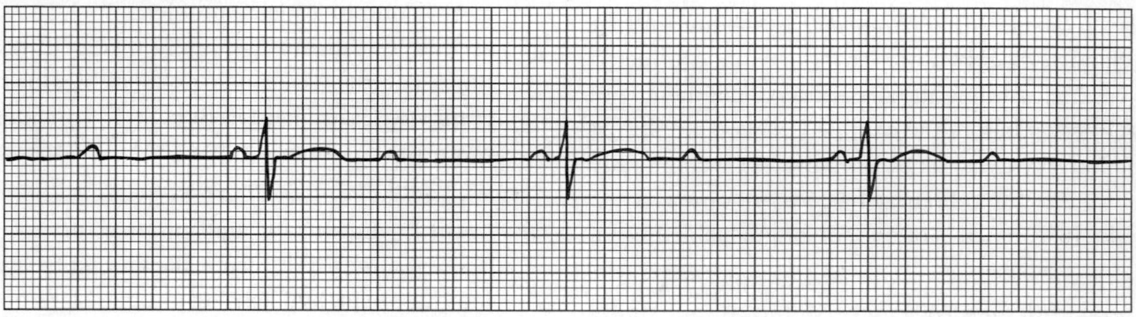

FIGURE 2-49 2:1 AV block.

2:1 AV Block

Description A *2:1 AV block* is a type of second-degree AV block in which there are two P waves for each QRS complex. The first P wave of each pair of P waves is blocked. A 2:1 AV block can result from either a Mobitz I (Wenckebach) or Mobitz II AV block.

Etiology Second-degree 2:1 AV block is usually associated with acute myocardial infarction and septal necrosis.

Rules of interpretation/lead II monitoring (Figure 2-49):

Rate—atrial rate is unaffected; ventricular rate is usually bradycardic

Rhythm—regular

Pacemaker site—SA node or atria

P waves—2 P waves for each QRS complex

PR interval—constant for conducted beats; may be greater than 0.20 second

QRS complex—may be normal; however, it is often greater than 0.12 second because of abnormal ventricular depolarization sequence.

Clinical significance A 2:1 AV block can compromise cardiac output, causing problems such as syncope and angina if beats are frequently dropped. This block is often associated with cell necrosis resulting from myocardial infarction. A 2:1 AV block can develop into full AV block (third-degree AV block).

Treatment Treatment is generally unnecessary unless signs of poor perfusion (e.g., acute altered mental status, ongoing chest pain, hypotension or other signs of shock) are present. If there are signs of poor perfusion, prepare for transcutaneous pacing. Consider administering a 0.5-mg bolus of atropine sulfate. Repeat every 3 to 5 minutes until you have obtained a satisfactory rate or have given 3.0 mg of the drug. If atropine fails, consider transcutaneous cardiac pacing (TCP) or catecholamine infusion.

Third-Degree AV Block

Description A *third-degree AV block,* or *complete block,* is the absence of conduction between the atria and the ventricles, resulting from complete electrical block at or below the AV node. The atria and ventricles subsequently pace the heart independently of each other. The sinus node often functions normally, depolarizing the atrial syncytium, while the escape pacemaker, located below the atria, paces the ventricular syncytium.

Etiology Third-degree AV block can result from acute myocardial infarction, digitalis toxicity, or degeneration of the conductive system, as occurs in the elderly.

Rules of interpretation/lead II monitoring (Figure 2-50):

Rate—atrial rate is unaffected. Ventricular rate is 40–60 if the escape pacemaker is junctional, less

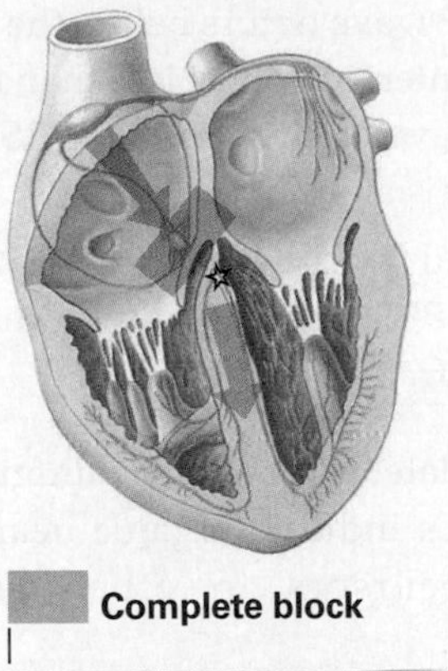

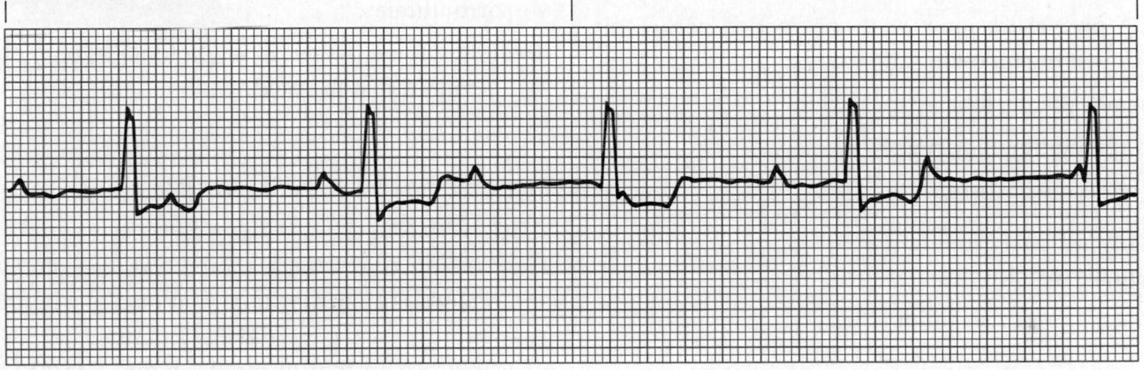

FIGURE 2-50 Third-degree AV block.

than 40 if the escape pacemaker is lower in the ventricles.

Rhythm—both atrial and ventricular rhythms are usually regular.

Pacemaker site—SA node and AV junction or ventricle

P waves—normal. P waves show no relationship to the QRS complex, often falling within the T wave and QRS complex.

PR interval—no relationship between P waves and R waves

QRS complex—greater than 0.12 second if pacemaker is ventricular; less than 0.12 second if pacemaker is junctional

Clinical significance Third-degree block can severely compromise cardiac output because of decreased heart rate and loss of coordinated atrial kick.

Treatment Treatment is generally unnecessary unless signs of poor perfusion (e.g., acute altered mental status, ongoing chest pain, hypotension or other signs of shock) are present. If there are signs of poor perfusion, prepare for transcutaneous pacing. Consider administering a 0.5-mg bolus of atropine sulfate. Repeat every 3 to 5 minutes until you have obtained a satisfactory rate or have given 3.0 mg of the drug. If atropine fails, consider transcutaneous cardiac pacing (TCP) or catecholamine infusion.

Arrhythmias Sustained or Originating in the AV Junction

Arrhythmias can originate within the AV node. The location of the pacemaker site will dictate the morphology of the P wave. Ischemia, hypoxia, and other factors have been identified as causes. Arrhythmias originating in the AV junction include:

- Premature junctional contractions
- Junctional escape complexes and rhythm
- Junctional bradycardia
- Accelerated junctional rhythm

All arrhythmias that originate in the AV junction have in common the following ECG features:

- Inverted P waves in lead II, resulting from retrograde depolarization of the atria. The P wave's relation to QRS depolarization depends on the relative timing of atrial and ventricular depolarization. The P wave can occur before the QRS complex if the atria depolarize first, after the QRS if the ventricles depolarize first, or during the QRS if the atria and ventricles depolarize simultaneously. Depolarization of the atria during ventricular depolarization masks the P wave. Some atrial complexes that originate near the AV junction can also result in inverted P waves.
- PR interval of less than 0.12 second
- Normal QRS complex duration

Premature Junctional Contractions

Description *Premature junctional contractions (PJCs)* result from a single electrical impulse originating in the AV node that occurs before the next expected sinus beat. A PJC can result in either a **compensatory pause** or noncompensatory pause, depending on whether the SA node is depolarized. A noncompensatory pause occurs if the premature beat depolarizes the SA node and interrupts the heart's normal cadence. A compensatory pause occurs only if the SA node discharges before the premature impulse reaches it.

Etiology A premature junctional contraction can result from any of the following conditions:

- Use of caffeine, tobacco, or alcohol
- Sympathomimetic drugs
- Ischemic heart disease
- Hypoxia
- Digitalis toxicity
- No apparent cause (idiopathic)

Rules of interpretation/lead II monitoring (Figure 2-51):

Rate—depends on the underlying rhythm

Rhythm—depends on the underlying rhythm; usually regular except for the PJC

Pacemaker site—ectopic focus in the AV junction

P waves—inverted; may appear before or after the QRS complex. P waves can be masked by the QRS complex or be absent.

PR interval—if the P wave occurs before the QRS complex, the PR interval will be less than 0.12 second; if the P wave occurs after the QRS complex, then technically it is an R-P interval.

QRS complex—usually normal; may be greater than 0.12 second if the PJC is abnormally conducted through partial refractory ventricles

Clinical significance Isolated PJCs are of minimal significance. Frequent PJCs indicate organic heart disease and may be precursors to other junctional arrhythmias.

Treatment If the patient is asymptomatic, only observation is required in the field.

Junctional Escape Complexes and Rhythms

Description A *junctional escape beat,* or *junctional escape rhythm,* is an arrhythmia that results when the rate of the primary pacemaker, usually the SA node, is slower than that of the AV node. The AV node then becomes the pacemaker. The AV node usually discharges at its intrinsic rate of 40 to 60 beats per minute. This is a safety mechanism that prevents cardiac standstill.

Etiology Junctional escape rhythm has several etiologies, including increased vagal tone, which can result in SA node slowing, pathological slow SA node discharge, or heart block.

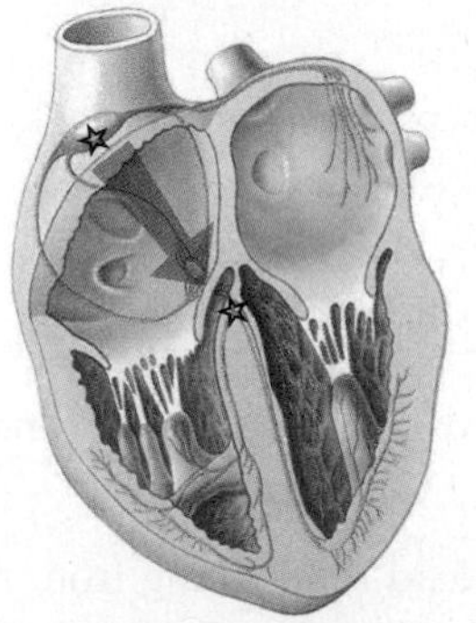

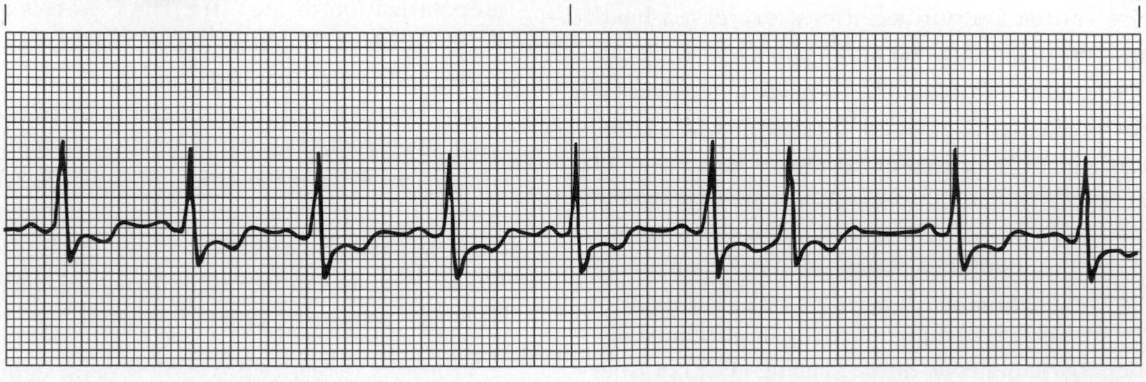

FIGURE 2-51 Premature junctional contractions.

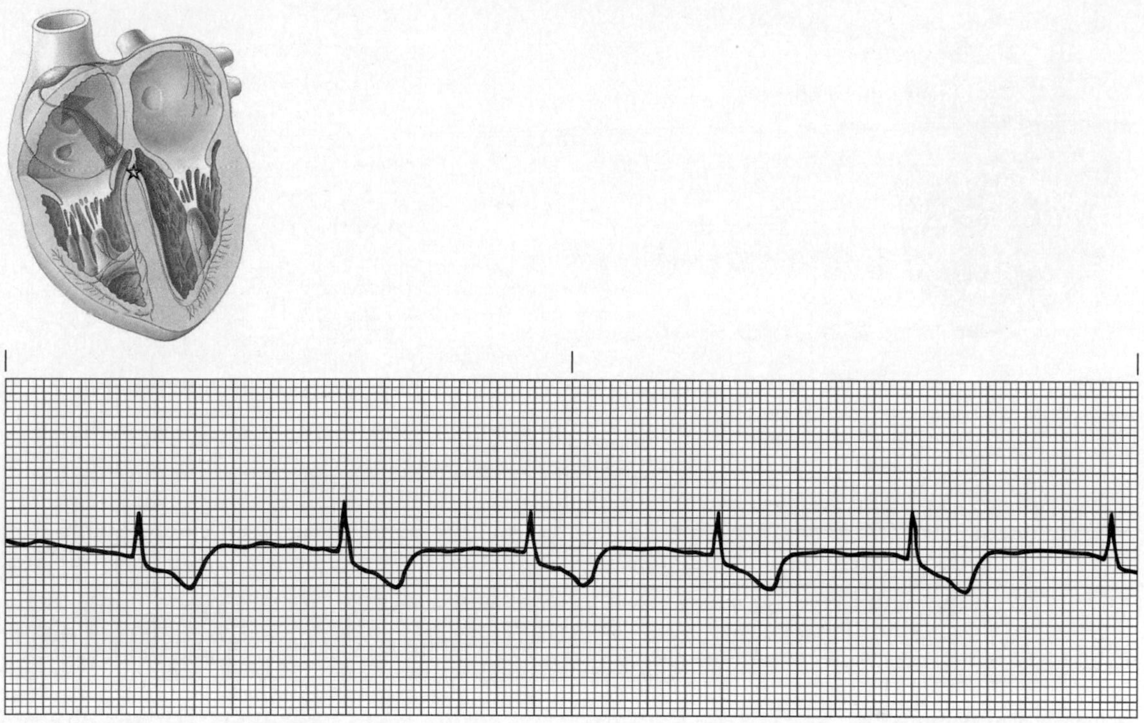

FIGURE 2-52 Junctional escape complex and rhythm.

Rules of interpretation/lead II monitoring (Figure 2-52):

Rate—40–60 per minute

Rhythm—irregular in single junctional escape complex; regular in junctional escape rhythm

Pacemaker site—AV junction

P waves—inverted; may appear before or after the QRS complex. The P waves can be masked by the QRS or be absent.

PR interval—if the P wave occurs before the QRS complex, the PR interval will be less than 0.12 second. If the P wave occurs after the QRS complex, technically it is an R-P interval.

QRS complex—usually normal; may be greater than 0.12 second

Clinical significance The slow heart rate can decrease cardiac output, possibly precipitating angina and other problems. If the rate is fairly rapid, the rhythm can be well tolerated.

Treatment Treatment is generally unnecessary unless signs of poor perfusion (e.g., acute altered mental status, ongoing chest pain, hypotension or other signs of shock) are present. If there are signs of poor perfusion, prepare for transcutaneous pacing. Consider administering a 0.5-mg bolus of atropine sulfate. Repeat every 3 to 5 minutes until you have obtained a satisfactory rate or have given 3.0 mg of the drug. If atropine fails, consider transcutaneous cardiac pacing (TCP) or catecholamine infusion.

Junctional Bradycardia

Description A *junctional bradycardia* is a junctional arrhythmia with a heart rate less than the intrinsic rate of the AV node (40 beats per minute). A slow rate can significantly compromise cardiac output.

Etiology Junctional bradycardias have several etiologies, including increased vagal tone, which can result in SA node slowing, pathological slow SA node discharge, or heart block. Intrinsic disease of the node can also be a cause.

Rules of interpretation/lead II monitoring (Figure 2-53):

Rate—less than 40 per minute

Rhythm—irregular in single junctional escape complex; regular in junctional escape rhythm

Pacemaker site—AV junction

P waves—inverted; may appear before or after the QRS complex. The P waves can be masked by the QRS or be absent.

PR interval—if the P wave occurs before the QRS complex, the PR interval will be less than 0.12 second. If the P wave occurs after the QRS complex, technically it is an R-P interval.

QRS complex—usually normal; may be greater than 0.12 second

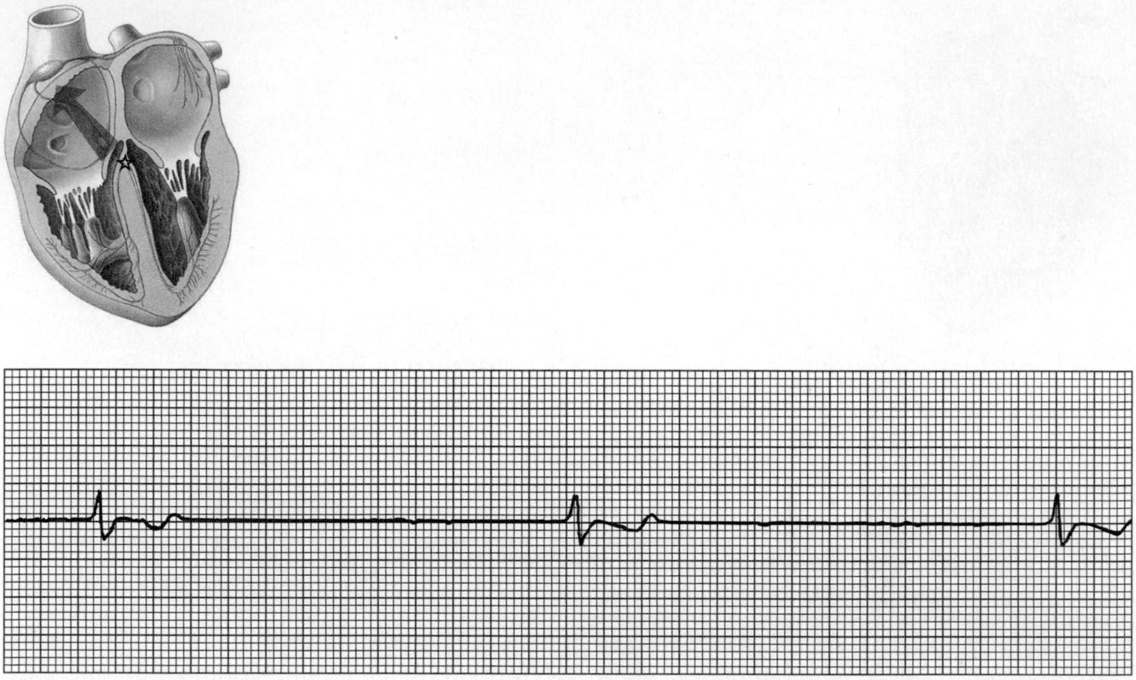

FIGURE 2-53 Junctional bradycardia.

Clinical significance The slow heart rate can decrease cardiac output, possibly precipitating angina and other problems.

Treatment Treatment is generally unnecessary unless signs of poor perfusion (e.g., acute altered mental status, ongoing chest pain, hypotension or other signs of shock) are present. If there are signs of poor perfusion, prepare for transcutaneous pacing. Consider administering a 0.5-mg bolus of atropine sulfate. Repeat every 3 to 5 minutes until you have obtained a satisfactory rate or have given 3.0 mg of the drug. If atropine fails, consider transcutaneous cardiac pacing (TCP) or catecholamine infusion.

Accelerated Junctional Rhythm

Description An *accelerated junctional rhythm* results from increased automaticity in the AV junction, causing the AV junction to discharge faster than its intrinsic rate. If the rate becomes fast enough, the AV node can override the SA node. Technically, the rate associated with an accelerated junctional rhythm is not a tachycardia. However, when compared to the intrinsic rate of the AV junctional tissue (40–60 beats per minute), it is considered accelerated.

Etiology Accelerated junctional rhythms often result from ischemia of the AV junction.

Rules of interpretation/lead II monitoring (Figure 2-54):

Rate—60–100 per minute

Rhythm—regular

Pacemaker site—AV junction

P waves—inverted; may appear before or after the QRS complex. P waves may be masked by the QRS or be absent.

PR interval—if the P wave occurs before the QRS complex, the PR interval will be less than 0.12 second. If it occurs after the QRS, technically it is an R-P interval.

QRS complex—normal

Clinical significance An accelerated junctional rhythm is usually well tolerated. However, because ischemia is often the etiology, the patient should be monitored for other arrhythmias.

Treatment Prehospital treatment generally is unnecessary.

Arrhythmias Originating in the Ventricles

Some arrhythmias originate within the ventricles. The pacemaker site will dictate the morphology of the QRS complex. Many factors, including ischemia, hypoxia, and medications, have been identified as causes. Arrhythmias originating in the ventricles include the following:

- Ventricular escape complexes and rhythms
- Accelerated idioventricular rhythm
- Premature ventricular contraction
- Ventricular tachycardia
- *Torsades de pointes*
- Ventricular fibrillation

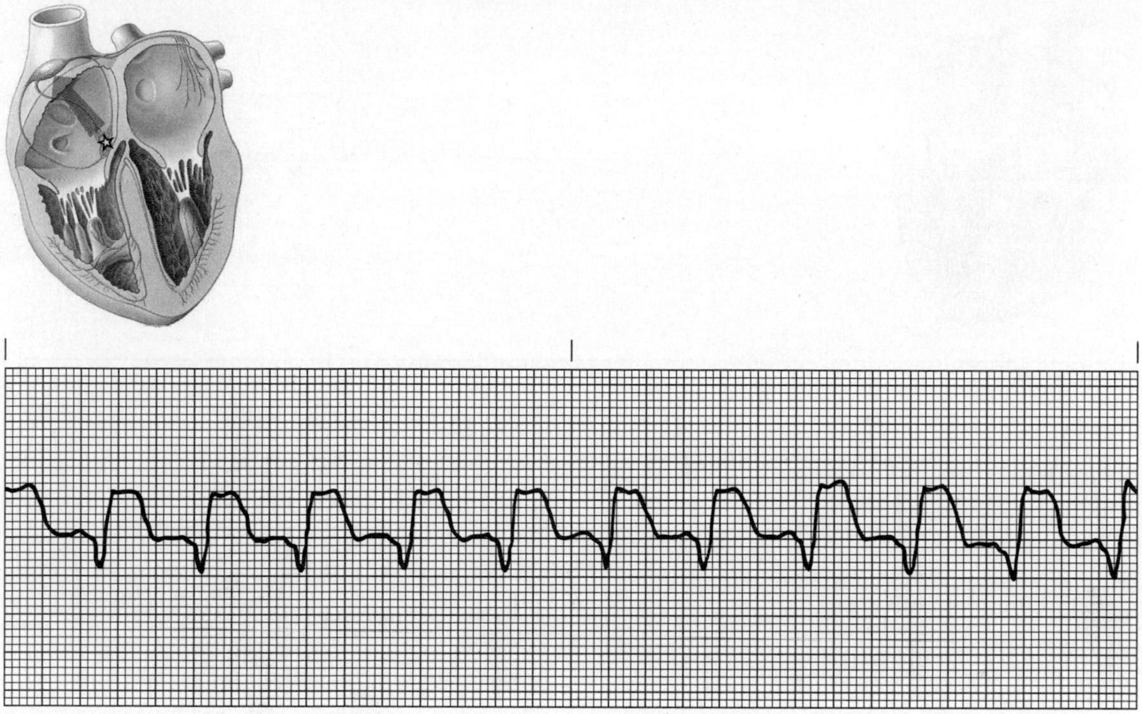

FIGURE 2-54 Accelerated junctional rhythm.

- Asystole
- Artificial pacemaker rhythm

ECG features common to all arrhythmias that originate in the ventricles are:

- QRS complexes of 0.12 second or greater
- Absent P waves

Ventricular Escape Complexes and Rhythms

Description A *ventricular escape beat* (*ventricular escape rhythm* or *idioventricular rhythm*) results either when impulses from higher pacemakers fail to reach the ventricles or when the discharge rate of higher pacemakers becomes less than that of the ventricles (normally 15–40 beats per minute). Ventricular escape rhythms serve as safety mechanisms to prevent cardiac standstill.

Etiology Ventricular escape complexes and ventricular rhythms have several etiologies, including slowing of supraventricular pacemaker sites or high-degree AV block. They are frequently the first organized rhythms seen following successful defibrillation.

Rules of interpretation/lead II monitoring (Figure 2-55):

Rate—15–40 per minute (occasionally less)

Rhythm—the rhythm is irregular in a single ventricular escape complex. Ventricular escape rhythms are usually regular unless the pacemaker site is low in the ventricular conductive system. Such placement makes regularity unreliable.

Pacemaker site—ventricle

P waves—none

PR interval—none

QRS complex—greater than 0.12 second and bizarre in morphology

Clinical significance The slow heart rate can significantly decrease cardiac output, possibly to life-threatening levels (Figure 2-56). The ventricular escape rhythm is a safety mechanism that you should not suppress. Escape rhythms can be perfusing or nonperfusing.

Treatment Treatment is generally unnecessary unless signs of poor perfusion (e.g., acute altered mental status, ongoing chest pain, hypotension or other signs of shock) are present. If there are signs of poor perfusion, prepare for transcutaneous pacing. Consider administering a 0.5-mg bolus of atropine sulfate. Repeat every 3 to 5 minutes until you have obtained a satisfactory rate or have given 3.0 mg of the drug. If atropine fails, consider transcutaneous cardiac pacing (TCP) or a catecholamine infusion. If the rhythm is slow and/or nonperfusing, follow the AHA cardiac arrest protocol. Direct treatment at correcting the primary problem (hypovolemia, hypoxia, cardiac tamponade, acidosis, or others). Consider a fluid challenge.

Accelerated Idioventricular Rhythm

Accelerated idioventricular rhythm is an abnormally wide ventricular arrhythmia that usually occurs during an acute myocardial infarction (Figure 2-57). It is a subtype

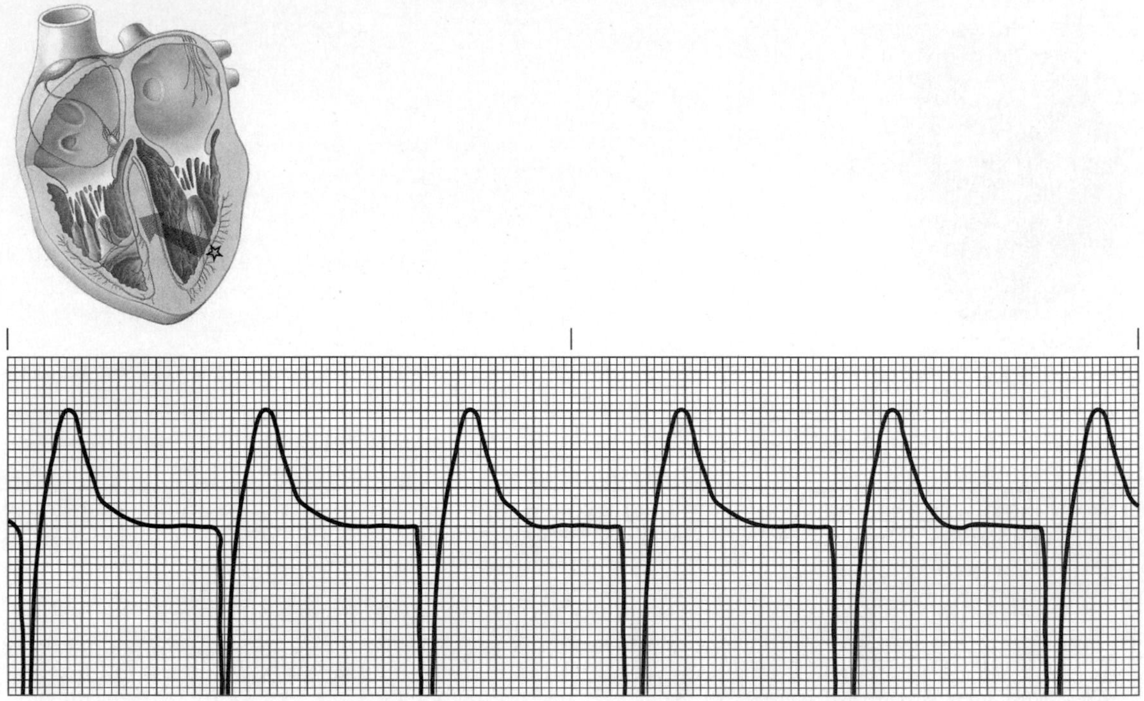

FIGURE 2-55 Ventricular escape rhythm (idioventricular rhythm).

of ventricular escape rhythm. Typically the rate is 60 to 110 beats per minute. The patient does not require treatment unless he becomes hemodynamically unstable. If this occurs, treat the ventricular focus with atropine or overdrive pacing. The principal action should be aggressive treatment of the underlying myocardial infarction as indicated, including appropriate prehospital care.

Premature Ventricular Contractions

Description A *premature ventricular contraction* (*PVC*, or *ventricular ectopic*) is a single ectopic impulse arising from an irritable focus in either ventricle that occurs earlier than the next expected beat (Figure 2-58). It may result from increased automaticity in the ectopic cell or a reentry mechanism. The altered sequence of ventricular depolarization results in a wide and bizarre

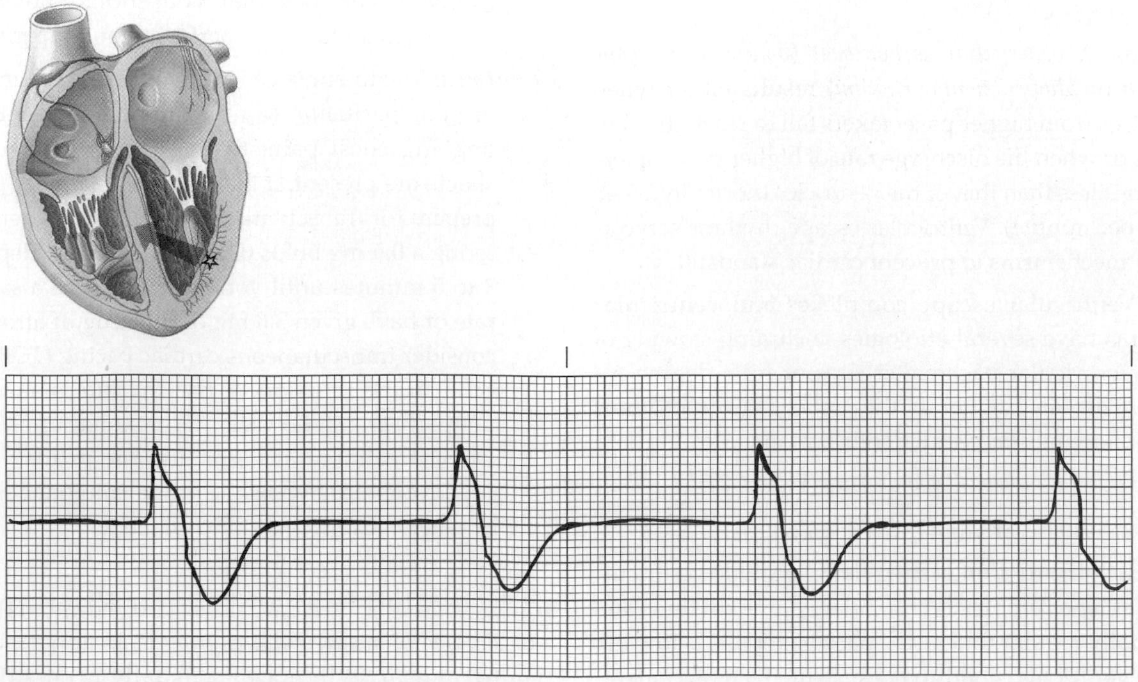

FIGURE 2-56 Idioventricular rhythm.

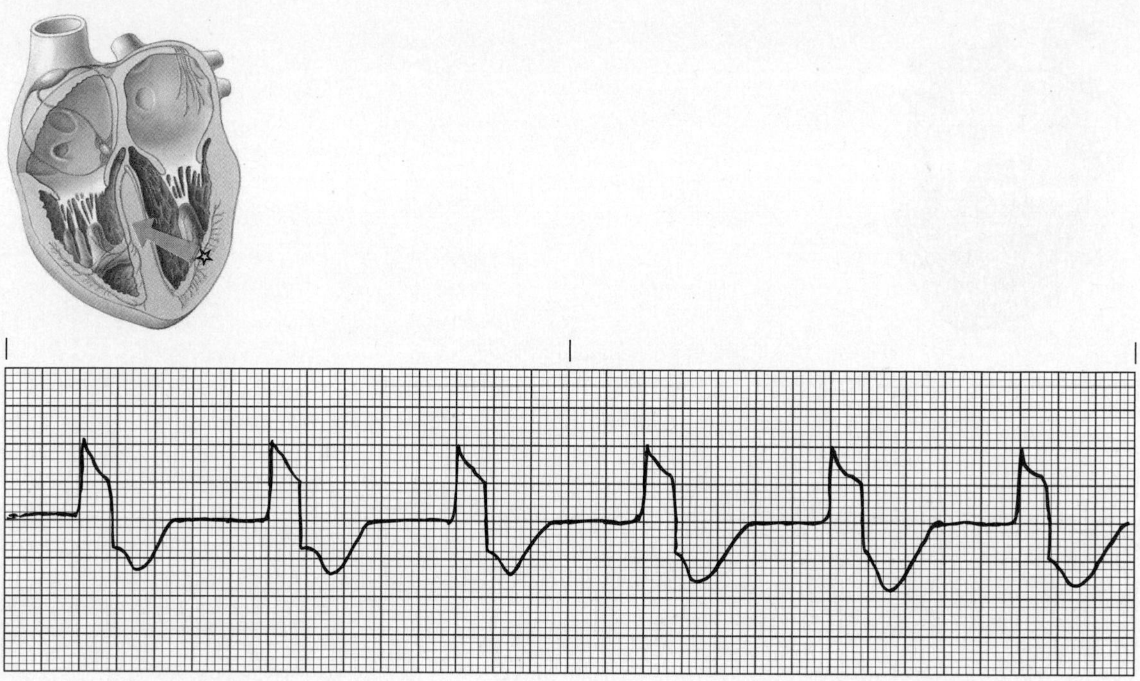

FIGURE 2-57 Accelerated idioventricular rhythm.

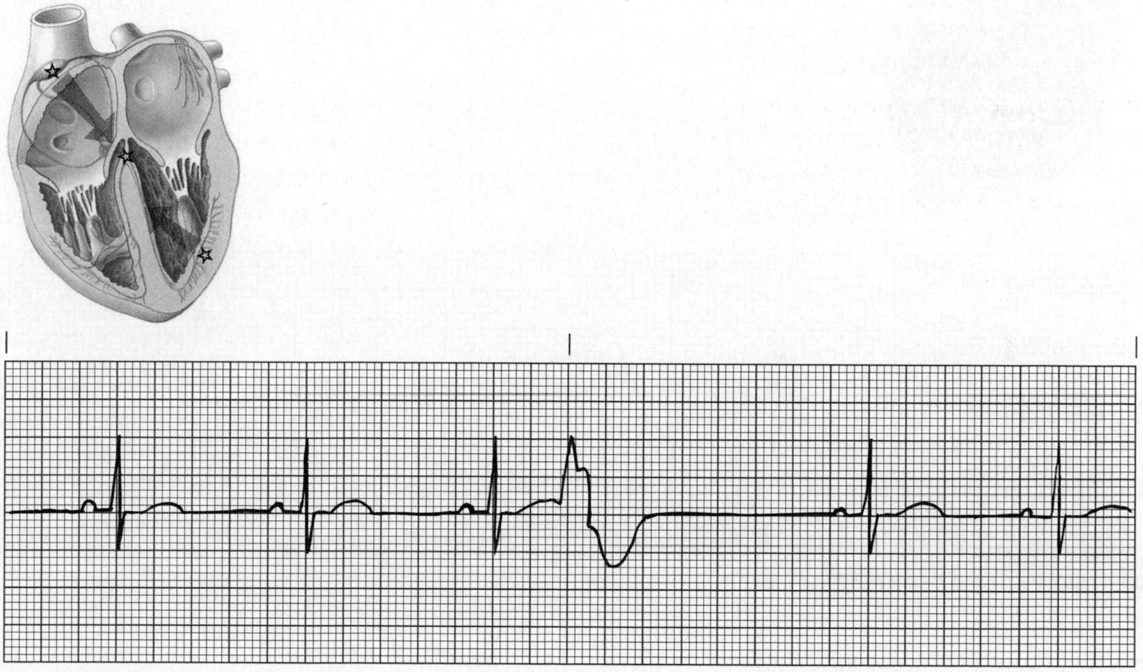

FIGURE 2-58 Premature ventricular contractions.

QRS complex and may additionally cause the T wave to occur in the direction opposite the QRS complex.

A PVC does not usually depolarize the SA node and interrupt its rhythm. That is, it does not interrupt the heart's normal cadence. The pause following the PVC is fully *compensatory*. Occasionally, an **interpolated beat** occurs when a PVC falls between two sinus beats without interrupting the rhythm.

If more than one PVC occurs, each can be classified as unifocal or multifocal (Figure 2-59). Because the PVC's morphology depends on the ectopic pacemaker's location, two PVCs of different morphologies imply two different

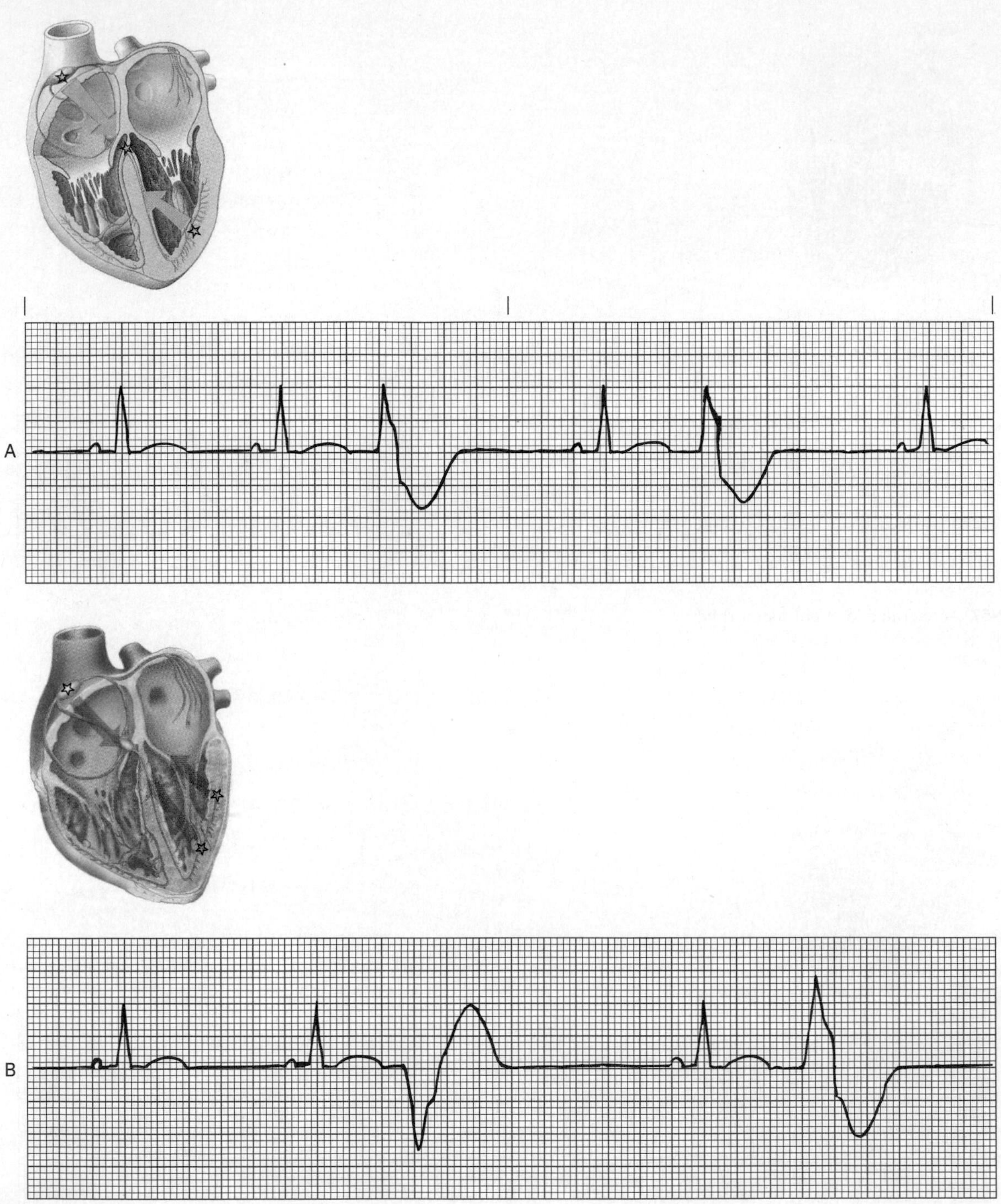

FIGURE 2-59 Unifocal (A) and multifocal (B) PVCs.

pacemaker sites (multifocal). PVCs with the same morphology imply one pacemaker site (unifocal). If the **coupling interval** (the distance between the preceding beat and the PVC) is constant, the PVCs are most likely unifocal.

PVCs often occur in patterns of group beating. These include:

- *Bigeminy*–every other beat is a PVC.
- *Trigeminy*–every third beat is a PVC.
- *Quadrigeminy*–every fourth beat is a PVC.

These terms can be applied to PACs and PJCs as well.

Repetitive PVCs are two consecutive PVCs without a normal complex in between. They can occur in groups of two (couplets) or three (triplets). More than three consecutive PVCs are often considered ventricular tachycardia.

PVCs can trigger lethal arrhythmias such as ventricular fibrillation if they fall within the relative refractory period (the so-called R on T phenomenon). They are often classified by their relationship to the previous normal complex.

Etiologies Etiologies for PVCs include:

- Myocardial ischemia
- Increased sympathetic tone

- Hypoxia
- Idiopathic causes
- Acid–base disturbances
- Electrolyte imbalances
- Normal variant

Rules of interpretation/lead II monitoring:

Rate—depends on underlying rhythm and rate of PVCs

Rhythm—interrupts regularity of underlying rhythm; occasionally irregular

Pacemaker site—ventricle

P waves—none; however, a normal sinus P wave (interpolated P wave) sometimes appears before a PVC.

PR interval—none

QRS complex—greater than 0.12 second and bizarre in morphology

Clinical significance Patients often sense PVCs as "skipped beats." In a patient without heart disease, PVCs may be insignificant. In patients with myocardial ischemia, PVCs may indicate ventricular irritability and may trigger lethal ventricular arrhythmias. PVCs are often classified as malignant or benign. Malignant PVCs have at least one of the following traits:

- More than six PVCs per minute
- R on T phenomenon
- Couplets or runs of ventricular tachycardia
- Multifocal
- Associated chest pain

With most PVCs, the ventricles do not fill adequately. Because of this, you will usually not feel a pulse during the PVCs themselves. Frequent PVCs may reduce cardiac output.

PVCs can be described in terms of the Lown grading system for premature beats. The higher the grade, the more serious the ectopy:

Grade 0 = No premature beats

Grade 1 = Occasional (<30 per hour) PVCs

Grade 2 = Frequent (≥30 per hour) PVCs

Grade 3 = Multiform (multifocal)

Grade 4 = Repetitive (couplets, salvos of three consecutive) PVCs

Grade 5 = R on T phenomenon

Treatment If the patient has no history of cardiac disease and no symptoms, and if the PVCs are nonmalignant, no treatment is required. Administer oxygen (if the patient is hypoxic) and place an IV line. Although it was once common practice to aggressively treat PVCs with antiarrhythmic drugs, research has shown that most treatments were ineffective or harmful. Today, PVCs are rarely treated, with the exception of PVCs that occur during reperfusion therapy, when the myocardium is extremely irritable. Even then, the use of antiarrhythmic drugs in these cases is extremely limited.

Ventricular Tachycardia

Description *Ventricular tachycardia (VT)* consists of three or more ventricular complexes in succession at a rate of 100 beats per minute or more. This rhythm overrides the heart's normal pacemaker, and the atria and ventricles are asynchronous. Sinus P waves may occasionally be seen, dissociated from the QRS complexes. In *monomorphic VT,* the complexes all appear the same; in *polymorphic VT,* they have different sizes and shapes. One example of a polymorphic VT is *torsades de pointes.*

Etiology As with PVCs, etiologies for ventricular tachycardia include:

- Myocardial ischemia
- Increased sympathetic tone
- Hypoxia
- Idiopathic causes
- Acid–base disturbances
- Electrolyte imbalances

Rules of interpretation/lead II monitoring (Figure 2-60):

Rate—100–250 (approximately)

Rhythm—usually regular; can be slightly irregular

Pacemaker site—ventricle

P waves—if present, not associated with the QRS complexes

PR interval—none

QRS complex—greater than 0.12 second and bizarre in morphology

Clinical significance Ventricular tachycardia usually results in poor stroke volume, which, coupled with the rapid ventricular rate, may severely compromise cardiac output and coronary artery perfusion. Whether ventricular tachycardia is perfusing or nonperfusing dictates the type of treatment. Ventricular tachycardia may eventually deteriorate into ventricular fibrillation.

Treatment The treatment of perfusing ventricular tachycardia has changed dramatically in recent years. Perfusing ventricular tachycardia that is causing hypotension, acutely altered mental status, signs of shock, ischemic chest pain, and/or acute heart failure should be treated with synchronized cardioversion. Perfusing

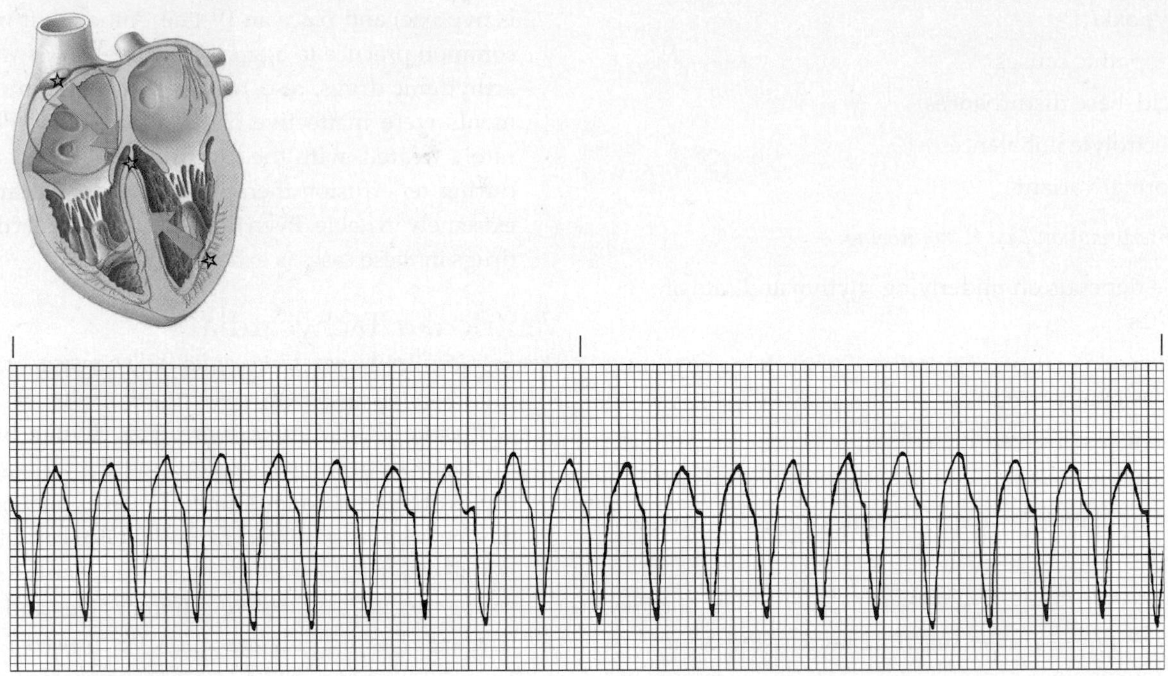

FIGURE 2-60 Ventricular tachycardia.

ventricular tachycardia that is not accompanied by the findings detailed above should be treated with adenosine (if regular and monomorphic) and/or an antiarrhythmic infusion (e.g., procainamide, amiodarone, sotalol). If the patient is nonperfusing, follow the protocol for ventricular fibrillation. Treatment includes defibrillation, epinephrine, and amiodarone.

TORSADES DE POINTES *Torsades de pointes* is a polymorphic ventricular tachycardia that differs in appearance and cause from ventricular tachycardia in general. It is more common in women than men. *Torsades de pointes* is most commonly caused by the use of certain antiarrhythmic drugs, including quinidine (Quinidex), procainamide (Pronestyl), disopyramide (Norpace), flecainide (Tambocor), sotalol (Betapace), and amiodarone (Cordarone). These agents' effects all seem to be exacerbated by the coadministration of certain nonsedating antihistamines, and, in addition, the azole antifungal agents and macrolide antibiotics: erythromycin, azithromycin (Zithromax), and clarithromycin (Biaxin). Any of these agents increase the likelihood of the patient's developing *torsades de pointes*.

The morphology of the QRS varies from beat to beat (hence the term *torsades de pointes*, which means "twisting on a point"). In addition, the QT interval is markedly increased, to 600 milliseconds or more. *Torsades de pointes* will usually occur in bursts that are not sustained. During the "breaks" from these bursts, you should examine the rhythm strip for a prolonged QT interval. The QRS rate is usually between 166 and 300 beats per minute, and the RR interval varies in an irregularly irregular pattern. The QRS complexes are wide and change in size over the span of several complexes (Figure 2-61). Attempting treatment of *torsades de pointes* with antiarrhythmics usually used for the treatment of ventricular tachycardia can have disastrous consequences. Therefore, recognition of *torsades de pointes* as a separate arrhythmia is essential. Treatment is 1 to 2 g of magnesium sulfate administered over 1 to 2 minutes. This can be repeated every 4 hours with close monitoring of the deep tendon reflexes. Ultimately, overdrive pacing may be required. Correct any underlying electrolyte problems, especially hyperkalemia.[4]

Ventricular Fibrillation

Description *Ventricular fibrillation* is a chaotic ventricular rhythm usually resulting from the presence of many reentry circuits within the ventricles. There is no ventricular depolarization or contraction.

Etiology A wide variety of causes have been associated with ventricular fibrillation. Most cases result from advanced coronary artery disease.

Rules of interpretation/lead II monitoring (Figure 2-62):

Rate—no organized rhythm

Rhythm—no organized rhythm

Pacemaker site—numerous ectopic foci throughout the ventricles

P waves—usually absent

PR interval—absent

QRS complex—absent

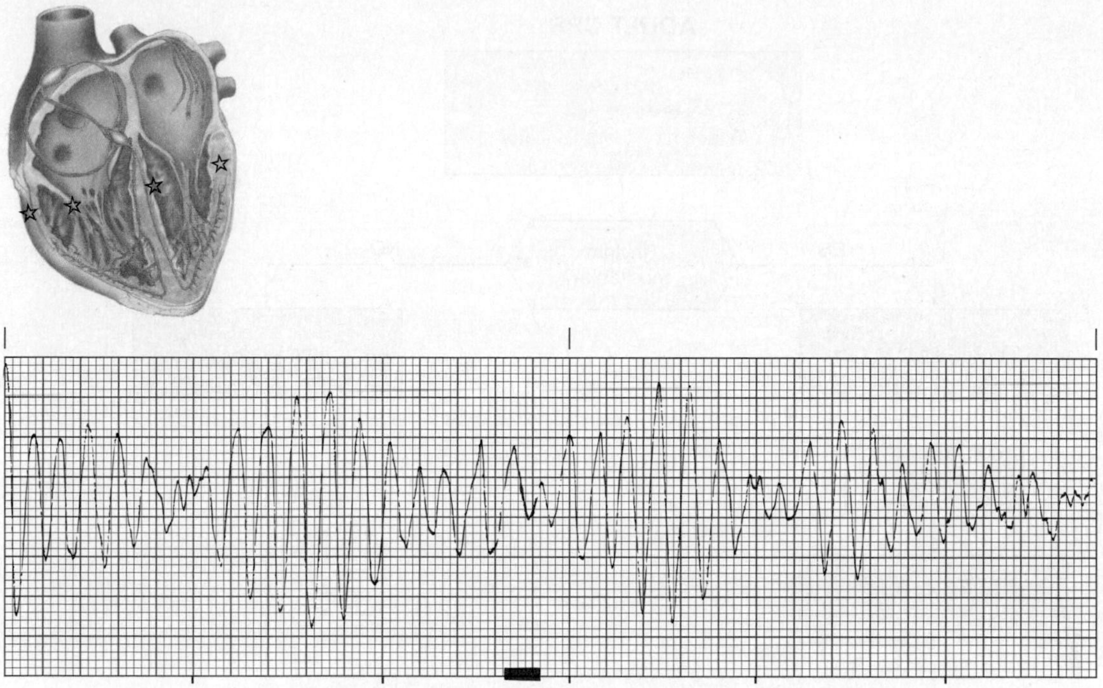

FIGURE 2-61 *Torsades de pointes.*

Clinical significance Ventricular fibrillation is a lethal arrhythmia. The absence of cardiac output or an organized electrical pattern results in cardiac arrest.

Treatment Ventricular fibrillation and nonperfusing ventricular tachycardia are treated identically (Figure 2-63).

Asystole

Description *Asystole (cardiac standstill)* is the absence of all cardiac electrical activity.

Etiology Asystole may be the primary event in cardiac arrest. It is usually associated with massive myocardial infarction, ischemia, and necrosis. Resulting from heart blocks when no escape pacemaker takes over, asystole is often the final outcome of ventricular fibrillation. Often, before all electrical activity is lost, occasional bizarre complexes are seen as the heart dies. This is often referred to as an *agonal rhythm* (Figure 2-64).

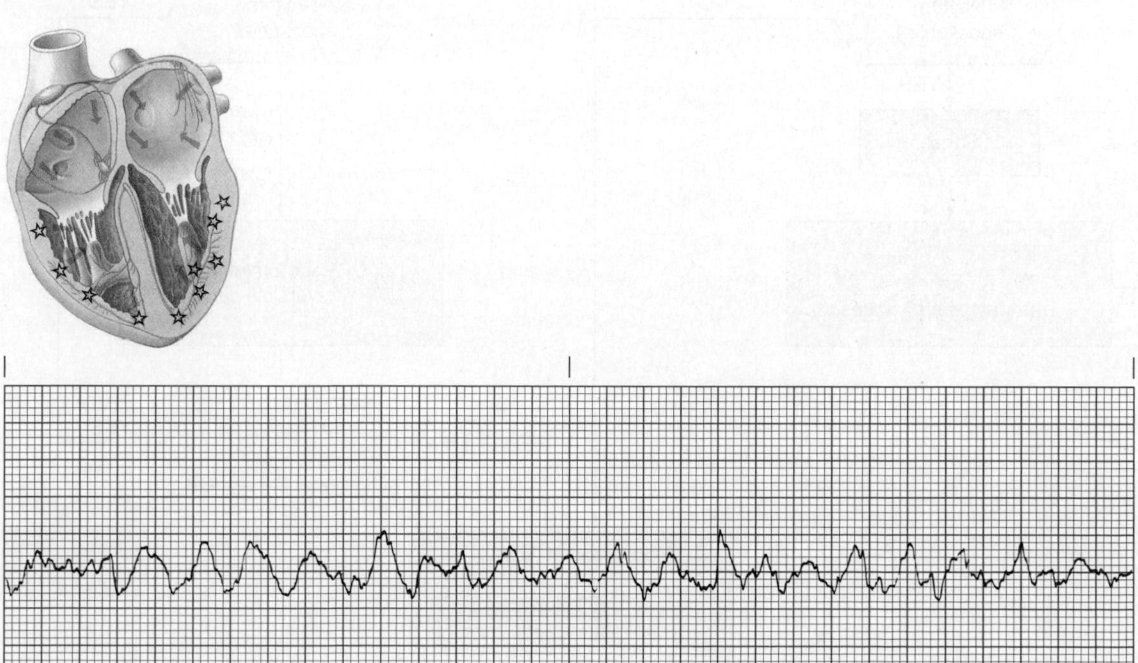

FIGURE 2-62 Ventricular fibrillation.

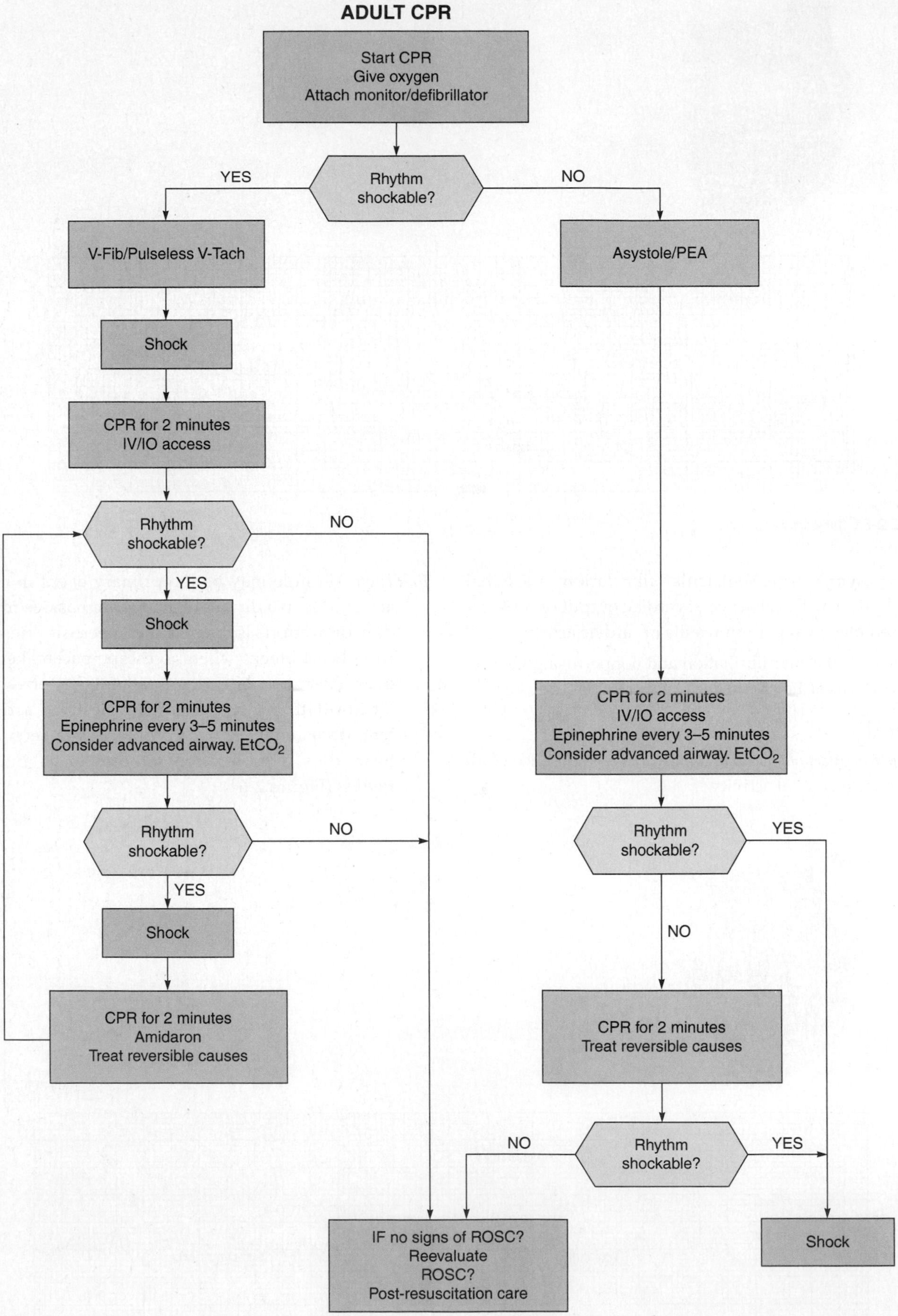

FIGURE 2-63 Treatment of cardiac arrest.

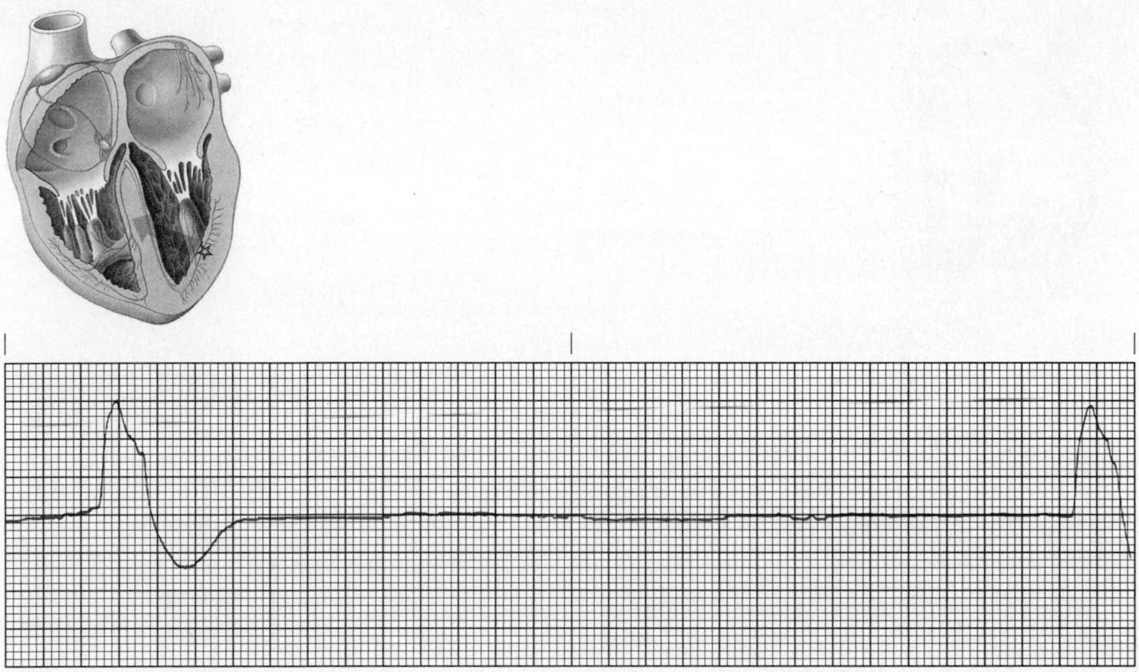

FIGURE 2-64 Agonal rhythm.

Rules of interpretation/lead II monitoring (Figure 2-65):

Rate—no electrical activity

Rhythm—no electrical activity

Pacemaker site—no electrical activity

P waves—usually absent, but in certain cases only P waves will be seen (no QRS complexes) (Figure 2-66).

PR interval—absent

QRS complex—absent

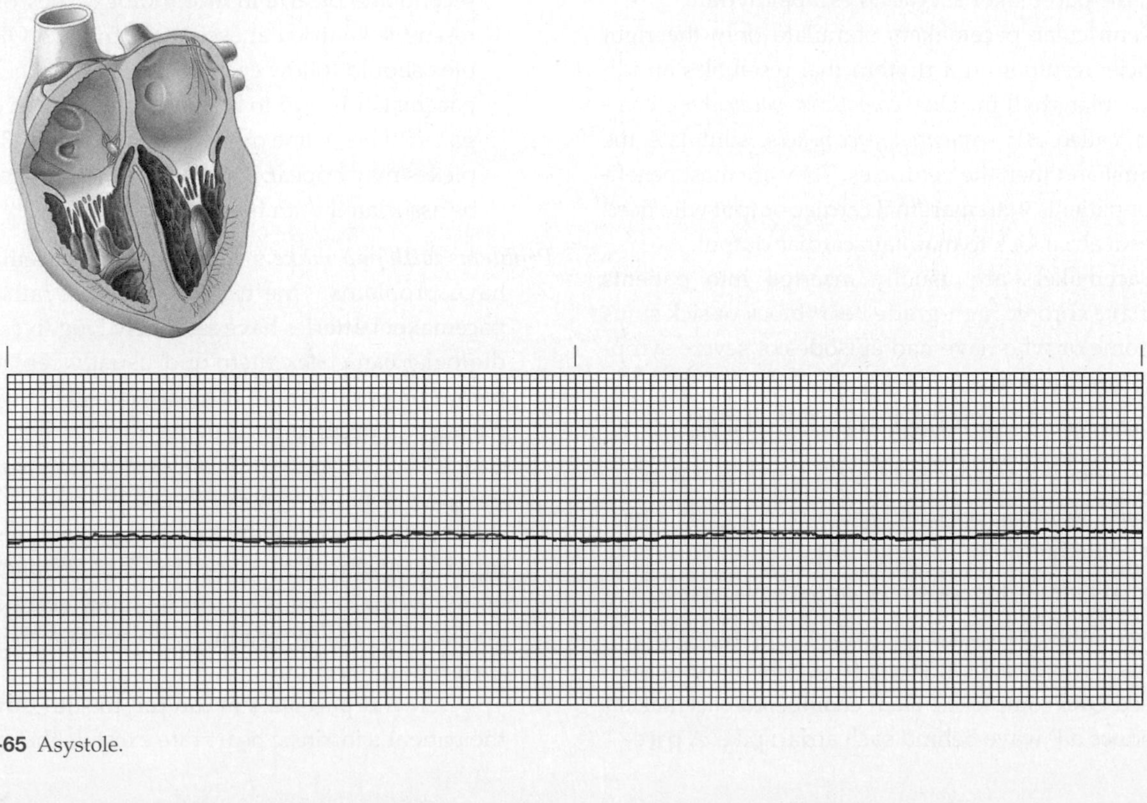

FIGURE 2-65 Asystole.

Clinical significance Asystole results in cardiac arrest. The prognosis for resuscitation is very poor.

Treatment Treat asystole as for all types of cardiac arrest. Look for and, if possible, treat the underlying cause.

Artificial Pacemaker Rhythm

Description An *artificial pacemaker rhythm* results from regular cardiac stimulation by an electrode implanted in the heart and connected to a power source. The pacemaker

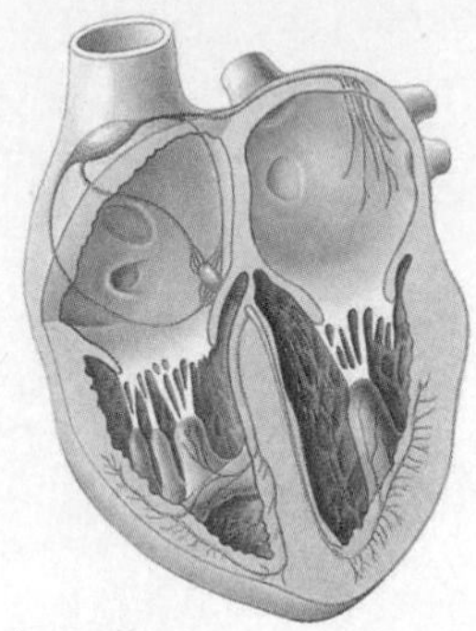

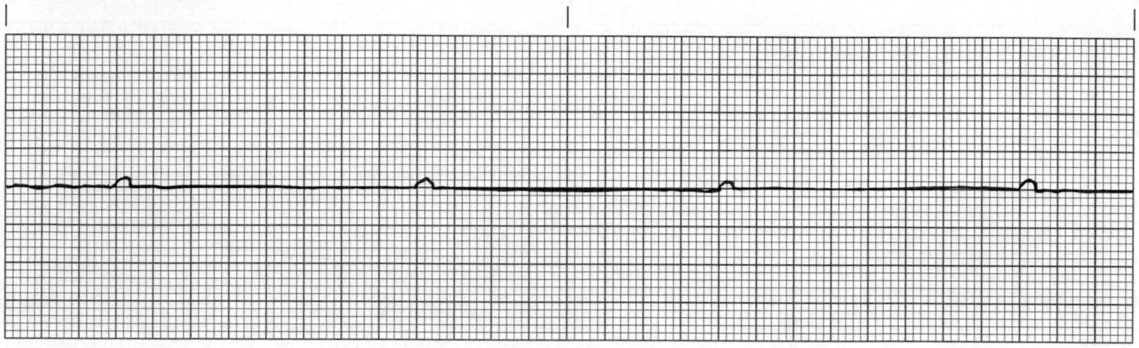

FIGURE 2-66 P wave asystole.

lead may be implanted in any of several locations in the heart, although it is most often placed in the right ventricle (ventricular pacemaker) or in both the right ventricle and the right atria (dual-chambered pacemaker).

Fixed-rate pacemakers fire continuously at a preset rate, regardless of the heart's electrical activity. *Demand pacemakers* contain a sensing device and fire only when the natural heart rate drops below a set rate. In these cases, the pacemaker acts as an escape rhythm.

Ventricular pacemakers stimulate only the right ventricle, resulting in a rhythm that resembles an idioventricular rhythm. *Dual-chambered pacemakers,* commonly called *AV sequential pacemakers,* stimulate the atria first and then the ventricles. They are most beneficial for patients with marginal cardiac output who need the extra atrial kick to maintain cardiac output.

Pacemakers are usually inserted into patients who have chronic high-grade heart block or sick sinus syndrome or who have had episodes of severe symptomatic bradycardia.

Rules of interpretation/lead II monitoring (Figure 2-67):

Rate—varies with the preset rate of the pacemaker

Rhythm—regular if pacing constantly; irregular if pacing on demand

Pacemaker site—depends on electrode placement

P waves—none produced by ventricular pacemakers. Sinus P waves may be seen but are unrelated to the paced QRS complexes. Dual-chambered pacemakers produce a P wave behind each atrial spike. A pacemaker spike is an upward or downward deflection from the baseline, which is an artifact created each time the pacemaker fires. The pacemaker spike tells you only that the pacemaker is firing. It reveals nothing about ventricular depolarization.

PR interval—if present, varies

QRS complex—the QRS complexes associated with pacemaker rhythms are usually longer than 0.12 second and bizarre in morphology. They often resemble ventricular escape rhythms. A QRS complex should follow each pacemaker spike. If so, the pacemaker is said to be "capturing." With demand pacemakers, some of the patient's own QRS complexes may appear. A pacemaker spike should not be associated with these complexes.

Problems with pacemakers Although rare, pacemakers can have problems. One cause is battery failure. Most pacemaker batteries have relatively long lives. The cardiologist can check them and usually replaces them before problems arise. If a battery fails, however, no pacing will occur and the patient's underlying rhythm, which may be bradycardic or asystolic, may return.

Occasionally, a pacemaker can *run away.* This condition, rarely seen with new pacemakers, results in a rapid discharge rate. A runaway pacemaker usually occurs when the battery runs low; newer models compensate for this by gradually increasing their rate as their batteries run low.

Demand pacemakers can fail to shut down when the patient's intrinsic heart rate exceeds the rate set for

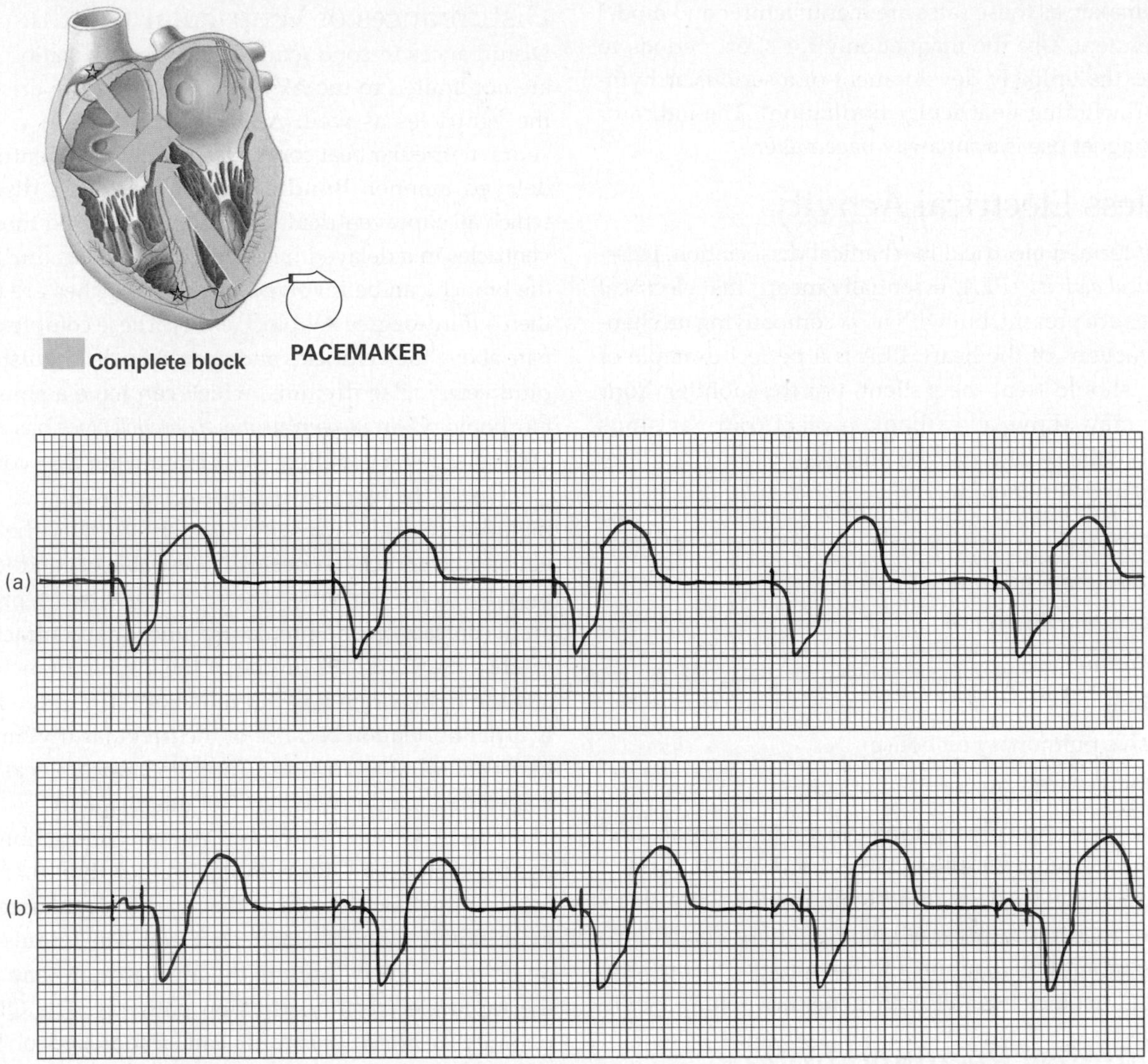

FIGURE 2-67 Artificial pacemaker rhythms: (a) ventricular pacing and (b) dual-chamber pacing.

the device. Thus, the pacemaker competes with the patient's natural pacemaker. Occasionally, a paced beat can fall in the absolute or relative refractory period, precipitating ventricular fibrillation.

Finally, pacemakers can fail to capture if the leads become displaced or the battery fails. In such cases, pacemaker spikes are usually present without P waves or QRS complexes. Bradycardia often results.

Considerations for management Always examine any unconscious patient for a pacemaker. Battery packs are usually palpable under the skin, often in the shoulder or axillary region. Treat bradyarrhythmias, asystole, and ventricular fibrillation from pacemaker failure as in any other patient. Defibrillate patients with pacemakers as usual, but do not discharge the paddles directly over the battery pack. If external cardiac pacing is available, you can use it until definitive care is available. Transport pacemaker failure patients promptly without prolonged field stabilization. Definitive care consists of battery replacement or temporary pacemaker insertion.

Most modern pacemakers can be "interrogated" for information about the device and patient incidents. These interrogations usually take place in a cardiologist's office or in the emergency department. Typically, a sensor or computer "wand" is placed over the pacemaker (on the skin), allowing communication between the device and an external computer. This provides important information such as battery usage and remaining battery life, as well as how often the pacemaker is used or not used. It also indicates whether the leads are still in the proper position and whether the lead wires are intact. It allows adjustment of the power level and other essential parameters.

Use of a magnet Applying a magnet over the pulse generator inhibits all sensing and sets the pacemaker to a predetermined rate (usually 70). The patient should carry a card with information about his particular pacemaker, as these rates are manufacturer and model dependent. Use the magnet only for short periods to avoid the unlikely development of a serious arrhythmia (including ventricular fibrillation). The indicator for magnet use is a runaway pacemaker.

Pulseless Electrical Activity

Formerly termed electrical mechanical dissociation, *pulseless electrical activity (PEA)* essentially means that electrical complexes are present, but with no accompanying mechanical contractions of the heart. PEA is a perfect example of why you should treat the patient, not the monitor. Your monitor may show a textbook perfect, normal sinus rhythm, but the patient may be pulseless.

Causes of PEA include:

- Hypovolemia
- Cardiac tamponade
- Tension pneumothorax
- Hypoxemia
- Acidosis
- Massive pulmonary embolism
- Ventricular wall rupture

Administer epinephrine 1 mg every 3 to 5 minutes and treat the underlying cause(s). Table 2-4 shows suggested treatment for the different underlying causes. Early treatment can potentially reverse some of these conditions; therefore, prompt recognition and initiation of therapy are essential. Outcomes from PEA are generally poor.[4]

Arrhythmias Resulting from Disorders of Conduction

Several arrhythmias result from improper conduction through the heart. The three general categories of conductive disorders are:

- Atrioventricular blocks (discussed earlier in a separate section)
- Disturbances of ventricular conduction
- Preexcitation syndromes

Table 2-4 Suggested Treatment for Underlying Causes of Pulseless Electrical Activity

Condition	Treatment (if allowed by local protocols)
Hypovolemia	Fluids
Cardiac tamponade	Pericardiocentesis
Tension pneumothorax	Needle thoracostomy
Hypoxemia	Intubation/oxygen
Acidosis	Ventilation, consider $NaHCO_3$

Disturbances of Ventricular Conduction

Disturbances in conduction of the depolarization impulse are not limited to the AV node. Problems can arise within the ventricles as well. **Aberrant conduction** is a single supraventricular beat conducted through the ventricles in a delayed manner. **Bundle branch block** is a disorder in which all supraventricular beats are conducted through the ventricles in a delayed manner. Either the left or right bundle branch can be involved. If both branches are blocked, then a third-degree AV block exists. These complexes originate above the ventricles and should be distinguished from pure ventricular rhythms, which can have a similar QRS morphology. An *incomplete bundle branch block* has a normal QRS complex; a complete block has a wide QRS complex.

One of the two known causes of ventricular conduction disturbances is ischemia or necrosis of either the right or left bundle branch, rendering it incapable of conducting the impulse to the ventricle. The second is either a premature atrial contraction or a premature junctional contraction that reaches the ventricles or one of the bundle branches, usually the right, when it is still refractory. This often happens in atrial fibrillation because of the irregular rhythm's varying speed of repolarization. (Bundle branch blocks are discussed in more detail in Part 3 of this chapter.)

The ECG features of ventricular conduction disturbances include a QRS complex longer than 0.12 second because the blocked side of the heart is depolarized much more slowly than the unaffected side. The impulse passes much more slowly through the myocardium than through the rapid electrical conduction pathway. The QRS morphology is often bizarre. It can be notched or slurred, reflecting rapid depolarization through the normal conductive system and slow depolarization through the myocardium on the blocked side.

Ventricular conduction disturbances sometimes complicate ECG rhythm strip interpretation. In these cases, supraventricular beats can have abnormally wide QRS complexes. If you suspect a conduction system disturbance relating to supraventricular beats, then it is prudent to inspect some of the other leads to determine the problems.

Although exceptions do occur, supraventricular tachycardias caused by disturbances in conduction usually differ in several ways from wide complex tachycardias originating in the ventricles:

- A changing bundle branch block suggests supraventricular tachycardia (SVT) with aberrancy.
- A trial of carotid sinus massage may slow conduction through the AV node and may terminate a reentrant SVT or slow conduction with other supraventricular tachyarrhythmias. These maneuvers will have no effect on ventricular tachycardias.
- AV dissociation, also known as AV block, indicates a ventricular origin of the arrhythmia.

- A full compensatory pause, usually seen after a ventricular beat, indicates ventricular tachycardia.
- Fusion beats suggest ventricular tachycardia.
- A QRS duration of longer than 0.14 second usually indicates VT.

The patient's history may also help to differentiate the etiologies of wide complex tachycardias. In older patients with a history of myocardial infarction, congestive heart failure, or coronary artery disease, these arrhythmias most likely have a ventricular origin.

When in doubt, treat the patient as if he has the more lethal arrhythmia: ventricular tachycardia. In either case, use cardioversion if the patient is unstable; it is effective for both ventricular and supraventricular tachycardias.

Preexcitation Syndromes

Preexcitation syndromes involve premature ventricular excitation by an impulse that bypasses the AV node. The most common of these is *Wolff-Parkinson-White (WPW) syndrome.* WPW occurs in approximately 3 of every 1,000 persons (Figure 2-68). It is characterized by a short PR interval, generally less than 0.12 second, and a long QRS duration, generally more than 0.12 second. Additionally, the upstroke of the QRS often has a slur, called the *delta wave* (Figure 2-69). In WPW, conduction of the depolarization impulse from the atria to the ventricles is abnormal. The **bundle of Kent**, an extra conduction pathway between the atria and ventricles, effectively bypasses the AV node, shortening the PR interval and prolonging the QRS complex. Most WPW patients are asymptomatic; however, the disorder is associated with a high incidence of tachyarrhythmias, usually through a reentry mechanism. WPW is also frequently associated with organic heart diseases, such as atrial septal defects or mitral valve prolapse. Base treatment on the underlying rhythm.

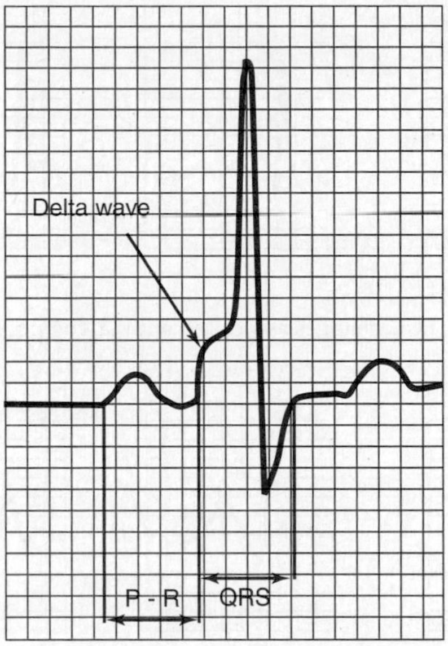

FIGURE 2-69 Delta wave characteristic of preexcitation (Wolff-Parkinson-White syndrome).

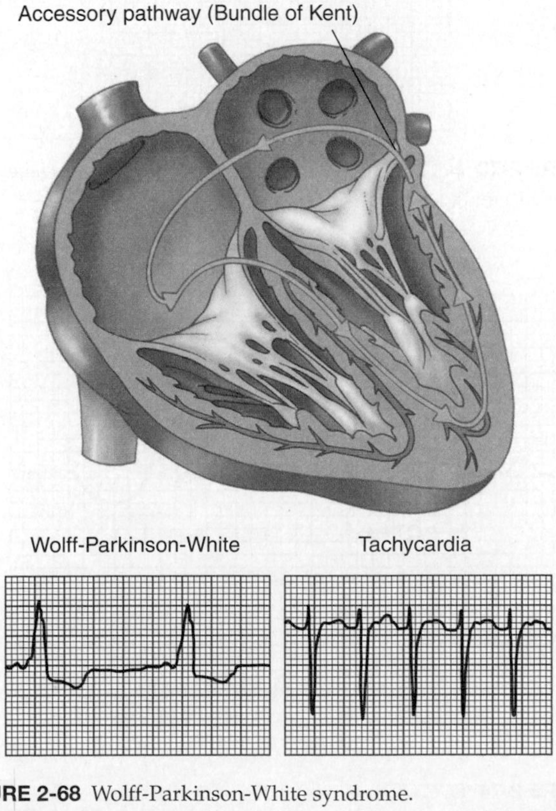

FIGURE 2-68 Wolff-Parkinson-White syndrome.

ECG Changes from Electrolyte Abnormalities and Hypothermia

Electrolyte imbalances can cause arrhythmias that will appear on ECG rhythm strips. The electrolytes most commonly associated with ECG disturbances are potassium and calcium.

- ***Hypokalemia.*** Hypokalemia is a condition in which the potassium level in the blood is low. Normal potassium levels are 3.5 to 5.0 mEq/L. Hypokalemia tends to cause a prominent U wave on the ECG and also tends to flatten the T wave. These changes result from the effect of low potassium levels on Phase 3 (repolarization) of the action potential (Figure 2-70).
- ***Hyperkalemia.*** Hyperkalemia is a condition in which the potassium level in the blood is elevated. Normal potassium levels are 3.5–5.0 mEq/L. As potassium levels start to rise, changes in the ECG can be seen. As potassium levels approach 6.0 to 6.5 mEq/L, a tall, pointed T wave will be seen. The T wave will become higher and more peaked as potassium levels approach 7.0 mEq/L. When levels approach 8.0 mEq/L the T wave begins to merge with the QRS forming a very wide QRS complex. At potassium levels of 9.0 mEq/L, the waveform becomes

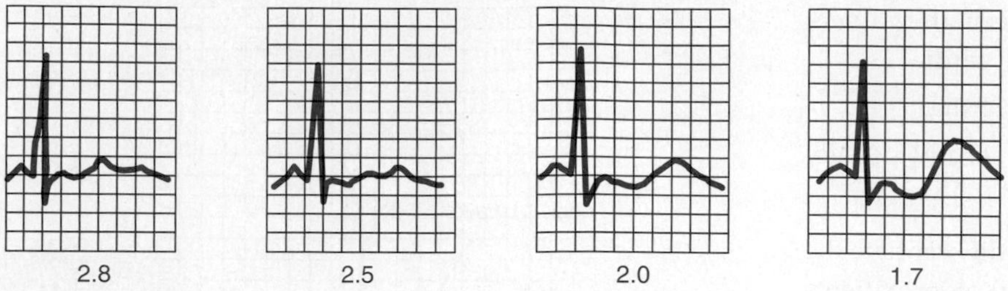

FIGURE 2-70 ECG changes associated with falling potassium levels (hypokalemia).

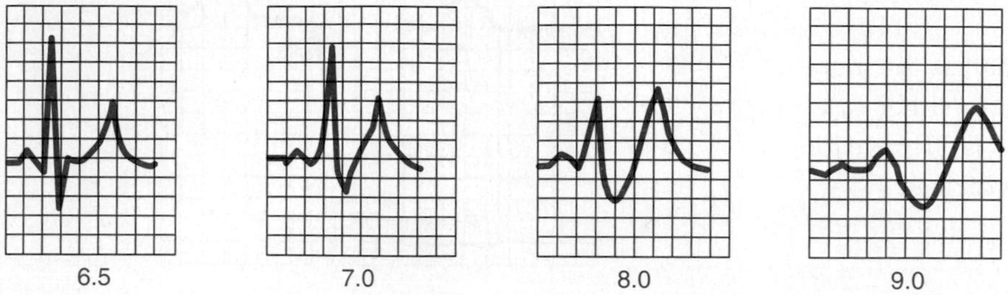

FIGURE 2-71 ECG changes associated with rising potassium levels (hyperkalemia).

almost sinusoidal. Potassium levels greater than 10 mEq/L are generally incompatible with life (Figure 2-71).

- ***Hypocalcemia.*** Hypocalcemia is a low serum calcium level and can be caused by the use of diuretics and certain endocrine conditions. Hypocalcemia prolongs repolarization and causes a prolonged ST segment and thus a prolonged QT interval (Figure 2-72).
- ***Hypercalcemia.*** Hypercalcemia is an abnormal elevation in serum calcium levels. It can be caused by adrenal insufficiency, hyperparathyroidism, kidney failure, or malignancies. Hypercalcemia shortens the repolarization phase, thus causing the ST segment to shorten—sometimes to the point at which the T wave seems to be almost on top of the QRS. The concomitant effects of hypercalcemia and digitalis can be quite detrimental (Figure 2-73).

Digitalis (Lanoxin) is sometimes used in the treatment of congestive heart failure and atrial fibrillation. It increases the force of cardiac contraction and slows AV conduction to slow ventricular response in atrial fibrillation. The effects of digitalis can often be seen on the ECG as a sagging or "scooping" of the ST segment. It can also prolong the PR interval because of slowing of AV conduction. Figure 2-74 illustrates the effects of digitalis on the ECG.

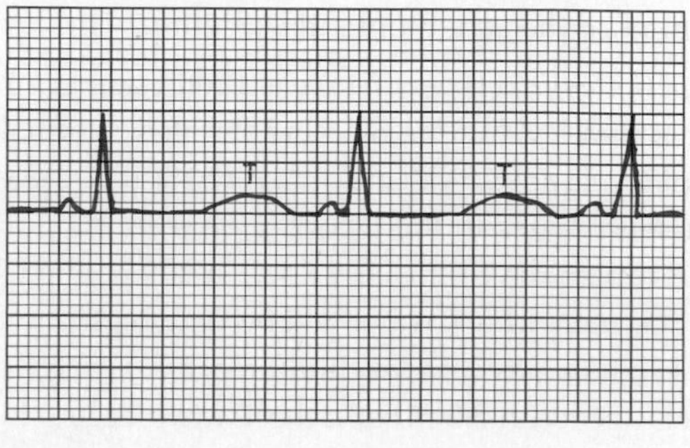

FIGURE 2-72 ECG changes associated with falling calcium levels (hypocalcemia).

In *hypothermia,* the Osborn wave, or J wave, is apparent. It is a slow, positive deflection at the end of the QRS complex (Figure 2-75). Other ECG changes may include:

- T wave inversion
- PR, QRS, QT prolongation
- Sinus bradycardia
- Atrial fibrillation or flutter
- AV block
- PVCs
- Ventricular fibrillation
- Asystole

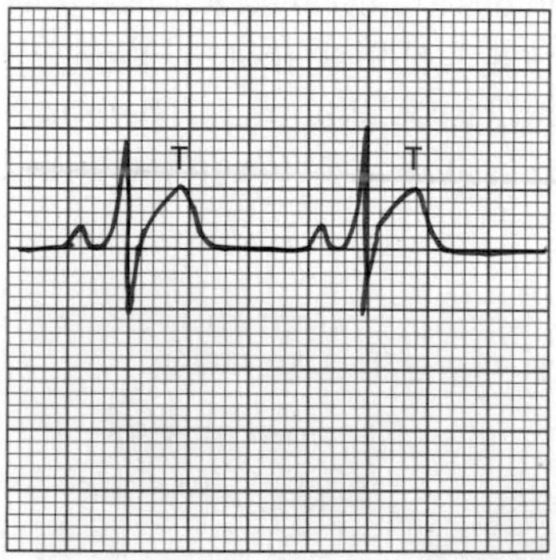

FIGURE 2-73 ECG changes associated with rising calcium levels (hypercalcemia).

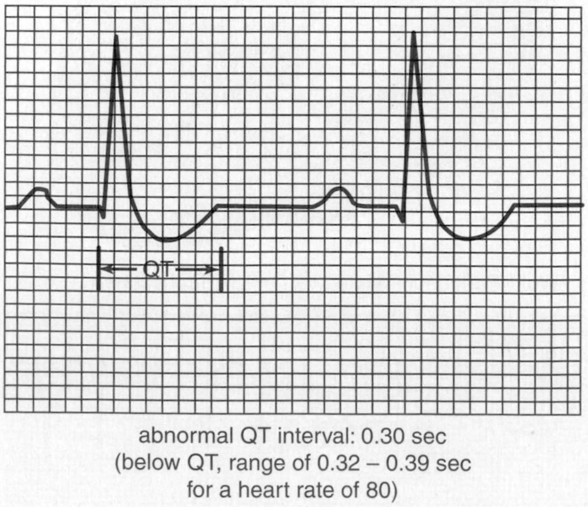

FIGURE 2-74 ECG changes associated with digitalis.

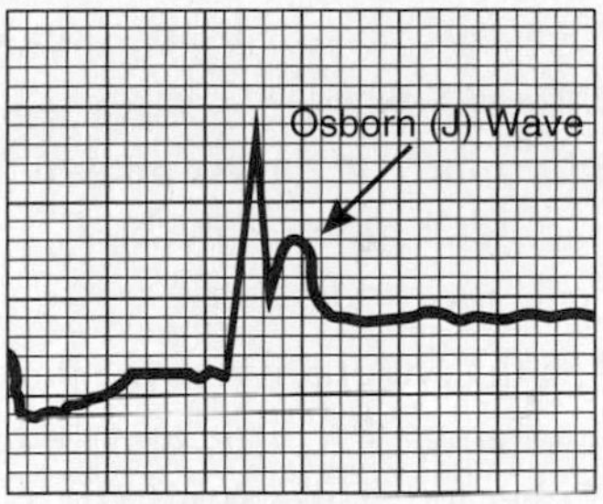

FIGURE 2-75 The Osborn ("J") wave.

PART 2: Assessment and Management of the Cardiovascular Patient

Assessment of the Cardiovascular Patient

The key to providing your cardiovascular patient with the best possible medical care is to take a systematic, step-by-step approach. When you initially contact your patient, always determine the most important problems first. Airway, breathing, circulatory problems, and shock are always the most critical issues during the first minute of patient care. What may have caused any life-threatening problems does not matter at this point. In some instances, such as cardiac arrest, your focus during prehospital care may never go beyond these four concerns.

After you have managed any life-threatening problems, the history and physical examination will help you form your field diagnosis. Cardiovascular diseases may affect the myocardium, the electrical conductive system, the pericardium, or the blood vessels. They may also involve a combination of these problems or problems associated with other systems, such as diabetes. Diseases of the myocardium include myocardial infarction, heart failure, and cardiogenic shock. In electrical conductive illnesses, the heart rate is either too fast or too slow. Although pericardial emergencies, such as pericarditis or pericardial tamponade, are usually diagnosed clinically by the physical examination findings, the history (blunt/penetrating trauma or recent infection, for example) may help you to recognize them. Vascular problems may include coronary artery occlusion, peripheral venous or arterial occlusion, or pulmonary embolism.

In your ongoing assessment, continually reevaluate your initial management. Based on the patient's needs, you will transport him in the appropriate mode to the appropriate facility. As with any patient, your management of the cardiac patient should include patient advocacy as well as communication and emotional support for the patient and his family. You must also effectively communicate the details of your assessment and management to the receiving staff. Additionally, your knowledge of nontransport criteria, education and prevention, proper documentation, and ongoing quality assurance will contribute to providing optimum care.

Your assessment of the patient with a cardiovascular emergency should vary according to the acuity of the situation. Patients with serious illnesses should have a limited, yet focused, exam. Patients who are less seriously ill should receive a more comprehensive assessment. It is important to remember that the cardiovascular system affects virtually every other body system. Signs of cardiac disease may initially be evident only in the respiratory system, as dyspnea. A comprehensive exam, however, will often reveal subtle findings that point to cardiovascular disease as the cause.

Scene Size-up and Primary Assessment

After ascertaining that the scene is safe, begin an initial cardiovascular primary assessment. This allows you to identify life-threatening problems and set transport priorities. First, determine the patient's level of responsiveness. Is he speaking with you or unresponsive? Then move on to the ABCs. Make sure his airway is patent and free of debris and blood. Suction the airway, if appropriate. Next, check the patient's rate and depth of breathing. Listen for the presence or absence of breath sounds. Certain breath sounds such as moist crackles (rales) should heighten your suspicion of cardiovascular disease. Note the effort or "work" of breathing. If the patient is not breathing, initiate manual ventilation and intubate as soon as possible. Check for the rate and quality of pulses. If no pulse is present, immediately begin cardiopulmonary resuscitation. The skin can indicate the degree of perfusion present. Look for:

- Color
- Temperature
- Moisture
- Turgor
- Mobility
- Edema

Finally, check the patient's blood pressure. Is he in shock? Is this a hypertensive issue? Treat all life-threatening conditions as you find them.

History

After you have completed your initial cardiovascular primary assessment and treated life-threatening conditions, proceed with your secondary assessment, including a history, using the SAMPLE format (symptoms, *a*llergies, *m*edications, *p*ast medical history, *l*ast oral intake, and *e*vents preceding the incident).

Common Symptoms

Cardiac disease can manifest itself in several ways. Common chief complaints and symptoms are as follows:

- Chest pain or discomfort
- Dyspnea
- Cough
- Syncope
- Palpitation

CHEST PAIN Chest pain or discomfort that may radiate to the shoulder, neck, jaw, or back is a common symptom of cardiac disease. Always remember, however, that not all patients who have cardiac disease will have chest pain. This is especially true in diabetic patients, who may have a myocardial infarction with no pain at all. Also, remember that chest pain can be benign and may have no association with cardiac disease. Differentiating benign from life-threatening chest pain is extremely difficult; do not attempt it in the field. If a cardiac etiology is even a remote possibility, treat the patient accordingly.

Follow the OPQRST mnemonic (*o*nset, *p*rovocation/palliation, *q*uality, *r*egion/radiation, *s*everity, *t*iming) to obtain the patient's description of the pain.

- ***Onset.*** Ask about the onset of the pain. When did it begin? What was the patient doing when it started? If the patient has had chest pain in the past, ask him to compare it to previous episodes. For instance, if he had a major heart attack in the past and tells you his current pain is the same, then strongly suspect that it is also from his heart. The time of pain onset is particularly important in the current era, as definitive interventions (i.e., fibrinolytics, percutaneous coronary intervention [PCI]) are extremely time sensitive and subject to an interventional window.
- ***Provocation/palliation.*** What provoked the pain? Is it exertional or nonexertional? The relationship of pain to exertion is very important. During exertion, the heart muscle needs more oxygen. If it does not receive the additional oxygen, the muscle becomes ischemic and the patient has pain (angina). He may tell you that he is now walking shorter distances before the pain begins, indicating lessening blood flow to the heart. Untreated, this may lead to pain at rest and, eventually, infarction. What alleviates the pain (palliation)? Is the pain related to movement or inspiration?
- ***Quality.*** Ask the patient to describe the quality of the pain. Ask open-ended questions and allow the patient to characterize this symptom in his own words. Common descriptive words include sharp, tearing, pressure, and heaviness.
- ***Region/Radiation.*** The patient may complain of pain radiating to other regions of his body, most commonly his arms, neck, jaw, and back.
- ***Severity.*** Ask the patient to rate the pain on a scale of 1 to 10, with 1 being very little and 10 being the worst pain he has ever felt. This can also be a useful gauge of your management's effectiveness. Some systems will use a pain scale of 1 to 5. Regardless of the scale, it is important that the scale used is standardized in the system. It can be problematic if a paramedic asks a patient to rate his pain on a scale of 1 to 5, but when the patient gets to the hospital, the nurse or doctor is using a scale of 1 to 10. Although seemingly trivial, this can significantly affect patient care.
- ***Timing.*** Check the timing of the pain. How long has the pain lasted? Always determine the time the pain began and record it. The onset and duration of pain directly affect decisions about the use of fibrinolytic drugs and PCI. Is the pain constant or intermittent? Is it getting worse? better? Does it occur at rest or with activity?

DYSPNEA Because of the heart's close relationship with the respiratory system, many cardiac patients have dyspnea (labored breathing). Dyspnea is often associated with myocardial infarction and in some patients may be the only symptom. Also, patients with congestive heart failure will experience increased dyspnea when lying down.

When confronted with a dyspneic patient, ask about the following:

- ***Duration.*** How long has it lasted? Is it continuous or intermittent?
- ***Onset.*** Was the onset sudden or rapid?
- ***Provocation/palliation.*** Does anything aggravate or relieve the dyspnea? Is it exertional or nonexertional?
- ***Orthopnea.*** Does sitting upright give relief?

COUGH Frequently, patients who cough have chest pain. Is the cough dry or productive? Did the patient pull a chest muscle during coughing? Try to determine whether the coughing results from congestive heart failure.

OTHER RELATED SIGNS AND SYMPTOMS Other related signs and symptoms to look for and ask about include:

- ***Level of consciousness.*** The level of consciousness indicates brain perfusion. An alteration in the level of consciousness can be due to problems within the cardiovascular system.
- ***Diaphoresis (perspiration).*** Cardiac problems significantly affect the autonomic nervous system. Stimulation

of the sympathetic nervous system can result in marked diaphoresis.

- *Restlessness and anxiety.* Restlessness and anxiety are among the earliest symptoms when a patient is experiencing *lowered* brain perfusion, whether due to decreased oxygenation, decreased blood supply, or both.
- *Feeling of impending doom.* The significant and massive stimulation of the sympathetic nervous system associated with severe cardiovascular emergencies can cause a feeling of impending doom. This is a part of the fight-or-flight response. A patient with a sensation of impending doom can be experiencing a significant cardiovascular event.
- *Nausea and/or vomiting.* Nausea and vomiting are common during cardiovascular events such as myocardial ischemia. This often results from slowed peristalsis due to sympathetic stimulation.
- *Fatigue.* Fatigue is a generalized finding associated with many diseases. In patients with cardiovascular disease, it can be caused by anemia, poor oxygenation, or poor overall cardiovascular system functioning.
- *Palpitations.* Palpitations are a sensation that the heart is beating fast or skipping beats. This can result from tachycardia or simply from increased awareness of the heart's normal function.
- *Edema.* Edema is the accumulation of fluid in third (interstitial) spaces. It accompanies poor cardiac function and often indicates chronic cardiovascular disease.
  - *Extremities.* Ambulatory patients usually will develop edema in the extremities, due to the effects of gravity.
  - *Sacral.* Sacral, or presacral, edema is seen in bedbound patients. Fluid collects in the lowest part of the patient's body, usually around the sacrum.
- *Headache.* Headache is a factor in cardiovascular disease for several reasons. First, decreased CNS perfusion can result in headaches. These are often severe. Many patients with established heart disease take nitroglycerin or other nitrate drugs. Excess administration of nitrates can cause a severe headache and may indicate worsening heart disease.
- *Syncope.* Syncope is a brief loss of consciousness due to a transient decrease in cerebral blood flow. It occurs in certain cardiac arrhythmias and in ischemic lesions where blood flow to the heart may be impaired, reducing cardiac output and interrupting CNS perfusion. Severe pain can also cause syncope, as well as other forms of psychic stress.
- *Behavioral change.* A behavioral change may very subtly indicate cardiovascular disease. More common in the elderly, it may point to either an acute or chronic decrease in cerebral blood flow.
- *Anguished facial expression.* The pain that accompanies myocardial ischemia can be quite severe. This, coupled with the effects of sympathetic nervous system stimulation, may cause the patient to exhibit anguished facial expressions.
- *Activity limitations.* Decreased cardiac performance can significantly limit a patient's physical activities. These limitations may develop slowly and be considered chronic or develop quickly and be considered acute.
- *Trauma.* Trauma, especially unexplained trauma, can be due to a temporary decrease in CNS perfusion. Unexplained facial injuries or bruises may indicate a cardiovascular problem.

Many of the signs and symptoms of cardiovascular disease can be subtle. Always assess for them and look for any sign or symptom patterns that point to cardiovascular disease.

Allergies

Ask about the patient's allergies. Is he allergic to any medications? Does he have an allergy to X-ray contrast (IVP dye)? Try to differentiate between true medication allergies and undesirable side effects of a particular medication. For instance, the patient who tells you he breaks out in hives and stops breathing if he takes penicillin is having an allergic reaction. The patient who says he gets abdominal upset from aspirin is, most likely, experiencing a side effect. If in doubt, withhold the medication and contact medical direction.

Medications

The patient's current use of prescription medications is important. What medications is he currently taking? Has he recently changed any medications? The following drugs may be especially significant:

- Antiarrhythmics
- Anticoagulants
- Antihypertensives
- Beta-blockers
- Calcium channel blockers
- Digitalis
- Diuretics
- Erectile dysfunction medications
- Lipid-lowering agents
- Nitrates
- Platelet aggregate inhibitors

Also question the patient in detail about his compliance with his medications. Does he take his medications? Does he take the right amount? Does he take them at the right time? With the high cost of medications and limited coverage by prescription plans, more and more patients are not taking their prescriptions. Some may even borrow a friend's medication—a dangerous practice, as it may be the wrong dosage or even the wrong drug.

The patient's use of nonprescription drugs is also important. Ask if he takes any over-the-counter medications. Numerous drugs interact, and you must be aware of all medications the patient is currently taking, prescription or otherwise. Try to bring all drug containers with you to the hospital if doing so will not adversely prolong transport time. This information is very important for the hospital staff.

Recreational drug use is another major problem. For example, cocaine causes vasoconstriction of the blood vessels and can lead to myocardial infarction and severe hypertension, often in the absence of coronary artery disease. These effects can last up to two weeks. Even though this question may make you or the patient uncomfortable, you must ask it.

Past Medical History

Avoid spending excessive time obtaining a cardiac patient's past medical history. If the patient's condition permits, however, a past medical history may help you determine whether his symptoms are attributable to a cardiac condition.

- Does the patient have a history of coronary artery disease, angina, or a previous myocardial infarction? Has he had an abnormal stress test or coronary angiogram? If so, chances are good that his symptoms are cardiac in origin. Comparing his prior symptoms to his present ones is helpful. If he tells you this pain is just like his previous heart attack, then he likely is experiencing another.
- Has the patient had any prior heart problems? Ask about the following:
  - Valvular disease (rheumatic heart disease)
  - Aneurysm
  - Previous cardiac surgery
  - Congenital cardiac anomalies
  - Pericarditis or other inflammatory cardiac disease
  - Congestive heart failure (CHF)
  - Prior cardiac catheterization and/or stress test
- What other medical problems does the patient have? Ask about the following:
  - Pulmonary disease/COPD
  - Diabetes mellitus
  - Renal (kidney) disease
  - Hypertension
  - Peripheral vascular disease
  - High cholesterol (lipids)
- Does anyone in the patient's family have cardiac disease? At what age did it first develop? Cardiac disease before the age of 50 in a close relative should heighten your concern about heart disease. If a family member had a cardiac event at a young age, especially sudden death, your patient is also at risk earlier in life. Has anyone in his family died of heart disease? At what age? Also ask if the family has a history of stroke, diabetes, or hypertension.
- Does the patient smoke? Does he know his cholesterol level? These are other modifiable risk factors for cardiac disease.

Last Oral Intake

When was the patient's last oral intake? If the patient ingested a meal high in saturated fats before the onset of symptoms, then gallbladder disease should be considered as a possible etiology. Also inquire if the patient has had an increase in caffeine intake and ask when he last drank a caffeinated beverage.

Events Preceding the Incident

What was the patient doing before the onset of symptoms? Was there emotional upset? Had he just completed a strenuous task, such as mowing the yard? Has he recently started a new exercise program? Did the symptoms begin while the patient was having sex? Does the patient take Viagra or another erectile dysfunction medication? The development of chest pain during sexual intercourse is not uncommon. However, patients often will not volunteer this information. Asking about intimate events such as this may be uncomfortable, but it is necessary for optimal patient care.

Physical Examination

After addressing any life-threatening problems you find in the primary assessment, begin the physical exam. Be systematic and thorough, and remember to look (inspect), listen (auscultate), and feel (palpate) while performing your detailed examination.

Inspection

During your inspection, look for:

- ***Tracheal position.*** The trachea should be midline. Movement toward a side may indicate a pneumothorax. Inspect the neck veins for evidence of jugular vein distention. The internal jugular veins are major vessels. Thus, jugular vein distention often evidences an increase in central venous pressure (Figure 2-76). Pump failure or cardiac tamponade can cause back pressure in the systemic circulation and jugular vein engorgement. Try to have the patient seated at a

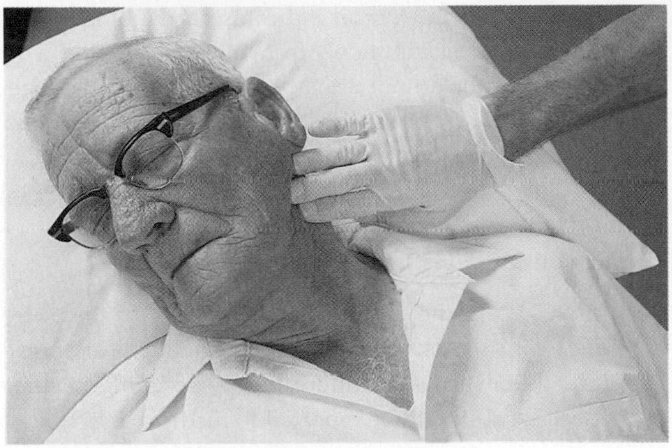

FIGURE 2-76 Look for the presence of jugular venous distention, ideally with the patient elevated at a 45° angle.

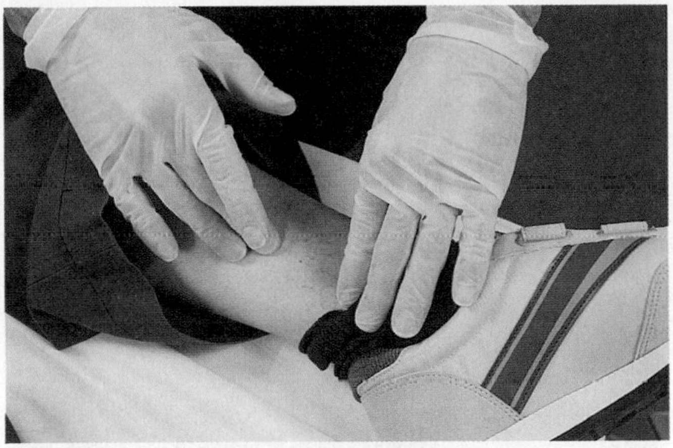

FIGURE 2-77 Check for peripheral edema.

45° angle, not lying flat, for this examination. Remember, however, that jugular vein distention is often difficult to assess in an obese patient.

- ***Thorax.*** Watch the patient breathe. To do this properly, expose the patient's chest wall, maintaining patient privacy if possible. Evidence of labored breathing includes retractions and accessory muscle use. Retractions are visible depressions in the soft tissues between the ribs that occur with increased respiratory effort. Accessory muscle use involves muscles of the neck, back, and abdomen. Normally, these muscles play a small role in breathing, but patients with labored breathing put them to greater use. A patient with chronic obstructive pulmonary disease (COPD) may have an increased anteroposterior (AP) diameter and may appear "barrel chested." Examination of the thorax can provide a great deal of information about the patient, including chronic problems such as COPD. The presence of a sternotomy scar, especially in an older patient, is a significant indicator of heart disease. Look for a generator (usually in the upper chest) for a pacemaker or an implanted defibrillator.
- ***Epigastrium.*** While the chest wall is exposed, inspect the epigastrium. Look for abdominal distention and visible pulsations. This may mean the patient has an aortic aneurysm with dissection or rupture.
- ***Peripheral and presacral edema.*** Chronic back pressure in the systemic venous circulation causes peripheral and presacral edema. These symptoms are most obvious in dependent parts such as the ankles (Figure 2-77). Often in bedridden patients you must inspect and palpate the sacral region for edema. Edema is generally classified as either mild or pitting. To distinguish between them, press firmly on the edematous part. If the depression remains after you remove pressure, the edema is pitting; otherwise it is mild.
- ***Skin.*** Several changes in the skin can be associated with cardiovascular disease. Pale and diaphoretic skin indicates peripheral vasoconstriction and sympathetic stimulation. It accompanies heart disease and other problems. A mottled appearance often indicates chronic cardiac failure.
- ***Subtle signs of cardiac disease.*** Look for subtle indicators of cardiac disease. Observe for signs that a patient is being treated for cardiac problems. These include midsternal scars from coronary artery bypass surgeries, pacemakers, or nitroglycerin skin patches.

Auscultation

During your inspection, listen for:

- ***Breath sounds.*** Assessing breath sounds in the cardiac patient is just as important as it is in the respiratory patient. Assess the lung fields for equality. Also listen for *adventitious sounds*—those that arise or occur sporadically or in unusual locations. Sounds such as crackles (rales), wheezes, or rhonchi (whistling or snoring sounds) may indicate pulmonary congestion or edema. Patients with pulmonary edema may also have foamy, blood-tinged sputum from the mouth and nose. In severe cases, this is audible from a distance as an ominous "gurgling" sound.
- ***Heart sounds.*** Avoid spending precious time auscultating heart sounds in the field. Background noise from traffic, family members, sirens, and other sources makes it difficult to hear heart sounds, and the information you obtain generally will not affect patient management. Nonetheless, become familiar with normal heart sounds and be able to distinguish abnormal from normal findings (Figure 2-78). The first heart sound (S_1) is produced by closure of the AV valves (tricuspid and mitral) during ventricular systole. The second heart sound (S_2) is produced by closure of the

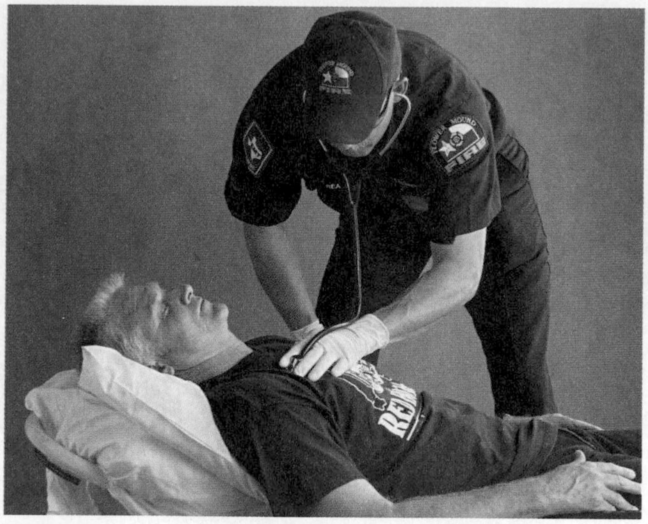

FIGURE 2-78 Auscultate the chest. Listen for heart sounds.

aortic and pulmonary valves. S_1 and S_2 are normal. Any extra heart sounds are abnormal. The third heart sound (S_3) is associated with congestive heart failure. Occasionally, the skilled listener can hear the fourth heart sound (S_4), which occurs immediately before S_1. It is associated with increased atrial contraction. Ideally, the heart should be examined from the four classic auscultatory sites: aortic, pulmonic, mitral, and tricuspid. The point on the chest wall where the heartbeat can best be heard or felt is known as the *point of maximum impulse* (PMI). (The PMI and examination of the heart are discussed in more detail in the chapter "Secondary Assessment.")

- ***Carotid artery bruit.*** Auscultation of the carotid arteries may reveal bruits (murmurs), which are a sign of turbulent blood flow through a vessel (Figure 2-79). They are audible over all major arteries, including the abdominal aorta. A bruit indicates partial blockage of the vessel, most commonly from atherosclerosis. If you detect a bruit, do not attempt carotid sinus massage. This procedure may dislodge plaque, resulting in stroke or other mishap.

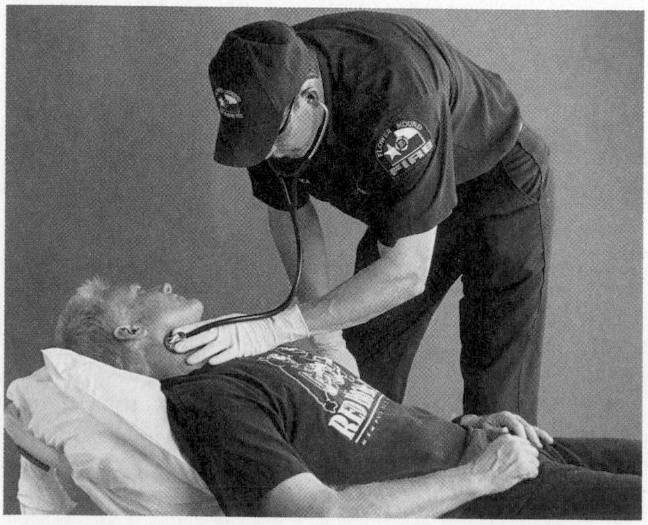

FIGURE 2-79 Listen to the carotid arteries. The presence of noisy blood flow is termed a *bruit* and may indicate underlying disease in the artery.

Palpation

During your examination, feel for:

- ***Pulse.*** Determine the rate and regularity of the pulse (Figure 2-80). Also note the pulse's equality. Any pulse deficit can indicate underlying peripheral vascular disease and should be reported to medical direction.
- ***Thorax.*** Palpation of the thorax is extremely important, as chest wall problems are quite common. These can be elicited only by palpation, which may reveal crepitus. *Crepitus* is a grating sensation that suggests the rubbing of broken bone ends or a "bubble wrap" crackling that suggests subcutaneous emphysema (air in the subcutaneous tissue). Palpitation may also reveal tenderness associated with a chest wall muscle strain, costochondritis (inflammation of the joint where the rib attaches to the sternum), or even rib fractures. It is important to remember that at least 15 percent of patients with acute myocardial infarction will have associated chest wall tenderness.
- ***Epigastrium.*** Also feel the abdomen for pulsations and distention, which may indicate an abdominal aortic aneurysm.

Physical examination of the chest is an essential aspect of comprehensive prehospital care. Employ the standard techniques of inspection, auscultation, palpation, and, occasionally, percussion. Together, these skills can provide a great deal of information about chronic problems as well as the ongoing acute episode.

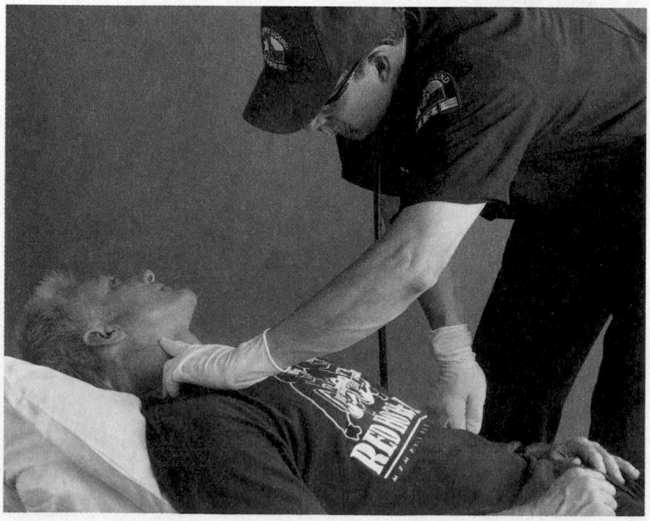

FIGURE 2-80 Check the patient's pulse for both strength and character.

Management of Cardiovascular Emergencies

The following section discusses management techniques frequently used in cardiac emergencies. You should also become familiar with your local protocols and procedures, as they vary from system to system.

Basic Life Support

Basic life support is the primary skill for managing serious cardiovascular problems. These include the basic airway maneuvers, as well as CPR. Review basic life support techniques frequently to keep your skills at their peak.[5]

Advanced Life Support

Most of the procedures that paramedics employ to manage cardiovascular emergencies are considered advanced life support. The number of skills will vary from system to system. Advanced prehospital skills used in managing cardiovascular emergencies include:

- ECG monitoring (3-lead and 12-lead)
- Vagal maneuvers (carotid sinus massage)
- Pharmacological therapy
- Defibrillation
- Synchronized cardioversion
- Transcutaneous cardiac pacing
- Diagnostic (12-lead) ECG (see Part 3 of this chapter)

Monitoring ECG in the Field

Most systems' primary tool for ECG monitoring in the field is a combination ECG monitor/defibrillator that operates on a direct current (DC) battery source (Procedure 2–1). It has the following parts:

- Defibrillator electrodes
- Defibrillator controls

Procedure 2-1 ECG Monitoring

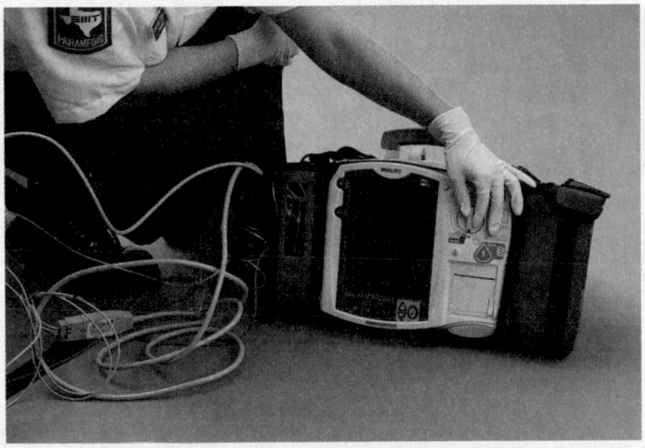

2-1a Turn on the machine.

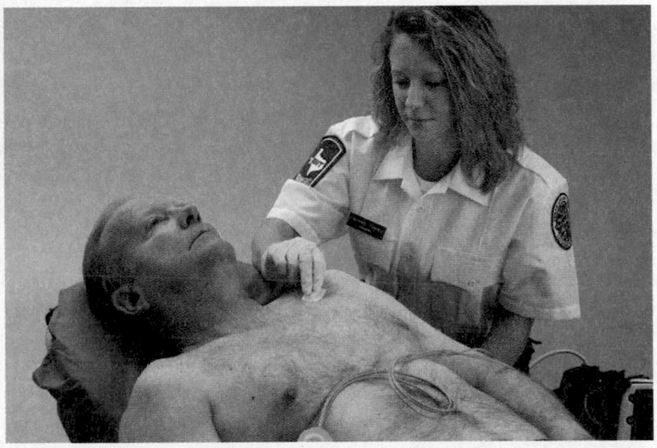

2-1b Prepare the skin.

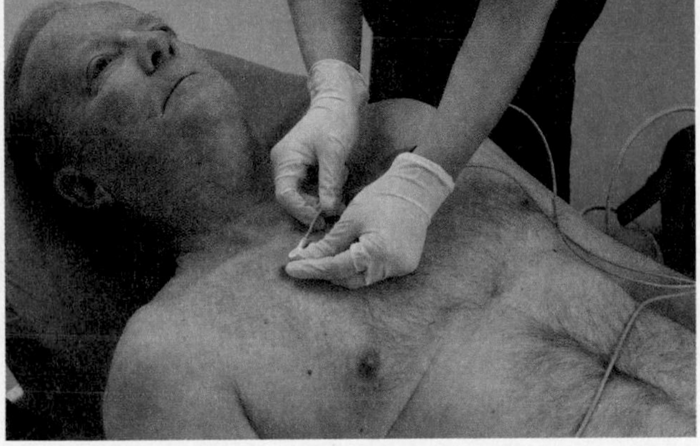

2-1c Apply the electrodes.

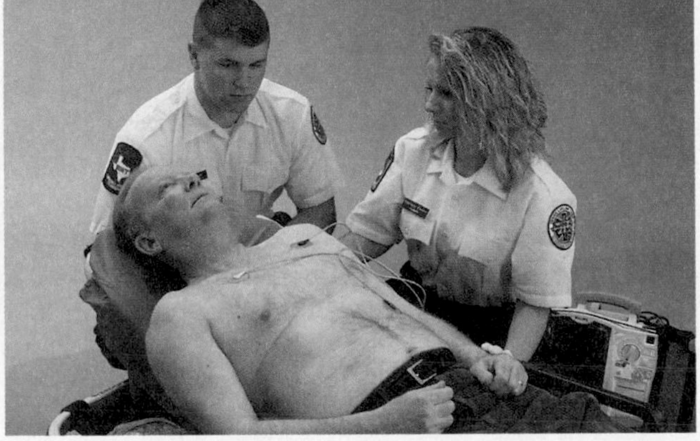

2-1d Ask the patient to relax and remain still.

(Continued)

Procedure 2-1 *Continued*

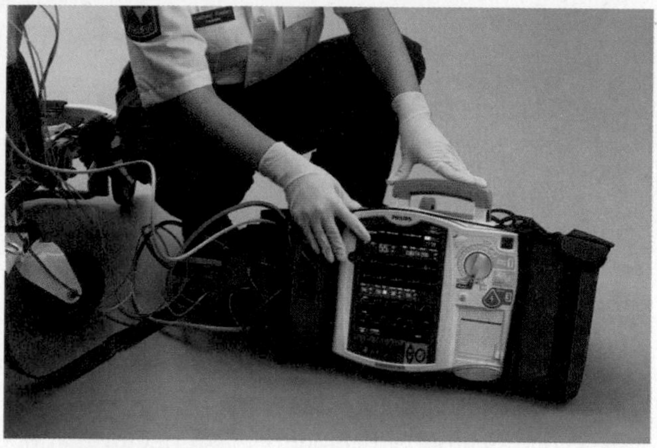

2-1e Check the ECG.

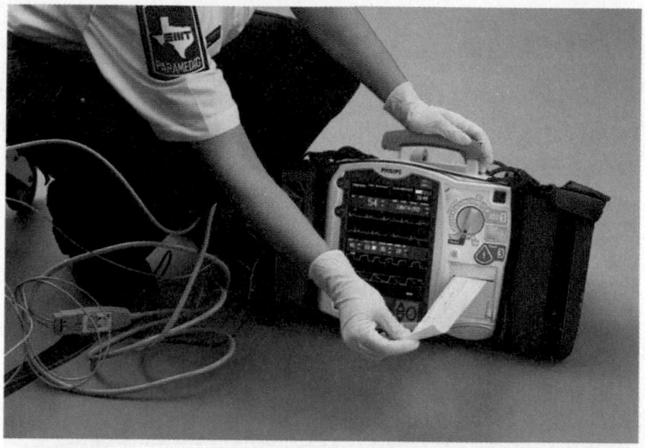

2-1f Obtain a tracing.

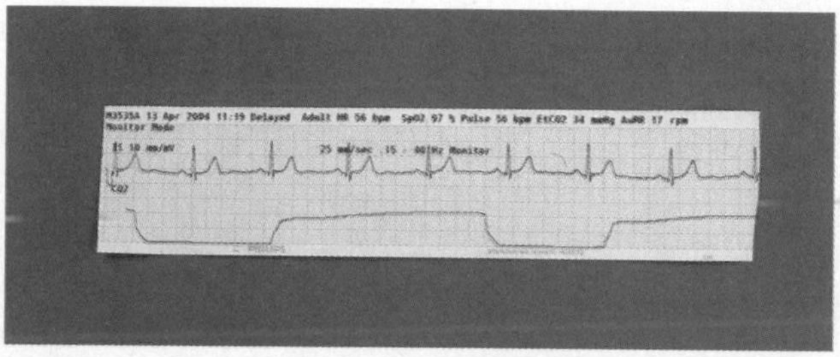

2-1g ECG strip.

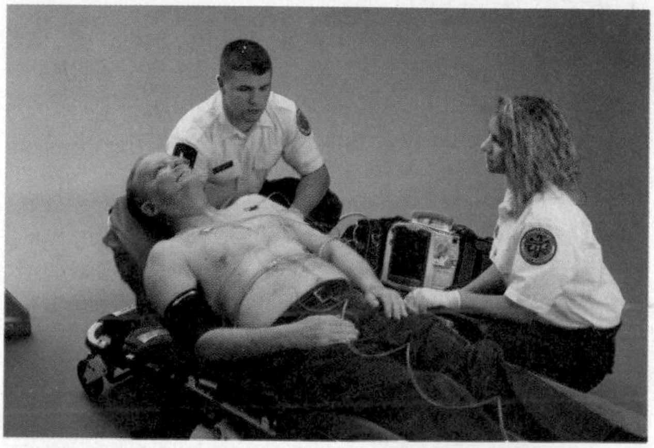

2-1h Continue ALS care.

- Synchronizer switch
- Graphic display
- Paper strip recorder
- Patient cable and lead wires
- Controls for monitoring
- Special features (such as data recorders)

Many prehospital ECG monitors are 12-lead ECG capable, and many have modules for capnography as well as temperature and hemodynamic monitoring.

To monitor your patient's ECG, you will place the three limb electrodes on the chest (in left arm, right arm, and left leg positions). Some manufacturers require a fourth lead on the right leg. By placing the three principal electrodes, you can monitor any of the bipolar leads (I, II, or III). On certain machines, you can also monitor the three augmented leads (aVR, aVL, or aVF) through these three electrodes. As a rule, lead II is usually monitored, as its axis is almost the same as that of the heart. Modified chest lead 1 (MCL_1) is used occasionally and is often better for determining the site of ectopic beats.

You can also monitor your patient through the defibrillator pads. These are more frequently used in cases of cardiac arrest, when there is no time to place chest electrodes. You can also use this system when the patient cable is inoperative.

To use defibrillation pads to monitor, follow these steps:

1. Turn on monitor power.
2. Clean the area of the chest where the pads will be applied.
3. Connect the electrodes (if not previously connected) to the monitor. Typically, the positive electrode is on the left lower chest and the negative electrode is on the right upper chest. This closely simulates lead II.
4. Observe the monitor and obtain a tracing if desired.

Chest electrodes vary among manufacturers. Usually, to mimic lead II, you will place the positive electrode on the patient's left lower chest and the negative electrode on his right upper chest. Placement of the ground wire varies. For MCL_1, place the positive electrode on the right lower chest wall and the negative electrode on the left upper chest wall. Again, placement of the ground wire varies. Place the electrodes to avoid large muscle masses, large quantities of chest hair, or anything that keeps the electrodes from resting flat on the skin. Also, avoid placing electrodes where you might have to place defibrillator paddles.

To place electrodes, follow these steps:

1. Cleanse the skin with alcohol or an abrasive pad to remove dirt and body oil, for better skin contact. If chest hair is thick, shave small amounts before placing the electrodes. If the patient is extremely diaphoretic, apply tincture of benzoin.
2. Apply electrodes to the skin surface.
3. Attach wires to the electrodes.
4. Plug the cable into the monitor.
5. Adjust gain or sensitivity to the proper level.
6. Adjust the QRS volume. (The continual beep of the ECG may disturb the patient.)
7. Obtain a baseline tracing.

Poor ECG signals are useless, so correct them. Their most common cause is faulty skin contact. When you spot a poor signal, check for the following possible causes:

- Excessive hair
- Loose or dislodged electrode
- Dried conductive gel
- Poor placement
- Diaphoresis

An initially poor tracing may improve as the conductive gel breaks down skin resistance. Other causes of poor tracings include:

- Patient movement or muscle tremor
- Broken patient cable
- Broken lead wire
- Low battery
- Faulty grounding
- Faulty monitor

Obtain a paper printout from each patient you monitor. Be sure to adjust the stylus heat properly. Calibrate each strip when you begin monitoring so that 1 mV deflects the stylus 10 mm (two large boxes).

Again, treat the patient and not the monitor. Always compare the rhythm you see on the monitor with the patient's signs and symptoms. A patient may have a perfect rhythm on the monitor but have no pulse or blood pressure.

Vagal Maneuvers

For a stable patient with symptomatic tachycardia, vagal maneuvers sometimes help slow the heart rate. Ask the patient to perform a Valsalva maneuver (bearing down as if attempting to have a bowel movement) or to cough deeply. If these are unsuccessful and the patient is eligible, consider carotid sinus massage. Do not attempt carotid sinus massage on patients with carotid bruits or known cerebrovascular or carotid artery disease, as it may precipitate a stroke. Carotid sinus massage is discussed in more detail later in this chapter.

Precordial Thump

The precordial thump, a blow to the midsternum with the heel of the fist, can stimulate depolarization within the heart. Although there is little support in the scientific literature regarding its effectiveness, there is no evidence of harm either. The precordial thump may be considered for termination of witnessed monitored unstable ventricular tachyarrhythmias when a defibrillator is not immediately ready for use. It should not delay CPR and shock delivery.

The precordial thump is most effective when performed immediately after the onset of ventricular fibrillation or pulseless ventricular tachycardia. On occasion, the precordial thump can cause depolarization of enough ventricular cells to allow resumption of an organized rhythm. Additionally, conversions from ventricular tachycardia, complete AV block, and, occasionally, ventricular fibrillation have been reported. If no defibrillator is immediately available, and the patient is monitored, you may attempt a precordial thump only one time. Because the amount of energy needed to convert ventricular fibrillation increases rapidly with time, a thump is likely to succeed only if delivered early. It is not recommended in pediatric patients.

To deliver a precordial thump, strike the midsternum with the heel of your fist from a distance of 10 to 12 inches (Figure 2-81). To avoid rib fractures and other

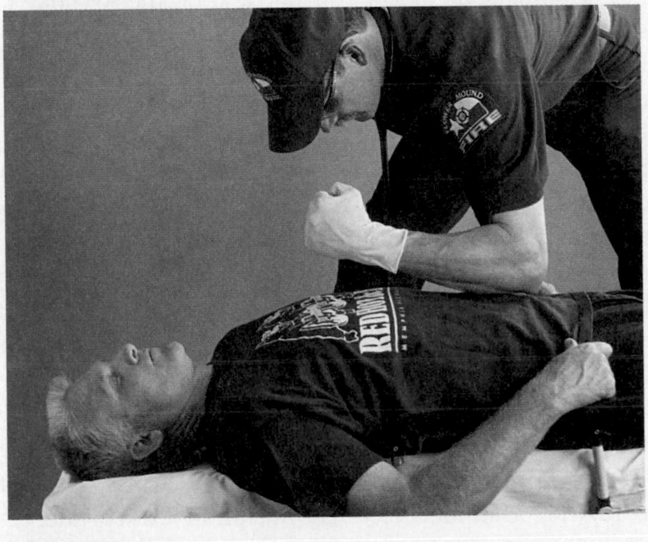

FIGURE 2-81 The precordial thump.

problems, keep your arm and wrist parallel to the sternum's long axis.[5]

Pharmacological Management

The drugs that you will use to manage cardiovascular emergencies generally fall into the categories of antiarrhythmics, sympathomimetics, and drugs used specifically for myocardial ischemia (including fibrinolytics), along with other prehospital medications, some of which are used only infrequently. For more detailed information on these types of drugs, see the chapter "Emergency Pharmacology."

Antiarrhythmics

Antiarrhythmic medications control or suppress arrhythmias. Among the more commonly used antiarrhythmics are atropine, lidocaine, adenosine, amiodarone, magnesium sulfate, and diltiazem.

ATROPINE SULFATE Atropine sulfate is a parasympatholytic agent used to treat symptomatic bradycardias, especially those arising in the atria. It is an anticholinergic. Side effects include blurred vision, dilated pupils, dry mouth, tachycardia, and drowsiness. It has no contraindications in the emergency setting. It is given by IV or IO bolus at a dose of 0.5 mg, repeated every 3 to 5 minutes for a total dose of 3.0 mg. It is no longer recommended for asystole.

ADENOSINE Adenosine is used to manage:

- Stable narrow-complex tachycardias.
- Unstable narrow-complex tachycardias while preparations are made for electrical cardioversion.
- Stable, regular monomorphic, wide-complex tachycardias as both a therapeutic and a diagnostic maneuver.

Adenosine is a naturally occurring nucleoside that acts on the sinus node to slow the rate and on the AV node to slow conduction and inhibit reentry pathways. Side effects include apprehension, burning sensation, heaviness in arms, hypotension, chest pressure, diaphoresis, numbness, tingling, dyspnea, tightness in the throat and/or groin pressure, headache, nausea, and vomiting. Adenosine is contraindicated in second- or third-degree blocks or in sick sinus syndrome unless a pacemaker is present. It is also contraindicated in patients with asthma. It is administered by IV rapid bolus, with the venous site as close to the heart as possible. Flush with saline rapidly, immediately after the adenosine, to ensure drug delivery. The initial dose is 6 mg (rapid push), followed by a 20-mL saline flush. If the tachyarrhythmia is not abolished, a second dose of 12 mg may be administered. If still ineffective, a third dose of 12 mg can be administered. The maximum dose of adenosine is 30 mg.

AMIODARONE Amiodarone (Cordarone) is an antiarrhythmic agent used in the management of:

- Cardiac arrest with shockable rhythm (ventricular fibrillation/tachycardia) unresponsive to CPR, defibrillation, and vasopressor therapy
- Stable narrow-complex tachycardia (atrial fibrillation)
- Stable narrow-complex tachycardia
- Rapid ventricular rate due to accessory pathway conduction in preexcited atrial arrhythmias

It is contraindicated in cardiogenic shock, marked sinus bradycardia, and high-degree heart blocks (second and third degree). Hypotension is the most common side effect. It can cause bradycardia and AV blocks. For pulseless ventricular fibrillation/tachycardia, the initial dose is 300 mg IV/IO. It can be followed by a single repeat dose of 150 mg IV/IO, if required. For other arrhythmias, the typical initial dose is 150 mg given over 10 minutes. If necessary, an amiodarone drip can follow at 1 mg/minute for 6 hours and then lowered to 0.5 mg/minute.

LIDOCAINE Once widely used in emergency cardiac care, lidocaine is now recommended only as an alternative agent to amiodarone for ventricular fibrillation and pulseless ventricular tachycardia. It is a weak sodium-channel blocker. The initial dose is 1.0 to 1.5 mg/kg IV/IO. It can be repeated if required, every 5 to 10 minutes, at 0.5 to 0.75 g/kg IV/IO to a maximum total dose of 3.0 mg/kg. Side effects include drowsiness, slurred speech, seizures, confusion, bradycardia, heart blocks, nausea, and vomiting.

DILTIAZEM Diltiazem is a calcium channel blocker that slows the heart rate in supraventricular tachycardias such as stable narrow-complex tachycardia if rhythm remains uncontrolled or unconverted by adenosine or vagal maneuvers or if supraventricular tachycardia is recurrent. It is also used for control of ventricular rate in patients with atrial fibrillation or atrial flutter.

Diltiazem is administered as an initial dose of 15 to 20 mg (0.25 mg/kg) IV over 2 minutes. If required, a repeat dose of 20 to 25 mg (0.35 mg/kg) IV can be given in 15 minutes. A maintenance infusion of 5 to 15 mg/hour IV (titrated to maintain a heart rate) can be used if required. For rate control, a slow IV bolus of 0.25 mg/kg, followed by a second dose of 0.35 mg/kg, can be given.

Vasopressor Agents

Vasopressor agents constrict blood vessels, thus increasing arterial pressure. Many vasopressor agents are *sympathomimetic agents* that are similar to the naturally occurring hormones epinephrine and norepinephrine. They duplicate or mimic sympathetic nervous system stimulation, acting on either the alpha- or beta-adrenergic receptors. Alpha receptor stimulation causes peripheral vasoconstriction. Beta receptor stimulation increases heart rate, cardiac contractile force, bronchodilation, and peripheral vasodilation. Commonly used sympathomimetic agents include epinephrine, norepinephrine, isoproterenol, dopamine, dobutamine, and vasopressin.

EPINEPHRINE Epinephrine, which acts on both alpha- and beta-adrenergic receptors, is the mainstay of cardiac arrest resuscitation. It is given by IV/IO bolus at a dose of 1 mg of a 1:10,000 solution given every 3 to 5 minutes. If given endotracheally, the dose should be increased to 2.0 to 2.5 mg.

NOREPINEPHRINE Norepinephrine is a sympathomimetic whose alpha-agonist properties are greater than those of epinephrine. It also acts on beta receptors to a lesser degree. In emergency cardiac care, it is used in the treatment of symptomatic bradycardias refractory to atropine. It is used in hemodynamically significant hypotension and cardiogenic and septic shock. Norepinephrine may be effective if total peripheral resistance is low, as in neurogenic shock. Side effects include anxiety, trembling, headache, dizziness, nausea, and vomiting. It can also cause bradycardia. Do not use norepinephrine in patients with hypotension from hypovolemia. The initial loading dose is 8 to 10 mcg/minute to obtain a blood pressure of 80–100 mmHg systolic. The maintenance dose is 2 to 4 mcg/minute.

DOPAMINE Dopamine (Intropin), a vasopressor, increases cardiac output. It stimulates both the alpha and beta receptors. In emergency cardiac care, it is used in the treatment of symptomatic bradycardias refractory to atropine. Side effects include nervousness, headache, arrhythmias, palpitations, chest pain, dyspnea, nausea, and vomiting. Dopamine is contraindicated for hypovolemic shock until fluid resuscitation has been completed. It is administered at 2 to 10 mcg/kg/minute.

DOBUTAMINE Like dopamine, dobutamine increases cardiac output by increasing stroke volume. It has little effect on heart rate and is occasionally used in isolated left-heart failure until other medications such as digitalis take effect. Its side effects are the same as dopamine. Do not use dobutamine as the sole agent in hypovolemic shock unless fluid resuscitation has been completed. Dobutamine is administered at a dose of 2 to 20 mcg/kg/minute, titrated to effect.

VASOPRESSIN Vasopressin is a naturally occurring hormone, commonly called *antidiuretic hormone (ADH)*, that is secreted by the posterior pituitary gland. High doses of vasopressin have sympathomimetic effects. When given during CPR, vasopressin appears to increase coronary perfusion pressure, vital organ blood flow, ventricular fibrillation (VF) median frequency, and cerebral oxygen delivery. It has been suggested that vasopressin be used in lieu of epinephrine. However, more recent human studies have shown it to be no more effective than epinephrine, and possibly less so. Because of this, vasopressin has been removed from current cardiac arrest management guidelines.[4]

Drugs Used for Myocardial Ischemia

Drugs used to treat myocardial ischemia and relieve its pain include oxygen, nitrous oxide, nitroglycerin, morphine sulfate, and fentanyl.

OXYGEN Oxygen is important in emergency cardiac care. It increases the blood's oxygen content and aids oxygenation of peripheral tissues. It is indicated in any situation in which hypoxia is present (as documented by pulse oximetry). It is important to administer only enough oxygen to correct hypoxia. Overoxygenation (hyperoxia) should be avoided, as this can cause oxidative stress. However, in cardiac arrest, 100 percent oxygen should be administered until return of spontaneous circulation (ROSC) occurs.

NITROUS OXIDE Nitrous oxide (Nitronox) is purely an analgesic, with no significant hemodynamic effects; however, delivery in fixed combination with 50 percent oxygen can increase myocardial oxygen supply. Nitrous oxide is self-administered by inhalation via a modified demand valve, to the desired effect. Its effects subside within 2 to 5 minutes. Side effects include CNS depression and potential respiratory depression. Do not give nitrous oxide to patients who cannot comprehend verbal instructions or who are intoxicated with alcohol or other drugs.

NITROGLYCERIN Nitroglycerin is an organic nitrate that dilates peripheral arteries and veins, thus reducing preload, afterload, and myocardial oxygen demand. It may cause some coronary artery dilation, increasing blood flow through the collaterals. Nitroglycerin administration often helps distinguish angina from MI. Nitroglycerin does not relieve MI symptoms, but it should be given before morphine, because it works in conjunction with morphine in an MI. Its side effects include headache, dizziness, weakness, hypotension, and tachycardia. Dosage for nitroglycerin is one tablet sublingually, repeated every 5 minutes, up to a total of three tablets. Monitor blood pressure before each dose. Nitroglycerin may be contraindicated in patients taking erectile dysfunction medications.

Note: Nitroglycerin starts losing potency as soon as the bottle is opened. Always use the nitroglycerin provided on the medical intensive care unit (MICU) and check the date before administration.

MORPHINE SULFATE The narcotic morphine is important in managing MI. It reduces myocardial oxygen demand by reducing preload and afterload. It also acts directly on the central nervous system to relieve pain, and it reduces sympathetic nervous system discharge, which can further decrease myocardial oxygen demand. Side effects include nausea, vomiting, abdominal cramping, respiratory depression, hypotension, and potential altered mental status. Toxic effects are apnea and severe hypotension. Dosage is 3- to 5-mg increments slow IV push, titrated to pain relief. Monitor blood pressure before each dose.

FENTANYL Fentanyl is a synthetic opiate analgesic chemically unrelated to morphine. It is considerably shorter acting than morphine and has a much better side-effect profile because of its short duration of action. Fentanyl is used in prehospital care with increasing frequency. The onset of action following the administration of fentanyl is immediate when given intravenously. Peak effects are seen in 3 to 5 minutes and effects last 30 to 60 minutes. A standard adult dose is 50 to 100 mcg.[6,7]

Fibrinolytic Agents

Definitive treatment of myocardial ischemia with fibrinolytic (also called thrombolytic) agents is one of the most important recent advances in medicine. In some instances, fibrinolytic therapy may be beneficial in the field. This is especially true in areas that have a long transport time to a definitive care facility. Fibrinolytic agents are very expensive, and their use requires a diagnostic 12-lead ECG.

ASPIRIN Although not a fibrinolytic, aspirin plays an important role in the treatment of cardiac ischemia. Aspirin inhibits the aggregation of platelets and is thus effective in the treatment of coronary ischemia and stroke. Its most common side effect is gastric upset, although bleeding can be a problem in selected patients. The standard dosage is one tablet (325 mg) orally. Some physicians prefer smaller doses. Baby aspirin is useful in that it can be chewed, thus more quickly reaching a therapeutic blood level.

ALTEPLASE (ACTIVASE) (tPA) Alteplase, commonly called tPA, is a potent fibrinolytic agent manufactured by recombinant DNA technology. Thus, the compound is identical to the human compound, which minimizes the chances of allergic reactions. tPA is effective if administered within 6 hours after the onset of coronary ischemia. It is given by a bolus dose followed by an infusion. The typical dose is 100 mg administered over 1.5 to 2 hours. Complications of tPA include hemorrhage, which can be fatal. Also, when reperfusion occurs, potentially life-threatening arrhythmias may develop.

TENECTEPLASE (TNKase) Tenecteplase is a newer-generation fibrinolytic that is more fibrin specific than tPA. The half-life of tenecteplase is longer than tPA, and the clinical outcomes are similar to those of tPA. The dose is typically 30 to 50 mg IV bolus over 5 seconds (based on weight).

Other Prehospital Medications

In some situations, medical direction or local protocol may recommend other medications. These may include furosemide, diazepam, promethazine, and sodium nitroprusside.

FUROSEMIDE Furosemide (Lasix) is a potent loop diuretic that relaxes the venous system. The prehospital use of furosemide has declined because it is a relatively slow diuretic, and most patients who need furosemide therapy are already taking a diuretic. Side effects include hypotension, ECG changes, chest pain, dry mouth, hypokalemia, hypochloremia, hyponatremia, and hyperglycemia. Furosemide should be used only in life-threatening emergencies in pregnancy, because it can cause fetal abnormalities. Dose is 40 mg slow IV push (40 mg/minute). If the patient is already taking furosemide, or another diuretic, you may need to double the dosage.

DIAZEPAM/LORAZEPAM You may administer diazepam or lorazepam if the patient is extremely apprehensive or agitated (after hypoxia and other causes have been addressed). Neither agent is an analgesic, but it will help with anxiety and apprehension.

ONDANSETRON Ondansetron (Zofran) is a centrally acting and highly effective antiemetic agent. It is generally non-sedating and well tolerated. The typical adult dose is 4 to 8 mg IV/IO/IM/PO.

Defibrillation

Defibrillation is the process of passing a current through a fibrillating heart to depolarize the cells and allow them to repolarize uniformly, thus restoring an organized cardiac rhythm. A critical mass of the myocardium must be depolarized to suppress all the ectopic foci. The critical mass is related to the size of the heart, but it cannot be calculated for a given individual or situation.

The *defibrillator* is an electrical capacitor that stores energy for delivery to the patient at a desired time. It consists of an adjustable high-voltage power supply, energy storage capacitor, and conductive pads. A current-limiting inductor connects the capacitor to the pads. Most modern defibrillators use a biphasic defibrillation waveform. It is thought that this waveform allows the use of less energy (thus decreasing possible tissue damage) and increases battery life. This technology evolved with the development of the compact automated external defibrillators (AEDs).

Most defibrillators use direct current (DC). Alternating current (AC) models should not be used. Direct current is more effective, more portable, and causes less muscle damage. It delivers an electrical charge of several thousand volts over a very short time, generally 4 to 12 milliseconds.

The shock's strength is commonly expressed in energy according to the following formula:

energy (joules) = power (watts) × duration (seconds)

The chest wall offers resistance to the electrical charge, which lowers the amount of energy actually delivered to the heart. Therefore, lowering the resistance pathway between the defibrillator pads and the chest is important. Factors that influence chest wall resistance include:

- Pad–skin interface
- Pad surface area

The following factors influence the success of defibrillation:

- ***Time from ventricular fibrillation onset.*** In conjunction with effective CPR, defibrillation begun within 4 minutes after the onset of fibrillation will yield significantly improved resuscitation rates, as compared with defibrillation begun within 8 minutes.
- ***Condition of the myocardium.*** Converting ventricular fibrillation is more difficult in the presence of acidosis, hypoxia, hypothermia, electrolyte imbalance, or drug toxicity. Secondary ventricular fibrillation (ventricular fibrillation that results from another cause) is more difficult to treat than primary ventricular fibrillation.
- ***Heart size and body weight.*** The effects of heart size and body weight on defibrillation are controversial. Pediatric and adult energy requirements differ, but whether size and energy level settings are related in adults is not clear.
- ***Pad size.*** Larger defibrillator pads are thought to be more effective and cause less myocardial damage. The ideal size for adults, however, has not been established. Generally, the pads should be 10 to 13 cm in diameter. In infants, 4.5-cm pads are adequate.
- ***Pad placement.*** For both adults and children in the emergency setting, place the pads on the chest according to the device manufacturer's recommendations. Generally, position one pad to the right of the upper sternum, just below the clavicle. Place the other to the left of the left nipple in an anterior axillary line immediately over the apex of the heart. Do not place pads over the sternum. Do not place pads over the generator of an implanted automatic defibrillator or pacemaker, which can damage or disable the device. Place the pads approximately 5 inches from the generator.
- ***Pad–skin interface.*** Pad–skin interface should have as little electrical resistance as possible. Greater resistance decreases energy delivery to the heart and increases heat production on the skin.
- ***Pad contact.*** The pads should be in maximum contact with the patient's skin. Make sure the pad is completely adhered prior to defibrillating.
- ***Properly functioning defibrillator.*** The machine should deliver the amount of energy that it indicates. Therefore, frequent inspection and testing of the machine are necessary. Change and cycle the batteries as the manufacturer directs.[8]

To perform defibrillation, use the following steps (Procedure 2–2):

1. Begin CPR while the defibrillator is being readied.
2. Ensure that the patient is in a safe environment if initially in contact with some electrically conductive material, such as metal or water.

Procedure 2-2 Defibrillation

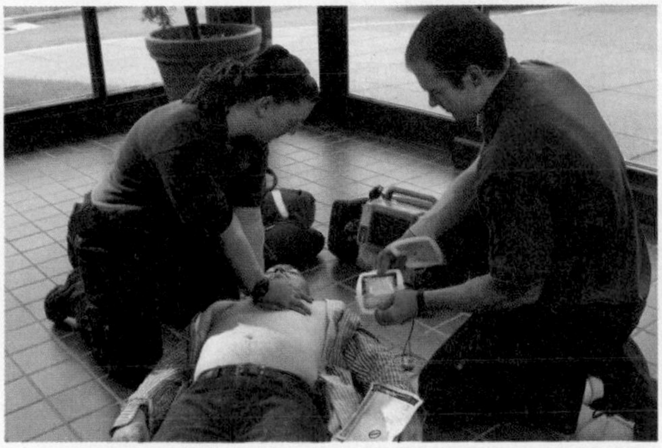

2-2a Begin CPR while the defibrillator is being readied.

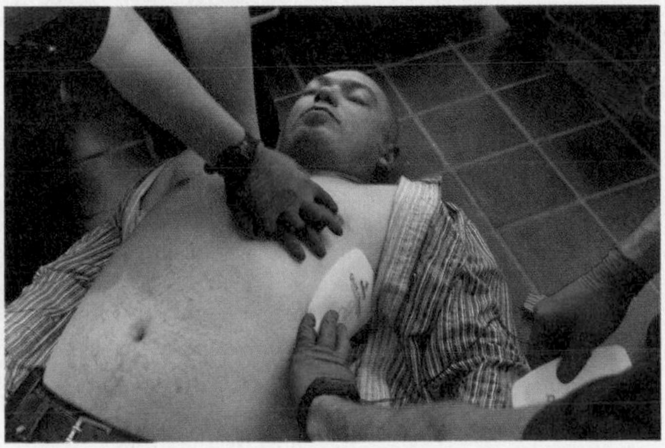

2-2b Continue CPR while the defibrillator pads are being applied.

(Continued)

Procedure 2-2 *Continued*

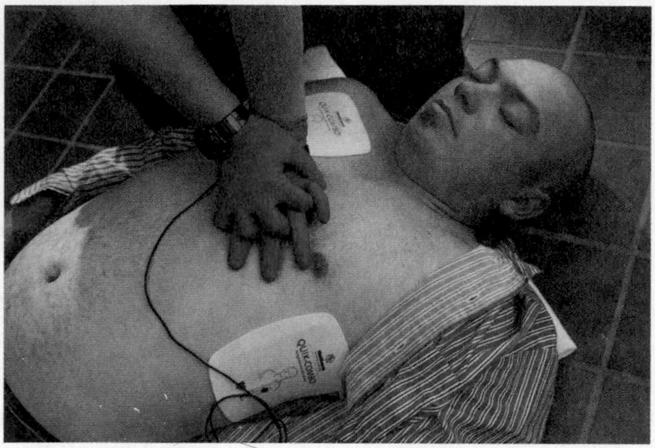

2-2c Continue effective CPR for at least 2 minutes while the pads are applied.

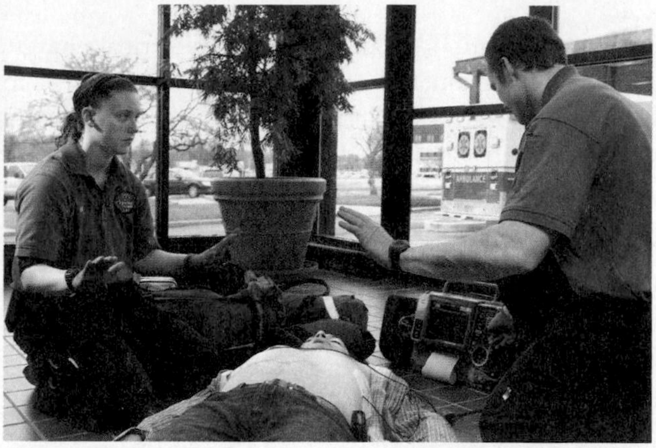

2-2d Ensure that no one is in contact with the patient.

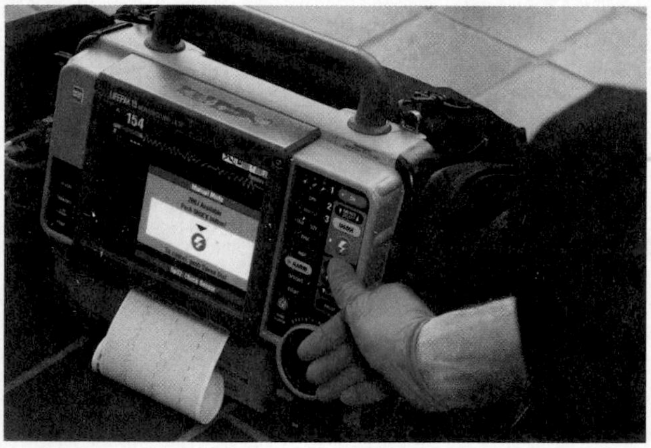

2-2e Check the rhythm.

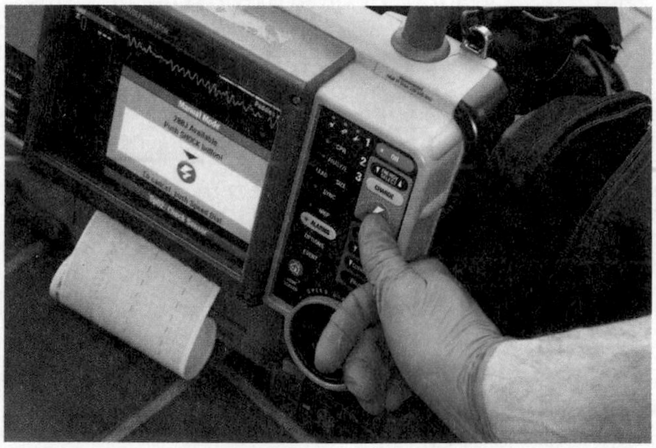

2-2f If a shockable rhythm is detected, administer a shock.

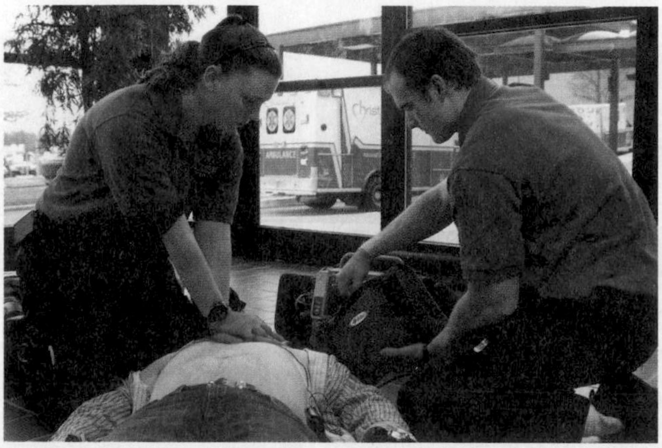

2-2g Resume CPR immediately after the shock without a pulse check. Administer appropriate medications. After 2 minutes of CPR, check the rhythm again. Apply next shock if indicated.

3. Continue effective CPR for at least 2 minutes while the defibrillator pads are applied to the patient's exposed chest.
4. Ensure that the pads are appropriately placed on the patient's thorax with proper pressure.
5. Ensure that no one else is in contact with the patient. Verbally and visually clear everyone, including yourself, before any defibrillation attempt.
6. Check the rhythm (or press analyze on AED).
7. If the rhythm is shockable (ventricular fibrillation/tachycardia), shock at maximum energy (typically 360 joules [monophasic] or 120 to 200 joules [biphasic]).
8. Resume CPR immediately after the shock (without a pulse check). Administer appropriate medications. After 2 minutes of CPR, check the rhythm again. If it is a shockable rhythm, continue CPR while the defibrillator is charging and administer a second shock.

The energy recommendations are machine specific. For monophasic machines, start at 360 joules. For manual biphasic machines, use the machine setting or 120 to 200 joules. For AEDs, use the machine setting.

Emergency Synchronized Cardioversion

Synchronized cardioversion is a controlled form of defibrillation for patients who still have organized cardiac activity with a pulse. A synchronizing circuit in the defibrillator interprets the QRS cycle and delivers the electrical discharge during the R wave of the QRS complex. This reduces the likelihood of delivering the cardioversion during the vulnerable period of the QRS cycle, which can precipitate ventricular fibrillation. Synchronizing also permits the use of lower energy levels and reduces the potential for secondary arrhythmias. Depending on the type of arrhythmia being treated, as little as 10 joules may be adequate, especially if the origin is atrial.

Indications for emergency synchronized cardioversion in an unstable patient include:

- Perfusing ventricular tachycardia
- Paroxysmal supraventricular tachycardia
- Rapid atrial fibrillation
- Atrial flutter

The procedure for synchronized cardioversion is the same as for defibrillation. Sedate conscious patients if at all possible. Turn on the synchronizer switch, and verify that the machine is detecting the R waves (Figure 2-82).

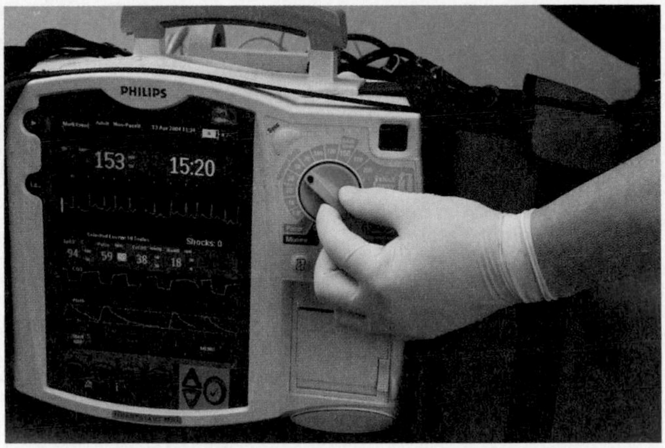

FIGURE 2-82 Activate the synchronizer.

If not, you may need to reposition the electrodes. Press and hold the discharge buttons until the machine discharges on the next R wave. Some models automatically turn off the synchronizer after a cardioversion and return to defibrillation mode. To give a second synchronized shock, depress the synchronizer button again. If ventricular fibrillation occurs, turn off the synchronizer switch and use the machine in the defibrillation mode, because the heart produces no R wave in ventricular fibrillation and the machine will not discharge. The procedure for synchronized cardioversion is summarized in Figure 2-83.

Transcutaneous Cardiac Pacing

Many of the newer cardiac monitor/defibrillators have a built-in cardiac pacing device that enables paramedic units to perform *transcutaneous* (external) cardiac pacing (TCP). Transcutaneous cardiac pacing allows electrical pacing of the heart through the skin via specially designed thoracic electrodes. Before the development of TCP, electrical cardiac pacing required placing an electrode through a major vein or directly into the chest. With TCP, pacing can now be provided in the prehospital setting. This is beneficial in such cases of symptomatic bradycardia as occur with high-degree AV blocks, atrial fibrillation with slow ventricular response, and other significant bradycardias (including asystole). Use transcutaneous pacing if pharmacological intervention has no effect and the patient is hypotensive or hypoperfusing. TCP can be painful for some patients. Consider administering an analgesic (e.g., fentanyl, morphine) or an anxiolytic (e.g., midazolam, diazepam) prior to or during TCP, if needed.

To perform external cardiac pacing, follow these steps (Procedure 2–3):

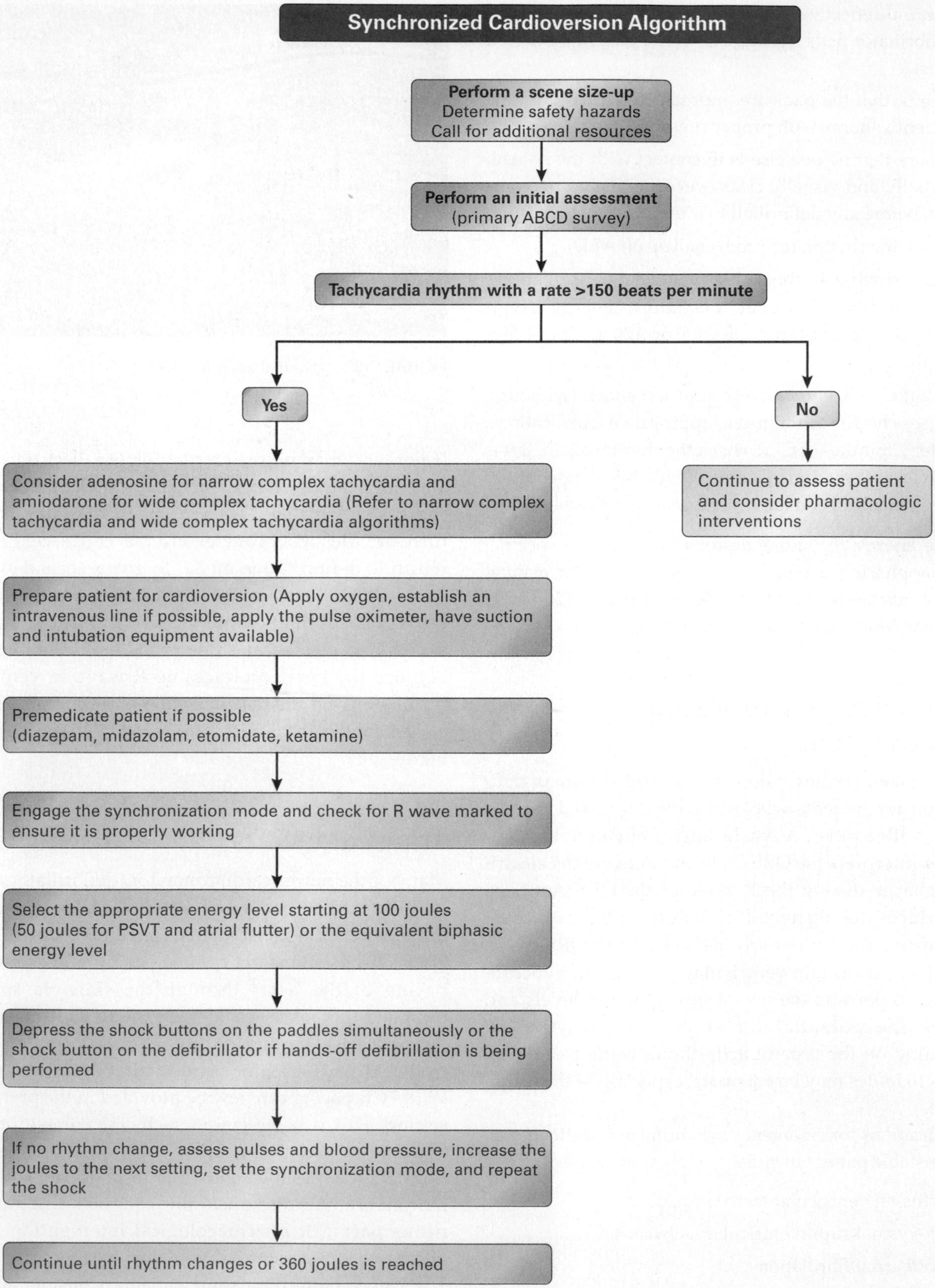

FIGURE 2-83 Electrical (synchronized) cardioversion.

Procedure 2-3 Transcutaneous Cardiac Pacing

External pacing is of benefit in bradycardias and heart blocks that are symptomatic. The electrodes are placed on the chest as shown. The desired heart rate is selected. The current is then adjusted until "capture" of the heart's conductive system is obtained.

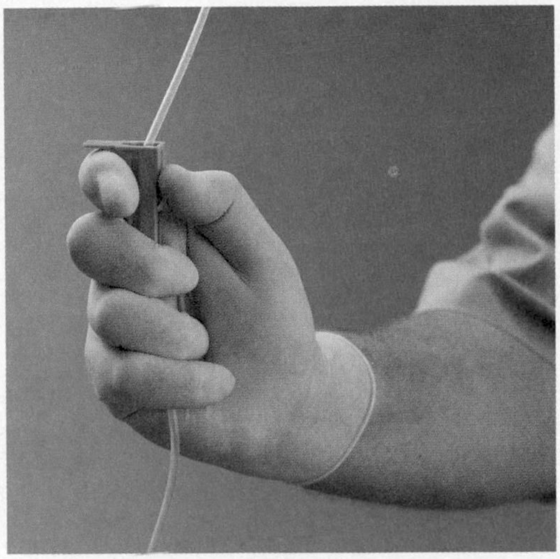

2-3a Establish an IV line.

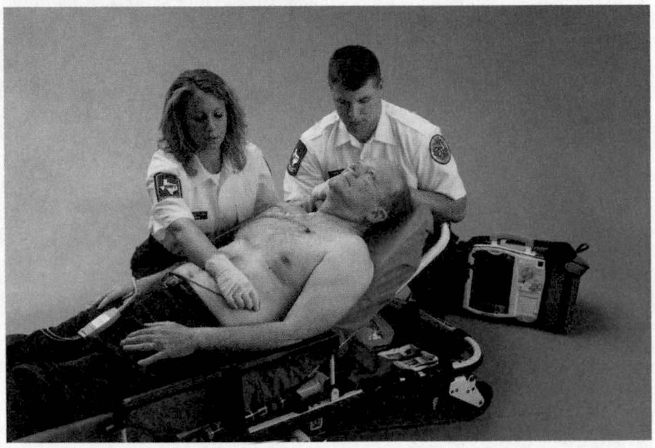

2-3b Place ECG electrodes.

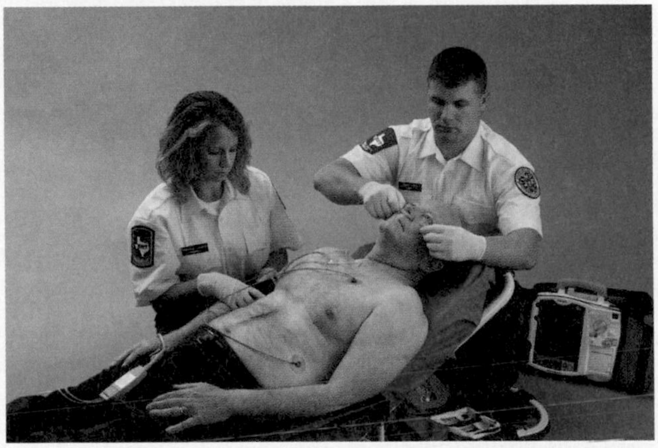

2-3c Carefully assess vital signs and place appropriate monitors.

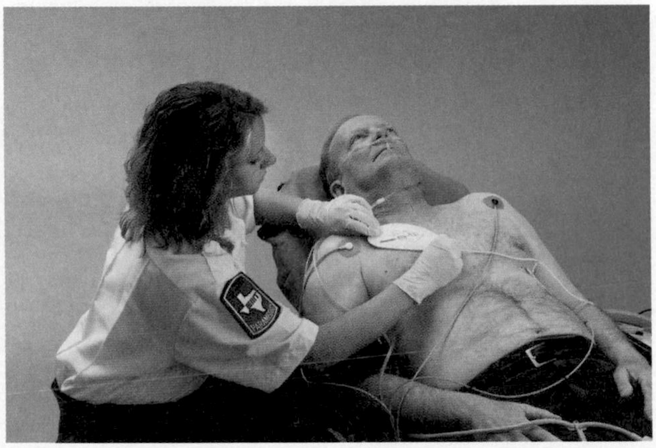

2-3d If transcutaneous cardiac pacing is indicated, apply the pacing electrodes according to the manufacturer's recommendations. Consider sedation or analgesia.

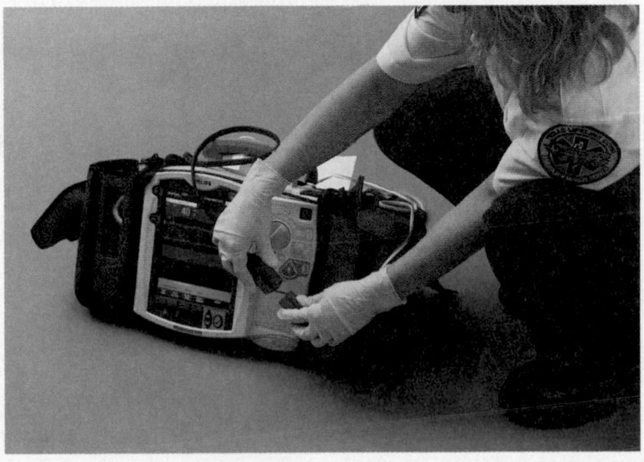

2-3e Connect the electrodes.

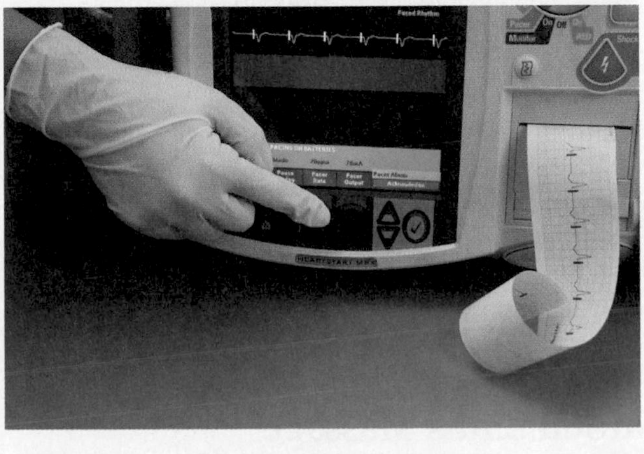

2-3f Select the desired pacing rate and current.

(Continued)

Procedure 2-3 *Continued*

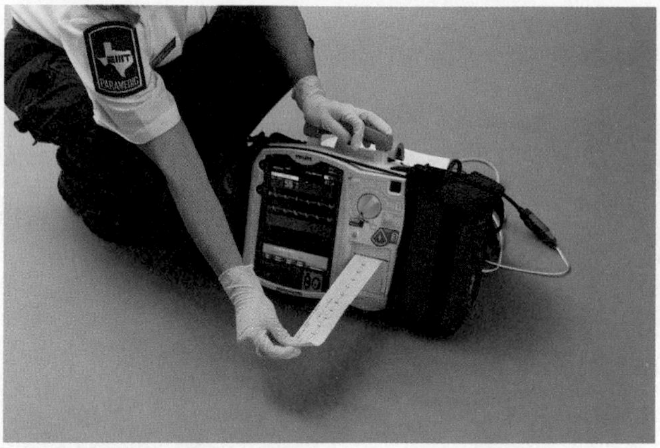

2-3g Monitor the patient's response to treatment.

1. Initiate IV, oxygen (if hypoxic), and ECG monitoring.
2. Place the patient supine.
3. Confirm symptomatic bradycardia and confirm medical direction order for external cardiac pacing.
4. Apply the pacing electrodes according to the manufacturer's recommendations, being sure that they interface well with the skin.
5. Connect the electrodes.
6. Set the desired heart rate on the pacemaker. This will typically range from 60 to 80 beats per minute.
7. Turn the output setting to zero.
8. Turn on the pacer.
9. Slowly increase the output until you note ventricular capture.
10. Check the pulse and blood pressure, and adjust the rate and amperage as medical direction orders.
11. Monitor the patient's response to treatment.

To manage patients in asystole, place the output on its maximum setting. Then decrease the output if capture occurs.

Overdrive pacing may deter recurrent tachycardia. This involves increasing the rate above the heart's current rate to suppress ventricular ectopy. This is particularly useful in *torsades de pointes.* Failure of transcutaneous pacing is similar to the failure of a permanent pacemaker, as discussed earlier in the section on artificial pacemaker rhythm.

Carotid Sinus Massage

Carotid sinus massage can convert paroxysmal supraventricular tachycardia into sinus rhythm by stimulating the baroreceptors in the carotid bodies. This increases vagal tone and decreases heart rate.

To perform carotid sinus massage, have atropine sulfate readily available and use the following technique (Procedure 2–4):

1. Initiate IV, oxygen (if the patient is hypoxic), and ECG monitoring.
2. Position the patient on his back, slightly hyperextending the head.
3. Gently palpate each carotid pulse separately. Auscultate each side for carotid bruits. Do not attempt carotid sinus massage if the pulse is diminished or if carotid bruits are present.
4. Tilt the patient's head to either side. Place your index and middle fingers over one artery, below the angle of the jaw and as high up on the neck as possible.
5. Firmly massage the artery by pressing it against the vertebral body and rubbing.
6. Monitor the ECG and obtain a continuous readout. Terminate massage at the first sign of slowing or heart block.
7. Maintain pressure no longer than 15 to 20 seconds.
8. If the massage is ineffective, you may repeat it, preferably on the other side of the patient's neck.

Complications of carotid sinus massage include arrhythmias such as asystole, PVCs, ventricular tachycardia, or fibrillation. In addition, this procedure can interfere with cerebral circulation, causing syncope, seizure, or stroke. Increased parasympathetic tone can cause bradycardias, nausea, or vomiting.[9]

Procedure 2-4 Carotid Sinus Massage

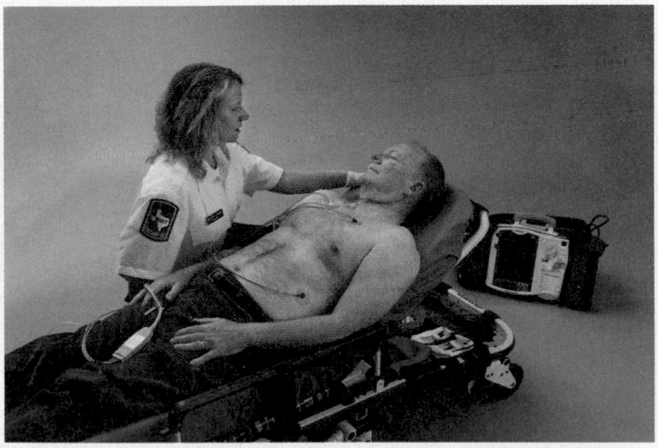

2-4A Assess the patient.

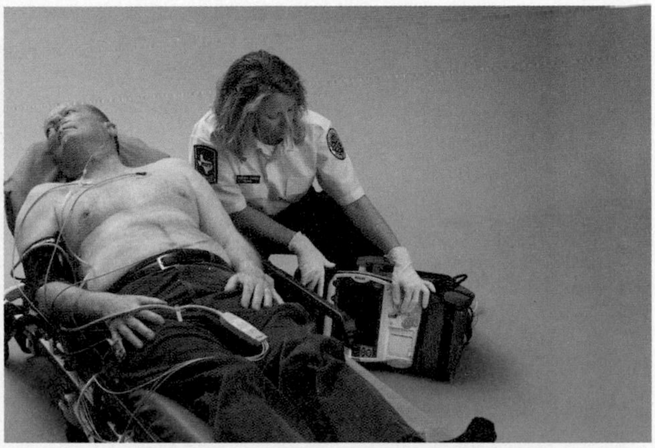

2-4b Turn on the monitor.

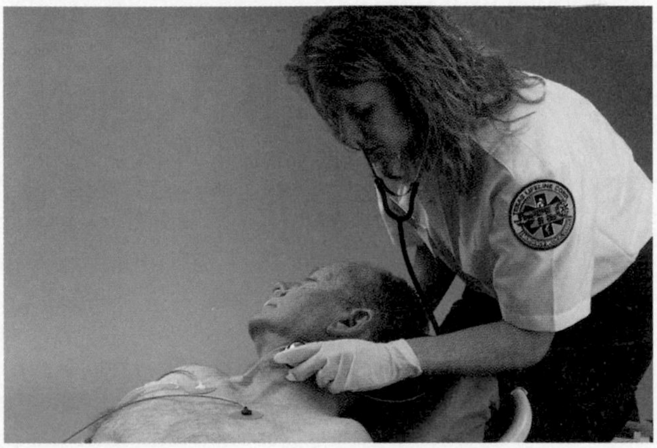

2-4c Listen to both carotids for the presence of bruits.

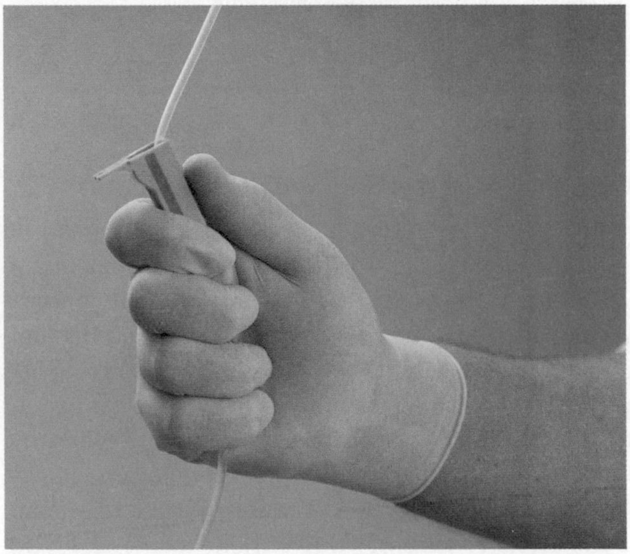

2-4d Start an IV line.

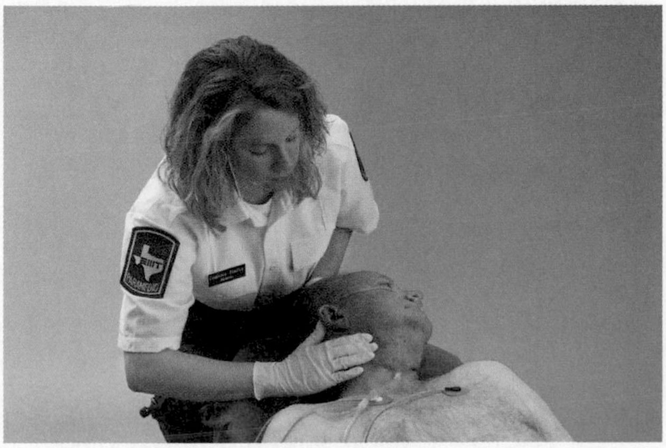

2-4e Rub either carotid. Wait.

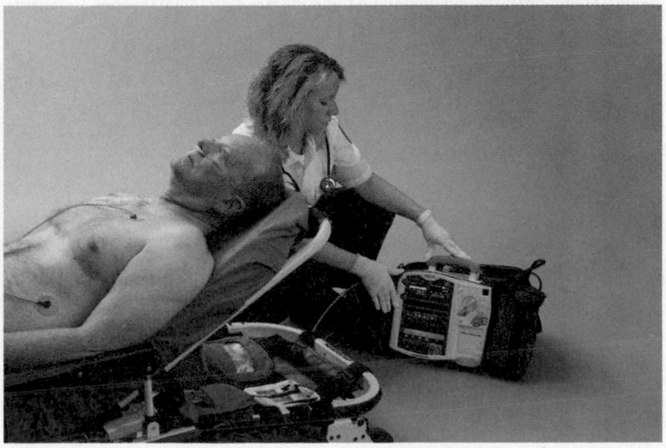

2-4f Check the rhythm.

(Continued)

Procedure 2-4 *Continued*

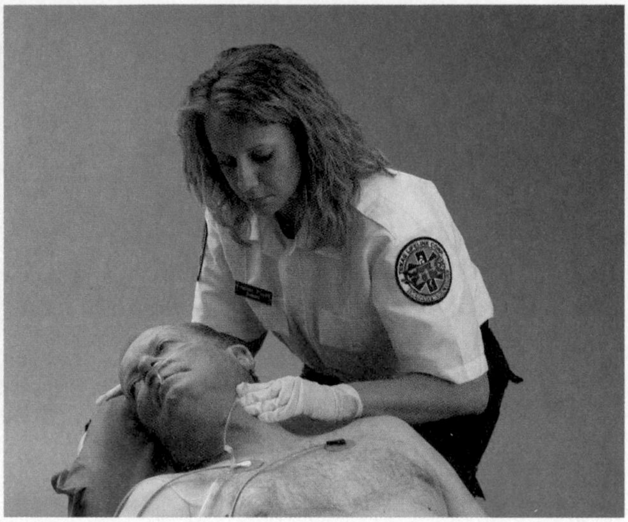

2-4g If unsuccessful, rub the other carotid.

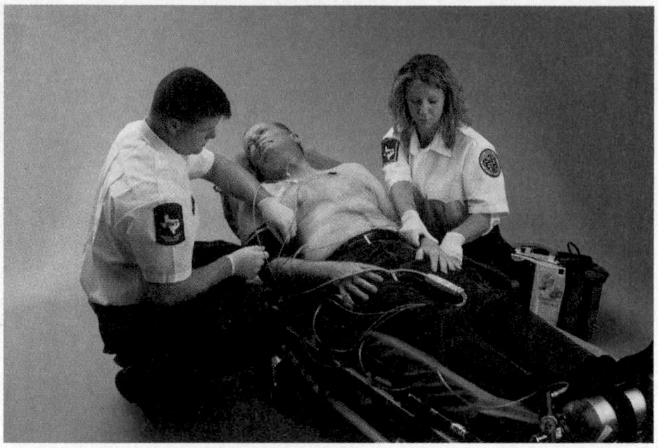

2-4h Reevaluate the patient.

Support and Communication

As with other emergencies, appropriate support and communication are an integral part of the treatment you provide for your cardiovascular patient. Time permitting, explain your treatment to the patient and his family and offer emotional support as indicated. When rapid transport is necessary, explain why. If the patient refuses transport, you will need to clearly explain the potential consequences, and use every available means to convince him of his need for appropriate treatment. As you transfer care of your patient to the receiving facility staff, you must clearly explain your findings to the receiving nurse or physician in a formal verbal briefing. This briefing should include the patient's vital information, chief complaint and history, physical exam findings, and any treatments rendered. In cardiovascular emergencies, any ECG findings will be especially important to the receiving staff.

Managing Specific Cardiovascular Emergencies

The following section details the pathophysiology of common cardiovascular emergencies. Each section covers epidemiology, morbidity and mortality, assessment, and management. Cardiovascular emergencies can present in many different ways. However, the most common presentation is chest pain. In fact, chest pain is the second most common reason that people seek care in hospital emergency departments.

It is important to remember that there are other causes of chest pain. Although cardiac ischemia is one of its major causes, chest pain can arise from problems in the cardiovascular, respiratory, gastrointestinal, and musculoskeletal systems. Causes of chest pain include:

- Cardiovascular causes
    - Cardiac ischemia
    - Pericarditis (viral or autoimmune)
    - Thoracic dissection of the aorta
- Respiratory causes
    - Pulmonary embolism
    - Pneumothorax
    - Pneumonia
    - Pleural irritation (pleurisy)
- Gastrointestinal causes
    - Cholecystitis
    - Pancreatitis
    - Hiatal hernia
    - Esophageal disease
    - Gastroesophageal reflux disease (GERD)
    - Peptic ulcer disease
    - Dyspepsia

- Musculoskeletal causes
  - Chest wall syndrome
  - Costochondritis
  - Acromioclavicular disease
  - Herpes zoster (shingles)
  - Chest wall trauma
  - Chest wall tumors

Diagnosing the cause of a patient's chest pain can be challenging in the hospital, let alone in the prehospital setting. As frequently occurs in emergency medicine, we look for the worst and hope for the best. Always be prepared to treat patients with chest pain as if they are suffering cardiac ischemia or another major disease process. Once you have excluded these possibilities, you can consider less critical causes.

Acute Coronary Syndrome

Acute coronary syndrome (ACS) includes a spectrum of coronary artery disease processes from myocardial ischemia and myocardial injury to myocardial infarction. The progressive narrowing of the lumen of the coronary arteries causes this spectrum of diseases, and the severity of clinical symptoms is dependent on the location and extent of narrowing. ACS includes the clinical entities of stable angina, unstable angina, and acute myocardial infarction.[10]

Stable angina is defined as transient, episodic chest discomfort resulting from myocardial ischemia. The discomfort is typically predictable and reproducible, with the frequency of attacks constant over time. The discomfort is frequently provoked by physical exertion or intense emotional stress. These episodes usually resolve with the use of palliative maneuvers such as rest or medications to open the coronary arteries and relieve the symptoms.

Unstable angina is defined as angina that meets any one of the following three presentations:

1. Angina at rest that lasts longer than 20 minutes
2. New onset angina
3. Crescendo (increasing) angina (more frequent or longer duration)

Acute myocardial infarction is now classified based on ECG findings:

- *Non-ST elevation myocardial infarction (NSTEMI)*
- *ST elevation myocardial infarction (STEMI)*

Acute myocardial infarction is defined as irreversible injury (necrosis) of the myocardium. Diagnosis typically relies on the combined presentation of three specific findings. These findings include a clinical history suggestive of coronary artery disease, evidence of ischemic changes on the electrocardiogram, and elevated myocardial enzymes in the blood (Figure 2-84).

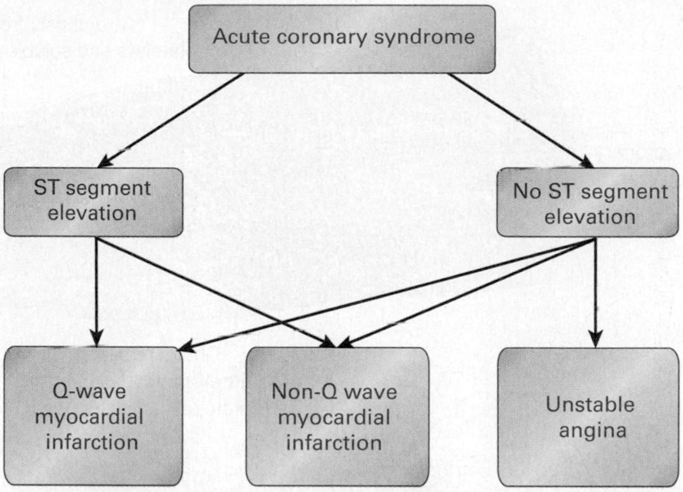

FIGURE 2-84 Differential diagnosis of acute coronary syndrome.

Pathophysiology

Coronary artery disease involves progressive narrowing of the lumen of the coronary arteries (atherosclerosis) caused by the development of thick, hard plaques (atheromas). As the narrowing of the coronary arteries progress, it leads to the clinical spectrum of myocardial ischemia, injury, and infarction. This spectrum of coronary occlusive disease is known as *acute ischemic coronary syndrome*.

Myocardial ischemia is caused by an imbalance of oxygen supply and demand—either a decreased oxygen supply or increased oxygen demand. Impairment of oxygen delivery is the primary contributor to decreased oxygen supply. Impaired oxygen delivery is caused by occlusion of the coronary arteries by spasm, stenosis, thrombus, or a combination of these. Other factors that might contribute to the decreased oxygen supply to the coronary arteries are any factors that produce low blood pressure, such as volume loss, drug effects, or infection. Physical exertion and emotional stress are factors that increase myocardial oxygen demand.

Thrombus formation is considered an integral factor in coronary artery disease. The process is usually initiated by endothelial damage, usually from disruption of an atherosclerotic plaque, which leads to platelet aggregation and thrombus formation. The resulting thrombus can occlude the vessel lumen, leading to myocardial ischemia, injury, and infarction. The consequences of coronary artery occlusion depend on the preexisting atherosclerotic plaque, the extent of occlusion by the thrombus formation, and the rate of development of the occlusion. Occlusions that occur more slowly give the body time to develop collateral circulation in an attempt to compensate for the decrease in blood flow to the area involved (Figure 2-85).

Angina Pectoris

Angina pectoris literally means "pain in the chest." This condition, however, is much more complicated than simple

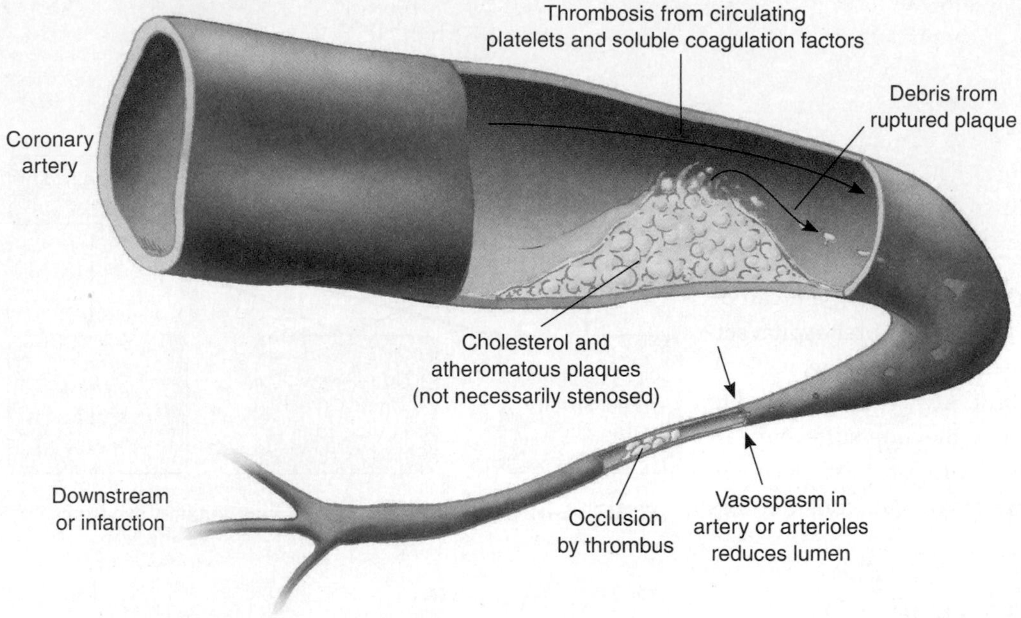

FIGURE 2-85 Acute coronary syndrome pathophysiology.

pain. Angina occurs when the heart's blood supply is transiently exceeded by myocardial oxygen demands. In other words, during periods of increased oxygen demand, the coronary arteries cannot deliver an adequate amount of blood to the myocardium. This can cause ischemia of the myocardium and chest pain.

As a rule, the reduced blood flow through the coronary arteries results from atherosclerosis. Atherosclerotic plaques can develop throughout the coronary circulation. Some patients may have atherosclerotic lesions that are isolated to one vessel, whereas others will have diffuse disease involving several vessels. Fixed blockages in the coronary arteries decrease blood flow. Remember that blood flow through a vessel is related to its diameter. Reducing the diameter of a vessel by one half, as can occur in atherosclerosis, drastically reduces the amount of blood that the vessel can transport.

In addition to atherosclerosis, angina can result from abnormal spasm of the coronary arteries. This disorder, commonly called **Prinzmetal's angina**, *vasospastic angina,* or *atypical angina,* can also lead to inadequate blood flow, causing pain. Approximately two-thirds of the people who have vasospastic angina also have atherosclerotic coronary artery disease. Spasm of the vessel on top of atherosclerotic blockage can cause ischemia. However, one-third of patients with vasospastic angina will have little or no coronary atherosclerosis.

Angina is generally classified as stable or unstable. *Stable angina* occurs during activity, when the heart's oxygen demands are increased. Attacks of stable angina are usually precipitated by physical or emotional stress. They are relatively brief and often respond readily to treatment. *Unstable angina,* on the other hand, occurs at rest and may not respond as readily to treatment. Because unstable angina often indicates severe atherosclerotic disease, it is also called *preinfarction angina*. Unstable angina usually indicates that the patient's disease process is worsening.

Angina is not a self-limiting disease. It results from underlying coronary artery disease. If it is untreated and its contributing factors are unchanged, the underlying problem remains even though the pain has resolved. Because of the nature of the episodes, angina is usually progressive; that is, it accelerates in frequency and duration. Myocardial infarction may follow a single episode of angina.

Field Assessment

When you assess an angina patient, remember that weak or absent peripheral pulses indicate potential or pending shock, which you should treat immediately. Changes in skin color, such as paleness or cyanosis, or changes in temperature, such as cold extremities, also suggest shock.

The typical angina patient's chief complaint is a sudden onset of chest discomfort. The pain may radiate, or it may be localized to the chest. Often, epigastric pain accompanies the chest pain. The patient with angina, however, often denies having chest pain, largely because he has dealt with this type of chest pain before. Although anginal episodes are common for the patient with a cardiac history, they should be considered significant when EMS is activated.

Angina usually lasts from 3 to 5 minutes, sometimes as long as 15 minutes, and is relieved with rest and/or nitroglycerin. Atypical, or Prinzmetal's, angina most often occurs at rest or without a precipitating cause. Prinzmetal's angina is often accompanied by ST segment elevation on the ECG, which can indicate myocardial tissue ischemia.

Labored breathing may or may not be present. After establishing the patency of the patient's airway, auscultate the lungs for congested breath sounds, particularly in the bases. Remember, however, that the lungs may be clear. The anginal patient's heart rate and rhythm may be altered. Peripheral pulses should be equal. Typically, the blood pressure will elevate during the episode and normalize afterward.

The contributing history may indicate that this is the patient's first recognized instance of angina, that it is a recurring event, or that the episodes are increasing in frequency or duration. A recurrence of angina or an increase in its frequency or duration is often the reason an anginal patient calls EMS. Any change in typical anginal pain is significant.

Without prolonging scene time, obtain an ECG tracing. If feasible, a 12-lead ECG is preferred for its additional diagnostic detail. After obtaining and interpreting the tracing, transmit it to the medical facility or medical direction. Typical 12-lead findings in the patient with angina are limited to patterns of ischemia: ST depression and/or T wave inversion. After relief of pain, the ST depression and T wave inversion generally will return to normal. This can take a few minutes or several hours. Occasionally, the patterns may not return to normal.

Many 12-lead monitors have internal computerized pattern identification programs that will identify baseline, certain arrhythmias, and anomalies that you might otherwise miss. These devices are most often accurate, but they do not always identify everything that may be pertinent. For example, patients experiencing Prinzmetal's angina can have ST segment elevation that dissipates after the pain has been relieved. Never trust the computer interpretation. Always overread the tracing for accuracy or telemeter it to the emergency department. The most common ECG finding in the angina patient is ST segment depression. ST segment changes often are not specific, however, and arrhythmias and ectopy may not be present when the tracing is obtained.

Management

The patient experiencing angina is often apprehensive. Place him at rest in a position of physical and emotional comfort to decrease myocardial oxygen demand. Administer enough oxygen to treat hypoxia. Avoid hyperoxia. Establish an IV either on scene, without delaying transport, or en route. If possible, and again without prolonging scene time, obtain and record a 12-lead or 3-lead ECG tracing. This is important because the ECG findings may be normal once the patient is pain free. Measure any ST segment changes and communicate them to the receiving facility. Because a single anginal episode can be a precursor to a myocardial infarction, anticipate ECG changes such as arrhythmias and ST segment elevation.

Administer nitroglycerin sublingually, either as a tablet or a spray. Nitroglycerin patches/ointment are effective if the patient is not hypotensive. Nitroglycerin decreases myocardial work and, to a lesser degree, dilates coronary arteries. If the patient's symptoms persist after one or two doses of nitroglycerin, assume something more serious than angina, such as myocardial infarction. Calcium channel blockers, another class of vasodilator, are now being used, in addition to nitroglycerin, to manage angina. Consider morphine sulfate or fentanyl for chest pain that does not respond to nitrates or calcium channel blockers. It is often difficult, especially early in treatment, to determine whether the patient is suffering stable or unstable angina. Thus, it may be prudent to administer a single aspirin to patients who are not allergic to the drug.

Patients with first episodes of angina or episodes that medication does not relieve are usually admitted to the hospital for evaluation. There is often a fine line between unstable angina and early myocardial infarction. Immediate transport is indicated if the patient does not feel relief after receiving oxygen and/or nitrates. The absence of relief indicates that the patient's underlying disease process may be worsening. If the event is the beginning of a myocardial infarction, *reperfusion* (restoring blood flow to the ischemic tissue) is crucial. Hypotension can occur, especially if the patient has taken nitroglycerin. Its presence indicates transport, because it may lead to hypoperfusion of myocardial tissue. ST segment changes, especially ST segment elevation, indicate rapid transport.

Sometimes, the patient experiencing anginal chest pain will call EMS and then refuse transport after his chest pain is relieved. This may be due to a number of reasons, from denial to the patient's having taken older nitrates, which take longer to work. In any case, strongly encourage immediate evaluation because of the potentially serious complications such as MI. Document patient refusal and be sure the patient signs the refusal and understands the potential risks. Encourage the patient to see his cardiologist or private care physician as soon as possible for follow-up.

Explain to the patient and family the reason and necessity for rapid transport, if indicated. Time permitting, also explain your treatment. On arrival at the emergency department, inform the physician of your findings—past history, vital signs, labored breathing, relief of pain, no relief of pain, and ECG findings, especially ST segment findings.

Myocardial Infarction

Myocardial infarction (MI) is the death of a portion of the heart muscle from prolonged deprivation of oxygenated arterial blood. MI can also occur when the heart's oxygen demand exceeds its supply over an extended time. Myocardial infarction is most often associated with *atherosclerotic heart disease (ASHD).* The precipitating event is commonly the formation of a *thrombus,* or blood clot, in a coronary artery already diseased from atherosclerosis. Atherosclerosis places many anginal patients at high risk for a myocardial infarction, especially those suffering from persistent or unstable angina. Myocardial infarction can also result from coronary artery spasm, microemboli (as seen with the recreational use of cocaine), acute volume overload, hypotension (from any cause), or from acute respiratory failure (acute hypoxia). Trauma can also cause myocardial infarction.

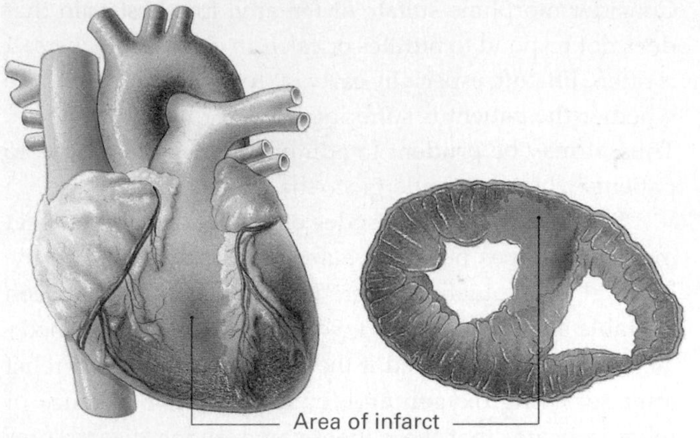

FIGURE 2-86 Myocardial infarction.

The location and size of the infarction depend on the vessel involved and the site of the obstruction (Figure 2-86). Most infarctions involve the left ventricle. Obstruction of the left coronary artery may result in anterior, lateral, or septal infarcts. Right coronary artery occlusions usually result in infarctions of the inferior wall, posterior wall, or the right ventricle.

The actual infarction is often classified as either transmural or subendocardial. In a **transmural infarction**, the entire thickness of the myocardium is destroyed. This lesion is associated with Q wave changes on the ECG and is occasionally called a pathological Q wave infarction. Unfortunately, Q waves can appear fairly late in transmural infarctions. However, ST segment elevation occurs almost immediately. Because of this, the current practice is to refer to a transmural (Q wave) infarction as a **ST-segment elevation myocardial infarction (STEMI)**. A **subendocardial infarction** involves only the subendocardial layer.

When looking for the presence of STEMI, it is important to look at the J point in the ECG. The J point is the junction between the termination of the QRS complex and the beginning of the ST-segment (Figure 2-87). ST-segment elevation with an upward convexity is usually benign, especially when seen in healthy, asymptomatic individuals (early repolarization). ST segment elevation with a downward concavity is more likely to be due to acute coronary syndrome (STEMI).

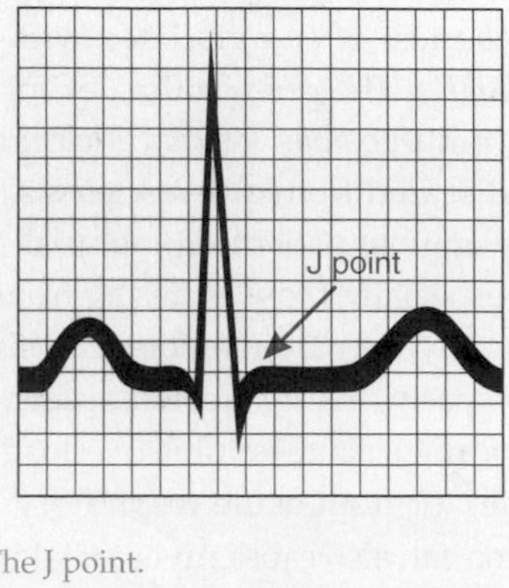

FIGURE 2-87 The J point.

Although both ST-segment elevation with an upward concavity and J-point notching commonly are normal variants, this is only true if the patient is asymptomatic. The same ST pattern in a patient with chest pain is assumed to be due to acute coronary syndrome until proven otherwise.

Because Q wave changes on ECG usually do not accompany this type of infarction, it is often called a *non–Q wave infarction*. The trend in terminology is to refer to a subendocardial infarction (non–Q-wave infarction) as a **non–ST-segment elevation myocardial infarction (NSTEMI)**. Although frequently used, this nomenclature is not entirely accurate, as approximately half of non–Q-wave infarctions present with STEMI, yet fail to develop Q waves later (Figure 2-88).

Myocardial infarction causes varying degrees of tissue damage. First, following occlusion of the coronary artery, the affected tissue develops ischemia. If the blockage is not relieved and collateral circulation is inadequate, the tissue will infarct and die. In trauma, the usual cause of occlusion is plaque that has broken loose. The infarcted tissue becomes necrotic and eventually forms scar tissue. A ring of ischemic tissue that surrounds the area of infarcted myocardium survives primarily because of collateral circulation. This ischemic area is the original site of many arrhythmias. Cardiogenic shock can develop, typically appearing first as ischemia on the 12-lead ECG (ST depression or T wave inversion), followed by injury (ST elevation), and finally infarction (sometimes a pathological Q wave) (see Table 2-5).

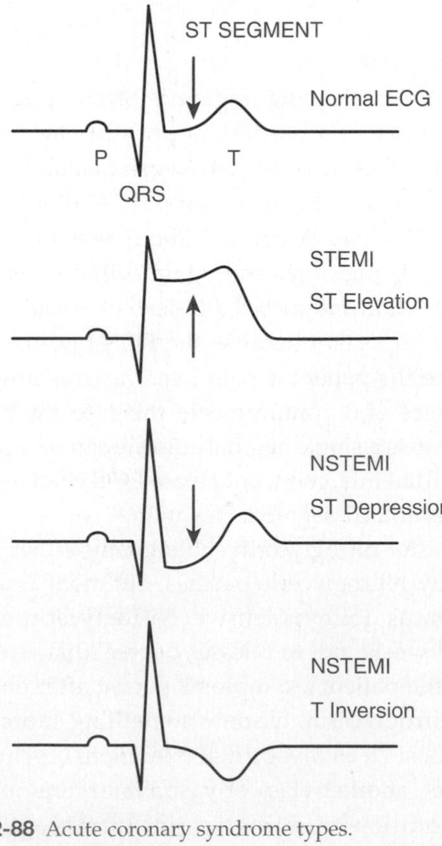

FIGURE 2-88 Acute coronary syndrome types.

Table 2-5 Evolution of a STEMI

Time	Age of STEMI	ECG	ECG Change	Implication
Pre-STEMI	None	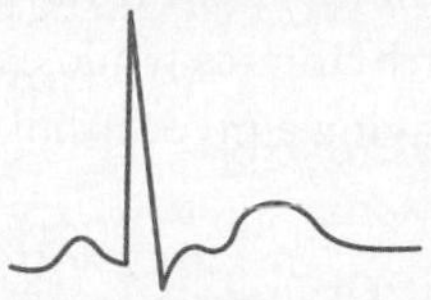	Normal ECG	Normal ECG
Within Minutes of Vessel Occlusion	Acute	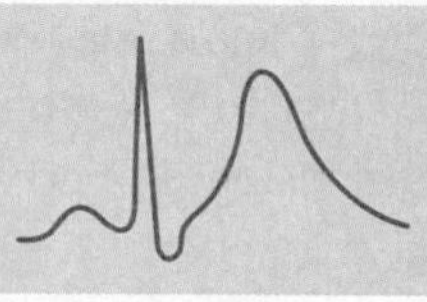	T wave changes: • Hyperacute T wave • T wave inversion	Cardiac tissue is ischemic but not yet injured.
Minutes to Hours	Acute	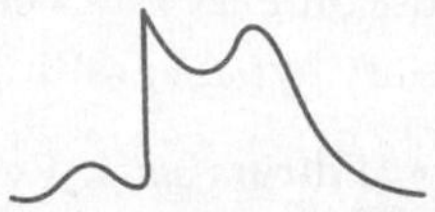	• ST segment elevation • Upright T wave	Tissue injury (ischemia) has begun.
Hours	Acute	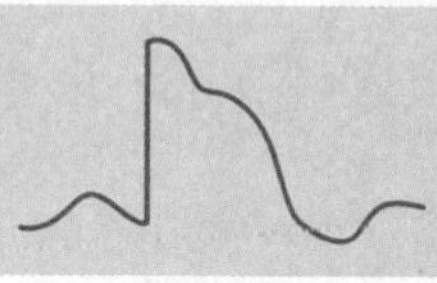	• Significant Q wave • ST segment elevation • Upright T wave	Myocardial death (infarction) has begun, while other tissue remains injured.
Hours to Days	Acute	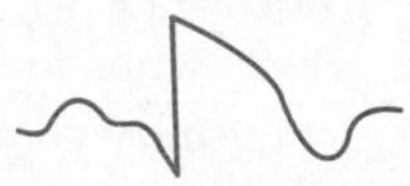	• Significant Q wave • Less ST segment elevation • Marked T wave inversion	Infarction near complete. Some ischemia/infarct persists at the infarct edges.
Days to Weeks	Age indeterminate	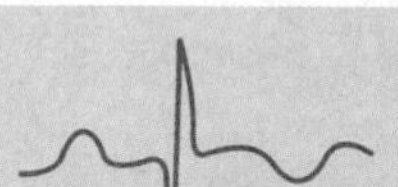	• Significant Q wave • T wave inversion	Infarction is complete. There is no more ischemic tissue (or it has recovered or died).
Weeks, Months, Years Later	Old	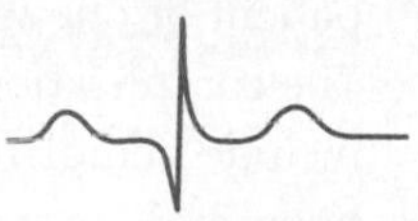	• Significant Q wave only	Permanent tissue death (Q wave)

Arrhythmias are the most common complications of myocardial infarction. They are also the most common direct cause of death resulting from myocardial infarction. Life-threatening arrhythmias can occur almost immediately and can result in sudden death or death within 1 hour after the onset of symptoms. Ventricular fibrillation or ventricular tachycardia may present early with myocardial infarction.

In addition to arrhythmias, the destruction of a portion of the myocardial muscle mass can cause congestive heart failure. Such patients may have right heart failure, left heart failure, or both. *Heart failure* exists if the heart's pumping ability is impaired but the heart can still meet the demands of the body. That is, the heart is inefficient but adequate. If the heart cannot meet the body's oxygen demands, *inadequate tissue perfusion* results in cardiogenic shock. In cardiogenic shock, the heart is both inefficient and inadequate. Another cause of death from MI is *ventricular aneurysm* of the myocardial wall. The damaged portion of the wall weakens and, in some cases, bursts, resulting in sudden death. *Pump failure* resulting from extensive myocardial damage can also result in death.

The primary strategies in managing a myocardial infarction are pain relief and reperfusion. For reperfusion to be effective, rapid and safe transport is paramount. Maximum efficiency on scene and in transit is the most important care you can provide for the patient suffering an MI.

Field Assessment

The patient's breathing may or may not be labored. Look for evidence of shock. Check for regularity of the peripheral pulses, which should be equal in the patient experiencing cardiac ischemia. Take the blood pressure; it usually elevates during the episode and normalizes afterward.

The most common chief complaint in MI is chest pain. Use the OPQRST mnemonic to determine specifics about the chest pain. Typically, the onset of the chest pain is acute, severe, constant, and unrelenting. Unlike the angina patient, the MI patient's discomfort usually lasts longer than 30 minutes. The pain can radiate to the arms (primarily left), the neck, posterior to the back, or down to the epigastric region of the abdomen. Have the patient rate his pain on a scale of 1 to 10. Patients with true myocardial ischemia can have severe pain and may rate their chest pain with high numbers such as 8, 9, 10, or above 10. Often, they will confirm an acute onset of nausea and vomiting. Neither nitroglycerin nor rest offers much pain relief.

Atypically, a patient may have mild symptoms or minimize his symptoms during your assessment. This is more common in diabetics. The patient can be vague when describing chest pain and may complain of generally not feeling well. You might easily mistake this for angina. This patient generally does not complain of vomiting and may or may not have nausea. He also will rate his pain low on a scale of 1 to 10. His vague, general descriptions may arise from many pathological causes. One is that myocardial infarctions generally evolve over 48 to 72 hours. If the patient is more than 24 hours into the infarction, the pain can be different than it was 12 to 24 hours after onset.

The patient experiencing chest pains tends to be very frightened, although this is not always the case. "A feeling of impending doom" describes the patient's fright and pain. This pain is so severe and intense that the patient fears death, especially if he is experiencing chest pain for the first time. Ask if this is the patient's first recognized episode of chest pain or a recurring event. A patient who has suffered infarction before or who has chronic angina may be less concerned with his current pain. If it is recurring, are the episodes increasing in frequency or duration? These patients often have angina-like pain with increasing frequency and/or duration. Denial is common among both the patient with a significant cardiac history and the first-time chest pain sufferer.

After ensuring the patient's airway, auscultate lung sounds. They may present clear or with congestion in the bases. The patient suffering a myocardial infarction usually presents with pallor and diaphoresis. Temperature may vary from the norm. Cold skin or extremities indicate shock. Check the heart rate and rhythm, which may be irregular, and check the peripheral pulses for equality, which MI usually does not affect. The patient's blood pressure may be elevated, normal, or lower than normal.

Apply the ECG. First, examine the underlying rhythm and potential arrhythmias. If you are using a 12-lead monitor, examine the ST segment and Q waves. Check the ST segment for height, depth, and overall contour. Note changes such as ST depression, which suggests ischemia or reciprocal changes, or elevation, which suggests injury. A *pathological Q wave*—deeper than 5 mm or wider than 0.04 seconds—can indicate infarcted tissue (necrosis) or extensive transient ischemia.

Cardiac arrhythmias are the greatest threat to the patient before he arrives at the emergency department. Of the many potential arrhythmias, the most serious are asystole (confirmed in two leads), pulseless electrical activity (PEA), ventricular fibrillation, and ventricular tachycardia. Other arrhythmias include narrow or wide-complex tachycardia, heart block, sinus bradycardia, and sinus tachycardia with or without ectopy. Remember, life-threatening arrhythmias are the leading cause of death among myocardial infarction patients. Anticipate such arrhythmias while caring for any patient you suspect to be having a myocardial infarction.

Reperfusion Therapies

After reviewing the patient's ECG tracing, determine whether he is a likely candidate for rapid transport and reperfusion. Reperfusion can occur via various methods. These include administration of fibrinolytics, percutaneous coronary intervention (PCI), and occasionally coronary artery bypass grafting.

- ***Fibrinolysis.*** Reperfusion uses fibrinolytics such as streptokinase or rtPA (Activase) to stop further injury. Used properly, fibrinolytics can reperfuse all ischemic tissue and much of the injured myocardial tissue, thus reducing the total damage of a myocardial infarction. They work by destroying blood clots—all clots—which, when lodged in arteries congested with plaque, are the most common cause of acute myocardial infarction. The window of time in which a fibrinolytic can be given and be effective is generally considered to be 6 hours from the onset of symptoms. Occasionally, the window will be expanded for a particularly young patient or one who is suffering serious complications. The complications associated with giving fibrinolytics include hemorrhage (which can be fatal), allergic reactions, and reperfusion arrhythmias. Unfortunately, not all myocardial infarctions are caused by blood clots. In addition, many patients have conditions that preclude them from receiving fibrinolytics. These include bleeding or clotting disorders, possible blood in the stool, uncontrolled hypertension, recent trauma, recent hemorrhagic stroke, or recent surgery.[11]
- ***Percutaneous coronary intervention.*** The increased availability of cardiac catheterization labs and the development of STEMI teams now allow MI patients to be immediately taken to the lab for diagnosis and treatment via percutaneous coronary intervention (PCI). A catheter is placed into an artery (usually the femoral) and advanced to the heart. Radiographic contrast dye is administered into the coronary arteries and their anatomy is visualized. This process, called a coronary arteriogram (or coronary angiogram) will detail any blockages or lesions that might be causing the patient's problem (Figure 2-89a). If the lesions can be treated in the lab, they are immediately treated with angioplasty (properly referred to as percutaneous transluminal coronary angioplasty [PTCA] [Figure 2-89b]). A balloon is advanced into the affected coronary artery to the point of the lesion. The balloon is inflated and

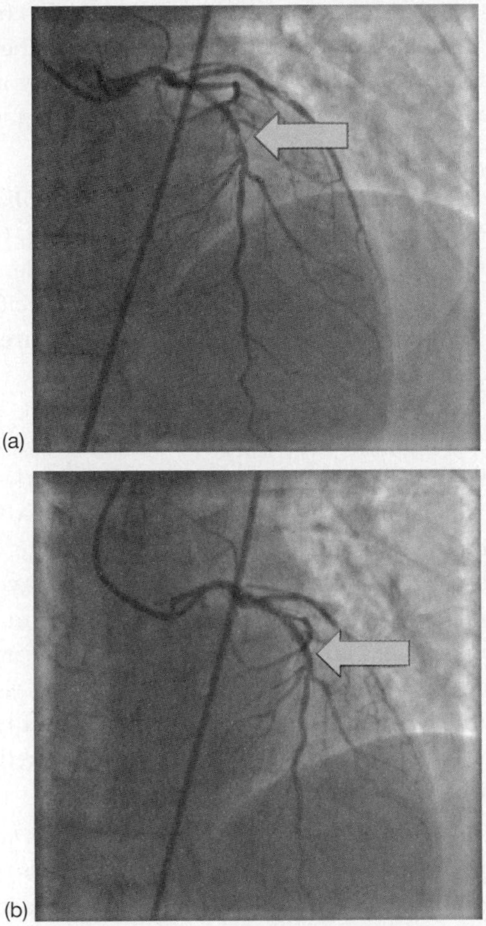

FIGURE 2-89 Coronary angiography. (a) Before treatment: Left anterior descending artery (LAD) blockage. (b) After treatment: Emergency stent placement to open the artery on an ST-segment elevation MI (STEMI).

(Both photos: © Edward T. Dickinson, MD)

the artery dilated. Often the artery will remain dilated after angioplasty. Sometimes it does not. When it does not, a stent is placed to keep the artery open. This procedure, called *primary coronary stenting*, is commonly employed.

- ***Coronary artery bypass grafting.*** Coronary artery bypass grafting (CABG), also referred to as *aortocoronary grafting*, is used when the patient has disease that is extensive or not amenable to PCI techniques. This procedure is rarely done emergently. Instead, the patient is medically stabilized and then taken to surgery. In the CABG procedure, the chest is opened and the heart exposed. Often the patient is placed on a cardiopulmonary bypass pump and the heart temporarily stopped for the procedure. The trend is to do more of these procedures "off pump" with the heart still beating, which tends to minimize some of the complications. In a CABG, the saphenous vein from one leg is harvested and used for the actual bypass graft. In younger patients, the internal mammary artery may be detached from the chest wall and grafted to the coronary artery distal to the lesion. Recently, technology has evolved to the point where some bypass grafts can be performed endoscopically. These require only small "keyhole" incisions instead of the classic sternotomy, thus markedly decreasing the pain and recovery time. Patients whose disease is either too mild or too severe may not be candidates for surgery. These patients are managed with medication alone.

Signs of STEMI or pathological Q waves indicate rapid transport for reperfusion, if symptoms began within 6 hours. Ascertain as near as possible the exact time when the symptoms started, the locations of the ischemia and of the infarction if evidenced on the 12-lead ECG, and any ST segment changes occurring on the 12-lead ECG. This will help the physician determine quickly whether the patient is a candidate for reperfusion. If you are not certain that the patient meets local criteria for fibrinolytic therapy, assume that he does.

After analyzing the patient's rhythm, prepare him for transport. Because reperfusion is the ultimate goal, time is of the utmost importance. Expediently treat any signs of acute ischemia, injury, or infarction. Carefully weigh treating the patient's pain while on scene against rapid transport. When practical, treat the patient suffering from a myocardial infarction in transit.

Many EMS systems have a checklist similar to those that emergency departments use to determine whether a patient qualifies for fibrinolytic therapy. Although these checklists vary from area to area, their use has reduced the waiting time for patients who meet the clinical criteria for fibrinolytic therapy. Standard information that should be relayed to the emergency physician or staff includes the time of the pain's onset, ST segment elevation, and the location of ischemia and infarction on a 12-lead ECG.

Management

PREHOSPITAL MANAGEMENT OF MI Keep in mind that the patient experiencing myocardial infarction is often apprehensive. Place him at rest in a position of physical and emotional comfort to decrease myocardial oxygen demand. Administer an adequate amount of oxygen to correct hypoxia. Avoid hyperoxia. Establish IV access, taking great care not to miss the vein or to have multiple misses, which could jeopardize a patient's chance of receiving fibrinolytics.

Administer medications according to written protocols or on order of medical direction. Remember; always ask the patient if he is allergic to any medication before giving any drug. Medications typically indicated for the patient suspected of myocardial infarction include:

- Aspirin
- Nitroglycerin

- Morphine sulfate
- Fentanyl

Medications that might be indicated include:

- Clopidogrel (Plavix)
- Heparin (or low-molecular-weight heparin)
- Beta-blockers
- Glycoprotein IIb/IIIa inhibitors (tirofiban [Aggrastat], eptifibatide [Integrilin])

Monitor the ECG constantly. Life-threatening arrhythmias are possible. The patient may need rapid defibrillation or synchronized cardioversion at any moment. Plan to quickly provide defibrillation, cardioversion, or transcutaneous pacing, if needed.

Transport the patient you suspect of a myocardial infarction without delay. Because most myocardial infarction patients are very apprehensive and frightened, transport the normotensive patient without lights and sirens. Rapid transport is indicated if the ST segment has any changes, such as depression or elevation, or if pathological Q waves are present on the 12-lead ECG. If a patient exhibits ST or Q wave anomalies, has signs and symptoms less than 3 hours in duration, or has no relief from medications, then consider him a candidate for fibrinolytic therapy. Hypotension indicates immediate transport, especially if the patient has taken nitroglycerin, because the potential hypoperfusion of myocardial tissue can compound the problem. Other factors that indicate rapid transport are any rhythm abnormalities and the presentation within 6 hours of the pain's onset.

If the patient is in the early stages of a myocardial infarction, the outcome of refusing transport is likely to be devastating, ranging from extensive, unnecessary myocardial damage to death. Avoid refusal at all cost, using every means at your disposal to convince the patient to be transported. If the patient still refuses, document the fact that the patient was repeatedly warned of the possible outcome and was also aware of the potential for severely decreased lifestyle or death. Have the patient sign to the fact that he understands the implications, and if at all possible, have a witness sign as well.

Explain to the patient and his family the reason and necessity for rapid transport, if indicated, and inform them of your treatment, time permitting. On arrival at the emergency department, inform the physician of your findings—past history, vital signs, labored breathing, relief of pain, no relief of pain, and ECG readings, especially ST segment results.

CARDIAC ENZYMES Cardiac enzymes are certain chemicals that are released by the heart when myocardial cells are damaged. Thus, an increase in these specific cardiac enzymes is an indicator of myocardial damage. For the most part, measurement of cardiac enzymes has been limited to in-hospital settings. However, with the advent of rapid enzyme assays, it is possible to quickly measure some cardiac enzymes in the prehospital setting. Cardiac enzymes routinely monitored include:

- ***Creatine kinase (CK) or creatine phosphokinase (CPK).*** This enzyme (CK is the newer term, CPK the older term) can be found in the heart muscle, skeletal muscle, and the brain. However, each specific form (isoenzyme) is different and can be measured separately. For example, CK from the brain is called CK-BB, CK from skeletal muscle is called CK-MM, and CK from the heart is called CK-MB. Thus, an elevation in total CK tells you nothing about the heart. When CK is fractionated, however, any elevation in the MB isoenzyme fraction indicates myocardial damage. An elevated CK-MB is seen in about 90 percent of myocardial infarctions. The CK begins to rise 4 to 6 hours postinfarction, peaks at 24 hours, and returns to near normal levels in 3 to 4 days. The CK-MB fraction rises and returns to normal faster than the total CK. It typically begins to rise within 3 to 4 hours postinfarction and returns to normal within 2 days.
- ***Lactic dehydrogenase (LDH).*** Also called *lactate dehydrogenase*, LDH can be found in heart muscle, skeletal muscle, the liver, erythrocytes, kidneys, and some types of tumors. It is increased in more than 90 percent of myocardial infarctions. However, increases in LDH can also be seen in other disease processes. The LDH will tend to rise within 24 hours after a myocardial infarction, reach a peak level in 3 days, and return to normal in 8 to 9 days. Isoenzyme forms of LDH can be assayed separately. They are as follows:
  - LD_1 = heart, erythrocytes, renal cortex
  - LD_2 = reticuloendothelial system
  - LD_3 = lung tissue
  - LD_4 = placenta, kidney, liver
  - LD_5 = skeletal muscle, liver

A reversal of the LD_1/LD_2 ratio suggests myocardial infarction with a sensitivity of 80 to 85 percent.

- ***Myoglobin.*** Myoglobin is chemically similar to hemoglobin, but it is found exclusively within striated (skeletal and cardiac) muscle. It is released into the circulation when skeletal or cardiac muscle is damaged. Myoglobin levels begin to rise within 2 hours after myocardial infarction, peak at 6 to 8 hours, and return to normal within 20 to 36 hours. False positive myoglobin levels can be associated with skeletal muscle injury and renal failure.
- ***Troponin.*** Troponins are proteins within the contractile regions of the cardiac fibers. There are three isoforms

of troponin: troponin I (TnI), troponin T (TnT), and troponin C (TnC). Troponin I is the form most frequently assessed. It is very specific for cardiac injury and is not found in the serum of healthy people. TnI begins to rise within 4 to 6 hours after injury, peaks in 12 to 16 hours, and stays elevated for up to 10 days.

Cardiac enzymes are just one tool in the diagnosis and management of acute coronary syndrome (Figure 2-90). They should always be used in conjunction with physical exam findings, ECG findings, and other diagnostic testing (e.g., stress tests, coronary angiography).

IN-HOSPITAL MANAGEMENT OF MI Your understanding of the management of the MI patient after you have delivered him to the emergency department is important. This is especially true if you belong to an EMS system whose paramedics also regularly staff emergency departments. Because the interventional window for STEMI is so short, many EMS systems and hospitals now allow activation of the PCI/STEMI team from the field setting. In such systems, the patient often bypasses the emergency department and is immediately taken to the cardiac catheterization lab.

With the advent of fibrinolytic therapy and STEMI teams, many hospitals have opened specially designed chest-pain units. These facilities specialize in diagnosing and observing patients with chest pain. In addition to 12-lead ECGs, obtaining cardiac enzyme levels in chest pain patients, as discussed, is routine.

In many chest pain patients, the diagnosis will be readily evident. In many others, however, it will remain unclear. These patients are commonly stratified according to risk. Patients with a low likelihood of cardiac ischemia may be discharged with instructions for follow-up care, which may include diagnostic tools such as stress tests. Patients with a higher likelihood of having myocardial ischemia are usually admitted to the hospital and are typically observed for 24 hours. During the patient's hospitalization, his cardiac enzyme levels are obtained several times, as is his

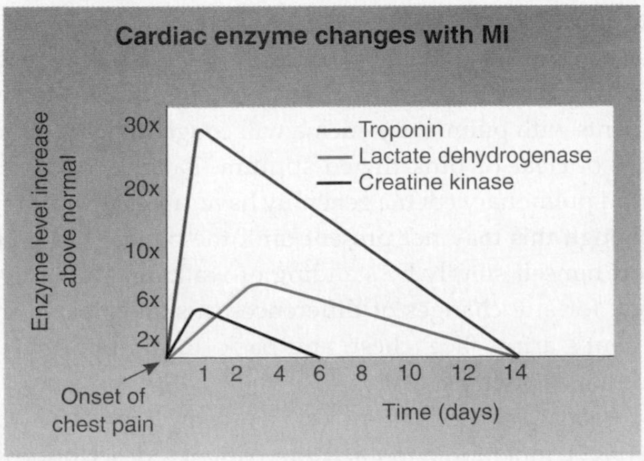

FIGURE 2-90 Cardiac enzyme changes with myocardial infarction.

ECG. If the tests all remain negative, the patient will usually see a cardiologist and have a stress test before going home. If the stress test is negative, the cardiologist will work up the problem as an outpatient. If the stress test is positive, additional testing is done prior to discharge. This testing includes nuclear medicine cardiac imaging (Cardiolyte) and, possibly, coronary angiography. Usually, cardiology immediately sees patients who have a high likelihood of cardiac ischemia but nondiagnostic ECGs and enzymes. These patients ordinarily are not observed but are taken directly to the cardiac lab for an angiogram.

Heart Failure

Heart failure is a clinical syndrome in which the heart's mechanical performance is compromised so that cardiac output cannot meet the body's needs. Heart failure is generally divided into left ventricle or right ventricle failure. Its many etiologies include valvular, coronary, or myocardial disease. Arrhythmias can also cause or aggravate heart failure. Many other factors can contribute to heart failure, such as excess fluid or salt intake, fever (sepsis), hypertension, pulmonary embolism, or excessive alcohol or drug use. It can manifest with exertion in the patient who has an underlying disease or as a progression of the underlying disease.

Types and Eiologies of Heart Failure

LEFT VENTRICULAR FAILURE Left ventricular failure occurs when the left ventricle fails as an effective forward pump, causing back pressure of blood into the pulmonary circulation, which often results in pulmonary edema (Figure 2-91). Its causes include various types of heart disease such as MI, valvular disease, chronic hypertension, and arrhythmias. In left ventricular failure, the left ventricle cannot eject all the blood that the right heart delivers to it via the lungs. Left atrial pressure rises and is subsequently transmitted to the pulmonary veins and capillaries. When pulmonary capillary pressure becomes too high, it forces the blood plasma into the alveoli, resulting in pulmonary edema. Progressive fluid accumulation in the alveoli decreases the lungs' oxygenation capacity and can cause death from hypoxia. Because MI is a common cause of left ventricular failure, consider that all patients with pulmonary edema may have had an MI.

RIGHT VENTRICULAR FAILURE In right ventricular failure, the right ventricle fails as an effective forward pump, resulting in back pressure of blood into the systemic venous circulation and venous congestion (Figure 2-92). The most common cause of right ventricular failure is left ventricular failure, because myocardial infarction is more common in the left ventricle than in the right and because chronic hypertension affects the left ventricle more adversely than the right. Right ventricular failure is also caused by systemic

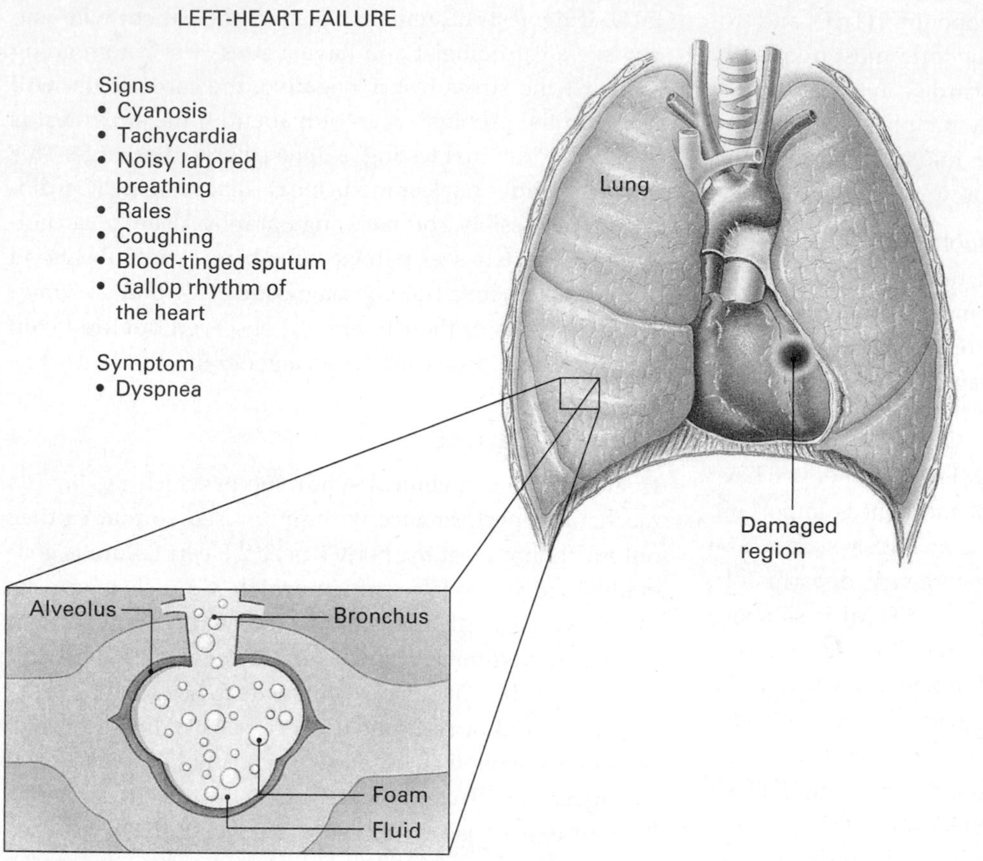

FIGURE 2-91 Left-heart failure.

hypertension, which can affect both sides of the heart and can cause pure right ventricular failure. Pulmonary hypertension and *cor pulmonale* (heart failure due to pulmonary disease) result from the effects of chronic obstructive pulmonary disease (COPD). These problems are related to increased pressure in the pulmonary arteries, which results in right ventricular enlargement, right atrial enlargement, and, if untreated, right-heart failure.

Pulmonary embolism (PE), a blood clot in one of the pulmonary arteries, also can cause right heart failure. If the clot is large enough to occlude a major vessel, the pressure that the right ventricle must pump against increases. This can throw the right ventricle into failure in much the same manner as pulmonary hypertension. In fact, it can be considered an acute form of pulmonary hypertension. Infarct of the right atrium or ventricle, although rare, is another cause of right ventricular failure.

Starling's law of the heart enables heart failure patients to compensate, at least for a time. As you will recall from earlier in this chapter, Starling's law states that the more the myocardial muscle is stretched, the greater will be its force of contraction. Thus, the greater the preload (the volume of blood filling the chamber), the farther the myocardial muscle stretches and the more forceful the cardiac contraction. This has its limits, however. If myocardial muscle is stretched too far, it will not contract properly and the contraction will be weaker. Afterload (the resistance against which the ventricle must contract) also affects stroke volume. An increase in peripheral vascular resistance will decrease stroke volume. The reverse is also true: Stroke volume will increase as peripheral vascular resistance decreases.

CONGESTIVE HEART FAILURE In **congestive heart failure (CHF)**, the heart's reduced stroke volume causes an overload of fluid in the body's other tissues. This presents as edema, which can be pulmonary, peripheral, sacral, or ascites (peritoneal edema). Congestive heart failure can manifest in an acute setting as pulmonary edema, pulmonary hypertension, or myocardial infarction. In the chronic setting, it can manifest as cardiomegaly (enlargement of the heart), left ventricular failure, or right ventricular failure. Heart failure can present in a first-time event, as in myocardial infarction, or in multiple events, as in left heart failure. CHF is one of the few diseases still on the rise in America. Approximately 400,000 new cases are diagnosed each year. CHF also is the most common cause of hospitalization in patients over age 65, accounting for approximately 900,000 admissions each year. Mortality is only 5 years in 50 percent of CHF patients. The end stage of this disease involves pulmonary edema and respiratory failure, followed by death. When the CHF patient calls EMS, one thing is clear: Starling's law is no longer allowing the patient to compensate.

Field Assessment

As in all cardiac emergencies, begin your assessment by checking the ABCs and managing any life threats. Often, patients with pulmonary edema will cough up large quantities of clear or pink-tinged sputum. Patients with profound pulmonary edema generally have labored breathing, although this may not present until the patient begins to exert himself simply by standing or walking a few steps. Look for any changes or differences in skin color on the patient's arms, face, chest, and back. In profound CHF, mottling is often present.

Focus on the patient's chief complaint. Use the OPQRST mnemonic to elicit the patient's description of symptoms. Patients with pulmonary edema will complain

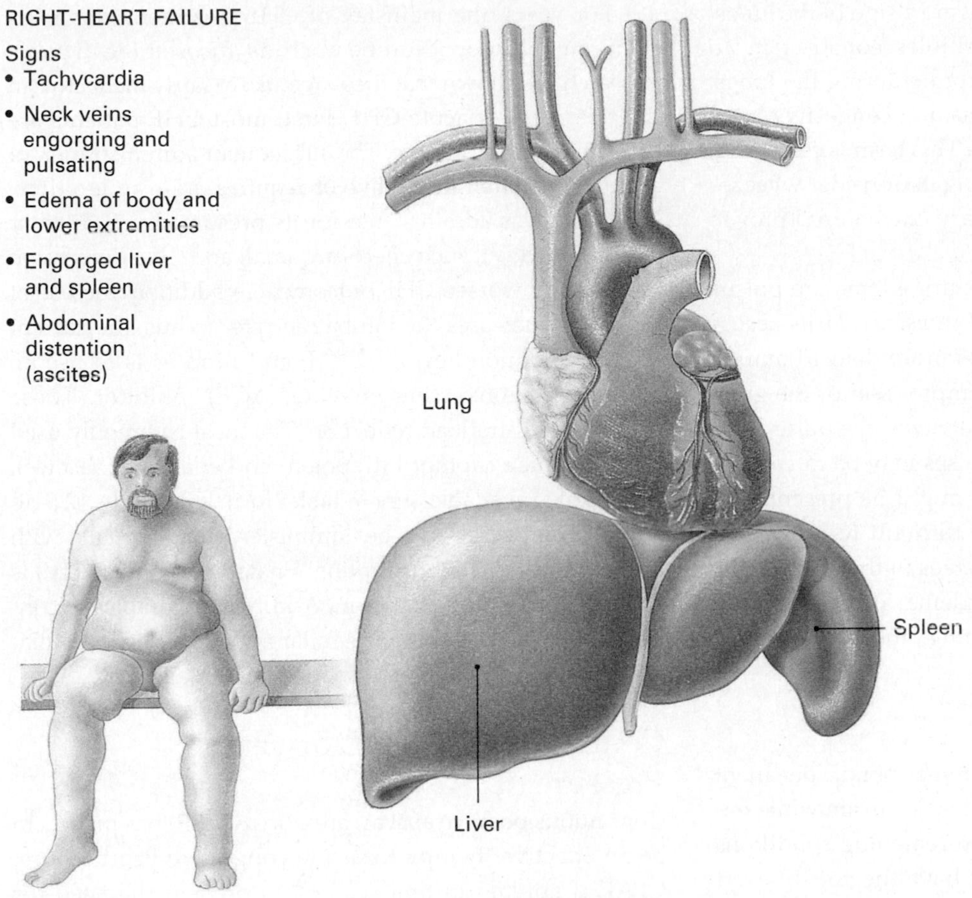

FIGURE 2-92 Right-heart failure.

of progressive or acute shortness of breath and will confirm being awakened by shortness of breath (**paroxysmal nocturnal dyspnea [PND]**). If the patient's episodes of PND are becoming more frequent, the disease process usually is worsening.

Often, the heart failure patient will confirm progressive accumulation of edema or weight gain over a short time. Because many heart failure patients have an underlying cardiac or prior MI history, they may complain of mild chest pain or generalized weakness. This may be due to a weakened myocardial muscle mass, myocardial ischemia, or current MI.

Determine the patient's current medications. CHF patients are generally prescribed a loop diuretic such as furosemide (Lasix) or bumetanide (Bumex) and/or hypertension medication. Many are prescribed digoxin (Lanoxin), which increases the heart's contractile force; many are oxygen dependent and may be on home oxygen. Angiotensin-converting enzyme (ACE) inhibitors are often used in CHF to decrease afterload. Find out whether the patient has been compliant in taking medications; if not, determine how long he has been off medications. Also record and report any over-the-counter or herbal medications that the patient is taking, as well as any prescription medications borrowed from someone else.

Unconsciousness or an altered level of consciousness indicates pending respiratory failure. If the patient shows any sign of respiratory failure, immediately assist his breathing with 100 percent oxygen by BVM and prepare to intubate if clinically warranted.

Next, assess the patient's breathing. Often, labored breathing, dyspnea, and productive cough appear. Labored breathing is the most common symptom of CHF, and it generally worsens with activity. CHF patients frequently assume the tripod position, sitting upright with both arms supporting the upper body, and confirm PND and pillow orthopnea, the inability to recline in bed without a pillow. Ask the patient how many pillows he sleeps on at night. As a rule, the more pillows, the worse the problem.

Check the skin. CHF patients present with changes in skin color, such as pallor, diaphoresis, mottling, or signs of cyanosis. Check the peripheral pulses for quality and rhythm. Also check for edema. Edema is usually found in the lower extremities, localized from the ankles to the mid-calf or the knees. Sometimes, the edema will be so severe that it obliterates the distal pulses. Check the edematous area for pitting and record its severity on a scale from 0 to 4+. Edema may also be present in the sacral area of the back, especially in the bed-bound, or in the upper quadrants of the abdominal cavity. Ascites (abdominal cavity edema or swelling) is difficult to assess accurately without X-ray or ultrasound. Blood pressure may be elevated in the CHF patient, due to the body's attempt to compensate for decreased cardiac output, but this can change quickly. A decompensating patient can have a normal blood pressure that drops quickly.

The most serious complication of heart failure is pulmonary edema. Untreated pulmonary edema can quickly lead to respiratory failure, because the abundant serum fluid in a large portion of the alveoli inhibits oxygen exchange in the lungs and hypoxia ensues. Respiratory failure will quickly lead to death. Patients with severe pulmonary edema present with tachypnea and adventitious lung sounds. Pulmonary edema can present as crackles (rales) at both bases. Rhonchi, which indicate fluid in the larger airways of the lungs, is a sign of severe pulmonary edema. Wheezes in the CHF patient are a sign of the lungs' protective mechanisms, as bronchioles constrict in an attempt to keep additional fluid from entering the lungs. This wheezing in pulmonary edema and congestive heart failure is often called *cardiac asthma*. This term is confusing, however, and you should avoid using it. Consider wheezes in a geriatric patient to be pulmonary edema until proven otherwise.

Other complications of pulmonary edema are pulsus paradoxus and pulsus alternans. *Pulsus paradoxus* occurs when systolic blood pressure drops more than 10 mmHg with inspiration. This is due to compression of the great vessels or the ventricles. In *pulsus alternans,* the pulse alternates between weak and strong. Pulses may be thready or weak, and jugular vein distention might be present. The apical pulse may be abnormal or difficult to auscultate because of abnormalities such as bulges in the heart, a displaced apex, or severe pulmonary edema. The patient may produce frothy sputum with coughing, and cyanosis may present in the late stages of CHF.

Management

In severe CHF with pulmonary edema, obtain pertinent medical history and complete the physical exam while initiating treatment. Reassess all life-threatening conditions and treat them accordingly. Do not have the patient exert himself in any way, including standing up or walking. Do not have the patient lie flat at any time. Seat him with his feet dangling. This will promote venous pooling, thus decreasing preload.[12,13]

Administer an adequate amount of oxygen to correct hypoxia as soon as possible and apply all monitors (ECG, pulse oximetry, capnography). As soon as possible, administer nitroglycerin. Nitroglycerin paste works quite well and has a prolonged duration of effect. Typically, 0.5 to 1 inch of paste is adequate. If nitroglycerin tablets or spray is used, it can be readministered when the beneficial effects wear off. While administering the nitroglycerin, have another team member prepare the CPAP unit. As soon as it is ready, begin administration of CPAP. Begin with a PEEP of 5 cm H_2O. Monitor the patient for changes following the initiation of CPAP therapy.[14,15] Generally, most patients will improve markedly with CPAP. If the patient fails to improve, consider increasing the PEEP to 7.5 to 10 cm H_2O and reassess. When possible, establish IV access. Limiting fluids is imperative. If the patient remains anxious, consider small doses of an anxiolytic (e.g., diazepam, lorazepam, or midazolam).

Administer medications according to written protocols or on the order of the medical director. Some left ventricular failures result from very rapid arrhythmias. If you suspect that an arrhythmia as a cause, treat it according to established protocols. Before giving the patient any drug, ask him or his family if he is allergic to any medication.

For years, the mainstay of CHF treatment was morphine and a loop diuretic such as furosemide (Lasix). Research has shown that these agents are fairly ineffective in the treatment of acute CHF. First, most CHF patients are already taking a diuretic. The subsequent administration of a diuretic is often ineffective or requires quite a high dose. Morphine was administered for its presumed vasodilatory effects. However, such effects are small and CNS depression can actually worsen CHF outcomes. In addition, the use of morphine increases the intubation rate.[16] Thus, the current recommendation beyond CPAP and nitrates is to use an angiotensin-converting enzyme (ACE) inhibitor. These agents cause afterload reduction. The most commonly used agents include captopril (Capoten) and enalapril (Vasotec). Captopril is available only in tablet form. Generally, 12.5- to 25-milligram tablets can be administered sublingually with a fairly rapid rate of absorption. Enalaprilat (Vasotec IV) is available in an injectable form. Additional therapies to consider include albuterol (or a similar adrenergic bronchodilator) and a pressor (dobutamine or dopamine).

Continuous Positive Airway Pressure (CPAP)

Continuous positive airway pressure (CPAP) has proven to be an effective therapy for acute congestive heart failure. CPAP, if applied in time, can often prevent the need for endotracheal intubation and mechanical ventilation. CPAP maintains a constant pressure within the airway throughout the respiratory cycle via a tight-fitting mask that is applied to the mouth and nose (Figure 2-93).

In congestive heart failure, the left ventricle begins to fail as an effective forward pump. When this occurs, pulmonary venous pressures begin to rise, resulting in fluid being forced from the pulmonary capillaries into the interstitial spaces between the capillaries and the alveoli. If allowed to progress, fluid will eventually enter and even fill the alveoli. This inhibits pulmonary gas exchange, thus leading to hypoxemia and hypercarbia. Hypercarbia can cause CNS

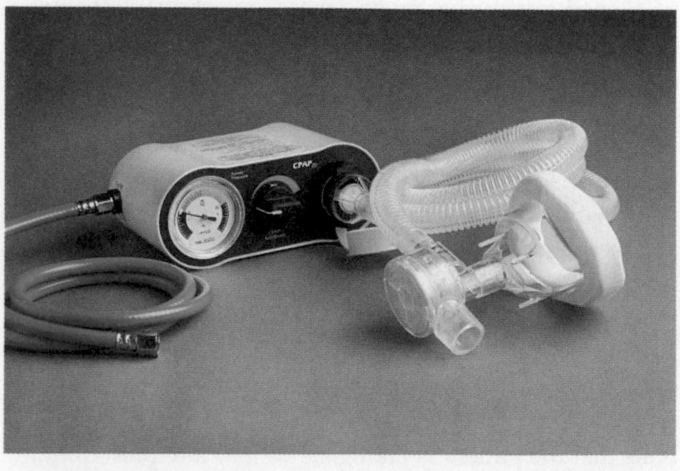

FIGURE 2-93 CPAP device.

depression, which slows respiratory drive and the ventilation rate. CPAP, by increasing continuous pressure throughout the respiratory tree, will force excess fluid out of the alveoli and back into the pulmonary capillaries. It will also help to fill atelactatic (airless) portions of the lungs. CPAP basically buys time so that other medications used in the acute treatment of CHF are allowed to work.

CPAP is often confused with positive end-expiratory pressure (PEEP). The difference is that PEEP is applied only during expiration, whereas CPAP is applied during the entire respiratory cycle. For this reason, CPAP is the preferred modality for CHF. Both CPAP and PEEP pressures are measured in centimeters of water (cm H_2O). Normally, a pressure of 2.5 to 5 cm H_2O is adequate. When pressures exceed 10 cm H_2O, the risk of barotrauma (pneumothorax, pneumomediastinum) begins to rise. Also, when CPAP or PEEP pressures become excessive, the increased pressure within the chest can inhibit ventricular filling and thus worsen cardiac output. Because of these possible adverse effects, it is important to use the lowest effective pressure when applying CPAP.

The indications for CPAP include any patient who is in respiratory distress with signs and symptoms consistent with asthma, COPD, pulmonary edema, CHF, or pneumonia *and* who is:

- Awake and able to follow commands
- >12 years old and is able to fit the CPAP mask
- Able to maintain an open airway
- *And* exhibits two or more of the following:
  - A respiratory rate greater than 25 breaths per minute
  - SpO_2 of less than 94 percent at any time
  - Use of accessory muscles during respirations

The contraindications for CPAP include any patient who is in respiratory arrest or apnea, who is suspected of having a pneumothorax or has suffered trauma to the chest, who has a tracheotomy, or who is actively vomiting or has upper GI bleeding.

The procedure for administering CPAP is as follows (see Procedure 2–5):

1. Explain the procedure and the device to the patient.
2. Ensure adequate oxygen supply to the device.
3. Place the patient on continuous pulse oximetry.
4. Place the patient on the appropriate monitors (oximetry, capnography, ECG, blood pressure) and record rhythm strips with vital signs.
5. Place the CPAP mask over the mouth and nose.
6. Secure the mask with provided straps or other provided devices.
7. Use 5 cm H_2O of PEEP valve.
8. Check for air leaks.
9. Monitor and document the patient's respiratory response to treatment.
10. Check and document vital signs every 5 minutes.
11. Administer appropriate medication as certified (continuous nebulized albuterol for COPD/asthma and repeated administration of nitroglycerin spray or tablets for CHF).
12. Continue to coach patient to keep mask in place and readjust as needed.
13. If respiratory status deteriorates, increase PEEP to 7.5 to 10 cm H_2O.
14. If deterioration continues, remove device and consider intermittent positive pressure ventilation via BVM and placement of an airway.

Do not remove the CPAP until hospital therapy is ready to be placed on the patient. Always monitor the patient for gastric distention, which can result in vomiting. For the most part, CPAP is not considered a resuscitative device and may be used on patients who have a Do Not Resuscitate (DNR) order. It is important to remember that CPAP can cause changes in preload and afterload therapy. Because of this, a complete set of vital signs must be obtained every 5 minutes.

Cardiac Tamponade

In **cardiac tamponade**, excess fluid accumulates inside the pericardium. (The normal amount of fluid between the visceral pericardium and the parietal pericardium is approximately 25 mL.) This excess fluid causes an increase in intrapericardial pressure that impairs diastolic filling and drastically decreases the amount of blood the ventricles can expel with each contraction. Chest pain or dyspnea is the chief complaint; depending on the underlying cause, the chest pain may be dull or sharp and severe.

The onset of cardiac tamponade may be gradual, as in pericarditis or as in a neoplasm such as benign or malignant cancer; or it may be acute, as in MI or trauma. All forms of cardiac tamponade involve pericardial effusion of air, pus, serum, blood, or any combination of these four. Gradual onset usually results from an underlying condition. Overlooking or misdiagnosing the tamponade is easy. Renal disease and hypothyroidism can cause cardiac tamponade, although such instances are rare. Traumatic causes can include CPR and penetrating or nonpenetrating injuries. Whether onset is gradual or acute, cardiac tamponade can lead to death.

Field Assessment

Perform your primary assessment, including the patient's airway, breathing, and circulation. If you suspect cardiac tamponade, limit your history taking to determining the

Procedure 2-5 CPAP Procedure

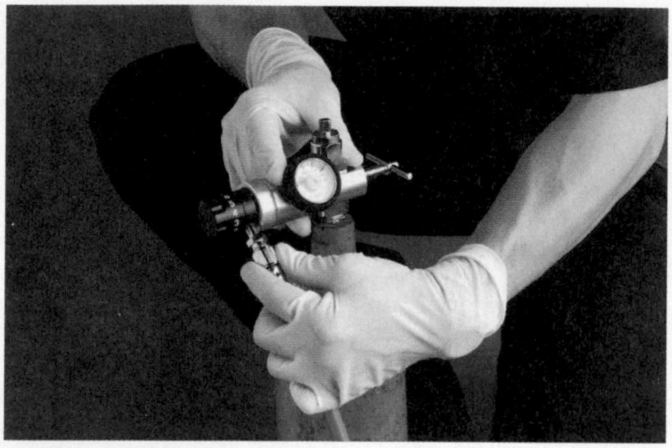

2-5a Attach CPAP unit to suitable oxygen source.

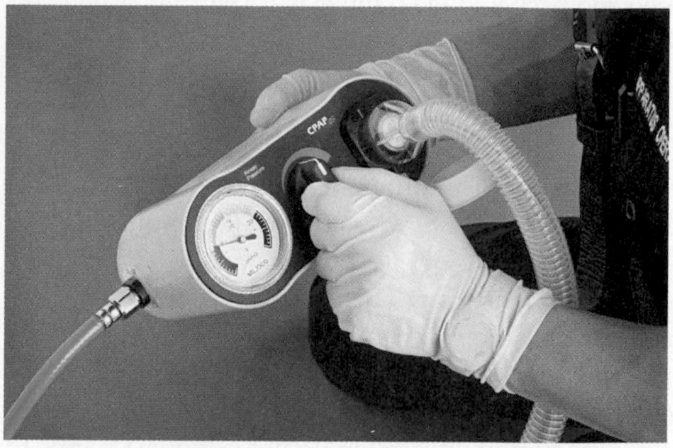

2-5b Set airway pressure to initial setting.

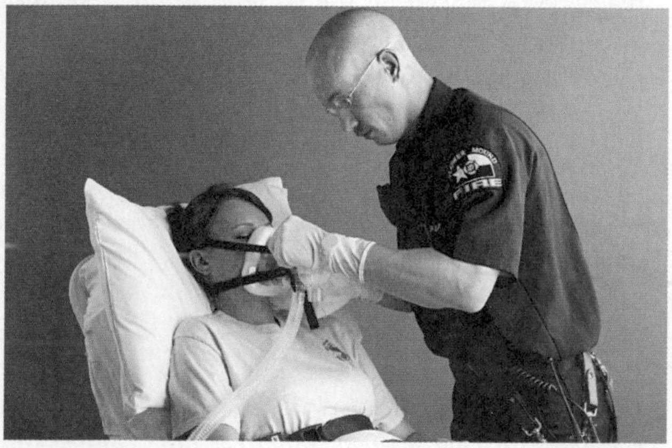

2-5c Secure CPAP to patient per manufacturer's recommendations.

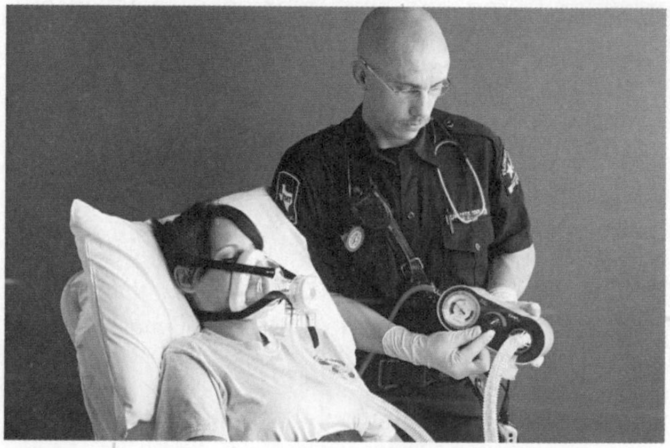

2-5d Increase airway pressure to desired setting.

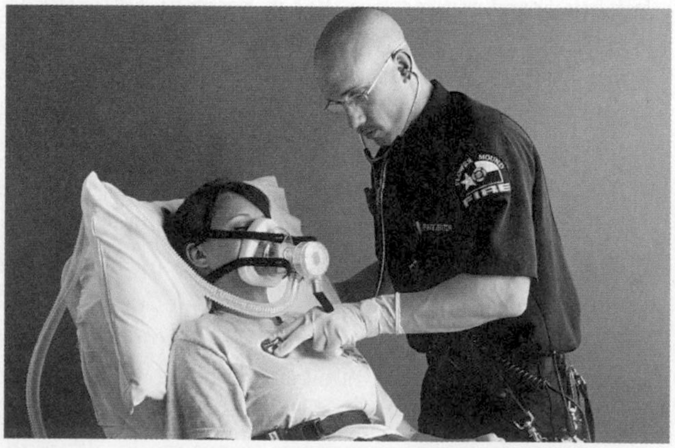

2-5e Reassess patient for response to CPAP therapy.

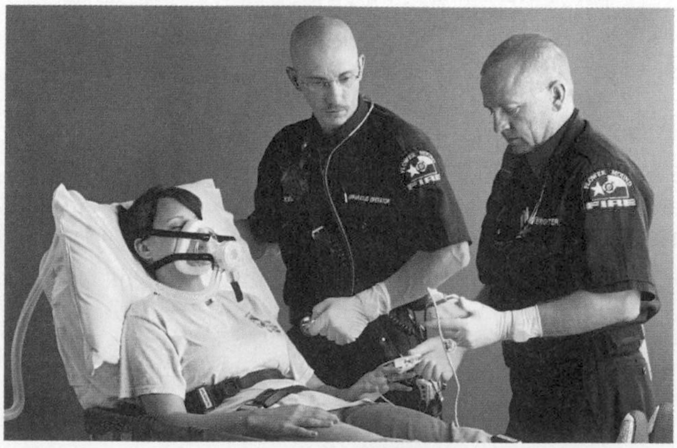

2-5f Continue to monitor patient and adjust airway pressure as indicated.

precipitating cause(s). Determine whether the cause might be acute trauma, such as penetrating or blunt trauma. Has the patient sustained recent trauma, including recent CPR? If you suspect a gradual onset, determine whether the patient has recently had an infection or MI. Is he currently having an MI? Does he have a history of renal disease or hypothyroidism? Has he been ill? Use the OPQRST mnemonic to obtain information about the patient's symptoms.

The patient generally will present with dyspnea and orthopnea. Anterior and posterior lung sounds are usually clear. Typically, the pulse is rapid and weak. In the early stages, venous pressures are often elevated, as evidenced by jugular vein distention. Blood pressure readings show a decrease in systolic pressure, pulsus paradoxus, and narrowing pulse pressures. Heart sounds are normal early on but then become muffled or faint.

Do not use the ECG, whether monitor quality or 12-lead, to diagnose cardiac tamponade; rather, consider it a tool to support your clinical suspicions. The ECG is generally inconclusive, but ectopy is usually a late sign of cardiac tamponade, because an effusion easily irritates the heart's epicardial tissue. QRS and T wave voltages are low, and nonspecific T wave changes occur. ST segments may elevate. Electrical alternans (weak voltage, then normal) may appear in the P, QRS, T, and ST segments.

Management

Initiate treatment while obtaining any pertinent medical history and completing the physical exam. Management of cardiac tamponade is primarily supportive, except when you detect shock or low perfusion. Maintain a patent airway and deliver high-concentration oxygen. If clinically indicated, secure the patient's airway with endotracheal intubation and maintain the patient's circulation with IV support, pharmacological agents, or CPR. Before administering any medication, ask the patient or family if he is allergic to any medications. Medications used in the treatment of cardiac tamponade include:

- Dobutamine (Dobutrex)
- Dopamine (Intropin)
- Furosemide (Lasix)
- Morphine sulfate

Rapid transport is indicated for patients with cardiac tamponade. Remember to be supportive of the patient and family throughout your care. On arrival at the emergency department, inform the physician of your findings—past history, medications, vital signs, labored breathing, ECG readings, pulsus paradoxus, and shock. The therapy of choice is invasive *pericardiocentesis,* which involves aspirating fluid from the pericardium with a cardiac needle. Unless you have adequate training and local protocol permits you to do so, a physician should perform this procedure.[17]

Hypertensive Emergencies

Hypertension is a chronic disease. However, in some patients, the disease is not well controlled and will sometimes result in a life-threatening elevation in blood pressure. These elevations are usually classified as a **hypertensive emergency** or as a *hypertensive urgency*. A hypertensive emergency is a life-threatening elevation of blood pressure and is quite rare—occurring in 1 percent or less of patients with hypertension, usually when the hypertension is poorly controlled or untreated. The different types of hypertensive problems are detailed in Table 2-6. A hypertensive emergency is characterized by an increase in blood pressure accompanied by end- or target-organ changes. It often occurs with **hypertensive encephalopathy**, a condition of acute or subacute consequence of severe hypertension characterized by altered mental status, vomiting, visual disturbances (including transient blindness), paralysis, seizures, stupor, and coma. On occasion, this condition may cause left ventricular failure, pulmonary edema, or stroke.[18–20]

A prior history of hypertension is the precipitating cause of most hypertensive emergencies. In many cases, the patient has not complied with his hypertensive medication or other prescribed drugs. Another cause of hypertensive crisis is preeclampsia or eclampsia. A precursor (elevated blood pressure) called *pregnancy-induced hypertension* can appear at any time between the 20th week of pregnancy and term delivery. It occurs in 5 percent of pregnancies and is defined as a blood pressure of at least 140/90 mmHg. Hypertension is a sign of toxemia, not the cause. Preeclampsia poses a high risk of abruptio placentae and generally progresses to eclampsia (coma and seizures). Left untreated, it progresses to eclampsia and death for the mother and unborn fetus.[21]

Experts estimate that more than 50 million people in the United States are hypertensive patients. Its prevalence increases with age, and it has a higher incidence, as well as a higher mortality and morbidity, among blacks. With modern medications, hypertensive encephalopathy has become rare, yet it is still seen in the prehospital setting. Ischemic and hemorrhagic stroke are more common results of severe hypertension. Both hypertensive encephalopathy and stroke (ischemic or hemorrhagic) can have devastating consequences.

Field Assessment

After making your primary assessment, including airway, breathing, and circulation, conduct your history and physical examination. Generally, hypertensive patients have a chief complaint of headache, accompanied by nausea and/or vomiting, blurred vision, shortness of breath, chest pain, epistaxis (nosebleed), and vertigo (dizziness). However, any one of these symptoms might be the patient's only complaint. The patient may have altered mental status, be

Table 2-6 Hypertensive Conditions

Condition	Definition	Symptoms	Treatment Goals	Medications
Hypertensive Emergency	Severe elevation in BP (>180/120 mmHg) complicated by evidence of impending or progressive target organ dysfunction: • Hypertensive encephalopathy • Intracerebral hemorrhage • Acute myocardial infarction • Acute left ventricular failure with pulmonary edema • Unstable angina • Dissecting aortic aneurysm	• Confusion • Loss of consciousness • Focal neurologic findings (stroke-like symptoms) • Seizures • ECG changes • Pulmonary edema	Reduce BP (not necessarily to normal) to limit target organ damage. Initial goal is to reduce mean arterial pressure (MAP) by no more than 25% (within minutes to 1 hour). Then, if stable, reduce to 160/100–110 mmHg within the next 2–6 hours. Excessive drops in BP should be avoided to avoid renal, cerebral, and coronary ischemia. Exceptions: • Patients with an ischemic stroke where there is no clear evidence to support the use of immediate antihypertensive treatment • Patients with aortic dissection who should have their systolic BP lowered to 100 mmHg, if tolerated.	• Sodium nitroprusside (Nipride) • Nicardipine (Cardene) • Esmolol (BreviBloc) • Labetalol (Trandate; Normodyne) • Fenoldopam (Corlopam) • Clevidipine (Cleviprex)
Hypertensive Urgency	Severe elevation in BP without progressive target organ dysfunction	• Headache • Dyspnea • Nosebleed • Severe anxiety • Chest pain	• No prehospital treatment is required. • Hospital treatment may include use of short-acting oral agents (usually, reinstitution of antihypertensive therapy).	None in the prehospital setting.
Hypertension in Pregnancy • Preeclampsia • Eclampsia	• Generalized edema/swelling • Headaches • Blurred vision • Photophobia • Fatigue • Nausea/vomiting • Reduced urine output • Right upper quadrant pain • Dyspnea • Increased bruising	• Visual disturbances • Headaches • Epigastric pain • Lower extremity edema • Rapid weight gain • Elevated BP • Seizures	Maintain BP at a systolic BP <160 mmHg and diastolic BP <110 mmHg.	• Labetalol • Hydralizine • Nifedipine • Magnesium sulfate (for eclampsia) Avoid: • Esmolol • ACE inhibitors

unresponsive, or be seizing. In pregnancy, the hypertensive expectant mother usually has edema of the hands or face. Photosensitivity and headache are common complaints.

Determine whether the patient has a history of hypertension and whether he has been taking medications as prescribed. Often he has been noncompliant, taking medicines only occasionally or not at all. In some situations, the patient will borrow someone else's medications or take over-the-counter products, such as herbal medications.

If left ventricular failure accompanies the hypertension, the lung sounds generally present with pulmonary edema; otherwise, they are clear. Often, the pulse is strong and at times may be bounding. By definition, hypertension is a systolic pressure greater than 160 mmHg and a diastolic pressure greater than 90 mmHg.

The hypertensive patient's level of consciousness may be normal or altered, or he may be unconscious. His skin may be pale, flushed, or normal; cool or warm; moist or dry. Look for edema, either pitting or nonpitting. The patient may confirm PND, orthopnea, vertigo, epistaxis, tinnitus (ringing of the ears), nausea or vomiting, or visual acuities. In addition, he may have seizures or motor/sensory deficits in parts of the body or on one side. ECG findings are generally inconclusive unless the patient has an underlying cardiac condition such as angina or MI.

Management

Place the patient in a position of comfort, unless a potential exists for airway compromise, as in stroke. Provide airway and ventilatory support, if clinically indicated. Provide oxygen if hypoxia is noted. Place a saline lock. Do not prolong on-scene time to establish an IV. Place pregnant patients on their left side and transport as smoothly and quietly as possible.

The next step is to determine whether or not the patient truly has a hypertensive emergency. Again, a hypertensive emergency is characterized by target-organ changes (e.g., confusion, seizures, ECG changes). Headache, shortness of breath, and chest pain (unless accompanied by ECG changes or suspicion of aortic dissection) do not constitute a hypertensive emergency. If it is determined that a hypertensive emergency exists, then treat according to local protocols. If the patient is having a hypertensive urgency (e.g., chest pain, headache, shortness of breath), then supportive care and reassurance are all that is required. Always follow your local protocols.

Cardiogenic Shock

Cardiogenic shock, the most severe form of pump failure, is shock that remains after existing arrhythmias, hypovolemia, or altered vascular tone have been corrected. It occurs when left ventricular function is so compromised that the heart cannot meet the body's metabolic demands and the compensatory mechanisms are exhausted. This usually happens after extensive myocardial infarction, often involving more than 40 percent of the left ventricle, or with diffuse ischemia.

A variety of mechanisms can cause cardiogenic shock, and its onset may be acute or progressive. Among the more common mechanical causes are tension pneumothorax and cardiac tamponade. Both affect ventricular filling, or preload, and tend to manifest acutely. Interference with ventricular emptying, or afterload, as in pulmonary embolism and prosthetic valve malfunction, can also cause cardiogenic shock. Impairments in myocardial contractility, as seen in MI, myocarditis, and recreational drug use, can manifest either progressively or acutely. Trauma, too, can cause cardiogenic shock, secondary to hypovolemia or to significant underlying disease processes such as neurologic, gastroenterologic, renal, or metabolic disorders.

In cardiogenic shock, the body tries to compensate either by increasing the contractile force, by improving preload, by reducing the peripheral resistance, or by all three. In the early stages, a conscious patient presents with obvious signs of shock (cold extremities, weak pulses, and low blood pressure). As Starling's law loses effect, the patient's mental status diminishes and his radial pulses are no longer palpable. Finally, when preload, afterload, and contractility fail to meet vital organ demands, unconsciousness occurs and, if left untreated, the patient will die.

Cardiogenic shock can occur at any age, but it is most often seen as an end-stage event in the geriatric patient, with significant underlying disease(s). Cardiogenic shock's mortality rate is high for geriatric patients following massive MI or septic shock, because end-organ damage is so severe or multiple end-organ damage reaches the point that life cannot be sustained.

Field Assessment

After conducting your primary assessment, including airway, breathing, and circulation, perform your history and physical exam. The chief complaint may range from acute onset of chest pain to shortness of breath, altered mental status or unconsciousness, or general weakness; onset may be acute or progressive. Ask about the patient's past medical history and determine whether he has had any recent trauma. Look for evidence of a hypovolemic cause, such as a gastrointestinal bleed, septic shock, or traumatic or nontraumatic internal hemorrhage. Has the patient recently suffered a myocardial infarction? Cardiogenic shock is most often associated with large anterior infarction and/or loss of 40 percent or more of the left ventricle.

The patient's medication history may be important. Large amounts of different cardiac medications may indicate that the patient has significant preexisting damage or a compromised but adequate cardiac output. Noncompliance with prescribed medications can further insult a preexisting weakened cardiac state, and the use of borrowed or over-the-counter medications can have unpredictable effects.

The altered mental status secondary to decreased cardiac output and unconsciousness common in cardiogenic shock may begin as restlessness and progress to confusion, ending in coma. Airway findings include dyspnea, productive cough, or labored breathing. Paroxysmal nocturnal dyspnea, tripoding, adventitious lung sounds, and retractions on inspiration are also common findings. Typical ECG findings include tachycardia and atrial arrhythmias such as atrial tachycardias. Ectopy is also common.

Myocardial infarction often precedes cardiogenic shock, and symptoms are initially the same as expected with MI; however, as cardiogenic shock develops and compensatory mechanisms fail, hypotension develops. The systolic blood pressure is often less than 80 mmHg. The usual heart rhythm is sinus tachycardia—a reflection of the cardiovascular system's attempts to compensate for the decreased stroke volume. If serious arrhythmias are present, determining whether they are the cause of the hypotension or the result of the cardiogenic shock may be difficult; therefore, you must correct any major arrhythmias.

The patient's skin is usually cool and clammy, reflecting peripheral vasoconstriction. Tachypnea is often present, as pulmonary edema is a common complication. Pitting or nonpitting peripheral edema may be present in the lower extremities or in the sacral area and may obliterate peripheral pulses.

Management

To manage the cardiogenic shock patient, place him in a position of comfort if he is hemodynamically stable. If any pulmonary edema is present, the patient may prefer sitting upright, with both legs hanging off the stretcher. Treatment of cardiogenic shock (Figure 2-94) consists mostly of treating the underlying problem (such as MI and CHF) or treating the patient supportively. Medical therapy is only a temporary remedy. The patient needs emergent revascularization and reperfusion.

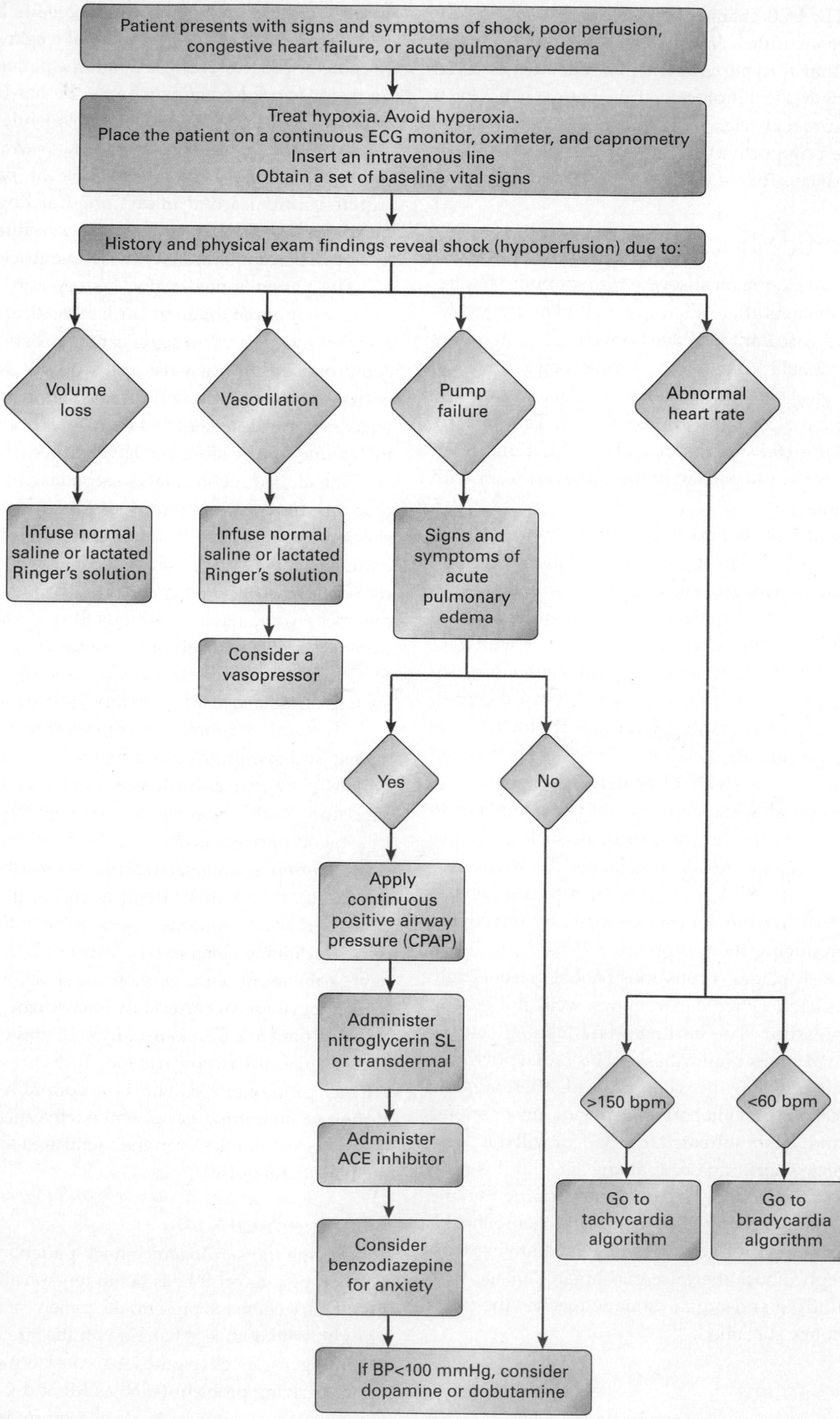

FIGURE 2-94 Management of cardiogenic shock.

Prehospital treatment should include CPAP and adequate oxygenation. Consider the use of a pressor (dopamine, dobutamine, norepinephrine) for pressure support. The most important factor in prehospital care is getting the patient rapidly to a facility with interventional cardiology capabilities.[22]

Cardiac Arrest

Cardiac arrest and sudden death accounts for 60 percent of all deaths from coronary artery disease. **Cardiac arrest** is the absence of ventricular contraction that immediately results in systemic circulatory failure. **Sudden death** is any death that occurs within 1 hour of symptom onset. At autopsy, actual infarction often is not present. Because severe atherosclerotic disease is common, authorities usually believe that a lethal arrhythmia is the mechanism of death. The risk factors for sudden death are basically the same as those for atherosclerotic heart disease (ASHD) and coronary artery disease (CAD). In a large number of patients, cardiac arrest is the first manifestation of heart disease.[4] Other causes of sudden death are:

- Acid–base disturbances
- Arrhythmias
- Drowning
- Drug intoxication/overdose
- Electrocution
- Electrolyte imbalance
- End-stage renal disease
- Hyperkalemia (high levels of potassium)
- Hypothermia
- Hypoxia
- Pulmonary embolism
- Stroke
- Trauma

Pathophysiology of Cardiac Arrest

It has been shown that people who suffer a cardiac arrest (clinical death), particularly due to ventricular fibrillation, go through several phases leading up to biological death. The type of prehospital intervention required is dependent on the particular phase the patient is in. The three phases are (Figure 2-95):

- Electrical phase (0–4 minutes post-arrest)
- Circulatory phase (4–10 minutes post-arrest)
- Metabolic phase (>10 minutes post-arrest)

To understand current treatment regimens for cardiac arrest, it is first necessary to understand the pathophysiology of cardiac arrest and sudden death.[23,24]

ELECTRICAL PHASE The electrical phase is the time interval beginning at the time of the cardiac arrest and ending at approximately 3 to 4 minutes post-arrest. During this phase, several factors must be considered. Generally, at this point in time, the myocardium is in fairly good shape. There is adequate oxygen at the level of the myocardial cells. This results from the fact that the body has oxygen stores. Oxygen is stored in the tissues in the form of **myoglobin**. Myoglobin is similar to hemoglobin except that it has only 2 subunits instead of 4. Myoglobin provides oxygen to the muscle cells during periods of extreme demand. In addition, if cardiac compressions are provided immediately, the circulating blood still may have some oxygen bound to hemoglobin. Many patients who suffer a cardiac arrest might continue to breathe for a brief period of time, which may contribute to increased oxygen availability. Thus, except in extremely diseased hearts, there is some oxygen available during the first few minutes after cardiac arrest. Because there is adequate oxygen, the cells are able to maintain energy production through normal metabolic pathways (aerobic metabolism). Thus, there is not yet an accumulation of acids and the pH is relatively normal. Finally, during this phase, the body's energy stores (primarily adenosine triphosphate [ATP]) are adequate to temporarily support the various biochemical processes occurring. In addition to adequate oxygen and energy stores, neither myocardial ischemia nor myocardial infarction has yet occurred.

The primary problem during the electrical phase is disordered electrical conduction in the heart (e.g., ventricular fibrillation, ventricular tachycardia). In this phase, the only beneficial treatment is immediate defibrillation. The myocardium is as prepared as it can be for application of a defibrillation shock. The administration of defibrillation during this phase can result in survival rates approaching 50 percent. Of course, the sooner the defibrillation is applied, the better will be the survival rate (Figure 2-96). Chest compressions and ventilations are not as important in this phase. However, they are extremely important for subsequent phases and should be addressed as soon as possible.

CIRCULATORY PHASE The circulatory phase is the time interval beginning approximately 4 minutes after cardiac arrest and extending to approximately 10 minutes post-arrest. During this phase, several factors must be considered. First, at this point in time, the myocardium is in distress. By now, there are inadequate oxygen levels in the myocardial cells. This results in a shift from aerobic to anaerobic metabolism. The use of anaerobic metabolism results in a marked decrease in energy production by the cells. ATP and other energy stores are now inadequate to power the cells' various biochemical processes. Anaerobic metabolism also results in the production of lactic acid that will eventually cause a fall in pH (acidosis). During the circulatory phase, myocardial infarction has not yet occurred but myocardial ischemia is possible.

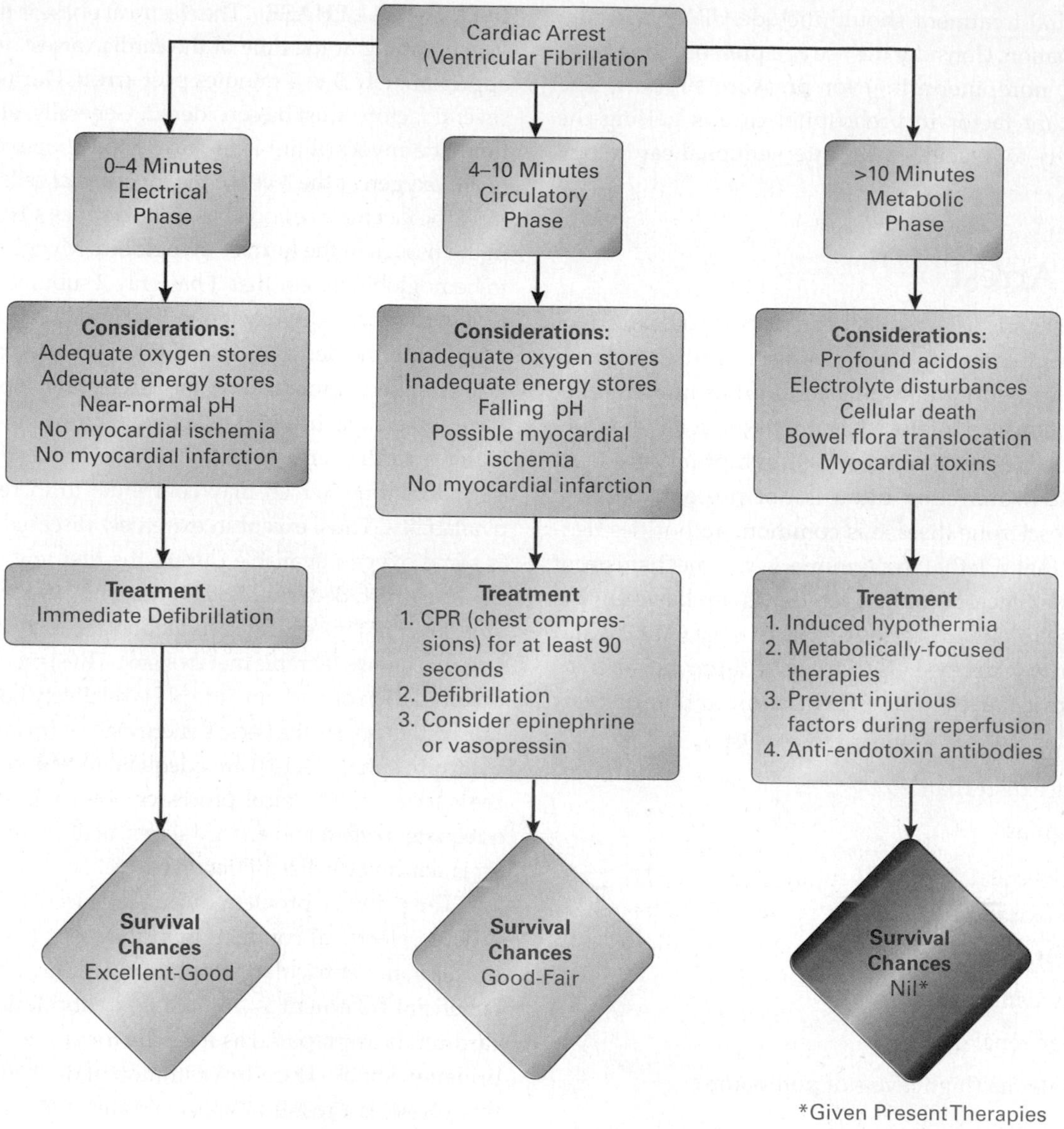

FIGURE 2-95 Three-phase model of cardiac arrest.

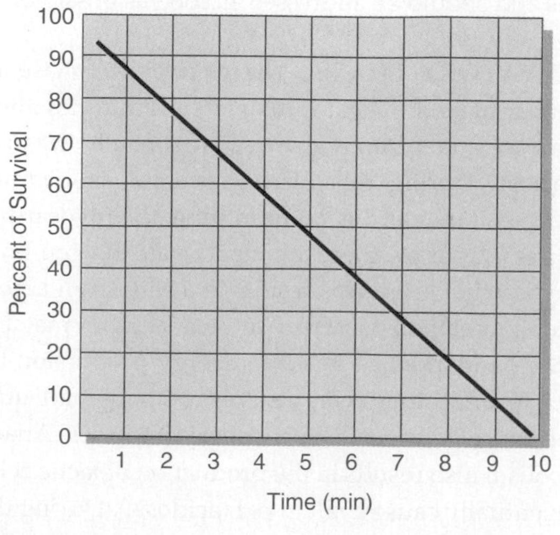

FIGURE 2-96 Survival rates based on time of emergency intervention (defibrillation).

The literature has demonstrated that immediate defibrillation during the circulatory phase may be detrimental. Several recent studies have shown that survival from cardiac arrest during this phase is better if at least 90 seconds of CPR is provided before the application of defibrillation. Unlike the electrical phase, the heart in the circulatory phase is not prepared for a defibrillator shock. Instead, the myocardium must be prepared, as best possible, for a shock. Preparation includes application of chest compressions and ventilation. Some studies have shown that the administration of epinephrine during this phase is beneficial.

METABOLIC PHASE The metabolic phase is the interval beginning approximately 10 minutes after the onset of cardiac arrest. Survival rates for this phase of cardiac arrest are quite low. As with the circulatory phase, the metabolic phase is characterized by severe hypoxia, severe acidosis, inadequate energy substrates, and possibly myocardial ischemia and infarction.

Several adverse events begin to occur during the metabolic phase. Among the most important of these is failure of the sodium–potassium pump. The sodium–potassium pump is responsible for maintaining sodium and potassium levels across cell membranes. When the pump fails, extracellular sodium begins to diffuse into the cell. Water ultimately follows sodium into the cell, resulting in cellular swelling. If allowed to progress untreated, the cell will rupture and die. This is a major mechanism for cell death following cardiac arrest. When a significant mass of cells dies, the organ will ultimately die even though blood flow has been restored.

Derangements in the gastrointestinal (GI) tract further contribute to problems during the metabolic phase. The GI tract provides an efficient barrier between its contents and the outside world. Everything inside the GI tract is kept from contact with the rest of the body through the protective nature of the GI tract. However, when the sodium–potassium pumps in cells lining the GI tract start to fail, a sodium influx occurs that is followed by water. As the cells swell and rupture, the barrier between the inside of the GI tract and the rest of the body is lost. The bacteria that normally reside in the GI tract can then enter the body. Many of these bacteria are of a specific type (Gram negative) and have certain characteristics and harmful effects. When certain Gram-negative bacteria die, they release various toxic chemicals, including endotoxins and cytokines. Both endotoxins and cytokines suppress myocardial function and interfere with other physiologic functions. These chemicals can further suppress an already highly dysfunctional heart. Even if the patient in this phase is resuscitated, reperfusion can cause the widespread distribution of harmful chemicals (endotoxins, cytokines, and others) and metabolic acids (lactic acid). These substances can cause diminished organ function independent of that caused by ischemia.

Current resuscitative measures do not improve survival during the metabolic phase. Stated another way, presently there is little we can do for persons in the metabolic phase. For example, epinephrine, though possibly beneficial during the circulatory phase, can be detrimental during the metabolic phase. Epinephrine shunts blood away from nonessential organs (such as the GI tract) to the brain, heart, and kidneys. A decrease in blood supply to the GI tract can result in earlier, and perhaps more severe, translocation of bacteria and perhaps increased amounts of harmful substances such as endotoxins.

The ability to resuscitate individuals who are still pulseless at the metabolic phase will involve controlling injurious factors during reperfusion. Several strategies are being considered. These include the induction of hypothermia (no longer recommended in the prehospital setting), the use of metabolically focused therapies to correct electrolyte (primarily sodium and potassium) problems, and administration of various buffers. The detrimental effects of endotoxins (the major causative factor in septic shock) may be minimized by the administration of antiendotoxin antibodies. Inflammation remains a problem and anti-inflammatory agents might be administered. However, until such therapies are available and tested, cardiac arrest survival beyond 10 minutes (with the exception of hypothermia and pediatrics) will be extremely limited.

Unusual Causes of Cardiac Arrest

Cardiac arrest can occur in patients without significant coronary artery disease. Many of these conditions are hereditary and involve the cardiac conductive system. Examples of these conditions include:

- ***Brugada syndrome.*** Brugada syndrome is a hereditary condition that is associated with high risk of sudden cardiac death. It is characterized by typical ECG abnormalities: a right bundle branch block (RBBB) and ST segment elevation in the precordial leads (V1–V3). Cardiac arrest and syncope in Brugada syndrome are usually caused by fast polymorphic ventricular tachycardia. If one of the two parents is affected by the disease, each child (whether male or female) has a 50 percent chance of inheriting the disease. Males are more often symptomatic than females. The arrhythmias usually occur in patients between 30 and 40 years of age. Prehospital treatment is identical to that for other forms of cardiac arrest. Patients who are diagnosed early may have an automated internal cardiac defibrillator (AICD) placed.
- ***Long QT syndrome (LQTS).*** Long QT syndrome (LQTS), also called prolonged QT syndrome (PQTS), is a group of disorders that increase the risk for sudden death from an arrhythmia. LQTS can be inherited or acquired. It is somewhat more common in women. In LQTS, QT interval prolongation can lead to polymorphic ventricular tachycardia, or *torsades de pointes*, which itself may lead to ventricular fibrillation and sudden cardiac death. Drug-induced QT prolongation may also increase the risk of ventricular tachyarrhythmias (e.g., *torsades de pointes*) and sudden cardiac death. Some medications (antipsychotics, certain antibiotics, and others) can cause QT interval prolongation and increase the risk of arrhythmias.
- ***Hypertrophic cardiomyopathy (HCM).*** Hypertrophic cardiomyopathy (HCM) is a disease in which the myocardium thickens and stiffens—especially in the ventricles and septum. HCM can be inherited or acquired. Most acquired cases are related to hypertension and aging. In some instances, the cause is unknown. HCM is the leading cause of sudden death in young athletes. Younger patients are more likely to have more significant disease. HCM is frequently asymptomatic until sudden cardiac death occurs.

- ***Commotio cordis.*** *Commotio cordis* typically affects young, otherwise healthy male athletes who sustain a sudden, blunt, nonpenetrating, and innocuous-appearing blow to the anterior chest (e.g., from a baseball or hockey puck) that results in immediate cardiac arrest/sudden death from ventricular fibrillation. Ventricular fibrillation in *commotio cordis* appears to be triggered by chest wall impact only over the heart (predominantly over the center of the left ventricle). CPR and early defibrillation (i.e., in the electrical phase) can be an effective treatment.

Field Assessment

A cardiac arrest patient is unresponsive, apneic, and pulseless. Peripheral pulses are absent. After initiating CPR, place ECG leads. Arrhythmias found in the cardiac arrest patient include ventricular fibrillation, ventricular tachycardia, asystole, or PEA (e.g., idioventricular rhythms). If you find asystole, you should confirm it in two or more leads.

Center questions on events prior to the arrest. Did bystanders or EMS personnel witness the arrest? Did bystanders start CPR? How much time passed from the discovery of the arrest until CPR was initiated? From discovery until EMS was activated? These questions all focus on **downtime**, the duration from the beginning of the cardiac arrest until effective CPR is established. Often physicians want to know the **total downtime**, which is the time from the beginning of the arrest until you deliver the patient to the emergency department. If possible, obtain the patient's past history and medications.

Management

To manage the cardiac arrest patient properly (review Figure 2-63), you must understand the terms *resuscitation, return of spontaneous circulation,* and *survival.*

- **Resuscitation** is the provision of efforts to return a spontaneous pulse and breathing to the patient in cardiac arrest.
- **Return of spontaneous circulation (ROSC)** occurs when resuscitation results in the patient's having a spontaneous pulse. ROSC patients may or may not have a return of breathing, and may or may not survive.
- **Survival** means that the patient is resuscitated and survives to be discharged from the hospital. Many resuscitated patients reach ROSC, but not all resuscitated patients survive.

CONTENT REVIEW

- "CAB" for Management of Cardiac Arrest
  - Circulation (compressions)
  - Airway
  - Breathing
- Begin management of cardiac arrest with chest compressions. Push hard, push fast, and avoid interruptions.
- Remember that basic life support is the mainstay of treatment for cardiac arrest.

RESUSCITATION The mnemonic "ABCs" (airway, breathing, circulation) has been the rule regarding the preferred sequence of primary assessment and management of an emergency patient. However, based on more recent science (such as was discussed earlier in regard to the three-phase model of cardiac arrest), circulation (chest compressions) now has priority over airway and breathing for a patient in apparent cardiac arrest, as indicated by the revised mnemonic that applies to this situation: "CAB" (circulation, airway, breathing). Begin management of cardiac arrest with chest compressions. Push hard, push fast, and avoid interruptions. Airway and breathing come later. Remember that basic life support is the mainstay of treatment for cardiac arrest.

As soon as chest compressions are initiated, a second rescuer should administer high-concentration oxygen and apply a defibrillator monitor or AED. After 2 minutes of uninterrupted CPR, check the rhythm. If it is a shockable rhythm (i.e., ventricular fibrillation, ventricular tachycardia), provide a shock and immediately resume CPR (without a pulse check). While CPR continues, a second rescuer should place an IV or IO. Then, following 2 minutes of CPR, quickly stop CPR and again check for a shockable rhythm. If present, deliver a shock and immediately resume CPR. During the next CPR interval, administer epinephrine and consider placing an advanced airway. Continue resuscitation measures per local protocols. See the AHA cardiac arrest algorithm (http://circ.ahajournals.org/content/122/18_suppl_3.toc [Part 8 Fig 1, page 736]).

RETURN OF SPONTANEOUS CIRCULATION (ROSC) AND POST-CARDIAC ARREST CARE Ideally, when successful, CPR will result in a return of spontaneous circulation (ROSC). Although ROSC is an important benchmark in cardiac arrest care, there is considerably more to do, and the patient's survival is still uncertain. Following a ROSC, post-arrest care is almost as important as pre-arrest care.[25]

Management of the successful post-cardiac arrest patient generally presents an unusual situation. The patient's blood pressure can return at low, normal, or high readings because of the drugs used in resuscitation. In addition, the pulse can return at bradycardic, normal, or tachycardic rates. The ideal range of the systolic blood pressure is 80 to 100 mmHg in the post-arrest patient. Do not be concerned if the post-arrest patient does not show any signs of response. He has endured a very harsh environment, and recovery, if any, can be slow. The post-arrest setting can be unnerving, with the patient's vitals and ECG changing every minute. Approach problems one at a time, and do not be fooled by a return in pulse that fades away while the monitor still has a rhythm (PEA).

It has now become common practice to cool survivors of cardiac arrest in the immediate post-resuscitation period. This procedure, called **induced therapeutic hypothermia (ITH)**, has been shown to improve survival and neurologic outcome in cardiac arrest survivors. The cooling process helps to slow metabolism and minimize the effects of hypoxic injury and oxidative stress (reperfusion injury), thus providing some degree of neuroprotection. The patient is typically cooled with chilled IV fluids and ice packs to a temperature of 32° to 36°C (90.0° to 96.8°F). Once cooled, the patient is usually maintained in the hypothermic state for at least 24 to 48 hours. Problems detected (e.g., STEMI) can be addressed during the hypothermic interval.[26,27]

Studies have indicated that prehospital induction of therapeutic hypothermia is difficult and generally ineffective. Because of this, current guidelines recommend against the use of prehospital ITH. Instead, patients with a ROSC should be transported to a designated facility where ITH may be a part of the bundle of post-resuscitation care strategies.

Withholding Resuscitation

In some situations, the certainty that the patient will not survive indicates not initiating resuscitation efforts. Rigor mortis, fixed dependent lividity (pooling of the blood), decapitation, decomposition, and incineration are all situations in which you should withhold resuscitation.

In addition, withhold resuscitation efforts if the patient has an out-of-hospital advance directive. A physician must sign and date the advance directive, and it must state conditions that apply to the patient at the time of the arrest. For example, the directive may state that resuscitation should be withheld if the patient has an end-stage terminal illness. Each state and many local regions treat advance directives differently. Review local protocol and medical direction before you might have to decide whether to honor an advance directive.

Field Termination of Resuscitation

In other instances, poor prognosis and survivability of many nontraumatic cardiac arrest patients makes termination of resuscitation in the field a consideration. Some of the *inclusion* criteria for termination of resuscitation are:

- 18 years or older
- Arrest is presumed to be nontraumatic in origin and not associated with a treatable cause such as hypothermia, overdose, or hypovolemia
- Successful definitive airway management and ventilation
- ACLS standards have been applied throughout the arrest
- On-scene ALS efforts have been sustained for 25 minutes, or the patient remains in asystole through four rounds of ALS drugs
- Patient's rhythm is asystolic or agonal when the decision to terminate is made, and this rhythm persists until the resuscitation efforts are actually terminated

Depending on local protocol, the *exclusion* criteria for termination of resuscitation may include:

- Under 18 years old
- Etiology that could benefit from in-hospital treatment (such as hypothermia)
- Transient return of a pulse
- Signs of neurologic viability

Criteria that should *not* be considered as either inclusionary or exclusionary:

- The patient's age, if 18 or over (for example, geriatric patient)
- Downtime before EMS arrival
- Presence of a nonofficial Do Not Resuscitate (DNR) order
- Quality-of-life evaluations by EMS

Review local protocol and medical direction before attempting termination of resuscitation. Most systems use documented protocols and direct communication with an on-line medical director or physician to approve or deny termination of resuscitation. The medical director or physician may base his or her decision on the following information:

- Medical condition of the patient
- Known etiological factors
- Therapy rendered
- Family's presence and appraisal of the situation
- Communication of any resistance or uncertainty on the part of the family
- Continuous documentation, including the ECG

The family should receive grief support. This requires EMS personnel or a community agency to be in place soon after termination of resuscitation. EMS personnel deal not only with the living or viable, but also with the families of lost loved ones, especially when they have witnessed the death. Many systems employ assigned personnel to support the family after termination of resuscitation. In other systems, paramedics on the scene provide support until a predetermined person from another local agency can arrive. Although this supportive role can be uncomfortable, it will be part of your job.

Law enforcement regulations require that all local, state, or federal laws pertaining to a death be followed. These, too, may vary from region to region, but their basic principles are the same. The officer discusses the death certificate with the attending physician. He will determine whether the event or patient requires assignment to a medical examiner, whether the nature of the death is suspicious in any way, or whether the physician is at all hesitant to sign the death certificate. The officer also may be required to assign the patient to a medical examiner if he does not have a physician. Check with local law enforcement agencies to determine their protocol.[28,29]

Peripheral Vascular and Other Cardiovascular Emergencies

In addition to cardiac arrest, MI, and hypertension emergencies, other common cardiovascular emergencies involve the arterial and venous systems. Such disorders are generally classified as traumatic or nontraumatic. Nontraumatic vascular emergencies typically arise from preexisting conditions or from a disease process.

Atherosclerosis

The major underlying factor in many cardiovascular emergencies is **atherosclerosis**, a progressive degenerative disease of the midsize and large arteries. Atherosclerosis affects the aorta and its branches, the coronary arteries, and the cerebral arteries, among others. It results from fats (lipids and cholesterol) deposited under the tunica intima (inner lining) of the involved vessels. The fat causes an injury response in the tunica intima, which subsequently damages the tunica media (middle layer) as well. Over time, calcium is deposited, causing plaques, where small hemorrhages can occur. These hemorrhages, in turn, lead to scarring, fibrosis, larger plaque buildup, and aneurysm. The involved arteries can become completely blocked, either by additional plaque, by a blood clot, or by an aneurysm that results from tearing in the arterial wall.

The results of atherosclerosis are evident in many disease processes. First, disruption of the vessel's intimal surface destroys the vessel's elasticity. This condition, **arteriosclerosis**, can cause hypertension and other related problems. Second, atherosclerosis can reduce blood flow through the affected vessel; common manifestations include angina pectoris and intermittent **claudication**. Frequently, thrombosis will develop, totally obstructing the vessel or the tissues it supplies. Myocardial infarction is a classic example of this process.

Aneurysm

Aneurysm is a nonspecific term meaning "dilation of a vessel." The types of aneurysm are:

- Atherosclerotic
- Dissecting
- Infectious
- Congenital
- Traumatic

Most aneurysms result from atherosclerosis and involve the aorta, because the blood pressure there is the highest of any vessel in the body. An aneurysm occurs when blood surges into the aortic wall through a tear in the aortic tunica intima. Infectious aneurysms are most commonly associated with syphilis and are rare. Congenital aneurysms can occur with several disease states such as Marfan's syndrome, a hereditary disease that affects the connective tissue. Aortic aneurysm occurs in people with this disease because it involves the connective tissue within the vessel wall. Those affected may experience sudden death, usually from spontaneous rupture of the aorta, often at a fairly young age.

ABDOMINAL AORTIC ANEURYSM **Abdominal aortic aneurysm** commonly results from atherosclerosis and occurs most frequently in the aorta, below the renal arteries and above the bifurcation of the common iliac arteries (Figure 2-97). It is 10 times more common in men than in women and most prevalent between ages 60 and 70.

Signs and symptoms of an abdominal aneurysm are:

- Abdominal pain
- Back and flank pain
- Hypotension
- Urge to defecate, caused by the retroperitoneal leakage of blood

DISSECTING AORTIC ANEURYSM Degenerative changes in the smooth muscle and elastic tissue of the aortic media cause most **dissecting aortic aneurysms**. This can result in a hematoma and, subsequently, aneurysm. The original tear often results from **cystic medial necrosis**,

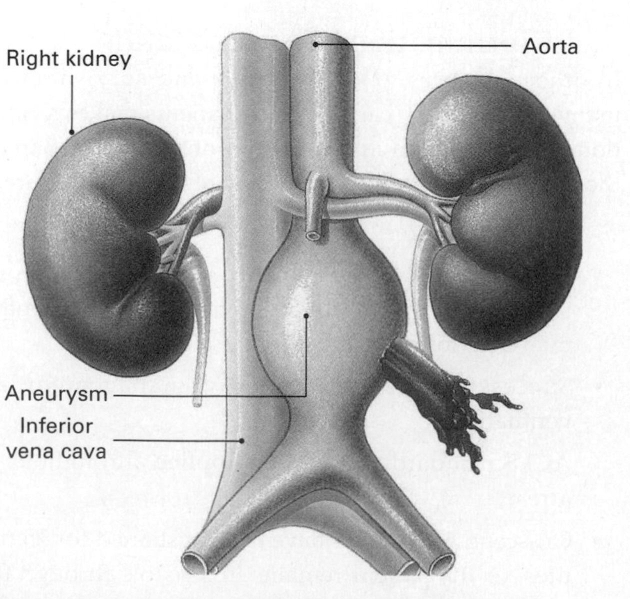

FIGURE 2-97 Rupture of an abdominal aortic aneurysm.

a degenerative disease of connective tissue often associated with hypertension and, to a certain extent, aging. Predisposing factors include hypertension, which is present in 75 to 85 percent of cases. It occurs more frequently in patients older than 40 to 50, although it can occur in younger individuals, especially pregnant women. A tendency for this disease also runs in families.

Of dissecting aortic aneurysms, 67 percent involve the ascending aorta. Once dissection has started, it can extend to all of the abdominal aorta as well as its branches, including the coronary arteries, aortic valve, subclavian arteries, and carotid arteries. The aneurysm can rupture at any time, usually into the pericardial or pleural cavity.

Acute Pulmonary Embolism

Acute pulmonary embolism occurs when a blood clot or other particle lodges in a pulmonary artery and blocks blood flow through that vessel. Pulmonary emboli may be composed of air, fat, amniotic fluid, or blood clots. Factors that predispose a patient to blood clots include prolonged immobilization, *thrombophlebitis* (inflammation and clots in a vein), use of certain medications, and atrial fibrillation.

When a pulmonary embolism blocks the blood flow through a vessel, the right heart must pump against increased resistance, which, in turn, increases pulmonary capillary pressure. The area of the lung supplied by the occluded vessel then stops functioning, and gas exchange decreases.

The signs and symptoms of pulmonary embolism depend on the size of the obstruction. The patient suffering acute pulmonary embolism may report a sudden onset of severe and unexplained dyspnea that may or may not be associated with chest pain. He may have a recent history of immobilization from a hip fracture, surgery, or other debilitating illness.[30]

Acute Arterial Occlusion

An **acute arterial occlusion** is the sudden occlusion of arterial blood flow due to trauma, thrombosis, tumor, embolus, or idiopathic means. Emboli are probably the most common cause. They can arise from within the chamber (*mural emboli*), from a thrombus in the left ventricle, from an atrial thrombus secondary to atrial fibrillation, or from a thrombus caused by abdominal aortic atherosclerosis. Arterial occlusions most commonly involve vessels in the abdomen or extremities.

Vasculitis

Vasculitis is an inflammation of blood vessels. Most vasculitis stems from a variety of rheumatic diseases and syndromes. The inflammatory process is usually segmental, and inflammation within the media of a muscular artery tends to destroy the internal elastic lamina. Necrosis and hypertrophy (enlarging) of the vessel occur, and the vessel wall has a high likelihood of breaching, leaking fibrin and red blood cells into the surrounding tissue. This, potentially, can lead to partial or total vascular occlusion and subsequent necrosis.

Noncritical Peripheral Vascular Conditions

Several peripheral vascular conditions are not immediately life threatening but often require prehospital care. They include peripheral arterial atherosclerotic disease, deep venous thrombosis, and varicose veins.

PERIPHERAL ARTERIAL ATHEROSCLEROTIC DISEASE **Peripheral arterial atherosclerotic disease** is a progressive degenerative disease of the midsize and large arteries. It affects the aorta and its branches, the brachial and femoral peripheral arteries, and the cerebral arteries. For reasons unknown, it does not affect coronary arteries. It is a gradual, progressive disease, often associated with diabetes mellitus. In extreme cases, significant arterial insufficiency may lead to ulcers and gangrene. Occlusion of the peripheral arteries causes chronic and acute ischemia.

In the chronic setting, intermittent claudication (diminished blood flow in exercising muscle) produces pain with exertion. It occurs most commonly with the calf, but can affect any leg muscle. Rest initially relieves this pain. When the disease progresses, however, the pain presents even at rest. The extremity usually appears normal, but pulses will be reduced or absent. As the ischemia worsens, the extremity becomes painful, cold, and numb, and ulceration, gangrene, and necrosis may be present. There is no edema.

In the acute setting, arterial occlusion from an embolus, aneurysm, or thrombosis occurs. The patient experiences a sudden onset of pain, coldness, numbness, and pallor. Pulses are absent distal to the occlusion. Acute occlusion may cause severe ischemia with motor and sensory deficits. Edema is not present.

DEEP VENOUS THROMBOSIS **Deep venous thrombosis** is a blood clot in a vein. It most commonly occurs in the larger veins of the thigh and calf. Predisposing factors include a recent history of trauma, inactivity, pregnancy, or varicose veins.

The patient frequently complains of gradually increasing pain and calf tenderness. Often, the leg and foot are swollen because of occluded venous drainage. Leg elevation may alleviate the signs and symptoms. In some cases, the patient may be asymptomatic. Gentle palpation of the calf and thigh may reveal tenderness and, on occasion, cordlike clotted veins. Dorsiflexion of the foot may cause Homan's sign, discomfort behind the knee, as associated with deep venous thrombosis. The skin may be warm and red.

VARICOSE VEINS **Varicose veins** are dilated superficial veins, usually in the lower extremities. Predisposing factors include pregnancy, obesity, and genetics. Signs and symptoms include the visible distention of the leg veins, lower leg swelling and discomfort (especially at the end of the day), and skin color and texture changes in the legs and ankles. If the condition is chronic, venous stasis ulcers, a noncritical condition, can develop. Venous stasis ulcers can rupture, but direct pressure usually can control the bleeding, which occasionally is significant.

General Assessment and Management of Vascular Disorders

Occlusion of any vessel can result in ischemia, injury, and necrosis of the affected tissue. Depending on the tissue or organ involved, untreated occlusion can cause severe disability or death. In pulmonary occlusion, hypotension and cardiac collapse can ensue quickly, and death can occur rapidly. In cerebral occlusion, debilitating seizures, paralysis, or death can occur. Mesenteric occlusion can cause necrosis, giving rise to sepsis; or it can affect vital organs, causing a slow and agonizing death. Pulmonary embolus, aortic aneurysm, and some acute arterial occlusions can produce a hypoperfusion state, and death can be rapid.

ASSESSMENT Begin your assessment by checking airway, breathing, and circulation. Breathing is usually not affected, except in pulmonary embolus and a decompensated state of shock. In decompensated shock resulting from aneurysm, arterial occlusion, or pulmonary embolus, breathing may be labored. Circulation may be compromised or absent distal to the affected area. Check circulation for the five *P*s:

- Pallor
- Pain
- Pulselessness
- Paralysis
- Paresthesias

Check the skin for pallor or mottling distal to the affected area. Skin temperature may appear normal systemically but cool or cold at the affected area or it may be systemically cool and clammy, as occurs in decompensated shock.

CONTENT REVIEW

➤ The Five *P*s of Vascular Disorder Assessment
- Pallor
- Pain
- Pulselessness
- Paralysis
- Paresthesia

Determine the patient's chief complaint. Depending on the type of vascular emergency, the patient may complain of a sudden or gradual onset of discomfort, and the pain may be localized. Use the OPQRST acronym to elicit the patient's description of symptoms and pain. Is the pain in the chest, abdomen, or extremity? Does it radiate, or is it localized? Was its onset gradual or sudden? If there is claudication, is it relieved with rest?

Conduct your history and physical exam. Determine the contributing history. This may well be the patient's first recognized event, or it may be a recurrence. Patients with a prior vascular emergency are prone to reoccurrences. They may report an increase in the frequency or duration of events. Breath sounds may be clear to auscultation. Alterations in the heart rate and rhythm may occur with pulmonary embolus and aortic aneurysm. Unequal bilateral blood pressures may indicate a high thoracic aneurysm. Peripheral pulses may be diminished or absent in the affected extremity with arterial occlusion or peripheral arterial atherosclerotic disease. Bruits may be audible over the affected carotid artery. The skin may be cool, moist, or dry, reflecting diminished circulation to the affected area or extremity. ECG findings generally do not contribute to vascular emergency treatment. If arrhythmias or ectopy are present, treat them accordingly.

MANAGEMENT Managing the patient with a vascular emergency is mostly supportive. Place the patient in a position of comfort. Give oxygen by nonrebreather mask (if the patient is hypoxic) if you suspect pulmonary embolus, aortic aneurysm, or arterial occlusion or if any hypotension or a hypoperfusion state presents.

Before administering any drug, ask the patient or his family whether he is allergic to any medications. Pharmacological agents that might be used in a vascular emergency include:

- Nitrous oxide (Nitronox)
- Morphine sulfate
- Fentanyl

Transport the patient as soon as possible. Indications for rapid transport with lights and sirens include any situation in which medications do not relieve the patient's symptoms or in which you suspect pulmonary embolism, aortic aneurysm, or arterial occlusion. Also consider any presentation of hypotension or hypoperfusion to be an emergency and transport the patient rapidly. Report your findings to the emergency department staff.

If the patient refuses transport, advise him that serious complications are likely to occur without further medical attention. Vascular emergencies can reach a point at which the patient permanently loses a limb or quickly decompensates into irreversible shock. Some patients will attempt to refuse transport because they have received relief from pain medications. Use every means at your disposal to convince them to be transported. Document refusals according to general guidelines.

PART 3: 12-Lead ECG Monitoring and Interpretation

An electrocardiogram (ECG) is a graphic recording of the electrical activity of the heart. For years, routine single-lead monitoring has been an intrinsic part of prehospital care. Now, with the advent of portable 12-lead ECG monitors, multilead monitoring is available to prehospital providers.

Single-lead ECG monitoring was designed principally to detect cardiac arrhythmias. It did not allow for diagnosis of acute myocardial infarction, conduction abnormalities, or other electrophysiologic problems. With the advent of fibrinolytic therapy, however, early detection of acute myocardial infarction has become very important. The window of time from the onset of symptoms to beginning fibrinolytic therapy is limited. In many instances, early diagnosis of acute myocardial infarction can be obtained in the field and fibrinolytic therapy initiated either in the field or on arrival at the emergency department.

This part of the chapter will examine the use of 12-lead ECG monitoring in prehospital care, including relevant electrophysiology, interpretation, and techniques.

Reviewing the Cardiac Conductive System

The cardiac conductive system was discussed in detail earlier in the chapter. It consists of conductive fibers that transmit the depolarization potential rapidly through the heart. Transmission through these specialized conductive fibers is much faster than if the impulse were transmitted through regular myocardial cells.

The purpose of the cardiac conductive system is to stimulate the atria and the ventricles to contract in the proper direction and at the proper time. The mass of atrial tissue functions together as the atrial syncytium. That is, when one cell of atrial muscle becomes excited, the action potential will spread rapidly across the entire group of cells, resulting in coordinated depolarization and subsequent contraction. Likewise, the mass of ventricular tissue functions together as the ventricular syncytium. Once stimulated, the action potential quickly spreads across the entire group of cells, resulting in coordinated depolarization and contraction.

Knowledge of the cardiac conductive system is essential to understanding and interpreting 12-lead ECG tracings (review Figure 2-16). Internodal pathways connect the SA (sinoatrial) node, located high in the right atrium, to the AV (atrioventricular) node. The internodal pathways conduct the depolarization impulse from the SA node to the atrial muscle mass and, through the atria, to the AV junction. The impulse is slowed at the AV junction, allowing time for ventricular filling. Then, as the impulse passes through the AV junction, it enters the AV node. The AV node is connected to the AV fibers, which conduct the impulse from the atria to the ventricles. The AV fibers then become the bundle of His, which transmits the impulse through the interventricular septum.

The bundle of His subsequently divides into the right and left bundle branches. The right bundle branch delivers the impulse to the apex of the right ventricle, where it is spread across the myocardium by the Purkinje system. At the same time, the impulse is carried into the left bundle branch. The left bundle branch divides into the anterior and posterior fascicles, which ultimately terminate into the Purkinje system. As the impulse is transmitted to the right ventricle, the Purkinje system simultaneously spreads it across the mass of the myocardium. Repolarization occurs predominantly in the opposite direction. This normal series of electrophysiologic events results in the normal ECG tracing (review Figure 2-18).

ECG Recording

An ECG machine records the electrical activity of the heart as detected by the various leads attached to the body. A minimum of two electrodes is required to detect the electrical activity of the heart, so each lead consists of a pair of electrodes. Typically, one electrode is positive and the other negative, or one electrode is positive and the other electrode functions as a reference point. (This is explained in more detail later.) Passage of electrical current toward the positive electrode will cause a positive deflection on the recorder. A positive deflection will cause the marker or stylus to move upward. Likewise, passage of an electrical current away from the positive electrode will cause a negative deflection on the recorder. A negative deflection will cause the marker or stylus to move downward on the recorder.

The stronger the current, the greater will be the deflection of the stylus on the ECG recorder. Electrical current that flows directly toward the positive electrode will cause a greater deflection than electrical current that flows obliquely toward the positive electrode (Figure 2-98). If current flow is exactly perpendicular to the axis of the ECG lead, there will be no deflection on the graph, because the current is flowing neither toward nor away from the electrode. In the absence of current flow, there will be no deflection on the ECG monitor.

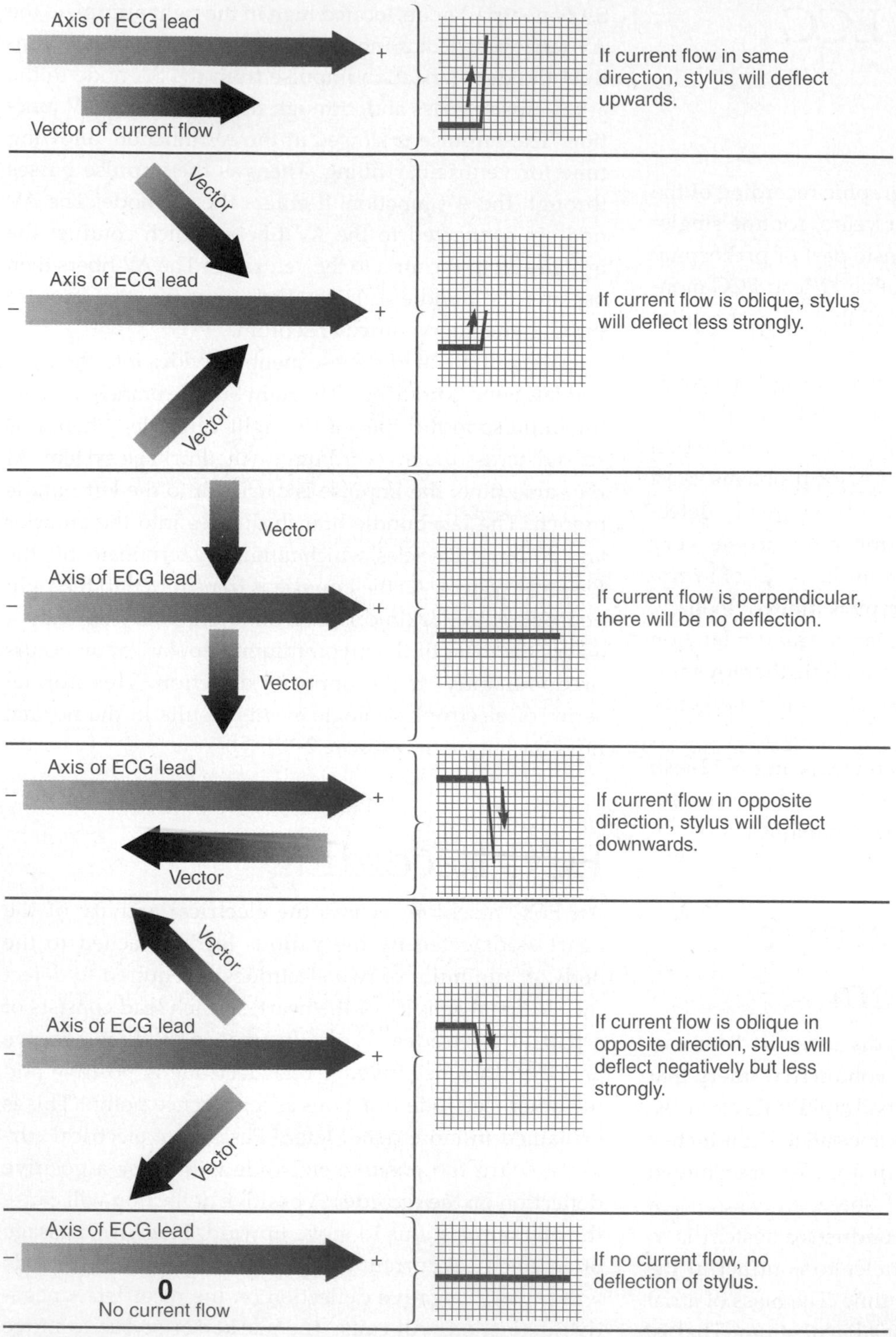

FIGURE 2-98 Results of relationships between current flow direction and ECG lead axis.

In summary, the electrical activity of the heart is a complex combination of positive and negative current flows that can be graphically recorded on paper or a monitor (Figure 2-99).

ECG Leads

The first ECG recording was reported by Willem Einthoven in 1903. Einthoven placed leads on the arms and legs in an effort to measure the electrical activity of the heart using a simple galvanometer. Today we still use some of the leads that Einthoven first used.

An ECG lead is not a single wire, but a combination of two wires and their electrodes that make a complete circuit with the electrocardiograph.

ECG leads may be bipolar, unipolar, or precordial. Leads I, II, and III are bipolar. Leads aVR, aVL, and aVF are unipolar. Together, leads I, II, III, aVR, aVL, and aVF constitute the frontal plane leads. That is, they record the electrical activity of the heart in the frontal plane of the body, using electrodes on the extremities. Developed in the 1930s, the precordial leads, or "chest leads," are designed to look at the heart in the horizontal plane. They are leads V_1, V_2, V_3, V_4, V_5, and V_6 (Figure 2-100). Additional information pertaining to the ECG leads is detailed in the following sections.

Bipolar Limb Leads

Leads I, II, and III are called bipolar limb leads because two electrodes of opposite polarity (positive and negative) are used. These leads record the difference in electrical potential between two limbs:

- *Lead I.* The negative electrode is placed on the right arm and the positive electrode is placed on the left arm. Thus, when the electrical current moves through the heart from the right arm toward the left arm, lead I will record a positive deflection.
- *Lead II.* The negative electrode is placed on the right arm and the positive electrode is placed on the left leg. Thus, when the electrical current moves through the heart from the right arm toward the left leg, lead II will record a positive deflection.
- *Lead III.* The negative electrode is placed on the left arm and the positive electrode is placed on the left leg.

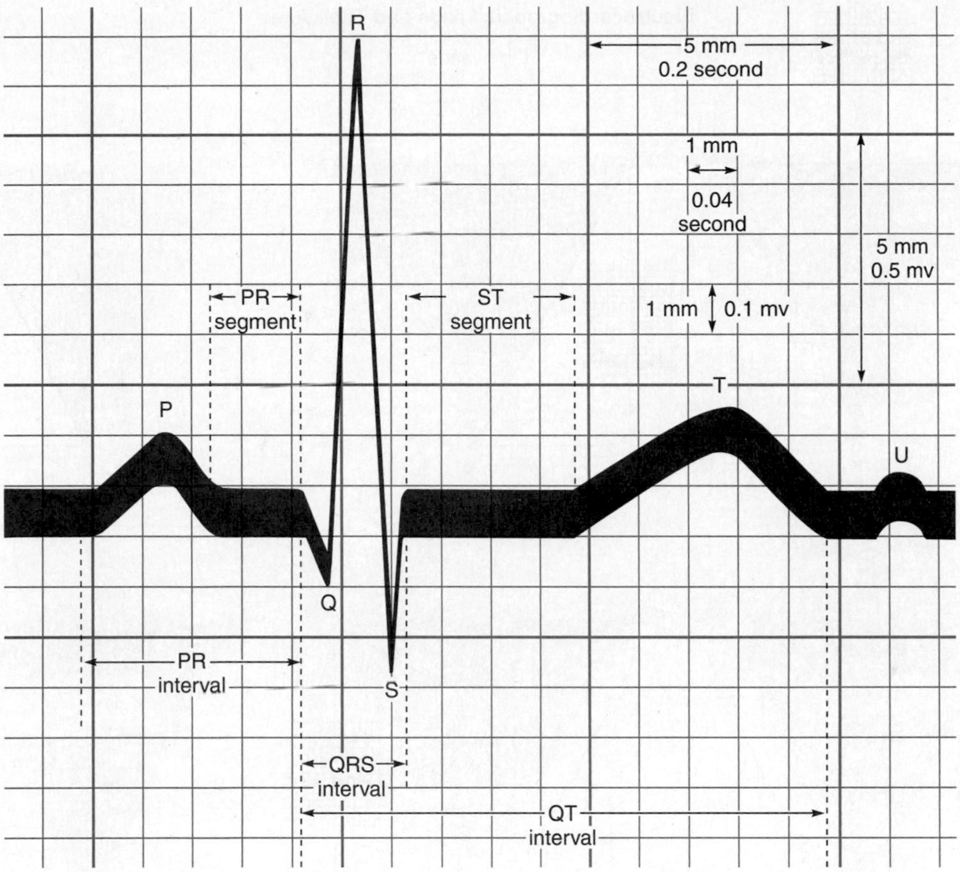

FIGURE 2-99 Electrocardiograph waves.

Thus, when the electrical current moves through the heart from the left arm toward the left leg, lead III will record a positive deflection.

These leads form Einthoven's triangle around the heart (Figure 2-101). The two arms and the left leg form the corners of the triangle. It is important to point out that electrodes are typically attached to both legs. The right leg is typically used as a ground or a spare, as recordings obtained from either leg are virtually identical. (Usually, the leads are placed on the chest wall rather than the limbs.)

Unipolar or Augmented Limb Leads

The unipolar, or augmented, limb leads use the same electrodes as the bipolar limb leads. These leads allow a different "look" at the heart by using two of the electrodes as a single electrode. To achieve this, two selected leads are combined in the ECG machine after each has been run through a resistor to reduce the current flow. This effectively provides a functional electrode halfway between the combined leads. The term *unipolar* refers to the resulting arrangement of one polarized (positive) electrode and the combined leads, which serve as a nonpolarized reference point. To increase the deflection's amplitude, the ground lead is disconnected, thus the term *augmented lead* (Figure 2-102):

- ***Lead aVR.*** The positive electrode is placed on the right arm. The negative electrode is a combination of the left arm and left leg electrode.
- ***Lead aVL.*** The positive electrode is placed on the left arm. The negative electrode is a combination of the right arm and left leg.
- ***Lead aVF.*** The positive electrode is placed on the left foot. The negative electrode is a combination of the right arm and the left arm.

All of the limb leads are in the frontal plane. If you superimpose the direction of each of these leads on a single diagram, the six leads will constitute a complete 360° circle (Figure 2-103). By established convention, the direction toward the left arm is considered to be 0°. Some systems will use the full 360° circle to describe the axis of the lead in question. The radials increase clockwise in this system. Other systems will divide the circle into positive and negative halves (semicircles). Using this system, moving

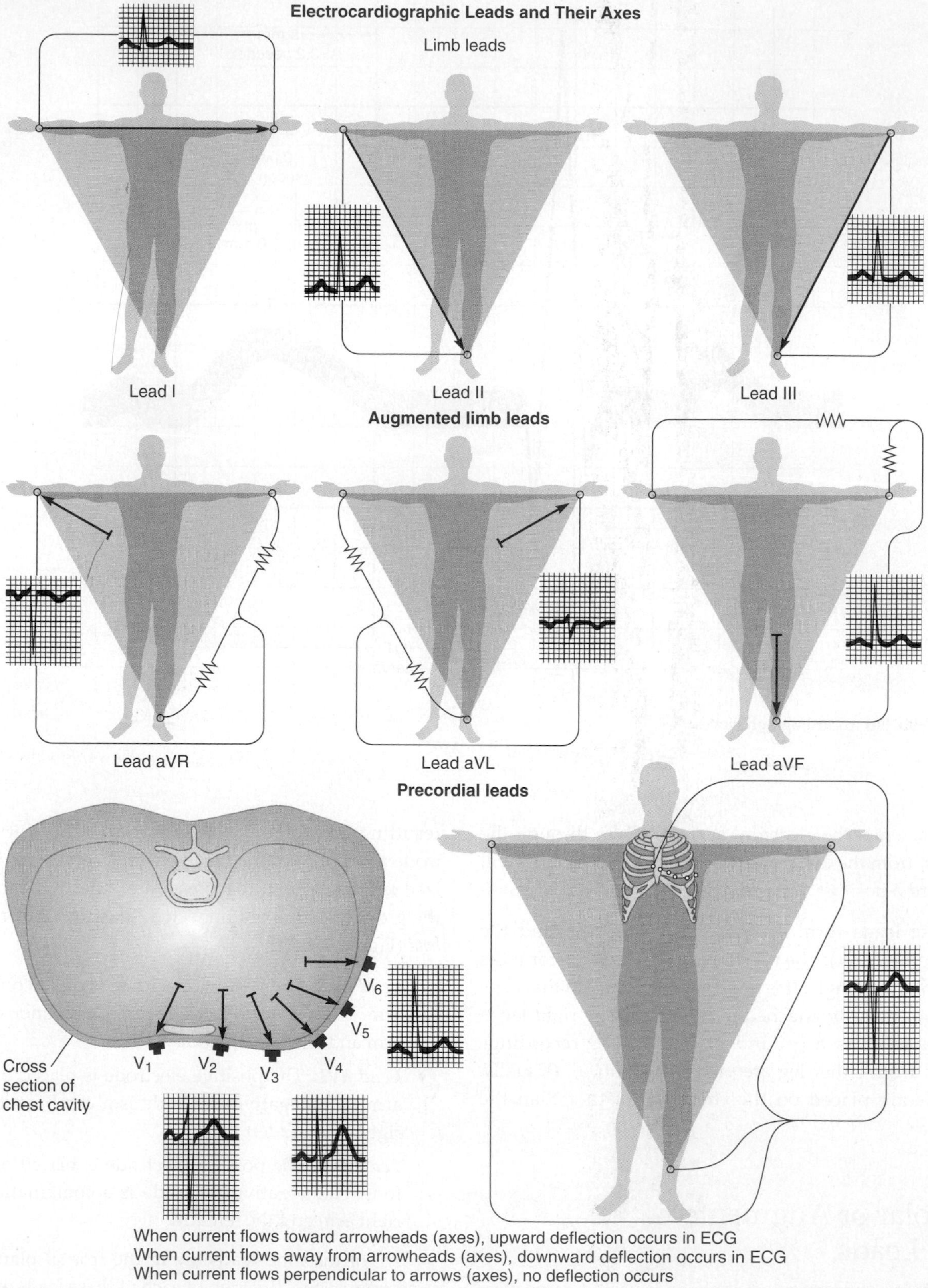

FIGURE 2-100 ECG leads and their axes.

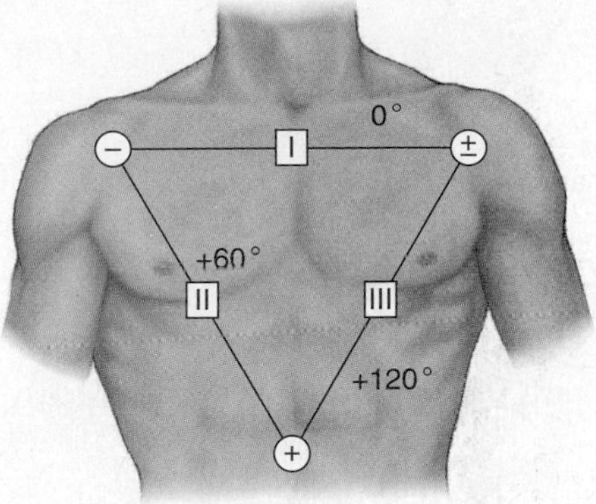

FIGURE 2-101 Einthoven's triangle as formed by the bipolar leads.

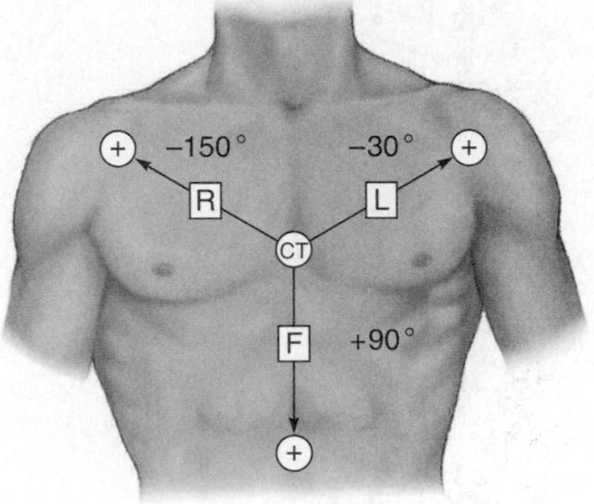

FIGURE 2-102 The pattern formed by the unipolar/augmented leads.

clockwise, the radial coordinates are positive up to 180°. Moving counterclockwise from 0°, the radial coordinates are negative up to 180°. Each lead can be measured on this coordinate system. Table 2-7 lists the limb leads and the direction in which they point.

This discussion will follow the semicircle system, which is more commonly used. Remember that both

Table 2-7 12-Lead Angles

Lead	Full Circle	Semicircle
Lead I	0°	0°
Lead II	60°	+60°
Lead III	120°	+120°
aVR	210°	
aVL	330°	−30°
aVF	90°	+90°

systems describe the same radials, but each uses a different frame of reference.

Precordial Leads

The precordial leads provide a look at the horizontal plane of the heart. The horizontal plane is the plane that results from a section taken from front to back, from the sternum to the spine. The negative pole for the precordial leads is a common ground arranged electronically within the ECG machine by connecting all limb leads together. The positive electrode is placed on the anterior surface of the chest in positions ranging from V_1 to V_6 (Figure 2-104).

- ***Lead V_1.*** Lead V_1 is obtained by placing the positive electrode to the right of the sternum at the fourth intercostal space.
- ***Lead V_2.*** Lead V_2 is obtained by placing the positive electrode to the left of the sternum at the fourth intercostal space.
- ***Lead V_3.*** Lead V_3 is obtained by placing the positive electrode in a line midway between lead V_2 and lead V_4.
- ***Lead V_4.*** Lead V_4 is obtained by placing the positive electrode at the midclavicular line at the fifth intercostal space.
- ***Lead V_5.*** Lead V_5 is obtained by placing the positive electrode at the anterior axillary line at the same level as V_4.
- ***Lead V_6.*** Lead V_6 is obtained by placing the positive electrode at the midaxillary line at the same level as V_4.

All 12 leads record exactly the same electrical events within the heart. Each lead, however, allows us to look at these events from a different perspective.

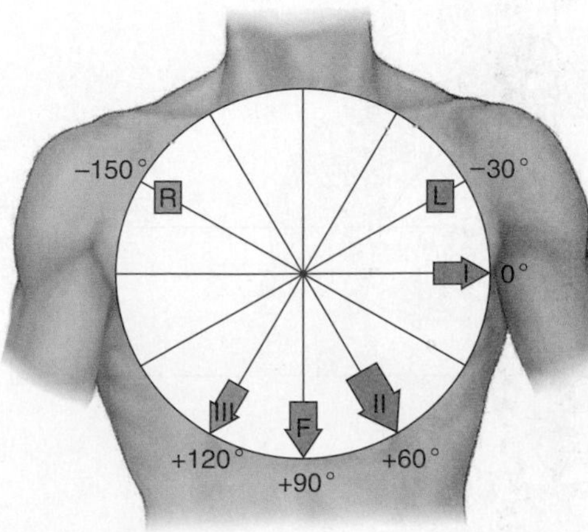

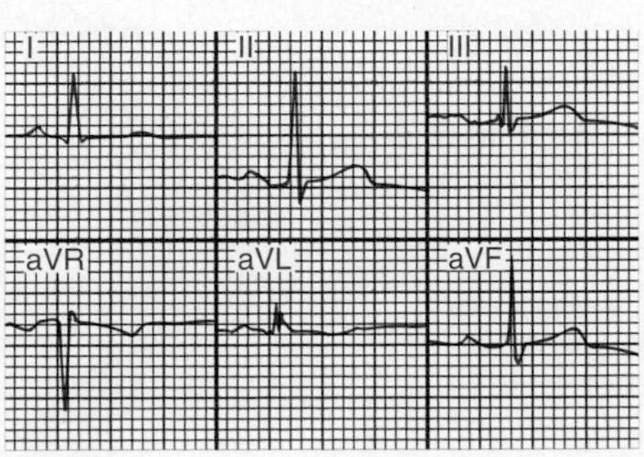

FIGURE 2-103 The hexaxial (six axes) reference system.

Mean QRS Axis Determination

The heart's electrical energy is the sum of the electricity generated by each individual cardiac muscle cell. This energy exhibits both magnitude and direction. Any force that has both magnitude and direction is a **vector**. In actuality, the electrical forces of the heart move in three dimensions simultaneously during the course of each cardiac cycle. However, these forces can be averaged together at any given point in time. This averaged vector is referred to as the *instantaneous vector*. Ultimately, we can combine all the instantaneous vectors occurring during the cardiac cycle into a single, averaged vector called the *resultant cardiac vector* or *mean cardiac vector*. This reduces all the electrical forces generated by the heart's millions of cardiac cells to a single vector represented by an arrow moving in a single plane, the **QRS axis**.

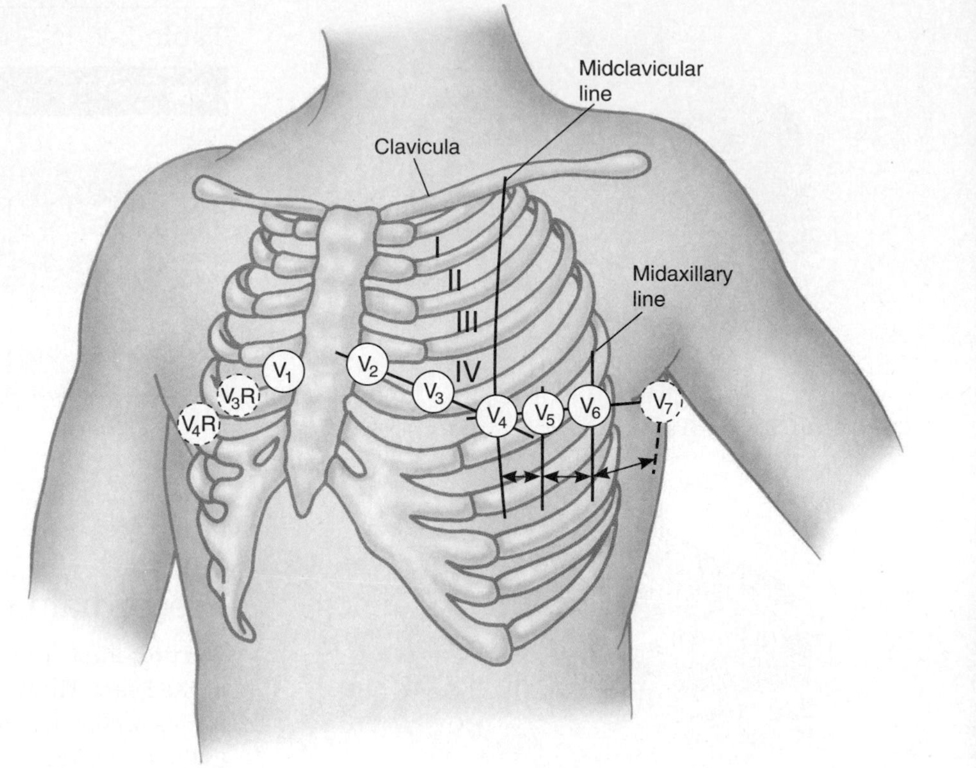

FIGURE 2-104 The precordial leads.

Axis Deviation

The heart's normal electrical axis is 59° (–29° to +105°). In the normal tracing, lead II should have the most positive deflection, as the axis of lead II is +60°. If the calculated axis of the heart falls outside normal, an axis deviation exists. Whenever the axis equals or exceeds +105°, the patient is said to have a **right axis deviation**. Right axis deviation is abnormal and often associated with chronic obstructive pulmonary disease and pulmonary hypertension. Whenever the axis of the heart is greater than or equal to –30°, a **left axis deviation** is said to exist. Left axis deviation can be associated with high blood pressure, valvular heart disease, and other disease processes.

To simplify matters, the frontal plane can be divided into quadrants (Figure 2-105). The quadrant from 0° to +90° is considered normal. The quadrant from +90° to +180° is considered right axis deviation (Figure 2-106). The quadrant from 0° to –90° is considered left axis deviation (Figure 2-107). Finally, the quadrant from –90° to –180° is considered **indeterminate axis**. Indeterminate axis is often considered extreme right axis deviation. Though not quite as accurate, this system is effective in detecting abnormal ECG axes.

Most modern 12-lead ECG machines will electronically calculate the axes of the various waves of the ECG (P, QRS, and T). These can be used to determine whether an axis deviation exists. In our discussion of cardiac axes, we have been referring to the QRS axis as it represents ventricular depolarization.

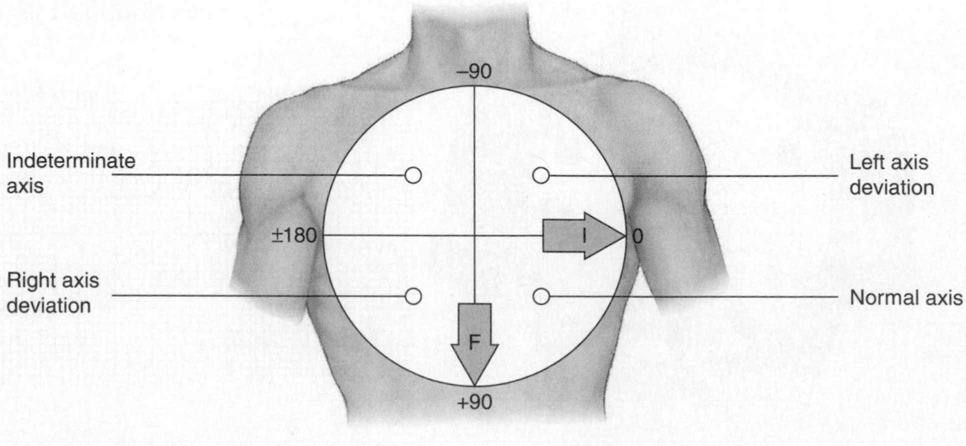

FIGURE 2-105 Axis determination.

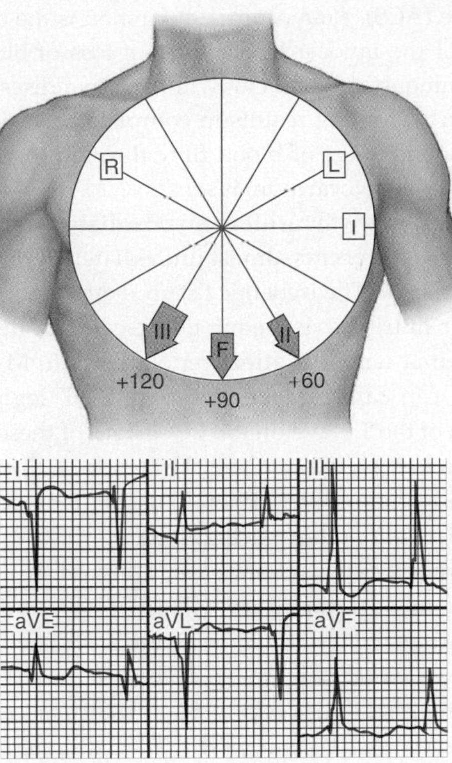

FIGURE 2-106 Right axis deviation.

When the machine does not calculate the QRS axis, it can be calculated based on leads I, II, and III (Figure 2-108). The heights of the QRS complexes can be measured and plotted on a triaxial reference system. Then, the cardiac axis

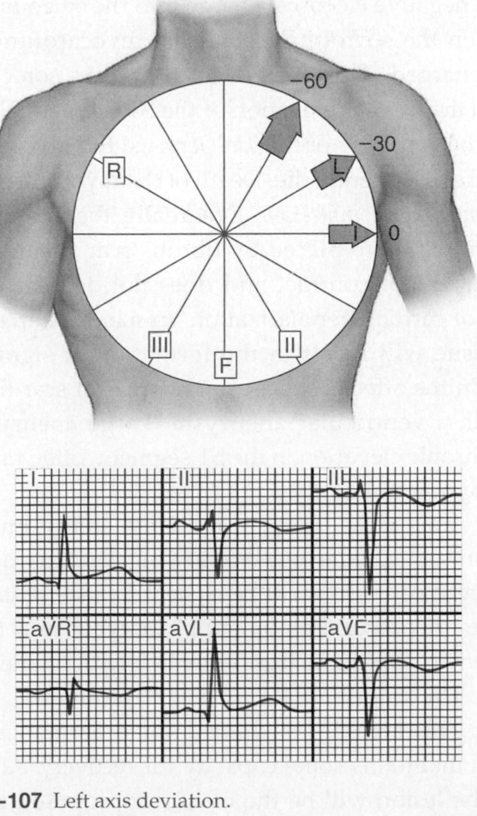

FIGURE 2-107 Left axis deviation.

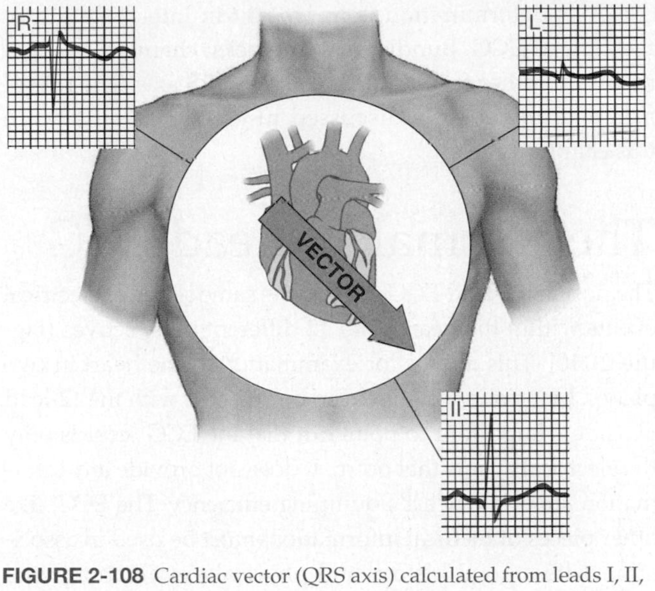

FIGURE 2-108 Cardiac vector (QRS axis) calculated from leads I, II, and III.

can be calculated. This system is of little use in the prehospital setting, as it is time consuming and requires calipers and graph paper. Alternatively, a practical system is available for rapidly estimating the electrical axis of the heart.

To rapidly determine the electrical axis of the heart, you must look at leads I, II, and III. The system follows these steps (Figure 2-109):

1. Look at the QRS in leads I, II, and III. If the QRS is *not* negative in any of these leads, the axis is within normal range.
2. Examine lead I. If the QRS is negative in lead I, look at leads II and III. If the QRS is negative in all three leads, the axis is indeterminate. If the QRS is variable in lead II (positive, intermediate, negative) and positive in lead III, then a right axis deviation is present.
3. Examine lead III. If the QRS is negative in lead III, look at lead II. If both lead II and III are negative, a left axis deviation is present.

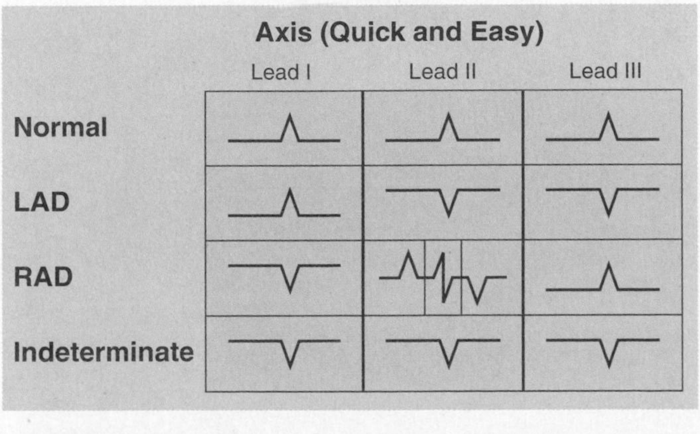

FIGURE 2-109 Rapid axis determination.

Axis determination is important in interpretation of the 12-lead ECG. Bundle branch blocks, chamber enlargement, and other factors can affect the QRS axis. The role of axis determination is discussed in greater detail later in this chapter.

The Normal 12-Lead ECG

The normal 12-lead ECG records the same series of electrical events within the heart from 12 different perspectives (Figure 2-110). This allows for examination of the heart in two planes. Many abnormalities can be detected with the 12-lead ECG. It is important to point out that the ECG records only the electrical events that occur. It does not provide any information about the heart's pumping efficiency. The ECG, like other pieces of medical information, must be used in association with a good history and physical examination, vital sign determination, and other ancillary testing and diagnostic equipment available for advanced prehospital care.

The 12-lead ECG can be presented several ways, depending on the machine being used. The most common 12-lead presentation is a three-channel machine that provides short strips of each lead (Figure 2-111). The most common format is to place the bipolar limb leads on the left with lead I at the top, lead II in the middle, and lead III at the bottom. To the right of this, in the second column, are the augmented limb leads with aVR at the top, aVL in the middle, and aVF at the bottom. To the right of the augmented limb leads are the precordial leads. Leads V_1 through V_3 are placed in the third column, and leads V_4 through V_6 in the fourth column. This system functionally groups the leads based on their view of the heart.

Disease Findings

Many disease processes can affect the ECG. Among the most important of these are myocardial ischemia, injury, and infarction, collectively referred to as acute coronary syndrome (ACS). A myocardial infarction is the death of a portion of the myocardium due to a loss of blood flow. Most commonly, a blood clot will form in a diseased coronary artery. This clot results in complete occlusion of the artery and stoppage of blood flow through that artery to the part of the myocardium it serves.

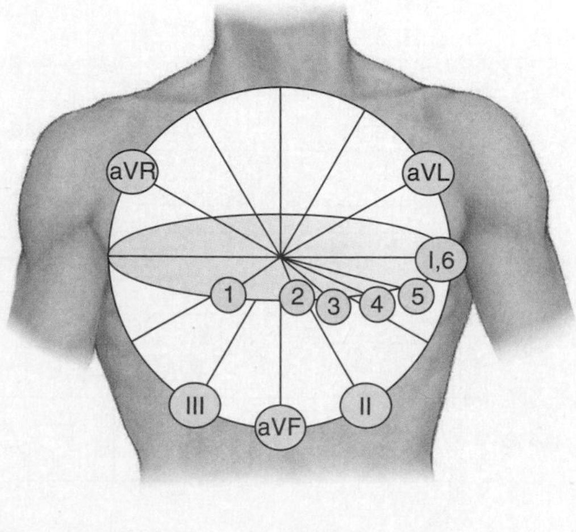

FIGURE 2-110 12-lead ECG perspectives.

Initially, this will result in **myocardial ischemia**. Myocardial ischemia occurs almost immediately following loss of blood supply. The ischemic tissue is deprived of oxygen and other nutrients. Ischemic tissue can still depolarize, but ischemia tends to affect repolarization. Myocardial ischemia can cause depression of the ST segment and inversion of the T wave on the ECG. Both of these findings are due to abnormalities of repolarization. If blood supply is restored promptly to ischemic tissue, then permanent myocardial injury often can be avoided.

If myocardial ischemia is allowed to progress untreated, **myocardial injury** will occur. Myocardial injury reflects actual injury to the myocardium. The degree of injury depends on how quickly blood supply is restored. Injured myocardium tends to be partially or completely depolarized. This tissue, often called stunned myocardium, does not contract and does not contribute to the heart's pumping ability. In addition, injured myocardium can be very irritable and a source of serious and potentially life-threatening arrhythmias. With myocardial injury, current flows between the pathologically depolarized area and the normally depolarized areas. This is referred to as a **current of injury**, or **injury current**. Thus, with myocardial injury, the injured tissue remains depolarized. It effectively emits a negative electrical charge into the surrounding fluids when the surrounding normal myocardium is positively charged. This current of injury can sometimes be seen on the ECG as elevation of the ST segment (STEMI).

If the coronary occlusion persists, the myocardial tissue will subsequently die. Death of the myocardial tissue is called *myocardial infarction*. Eventually, the infarcted myocardium will be replaced by fibrous scar tissue. The scar tissue does not contract and does not depolarize in the course of cardiac depolarization. In major infarctions, the scar tissue will result in the formation of significant Q waves in the affected leads. Large areas of scar tissue can result in a ventricular aneurysm. Large aneurysms can cause chronic elevation in the ST segment, often mimicking acute myocardial injury.

All three areas (areas of ischemia, injury, and infarction) can typically be found following coronary occlusion. The outermost tissue will be ischemic (zone of ischemia). Because of collateral blood supply, oxygen and nutrients are often resupplied to this tissue before permanent injury occurs. The intermediate area will be injured (zone of injury). This area has sustained some permanent injury but still maintains some capacity for recovery. At the center of the lesion will be the most compromised tissue, or

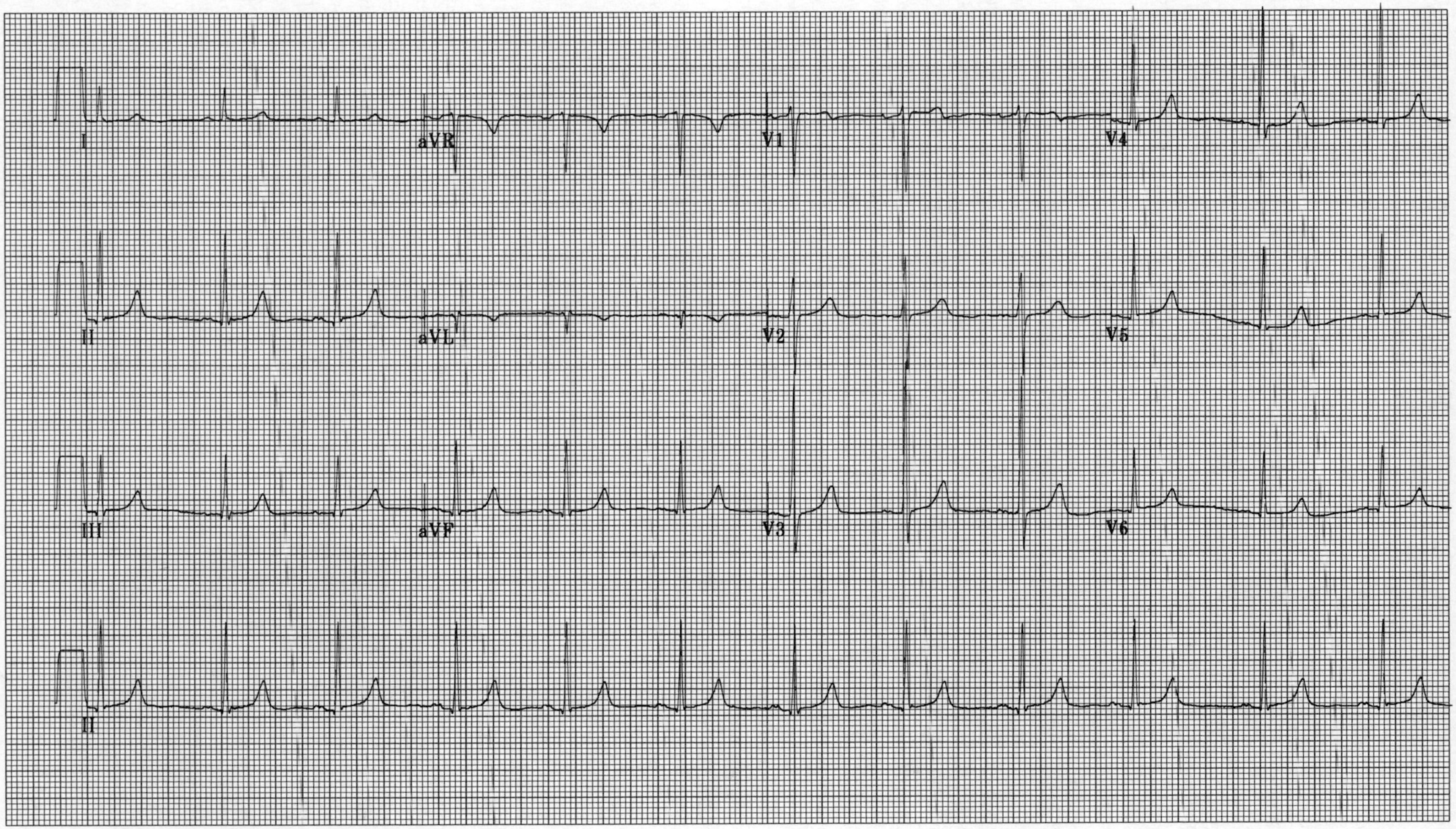

FIGURE 2-111 Normal 12-lead ECG.

infarcted tissue (zone of infarction). This part of the myocardium will die and eventually be replaced by scar tissue. Figure 2-112 illustrates the effects of myocardial ischemia, injury, and infarction. It also illustrates the ECG changes commonly associated with each.

Myocardial infarctions may involve the whole thickness of the myocardium or only a partial thickness. The coronary arteries lie on the surface of the heart (at the epicardial level). Interruption of blood supply threatens the deeper layers (subendocardium) of the myocardium more than the superficial layers.

A myocardial infarction that affects only the deeper part of the myocardium is called a *subendocardial infarction*. The amount of tissue affected in a subendocardial infarction is typically less than in full-thickness infarctions. Subendocardial infarctions usually do not result in the development of a significant Q wave in the affected lead. Because of this, subendocardial infarctions are often called non–Q-wave infarctions. An infarction that affects the full thickness of the myocardium is called a *transmural infarction*.

Both types of infarction can result in permanent myocardial death if appropriate intervention, such as fibrinolytic therapy or percutaneous transluminal coronary angioplasty (PTCA), is not completed early in the course of the event. Transmural infarctions almost always result in the formation of a significant Q wave in the affected leads.

The goal of emergency care is to identify myocardial ischemia long before it becomes myocardial injury and infarction.[31]

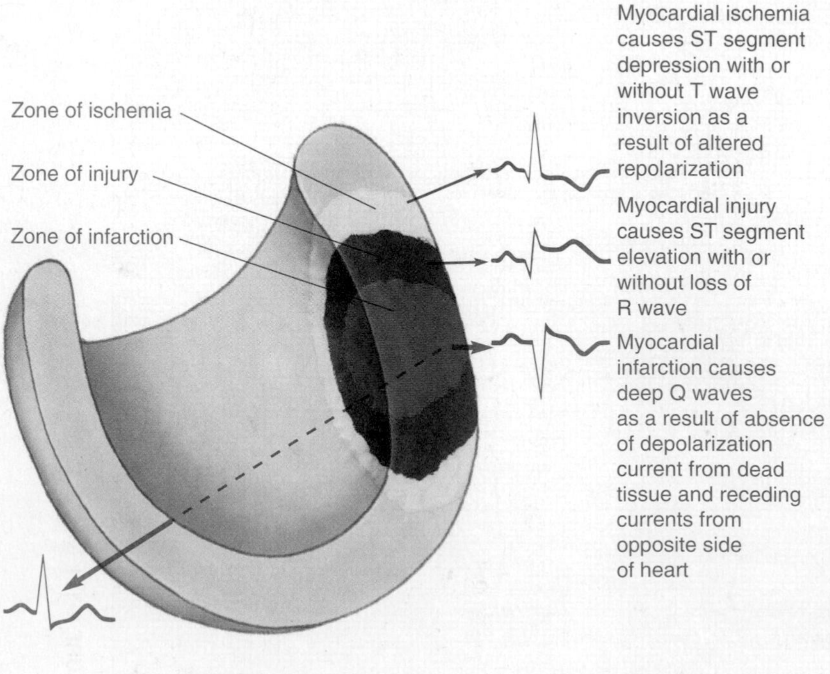

FIGURE 2-112 The effects of myocardial ischemia, injury, and infarction.

Evolution of Acute Coronary Syndrome

The precipitating event in acute coronary syndrome is occlusion of a coronary artery and interruption of blood flow to a portion of the myocardium it supplies. At this precise moment the clock starts running. In the field of emergency care, time is myocardium!

The evolution of acute coronary syndrome has been extensively studied. Figures 2-113 and 2-114 illustrate the events that occur in transmural and subendocardial myocardial infarctions. The following description details the evolution of a transmural myocardial infarction.

Initially, following coronary occlusion, the affected tissue will become deprived of oxygen and other nutrients and will become ischemic. Myocardial ischemia can often be demonstrated on the ECG as ST segment depression and T wave inversion in the affected leads. ST segment depression and T wave inversion may not be present at the same time. As a rule, as the quantity of ischemic tissue increases, the ECG findings will become more significant.

If allowed to progress untreated, tissue at the center of the myocardial injury will transition from ischemia to injury. When a critical mass of tissue is affected, the ST segments will become elevated in the affected leads. In addition, T waves in the affected leads will become more peaked.

If blood supply has not been restored, the injured tissue will begin to die after approximately 6 hours. This infarcted tissue is lost. The ST segment will remain elevated (because of the adjoining zone of injury) and the R wave amplitude will diminish. As the infarction becomes complete over the next 48 to 72 hours, most ischemia and injury will have been replaced by infarcted tissue or will have been reperfused. This results in a decrease in ST segment elevation. However, a significant Q wave will also develop. A significant Q wave has a width greater than or equal to 0.04 second (one small box) or amplitude (depth) greater than or equal to one-fourth of the R wave in the same lead. T wave inversion will continue. After several months, the infarcted tissue will be replaced with a fibrous scar. By this time, the ST segment will usually return to normal and some R wave may return. T wave inversion often persists. A significant Q wave usually persists and is an indicator of an old transmural infarction.

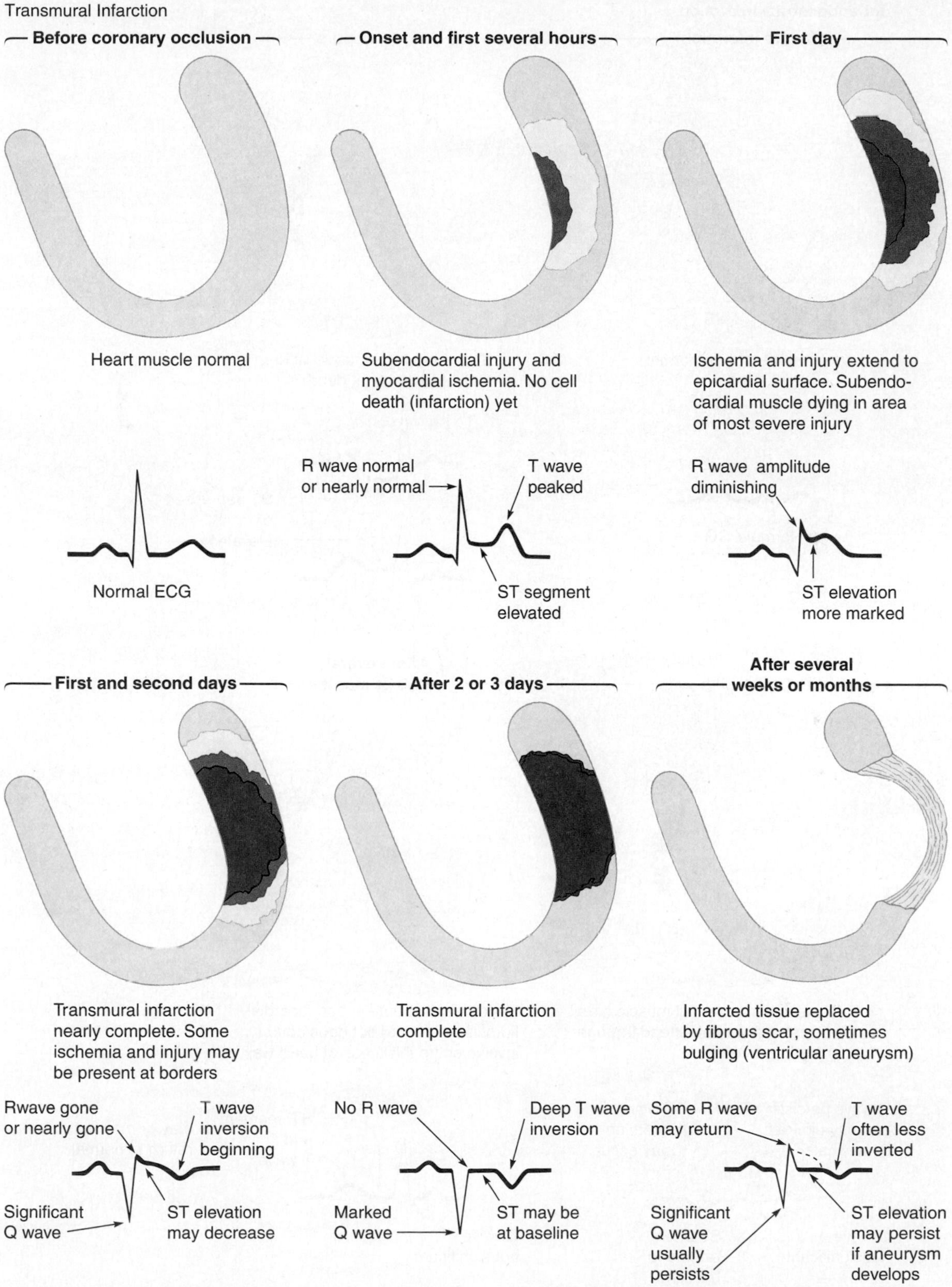

FIGURE 2-113 STEMI (transmural) infarction.

The evolution of a subendocardial infarction is similar to that described for a transmural infarction. However, significant Q waves typically do not occur. In addition, as the lesion heals, the ECG may return to normal, leaving no indication of a prior infarct.[32]

Localization of Acute Myocardial Infarction

Each ECG lead is designed to visualize a particular part of the heart. Whereas the bipolar and augmented limb leads

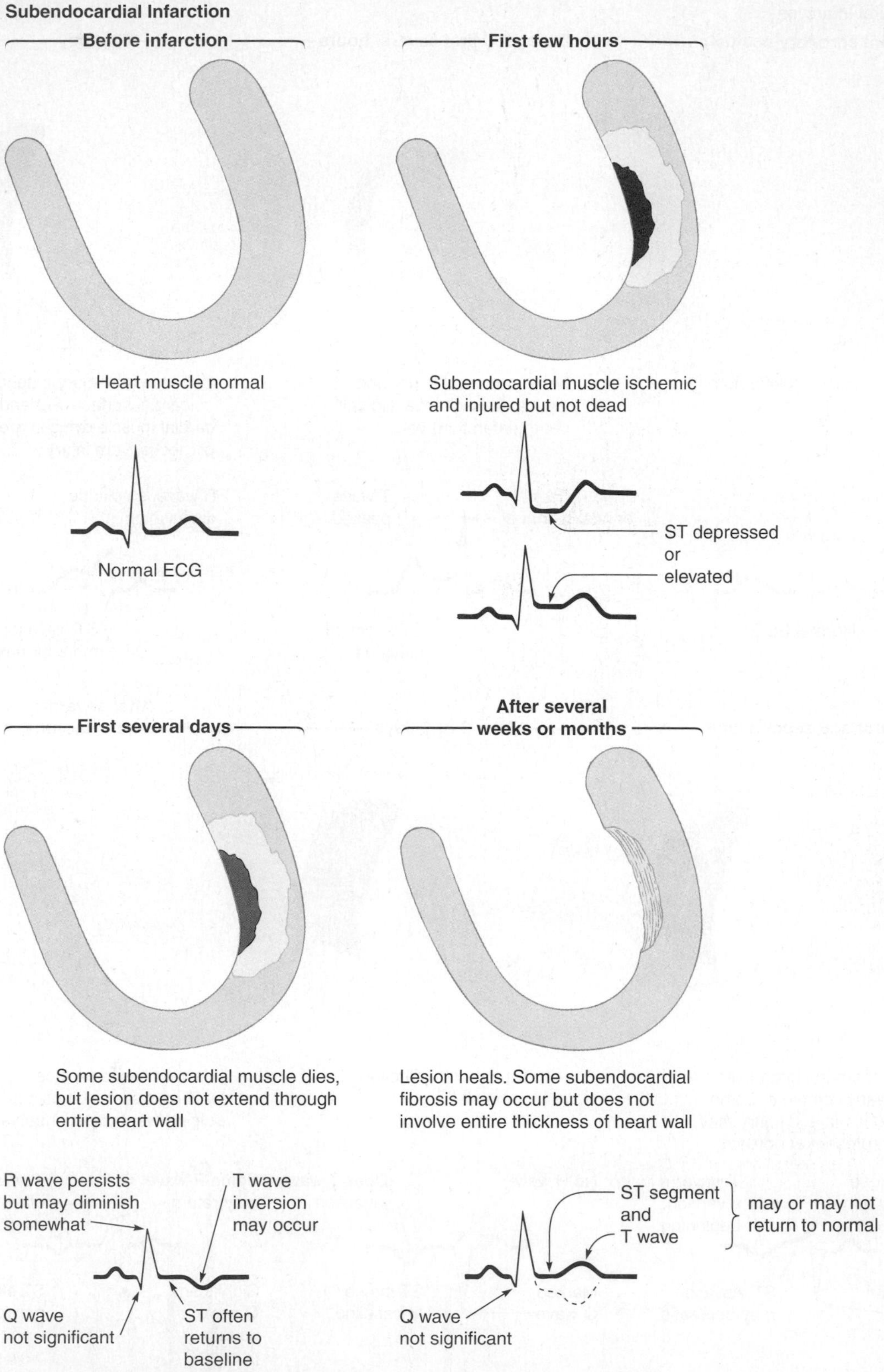

FIGURE 2-114 NSTEMI (subendocardial) infarction.

evaluate the heart from the frontal plane, the precordial leads look at the heart from a horizontal plane.

Various ECG leads look at a specific part of the myocardium. Abnormalities of the ECG in certain leads, with a few exceptions, indicate problems in the part of the heart those leads visualize. The following is a generalized description of the various ECG lead groupings associated with various locations of acute myocardial infarction (Table 2-8 and Figure 2-115). These descriptions are generalized and some overlapping may occur.

I **Lateral** Left circumflex artery	aVR *Generally ignored* Left coronary artery	V_1 **Septal*** Left anterior descending coronary artery	V_4 **Anterior** Left anterior descending coronary artery
II **Inferior** Right coronary artery	aVL **Lateral** Left circumflex artery	V_2 **Septal*** Left anterior descending coronary artery	V_5 **Lateral** Left circumflex artery
III **Inferior** Right coronary artery	aVF **Inferior** Right coronary artery	V_3 **Anterior** Left anterior descending coronary artery	V_6 **Lateral** Left circumflex artery

*- Posterior if mirror image (Left circumflex or right coronary artery)

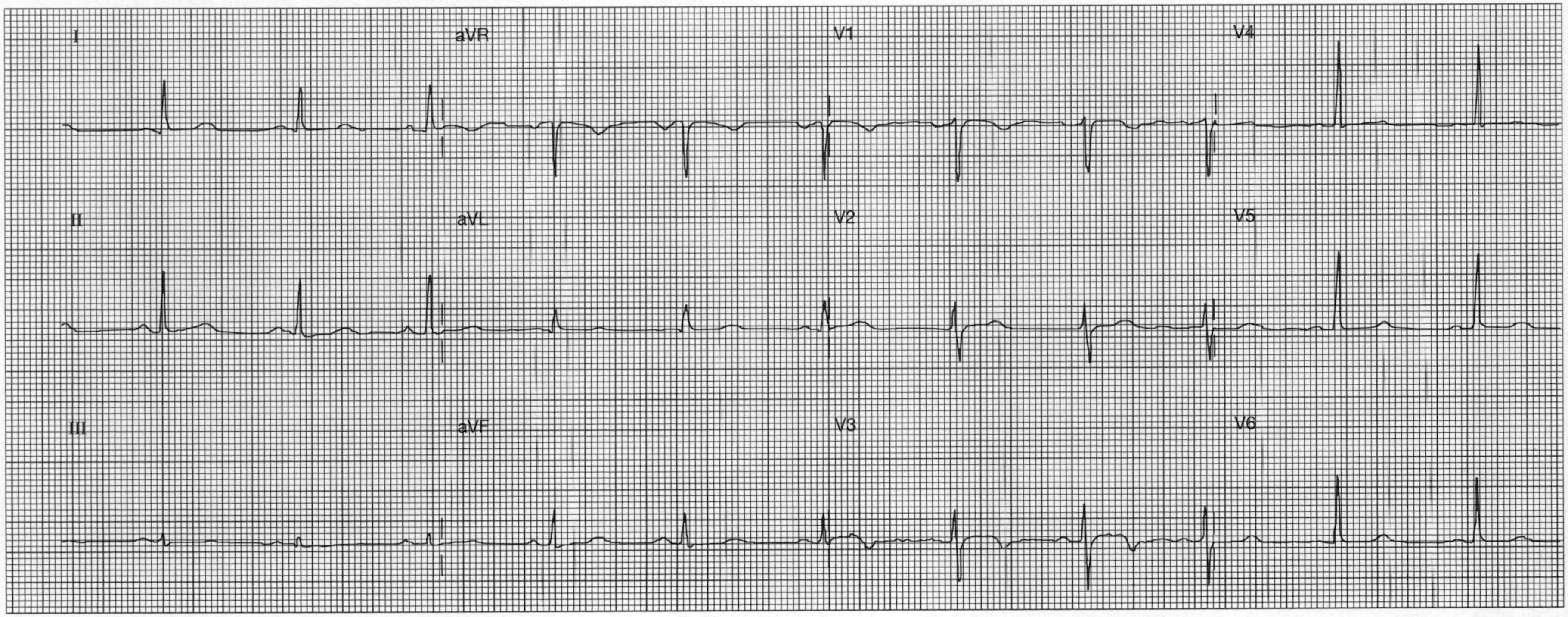

FIGURE 2-115 Infarction localization grid.

Table 2-8 Location of Myocardial Ischemia/Infarction

Location	Occluded Artery	Ischemic Leads	Reciprocal Leads
Anterior	Left anterior descending	V_2, V_3, and V_4	II, III, and aVF
Anterolateral	Left anterior descending	I, aVL, V_5, and V_6	II, III, aVF, V_1, and V_2
Septum	Left anterior descending Septal	V_1 and V_2	V_5 and V_6
Lateral	Left circumflex	V_5 and V_6	II, III, and aVF
High lateral	Left anterior descending Left circumflex	I and aVL (often with V_5, V_6)	II, III, aVF, V_1, and V_2
Inferior	Right coronary artery (90%) Left circumflex	II, III, and aVF	Varies (I and aVL)
Inferolateral	Right coronary artery Left circumflex	II, III, aVF, and V_6	V_1 and V_2
True posterior	Left circumflex Posterior descending	V_8 and V_9	V_1 and V_2
Right ventricle	Right coronary artery Left circumflex (rarely)	V_1 and V_1R	I and aVL

- ***Anterior.*** Leads I, V_2, V_3, and V_4 are immediately over the anterior surface of the heart. ST segment elevation, T wave inversion, and the development of significant Q waves in these leads indicate myocardial infarction involving the anterior surface of the heart (Figure 2-116). Leads V_2 and V_3 overlie the ventricular septum. Ischemic changes in these leads, and possibly in the adjoining precordial leads, are often referred to as septal infarctions.
- ***Anterolateral.*** Leads I, aVL, V_5, and V_6 examine the anterior and lateral surface of the heart. ST segment elevation, T wave inversion, and the development of significant Q waves in these leads indicate myocardial

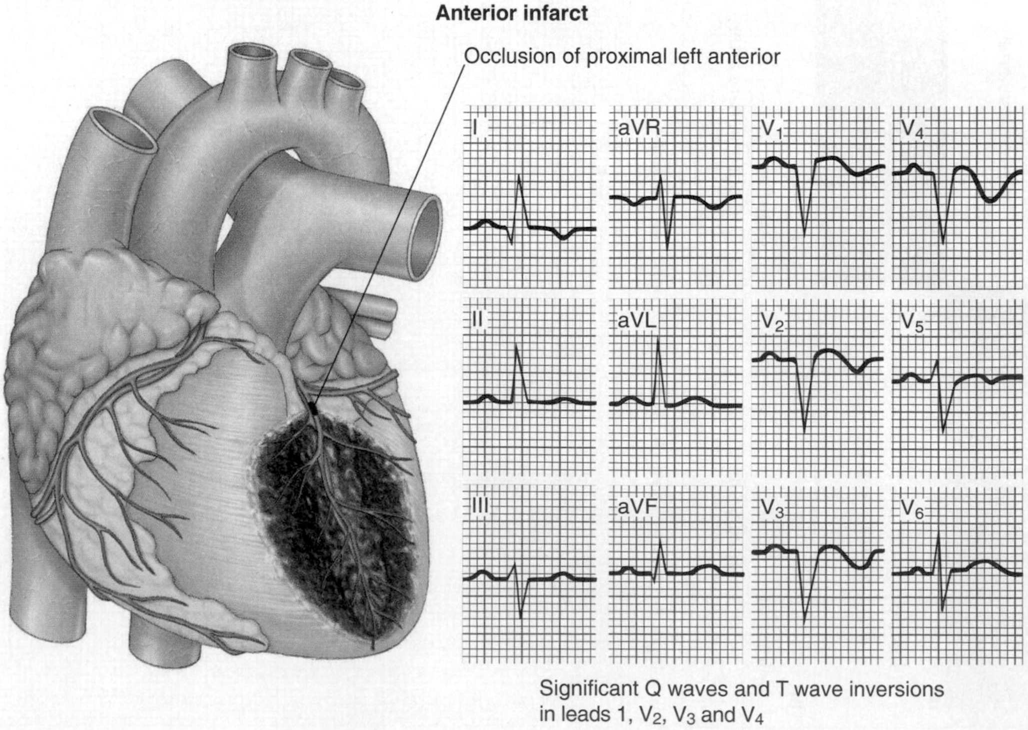

FIGURE 2-116 Anterior infarct.

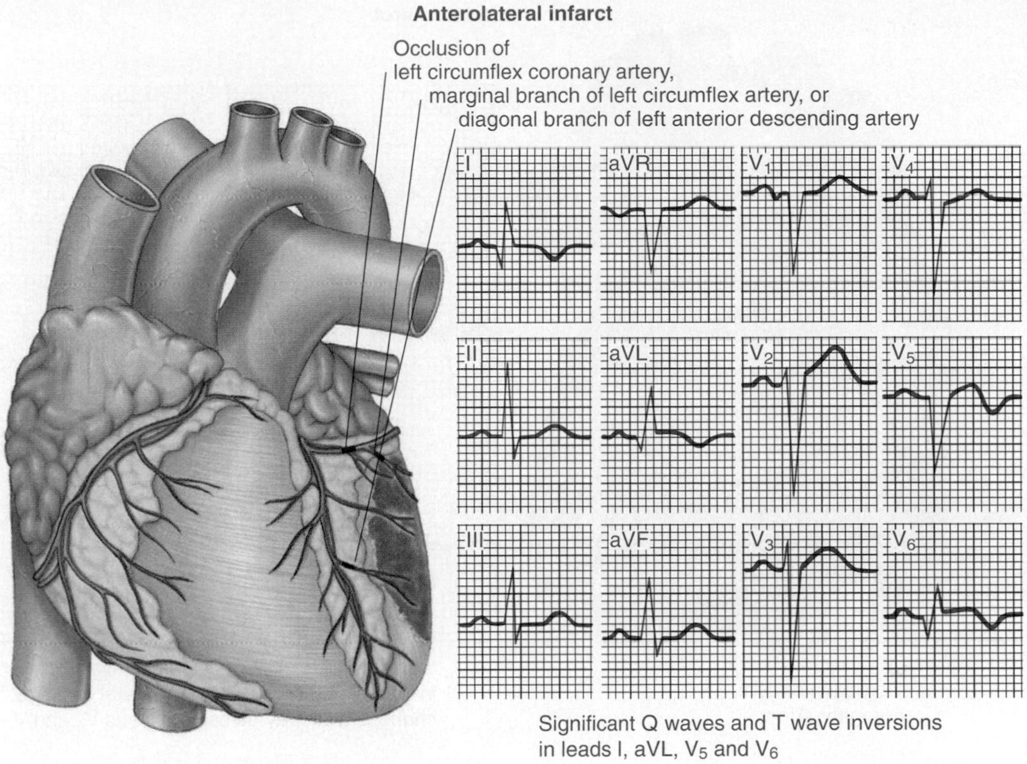

FIGURE 2-117 Anterolateral infarct.

infarction involving the anterolateral surface of the heart (Figure 2-117).

- ***Lateral.*** Leads V_5 and V_6 visualize the lateral surface of the heart. ST segment elevation, T wave inversion, and the development of significant Q waves in these leads indicate myocardial infarction involving the lateral surface of the heart.
- ***High lateral.*** Leads I and aVL visualize the high lateral surface of the heart. Changes in these leads can often be seen in the other lateral leads (V_5 and V_6). ST segment elevation, T wave inversion, and the development of significant Q waves in these leads indicate myocardial infarction involving the high lateral surface of the heart.
- ***Inferior.*** Leads II, III, and aVF visualize the inferior (diaphragmatic) surface of the heart. ST segment elevation, T wave inversion, and the development of significant Q waves in these leads indicate myocardial infarction involving the inferior surface of the heart (Figure 2-118). Inferior infarcts can sometimes primarily affect the right ventricle, causing right ventricular failure and elevated right ventricular filling pressures. These occur despite relatively normal left ventricular filling pressures. The classic clinical triad of right ventricular infarction includes distended neck veins, clear lung fields, and hypotension. All patients with inferior wall myocardial infarction should have a right-sided ECG performed. ST-segment elevation in lead V_4R is the single most powerful predictor of right ventricular infarction. Patients with this finding (right ventricular infarctions) are a high-risk group of patients in the setting of inferior wall myocardial infarction.
- ***Inferolateral.*** Leads II, III, aVF, and V_6 visualize the inferolateral portion of the heart. ST segment elevation, T wave inversion, and the development of significant Q waves in these leads indicate myocardial infarction involving the inferolateral surface of the heart.
- ***True posterior.*** There are no ECG leads over the posterior surface of the heart. True posterior infarctions, although rare, can be diagnosed by looking for **reciprocal** changes in the anterior leads (V_1 and V_2). Normally, the R wave in leads V_1 and V_2 is principally negative. An unusually large R wave in lead V_1 and V_2 can actually be a reciprocal of a posterior Q wave. Likewise, an upright T wave in these leads would be a reciprocal of posterior T wave inversion (Figure 2-119). These findings are subtle and require practice to learn. Alternatively, posterior leads (V_7 through V_{12}) can be applied to the back to confirm the presence of a true posterior myocardial infarction.

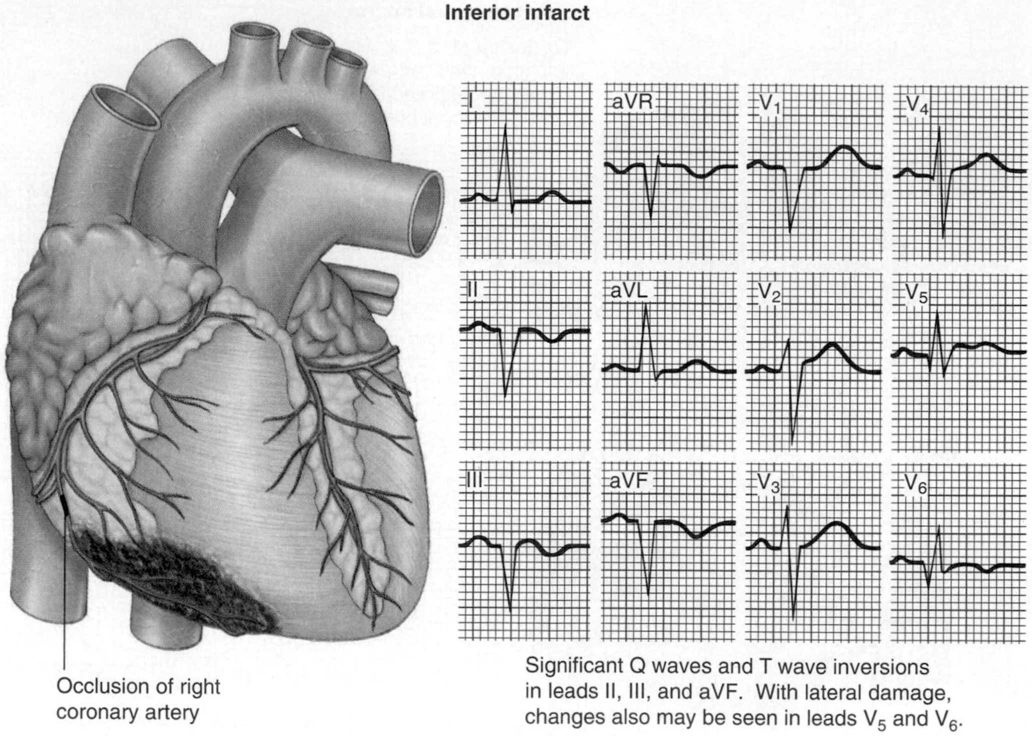

FIGURE 2-118 Inferior infarct.

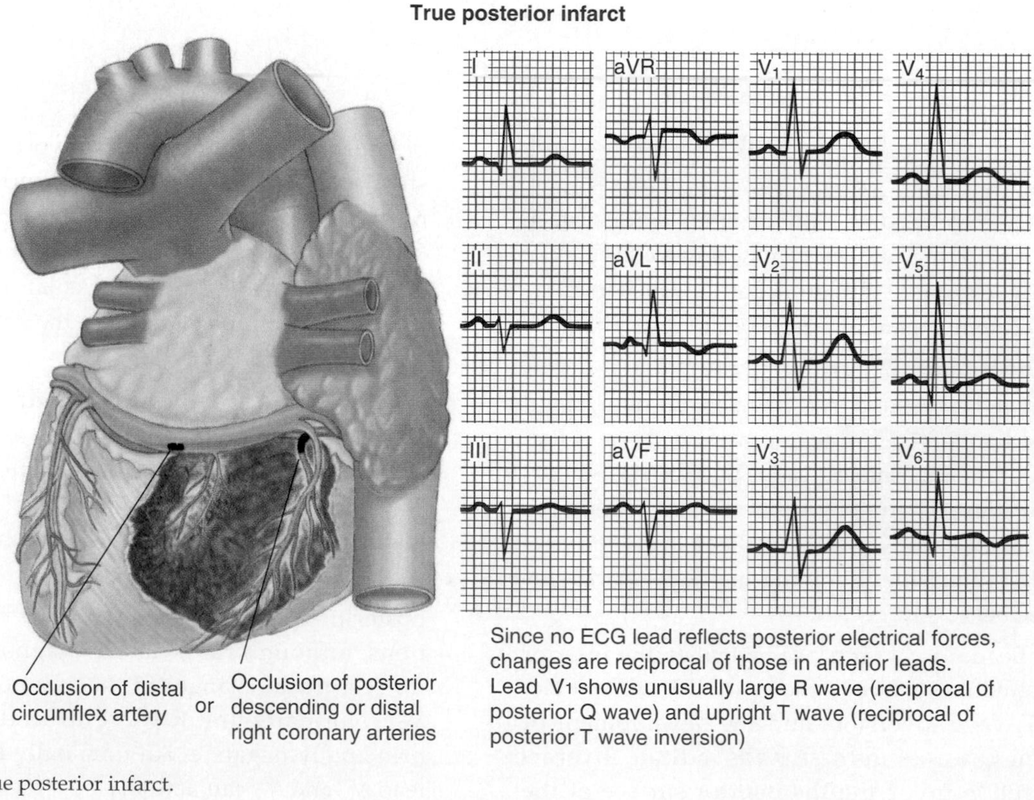

FIGURE 2-119 True posterior infarct.

It is important to point out that the guidelines just stated are generalized. Individual ECG tracings will vary owing to variances in body structure, underlying heart and lung disease, and other factors that can affect the ECG tracing. Thus, abnormal findings may overlap somewhat in various leads. Figure 2-120 is an actual 12-lead tracing from a patient suffering an acute anterior wall myocardial infarction. Figure 2-121 is an actual 12-lead ECG from a patient with an acute anterior wall myocardial infarction with lateral extension of the infarction (anterolateral MI). Finally, Figure 2-122 is an actual 12-lead tracing taken from a patient suffering an acute inferior wall (diaphragmatic)

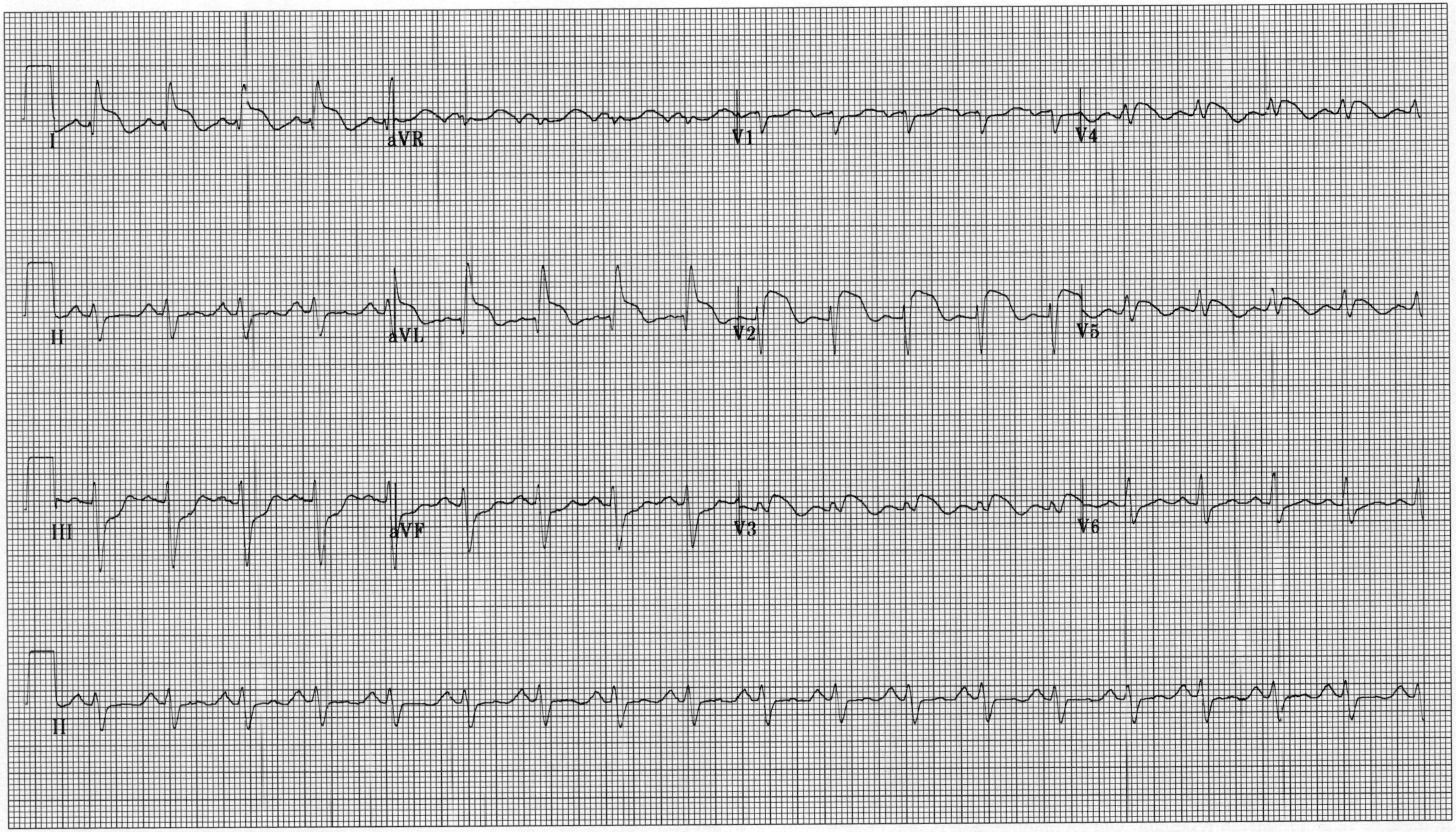

FIGURE 2-120 Tracing from patient with acute anterior wall infarct.

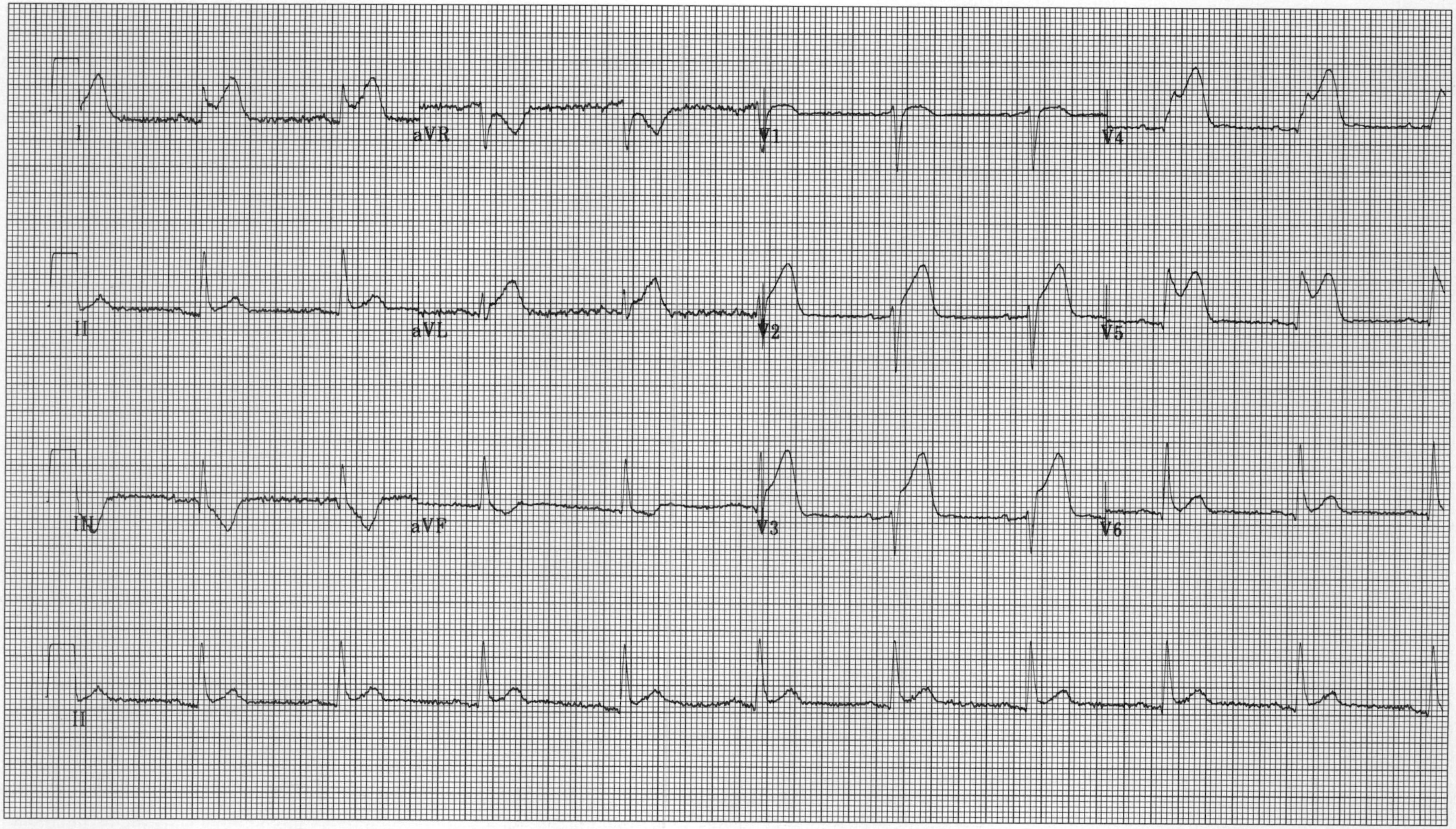

FIGURE 2-121 Tracing from patient with acute anterior wall infarct with lateral extension of the infarction (anterolateral infarct).

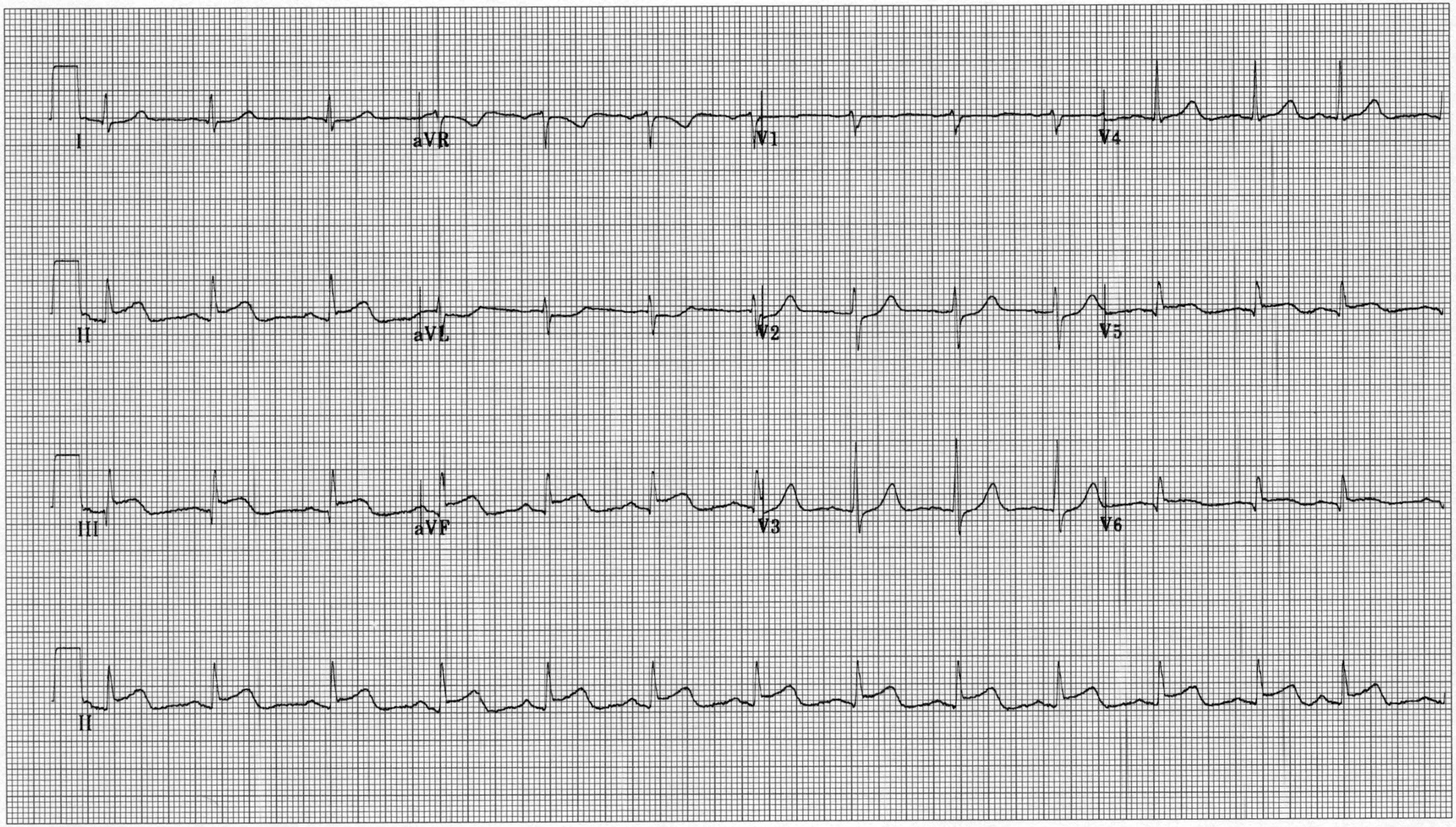

FIGURE 2-122 Tracing from a patient with acute inferior wall (diaphragmatic) infarct.

myocardial infarction. It is important to study and periodically review actual patient ECG tracings to learn the various pathological changes described in this text.

Right Ventricular Infarctions

Isolated infarction of the right ventricle is an extremely rare event. However, when it does occur, it must be managed differently from a left ventricular infarction. Most commonly, right ventricular infarction is associated with an inferior wall myocardial infarction. The incidence of right ventricular infarction in such cases ranges from 10 to 50 percent, depending on the study.

The right ventricle has a much thinner wall than the left ventricle and functions at lower pressure and lower oxygen demands. Unlike the left ventricle, it is perfused in both systole and diastole. Its ability to extract oxygen is increased during hemodynamic stress. All these factors make the right ventricle less susceptible than the left ventricle to infarction.

The posterior descending branch of the right coronary artery usually supplies the inferior and posterior walls of the right ventricle. The marginal branches of the right coronary artery supply the lateral wall of the right ventricle. The anterior wall of the right ventricle usually has a dual blood supply arising from the conus branch of the right coronary artery and the moderator branch artery (which is derived from the left anterior descending artery).

The right ventricle is considered to be a low-pressure volume pump. Thus, its contractility is highly dependent on the patient's diastolic pressure. When cardiac contractility is impaired and diastolic dysfunction develops secondary to right ventricular infarction, the right ventricular diastolic pressure increases substantially and systolic pressure decreases. This increases right ventricular afterload and can decrease right ventricular output dramatically. In many cases, the only remaining force driving right ventricular output is an elevated right atrial pressure. Thus, blood flow from the right ventricle to the pulmonary artery is impaired.

ASSESSMENT A right ventricular infarct should be considered in all patients who present with an acute inferior wall myocardial infarction, especially in the setting of a low cardiac output. The patient may report symptoms consistent with hypotension. Often these patients are extremely sensitive to preload-reducing agents such as nitroglycerin and morphine. Patients with a right ventricular infarction will often present with the following classic triad:

- Distended neck veins
- Clear lung fields
- Hypotension

Right ventricular infarction should always be suspected in any patient who presents with an inferior wall myocardial infarction and has associated hypotension, especially in the absence of crackles (rales). A 15-lead or 18-lead ECG, as discussed in the section following "Management," can be helpful in detecting the presence of a right ventricular infarct.

MANAGEMENT The management goals of a right ventricular infarction are:

- Maintenance of right ventricular preload
- Inotropic support
- Afterload reduction
- Early reperfusion

The patient should receive supplemental oxygen to correct hypoxia, and continuous monitors should be applied. Patients suffering a right ventricular infarction (RVI) may require different management for hypotension and pain control.

If the RVI patient exhibits hypotension, fluid therapy, which increases preload and improves the pumping function of the right ventricle, may be warranted. Many patients with right ventricular infarction and hypotension will respond to a fluid bolus of isotonic normal saline. If hypotension persists, consider inotropic support with dobutamine. However, dobutamine should be used with caution because the hemodynamic effects are often unpredictable. Therapies that reduce preload (morphine, nitroglycerin) should be used with caution when a right ventricular infarction is suspected.

The patient should be transported to a facility where immediate intervention can be provided (fibrinolysis, PCI).[33]

15-LEAD AND 18-LEAD ECGS IN RIGHT VENTRICULAR AND LEFT VENTRICULAR POSTERIOR WALL INFARCTIONS The classic 12-lead ECG is designed to detect the most common types of cardiac problems—usually those involving the left side of the heart and the left anterior descending coronary artery. However, problems that arise in the right ventricle and the posterior wall of the left ventricle may not be readily visible on the standard 12 leads. Because of this, some clinicians recommend the use of a 15-lead or 18-lead ECG to increase the sensitivity of the test. These supplemental leads specifically look at the right ventricle and the posterior wall of the left ventricle.

To the standard 12 leads (I, II, III, aVR, aVL, aVF, and V_1 through V_6), the 18-lead ECG adds three right-sided chest leads (V_4R, V_5R, and V_6R) and three posterior leads (V_7, V_8, and V_9) (Figure 2-123). The 15-lead ECG is a subset of the 18-lead ECG, using V_4R, V_8, and V_9 as additional leads to the standard 12-lead ECG. Placement of the right chest electrodes mirrors left chest placement. The V_4R electrode is placed in the fifth intercostal space at the right midclavicular line. V_5R is placed level with V_4R at the right

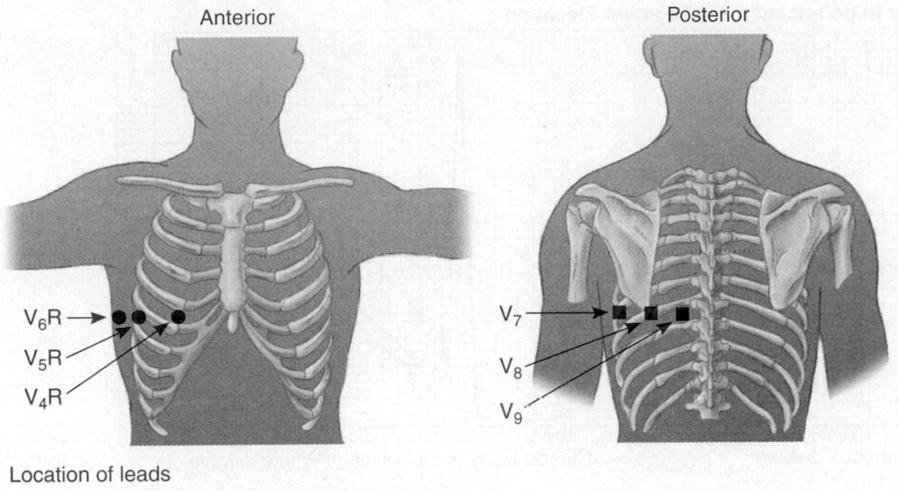

FIGURE 2-123 Supplemental lead placements for an 18-lead ECG.

anterior axillary line. V_6R is placed level with V_5R at the right midaxillary line. The V_7 to V_9 electrodes extend in a horizontal line from V_6. V_7 is placed lateral to V_6 at the posterior axillary line. V_8 is placed at the level of V_7 at the midscapular line. V_9 is placed at the level of V_8 at the paravertebral line.

Early Repolarization Versus STEMI

Several phenomena can look similar to STEMI patterns on ECG. One of the most common is **early repolarization** (Figure 2-124a). Early repolarization is ST-segment elevation without underlying disease and is generally considered a benign variance. It occurs in about 1 to 2 percent of the population and is often seen in young men (<50 years). Unfortunately, the physiologic basis for early repolarization is poorly understood. Early repolarization is suggested by:

- Widespread concave ST-segment elevation (most prominent in leads V_2–V_5)
- Notching or slurring at the J point
- Prominent slightly asymmetric T waves that are in the same direction as the QRS complexes
- Degree of ST-segment elevation is small compared to the T wave amplitude (<25% of the T-wave height in lead V_6)
- ST-segment elevation <2 mm in the precordial leads and <0.5 mm in the limb leads
- No reciprocal ST depression
- ST changes are stable over time (no progression on serial ECGs)

Although early repolarization is a benign finding, it should be distinguished from pathological ST-segment elevation (Figure 2-124b) seen during myocardial infarction and pericarditis.

Conduction Abnormalities

Conduction abnormalities occur when there is a delay or blockage of a part or parts of the cardiac conductive system. Conduction abnormalities can be caused by disease, drugs, and various electrolyte abnormalities.

AV Blocks

AV heart blocks are some of the more common types of conduction abnormalities. AV blocks result from a delay in impulse transmission through the AV node from the atria to the ventricles.

- ***First-degree AV block.*** The simplest type of AV heart block is a first-degree AV block. In a first-degree AV block, there is a delay in transmission of the electrical impulse from the atria to the ventricles. This can be detected on the ECG by noting a PR interval of greater than 0.20 second. In a first-degree block, there is not a complete blockage of AV transmission, only a slowing of the impulse in the AV node.
- ***Second-degree AV block (Mobitz I).*** The next type of heart block is a second-degree AV block (Mobitz I). This unique type of block, also referred to as a Wenckebach phenomenon, involves a delay of impulse conduction at the AV node. Each impulse arriving at the AV junction is progressively delayed until, eventually, AV conduction is completely blocked. This results in failure of the impulse to be transmitted through to the ventricles. Typically, following the dropped beat, the cycle will repeat itself.
- ***Second-degree AV block (Mobitz II).*** A more severe form of AV heart block is a second-degree AV block (Mobitz II). In this block, certain impulses are conducted through the AV node while others are blocked. There is usually a recognized pattern in that one, two, or three impulses are conducted, and then one is blocked.
- ***Third-degree AV block.*** The most serious type of AV heart block is a third-degree AV block, also called a complete heart block. In a third-degree heart block, none of the impulses originating in the atria are conducted into the ventricles. This results in the atria and ventricles each having their own intrinsic rate. This can lead to severe bradycardia, heart failure, and, in certain situations, cardiac arrest.

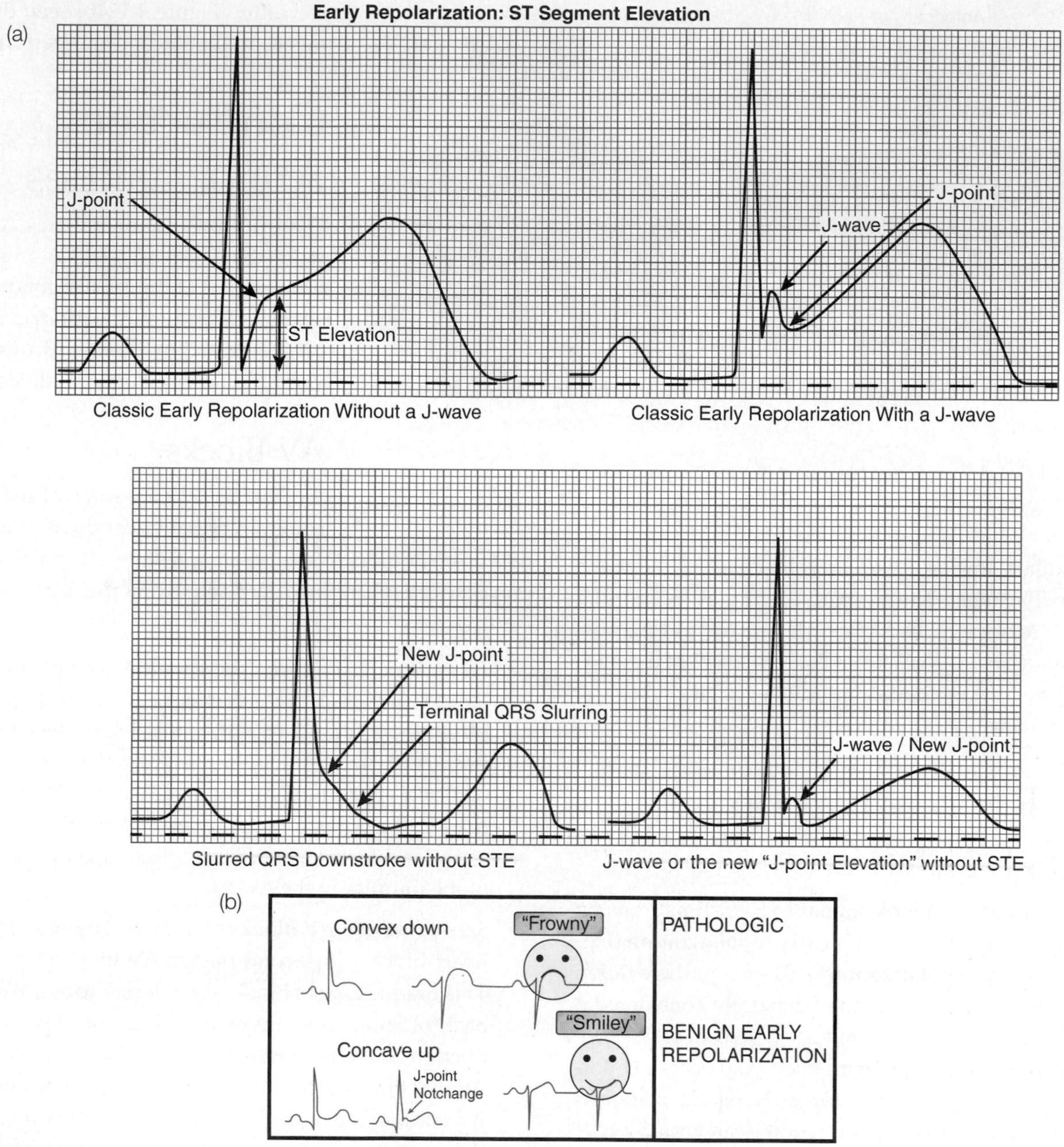

FIGURE 2-124 (a) Early repolarization is characterized by an upward convex ST-segment and notching. (b) Emoticons are sometimes used to compare pathological ST-segment elevation ("Frowny" emoticon) with benign early repolarization ST-segment elevation ("Smiley" emoticon).

Bundle Branch Blocks

Conduction abnormalities are not limited to the AV node. Conduction defects can also occur in the right bundle branch, the left bundle branch, or even in one of the fascicles of the left bundle branch. AV blocks can be detected by single-lead monitoring. Bundle branch blocks, on the other hand, can be diagnosed only with a 12-lead tracing.

In a bundle branch block, ventricular depolarization is abnormal. The impulse will originate in the SA node, be transmitted through the internodal pathways, through the AV node, and into the bundle of His. After entering the bundle of His, the impulse is transmitted into the left and right bundle branches, and then into the Purkinje system. If the right bundle branch is blocked, the impulse will proceed down the left bundle branch. The block will prevent transmission of the impulse through the right bundle branch. The impulse must then spread from the left bundle branch through the myocardial cells of the interventricular septum and into the right ventricle. Likewise, blockage of the left bundle branch will cause the impulse to be spread from the right bundle branch through the interventricular septum and into the left ventricle.

In the case of a bundle branch block, the electrical forces traveling across the interventricular septum cannot use the rapid fibers of the ventricular conductive system. Because the impulse must be transmitted through the interventricular septum itself, from the functioning bundle branch to the side with the nonfunctioning bundle branch, depolarization of the affected ventricle will be delayed. This can be detected on the ECG as prolongation of the QRS complex of greater than or equal to 0.12 second. In addition, the delay in depolarization of the ventricle on the affected side can result in abnormal formation of the QRS complex.

The following discussion will address the common bundle branch blocks and hemiblocks:

- ***Right bundle branch block.*** A right bundle branch block results from blockage of some portion of the right bundle branch. In this case, the impulse must continue down the left bundle branch and spread through the interventricular septum until the right ventricle is depolarized. This results in a delay of impulse transmission into the right ventricle, causing a prolongation of the QRS complex (greater than or equal to 0.12 second). The right ventricle is a low-pressure pump. Because of this, the right ventricular muscle mass is considerably smaller than the left. In the normal ECG, the electrical forces of the right ventricle are overshadowed by the more massive forces of the left ventricle. In the case of a right bundle branch block, right ventricular depolarization occurs after left ventricular depolarization. The vector of the right ventricular depolarization is rightward and anterior as compared to the left, because the impulse is spreading from the left ventricle to the right ventricle instead of the normal scenario where the right ventricle is stimulated by the right bundle branch.

  A complete right bundle branch block is typically characterized by a prolonged QRS complex of greater than or equal to 0.12 second. In addition, an abnormal late portion of the QRS is directed toward the right ventricle and away from the left ventricle. This typically appears as a broad S wave in lead I. Also, a characteristic RSR′ (R-S-R prime) complex will be seen in lead V_1 (Figure 2-125). The RSR′ (also called a "rabbit ear") reflects the abnormal septal depolarization and subsequent right ventricular depolarization. Lead V_1 lies immediately over the right ventricle and is a good lead for detecting right ventricular abnormalities.

- Right bundle branch block is a rather common finding. It is a relatively thin bundle of fibers compared to the left bundle branch and is thus more susceptible to injury. Right bundle branch block can result from acute MI, drugs, electrolyte abnormalities, or general age-related deterioration of the cardiac conductive system.
- ***Left bundle branch block.*** The left bundle branch is derived from the bundle of His. It subsequently divides into the anterior and posterior fascicles before it terminates in the Purkinje system of the left ventricle. When a left bundle branch block occurs, the left ventricle cannot be depolarized normally. Thus, the electrical impulse must be transmitted from the right ventricle, through the interventricular septum, and then into the left ventricle. As with a right bundle branch block, the depolarization impulse must spread through the interventricular septum without the aid of

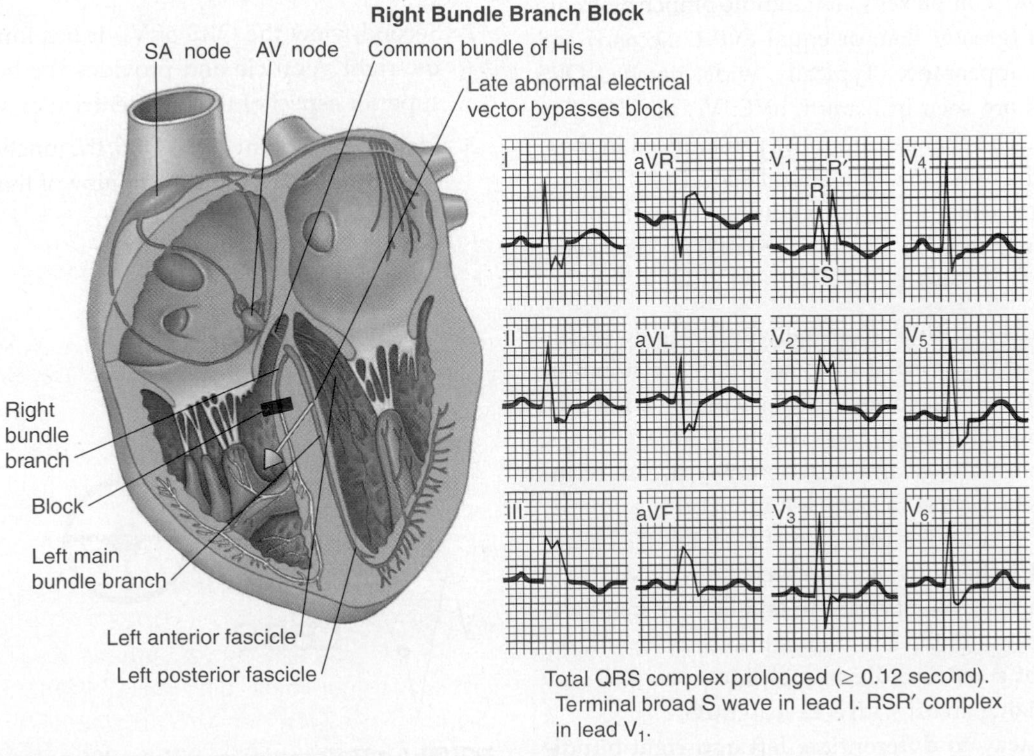

FIGURE 2-125 Right bundle branch block.

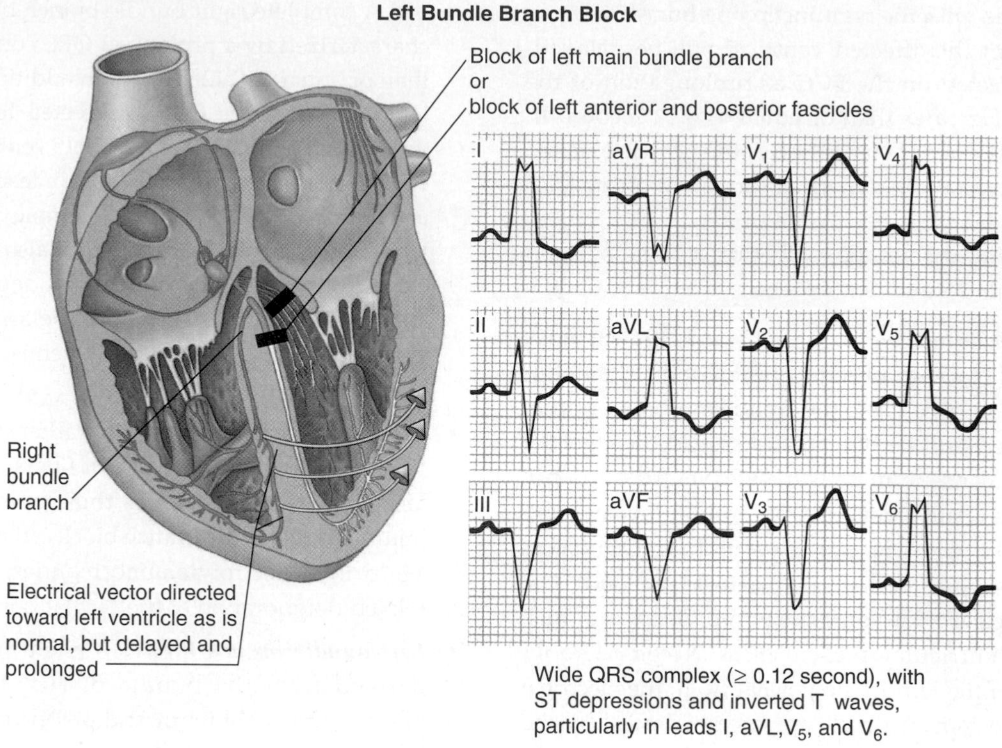

FIGURE 2-126 Left bundle branch block.

specialized conductive fibers. This causes a delay in impulse transmission through the interventricular septum and results in a prolongation of the QRS complex. Unlike a right bundle branch block, the direction of the forces in a left bundle branch block is from right to left, nearly the same as in the normal heart.

The QRS complexes in left bundle branch block are prolonged (greater than or equal to 0.12 second) and bizarre in appearance. Typically, wide, notched QRS complexes are seen in leads I, aVL, V_5, and V_6 (Figure 2-126). The changes are more pronounced in these leads, as they visualize the lateral aspect of the heart, which is principally the left ventricle. Deep S waves can be seen in lead V_1, V_2, or V_3 or tall R waves seen in leads I, aVL, V_5, and V_6 (as described previously).

A left bundle branch block usually indicates significant and widespread myocardial disease (although it can be seen in patients who have had cardiac surgery). Like the right bundle branch block, it too results from MI, drugs, electrolyte abnormalities, and degenerative disease of the conductive system. Most myocardial infarctions primarily affect the left ventricle. The presence of a left bundle branch block will mask ischemic changes associated with MI. Thus, a patient can suffer a significant MI, and ECG changes will not be seen because of the left bundle branch block. In fact, the presence of a left bundle branch block negates any chance of localizing an MI with a 12-lead ECG.[34]

An easier way to differentiate left and right bundle branch blocks is to apply the four steps of the turn-signal rule, which parallels the action of a vehicle's turn signal (Figure 2-127):

1. Determine that the QRS complex is consistently greater than 0.12 second throughout the ECG. You often can do this best by viewing the QRS duration of the precordial leads (V_1 through V_6).
2. Second, view the QRS of V_1. It lies immediately over the right ventricle and provides the best view of the superior aspect of the interventricular septum.
3. Identify the J point of the QRS, the junction between the end of the QRS and the beginning of the ST segment.

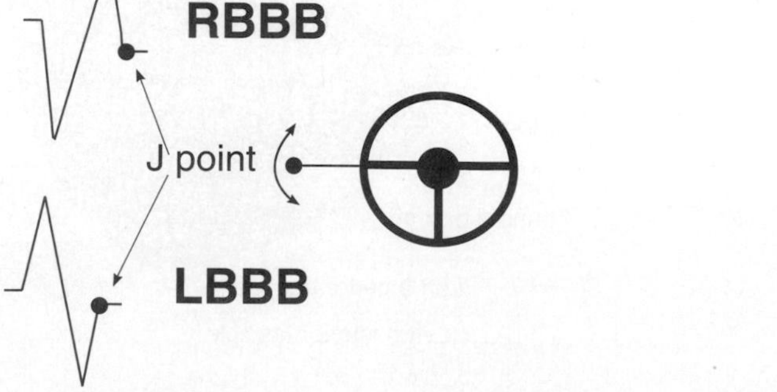

FIGURE 2-127 The turn-signal rule for differentiating right and left bundle branch blocks.

4. Draw a horizontal line from the J point to an intersecting line of the QRS, or to the beginning of the QRS. This will produce a triangle pointing either up or down. If the triangle points up, it indicates a right bundle branch block. (If you push up a vehicle's turn signal, the signal lights indicate a right turn.) If the triangle points down, it indicates a left bundle branch block. (If you push down the turn signal lever, the lights indicate a left turn.)

Detecting bundle branch blocks is important because left bundle branch blocks can mask ischemic changes associated with MI. Also, some ST elevation usually appears in the precordial leads with left bundle branch blocks, thus rendering 12-lead tracings useless in determining or localizing an MI.

- ***Hemiblocks.*** The left bundle branch divides into the left anterior and left posterior fascicles. Blocks can occur in either of these fascicles and are a fairly common finding.
- ***Left posterior hemiblock.*** A left posterior hemiblock, also called a *left posterior fascicular block*, results from blockage of the left posterior fascicle. Blockage of the left posterior fascicle results in a delay in depolarizing the portion of the left ventricle it innervates. A left posterior hemiblock does not typically prolong the QRS interval. In addition, the shape of the QRS complex remains relatively normal. The principal finding in a left posterior hemiblock is a rightward shift in the QRS axis. This is often difficult to diagnose, particularly if there is underlying right ventricular or pulmonary disease. Generally, the QRS axis must be greater than or equal to 120° to consider a left posterior hemiblock (Figure 2-128). Left posterior hemiblock is usually due to degenerative disease of the conductive system or ischemic heart disease.
- ***Left anterior hemiblock.*** A left anterior hemiblock, also called a *left anterior fascicular block*, results from blockage of the left anterior fascicle. This block is similar to a bundle branch block, but it does *not* result in a delay in ventricular depolarization. Thus, the QRS complex is of normal duration and is generally of normal shape, without the unusual notching seen in the bundle branch blocks. The principal abnormality in a left anterior hemiblock is a shift in the QRS axis far to the left (typically more negative than −30°). This results in a negative QRS complex in leads II, III, and aVF (Figure 2-129). A left anterior hemiblock is usually caused by degeneration of the cardiac conductive system or ischemic heart disease. It is usually a benign finding.

Figure 2-130 is an actual tracing from a patient with a left bundle branch block. Figure 2-131 is an actual tracing from a patient with a complete right bundle branch block. Both are common findings in 12-lead ECG interpretation. Remember, a left bundle branch block renders the ECG relatively useless for detecting injury or ischemia.

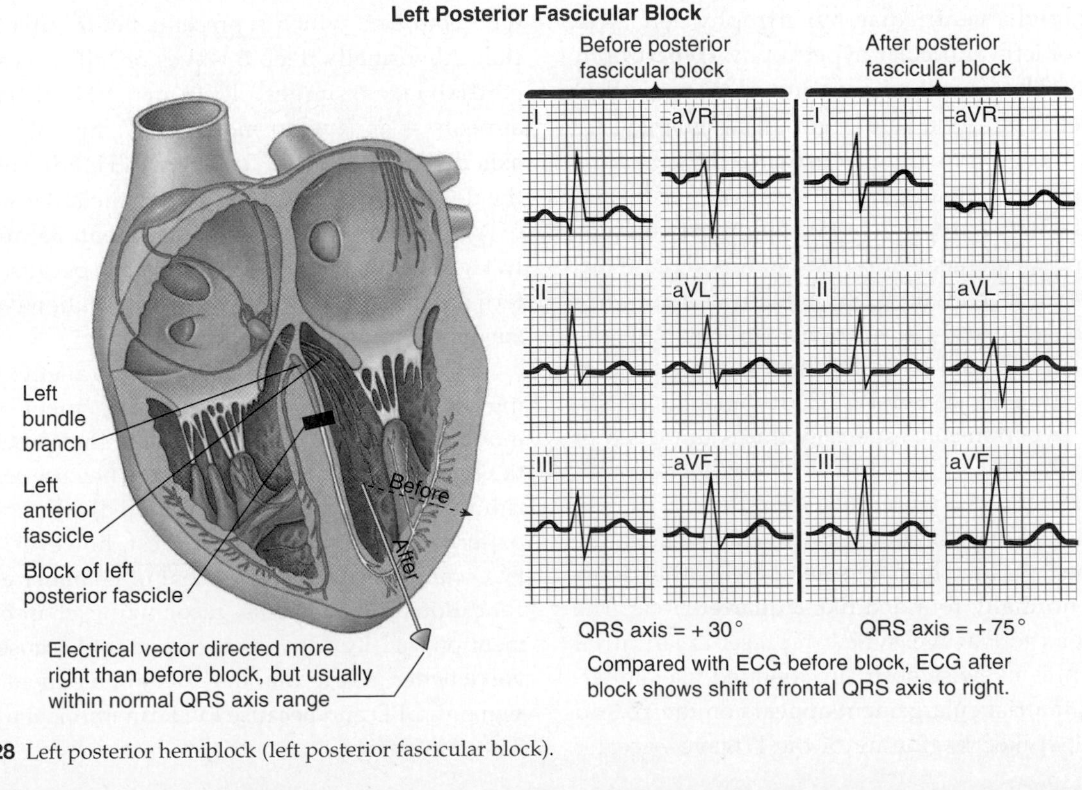

FIGURE 2-128 Left posterior hemiblock (left posterior fascicular block).

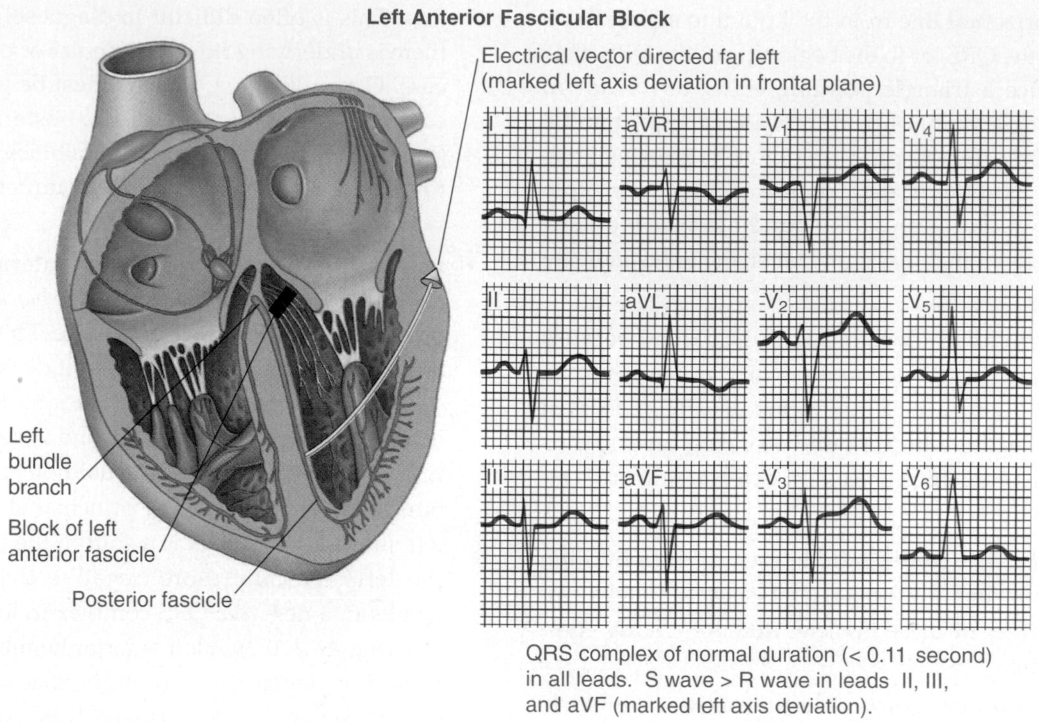

FIGURE 2-129 Left anterior hemiblock (left anterior fascicular block).

Chamber Enlargement

Although chamber enlargement rarely affects prehospital care, you should understand the condition's basic pathophysiology because it often can appear on a 12-lead ECG tracing and cause misleading patterns of ischemia.

Chamber enlargement may involve right atrial enlargement, right ventricular hypertrophy, left atrial enlargement, or left ventricular hypertrophy. **Hypertrophy** simply means enlargement without any additional cells—basically, stretching. As a rule, right atrial enlargement (RAE) is a precursor to right ventricular hypertrophy (RVH), and left atrial enlargement (LAE) is a precursor to left ventricular hypertrophy (LVH). The most common cause of chamber enlargement is disease. Any disease that causes long-term increased pressure in any of the heart's four chambers can cause chamber enlargement. RAE and RVH are usually caused by pulmonary disease such as COPD or emphysema. LAE and LVH are generally caused by long-term hypertension, especially if it is untreated or poorly managed.

Because the P wave represents atrial depolarization, atrial enlargement appears in the P wave formation. The first half of the P wave, which represents right atrial depolarization, is normally rounded like a quarter-circle. The second half of the P wave, which represents left atrial depolarization, is likewise normally rounded like a quarter-circle. Right atrial enlargement appears on the 12-lead ECG as a tall, spiked beginning of the P wave—greater than 2 mm (two small boxes). Left atrial enlargement appears as a biphasic, widened P wave of 2.5 mm (two and one-half small boxes). Leads II, aVL, V_1, and V_2 offer the best views of both right and left atrial enlargement (Figure 2-132).

Ventricular chamber enlargement appears in the QRS complex, which represents ventricular depolarization. Abnormally deep S waves or tall waves in the precordial leads suggest RVH or LVH. RVH generally appears as an R wave more than 7 mm tall, with a right axis deviation (RAD). To detect LVH, add the heights of the deeper S wave of V_1 or V_2 and the taller R wave of V_5 or V_6. A sum equal to or greater than 35 mm indicates LVH. Recognizing LVH is important because its ST pattern often mimics the ST segment elevation pattern of tissue injury (Figure 2-133).

Echocardiography is the standard method for detecting and diagnosing chamber enlargement, but 12-lead monitors programmed with internal interpretive capabilities often will detect this condition. They use complex algorithms to detect numerous, detailed, and specific wave patterns in multiple leads. At best, however, the 12-lead ECG can detect only 50 percent of chamber enlargement conditions. Nonetheless, recognizing chamber enlargement on a 12-lead tracing is important because it can give you a better insight into the extent of a patient's hypertension or COPD and because LVH can mimic the ST segment pattern of injury.

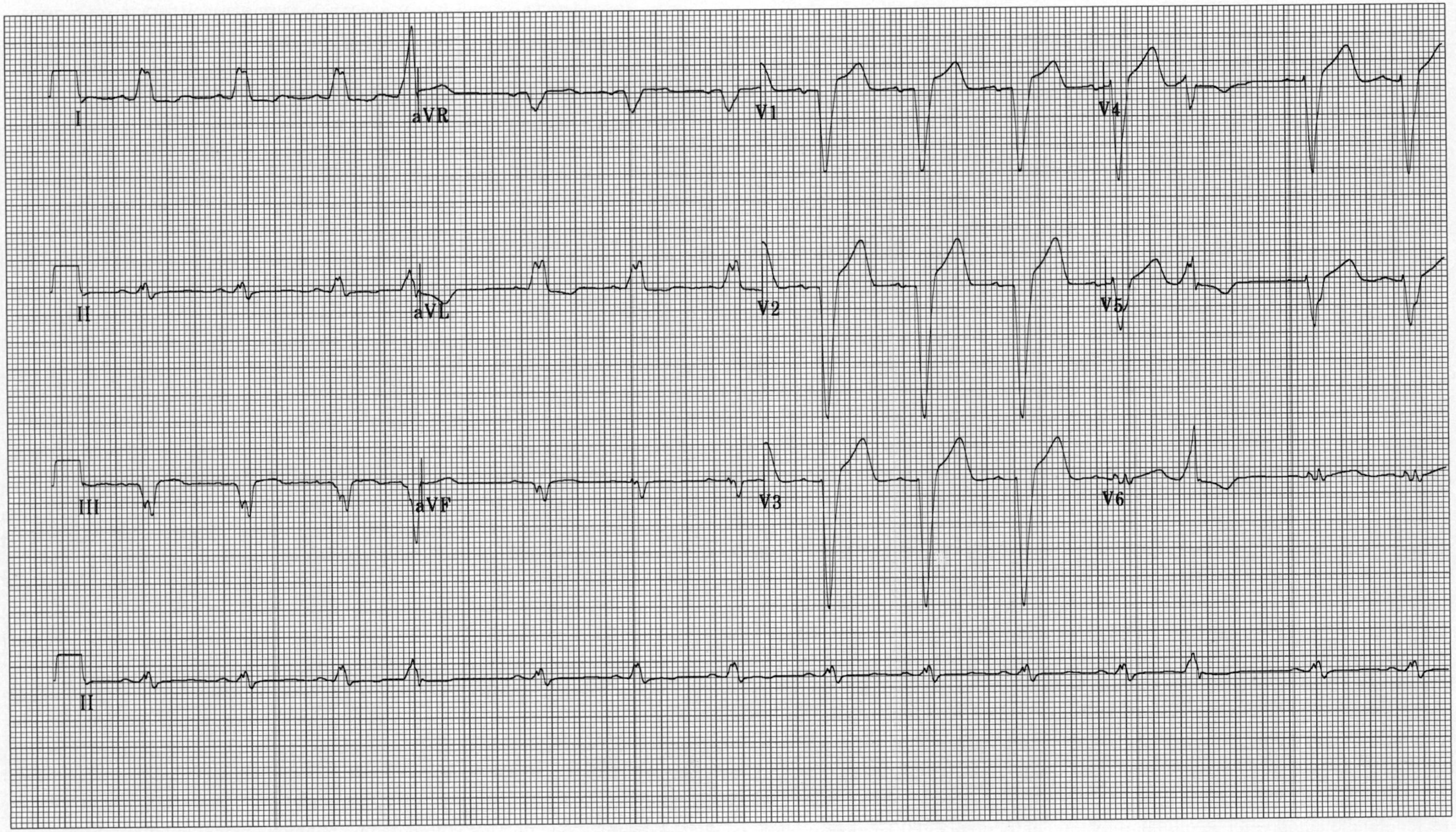

FIGURE 2-130 Tracing from a patient with a left bundle branch block.

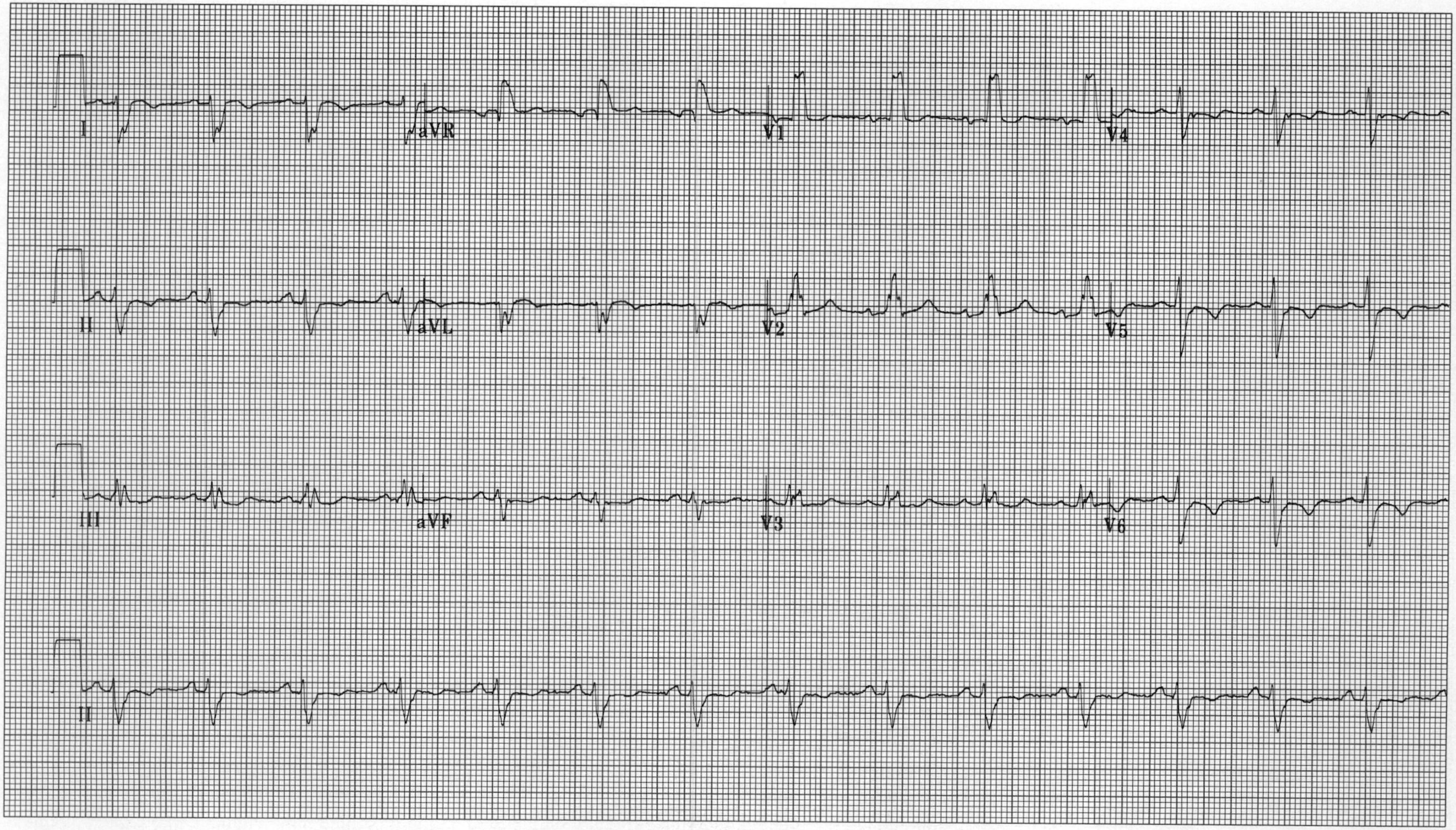

FIGURE 2-131 Tracing from a patient with a complete right bundle branch block.

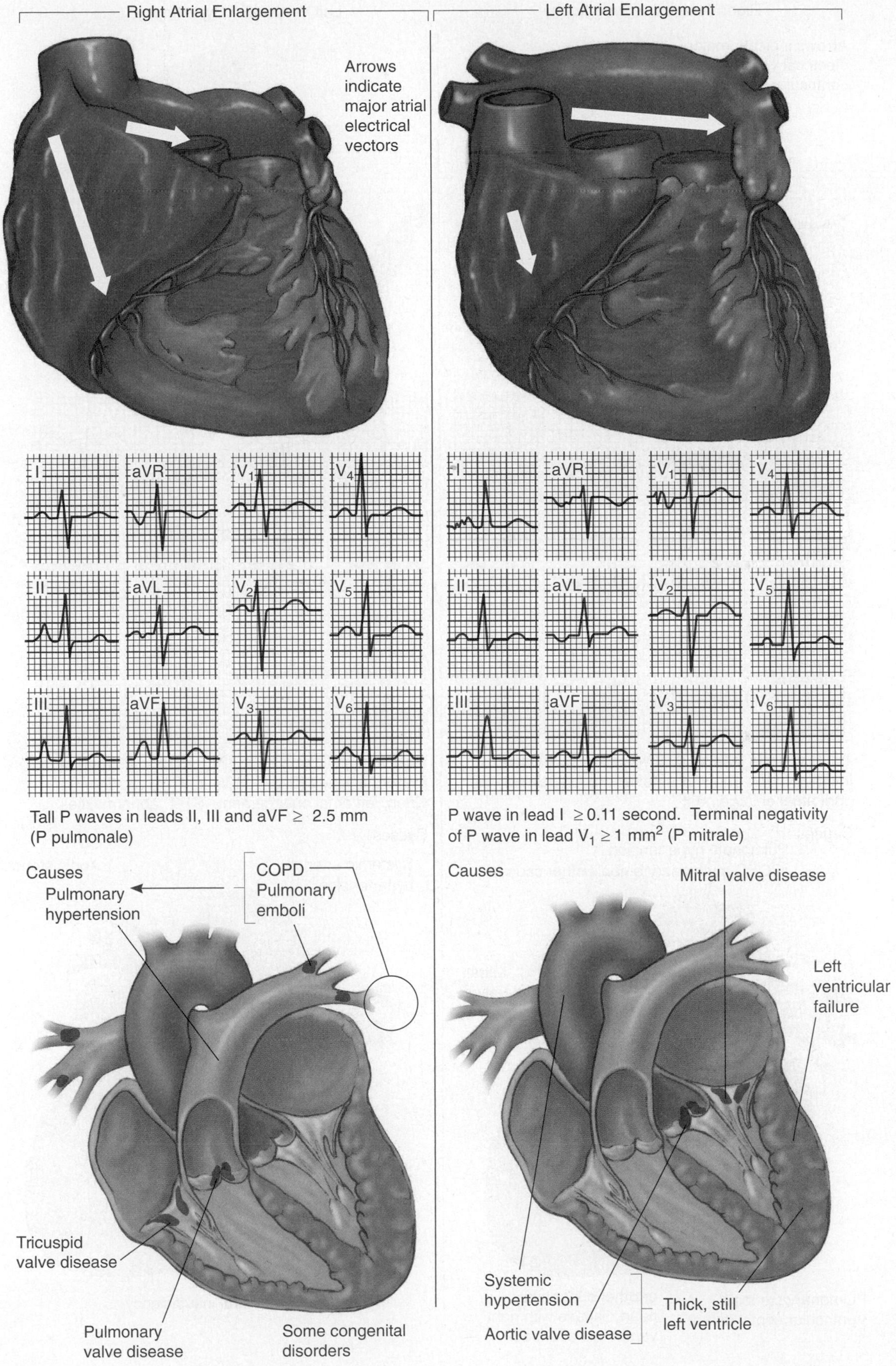

FIGURE 2-132 Findings in atrial enlargement.

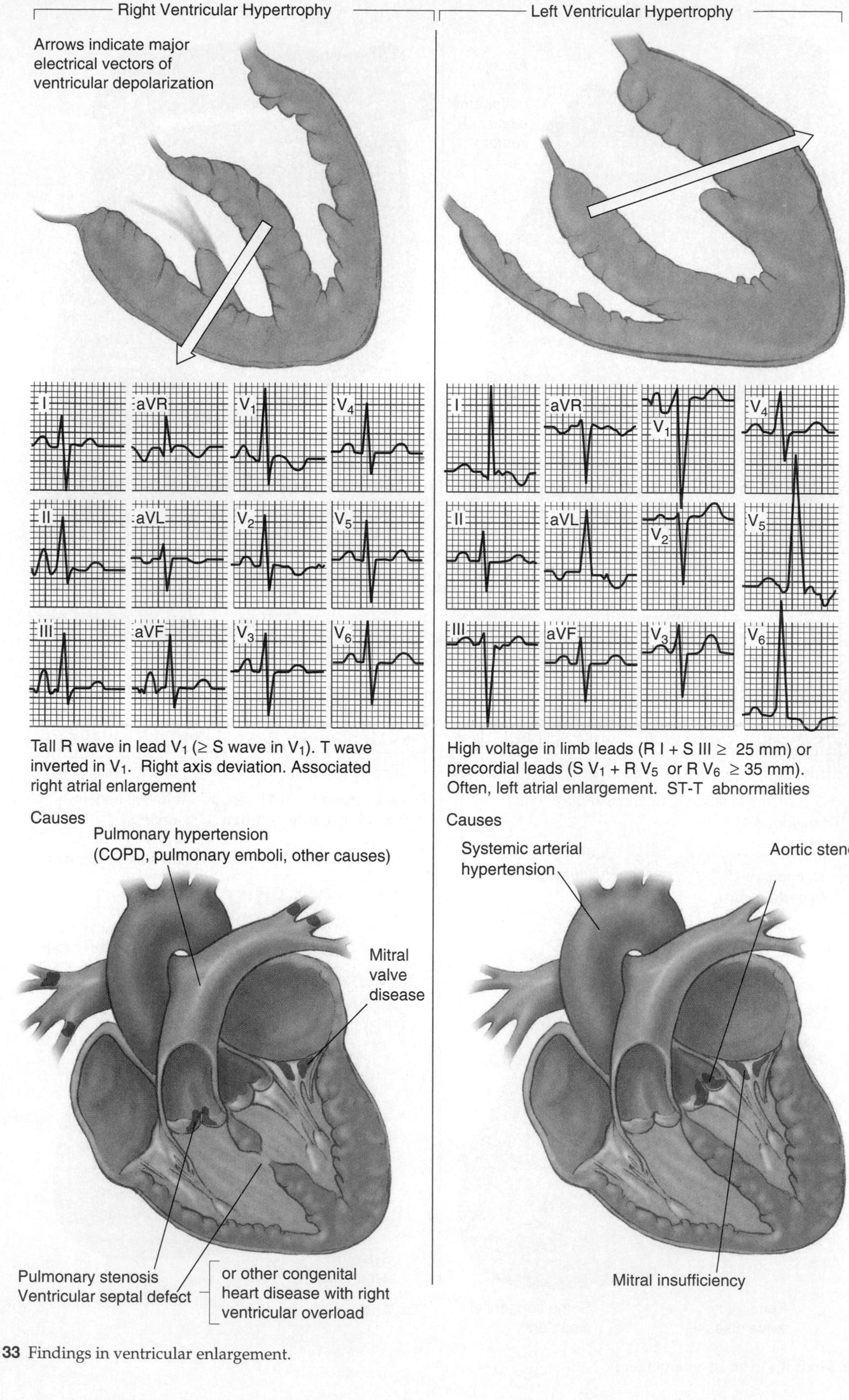

FIGURE 2-133 Findings in ventricular enlargement.

Prehospital ECG Monitoring

Technology has evolved to a point where portable 12-lead ECG monitoring is readily available. Many manufacturers now make 12-lead machines for prehospital care. Most machines have sophisticated electronics, many with ECG diagnostic packages. Some now have a defibrillator/pacer unit (Figure 2-134). The principles of 12-lead monitoring are similar to those for routine ECG monitoring described earlier in this chapter.

Prehospital 12-Lead ECG Monitoring

The following skill sequence details 12-lead prehospital ECG monitoring.

1. Explain what you are going to do to the patient. Reassure him that the machine will not shock him.
2. Prepare all the equipment and ensure that the cable is in good repair. Check to make sure there are adequate leads and materials for prepping the skin.
3. Prep the skin (Procedure 2–6). Dirt, oil, sweat, and other materials on the skin can interfere with obtaining

Procedure 2-6 12-Lead Prehospital ECG Monitoring

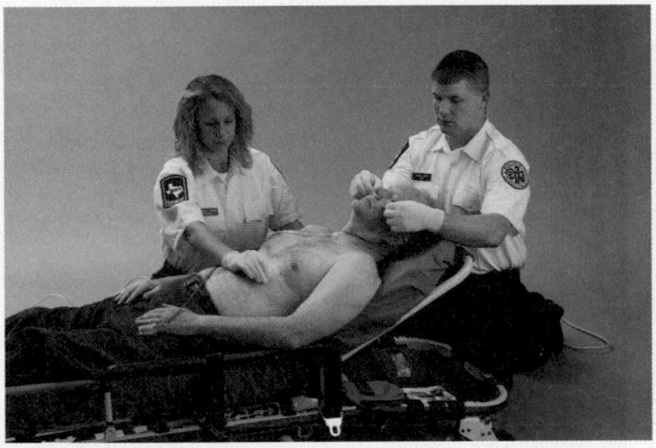

2-6a Prep the skin.

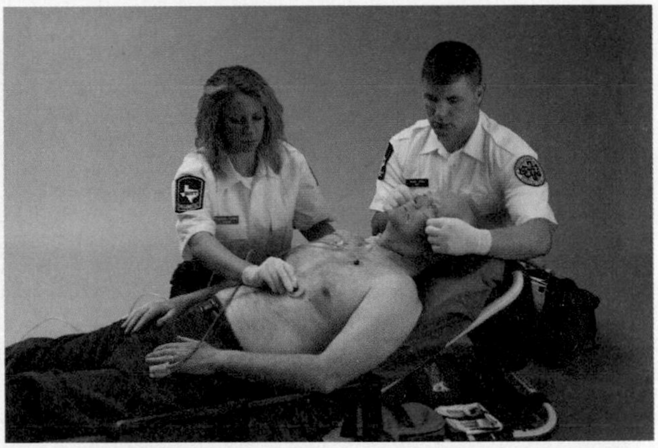

2-6b Place the four limb leads according to the manufacturer's recommendations.

Lead V_1 The electrode is at the fourth intercostal space just to the right of the sternum.
Lead V_2 The electrode is at the fourth intercostal space just to the left of the sternum.
Lead V_3 The electrode is at the line midway between leads V_2 and V_4.
Lead V_4 The electrode is at the midclavicular line in the fifth interspace.
Lead V_5 The electrode is at the anterior axillary line at the same level as lead V_4.
Lead V_6 The electrode is at the midaxillary line at the same level as lead V_4.

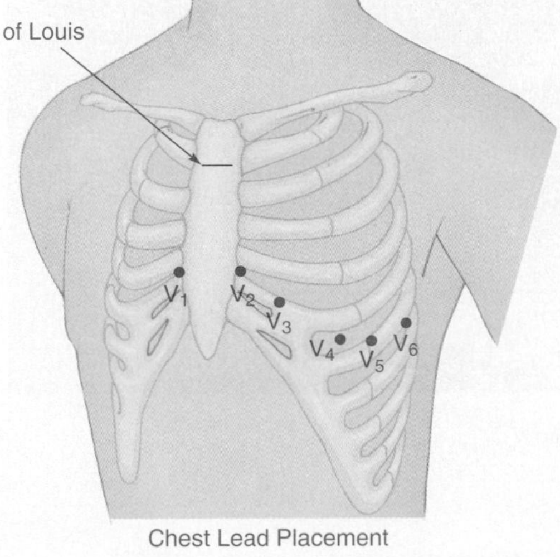

2-6c Proper placement of the precordial leads.

(Continued)

Procedure 2-6 *Continued*

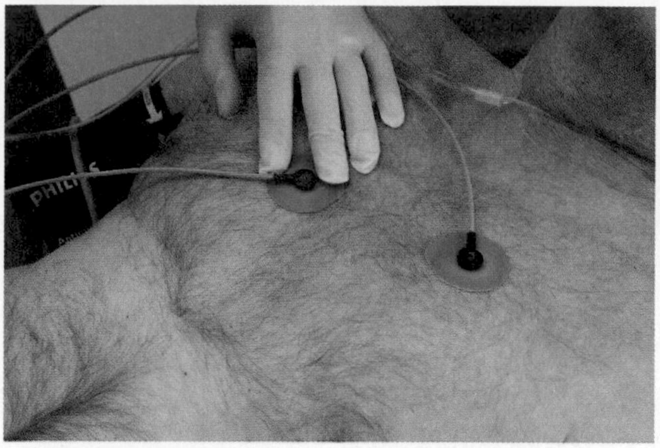

2-6d Place lead V_1.

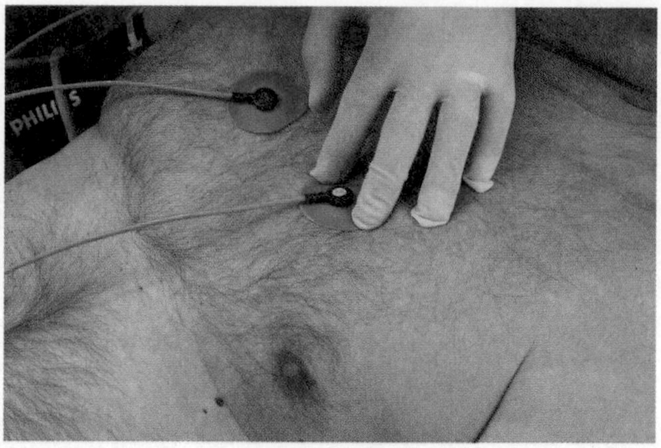

2-6e Place lead V_2.

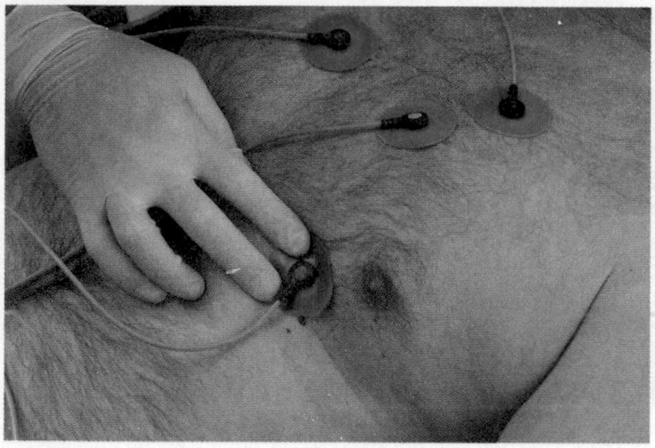

2-6f Place lead V_4.

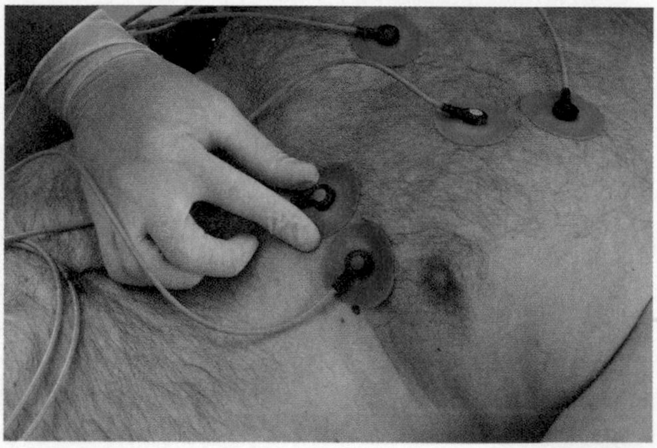

2-6g Place lead V_3.

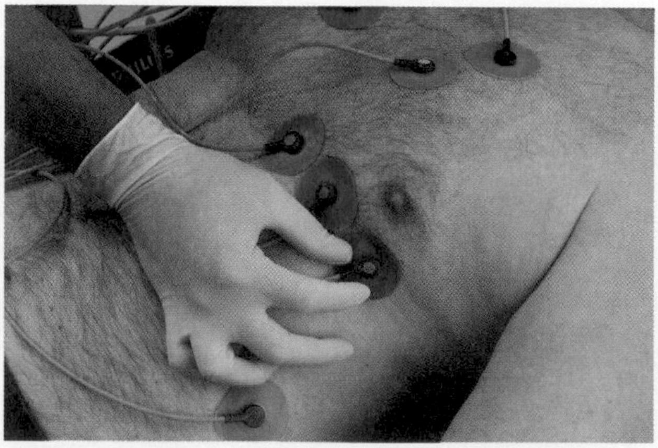

2-6h Place lead V_5.

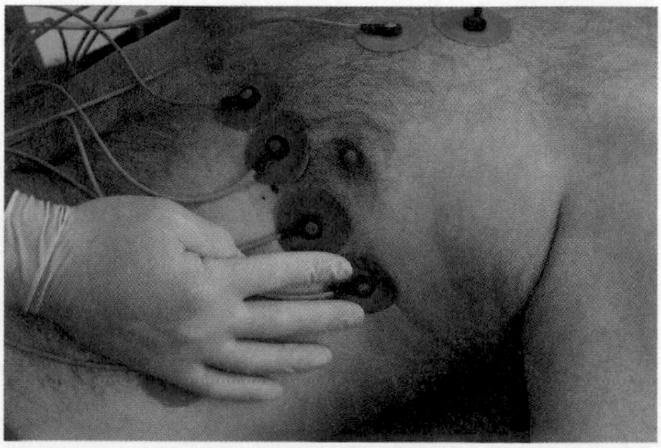

2-6i Place lead V_6.

Procedure 2-6 *Continued*

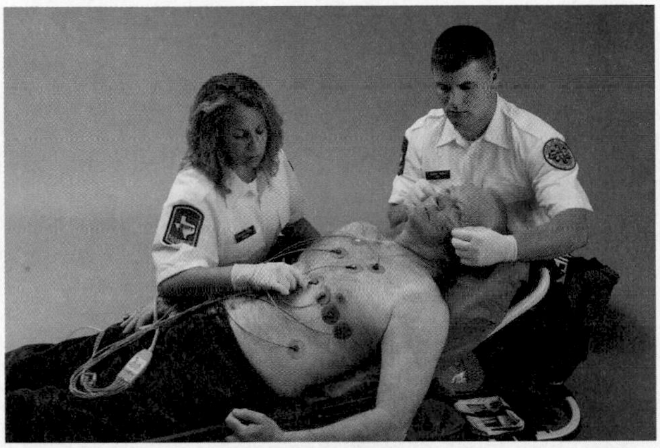

2-6j Ensure that all leads are attached.

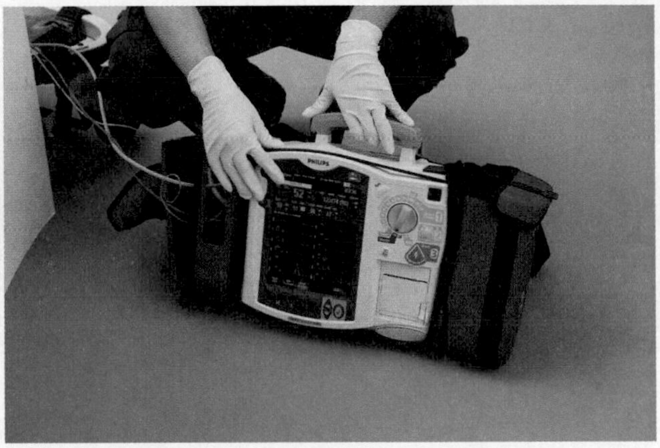

2-6k Turn on the machine.

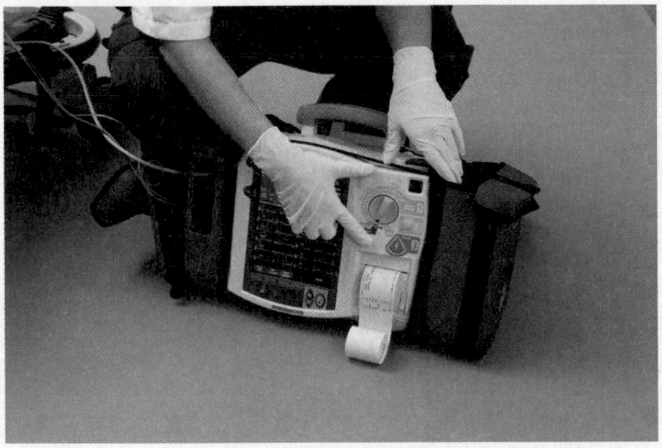

2-6l Check the quality of the tracing being received from each channel.

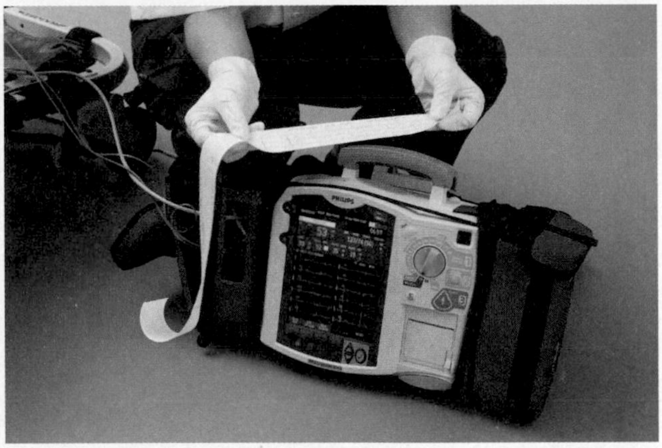

2-6m Record the tracing.

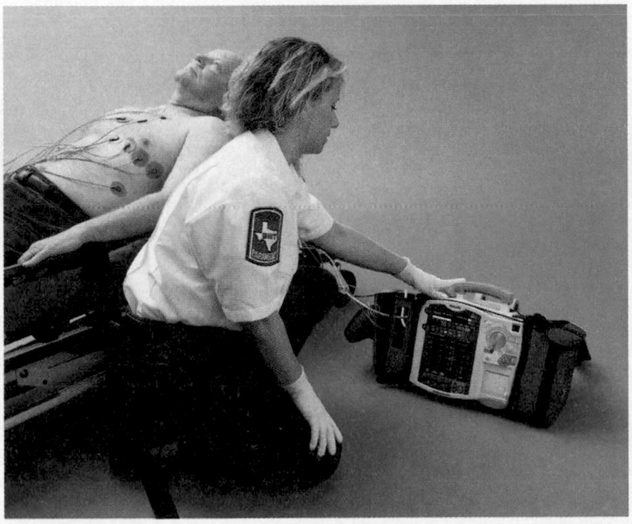

2-6N Examine the tracing.

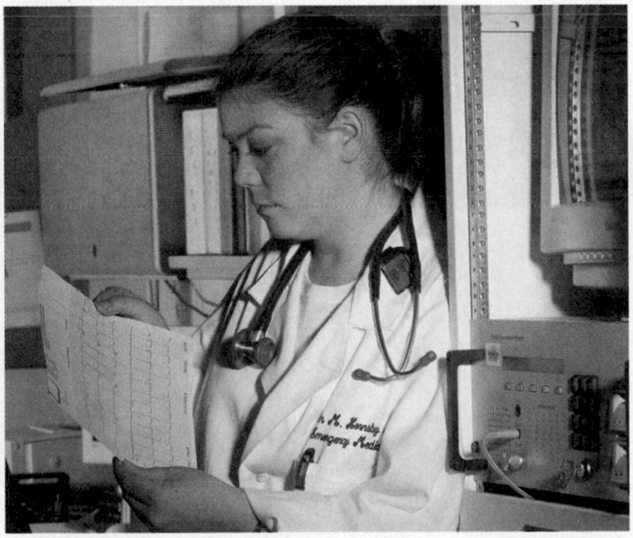

2-6o Transmit the tracing to the receiving hospital.

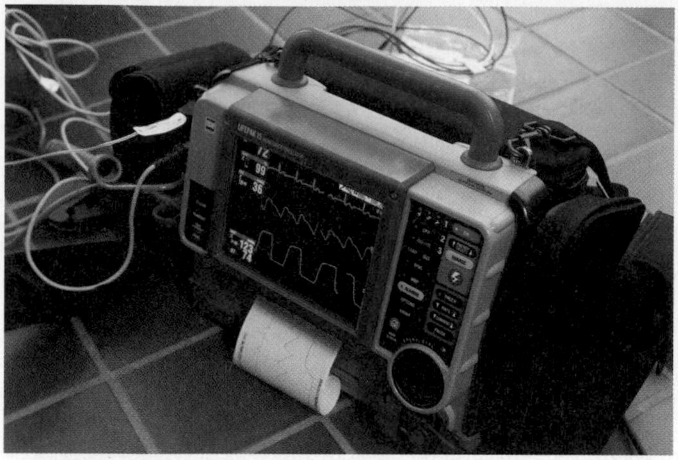

FIGURE 2-134 Prehospital 12-lead monitor.

a quality tracing. The skin should be cleansed with an appropriate substance. If the patient is diaphoretic, dry the skin with a towel. On very hot days or if the patient is very diaphoretic, tincture of benzoin can be applied to the skin before attaching the electrode. Occasionally, it may be necessary to slightly abrade the skin to obtain a good interface. Patients with a lot of body hair may need to have the area immediately over the electrode site shaved to ensure good skin/electrode interface.

4. Place the four limb leads according to the manufacturer's recommendations (Procedure 2–6b).
5. Following placement of the limb leads, prepare for placement of the precordial leads. Procedure 2–6c illustrates proper placement of the precordial leads.
6. First, place lead V_1 by attaching the positive electrode to the right of the sternum at the fourth intercostal space (Procedure 2–6d).
7. Next, place lead V_2 by attaching the positive electrode to the left of the sternum at the fourth intercostal space (Procedure 2–6e).
8. Next, place lead V_4 by attaching the positive electrode at the midclavicular line at the fifth intercostal space (Procedure 2–6f).
9. Next, place lead V_3 by attaching the positive electrode in a line midway between lead V_2 and lead V_4 (Procedure 2–6g).
10. Next, place lead V_5 by attaching the positive electrode at the anterior axillary line at the same level as V_4 (Procedure 2–6h).
11. Finally, place V_6 by attaching the positive electrode at the midaxillary line at the same level as V_4 (Procedure 2–6i).
12. Ensure that all leads are attached (Procedure 2–6j).
13. Turn on the machine (Procedure 2–6k).
14. Ensure that all leads are properly attached and a good tracing is being received from each channel (Procedure 2–6l).
15. Record the tracing (Procedure 2–6m).
16. Examine the tracing. Do not completely rely on the machine's interpretation of the tracing. If necessary, confirm with medical direction (Procedure 2–6n).
17. Provide the tracing to the receiving hospital (Procedure 2–6o). If you do not start fibrinolytic therapy in the field, you can reduce the door-to-needle time by providing a quality 12-lead tracing to the emergency staff as soon as the patient arrives.
18. Perform patient pass-off to the hospital personnel.
19. Restock equipment for the next call.
20. Compare field interpretation with emergency department and cardiology interpretation.

Summary

Cardiovascular disease is the number-one cause of death in the United States and Canada. Many deaths from heart attack occur within the first 24 hours—frequently within the first hour. The longer cardiac ischemia continues, the more heart muscle is lost.

Cardiac care has improved by leaps and bounds over the past decade. Fibrinolytic therapy and cardiac catheterizations are saving more and more hearts and lives every day. Because 12-lead ECGs have become mainstream EMS tools, identification of cardiac ischemia and subsequent notification of the receiving hospital is happening at breakneck speeds. ST-segment elevation myocardial infarction (STEMI) protocols have progressed to the point at which EMS activation of cardiac catheter lab teams has become routine practice. The overall goal is to reduce the amount of time the patient spends in routine care before receiving the definitive treatment of a cardiac catheterization or thrombolysis. Time is of the essence; time equals heart muscle.

With technological advances, cardiac care in EMS has all but put the physicians on the scene with a cardiac patient. As you assess your patient and obtain a 12-lead ECG, you can quickly send a copy of the ECG and vitals to the receiving hospital. In some cases, the cardiologist on call instantly receives the ECG on a smartphone and is able to review the ECG for abnormalities and even contact you to give further orders. In some cases, and some services, the cardiologist can order thrombolytics to be started in the field or may direct EMS to go straight to the catheter lab rather than stop in the emergency department. All of these help expedite treatment for the patient and save heart muscle.

Cardiac care is an area in which EMS can truly make the difference between life and death for a patient.

You Make the Call

You and your partner on Medic 3 are dispatched to a well-kept residence about three blocks from the station. The dispatch information relates the nature of the call as chest pain. On your arrival at the residence, the patient's wife meets you and shows you to a back room. The patient is a man who appears to be in his late 60s. He is complaining of chest pain that began approximately 30 minutes ago while he was at rest. He thinks it may be due to some light yard work he did earlier in the day. The patient appears in severe distress, however, and is sweaty and diaphoretic.

You move to your history and physical exam. The patient has a history of hypertension and of diabetes that is controlled by diet. He has been in good health until the current episode. Physical exam reveals the patient to be pale and diaphoretic. The heart rate is 40, the blood pressure is 110/70 mmHg, and respirations are 20. The patient describes the pain as a "weight on my chest" that does not improve with a change in position. He states that his left arm feels heavy, and it is getting difficult to get a deep breath. You quickly place the 12-lead ECG, obtain a tracing, and send it ahead to the receiving facility. The 12-lead shows ST-segment elevation of 4 mm in leads II, III, and aVF and ST-segment depression of 2 mm in leads I, aVL, and V_5.

1. What is your assessment of the patient's condition?
2. What prehospital care should be provided?
3. What additional orders or directions could you expect to receive from medical direction?

See Suggested Responses at the back of this book.

Review Questions

1. What is the name of the protective sac surrounding the heart that consists of two layers, visceral and parietal?
   a. Myocardium
   b. Pericardium
   c. Mesocardium
   d. Endocardium
2. What is the name of the outermost lining of the walls of arteries, described as a fibrous tissue covering that gives the vessel strength to withstand the pressures generated by the heart's contractions?
   a. Tunica media
   b. Tunica intima
   c. Tunica adventitia
   d. Visceral media
3. Which law states that the more the myocardial muscle is stretched, the greater its force of contraction will be?
   a. Cushing's law
   b. Starling's law
   c. Poiseuille's law
   d. Newton's law
4. Which term refers to the strength of a cardiac muscular contraction?
   a. Atropy
   b. Inotropy
   c. Dromotropy
   d. Chronotropy

5. Which cellular property, possessed by certain cells of the myocardium, allows the conductive system to depolarize without any impulse from an outside source?
   a. Excitability
   b. Conductivity
   c. Automaticity
   d. Contractility
6. Which ECG rhythm will most likely result from an increased rate of SA node discharge?
   a. Sinus bradycardia
   b. Sinus tachycardia
   c. Sinus arrhythmia
   d. Atrial tachycardia
7. Which ECG finding is the result or a single electrical impulse originating in the atria outside the SA node, which in turn causes a premature depolarization of the ventricles before the next expected sinus beat?
   a. Premature atrial contractions
   b. Wandering atrial pacemaker
   c. Multifocal atrial tachycardia
   d. Multifocal atrial bradycardia
8. Which ECG arrhythmia results from a rapid atrial reentry circuit and an AV node that physiologically cannot conduct all impulses through to the ventricles?
   a. Atrial flutter
   b. Atrial fibrillation
   c. Wandering atrial pacemaker
   d. Paroxysmal atrial tachycardia
9. Which ECG dysrhythmia is an intermittent block at the level of the AV node that produces a characteristic cyclic pattern in which the PR intervals become progressively longer until an impulse is blocked?
   a. Mobitz I
   b. Mobitz II
   c. First-degree block
   d. Third-degree block
10. Which emergency medication is relatively safe and highly effective in terminating PSVT, especially if its etiology is reentry in nature?
    a. Valium
    b. Atropine
    c. Adenosine
    d. Dopamine
11. In this pattern of group beating, if every fourth beat is a PVC, the term used to describe this is ________
    a. bigeminy.
    b. trigeminy.
    c. quadrigeminy.
    d. interpolated.
12. Ventricular tachycardia with no pulse and what other ventricular dysrhythmia are treated identically by the paramedic?
    a. Atrial fibrillation
    b. Paroxysmal supraventricular tachycardia
    c. Premature ventricular contractions
    d. Ventricular fibrillation
13. What is the name of the first heart sound, which is produced by closure of the AV valves (tricuspid and mitral) during ventricular systole?
    a. S_1
    b. S_2
    c. S_3
    d. S_4
14. What is the most common cause of poor ECG signals?
    a. Weak batteries
    b. Loose lead connection
    c. Faulty skin contact
    d. Radio signal interference
15. Which narcotic medication is used during the prehospital management of a myocardial infarction?
    a. Codeine
    b. Morphine
    c. Alteplase
    d. Diazepam
16. What is the most common 12-lead ECG finding in the angina patient?
    a. PR prolongation
    b. J waves
    c. T wave elevation
    d. ST segment depression
17. What is the most common chief complaint of a patient experiencing a myocardial infarction?
    a. Dyspnea
    b. Weakness
    c. Chest pain
    d. Diaphoresis

18. Which pathology is the most common cause of hospitalization in patients over age 65 each year?
    a. CHF
    b. CVA
    c. Hypertension
    d. Diabetes

19. Inclusion criteria for termination of resuscitation include all of the following *except* ___________
    a. age 16 years and older.
    b. successful and maintained endotracheal intubation.
    c. ACLS standards have been applied throughout the arrest.
    d. victims of blunt trauma who present and remain in asystole.

20. Which of the following medications would not be used during the management of an arrested patient who started out in ventricular fibrillation, but eventually became asystolic prior to termination of efforts?
    a. Amiodarone
    b. Epinephrine
    c. Lidocaine
    d. Atropine

See Answers to Review Questions at the back of this book.

References

1. Nichol, G., E. Thomas, C. W. Callaway, et al. "Regional Variation in Out-of-Hospital Cardiac Arrest Incidence and Outcome." *JAMA* 300 (2008): 1423–1431.
2. Clerico, A., A. Giannoni, S. Vittorini, and C. Passino. "Thirty Years of the Heart as an Endocrine Organ: Physiological Role and Clinical Utility of Cardiac Natriuretic Hormones." *Am J Physiol Circ Physiol* 6 (2011).
3. Hurst, J. W. "Naming of the Waves in the ECG, with a Brief Account of Their Genesis." *Circulation* 98 (1998): 1937–1942.
4. Link, M. S., L. C. Berkow, P. J Kudenchuk, et al. "Part 7: Adult Advanced Cardiovascular Life Support: 2015 American Heart Association Guidelines for Cardiopulmonary Resuscitation and Emergency Cardiovascular Care." *Circulation* 132 (2015): S444–S464.
5. Kleinman, M. E., E. E. Brennan, Z. D. Goldberger, et al. "Part 5: Adult Basic Life Support: 2015 American Heart Association Guidelines for Cardiopulmonary Resuscitation and Emergency Cardiovascular Care." *Circulation* 132 (2015): S414–S435.
6. Kanowitz, A., T. M. Dunn, E. M. Kanowitz, W. W. Dunn, and K. Vanbuskirk. "Safety and Effectiveness of Fentanyl Administration for Prehospital Pain Management." *Prehosp Emerg Care* 10 (2006): 1–7.
7. Galinski, M., F. Dolveck, S. W. Borron, et al. "A Randomized, Double-Blind Study Comparing Morphine with Fentanyl in Prehospital Analgesia." *Am J Emerg Med* 23 (2005): 114–119.
8. Link, M. S., D. L. Atkins, R. S. Passman, et al. "Part 6: Electrical Therapies: Automated External Defibrillators, Defibrillation, Cardioversion, and Pacing: 2010 American Heart Association Guidelines for Cardiopulmonary Resuscitation and Emergency Cardiovascular Care." *Circulation* 122 (2010): S706–S719.
9. Smith, G., A. Morgans, and M. Boyle. "Use of Valsalva Manoeuvre in the Prehospital Setting: A Review of the Literature." *Emerg Med J* 26 (2009): 8–10.
10. O'Connor, R. E., W. Brady, S. C. Brooks, et al. "Part 10: Acute Coronary Syndromes: 2010 American Heart Association Guidelines for Cardiopulmonary Resuscitation and Emergency Cardiovascular Care." *Circulation* 122 (2010): S787–S817.
11. Welsh, R. C., J. Ornato, and P. W. Armstrong. "Prehospital Management of Acute ST-Elevation Myocardial Infarction: A Time for Reappraisal in North America." *Am Heart J* 145 (2003): 1–8.
12. Marik, P. E. and M. Flemmer. "Narrative Review: The Management of Acute Decompensated Heart Failure." *J Intensive Care Med* (May 26 2011). PubMed: 21616957.
13. Mosesso, V. N., J. Dunford, T. Blackwell, and J. K. Griswell. "Prehospital Therapy for Acute Congestive Heart Failure: State of the Art." *Prehosp Emerg Care* 7 (2003): 13–23.
14. Kallio, T., M. Kuisma, A. Alaspää, and P. H. Rosenberg. "The Use of Prehospital Continuous Positive Airway Pressure Treatment in Presumed Acute Severe Pulmonary Edema." *Prehosp Emerg Care* 7 (2003): 209–213.
15. Hubble, M. W., M. E. Richards, R. Jarvis, T. Millikan, and D. Young. "Effectiveness of Prehospital Continuous Positive Airway Pressure in the Management of Acute Pulmonary Edema." *Prehosp Emerg Care* 10 (2006): 430–439.
16. Vismara, L. A., D. M. Leaman, and R. Zelis. "The Effects of Morphine on Venous Tone in Patients with Acute Pulmonary Edema." *Circulation* 54 (1976): 335–337.
17. Khandaker, M. H., R. E. Espinosa, R. A. Nishimura, et al. "Pericardial Disease: Diagnosis and Management." *Mayo Clin Proc* 85 (2010): 572–593.
18. Levy, P. D. and D. Cline. "Asymptomatic Hypertension in the Emergency Department: A Matter of Critical Public Health Importance." *Acad Emerg Med* (Nov 16, 2009): 1251–1257.
19. Kessler, C. S. and Y. Joudeh. "Evaluation and Treatment of Severe Asymptomatic Hypertension." *Am Fam Physician* 81 (2010): 470–476.
20. Chobanian, A. V., G. L. Bakris, H. R. Black, et al. "Seventh Report of the Joint National Committee on Prevention, Detection, Evaluation, and Treatment of High Blood Pressure." *Hypertension* 42 (2003): 1206–1252.
21. Barton, J. R. "Hypertension in Pregnancy." *Ann Emerg Med* 51 (2008): S16–S17.
22. Reynolds, H. R. and J. S. Hochman. "Cardiogenic Shock: Current Concepts and Improving Outcomes." *Circulation* 117 (2008): 686–697.
23. Weisfeldt, M. L. and L. B. Becker. "Resuscitation after Cardiac Arrest: A 3-Phase Time-Sensitive Model." *JAMA* 288 (2002): 3035–3038.
24. Vilke, G. M., T. C. Chan, J. V. Dunford, et al. "The Three-Phase Model of Cardiac Arrest as Applied to Ventricular Fibrillation in a Large, Urban Emergency Medical Services System." *Resuscitation* 64 (2005): 341–346.
25. Peberdy, M. A., C. W. Callaway, R. W. Neumar, et al. "Part 9: Post-Cardiac Arrest Care: 2010 American Heart Association Guidelines for Cardiopulmonary Resuscitation and Emergency Cardiovascular Care." *Circulation* 122 (2010): S768–S786.

26. Arrich, J., M. Holzer, H. Herkner, and M. Müllner. "Hypothermia for Neuroprotection in Adults after Cardiopulmonary Resuscitation." *Cochrane Database Syst Rev* (2009): CD004128.
27. Bernard, S. A., K. Smith, P. Cameron, et al. "Induction of Therapeutic Hypothermia by Paramedics after Resuscitation from Out-of-Hospital Ventricular Fibrillation Cardiac Arrest: A Randomized Controlled Trial." *Circulation* 122 (2010): 737–742.
28. Morrison, L. J., G. Kierzek, D. S. Diekema, et al. "Part 3: Ethics: 2010 American Heart Association Guidelines for Cardiopulmonary Resuscitation and Emergency Cardiovascular Care." *Circulation* 122 (2010): S665–S675.
29. Morrison, L. J., B. L. Bigham, A. Kiss, and P. R. Verbeek. "Termination of Resuscitation: A Guide to Interpreting the Literature." *Resuscitation* 79 (2008): 387–390.
30. Agnelli, G. and C. Becattini. "Acute Pulmonary Embolism." *N Engl J Med* 363 (2010): 266–274.
31. Achar, S. A., S. Kundu, and W. A. Norcross. "Diagnosis of Acute Coronary Syndrome." *Am Fam Physician* 72 (2005): 119–126.
32. Nable, J. V. and W. Brady. "The Evolution of Electrocardiographic Changes in ST-Segment Elevation Myocardial Infarction." *Am J Emerg Med* 27 (2009): 734–746.
33. Haji, S. A. and A. Movahed. "Right Ventricular Infarction—Diagnosis and Treatment." *Clin Cardiol* 23 (2000): 473–482.
34. Brady, W. J., B. Lentz, K. Barlotta, R. A. Harrigan, and T. Chan. "ECG Patterns Confounding the ECG Diagnosis of Acute Coronary Syndrome: Left Bundle Branch Block, Right Ventricular Paced Rhythms, and Left Ventricular Hypertrophy." *Emerg Med Clin North Am* 23 (2005): 999–1025.

Further Reading

Beasley, B. M. *Understanding 12-Lead EKGs: A Practical Approach.* 3rd ed. Hoboken, NJ: Pearson/Prentice Hall, 2013.

Beasley, B. M. *Understanding EKGs: A Practical Approach.* 4th ed. Hoboken, NJ: Pearson/Prentice Hall, 2014.

Bledsoe, B. E. and D. E. Clayden. *Prehospital Emergency Pharmacology.* 7th ed. Upper Saddle River, NJ: Pearson/Prentice Hall, 2012.

Ellis, K. M. *EKG: Plain and Simple.* 2nd ed. Upper Saddle River, NJ: Pearson/Prentice Hall, 2007.

Garcia, T. B. and N. E. Holtz. *12-Lead ECG: The Art of Interpretation.* 2nd ed. Burlington, MA: JB Learning, 2015.

Hall, J. E. *Textbook of Medical Physiology.* 13th ed. Philadelphia: W.B. Saunders, 2015.

Page, B. *12-Lead ECG for Acute and Critical Care Providers.* Upper Saddle River, NJ: Pearson/Prentice Hall, 2005.

Peacock, W. F. and B. R. Tiffany. *Cardiac Emergencies.* New York, NY: McGraw-Hill, 2006.

2015 American Heart Association Guidelines for Cardiopulmonary Resuscitation and Emergency Care, *Circulation* 132 supp. 2) 2015, October 15, 2015. Available at http://circ.ahajournals.org/content/132/18_suppl_2/S444.full.

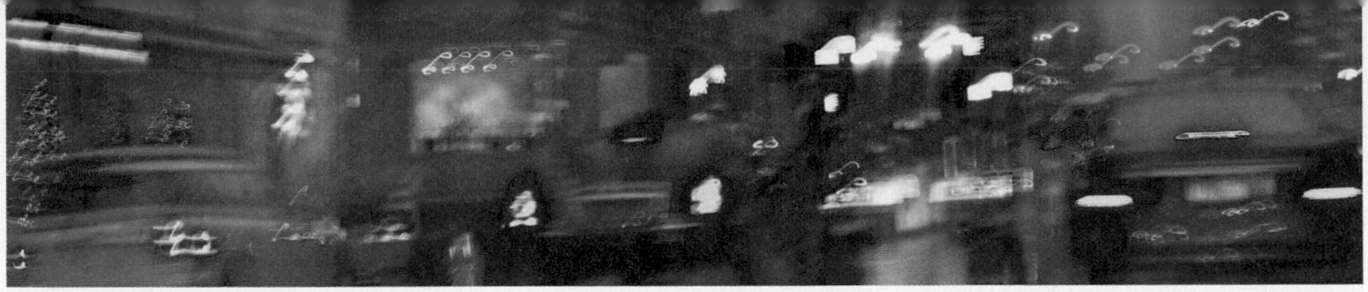

Chapter 3

Neurology

Bryan Bledsoe, DO, FACEP, FAAEM, EMT-P

STANDARD

Medicine (Neurology)

COMPETENCY

Integrates assessment findings with principles of epidemiology and pathophysiology to formulate a field impression and implement a comprehensive treatment/disposition plan for a patient with a medical complaint.

Learning Objectives

Terminal Performance Objective: After reading this chapter, you should be able to integrate patient assessment findings, patient history, and knowledge of anatomy, physiology, pathophysiology, and basic and advanced life support interventions to recognize and manage patients with neurologic disorders.

Enabling Objectives: To accomplish the terminal performance objective, you should be able to:

1. Define key terms introduced in this chapter.
2. Describe the epidemiology and demographics of neurologic disorders in the United States.
3. Review the anatomy and physiology of the nervous system.
4. Describe the general pathophysiological changes of nontraumatic neurologic emergencies, and relate this to disturbances in normal neurological physiology.
5. Adapt the scene size-up, primary assessment, history, secondary assessment, and use of monitoring technology to arrive at a field impression and differential diagnoses for neurologic emergencies.
6. Use a process of clinical reasoning to guide and interpret the patient assessment findings and develop a management plan for patients with neurologic disorders in the prehospital environment.
7. Differentiate between multiple causes of altered mental status.
8. List and describe the pathophysiology of various cardiovascular disorders commonly seen in the prehospital environment by the paramedic.
9. Given a variety of scenarios, discuss the integration of assessment and management guidelines as they relate to neurological emergencies.

KEY TERMS

absence seizure, p. 221
afferent, p. 203
Alzheimer's disease, p. 228
amyotrophic lateral sclerosis (ALS), p. 230
apneustic respiration, p. 209
arachnoid membrane, p. 200
ataxic respiration, p. 209
aura, p. 220
autonomic nervous system, p. 197
Bell's palsy, p. 225
brain abscess, p. 228
brainstem, p. 200
cauda equina syndrome, p. 232
central nervous system (CNS), p. 197
central neurogenic hyperventilation, p. 209
central pain syndrome, p. 230
cerebellum, p. 200
cerebrospinal fluid, p. 200
cerebrum, p. 200
Cheyne-Stokes respirations, p. 209
clonic phase, p. 220
coma, p. 206
complex partial seizure, p. 221
cranial nerves, p. 203
Creutzfeldt-Jakob disease (CJD), p. 228
Cushing's triad, p. 212
decerebrate posturing, p. 210
decorticate posturing, p. 210
degenerative neurologic disorders, p. 228
dermatomes, p. 203
diencephalon, p. 200
dura mater, p. 200
dystonias, p. 229
efferent, p. 203
generalized seizures, p. 220
Glasgow Coma Scale (GCS), p. 211
Guillain-Barré syndrome, p. 229
Huntington's disease, p. 228
Korsakoff's psychosis, p. 214
Kussmaul's respirations, p. 209
medulla oblongata, p. 200
meninges, p. 200
mesencephalon, p. 200
multiple sclerosis (MS), p. 229
muscular dystrophy (MD), p. 229
myoclonus, p. 230
neoplasm, p. 226
neuron, p. 198
neurotransmitter, p. 198
parasympathetic nervous system, p. 198
Parkinson's disease, p. 229
partial seizures, p. 220
peripheral nervous system (PNS), p. 197
peripheral neuropathy, p. 206
pia mater, p. 200
Pick's disease, p. 228
poliomyelitis (polio), p. 230
pons, p. 200
reticular activating system, p. 202
seizure, p. 220
simple partial seizure, p. 221
somatic nervous system, p. 197
spina bifida (SB), p. 230
status epilepticus, p. 222
stroke, p. 214
sympathetic nervous system, p. 198
syncope, p. 223
tonic phase, p. 220
tonic–clonic seizure, p. 220
transient ischemic attack (TIA), p. 217
Wernicke's syndrome, p. 214

Case Study

Paramedic Engine Company 201 and Ambulance 68 receive a call for a "possible stroke patient." Dispatch reports that the patient is a man in his 60s with reported right-sided weakness and inability to speak. He is being assisted by bystanders in the lobby of a local bank. The response time is approximately 3 minutes. On arrival, the bank manager leads paramedics Jack Tory and Linda Alvarez to a corner area of the lobby, where they see an elderly man sitting in a chair and being held upright by bystanders.

Jack and Linda quickly perform a primary assessment. Although he is unable to speak, the patient appears to be alert and cooperative. His airway is patent. His respiratory rate is 18 breaths per minute and regular. His pulse is 88 beats per minute and strong. The blood pressure is 160/90 mmHg taken in the left arm (because of the weakness in his right arm). The patient's skin is warm and dry, yet pale. The blood glucose level is 80 mg/dL. He has marked right-sided weakness but otherwise appears to be well nourished and in good overall health. Linda rates the patient's exam findings with the Cincinnati Prehospital Stroke Scale. The patient has right-sided arm weakness and drift, as well as slurred speech. Based on these findings, a stroke appears likely as the cause for the patient's symptoms.

Jack quickly provides supplemental oxygen while Linda obtains a more detailed medical history from the patient's family. Linda places a saline lock in the patient's left forearm while Jack places the ECG leads and turns on the monitor. The patient exhibits atrial fibrillation with a rate of 90. Linda applies the pulse oximeter. The patient appears well oxygenated, with a SpO_2 of 99 percent, and the supplemental oxygen is tapered to avoid hyperoxia. Jack and Linda move the patient to a stretcher, being careful to protect the paralyzed extremity. They load the patient into the ambulance and transport him to the nearest emergency department with a "stroke team."

On arrival at the emergency department, the patient's condition remains unchanged. His airway remains patent and his symptoms persist. A routine laboratory profile is normal. Because the patient has a hemiparesis and is unable to speak, the stroke team physician orders a computed tomography (CT) scan of the brain. A neuroradiologist reads the CT scan and reports no evidence of hemorrhage in the brain. An interventional neurologist is consulted and administers intravenous fibrinolytic therapy. The patient is then admitted to the neurologic intensive care unit.

Following fibrinolytic therapy, the patient recovers his speech, and most of his right-sided weakness is alleviated. Several days later, the patient is discharged to the rehabilitation unit.

Introduction

Nervous system conditions and diseases affect millions of lives in the United States. Strokes attack 795,000 people every year, of whom 150,000 die.[1] Epilepsy affects 3 million people, or approximately 1 percent of the U.S. population.[2] An additional 60,000 Americans are diagnosed with Parkinson's disease each year.[3] These are only a few examples of the impact of nervous system disorders. Millions of people are also affected by headache, multiple sclerosis, syncope, neoplasm, and other nervous system emergencies, all of which you will learn about in this chapter.

Many conditions, diseases, and injuries can cause nervous system disorders. Such disorders may be caused by internal or external factors. Modern advances and clinical studies continue to yield new medications and treatments for many conditions. Paramedics should maintain a solid knowledge of the nervous system and remain familiar with current trends and advancements in treating the neurologic patient.

This chapter provides an overview of the common neurologic conditions that may be encountered in the prehospital setting. It discusses the relevant anatomy and physiology of the nervous system, assessment techniques, and the recommended prehospital management.

Anatomy and Physiology

The nervous system is the body's principal control system. This network of cells, tissues, and organs regulates nearly all bodily functions via electrical impulses transmitted through nerves, all of which are highly susceptible to hypoxia. The endocrine system is closely related to the nervous system. It exerts bodily control via hormones. (You will learn more about this system in the "Endocrinology" chapter.) A third system, the circulatory system, assists in regulatory functions by distributing hormones and other chemical messengers.

The nervous system consists of two main divisions—the central nervous system and the peripheral nervous system. The **central nervous system (CNS)** consists of the brain and the spinal cord. **The peripheral nervous system (PNS)** is somewhat more complex. As you look at Figure 3-1, note that the peripheral nervous system is divided into two major subdivisions—the **somatic nervous system**, which governs voluntary functions (those we control consciously), and the **autonomic nervous system**, which has two subdivisions—the

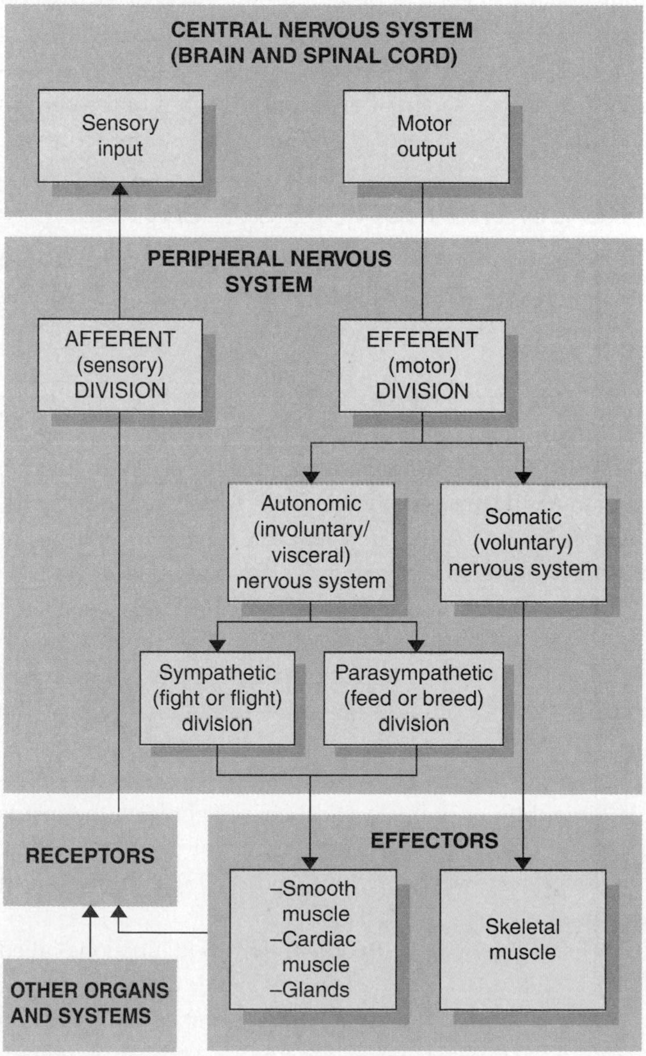

FIGURE 3-1 Overview of the nervous system.

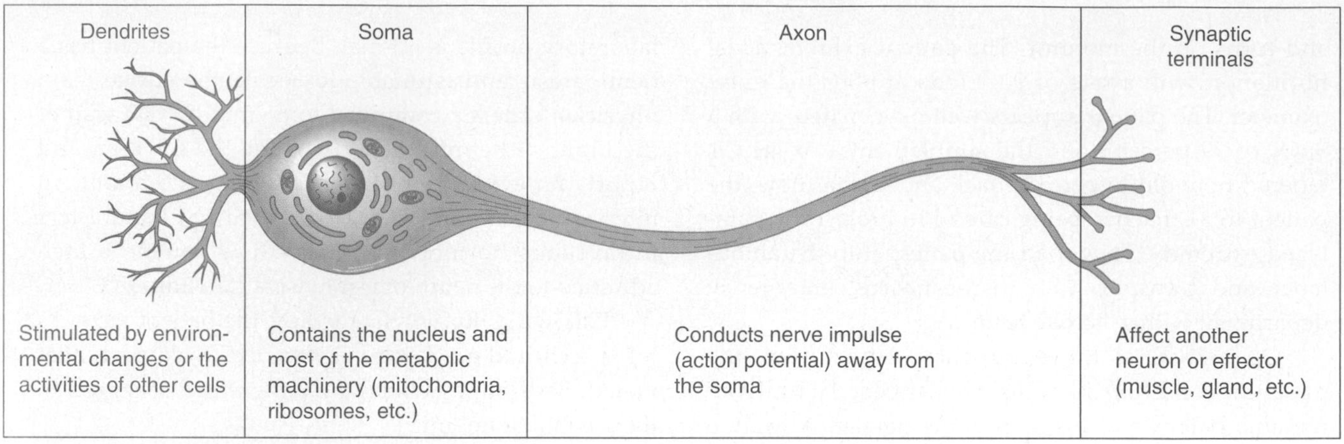

FIGURE 3-2 Anatomy of a neuron.

sympathetic nervous system and the **parasympathetic nervous system**. These two subdivisions of the autonomic nervous system work together to carry out involuntary physiologic processes such as regulation of blood pressure, heart rate, and digestion.

You will learn more about these divisions of the nervous system as you continue through this chapter. As you read, it will be helpful if you think of the nervous system as a "living computer." The central nervous system is the central processing unit and the various divisions of the peripheral nervous system carry on the input and output processes.

The Central Nervous System

Knowledge of the anatomy and physiology of the central nervous system is essential to understanding and treating nervous system emergencies.

Basic Unit—The Neuron

The fundamental unit of the nervous system is the nerve cell, or **neuron**. The neuron includes the *cell body* (soma), containing the nucleus; the *dendrites*, which transmit electrical impulses to the cell body; and the *axons*, which transmit electrical impulses away from the cell body (Figure 3-2).

The transmission of impulses in the nervous system resembles the conduction of electrical impulses through the heart. In its resting state, the neuron is positively charged on the outside and negatively charged on the inside. When electrically stimulated, sodium rapidly surges into the cell and potassium rapidly leaves it to eliminate the difference in electrical charge between the inside and the outside. This "depolarization," or loss of the charge difference, is subsequently transmitted down the neuron at an extremely high rate of speed.

The neuron joins with other neurons at junctions called *synapses* (Figure 3-3). The neurons never come into direct contact with one another at these synapses. Instead, on reaching the synapse, the axon causes the release of a chemical **neurotransmitter**. This neurotransmitter, either acetylcholine or norepinephrine, then crosses the gap between the axon of the depolarized neuron and the dendrite of the adjacent neuron. The neurotransmitter stimulates the postsynaptic membrane of the connecting nerve. Acetylcholine is the neurotransmitter of the parasympathetic and voluntary (somatic) nervous systems. Norepinephrine is found in the synaptic terminals of sympathetic nerves.

Protective Structures

Most of the central nervous system is protected by bony structures. The brain lies within the cranial vault, protected by the skull. Covered by the scalp, the cranium consists of the bones of the head, excluding the facial bones. Bones composing the cranium include two single bones—the frontal and occipital bones—and a series of paired bones—the parietals, temporals, sphenoids, and ethmoids (Figure 3-4).

A total of 33 bones constitute the spine. They include 7 cervical vertebrae, 12 thoracic vertebrae, 5 lumbar vertebrae, 5 sacral vertebrae, and 4 coccygeal vertebrae. The spinal cord is housed inside and is protected by the "spinal canal" formed by these bones (Figure 3-5).

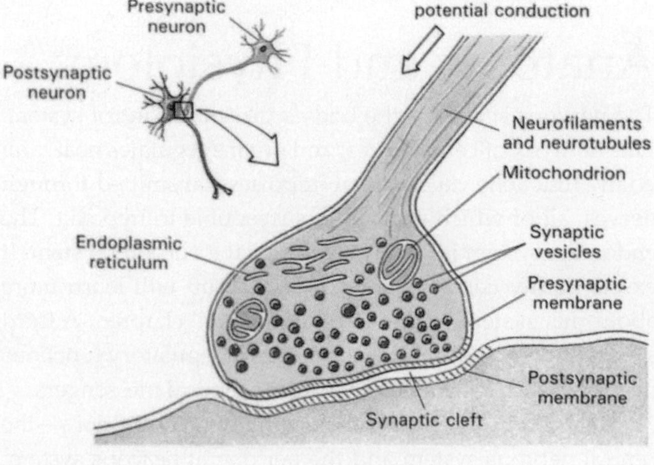

FIGURE 3-3 The synapse.

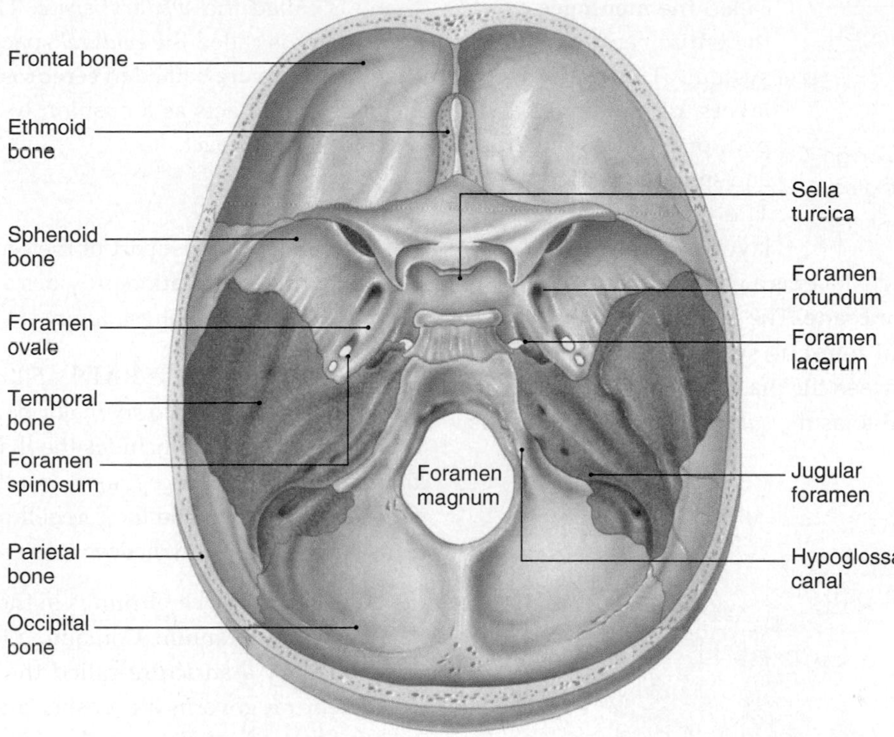

FIGURE 3-4a The bones of the skull (cross section).

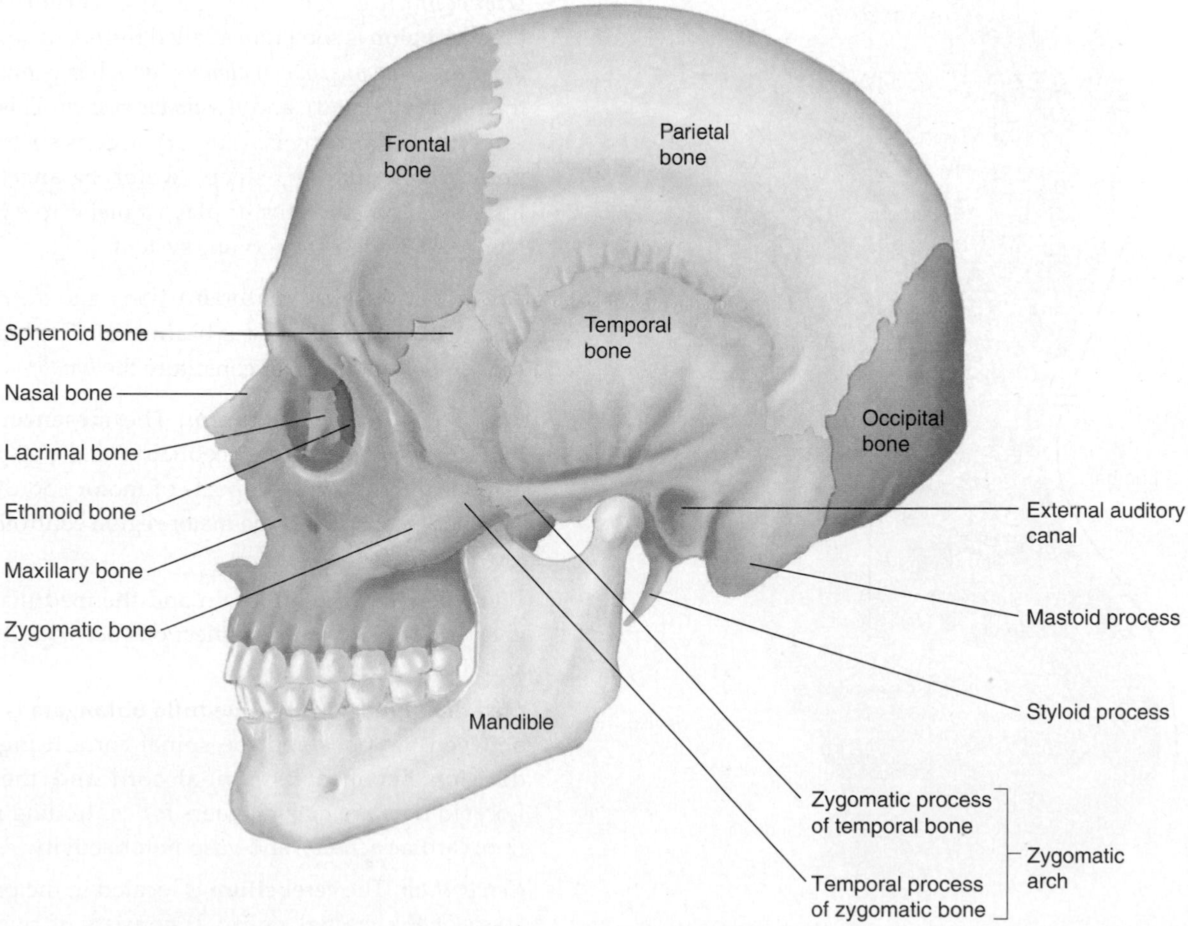

FIGURE 3-4b The bones of the skull (profile).

CONTENT REVIEW
- ➤ Central Nervous System
  - Brain
  - Spinal cord
- ➤ An alteration in mental status is the hallmark sign of central nervous system (CNS) injury or illness.

Protective membranes called the **meninges** cover the entire central nervous system. There are three layers of meninges that pad, or cushion, the brain and spinal cord (Figure 3-6). The durable, outermost layer is referred to as the **dura mater**. The middle layer is a weblike structure known as the **arachnoid membrane**. The innermost layer, directly overlying the central nervous system, is called the **pia mater**. The space between the pia mater and the arachnoid membrane is referred to as the *subarachnoid space*, whereas the space between the dura mater and the arachnoid membrane is called the *subdural space*. The space outside the dura mater is called the *epidural* space. Both the brain and the spinal cord are bathed in **cerebrospinal fluid**, a watery, clear fluid that acts as a cushion to protect these organs from physical impact.

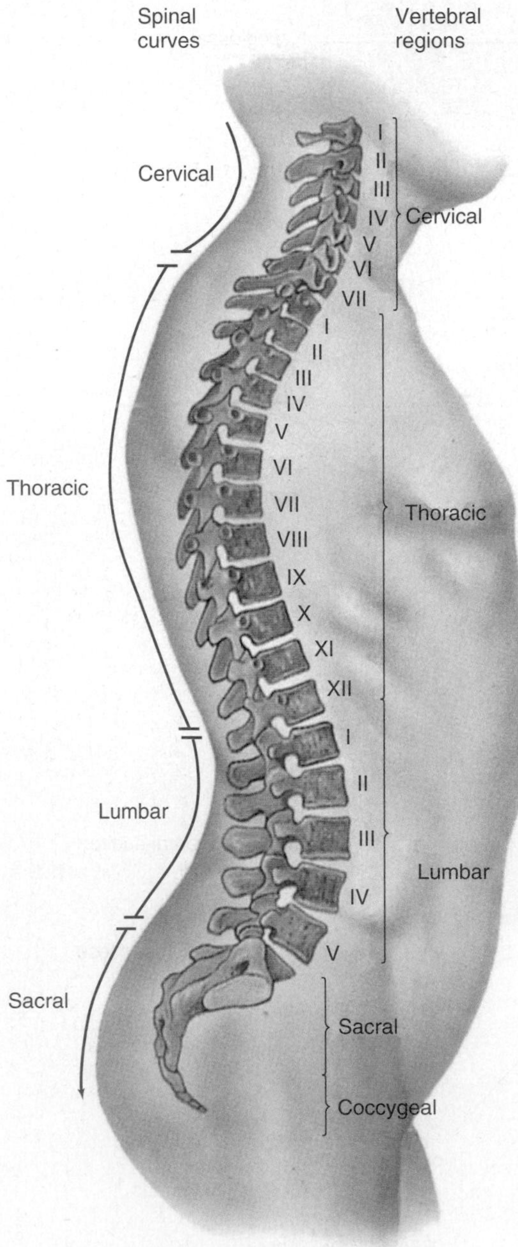

FIGURE 3-5 The vertebral column.

The Brain

The brain is the largest part of the central nervous system. The following information provides a general profile of the brain's anatomy and physiology.

DIVISIONS OF THE BRAIN Filling the cranial vault, the brain is divided into six major parts: the cerebrum, the diencephalon (which includes the thalamus and the hypothalamus), the mesencephalon (midbrain), the pons, the medulla oblongata, and the cerebellum (Figure 3-7).

The cerebrum and diencephalon constitute the *forebrain*:

- ***Cerebrum.*** The **cerebrum** is in the anterior and middle area of the cranium. Containing two hemispheres, it is joined by a structure called the *corpus callosum*. The cerebrum governs all sensory and motor actions. It is the seat of intelligence, learning, analysis, memory, and language. The *cerebral cortex* is the outermost layer of the cerebrum.
- ***Diencephalon.*** Covered by the cerebrum, the **diencephalon** is sometimes called the *interbrain*. Inside it are the *thalamus*, *hypothalamus* (which is connected to the pituitary gland), and the *limbic system*. This area is responsible for many involuntary actions such as temperature regulation, sleep, water balance, stress response, and emotions. It plays a major role in regulating the autonomic nervous system.

The mesencephalon (midbrain), pons, and the medulla oblongata collectively form the **brainstem**. The brainstem and the cerebellum together constitute the *hindbrain:*

- ***Mesencephalon, or midbrain.*** The **mesencephalon**, located between the diencephalon and the pons, is responsible for certain aspects of motor coordination. The mesencephalon is the major region controlling eye movement.
- ***Pons.*** Between the midbrain and the medulla oblongata, the **pons** contains connections between the brain and the spinal cord.
- ***Medulla oblongata.*** The **medulla oblongata** is located between the pons and the spinal cord. It marks the division between the spinal cord and the brain. Located here are major centers for controlling respiration, cardiac activity, and vasomotor activity.
- ***Cerebellum.*** The **cerebellum** is located in the posterior fossa of the cranial cavity. It consists of two hemispheres closely related to the brainstem and higher

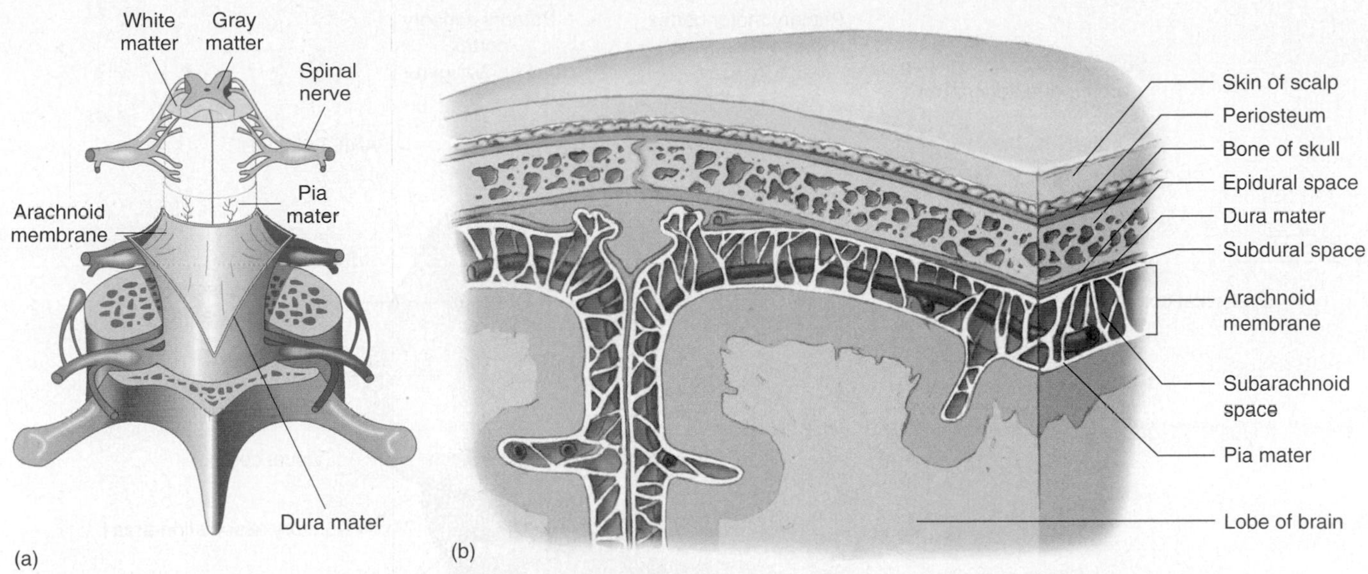

FIGURE 3-6 The meninges: (a) posterior view of the spinal cord showing the meningeal layers; (b) the meninges of the brain.

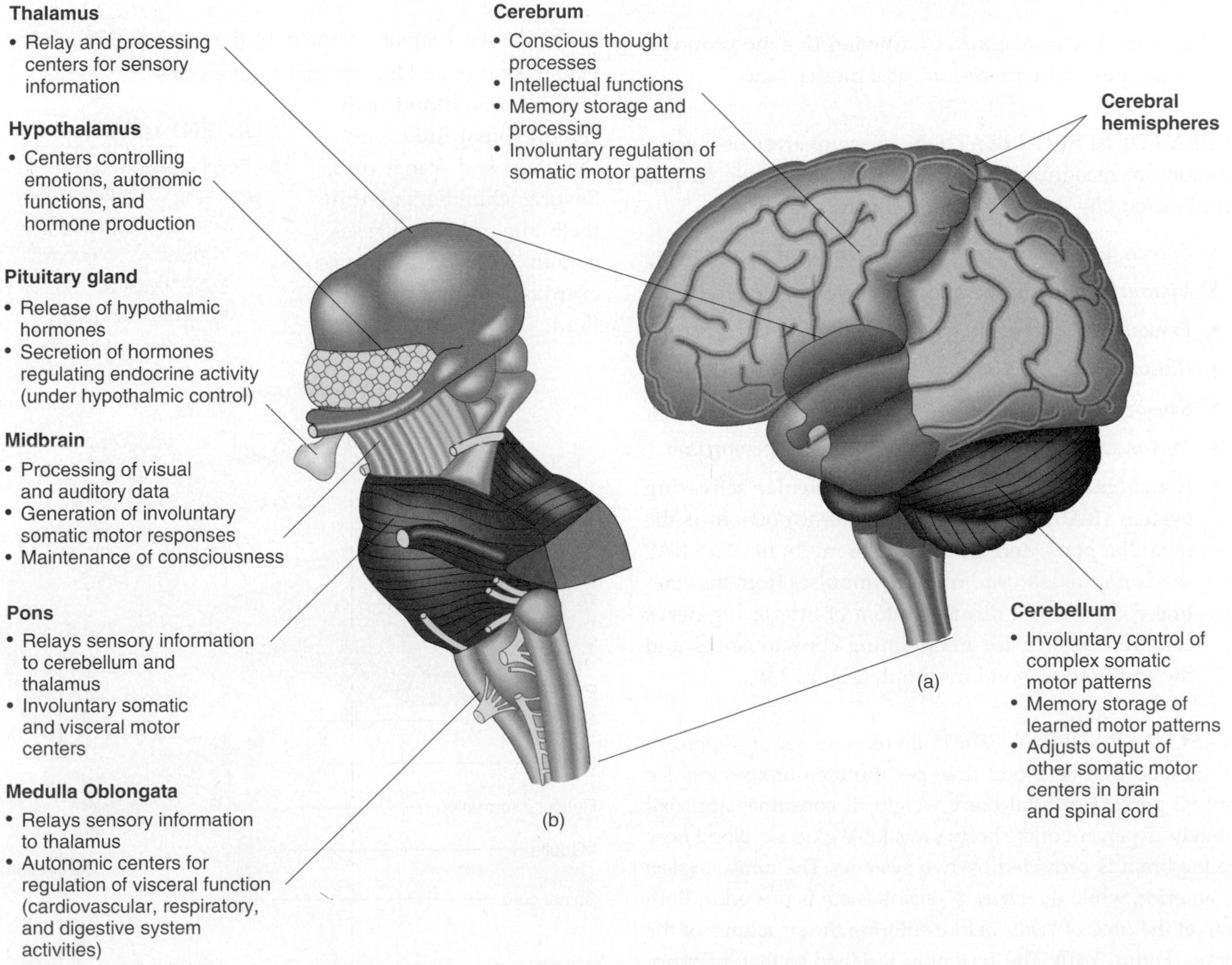

FIGURE 3-7 The human brain: (a) superficial view of the brain; (b) components of the brainstem.

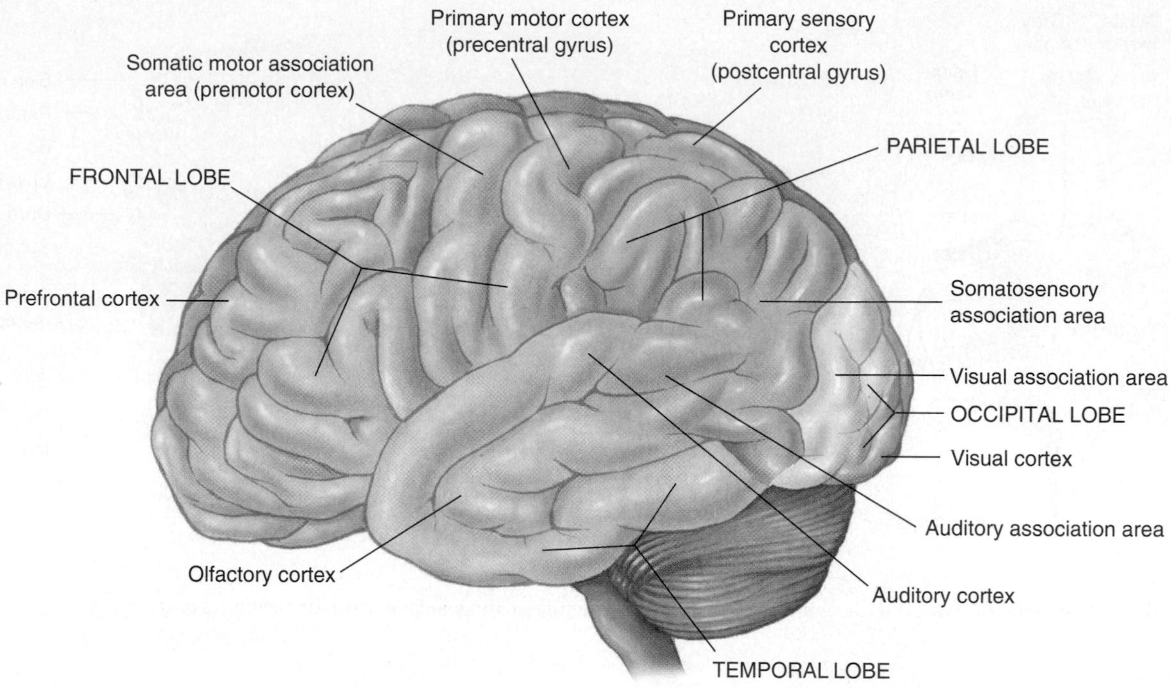

FIGURE 3-8 External anatomy of the brain.

centers. The cerebellum coordinates fine motor movement, posture, equilibrium, and muscle tone.

AREAS OF SPECIALIZATION Several areas of specialization are recognized within the brain and have clinical application (Figure 3-8). These include:

- ***Speech.*** Located in the temporal lobe of the cerebrum.
- ***Vision.*** Located in the occipital cortex of the cerebrum.
- ***Personality.*** Located in the frontal lobes of the cerebrum.
- ***Balance and coordination.*** Located in the cerebellum.
- ***Sensory.*** Located in the parietal lobes of the cerebrum.
- ***Motor.*** Located in the frontal lobes of the cerebrum.
- ***Reticular activating system.*** The **reticular activating system (RAS)** operates in the lateral portion of the medulla, pons, and especially the midbrain. The RAS sends impulses to and receives impulses from the cerebral cortex. It is a diffuse system of interlacing nerve cells responsible for maintaining consciousness and the ability to respond to stimuli (Figure 3-9).

VASCULAR SUPPLY The brain receives about 20 percent of the body's total blood flow per minute but accounts for only 2 percent of total body weight. It consumes approximately 25 percent of the body's available glucose. Blood flow to the brain is provided by two systems. The *carotid system* is anterior, while the *vertebrobasilar* system is posterior. Both join at the *circle of Willis* before entering the structures of the brain (Figure 3-10). The system is designed so that interruption of any part will not cause significant loss of blood flow to the tissues. Venous drainage of the brain is through the venous sinuses and the internal jugular veins.

Besides blood flow, cerebrospinal fluid bathes the brain and spinal cord. Several chambers within the brain, called ventricles, contain most of the intracranial volume of this fluid.

CONTENT REVIEW

- ➤ Peripheral Nervous System
  - Voluntary (somatic)
  - Involuntary (autonomic)
    - Sympathetic
    - Parasympathetic

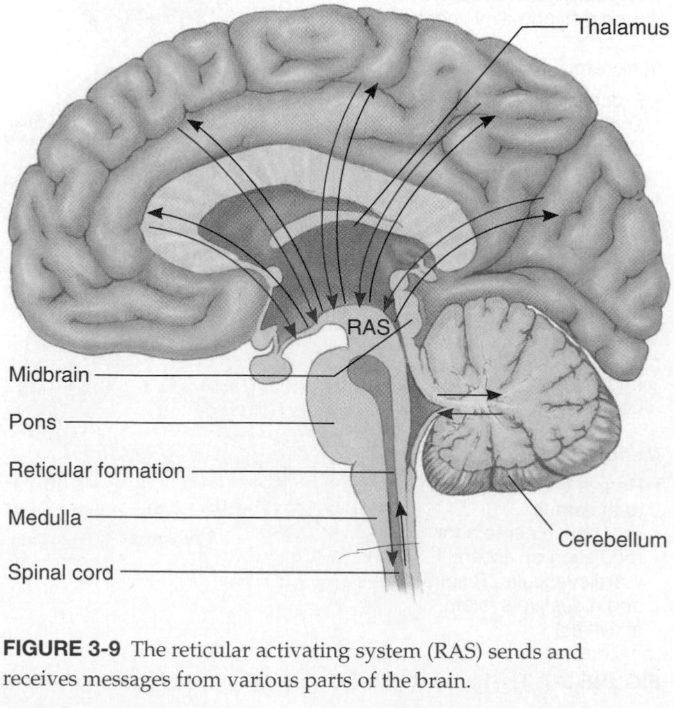

FIGURE 3-9 The reticular activating system (RAS) sends and receives messages from various parts of the brain.

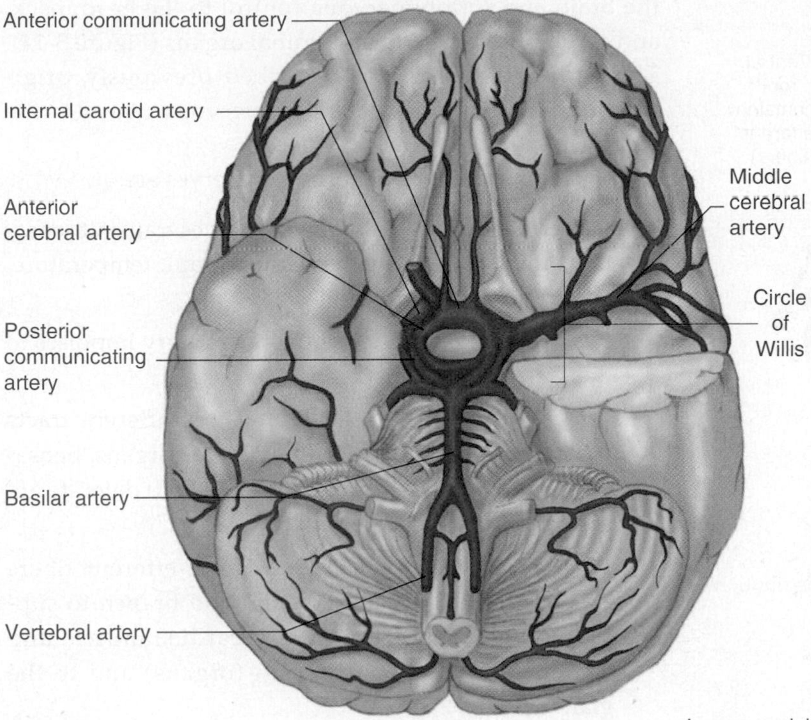

FIGURE 3-10 An inferior view of the brain showing the circle of Willis, which is formed by the anterior and posterior communicating arteries.

The Spinal Cord

The spinal cord is 17 to 18 inches long in the average adult. It leaves the brain at the medulla and proceeds, through an opening called the *foramen magnum*, down the spinal canal. The spinal cord, ending near the level of the first lumbar vertebra, is responsible for conducting impulses to and from the peripheral nervous system and for reflexes.

Thirty-one pairs of nerve fibers exit the spinal cord as it descends and enters the peripheral nervous system (Figure 3-11). The dorsal roots contain afferent fibers, and the ventral roots contain efferent fibers. **Afferent** (sensory) fibers transmit impulses to the central nervous system from the body. **Efferent** (motor) fibers carry impulses from the central nervous system to the body (Figure 3-12). Each nerve root has a corresponding area of the skin, called a **dermatome**, to which it supplies sensation (Figure 3-13). Sensory deficits in a dermatomal distribution can indicate the level of a spinal cord problem. Spinal cord injury can result in damage to afferent or efferent pathways, or both. The nearer to the brainstem, the more serious the effects are likely to be.

Reflexes are protective. If a peripheral sensory nerve senses harm, such as intense heat, it sends an impulse to the spinal cord. The spinal cord then stimulates the appropriate muscles to remove the part of the body closest to the perceived threat. This process saves time, as impulses do not have to go to the brain for processing. Because they are mediated in the spinal cord, reflex actions lack fine motor control.

The Peripheral Nervous System

Consisting of the cranial and the peripheral nerves, the peripheral nervous system has both voluntary and involuntary components. The 12 pairs of **cranial nerves** originate in

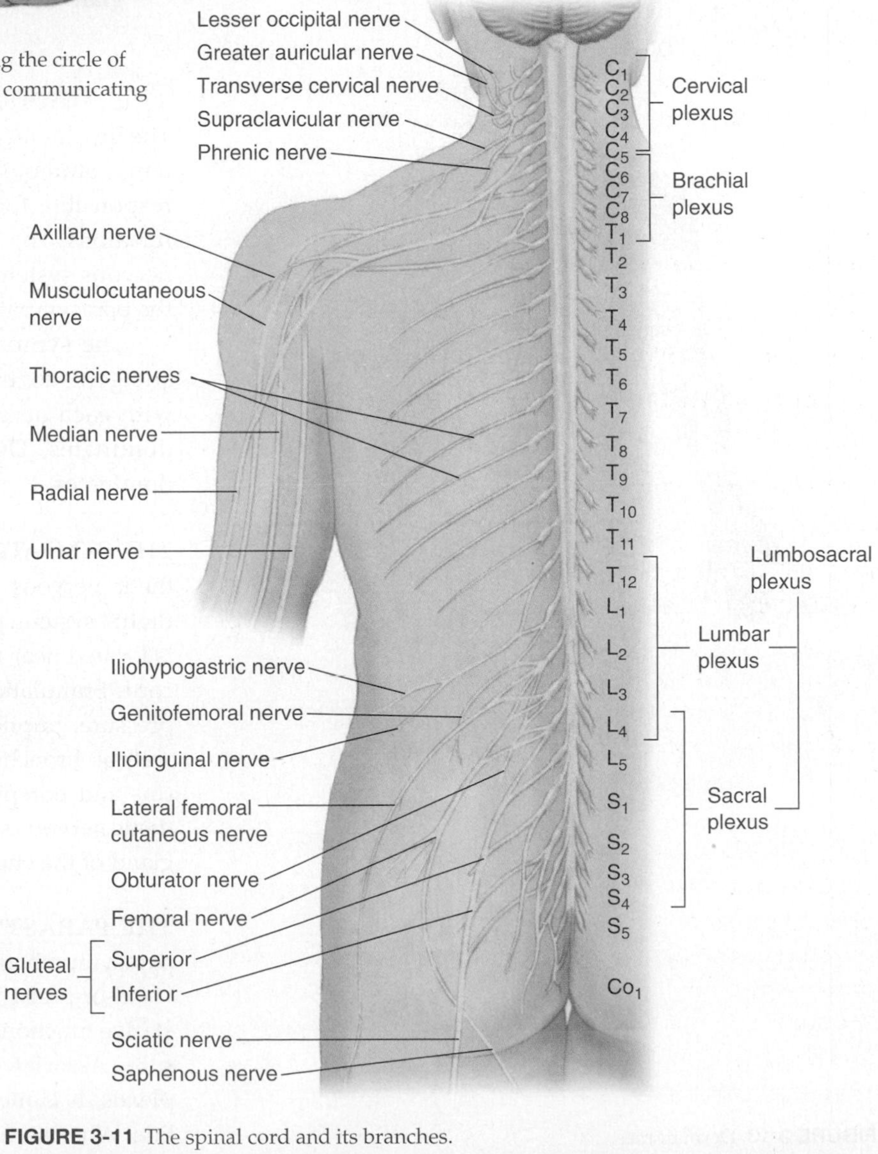

FIGURE 3-11 The spinal cord and its branches.

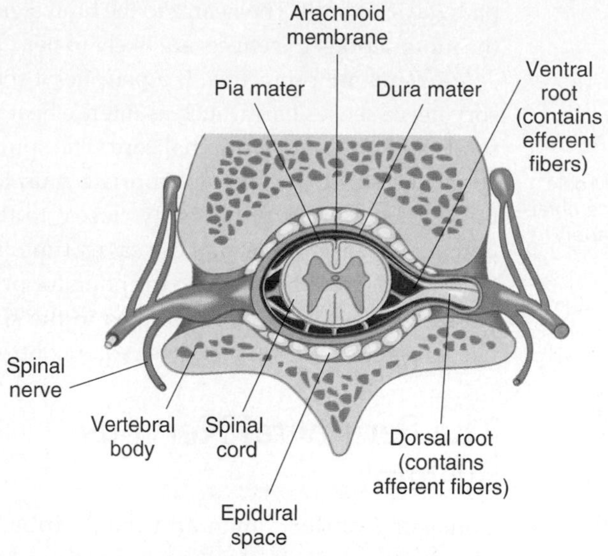

FIGURE 3-12 Sectional view of the spinal cord showing distribution of spinal nerves.

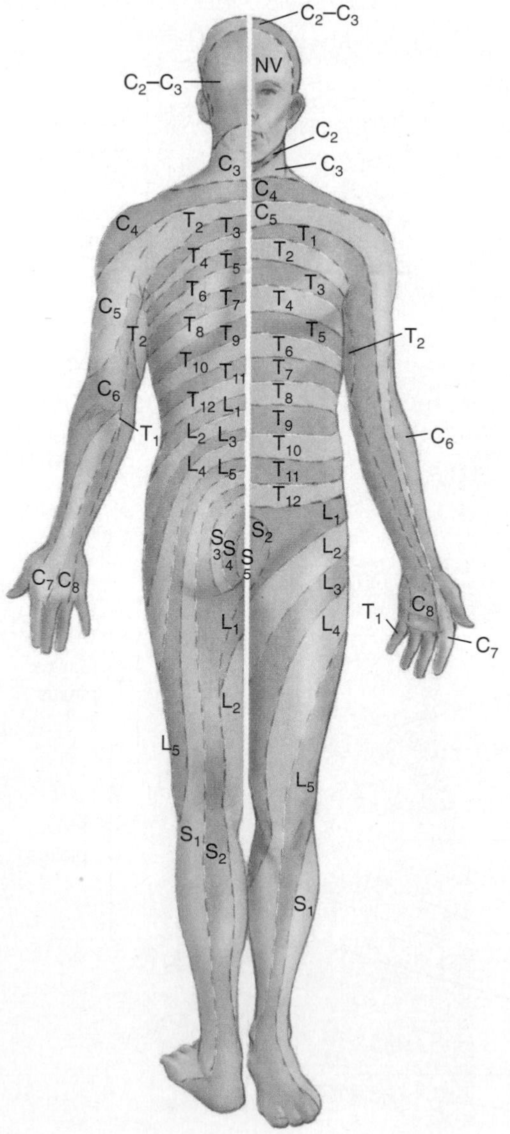

FIGURE 3-13 Dermatomes.

the brain and supply nervous control to the head, neck, and certain thoracic and abdominal organs (Figure 3-14). The peripheral nerves, as described previously, originate in the spinal cord and supply nervous control to the periphery.

The four categories of peripheral nerves are:

- ***Somatic sensory.*** These afferent nerves transmit sensations involved in touch, pressure, pain, temperature, and position (proprioception).
- ***Somatic motor.*** These efferent fibers carry impulses to the skeletal (voluntary) muscles.
- ***Visceral (autonomic) sensory.*** These afferent tracts transmit sensations from the visceral organs. Sensations such as a full bladder or the need to defecate are mediated by visceral sensory fibers.
- ***Visceral (autonomic) motor.*** These efferent fibers exit the central nervous system and branch to supply nerves to the involuntary cardiac muscle and smooth muscle of the viscera (organs) and to the glands.

The Autonomic Nervous System

The involuntary component of the peripheral nervous system, commonly called the *autonomic nervous system,* is responsible for the unconscious control of many body functions. The two functional divisions of the autonomic nervous system are the sympathetic nervous system and the parasympathetic nervous system.

The sympathetic and parasympathetic systems are antagonistic. In their normal state, they exist in balance with each other. During stress, the sympathetic system dominates. During rest, the parasympathetic system dominates.

THE SYMPATHETIC NERVOUS SYSTEM The sympathetic nervous system, often referred to as the "fight-or-flight" system, prepares the body for stressful situations. It is located near the thoracic and lumbar parts of the spinal cord. Stimulation causes increased heart rate and blood pressure, pupillary dilation, a rise in the blood sugar, as well as bronchodilation. The neurotransmitters epinephrine and norepinephrine mediate its actions. The sympathetic nervous system is closely associated with the adrenal gland of the endocrine system.

THE PARASYMPATHETIC NERVOUS SYSTEM The parasympathetic nervous system, sometimes called the "feed-or-breed" system, is responsible for controlling vegetative functions, such as normal heart rate and blood pressure. Associated with the cranial nerves and the sacral plexus, it is mediated by the neurotransmitter acetylcholine. When stimulated, it causes a decrease in heart rate, an

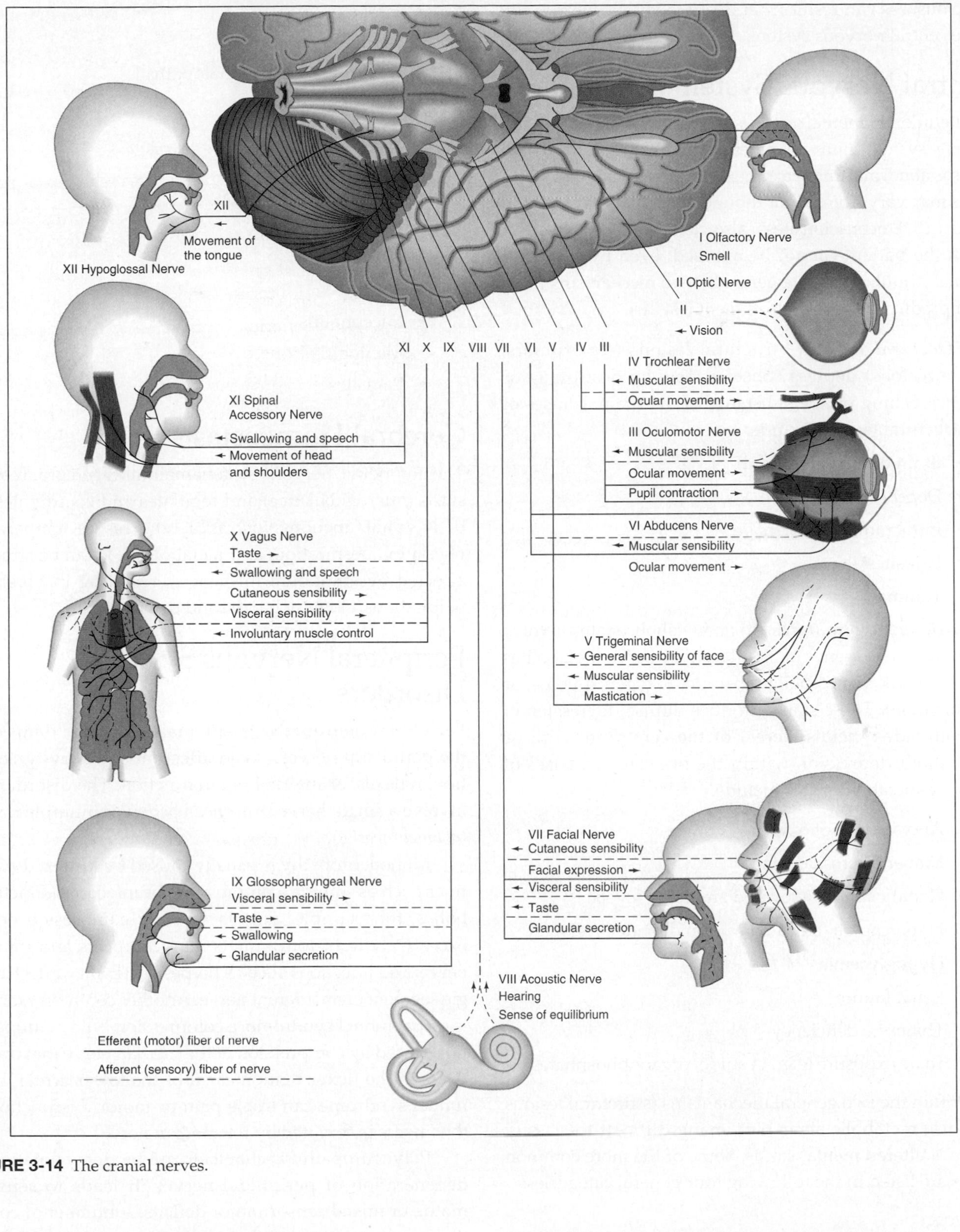

FIGURE 3-14 The cranial nerves.

increase in digestive activity, pupillary constriction, and a reduction in blood glucose.

Pathophysiology

A firm grasp of the pathophysiology of nontraumatic neurologic emergencies is essential for the paramedic to provide appropriate and timely emergency care.

Alteration in Cognitive Systems

Consciousness is a condition in which an individual is fully responsive to stimuli and demonstrates awareness of the environment. The ability to respond to stimuli is dependent on an intact reticular activating system. Cognition and the ability to respond to the environment rely on an intact cerebral cortex. Therefore, altered forms of consciousness can result from dysfunction or interruption of the central nervous system.

Central Nervous System Disorders

An alteration in mental status is the hallmark sign of central nervous system injury or illness. Any alteration in mental status is abnormal and warrants further examination. Alterations may vary from minor thought disturbances to unconsciousness. Unconsciousness, also called **coma**, is a state in which the patient cannot be aroused, even by powerful external stimuli. There are generally two mechanisms capable of producing alterations in mental status:

- ***Structural lesions.*** Structural lesions (e.g., tumors, contusions) depress consciousness by destroying or encroaching on the substance of the brain. Causes of structural lesions include:
  - Brain tumor (neoplasm)
  - Degenerative disease
  - Intracranial hemorrhage
  - Parasites
  - Trauma
- ***Toxic-metabolic states.*** Toxic-metabolic states involve either the presence of circulating toxins or metabolites or the lack of metabolic substrates (oxygen, glucose, or thiamine). These states produce diffuse depression of both sides (hemispheres) of the cerebrum, with or without depression within the brainstem. Causes of toxic-metabolic states include:
  - Anoxia (lack of oxygen)
  - Diabetic ketoacidosis
  - Hepatic failure (elevated ammonia levels)
  - Hypercapnia (elevated carbon dioxide levels)
  - Hypoglycemia
  - Renal failure
  - Thiamine deficiency
  - Toxic exposure (e.g., cyanide, organophosphates)

Within the two general mechanisms (structural lesions and toxic-metabolic states) are many difficult-to-classify causes of altered mental status. Some of the more common causes are listed in the following four general categories:

- Drugs
  - Depressants (including alcohol)
  - Hallucinogens
  - Narcotics
- Cardiovascular
  - Anaphylaxis
  - Cardiac arrest
  - Stroke
  - Arrhythmias
  - Hypertensive encephalopathy
  - Shock
- Respiratory
  - COPD
  - Inhalation of toxic gas
  - Hypoxia
- Infectious
  - AIDS
  - Encephalitis
  - Meningitis
  - Parasites

Cerebral Homeostasis

The autonomic nervous system maintains cerebral homeostasis (internal balance) and regulates and coordinates the body's vital functions, such as blood pressure, temperature regulation, respiration, and metabolism. It can be strongly affected by emotional influences, resulting in blushing, palpitations, clammy hands, and dry mouth.

Peripheral Nervous System Disorders

Peripheral neuropathy is any malfunction or damage of the peripheral nerves. It can affect muscle activity, sensation, reflexes, or internal organ function. The disorder can involve a single nerve (*mononeuropathy*) or multiple nerves (*polyneuropathy*).

Mononeuropathy is usually caused by localized conditions such as trauma, compression, or infections. Fractured bones, for example, may lacerate or compress a nerve; excessively tight tourniquets may compress and injure a nerve; and infections such as herpes zoster may affect a single segment of an afferent nerve. Another common example is carpal tunnel syndrome, a compression-type neuropathy. It is caused by compression of the median nerve that travels through the flexor tendon canal of the lower arm. Carpal tunnel syndrome can cause pain or motor dysfunction in the fingers innervated by the median nerve.

Polyneuropathy is characterized by demyelination or degeneration of peripheral nerves. It leads to sensory, motor, or mixed sensorimotor deficits. A number of conditions, such as immune disorders, toxic agents, and metabolic disorders, are known causes of polyneuropathy. One example of a polyneuropathy is Guillain-Barré syndrome, which is characterized by rapidly worsening muscle weakness of the limbs that can sometimes lead to paralysis. Diabetes is one of the major causes of peripheral neuropathy. It usually affects the distal nerves of the hands and feet in the classic "stocking and glove" distribution.

Autonomic Nervous System Disorders

Disorders affecting the ANS are frequently a result of another condition. Because the control of the body's internal environment is vested in the ANS, most conditions that affect the integrity of an individual are accompanied by some changes in autonomic nervous system functioning.

General Assessment Findings

Assessment of the neurologic system is often difficult. Many of the signs and symptoms of nervous system dysfunction are subtle. As you conduct the scene size-up and begin the primary assessment, form a general impression of the patient and evaluate mental status before assessing the ABCs. If your primary assessment causes you to suspect nervous system dysfunction, this will prompt you to place particular emphasis on the neurologic examination during the secondary assessment.

Scene Size-Up and Primary Assessment

A great deal of crucial information can be obtained while approaching the patient. Size up the scene and the surroundings, as well as the patient, to form a general impression. Is there evidence of toxic exposure or trauma? Look for clues that can indicate a patient's condition, such as:

- *General Appearance*
  - Is the patient conscious?
  - Alert?
  - Confused?
  - Sitting upright?
- *Speech*
  - Can the patient speak?
  - Clear and coherent?
  - Full sentences?
  - Slurred speech?
- *Skin*
  - Color (pink, pale, cyanotic?)
  - Temperature (warm, hot, cool?)
  - Moisture (diaphoretic, clammy?)
  - Facial drooping present?
- *Posture/Gait*
  - Upright?
  - Leaning?
  - Staggered?
  - Steady gait?

Next, quickly check the patient's mental status through the "AVPU" method.

- *A* = The patient is alert and aware of his surroundings. A patient who is alert and oriented to person, place, and time is said to be "alert and oriented times three." Remember, no patient is "oriented" unless he has answered the questions that the paramedic has to ask.
- *V* = The patient responds to verbal stimuli. The patient responds when talked to, perhaps in a loud voice. Note if the patient delivers the answers normally or sluggishly. Also observe whether the patient has purposeful or uncoordinated movements.
- *P* = The patient responds to painful stimuli. The patient responds when tactile stimulation is used, such as a sternal rub, a squeeze of the trapezius muscle, or pinching the thenar (thumb) web space.
- *U* = The patient is unresponsive. The patient is not alert and does not respond to verbal or painful stimuli.

Assessment of cerebral functioning also includes assessing the patient's emotional status. If the patient is conscious, you can detect changes in the following:

- *Mood*
  - Is the patient's affect natural or is the patient irritable, anxious, or apathetic?
  - Does the patient appear depressed? manic? happy? solemn? reserved?
- *Thought*
  - What is the patient's thought pattern? Is it logical? appropriate? scattered?
- *Perception*
  - How does the patient perceive his surroundings? Are his interactions appropriate?
- *Judgment*
  - Is the patient using reasonable and sound judgment? Is he logical?
- *Memory and Attention*
  - Is short-term memory present? long-term memory? Question family members or caregivers to obtain this information.
  - Does the patient maintain conversation? pay attention? repeatedly ask or answer questions?

Any alteration from the patient's normal mental status or mood should be considered significant and warrants additional assessment.

Once a patient's level of consciousness has been determined, place the greatest emphasis on maintenance of the airway. If the patient is unconscious, assume that a cervical spine injury exists and treat it appropriately. Use the modified jaw-thrust maneuver to open the airway. Once the airway has been opened, insert the appropriate airway adjunct. In unresponsive patients, the tongue may be occluding the airway. In such cases, you may need only to place an oropharyngeal or nasopharyngeal airway to maintain patency. If the patient tolerates an oropharyngeal airway, consider intubation.

Vigilantly monitor the airway in any patient with central nervous system injury. It is essential to observe for respiratory arrest that can result from increased intracranial pressure. Remain alert for an absent gag reflex and vomiting. In addition, blood from facial injuries and possible aspiration of gastric contents further threaten the patient's airway.

Observe the patient for any signs and symptoms of inadequate or impaired breathing or the presence of any abnormal respiratory patterns. Remember, the body's "breathing center" is located in the brain. Certain neurologic conditions can cause these areas to malfunction and limit the patient's ability to breathe.

Complete assessment of the body's circulatory status is also a crucial part of the primary assessment. Evaluation of the heart rate, rhythm, and ECG pattern can shed light on the body's overall state of perfusion. Observe the patient's skin color, temperature, and moisture for abnormal findings such as cyanosis and moisture. A healthy adult's skin is usually warm, dry, and pink.

Secondary Assessment

Following completion of the primary assessment and correction of any immediate threats to the patient's life, turn your attention to the secondary assessment. This assessment should include an accurate history and a physical exam, including vital signs. Remember that any indications of nervous system dysfunction should cause you to place particular emphasis on neurologic evaluation. Neurologic evaluation is detailed under "Nervous System Status" later in this chapter.

History

A thorough, accurate history of a patient is crucial in determining the current problem and subsequent treatment of a patient. One of the first steps in obtaining a thorough history involves attempting to determine whether the neurologic problem is traumatic or medical. Clarification will help determine the plan for subsequent prehospital treatment. The initial history may not be easy to obtain because of the patient's altered mental status. In these cases, it is critical for you to obtain information from family, friends, or other bystanders, if available.

If the neurologic emergency is due to trauma, ask the following questions:

- When did the incident occur?
- How did the incident occur, or what is the mechanism of injury?
- Was there any loss of consciousness?
- Was there evidence of incontinence? (Incontinence suggests loss of consciousness.)
- What is the patient's chief complaint?
- Has there been any change in symptoms?
- Are there any complicating factors?

If there is no evidence of a traumatic cause of the neurologic emergency, ask the following questions to determine the nature of the illness:

- What is the chief complaint?
- What are the details of the present illness, or the nature of the illness?
- Is there a pertinent underlying medical problem such as:
  - Cardiac disease
  - Chronic seizures
  - Diabetes
  - Hypertension
- Have these symptoms occurred before?
- Are there any environmental clues? These may include:
  - Evidence of current medications
  - Medic-Alert identification
  - Alcohol bottles or drug paraphernalia
  - Chemicals, hazardous materials

Physical Examination

The physical examination of a patient with a neurologic emergency should include the standard head-to-toe examination and a more detailed neurologic assessment. Pay particular attention to the pupils, respiratory status, and spinal evaluation.

FACE A patient's ability to smile, frown, and wrinkle his forehead indicates an intact facial nerve (cranial nerve VII). If the patient is conscious, test these abilities. Note any drooping or facial paralysis.

EYES The pupils are controlled by the oculomotor nerve (cranial nerve III). This nerve follows a long course through the skull and is easily compressed by brain swelling. Although slight pupillary inequality is normal, abnormal pupils can be an early indicator of increasing intracranial pressure. If both pupils are dilated and do not react to light, the patient probably has a brainstem injury or has suffered serious brain anoxia. If the pupils are dilated but still react to light, the injury may be reversible. However, the patient must be transported quickly to an emergency facility capable of treating central nervous system injuries. A unilaterally dilated pupil that remains reactive to light may be the earliest sign of increasing intracranial pressure. The patient with altered mental status who presents with or develops a unilaterally dilated pupil is in the "immediate transport" category. Constricted, or pinpoint, pupils suggest a toxic etiology for the altered mental status.

A common method of assessing extraocular movement is to have the patient follow finger movements. For example, ask the patient to follow your finger to the extreme left, then up, then down. Repeat the same motions to the extreme right. These positions are referred to as the *cardinal positions of gaze.* Because extraocular movements are controlled by cranial nerves III (oculomotor), IV (trochlear), and VI (abducens), inability to look in all directions with both eyes can be an early indication of a central nervous system problem. This is particularly important in the indication of facial trauma.

When examining a patient's pupils, it is important to check for contact lenses. Contact lenses, if present, should be removed and placed into their container or a saline solution and transported with the patient.

NOSE/MOUTH In the presence of facial paralysis, drooping of the patient's mouth may occur. Pay particular attention to any of these changes that may potentially compromise the patient's airway. A common way to assess for mouth droop is to ask the patient to smile. Also, ask the patient to "show your teeth." Both maneuvers will help determine whether there is any degree of facial drooping.

RESPIRATORY STATUS Respiratory derangement can occur with CNS illness or injury. Any of five abnormal respiratory patterns may commonly be observed (Figure 3-15):

- **Cheyne-Stokes respirations**. A breathing pattern characterized by a period of apnea lasting 10 to 60 seconds, followed by gradually increasing depth and frequency of respirations.
- **Kussmaul's respirations**. Rapid, deep respirations caused by severe metabolic and CNS problems.
- **Central neurogenic hyperventilation**. Hyperventilation caused by a lesion in the central nervous system, often characterized by rapid, deep, noisy respirations.
- **Ataxic respiration**. Poor respirations due to CNS damage, causing ineffective thoracic muscular coordination.
- **Apneustic respiration**. Breathing characterized by prolonged inspiration unrelieved by expiration attempts. This is seen in patients with damage to the upper part of the pons.

Several other respiratory patterns are also possible, depending on the injury. A patient's respirations can be affected by so many factors—fear, hysteria, chest injuries,

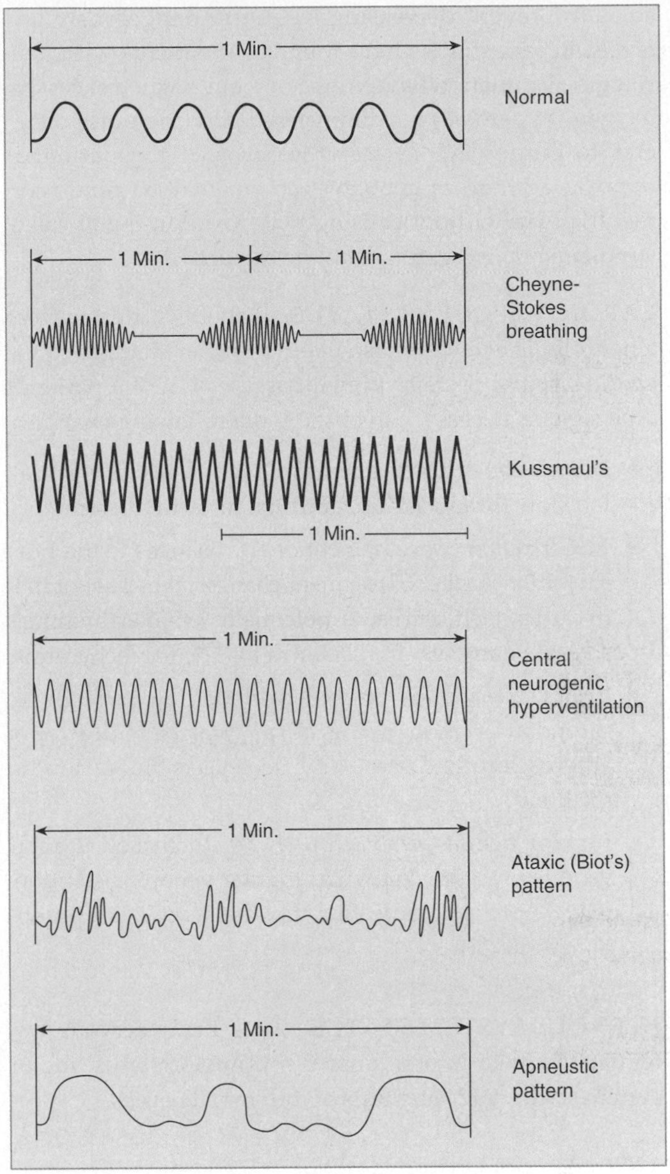

FIGURE 3-15 Respiratory patterns seen with CNS dysfunction.

spinal cord injuries, or diabetes—that they are not as useful as other signs in monitoring the course of CNS problems. Just before death, the patient may present with central neurogenic hyperventilation.

It is important to remember that the level of carbon dioxide ($PaCO_2$) in the blood has a critical effect on cerebral vessels. The normal blood $PaCO_2$ is 40 mmHg. Increasing the $PaCO_2$ causes cerebral vasodilation, whereas decreasing it results in cerebral vasoconstriction. If the patient is poorly ventilated, the $PaCO_2$ will increase, causing even further vasodilation, with a subsequent increase in intracranial pressure. Therefore, be careful to ventilate the patient who is suspected of having increased intracranial pressure at a rate of 10 to 12 breaths per minute. Use capnography to guide care. Generally speaking, an $ETCO_2$ level of 35 to 40 mmHg is a good target. It is important to avoid *excessively* hyperventilating a patient so as to prevent decreasing $ETCO_2$ to dangerously low levels. Recent studies have found that patients with neurologic dysfunction have worse outcomes when excessive oxygen (hyperoxia) is administered. Use the pulse oximeter to guide care. Assess the SpO_2. If the patient is hypoxic, administer enough supplemental oxygen to correct hypoxia without causing hyperoxia. In many cases, supplemental oxygen will not be required.[4]

CARDIOVASCULAR STATUS Patients suffering from a neurologic event are also likely to suffer changes to the cardiovascular system. Vigilant assessment of a patient's vital signs is necessary to observe the following changes:

- ***Heart rate.*** A heart rate may be too fast (tachycardia), too slow (bradycardia), or irregular (arrhythmias).
- ***ECG/rhythm.*** Development of any changes to the ECG rhythm including ST segment changes, the onset of bradycardia, tachycardia, or potentially lethal arrhythmias such as ventricular fibrillation or ventricular tachycardia.
- ***Bruits.*** The sound of turbulent blood flow through the carotid arteries, known as a *bruit,* may be indicative of atherosclerotic disease and decreased blood flow to the brain.
- ***Jugular venous distention (JVD).*** Increased jugular venous pressure, known as jugular venous distention, may be present, indicating that the heart is not pumping effectively.

NERVOUS SYSTEM STATUS To evaluate nervous system status, take into account sensorimotor status, motor system status, and the status of the cranial nerves.

Sensorimotor Evaluation The purpose of sensorimotor evaluation is to document loss of sensation and/or motor function. To initially assess the patient with a possible spinal injury, perform these steps:

1. If the patient is unconscious, determine the response to voice, gentle tactile stimulation, and then, if necessary, pain.
2. Evaluate the spine for pain and tenderness.
3. Observe for bruises on the spine.
4. Observe for deformity of the spine.
5. Note any incontinence.
6. Check for circulation, motor function, and sensation in each extremity. Does the patient have feeling in his hands and feet? Ask the patient to wiggle his toes and push them against resistance. Compare both sides. Check bilateral grip strength. If the patient is unconscious, pain response should be observed. If the unconscious patient withdraws or localizes to the pinching of fingers and toes, there sensation and motor function are intact. This is a sign of normal or only minimally impaired cortical function.

A patient with a suspected spinal cord injury will require full spinal immobilization on a long spine board. See the chapter "Head, Neck, and Spinal Trauma" for a discussion of traumatic spinal cord injury.

Both **decorticate posturing** (arms flexed, legs extended) and **decerebrate posturing** (arms and legs extended) are ominous signs of deep cerebral or upper brainstem injury (Figures 3-16 and 3-17). Flaccid paralysis usually indicates spinal cord injury.

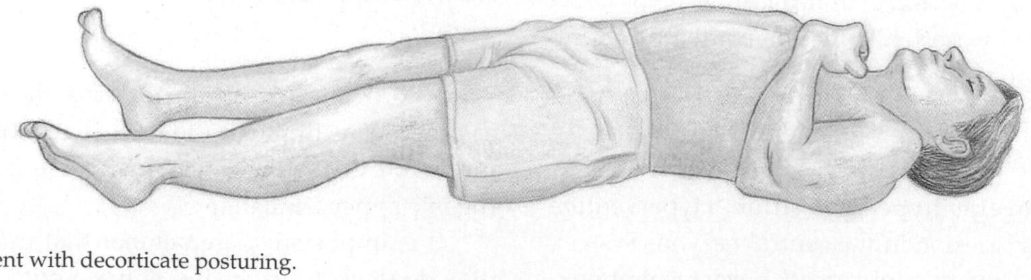

FIGURE 3-16 Patient with decorticate posturing.

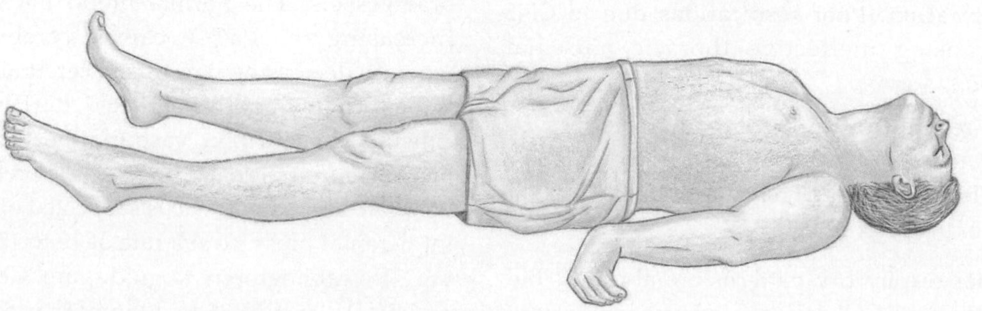

FIGURE 3-17 Patient with decerebrate posturing.

Motor System Status A thorough examination of the motor system of the body includes an assessment of muscle tone, strength, flexion, extension, coordination, and balance. Assess the patient for the following:

- ***Muscle tone.*** Are the patient's muscles firm? Or is atrophy present?
- ***Strength.*** Does the patient have adequate muscle strength? Or is weakness present? Does the patient have strong and equal grip strength?
- ***Flexion/extension.*** Can the patient flex, extend, and move extremities adequately?
- ***Coordination.*** Are the patient's gait and movements steady and smooth? Can the patient touch finger to nose?
- ***Balance.*** Can the patient stand or sit upright without becoming dizzy?

Cranial Nerves Status As you learned earlier, 12 pairs of cranial nerves extend from the lower surface of the brain. Each pair is designated by a Roman numeral, from I to XII. Proper and intact functioning of these nerves may be assessed during a complete neurologic examination, as detailed in the chapter "Secondary Assessment." Review Figure 3-14 in this chapter, which outlines the cranial nerves and their functions.

FURTHER MENTAL STATUS ASSESSMENT For patients with an altered mental status or those who are unresponsive, the **Glasgow Coma Scale (GCS)** is a simple tool that can be used to evaluate and monitor the patient's condition. Although it is used most commonly in trauma situations, the scale can also be a valuable tool for monitoring a medical patient's status (Figure 3-18). The scale includes three components:

- Eye opening
- Verbal response
- Motor response

A number is applied to each of the components based on the patient's condition. The total score can serve as an indicator of survival. The lowest GCS score possible is 3; the highest possible score is 15. The GCS can also be used as a predictor of long-term morbidity and mortality. The following are examples of the predictive value of the GCS system:

Glasgow Coma Scale: Adult		
EYE OPENING	Spontaneous	4
	To voice	3
	To pain	2
	None	1
BEST VERBAL RESPONSE	Oriented	5
	Confused	4
	Inappropriate words	3
	Incomprehensible words	2
	None	1
BEST MOTOR RESPONSE	Obeys commands	6
	Localizes pain	5
	Withdraws (to pain)	4
	Flexion (to pain)	3
	Extension (to pain)	2
	None	1
TOTAL SCORE		

Glasgow Coma Scale: Pediatric		
EYE OPENING	Spontaneous	4
	To speech	3
	To pain	2
	No response	1
BEST VERBAL RESPONSE	Oriented (Infant coos or babbles)	5
	Confused (Infant irritable, cries)	4
	Inappropriate words (Infant cries to pain)	3
	Incomprehensible sounds (Infant moans to pain)	2
	No response	1
BEST MOTOR RESPONSE	Obeys (Infant moves spontaneously/purposefully)	6
	Localizes (Infant withdraws to touch)	5
	Withdraws to pain	4
	Abnormal flexion to pain (decorticate)	3
	Extensor response to pain (decerebrate)	2
	No response	1
TOTAL SCORE		

INTERPRETATION
Possible Total: 3–15
Minor Head Injury: 13–15
Moderate Head Injury: 9–12
Severe Head Injury (Coma) (Confers Significant Mortality Risk): 8

FIGURE 3-18 Glasgow Coma Scale—adult and pediatric.

A Patient with a Total Score of:	Has an Estimated:
8 or better	94% favorable outcome
5, 6, 7	50% favorable (adult), 90% (children)
3, 4	10% favorable outcome
5, 6, 7 who drop a grade	0% favorable outcome
5, 6, 7 who improve to more than 7	80% favorable outcome

Vital Signs

Vital signs are crucial in following the course of neurologic problems. Such signs can indicate changes in intracranial pressure. Increased intracranial pressure is characterized by the following changes in vital signs, sometimes collectively referred to as **Cushing's triad**:

- Increased blood pressure
- Decreased pulse
- Irregular respirations

A patient in the early stages of increased intracranial pressure usually exhibits an increase in blood pressure, a decrease in pulse rate, and irregular respirations. There will also be an increase in temperature. Later, if the intracranial pressure continues to rise without correction, the blood pressure will fall and the pulse rate will increase. Respirations will remain irregular, and the body temperature will remain elevated. Arrhythmias may be seen with increased intracranial pressure. Continuous ECG monitoring, and pulse oximetry, if available, should be used to spot early signs of CNS lesions. Table 3-1 compares vital signs of a patient in shock with those of a patient with head injury and increased intracranial pressure. Remember, if you suspect that a patient has a CNS injury, take and record vital signs every 5 minutes.

Additional Assessment Tools

Additional technological tools may be useful in assessing and monitoring the neurologic patient. Such tools should be used as adjuncts to a complete patient assessment, and they should not be relied on as sole indicators of a patient's condition. Paramedics should continue to base their clinical decisions on a patient's entire presentation. Use such instruments as capnography, pulse oximeter, and blood glucose meter to gain further insight into a patient's condition. Remember that carbon monoxide (CO) poisoning can be an insidious cause of neurologic symptoms. Consider checking for elevated CO levels with a CO-oximeter.

Table 3-1 Comparison of Vital Signs in Shock and Increased Intracranial Pressure

Vital Signs	Shock	Increased ICP
Blood pressure	Decreased	Increased
Pulse	Increased	Decreased
Respirations	Increased	Decreased
Level of consciousness	Decreased	Decreased

CAPNOGRAPHY Capnography monitors the amount of carbon dioxide being exhaled by a patient while being ventilated. This device works on the premise that during exhalation, CO_2 should be detected. In the apneic patient with a suspected neurologic injury, the device can be used to monitor the effectiveness of the assisted ventilations. Monitoring the levels of CO_2 can ensure that the ventilation rate and quality are appropriate for decreasing the increased intracranial pressure.

PULSE OXIMETER The pulse oximeter is an effective tool for monitoring a patient's general state of perfusion. Any patient with a pulse oximetry reading of less than 90 percent is likely to be hypoxic. In a patient who has suffered a stroke, altered mental status, or syncope, the oximeter can be a useful adjunct in monitoring a patient's condition. It can also monitor the effectiveness of airway management techniques.

BLOOD GLUCOSE METER A common cause of an altered mental status or focal neurologic deficits is hypoglycemia. Determining the blood glucose level is often a crucial step in caring for the neurologic patient. Use the blood glucose meter to obtain an accurate blood glucose level. (See the chapter "Endocrinology" for a discussion of this procedure.) Documented hypoglycemia should be treated with a bolus of 50 percent dextrose.

CO-OXIMETRY Carbon monoxide (CO) poisoning is the most common cause of poisoning in industrialized countries. It has often been called "the great imitator" because the signs and symptoms are vague and mimic the signs and symptoms of other disorders. Detection of elevated CO levels is possible in the prehospital setting through the use of CO-oximetry.

Geriatric Considerations in Neurologic Assessment

The neurologic system of the geriatric patient is susceptible to systemic illness and is often affected by other body disorders. In addition, certain neurologic changes such as pupil sluggishness, loss of overall body strength, and muscle atrophy occur naturally with the aging process. Slowing of nerve conduction is another characteristic often seen in the geriatric patient. Such slowing may indicate that a little more time is necessary to obtain a complete neurologic history.

The level of consciousness and overall mental status of a geriatric patient is evaluated by assessing judgment, memory, affect, mood, orientation, speech, and grooming. Interviewing family members about the patient's normal state may reveal any change in mental status. Common neurologic problems of the older patient include headache, low back pain, dizziness, weakness, loss of balance, disorders such as Parkinson's disease, and vascular emergencies such as stroke.

Ongoing Assessment

Any patient suffering from a neurologic emergency should be reassessed every 5 minutes during your care and during transportation. Constantly reevaluate and monitor the patient's airway and neurologic system.

Management of Specific Nervous System Emergencies

The primary treatment for nervous system emergencies in the field is supportive. Most conditions will not be "cured" in the prehospital setting, but symptoms may be reduced or controlled. Make a strong effort to make the patient comfortable and to reduce any of the existing symptoms. Follow these steps:

- ***Airway and breathing.*** Properly position any patient who you suspect has a neurologic emergency and protect the airway. If there is known or possible trauma, maintain cervical spine stabilization (per local protocols). Administer supplemental oxygen if the patient is hypoxic—but only enough to correct hypoxia. Avoid hyperoxia. If the patient is breathing inadequately or is apneic, initiate ventilatory assistance. If an airway problem is detected, first apply basic airway maneuvers such as head positioning or the modified jaw-thrust maneuver. Intubate, if indicated.
- ***Circulatory support.*** Establish a saline lock. It is important to have an accessible route for medications.
- ***Pharmacological interventions.*** Medications are available to alleviate signs and symptoms in patients with neurologic emergencies. Medications include aspirin, dextrose, thiamine, naloxone, and diazepam.
- ***Psychological support.*** Patients suffering from a nervous system emergency, whether acute or chronic, are likely also to suffer anxiety. Neurologic deficits of any kind are frightening experiences. Provide the patient with emotional support and explain the treatment regimen. In most cases, it is appropriate to explain to the patient what is occurring and why. Careful explanation and emotional support will help allay anxiety and apprehension.
- ***Transport considerations.*** Assess, provide emergency care, and package the patient as quickly and safely as possible. Rapidly transport any patient with a neurologic deficit or altered mental status to an appropriate emergency department, equipped with a computed tomography (CT) or magnetic resonance imaging (MRI) scanner and facilities capable of managing strokes with fibrinolytic therapy. Modern medicine has seen the development of new advances in pharmacological and surgical interventions that are available only in the hospital setting.

There are numerous causes of nervous system emergencies. The more common nontraumatic nervous system emergencies encountered in the prehospital setting include altered mental status, seizures, stroke, transient ischemic attack (TIA), and headache. The following discussion details the assessment and management of these frequently encountered nontraumatic nervous system emergencies.

Altered Mental Status

When evaluating a patient, you may find mnemonic devices useful as assessment aids. A mnemonic that may help you remember some of the common causes of altered mental status is "AEIOU-TIPS."

A = Acidosis, alcohol

E = Epilepsy

I = Infection

O = Overdose

U = Uremia (kidney failure)

T = Trauma, tumor, toxin

I = Insulin (hypoglycemia or diabetic ketoacidosis)

P = Psychosis, poison

S = Stroke, seizure

Make an effort through history taking and patient assessment to determine the underlying cause of the altered level of consciousness. Often, however, a clear cause will not be evident and cannot be determined in the prehospital setting.

Assessment

Using the AVPU method discussed earlier, determine the patient's level of consciousness. Unresponsive patients require vigilant monitoring and protection of the airway. Use information from family, friends, or other bystanders to try to determine the underlying cause of unconsciousness. Perform a physical exam to uncover any hidden injuries, signs, or symptoms.

Management

Your initial priority is to ensure that the patient's airway is open and cervical spine is immobilized (in cases of suspected head/neck injury). Simultaneously secure the patient's airway and administer supplemental oxygen (if the patient is hypoxic). If the patient is breathing inadequately, support respirations. An unresponsive patient requires an appropriate airway adjunct. Then assess the patient's circulatory status. Evaluate the patient's heart rate and blood pressure, and monitor the cardiac rhythm.

After these steps are completed, perform the following steps:

- Establish an IV with a saline lock.
- Determine the blood glucose level using a reagent strip or glucometer. A serum glucose determination will assist in determining if the altered mental status is due to hypoglycemia.
- If the blood glucose level is low, administer 50 percent dextrose. This will mediate hypoglycemia, which may be the cause of the altered mental status. Elevated glucose levels are associated with worse outcomes from neurologic problems. If glucose is required, give only enough to arouse the patient. If possible, avoid giving the whole 25 grams of glucose found in the $D_{50}W$ syringe (or use a $D_{25}W$ solution). For the alcoholic patient who is hypoglycemic, the glucose may be lifesaving as well. (For more information on diabetic emergencies, see the chapter "Endocrinology.")
- Administer naloxone if the patient is suspected of having a narcotic overdose. Naloxone, a narcotic antagonist, has proven effective in the management and reversal of overdose caused by narcotics or synthetic narcotic agents. (For more information, see the chapter "Toxicology and Substance Abuse.")
- If the patient is a suspected alcoholic, consider the administration of 100 mg of thiamine (vitamin B_1). It is required for the conversion of pyruvic acid to acetyl-coenzyme-A (an important step in normal metabolism). Without this conversion, a significant amount of energy available in glucose cannot be obtained. The brain is extremely sensitive to thiamine deficiency. (For more information, see the chapter "Toxicology and Substance Abuse.")

CHRONIC ALCOHOLISM Chronic alcoholism interferes with the intake, absorption, and use of thiamine. A significant percentage of alcoholics have thiamine deficiency that can cause Wernicke's syndrome or Korsakoff's psychosis. **Wernicke's syndrome** is an acute but reversible encephalopathy (brain disease) characterized by ataxia, eye muscle weakness, and mental derangement. Of even greater concern is **Korsakoff's psychosis**, characterized by memory disorder. Once established, Korsakoff's psychosis may be irreversible. Paramedics should follow local protocols. If ordered by medical direction, administer 100 mg of thiamine IV, IM, or PO.

INCREASED INTRACRANIAL PRESSURE If an increase in intracranial pressure is likely, as occurs in a closed head injury, ventilate the patient at 10 to 12 breaths per minute. Maintaining a normal $ETCO_2$ (~35–40 mmHg) is the preferred practice. Use caution not to hyperventilate the patient, which could decrease CO_2 levels to dangerously low levels. If herniation of the brain is evident, hyperventilation (at a rate of 20 per minute) and medications (e.g., mannitol) may be indicated. Mannitol causes diuresis, eliminating fluid from the intravascular space through the kidneys. Many authorities believe that its oncotic effect also causes a fluid shift from the substance of the brain to the circulation, thus reducing brain edema. As with all medications, follow local protocols.

Stroke and Intracranial Hemorrhage

Stroke is a general term that describes injury or death of brain tissue usually due to interruption of cerebral blood flow. The term "brain attack" is occasionally used because it compares the physiology of a stroke with that of a heart attack. In both cases, oxygen deprivation causes damage to the affected tissue.

For many years, the treatment options for stroke patients were extremely limited. Prior to 1995, prehospital care of the stroke patient was considered primarily supportive. Since then, however, modern medicine has discovered new therapies and has realized the importance of early intervention. Now, early recognition and rapid transport to the hospital are identified as crucial to improving the outcome for stroke patients. The National Institute of Neurological Disorders and Stroke (NINDS) suggests transport to an emergency facility with the capability to respond to a stroke patient quickly, such as a facility equipped with computed tomography (CT) and neurologic services.

In addition, studies have proven that *tissue plasminogen activator (tPA)* and other fibrinolytic agents used in the treatment of heart attack are also effective in treating certain occlusive strokes. NINDS stresses that the use of fibrinolytic agents in strokes is approved by the Food and Drug Administration and is encouraged in a certain patient population. Stroke patients who may be candidates for the fibrinolytic therapy must receive definitive treatment within 4.5 hours of onset. Because of the possibility of intervention with fibrinolytics, it is crucial to determine the

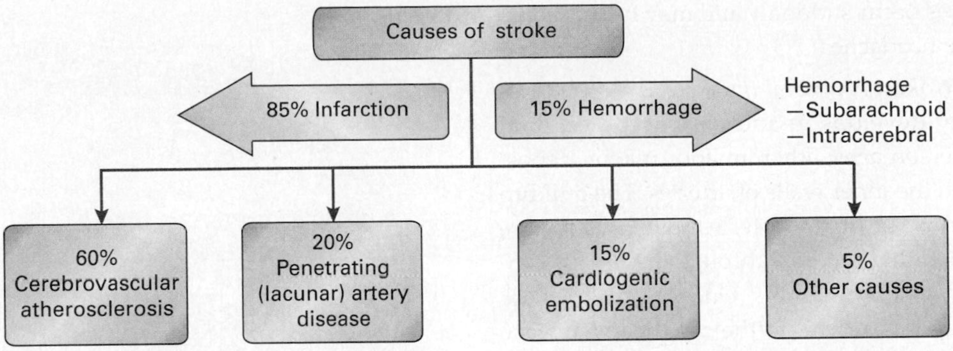

FIGURE 3-19 Causes of stroke.

exact time of the onset of symptoms as accurately as possible. In addition, it is essential that the public be aware of the signs and symptoms of stroke so that EMS can be notified. Therefore, extensive public education is necessary in achieving early recognition of symptoms and appropriate intervention and treatment. Transportation to an emergency facility is crucial in achieving the best possible outcome for these patients.

Strokes are the third most common cause of death and, in middle-aged and older patients, are a frequent cause of disability. Therefore, the public, particularly those with a history of atherosclerosis (hardening of the arteries), heart disease, or hypertension, should be educated on the signs and symptoms of stroke as well as the need to contact EMS at the outset of symptoms. Likewise, paramedics must understand stroke as a serious, potentially life-threatening condition that warrants rapid recognition and prompt transport.

Strokes can be divided into two broad categories: those caused by occlusion (blockage) of an artery and those caused by hemorrhage from a ruptured cerebral artery (Figures 3-19 and 3-20):

- ***Occlusive strokes.*** An occlusive stroke occurs when a cerebral artery is blocked by a clot or other foreign matter. This results in *ischemia,* an inadequate blood supply to the brain tissue, and progresses to *infarction,* the death of tissues as a result of cessation of blood supply. In infarction, the tissue that has died will swell, causing further damage to nearby tissues, which have only a marginal blood supply. If swelling is severe, *herniation* (protrusion of brain tissue from the skull through the foramen magnum, the narrow opening at the base of the skull) may result. Occlusive strokes are classified as either embolic or thrombotic, depending on the cause.
- ***Embolic strokes.*** An *embolus* is a solid, liquid, or gaseous mass carried to a blood vessel from a remote site. The most common emboli are clots (thromboemboli) that usually arise from diseased blood vessels in the neck (carotid) or from abnormally contracting chambers in the heart. Atrial fibrillation often results in atrial dilation, a precursor to the formation of clots. Other types of emboli that may cause occlusion in cerebral blood vessels are air, tumor tissue, and fat.

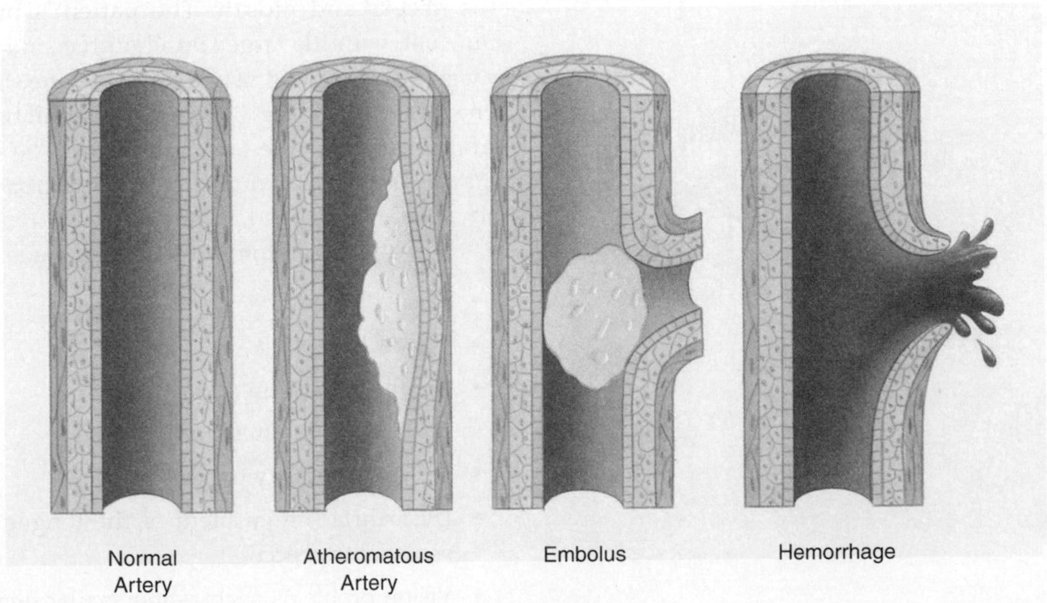

FIGURE 3-20 Etiologies of stroke.

Embolic strokes occur suddenly and may be characterized by severe headaches.

- ***Thrombotic strokes.*** A *cerebral thrombus* is a blood clot that gradually develops in and obstructs a cerebral artery. As a person ages, atheromatous plaque deposits can form on the inner walls of arteries. The buildup causes a narrowing of the arteries and reduces the amount of blood that can flow through them. This process is known as *atherosclerosis*. Once the arteries are narrowed, platelets adhere to the roughened surface and can create a blood clot that blocks the blood flow through the cerebral artery. This ultimately results in brain tissue death. Unlike the embolic stroke, the signs and symptoms of thrombotic stroke develop gradually. This type of stroke often occurs at night and is characterized by a patient awakening with altered mental status and/or loss of speech, sensory, or motor function.
- ***Hemorrhagic strokes.*** Hemorrhagic strokes are usually categorized as being within the brain (intracerebral) (Figure 3-21) or in the space around the outer surface of the brain (subarachnoid) (Figure 3-22). Onset is often sudden and marked by a severe headache. Most intracranial hemorrhages occur in the hypertensive patient when a small vessel deep within the brain tissue ruptures. Subarachnoid hemorrhages most often result from congenital blood vessel abnormalities or from head trauma. Congenital abnormalities include aneurysms (weakened vessels) and arteriovenous malformations (collections of abnormal blood vessels). Aneurysms tend to be on the surface and may hemorrhage into the brain tissue or the subarachnoid space. Arteriovenous malformations may be within the brain, in the subarachnoid space, or both. Hemorrhage inside the brain often tears and separates normal brain tissue.

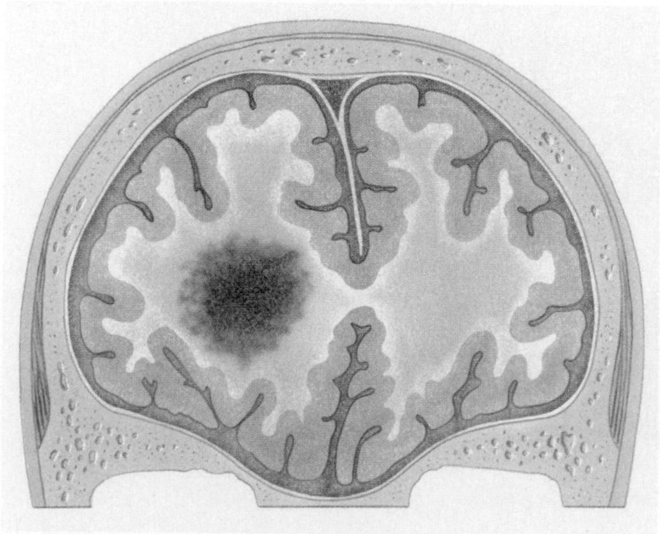

FIGURE 3-21 Intracerebral hemorrhage.

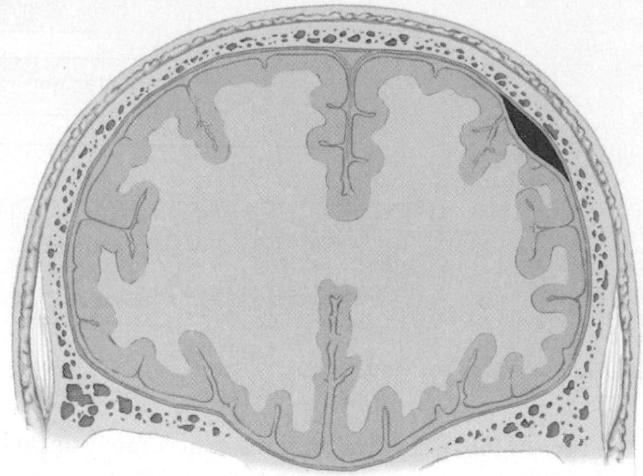

FIGURE 3-22 Subarachnoid hemorrhage.

The release of blood into the cavities within the brain that contain cerebrospinal fluid may paralyze vital centers. If blood in the subarachnoid space impairs drainage of cerebrospinal fluid, it may cause a rise in the intracranial pressure. Herniation of brain tissue may then occur.

Assessment

Signs and symptoms of a stroke will depend on the type of stroke and the area of the brain damaged (Table 3-2). Areas commonly affected are the motor, speech, and sensory centers. The onset of symptoms will be acute, and the patient may experience unconsciousness. There may be stertorous breathing (laborious breathing accompanied by snoring) due to paralysis of a portion of the soft palate. Respiratory expiration may be puffs of air out of the cheeks and mouth. The patient's pupils may be unequal, with the larger pupil on the side of the hemorrhage. Paralysis will usually involve one side of the face, one arm, and one leg. The eyes often will be turned away from the side of the body paralysis. The patient's skin may be cool and clammy. Speech disturbances, or aphasia, may also be noted.

Signs and symptoms of a stroke include:

- Facial drooping
- Headache
- Confusion and agitation
- Dysphasia (difficulty in speaking)
- Aphasia (inability to speak)
- Dysarthria (impairment of the tongue and muscles essential to speech)
- Vision problems such as monocular blindness (blindness in one eye) or double vision

Table 3-2 Stroke Syndromes

Stroke	Signs/Symptoms	Localization
	ANTERIOR CIRCULATION (CAROTID)	
Middle cerebral artery	Expressive aphasia	Dominant posterior frontal lobe
	Receptive aphasia	Dominant superior temporal lobe
	Leg/arm weakness	Contralateral parietal lobe
	Visual field cuts	Contralateral parietal lobe
Anterior cerebral artery	Leg weakness	Medial (parafalcine) parietal lobe
	POSTERIOR CIRCULATION (VERTEBRAL)	
	Vertigo, nystagmus, cranial nerve	Cerebellum
	Hemiparesis, hemisensory loss, difficulty swallowing	Brainstem
	LACUNAR	
	Pure motor stroke	Internal capsule
	Pure sensory stroke	Thalamus
	Ataxic hemiparesis	Pons
	Clumsy hand dysarthria	Pons
	Mixed motor/sensory stroke	Junction of thalamus/internal

- Hemiparesis (weakness on one side)
- Hemiplegia (paralysis on one side)
- Paresthesia (numbness or tingling)
- Inability to recognize by touch
- Gait disturbances or uncoordinated fine motor movements
- Dizziness
- Incontinence
- Coma

Predisposing factors that may contribute to the stroke include hypertension, diabetes, abnormal blood lipid levels, oral contraceptives, sickle cell disease, and some cardiac arrhythmias (e.g., atrial fibrillation).[5]

Prehospital Stroke Scoring Systems

Standardized scoring systems are now available to aid paramedics in making a field diagnosis of stroke. The two most commonly used are:

- ***Los Angeles Prehospital Stroke Screen (LAPSS).*** The Los Angeles Prehospital Stroke Screen (LAPSS) assesses blood glucose levels, facial droop (Figure 3-23), grip strength, and arm (pronator) drift (Figure 3-24). Patients meeting the LAPSS criteria should result in activation of the stroke team at the receiving hospital (Figure 3-25).[6]
- ***Cincinnati Prehospital Stroke Scale (CPSS).*** The Cincinnati Prehospital Stroke Scale (CPSS) evaluates facial droop, arm drift, and speech. An abnormal finding on any of these three parameters is associated with a 72% probability the patient has suffered a stroke (Figure 3-26).[7]

DISTINGUISHING TRANSIENT ISCHEMIC ATTACKS

Some patients may have transient stroke-like symptoms known as **transient ischemic attacks (TIAs)**. These indicate

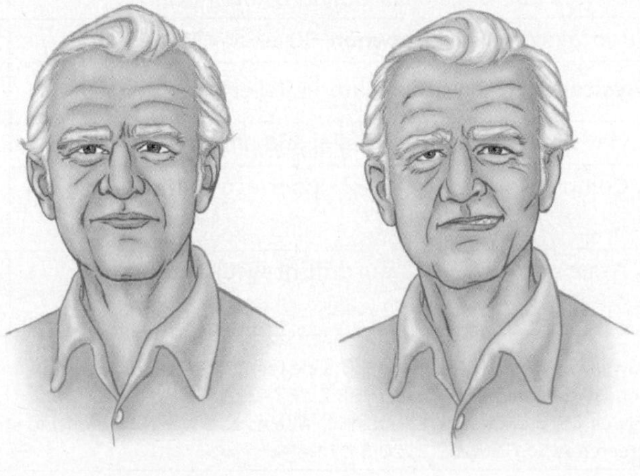

FIGURE 3-23 Facial droop.

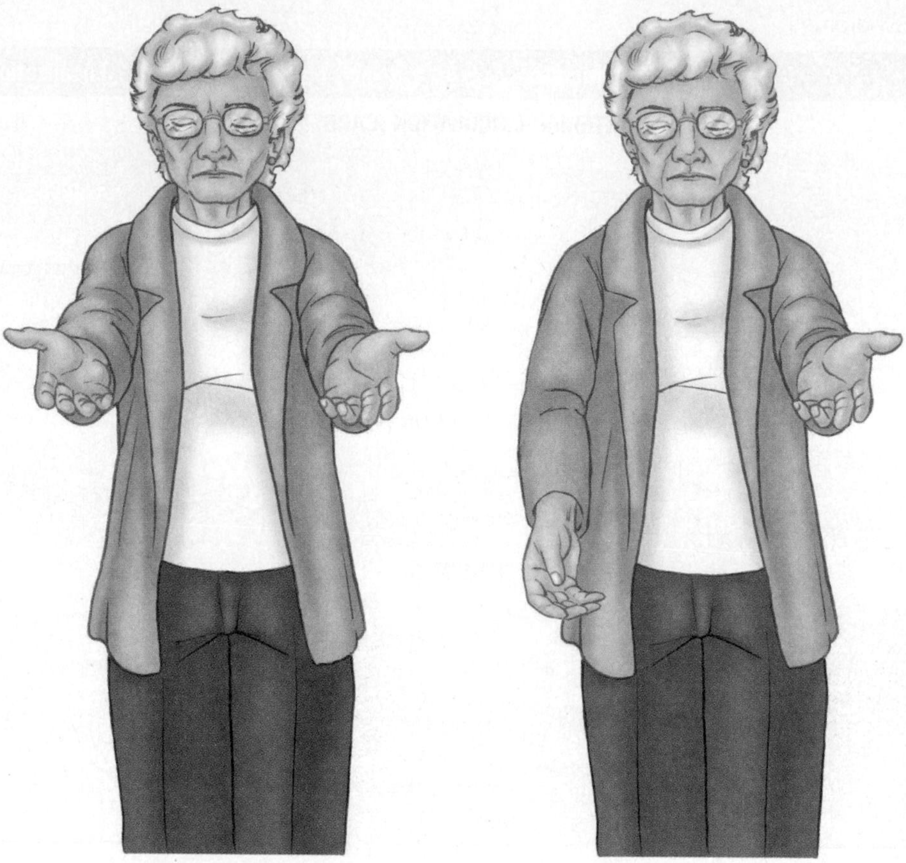

FIGURE 3-24 Arm drift.

Los Angeles Prehospital Stroke Screen (LAPSS)			
Considerations	**Yes**	**Unknown**	**No**
Age **greater than** 45 years			
No history of seizures or epilepsy			
Duration of symptoms is **less** than 24 hours			
Patient is **not** wheelchair bound or bedridden			
Blood glucose level **between 60 and 400 mg/dL**			
Physical exam to determine unilateral asymmetry	**Equal**	**R Weakness**	**L Weakness**
A. Have patient look up, smile, and show teeth		Droop	Droop
B. Compare grip strength of upper extremities		Weak grip No grip	Weak grip No grip
C. Assess arm strength for drift or weakness		Drifts down Falls rapidly	Drifts down Falls rapidly

Kidwell CS, Saver JL, Schubert GB, Eckstein M, Starkman S. Design and retrospective analysis of the Los Angeles Prehospital Stroke Screen (LAPSS). *Prehospital Emergency Care.* 1998;2:267–273.
Kidwell CS, Starkman S, Eckstein M, Weems K, Saver JL. Identifying stroke in the field: Prospective validation of the Los Angeles Prehospital Stroke Screen (LAPSS). *Stroke.* 2000;31:71–76.

FIGURE 3-25 Los Angeles Prehospital Stroke Screen (LAPSS).

Cincinnati Prehospital Stroke Scale		
Sign of Stroke	**Patient Activity**	**Interpretation**
Facial droop	Have patient look up at you, smile, and show his teeth.	*Normal:* Symmetry to both sides. *Abnormal:* One side of the face droops or does not move symmetrically.
Arm drift	Have patient lift arms up and hold them out with eyes closed for 10 seconds.	*Normal:* Symmetrical movement in both arms. *Abnormal:* One arm drifts down or asymmetrical movement of the arms.
Abnormal speech	Have the patient say, "You can't teach an old dog new tricks."	*Normal:* The correct words are used and no slurring of words is noted. *Abnormal:* The words are slurred, the wrong words are used, or the patient is aphasic.
Kothari RU, Pancioli A, Liu T, Broderick J. Cincinnati Prehospital Stroke Scale: Reproducibility and validity. *Annals of Emergency Medicine*. 1999;33:373–378.		

FIGURE 3-26 Cincinnati Prehospital Stroke Scale (CPSS).

temporary interference with the blood supply to the brain, producing symptoms of neurologic deficit. These symptoms may last for a few minutes or for several hours but usually resolve within 24 hours. After the attack, the patient will show no evidence of residual brain or neurologic damage. However, the patient who experiences a TIA may be a candidate for an eventual stroke. In fact, one-third of TIA patients suffer a stroke soon after the transient attack. These are considered high-risk events.[8,9]

The onset of a transient ischemic attack is usually abrupt. The specific signs and symptoms depend on the area of the brain affected. Any one or a combination of stroke symptoms may be present. In fact, it is virtually impossible to determine whether such a neurologic event is due to a stroke or to a TIA in the prehospital setting.

The most common cause of a TIA is carotid artery disease. Other causes can be a small embolus, decreased cardiac output, hypotension, overmedication with antihypertensive agents, or cerebrovascular spasm.

While obtaining the history of the patient suspected of sustaining a TIA, try to collect information on or take note of the following factors:

- Previous neurologic symptoms
- Initial symptoms and their progression
- Changes in mental status
- Precipitating factors
- Dizziness
- Palpitations
- History of hypertension, cardiac disease, sickle cell disease, or previous TIA or stroke

Management

Care for the stroke or TIA patient emphasizes early recognition, supportive measures, rapid transport, and notification of the emergency department. Aggressive airway management is a priority in caring for these patients. Field management of the stroke patient generally includes the following procedures:

- Ensure scene safety, including Standard Precautions.
- Establish and maintain an adequate airway. Have suction equipment readily available. Control of the patient's airway is a priority. Brain damage can affect a patient's ability to swallow and maintain an open airway.
- If the patient is apneic or if breathing is inadequate, provide positive pressure ventilations at a rate of 10 to 12 per minute. Avoid overzealous hyperventilation that may lower CO_2 levels to detrimentally low levels causing profound cerebral vasoconstriction. Use capnography.
- Check for hypoxia with pulse oximetry. If the patient is hypoxic, administer enough supplemental oxygen to correct hypoxia. Avoid hyperoxia.[10,11]
- Complete a detailed patient history.
- Perform a stroke assessment.
- Keep the patient supine or in the recovery position. If the patient has congestive heart failure, a semi-upright position may be necessary.
- If an altered mental status is present or there is potential for airway compromise, place the patient in the recovery position.
- Determine the blood glucose level.
- Place a saline lock. (Avoid dextrose solutions that may increase intracranial pressure due to increased osmotic effects.) If hypoglycemia is present, consider the judicious administration of 50 percent dextrose by slow intravenous push.

Patho Pearls

The Best Treatment for Stroke. Because strokes are so debilitating, a tremendous amount of research has been devoted to acute stroke care. Initially, fibrinolytic therapy was proposed—similar to treatment for ST-segment elevation MI (STEMI). However, strokes are harder to diagnose, and fibrinolytic therapy is useful only for some causes of stroke.

Second-phase research has concentrated on early identification of stroke and development of multidisciplinary stroke care facilities. Most stroke therapies must be initiated within 4.5 hours after onset of symptoms if brain tissue is to be salvaged, so a public awareness program has been developed to help lay people recognize stroke signs and symptoms early. In special hospital stroke centers, patients are rapidly assessed and appropriate therapy is provided for that patient's stroke type and location.

Hospitals that provide a lot of stroke care have been shown to have better outcomes than those that do not. Thus, most EMS systems now have protocols for the early identification of stroke and transport to an appropriate stroke center for definitive care. As a key part of the stroke care team, paramedics must stay abreast of evolving stroke care strategies.

- Monitor the cardiac rhythm, oximetry, and capnography.
- Protect the paralyzed extremities.
- Give the patient reassurance—all procedures should be explained. The patient may be unable to speak but still may be able to hear and understand.
- Rapidly transport without excessive movement or noise to an appropriate medical facility.

The American Heart Association algorithm "Adult Suspected Stroke" is available at http://circ.ahajournals.org/content/122/18_suppl_3.toc (Part 11, unnumbered figure, page S819).

Seizures and Epilepsy

A **seizure** is a temporary alteration in behavior due to the massive electrical discharge of one or more groups of neurons in the brain. Seizures in any individual may be caused by stresses to the body, such as hypoxia, or a rapid lowering of blood sugar. Febrile seizures can occur in young children with sudden elevations in body temperature. Structural diseases of the brain, such as tumors, head trauma, toxic eclampsia, and vascular disorders, also cause seizures. The most common cause is *idiopathic epilepsy*. The term *idiopathic* means "without a known cause." The terms *epilepsy* and *epileptic* indicate nothing more than the potential to develop seizures in circumstances that would not induce them in most individuals. Seizures can provoke a great deal of anxiety in both yourself and bystanders.

To assess seizures quickly under such conditions, you need to be thoroughly familiar with their various forms.

Types of Seizures

Seizures can be clinically classified as generalized or partial. **Generalized seizures** begin as an electrical discharge in a small area of the brain but spread to involve the entire cerebral cortex, causing widespread malfunction. **Partial seizures** may remain confined to a limited portion of the brain, causing localized malfunction, or may spread and become generalized.

GENERALIZED SEIZURES Generalized seizures include tonic–clonic and absence seizures. Another type, pseudoseizures, may mimic generalized seizures.

- *Tonic–clonic.* A **tonic–clonic seizure**, also known as a *grand mal seizure*, is a generalized motor seizure, producing a loss of consciousness. It typically includes a **tonic (increased tone) phase**, characterized by tensed, contracted muscles, and a **clonic phase**, characterized by rhythmic jerking movements of the extremities. During the seizure episode, a patient's intercostal muscles and diaphragm become temporarily paralyzed, interrupting respirations and producing cyanosis. The patient's neck, head, face, and eye muscles may also jerk. Once respirations resume, there may be copious amounts of oral secretions (frothing) present. Incontinence is also common during a seizure. Agitation or confusion, drowsiness, or coma may also follow the seizure.

  Tonic–clonic seizures have a specific progression of events. It is descriptively convenient to refer to this progression as ranging from warning phase to period of recovery. However, not all seizure patients experience all these events.

  - *Aura.* An **aura** is a subjective sensation preceding seizure activity. The aura may precede the attack by several hours or by only a few seconds. An aura may be of a psychic or a sensory nature, with olfactory, visual, auditory, or taste hallucinations. Some common types include hearing noise or music, seeing floating lights, smelling unpleasant odors, feeling an unpleasant sensation in the stomach, or experiencing tingling or twitching in a specific body area. Not all seizures are preceded by an aura.
  - *Loss of consciousness.* The patient will become unconscious at some point after the aura sensations, if any.
  - *Tonic phase.* This is a phase of continuous muscle tension, characterized by contraction of the patient's muscles.
  - *Hypertonic phase.* The patient experiences extreme muscular rigidity, including hyperextension of the back.
  - *Clonic phase.* The patient experiences muscle spasms marked by rhythmic movements. The

patient's jaw usually remains clenched, making airway management difficult.

- *Post-seizure.* The patient remains in a coma.
- *Postictal.* The patient may awaken confused and fatigued. He may complain of a headache and may experience some neurologic deficit. In many cases, patients will be in this postictal state when paramedic crews arrive. There may be evidence of incontinence, which supports the likelihood that seizure activity has taken place.
- *Absence.* An **absence seizure**, also called a *petit mal seizure,* is a brief, generalized seizure that usually presents with a 10- to 30-second loss of consciousness or awareness, eye or muscle fluttering, and an occasional loss of muscle tone. Loss of consciousness may be so brief that the patient or observers may be unaware of the episode. Absence seizures are idiopathic disorders of early childhood and rarely occur after age 20. Children who suffer frequent absence seizures are often accused of daydreaming or inattentiveness. Absence seizures may not respond to normal treatment modalities.
- *Pseudoseizures.* Pseudoseizures, also called "hysterical seizures," stem from psychological disorders. The patient presents with sharp and bizarre movements that can often be interrupted with a terse command, such as "stop it!" The seizure is usually witnessed, and there will not be a postictal period. Very rarely do patients experiencing a pseudoseizure injure themselves.

PARTIAL SEIZURES Partial seizures may be either simple or complex.

- *Simple partial seizures.* **Simple partial seizures**, also sometimes called focal motor, focal sensory, or Jacksonian seizures, are characterized by chaotic movement or dysfunction of one area of the body. When there is abnormal electrical discharge from a specific portion of the brain, only the functions served by that area will have dysfunction. Simple partial seizures involve no loss of consciousness and begin as localized tonic–clonic movements. They frequently spread and can progress to generalized tonic–clonic seizures. Therefore, it is crucial that you document how such seizures begin and the course that they subsequently take.

CONTENT REVIEW

➤ Types of Seizures
- Generalized seizures
  - Tonic–clonic
  - Absence
- Partial seizures
  - Simple partial seizures
  - Complex partial seizures

- *Complex partial seizures.* **Complex partial seizures**, sometimes called temporal lobe or psychomotor seizures, are characterized by distinctive auras. They include unusual smells, tastes, sounds, or the tendency of objects to look either very large and near or small and distant. Sometimes a seizure patient may visualize scenes that look very familiar (*déja vu*) or very strange. A metallic taste in the mouth is a common psychomotor seizure aura. These are focal seizures, lasting approximately 1 to 2 minutes. The patient experiences a loss of contact with his surroundings. Additionally, the patient may act confused, stagger, perform purposeless movement, or make unintelligible sounds. He may not understand what is said. The patient may even refuse medical aid. Some patients develop automatic behavior or show a sudden change in personality, such as abrupt explosions of rage.

Assessment

Your initial contact with the patient and bystanders will offer a unique opportunity to obtain a history that may influence your plan of management. What an untrained observer calls a seizure may be a simple fainting spell. Therefore, you need to ascertain exactly what the patient may recall or what bystanders witnessed.

Many other problems can mimic or suggest a seizure. These include migraine headaches, cardiac arrhythmias, hypoglycemia after exercise or drug ingestion, and the tendency to faint when rising from a supine or sitting position (orthostatic hypotension). Hyperventilation, meningitis, intracranial hemorrhage, or certain tranquilizers can cause stiffness of the extremities. Decerebrate movements, if present, may be caused by increased intracranial pressure. If you are unsure whether the patient has had a seizure, it may be more harmful than beneficial to administer an anticonvulsant medication.

It is also important to try to distinguish between syncope and true seizure (Table 3-3). Syncope patients sometimes have a short initial period of seizure-like activity (usually less than 1 minute), but this is not followed by a postictal state. The most common cause of fainting is vasovagal syncope associated with fatigue, emotional stress, or cardiac disease. Syncope will be discussed in greater detail later in this chapter.

CONTENT REVIEW

➤ Phases of a Generalized Seizure
- Aura
- Loss of consciousness
- Tonic phase
- Hypertonic phase
- Clonic phase
- Post-seizure
- Postictal phase

➤ The prime concerns in seizure management are control of the airway and prevention of injury.

Table 3-3 Differentiation between Syncope and Generalized Tonic–Clonic Seizure

Syncope	Seizure
Usually begins in a standing position	May begin in any position
Patient will usually remember a warning of fainting (feeling of weakness or dizziness)	May begin without warning or may be preceded by an aura
Jerking motions usually not present	Jerking motions present during unconsciousness
Patient regains consciousness almost immediately on becoming supine	Patient remains unconscious during seizure, remains drowsy during postictal period

When obtaining a history, remember to include the following points:

- History of seizures (This data should include length of any past seizure; whether it was generalized or focal; and the presence of auras, incontinence, or trauma to the tongue.)
- Recent history of head trauma
- Any alcohol and/or drug abuse
- Recent history of fever, headache, or stiff neck
- History of diabetes, heart disease, or stroke
- Current medications (most chronic seizure patients take anticonvulsant medication on a regular basis. Common anticonvulsant medications are phenytoin [Dilantin], phenobarbital, carbamazepine [Tegretol], ethosuxamide [Zarontin], gabapentin [Neurontin], lamotrigine [Lamictal], and valproic acid [Depakote].)

The physical examination of the seizure patient should include the following steps:

- Note any signs of head trauma or injury to the tongue.
- Determine the blood glucose level.
- Check for hypoxia (oximetry, physical examination).
- Note any evidence of alcohol and/or drug abuse.
- Document arrhythmias.

Management

Remember that seizures tend to provoke anxiety in patients, families, and paramedics. From a medical standpoint, however, most of these situations only require managing the airway and preventing the patient from injuring himself. Because the patient may become hypo- or hyperthermic if exposed, protecting body temperature is also crucial. Field management of the seizure patient generally includes the following procedures:

- Ensure scene safety.
- Maintain the airway. Do not force objects between the patient's teeth—this includes padded tongue blades. Pushing objects into the patient's mouth may cause him to vomit or to aspirate. It can also cause laryngospasm.
- Administer supplemental oxygen to correct hypoxia.
- Establish intravenous access.
- Determine the blood glucose level. If hypoglycemic, administer 50 percent dextrose.
- Never attempt to restrain the patient. This may injure him. However, protect the patient from hitting objects in the environment (Figure 3-27). (*Note:* If there is evidence of head trauma, cervical spine stabilization (based on local protocols) may be considered as in any other head injury.)
- Maintain body temperature.
- Position the patient on his left side after the tonic–clonic phase (Figure 3-28).
- Suction, if required.
- Monitor cardiac rhythm, oximetry, and capnography.
- If the seizure is prolonged (>5 minutes), consider an anticonvulsant.
- Provide a quiet, reassuring atmosphere.
- Transport the patient in the supine or lateral recumbent position.

Status Epilepticus

Status epilepticus is a series of two or more generalized motor seizures without an intervening return of consciousness. The most common cause in adults is failure to take prescribed anticonvulsant medications. Status epilepticus is a major emergency because it involves a prolonged period of apnea, which, in turn, can cause hypoxia of vital brain tissues. These seizures may result in respiratory arrest, severe metabolic and respiratory acidosis, extreme hypertension, increased intracranial pressure, serious elevations in body temperature, fractures of the long bones and spine, necrosis of the cardiac muscle, and severe dehydration.

The most valuable intervention is to protect the patient from airway obstruction and deliver 100 percent oxygen (if hypoxic). Preferably this should be accomplished by

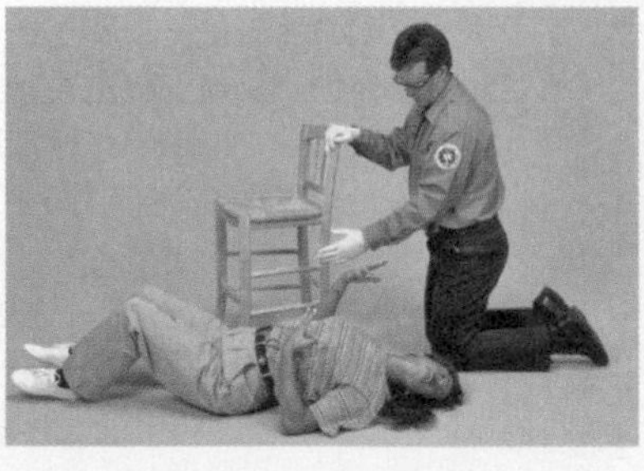

FIGURE 3-27 Protection of a seizing patient.

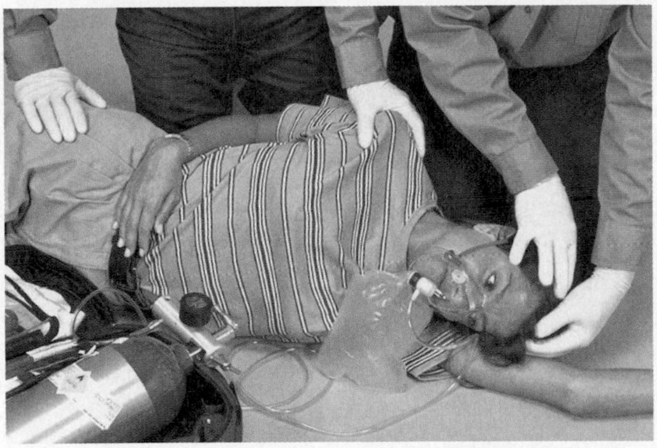

FIGURE 3-28 Place a seizing patient with no suspected spine injury on her left side.

bag-valve-mask assistance, as the normal ventilatory mechanisms of the patient are seriously impaired and air exchange is generally ineffective. Once the airway is maintained and ventilations are being assisted, take the following steps:

- Start an IV of normal saline at a keep-open rate.
- Monitor cardiac rhythm, oximetry, and capnography.
- Administer 25 g of 50 percent dextrose IV push (only if hypoglycemia is present).
- Administer 5 to 10 mg diazepam IV push for an adult. (Diazepam is a sedative and anticonvulsant that depresses the spread of seizure activity across the motor cortex of the brain.) Other benzodiazepines may be used as directed by system protocols and standing orders.
- Continue to monitor the airway. Some patients may require large doses of diazepam. Always have flumazenil (Romazicon) available in case it is needed to reverse any significant respiratory depression caused by diazepam. Remember, administration of flumazenil may result in the return of seizures. It should be used only when absolutely necessary.[12]

Syncope

As discussed earlier, **syncope** (fainting) is a neurologic condition characterized by the sudden, temporary loss of consciousness caused by insufficient blood flow to the brain, with recovery of consciousness almost immediately on becoming supine. Nearly half of all Americans will experience at least one episode of syncope during their lifetime. According to the National Institutes of Health, syncope accounts for 3 percent of all emergency department visits.

Assessment

Focus on what caused the patient to faint, or lose consciousness. The causes of syncope can be classified into four general categories:

- *Cardiovascular* conditions, such as arrhythmias or mechanical problems—A heart rate that is too fast or too slow, or an abnormally functioning heart valve, may trigger hypoxia in the brain and subsequent fainting.
- *Hypovolemia*, a decrease in total body fluid volume—This can cause syncope, especially when the patient moves from a seated or supine position to a standing position (orthostatic or positional syncope).
- *Noncardiovascular* disease, such as metabolic, neurologic, or psychiatric conditions—Hypoglycemia, a transient ischemic attack, or an anxiety attack can cause syncope.
- *Idiopathic*, or unknown, cause—Often, the cause of a patient's syncope remains unknown despite careful assessment and diagnostic tests.

Syncope can occur in patients of all ages. from the very young to the very old. Symptoms may include feeling faint, dizziness, light-headedness, or a loss of consciousness without warning. Keep in mind, however, that the definition of syncope includes rapid recovery of consciousness (usually less than a minute). If a patient does not spontaneously regain consciousness within a few moments, it is *NOT* syncope—it is something more serious.

Management

When caring for someone who has fainted, it is important to attempt to identify the underlying cause and treat it. If no cause can be identified, anyone who loses consciousness should be transported to an appropriate emergency department and evaluated. Field management of the syncopal patient generally includes the following procedures:

- Ensure scene safety.
- Establish and maintain an adequate airway.
- Administer supplemental oxygen to correct hypoxia. Avoid hyperoxia.
- Check circulatory status (heart rate, blood pressure, ECG).
- Check and continuously monitor mental status.
- Obtain IV access.
- Determine the blood glucose level.
- Monitor the ECG, oximetry, and capnography.
- Reassure the patient.
- Transport the patient to an emergency department.

Headache

Headache can seriously disrupt a person's life. Nearly 45 million Americans suffer from chronic headaches. Of these, approximately 17 million suffer migraine headaches.

An estimated $4 billion is spent annually on over-the-counter pain relievers for headache.[13]

Headache pain can be acute (sudden onset) or chronic (constant or recurring), generalized (all over) or localized (in one specific area), and can range from mild to severe. In some cases, the cause is known. In others, it is not. The most common types of headache can be classified into three categories:

- ***Vascular.*** Vascular headaches include migraines and cluster headaches. *Migraines* can last from several minutes to several days. They can be characterized by an intense or throbbing pain, photosensitivity (sensitivity to light), nausea, vomiting, and sweats. Migraines are frequently unilateral (on one side of the head) and may be preceded by an aura. *Cluster* headaches usually occur as a series of one-sided headaches that are sudden and intense, and may continue for 15 minutes to 4 hours. Symptoms may include nasal congestion, drooping eyelid, and an irritated or watery eye. Migraines occur more commonly in women, whereas cluster headaches generally occur in men.
- ***Tension.*** A significant percentage of headaches are tension headaches. Most personnel in the emergency medical field have, at one time or another, suffered from a tension headache. Sometimes such headaches occur on a daily basis. Sufferers often awake in the morning with a mild headache that gets worse during the course of the day. The tension headache produces a dull, achy pain that feels like a forceful pressure is being applied to the neck and/or head.
- ***Organic.*** A third, less common, category includes organically caused headaches. They occur in individuals suffering from tumors, infections (especially sinus infections), or other diseases of the brain, eye, or other body system.

A continuous throbbing headache (often predominantly over the occiput) with fever, confusion, and nuchal rigidity (stiffness of the neck) are classic signs and symptoms of *meningitis.* Be alert for these features while assessing patients complaining of headache, particularly those who have also been complaining of nausea, vomiting, or rash. (The chapter "Infectious Disease and Sepsis" provides further discussion on meningitis and other infectious diseases.)

Assessment

In addition to pain, those suffering from a headache of any type may also complain of nausea, vomiting, blurred vision, dizziness, weakness, or watery eyes. A complete and thorough history of the patient's headache is crucial to its treatment. Determine as much as you can about the pain, including:

- What was the patient doing during the onset of pain?
- Does anything provoke, or worsen, the pain? (Light, sound, or movement?)
- What is the quality of the pain? (Is it throbbing? crushing? tension?)
- Does the pain radiate to the neck, arm, back, or jaw?
- What is the severity of the pain? (On a scale of 0–10, how does the patient rate the pain?)
- How long has the headache been present? (Acute vs. chronic?)

Some headache-associated signs and symptoms are worrisome (Table 3-4). Headache of acute onset or of a changing pattern demands immediate attention. A sudden onset of pain, description of the pain as "the worst headache in my life," or changes in the pattern of pain should be considered characteristics of potentially serious conditions, such as intracranial hemorrhage.

Table 3-4 Worrisome Headache Signs and Symptoms

• Onset in persons older than 50 years or younger than 5 years.
• Change in previous headache pattern (increased frequency and/or severity).
• Onset of sudden "worst headache ever."
• Subacute headache that progressively worsens over time.
• Onset of headache with exertion, coughing, sneezing, or sexual activity.
• Unaccountable change in vital signs. Fever, raised systolic pressure with tachycardia, anxiety, pallor, or sweating. Diastolic pressure ≥120 mmHg.
• Drowsiness, confusion, memory impairment.
• Slurred speech.
• Ataxia, loss of coordination.
• Diplopia, abnormal pupillary reflexes, papilledema.
• Persistent tinnitus.
• Loss of sense of smell.
• Facial numbness, asymmetry, palsy.
• Stiff neck, occipital pain and tenderness.
• Handgrip power loss, tremor.
• Motor and/or sensory loss in extremities.
• Loss of deep tendon reflexes.
• Abnormal Babinski sign or other neurologic signs.
• Persistent headache following significant head trauma or whiplash injury.
• Chronic cough, lymphadenopathy, weight loss.
• History of malignancy, HIV infection, or other significant systemic disease.

Management

Treatment for a victim of headache is supportive. Field management of the headache patient generally includes the following:

- Ensure scene safety.
- Establish and maintain an adequate airway.
- Place the patient in a position of comfort. Patients will often place themselves in a position that best alleviates the symptoms, such as lying flat in a dark room.
- Administer supplemental oxygen to correct hypoxia. Avoid hyperoxia.
- Obtain IV access.
- Determine the blood glucose level.
- Monitor the ECG, oximetry, and capnography.
- Reassure the patient.
- Consider antiemetics or pain-control measures. Migraine headaches typically are accompanied by nausea and vomiting. Antiemetic medications, such as ondansetron (Zofran), have proven effective in treating headache-associated nausea and vomiting. Some medications will terminate specific headache types (primarily migraine). Generally, these are ergot derivatives or sumatriptan (Imitrex). Sumatriptan causes cerebral vasoconstriction and mitigates or terminates a migraine headache in certain patients. If these agents fail, then small doses of analgesics should be considered.
- Ensure a calm, quiet environment. Dimming the interior ambulance lights will help comfort the headache patient with photosensitivity.
- Transport the patient to an emergency department.

Cranial Nerve Disorders

The 12 pairs of cranial nerves innervate parts of the head, neck, and trunk. The function of these nerves can be sensory (touch, pain, hearing, taste, sight, and smell) or motor. A cranial nerve disorder is one that affects the connection between the cranial nerve centers of the brain and the particular tissues innervated by those nerves. The signs and symptoms of cranial nerve disorders depend on the nerve involved. Some cranial nerve disorders are common, but most are rare. The two most common cranial nerve disorders encountered in emergency medicine are Bell's palsy and trigeminal neuralgia.

- ***Bell's palsy.*** **Bell's palsy** is a sudden, unilateral weakness or paralysis of the facial muscles. It is due to a dysfunction of the seventh cranial nerve (facial nerve). The facial nerve controls some of the facial muscles, innervates the salivary and tear glands, and allows the front portion of the tongue to detect taste. In most cases, the cause of Bell's palsy is unknown, but it has been associated with a herpes simplex virus infection. Initially, the patient develops pain behind the ear. This may occur over days and then is followed by the rapid development of unilateral facial muscle weakness. This is often alarming for the patient, and many will seek emergency care, fearing that the condition is a stroke. The patient may complain of the face feeling numb or heavy. However, sensation remains unaffected. Some patients are unable to close the eye on the affected side. They also blink less often, causing dryness of the eye (Figure 3-29). In some instances, Bell's palsy may interfere with the normal production of saliva and/or tears, thus causing a dry eye or dry mouth. The diagnosis is made based on the history and physical exam. Treatment sometimes includes the use of antiviral drugs. In most instances, Bell's palsy resolves completely without any residual deficits.
- ***Trigeminal neuralgia.*** Trigeminal neuralgia, also called *tic doloureux*, is an extremely painful disorder that affects the fifth cranial nerve (trigeminal nerve). The trigeminal nerve is responsible for sensation in the face. Although primarily a sensory nerve, it also has some motor functions (e.g., biting and chewing). The trigeminal nerve has three branches: the ophthalmic nerve, the maxillary nerve, and the mandibular nerve. The pain associated with trigeminal neuralgia arises from the nerve (Figure 3-30). It is usually a condition of older adults but can be seen at any age. The signs and symptoms of trigeminal neuralgia include painful electrical–shock-type spasms and pain in the

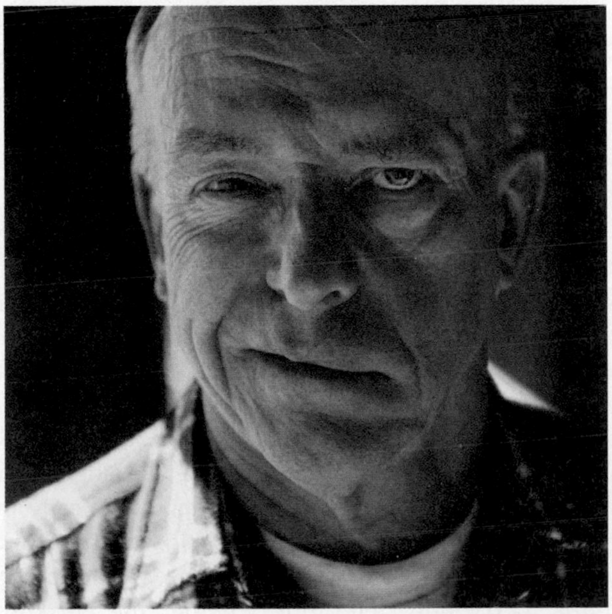

FIGURE 3-29 Bell's palsy.

(© Michal Heron)

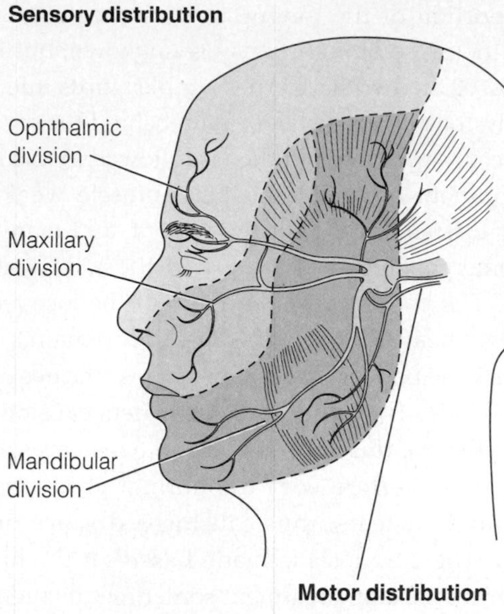

FIGURE 3-30 Trigeminal neuralgia.

distribution of the nerve. The pain is usually localized to one side of the face—often around the eyes, cheek, and lower part of the face. It is sometimes exacerbated by touch or loud sounds. Common activities of daily living, such as brushing one's teeth, chewing, or eating, can trigger trigeminal neuralgia. Trigeminal neuralgia tends to be a chronic condition. Various medications, especially antiseizure drugs, are used in treatment of this condition. In severe cases, surgery may be necessary.

"Weak and Dizzy"

A frequent problem that paramedics encounter is the patient who is "weak and dizzy" or "weak all over." Generalized weakness and dizziness, although vague, can be symptoms of many diseases. Furthermore, the feeling of being weak or the feeling of being dizzy can be quite disconcerting, especially to the elderly.

Assessment

Obtain a more detailed history of the illness. Has the patient ever had symptoms like this before? Has he had vomiting and/or diarrhea? Has there been a change in his medication regimen recently or has he taken a new medication in the past 72 hours?

Patients with weakness and/or dizziness should receive a focused assessment including a neurologic examination. Be alert for the presence of nystagmus (a constant, involuntary, cyclical motion of the eyeball), which can indicate a CNS or inner ear problem. Assess the various muscle groups to try and determine whether the weakness reported by the patient is localized or diffuse. Be alert for potential causes. These can be neurologic, respiratory, cardiovascular, endocrine, or infectious. Many viral illnesses will cause a feeling of malaise in the early stages. Inner ear infections (labyrinthitis) often will cause dizziness, especially with sudden movements of the head. Mild volume depletion (dehydration) can cause both weakness and dizziness. Sometimes the dizzy patient will become nauseated or may actually vomit.

Management

While assessing the patient, provide supportive care. This includes the following:

- Ensure scene safety.
- Establish and maintain an adequate airway.
- Place the patient in a position of comfort, generally with the head elevated. Avoid sudden or exaggerated movement of the head, as it can exacerbate symptoms.
- Administer supplemental oxygen to correct hypoxia. Avoid hyperoxia.
- Obtain IV access. Consider a fluid bolus if the patient appears dehydrated.
- Check the blood glucose level.
- Monitor the ECG, oximetry, and capnography.
- Consider the administration of an antiemetic. Often, antiemetics such as dimenhydrinate (Dramamine, Gravol) are helpful in treating dizziness and nausea. If the patient is nauseated or vomiting, consider ondansetron (Zofran) or a similar agent.
- Consider analgesic therapy with an opiate.
- Ensure a calm, quiet environment.
- Reassure the patient.
- Transport the patient to an emergency department.

Neoplasms

Brain and spinal cord tumors are abnormal growths of tissue found inside the skull or the bony spinal column. The term **neoplasm** is used to describe the new growth of a tumor (as contrasted to those present at birth, known as congenital tumors). Neoplasms that affect the central nervous system occur in 40,000 Americans per year.

Neurologic neoplasms can be divided into two main categories. *Benign* (noncancerous) *tumors* are composed of cells that grow similarly to normal cells, grow relatively slowly, and are confined to one location. *Malignant* (cancerous) *tumors* are those with growth very different from that of normal cells. They grow quickly and spread easily to other sites within the body.

Benign neoplasms in most parts of the body are not particularly harmful. Such tumors within the brain or spinal cord, however, pose a greater threat. Because the nervous system is contained within the rigid confines of the skull and spinal column, abnormal growth can place pressure on tissues and impair function. Any tumor located near any of the vital structures of the brain may seriously threaten the ability to breathe, move, or regulate other bodily functions.

Malignant tumors in most parts of the body have a tendency to spread, or *metastasize.* Most brain tumors are metastases from cancer that started somewhere else in the body. For example, breast cancers often metastasize to the brain. These metastases can grow in a single area of the brain or in several areas. However, tumors that originate in the brain or spinal cord rarely spread to other sites in the body. There are numerous types of brain tumors, which must be diagnosed in a medical facility through the use of CT or MRI scan. The cause of most tumors—and most cancers—remains poorly understood (Figure 3-31).

Assessment

Central nervous system neoplasms present with many signs and symptoms. The clinical manifestations a patient exhibits will depend on the size, type, and location of the tumor. As a paramedic, it is not your role to diagnose such new tumors. Instead, you will likely be called to care for someone with a previously diagnosed tumor. Or perhaps you will be asked to assess a patient with one or more of these common signs and symptoms of a neoplasm:

- Headache (often severe and recurring frequently)
- New seizures in an adult with no history of a seizure disorder
- Nausea
- Vomiting
- Behavioral or cognitive changes
- Weakness or paralysis of one or more limbs or a side of the face
- Change in sensation of one or more limbs or a side of the face
- Lack of coordination
- Difficulty walking or unsteady gait
- Dizziness
- Double vision

Be alert for any of the classic signs and symptoms of a brain or spinal cord tumor. Obtain a thorough medical history. In addition to the SAMPLE questions, ask about the following:

- What is the state of the patient's general health?
- Has the patient had any seizure activity, headache, or nosebleed?
- Ask about the type and timing of prior treatment, such as:
  - Surgery for removal of a tumor

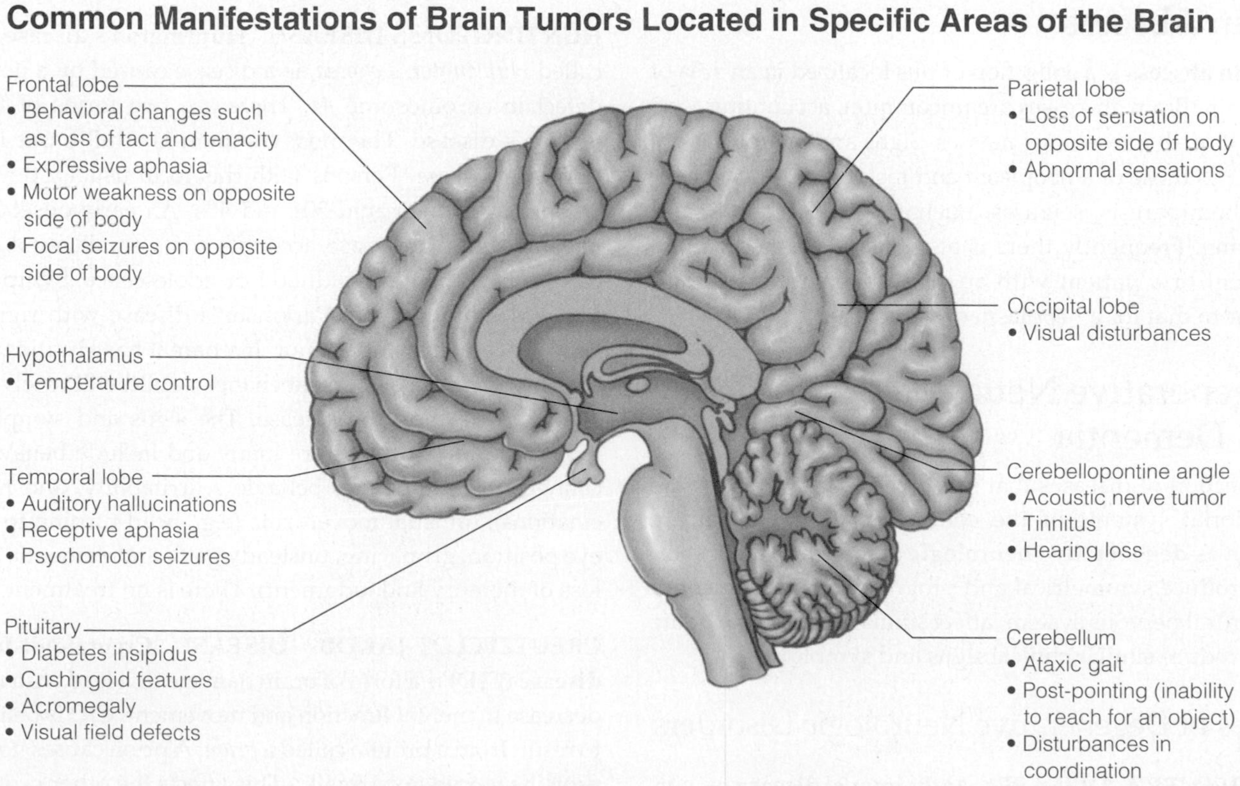

FIGURE 3-31 Locations and common manifestations of brain tumors.

- Chemotherapy
- Radiation therapy
- Holistic therapy
- Experimental treatments

Management

Treatment of a patient with a neoplasm is primarily supportive. You should attempt to alleviate the patient's anxiety and to reduce his symptoms. Field management of the patient with a neoplasm generally includes the following:

- Ensure scene safety.
- Establish and maintain an adequate airway.
- Place the patient in a position of comfort, generally with the head elevated.
- Administer supplemental oxygen to correct hypoxia. Assist ventilations when required.
- Obtain IV access.
- Monitor the ECG, oximetry, and capnography.
- Consider narcotic analgesia.
- Consider diazepam if seizure activity is present.
- Anti-inflammatories (dexamethasone) and diuretics may be requested by medical direction.
- Ensure a calm, quiet environment.
- Reassure the patient.
- Transport the patient to an emergency department.

Brain Abscess

A **brain abscess** is a collection of pus localized in an area of the brain. Brain abscesses are uncommon, accounting for 2 percent of all intracranial masses. Signs and symptoms are similar to those of a neoplasm and include headache, lethargy, hemiparesis, seizures, nuchal rigidity, nausea, and vomiting. Frequently there is also fever. Paramedic management of a patient with an abscess is supportive and similar to that for a neoplasm or meningitis.

Degenerative Neurologic Disorders and Dementia

A collection of diseases that selectively affect one or more functional systems of the central nervous system are known as **degenerative neurologic disorders**. They generally produce symmetrical and progressive involvement of the central nervous system, affect similar areas of the brain, and produce similar clinical signs and symptoms.

Types of Degenerative Neurologic Disorders

ALZHEIMER'S DISEASE **Alzheimer's disease** is perhaps the most important of all the degenerative neurologic disorders because of its frequent occurrence and devastating nature. It is the most common cause of dementia in the elderly. Alzheimer's disease results from death and disappearance of nerve cells in the cerebral cortex. This causes marked atrophy of the brain. Initially, patients will have problems with short-term memory. This will usually progress to problems with thought and intellect. The patient will develop a shuffling gait and will have stiffness of the body muscles. As the disease progresses, the patient will develop aphasia (inability to speak) and psychiatric disturbances. In the final stages the patient may become nearly decorticate, losing all ability to think, speak, and move.

PICK'S DISEASE **Pick's disease** is a permanent form of dementia that is similar to Alzheimer's disease. It differs from Alzheimer's in that it tends to affect only certain areas of the brain. People with Pick's disease have abnormal substances (called Pick bodies and Pick cells) inside the nerve cells in the damaged areas of the brain. These Pick bodies contain an abnormal form of a protein called tau. The exact cause of the disease is unknown, although it tends to occur in certain families. Pick's disease is rare. It can occur in people as young as 20, but usually begins between ages 40 and 60. People with Pick's disease tend to behave the wrong way in different social settings. The changes in behavior continue to get worse and are often one of the most disturbing symptoms of the disease. Some patients will have more prominent difficulty with decision making, complex tasks, or language (trouble finding or understanding words or writing). There is no specific treatment for Pick's disease.

HUNTINGTON'S DISEASE **Huntington's disease**, also called *Huntington's chorea,* is a disease caused by a genetic defect in chromosome #4. There are two forms of Huntington's disease. The most common is adult-onset Huntington's disease. Persons with this form usually develop symptoms in their mid-30s and 40s. An early-onset form of Huntington's disease accounts for a small number of cases and begins in childhood or adolescence. Symptoms may resemble those of Parkinson's disease with rigidity, slow movements, and tremor. If a parent has Huntington's disease, there is a 50 percent chance a child will receive the gene and develop the disease. The signs and symptoms of Huntington's disease are many and include behavioral changes (e.g., antisocial behaviors, irritability, and hallucinations), unusual movements (e.g., head turning to shift eye position, grimacing, unsteady gait), and dementia (e.g., loss of memory and judgment). There is no treatment.

CREUTZFELDT-JAKOB DISEASE **Creutzfeldt-Jakob disease (CJD)** is a form of brain damage that leads to a rapid decrease in mental function and movement. CJD is believed to result from a protein called a *prion*. A prion causes normal proteins to fold abnormally. This affects the other proteins' ability to function. CJD is very rare, occurring in about 1 out of 1 million people. It usually first appears between ages 20 and 70, with average age at onset of symptoms in the late 50s. Although classic CJD is not related to mad cow disease (bovine spongiform encephalitis), a new variant CJD (nvCJD) is an infectious form that *is* related to mad cow disease. The symptoms of CJD include dementia, ataxia, hallucinations, jerking, and general decline. CJD is rarely confused with other types of dementia (such as Alzheimer's disease), because in CJD, symptoms progress much more rapidly. There is no treatment.

MUSCULAR DYSTROPHY **Muscular dystrophy (MD)** refers to a group of genetic diseases characterized by progressive muscle weakness and degeneration of the skeletal or voluntary muscle fibers. The heart and other involuntary muscles are affected in some types of MD. There are several forms of MD, the most common of which is Duchenne. Some forms begin in childhood, whereas others do not appear until middle age. The prognosis of MD varies, depending on the type and progression of the disorder.

MULTIPLE SCLEROSIS **Multiple sclerosis (MS)** refers to an unpredictable disease of the central nervous system. MS involves inflammation of certain nerve cells followed by demyelination, or the destruction of the myelin sheath, which is the fatty insulation surrounding nerve fibers of the brain and spinal cord. When the myelin sheath is damaged, the nerves are unable to properly conduct impulses. An estimated 300,000 to 400,000 Americans are currently diagnosed with MS. Most MS sufferers are women and first experience symptoms between the ages of 20 and 40.

The disease is known to involve an autoimmune attack against myelin. Signs and symptoms include weakness of one or more limbs, sensory loss, paresthesias, and changes in vision. Symptoms can wax and wane over years, and range from mild to severe. Severe cases can be debilitating, rendering a patient unable to care for herself.

GUILLAIN-BARRÉ SYNDROME **Guillain-Barré syndrome** is a serious disorder that occurs when the body's defense (immune) system mistakenly attacks the peripheral nerves, leading to nerve inflammation that causes muscle weakness. It is an autoimmune disorder, but the exact triggering cause is unknown (although it often follows a minor infection). It can occur at any age, but is most common in people of both sexes between ages 30 and 50. The signs and symptoms of Guillain-Barré can get worse very quickly and include muscle weakness or paralysis. In most cases, the muscle weakness starts in the legs and then spreads to the arms (ascending paralysis). Mechanical ventilation is often required. There is no cure for Guillain-Barré syndrome. However, many treatments are available to help reduce symptoms, treat complications, and speed recovery.

DYSTONIAS The **dystonias** are a group of disorders characterized by muscle contractions that cause twisting and repetitive movements, abnormal postures, or freezing in the middle of an action. Such movements are involuntary and sometimes painful. They may affect a single muscle, a group of muscles, or the entire body.

Early symptoms of dystonia include a deterioration in handwriting, foot cramps, or a tendency of one foot to drag after walking or running. These initial symptoms can be mild and may be noticeable only after prolonged exertion, stress, or fatigue. In many cases, they become more noticeable and widespread over time. In other individuals, there is little or no progression.

PARKINSON'S DISEASE **Parkinson's disease** belongs to a group of conditions known as motor system disorders. James Parkinson, a British physician who published a paper on what he called "the shaking palsy," first described the disease in 1817. In his paper, Dr. Parkinson described the major symptoms of the disease that would later bear his name. Since then, scientists have been searching diligently for a cause and subsequent cure.

In the 1960s, researchers identified that a naturally occurring chemical crucial to muscle activity, dopamine, is lower in victims of Parkinson's. This discovery led to the first successful treatment of the disease.

Today, more than a half million Americans are affected with Parkinson's, with more than 50,000 new cases being reported every year. It affects men and women in almost equal numbers and it knows no social, economic, or geographic boundaries. The average age of onset is 60 years and it usually does not occur in patients less than 40 years old.

Parkinson's is a chronic and progressive disorder. It has four main characteristics:

- ***Tremor.*** Sometimes called "pill rolling," the typical tremor is a rhythmic back-and-forth motion of the thumb and forefinger. It usually begins in the hand and may progress to an arm, a foot, or the jaw.
- ***Rigidity.*** Most Parkinson's patients suffer rigidity, or resistance to movement. All muscles have an opposing muscle. In the healthy adult, one muscle contracts while the opposing muscle relaxes. In Parkinson's, the balance of this opposition is disturbed, leading to rigidity.
- ***Bradykinesia.*** Normal, spontaneous, and autonomic movement is slowed and sometimes lost. Such loss of movement is unpredictable. One moment the patient can move easily, and the next moment he cannot.
- ***Postural instability.*** Impaired balance and coordination cause patients to develop a forward or backward lean, stooped posture, and the tendency to fall easily.

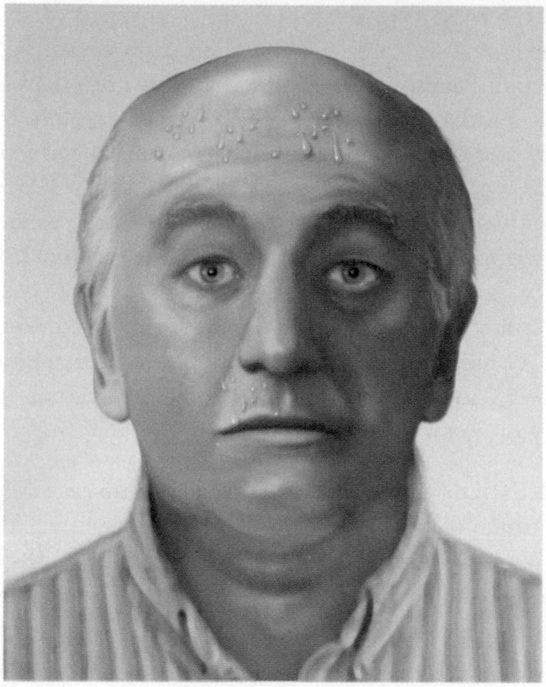

FIGURE 3-32 Typical facial appearance of a patient with Parkinson's disease.

Parkinson's patients may also be plagued with depression, a slowing or "shuffling" gait, a stiff or "stonelike" face, and dementia (Figure 3-32).

CENTRAL PAIN SYNDROME **Central pain syndrome** is a condition that results from damage or injury to the brain, brainstem, or spinal cord. It is characterized by intense, steady pain described as burning, aching, tingling, or a "pins and needles" sensation. The syndrome may develop weeks, months, or years after an injury to the CNS. It occurs in patients who have had strokes, multiple sclerosis, limb amputations, or spinal cord injuries. Pain medications generally provide no relief for victims of central pain syndrome. Patients rely on sedation and other methods to keep the central nervous system free from stress.

AMYOTROPHIC LATERAL SCLEROSIS **Amyotrophic lateral sclerosis (ALS)**, also known as Lou Gehrig's disease, is a progressive degeneration of specific nerve cells that control voluntary movement. Characterized by weakness, loss of motor control, difficulty speaking, and cramping, the disease eventually weakens the diaphragm, which leads to breathing problems. ALS belongs to a class of disorders known as motor neuron diseases. It affects 20,000 Americans, with 5,000 new cases being reported each year.

There is currently no cure for ALS. There is also no effective therapy. However, the FDA has approved riluzole, the first drug that has been shown to prolong the lives of ALS patients. The prognosis continues to be poor. Most patients die within 3 to 5 years of being diagnosed, usually as a result of pulmonary infection.

MYOCLONUS **Myoclonus** is a term that refers to the temporary, involuntary twitching or spasm of a muscle or group of muscles. It is generally considered not a diagnosis, but a symptom. It is usually one of several symptoms of a variety of nervous system disorders such as multiple sclerosis, Parkinson's, or Alzheimer's. Some simple examples of myoclonus include hiccups or muscle twitching. Pathologic myoclonus can distort normal movement and limit a person's ability to eat, walk, and talk.

Treatment of myoclonus consists of medications to reduce symptoms. Many of these drugs are also used to treat epilepsy, such as barbiturates, clonazepam, phenytoin, and sodium valproate.

SPINA BIFIDA **Spina bifida (SB)** is a neural defect that results from the failure of one or more of the fetal vertebrae to close properly during pregnancy. This leaves a portion of the spinal cord unprotected. The spinal opening can usually be repaired shortly after birth, but the nerve damage is permanent. Long-term effects include physical and mobility impairments, and most individuals also have some form of learning disability. The three most common types of SB are:

- *Myelomeningocele*—the severest form, in which the spinal cord and the meninges protrude from an opening in the spine.
- *Meningocele*—characterized by the normal development of the spinal cord, but the meninges protrude through a spinal opening.
- *Occulta*—the mildest form, in which one or more vertebrae are malformed and covered by a layer of skin.

There is currently no cure for spina bifida. Treatment includes surgery, medications, and physiotherapy. With proper care, most children with SB live into adulthood.

POLIOMYELITIS **Poliomyelitis (polio)** is an infectious, inflammatory viral disease of the central nervous system that sometimes results in permanent paralysis. It is characterized by fatigue, headache, fever, vomiting, stiffness of the neck, and pain to the hands and feet. New cases in the United States are rare. A vaccine developed in the 1950s caused the number of cases to decline from 50,000 to only a few per year. Thousands of prevaccine survivors of the disease are alive today. Many of these patients require supportive care.

Assessment of Degenerative Neurologic Disorders

When you encounter a patient with a degenerative neurologic disorder, use your assessment and history-taking skills to determine the patient's chief complaint. You may be called to treat someone with an exacerbation (flare-up) of one of the degenerative diseases, or someone with an unrelated complaint. In either case, it is important to conduct a primary assessment, correct any life-threatening problems, and find out exactly what prompted the call to EMS.

Management of Degenerative Neurologic Disorders

When caring for a patient with a degenerative neurologic disease, make treating the chief complaint a priority. Do not overlook the patient's underlying condition, but do not allow it to cloud a more serious problem. After performing a primary assessment and managing any life-threatening conditions, manage the chief complaint. While providing care, consider the following about patients who suffer from a degenerative neurologic disorder:

- ***Mobility.*** The ability to walk and move about freely is often taken for granted by many of us. Neurologic patients often lack this ability and require assistance.
- ***Communication.*** Certain neurologic disorders will affect a patient's ability to speak clearly and distinctly. Take the necessary time to ensure open communication. Speak with bystanders and family members to assist in gaining a thorough history.
- ***Respiratory compromise.*** Exacerbations of ALS and other conditions may affect the ability to breathe. Treat any breathing problem as a priority.
- ***Anxiety.*** Coping with a debilitating disease is a strenuous and taxing task. Dealing with the ongoing battles with a neurologic condition will cause stress—and anxiety. Approach the patient and his family with compassion and care.

The following steps may be appropriate, depending on the patient's chief complaint:

- Determine the patient's blood glucose level. A serum glucose determination will assist in determining whether an altered mental status is due to hypoglycemia.
- Obtain IV access.
- Monitor the ECG.
- Transport the patient to an emergency department.

Back Pain and Nontraumatic Spinal Disorders

Back pain is one of the most common reasons that people seek health care. Millions and millions of health care dollars are spent each year on the treatment of back pain. Back pain can be classified as either traumatic or nontraumatic in origin. Many patients will develop chronic back pain. Chronic back pain is a significant cause of disability and lost time from work. EMS is often called to treat persons with back pain. These calls can be due to a new injury or exacerbation of chronic back pain. In addition, some patients will develop back pain without an identifiable injury.

Low Back Pain

Back pain can be felt anywhere along the spinal column. However, low back pain (LBP) is the most common back pain complaint. It is a common, yet debilitating, condition. Low back pain is defined as back pain felt between the lower rib cage and the gluteal muscles, often radiating to the thighs.

Both chronic and new-onset low back pain are increasingly common. This complaint of low back pain is the cause of a great amount of lost work time in the United States. Between 60 and 90 percent of the population experience some form of low back pain at some time in their life. Men and women are equally affected, although women over 60 years of age report low back pain symptoms more often, most likely as a result of postmenopausal osteoporosis. Occupations that involve exposure to vibrations from vehicles or machinery and those that require repetitious lifting are often implicated in low back pain. As a paramedic, you yourself are particularly at risk for back problems.

About 1 percent of acute low back pain results from sciatica, which causes severe pain along the path of the sciatic nerve, down the back of the thigh and inner leg. This is sometimes accompanied by motor and sensory deficits, such as muscle weakness. Sciatica may be caused by compression or trauma to the sciatic nerve or its roots, often resulting from a herniated intervertebral disk or osteoarthritis of the lumbosacral vertebrae. It may also be caused by inflammation of the sciatic nerve from metabolic, toxic, or infectious causes.

Pain occurring at the level of L-3, L-4, L-5, and S-1 may be due to inflammation of the interspinous bursae. Low back pain may also result from inflammation or sprains or strains of the muscles and ligaments that attach to the spine or from vertebral fractures. Additional causes of back pain include tumors, inflammation of the synovial sacs, rising venous pressure, degenerative joint disease, abnormal bone pressure, problems with spinal mobility, and inflammation caused by infection (osteomyelitis).

In fact, however, most low back pain is idiopathic. That is, the cause may be difficult or impossible to diagnose, even by a physician or in a hospital setting. This makes treatment of many cases of low back pain frustrating and sometimes unsuccessful.

Causes of Nontraumatic Spinal Disorders and Back Pain

Spinal problems may be caused by trauma, but many spinal disorders have nontraumatic causes. Nontraumatic spinal injuries most often result from three causes:

- Degeneration or rupture of the disks that separate the vertebrae
- Degeneration or fracture of the vertebrae
- Cyst or tumor that impinges on the spine

The type and degree of pain that results from these conditions differs from person to person.

DISK INJURY The cartilaginous disks that separate the vertebrae may rupture as a result of injury or may rupture or degenerate as part of the process of aging. Degeneration may cause a narrowing of the disk that compromises spinal stability. Degenerative disk disease is more common in patients over 50 years of age.

A herniated disk occurs when the gelatinous center of the disk (the *nucleus pulposa*) extrudes through a tear in the tough outer capsule (the *anulus fibrosa*). The pain that results from these conditions usually results from pressure on the spinal cord or muscle spasm at the site. The intervertebral disks themselves have no innervation. Herniation may be caused by degenerative disk disease, trauma, or improper lifting. Improper lifting is the most common cause. Men aged 30 to 50 years are more prone to disk herniation than women. Herniation most commonly affects the disks at L-4, L-5, and S-1 but may also occur in C-5, C-6, and C-7.

VERTEBRAL INJURY The vertebrae themselves may break down (vertebral spondylolysis), especially the lamina or vertebral arch between the articulating facets (the areas where adjoining vertebrae contact one another). Heredity is thought to be a significant factor in the development of spondylolysis. Rotational fractures are common at these sites. Spinal fractures are frequently associated with osteoporosis (brittle bones), which tends to develop in many elderly persons.

CYSTS AND TUMORS A cyst or tumor along the spine or intruding into the spinal canal may cause pain by pressing on the spinal cord, by causing degenerative changes in the bone, or by interrupting blood supply. The specific manifestations depend on the location and type of cyst or tumor.

***CAUDA EQUINA* SYNDROME** *Cauda equina* **syndrome** is caused by a significant narrowing of the spinal canal that compresses the nerve roots below the level of the spinal cord (in the *cauda equina*). Numerous causes of *cauda equina* syndrome have been identified. These include trauma, disk herniation, spinal stenosis, spinal tumors (neoplasms), inflammation, infection (e.g., epidural abscess), and similar causes (e.g., spinal surgery).

The signs and symptoms of *cauda equina* syndrome include:

- Low back pain
- Unilateral or bilateral leg pain:
  - Localized back pain (due to swelling or infection)
  - Radicular symptoms (sciatica)
- Numbness/anesthesia in the groin or perineal region (saddle anesthesia)
- Bowel and/or bladder disturbances:
  - Incontinence
  - Hesitancy
  - Decreased sensation when urinating
  - Inability to urinate
  - Constipation
  - Loss of rectal tone
- Diminished lower extremity reflexes
- Lower extremity muscle weakness and loss of sensations

Cauda equina syndrome is a neurologic emergency. Prompt decompressive surgery is often necessary to avoid permanent injury to the *cauda equina* and associated structures.[14]

OTHER MEDICAL CAUSES Back pain can also be caused by medical conditions associated with neither traumatic nor nontraumatic spinal injury. For example, back pain may manifest as referred pain from disorders such as diabetic neuropathy, renal calculus, abdominal aortic aneurysm, and many other conditions, such as those discussed in this chapter. It would be a mistake to assume that all back complaints are related to the spinal cord, the vertebrae, the intervertebral disks, or the muscles and ligaments surrounding the vertebrae.

Assessment

Assessment of back pain is based on the patient's chief complaint, the history, and the physical exam. When the complaint is low back pain, a precise diagnosis is likely to be difficult. The preliminary diagnosis may be based on a history of risk factors, such as an occupation requiring repetitive lifting, exposure to vibrations from vehicles or industrial machinery, or a known history of osteoporosis.

The complaint of low back pain often involves radiation of the pain from the gluteus to the thigh, leg, and foot. Usually there is a history of slow onset over several weeks to months and the patient has called for your help secondary to an increase in pain and the lack of relief from warm compresses or over-the-counter analgesics. The patient may or may not recall a particular incident that has caused this "low back pain"; direct trauma is rarely a contributing factor in this type of pain.

Just because low back pain is a common complaint that can be hard to diagnose, do not dismiss this type of complaint as "not real pain." A complete history and physical exam by a physician are necessary to determine the cause of any back pain. Diagnosis will often depend on the results of a CT or MRI scan, electromyelography, or other in-hospital testing.

In the prehospital setting, the important task is to determine whether the patient's pain is caused by a life-threatening or a non-life-threatening condition. A good patient history will help in this determination. A history of work or play involving lifting or twisting and a sudden onset of pain, often associated with straining, coughing, or sneezing, may point to a mechanical type of muscle or ligament injury. A gradual onset of pain may point instead to a chronic condition such as degenerative disk disease or tumor development. The presence of an associated neurologic deficit may also point to a more serious underlying cause. When the complaint is back pain, be sure to inquire about prior back surgery, physical therapy, and time lost from work.

Location of the injury may be revealed by a limited range of motion in the lumbar spine; tenderness on palpation at the location of the injury; alterations in sensation, pain, and temperature at the site; and pain or paresthesia below the injury (in the upper extremities with cervical injury, symptoms increasing with neck motion, with possible slight motor weakness in the biceps and triceps; similar symptoms in the lower extremities with injury to the thoracic or lumbar spine).

Keep in mind that you are very unlikely to be able to determine the cause of your patient's back pain in the field. Primarily, you need to gather information from the history and physical exam that you will report to the receiving physician and that will help you determine what degree of immobilization, if any, will be necessary during transport.

Management

Prehospital management of back pain is aimed primarily at decreasing any pain or discomfort caused by moving the patient and keeping a watchful eye for signs and symptoms of any serious underlying disorder.

Should cervical spine stabilization measures be taken with the patient complaining of back pain? Should this patient be immobilized to a long backboard or a vacuum-type stretcher? These questions are best answered, "Generally not." First you must consider trauma as a possible cause of the patient's pain. If there is no recent mechanism of injury, consider whether the patient has a possible history of osteoporosis or another disease that might lead to spinal fracture. In these cases, consider immobilizing the patient.

If trauma and possible fracture are ruled out, you may still undertake C-spine precautions and immobilization, because the less movement a patient is put through, the more comfortable he will feel. Long-board or vacuum-stretcher immobilization may be the best mode of transportation. If in doubt, immobilize, remembering the injunction to "do no harm."

Some patients with back pain and back spasms may require parenteral analgesics and parenteral diazepam before they can even lie on the stretcher. Contact medical direction regarding analgesic and muscle relaxant therapy.

Conduct ongoing assessment en route with special attention to the airway, breathing, vital signs, and the possible presence or development of motor and sensory deficits that may indicate a critical condition and that can adversely affect the patient's breathing effort.

Summary

The nervous system can be thought of as the complex system of computer processors (central nervous system) and wiring (peripheral nervous system) that are responsible for the entirety of body functions. When an abnormality occurs in either the processor or the wiring, signs and symptoms will include a reduced ability or inability to complete a task or function that otherwise would normally occur.

Remember that the brain is the control center for all functions of the body. Whenever there is an interruption in blood supply to any part of the brain, the result will be an inability to perform the associated function or functions. Therein lies the reason that EMS personnel should know the 12 cranial nerves—or, at a minimum, how to assess each one. A thorough neurologic assessment of all 12 cranial nerves helps to quickly identify abnormalities and even the specific area of the brain that has been affected.

You will respond to neurologic emergencies varying from headaches to seizures and strokes. In all neurologic emergencies, it is imperative to address airway and oxygenation first, followed closely by a general assessment, making sure to use the diagnostic tools you have available.

Keep in mind that the brain is largely powered by glucose and oxygen. If the level of either of these becomes altered, the patient is likely to present with neurologic symptoms. Therefore, your first assessment tools should include blood glucose assessment and pulse oximetry. Always treat hypoglycemia in neurologically impaired patients, because often hypoglycemia is the cause and is easily corrected with dextrose.

Neurologic emergencies often present with an altered level of consciousness up to and including coma. Rapid identification and treatment of the possible causes (AEIOU-TIPS) with rapid transport to the closest appropriate facility is imperative. For neurologic impairment (especially for stroke), treatment is very time sensitive (definitive treatment must occur within 4.5 hours from onset). Rapid treatment is essential for the best possible outcomes.

To summarize: Whether you are treating a possible stroke, seizures, coma, or headache, your treatment must remain focused on assessing and maintaining the patient's airway, oxygen, and glucose levels. Rapid identification and early notification to your receiving facility are key in achieving successful recovery from strokes and other neurologic impairments.

Often, your care for the neurologic patient may simply be supportive, but in other cases, you will need to provide drug therapy or other interventions to limit or reduce the presenting symptoms. In every case, airway management remains your priority.

You Make the Call

You and your partner are called to 222 East 19th Street on an unknown medical problem. Dispatch reports that the call came from a neighbor and further information is not available.

On arrival at the scene, you find a 64-year-old woman sitting upright in a chair, complaining of a "terrible headache." As you begin to interview the patient, you discover that she is having difficulty breathing and has slurred speech. Your partner interviews the neighbor and the patient's niece, who has just arrived.

While you are taking the patient's pulse, the niece reports that her aunt is usually alert and able to speak complete sentences. Her blood pressure is 190/110 mmHg, pulse 90, and respiratory rate 18 breaths per minute. Blood glucose level is 92 mg/dL. SpO_2 is 97 percent on room air.

En route to the hospital, the patient sits up slightly and says, "I am feeling much better now." She reports that her headache has dissipated, and you notice that her speech is no longer slurred.

1. Based on the clinical symptoms present, what might be wrong with this patient?
2. What would account for the quickly dissipating symptoms?
3. What is the priority in managing this patient's care?
4. What are the appropriate steps in caring for this patient?

See Suggested Responses at the back of this book.

Review Questions

1. The sympathetic and parasympathetic nervous systems are two divisions of the __________
   a. central nervous system.
   b. automatic nervous system.
   c. autonomic nervous system.
   d. peripheral nervous system.
2. What is the neurotransmitter of the parasympathetic and voluntary (somatic) nervous systems?
   a. Acetylcholine
   b. Epinephrine
   c. Norepinephrine
   d. Dopamine

3. The innermost layer of meninges, directly overlying the central nervous system, is called the ____________
   a. pia mater.
   b. dura mater.
   c. arachnoid membrane.
   d. cerebrospinal membrane.

4. The area that is responsible for many involuntary actions such as temperature regulation, sleep, water balance, stress response, and emotions is the ________
   a. cerebrum.
   b. diencephalon.
   c. cerebral cortex.
   d. mesencephalon.

5. Which afferent nerves transmit sensations involved in touch, pressure, pain, temperature, and position (proprioception)?
   a. Somatic motor
   b. Somatic sensory
   c. Visceral motor
   d. Visceral sensory

6. Which clinical finding is the hallmark sign of central nervous system (CNS) injury or illness?
   a. Elevated heart rate
   b. Altered mental status
   c. Elevated blood pressure
   d. Diminished pulse oximetry value

7. A patient's ability to smile, frown, and wrinkle his forehead indicates an intact cranial nerve ____________
   a. IV.
   b. V.
   c. VI.
   d. VII.

8. What is the name for the respiratory pattern characterized by ineffective thoracic muscular coordination and inadequate air exchange?
   a. Ataxic respirations
   b. Apneustic respiration
   c. Kussmaul's respirations
   d. Cheyne-Stokes respirations

9. Which of the following is not included in the changes that characterize Cushing's triad?
   a. Decreased pulse
   b. Decreased body temperature
   c. Irregular respirations
   d. Increased blood pressure

10. Which pathology is the third most common cause of death in middle-aged and older patients?
    a. Cancer
    b. Strokes
    c. Diabetes
    d. Epilepsy

11. Which type of stroke often occurs at night and is characterized by a patient awakening with altered mental status and/or loss of speech, sensory, or motor function?
    a. Embolic
    b. Occlusive
    c. Thrombotic
    d. Hemorrhagic

12. In a child, a seizure characterized by a 10- to 30-second loss of consciousness or awareness, eye or muscle fluttering, and an occasional loss of muscle tone is known as what type of seizure?
    a. Absence
    b. Tonic–clonic
    c. Grand mal
    d. Simple partial

13. Which of the following headaches is a type of vascular headache?
    a. Tension
    b. Migraine
    c. Organic
    d. Throbbing

14. What was first described in 1817 and called "the shaking palsy"?
    a. Dystonia disorder
    b. Muscular dystrophy
    c. Parkinson's disease
    d. Alzheimer's disease

15. Most low back pain is ____________
    a. felt between the ribs and the waist.
    b. a result of sciatica.
    c. caused by inflammation of interspinous bursae.
    d. idiopathic.

16. You have a patient with an altered mental status secondary to a hypoglycemic episode. What would be the correct dose of dextrose for this situation?
    a. 2 g/kg
    b. 50 mg
    c. 25 g
    d. 50 mcg

17. A patient who is suspected to be alcoholic has an altered mental status. For this patient, the first intravenous medication would most likely be __________
    a. oxygen.
    b. thiamine.
    c. solumedrol.
    d. naloxone.
18. Which scale has been found most reliable for detecting a stroke in the prehospital environment?
    a. Chicago Stroke Scale
    b. Cincinnati Prehospital Stroke Scale
    c. Lewisburg Prehospital Stroke Scale
    d. Los Angeles Prehospital Stroke Screen
19. What would be the primary medication for stopping a seizure in an epileptic patient who has not taken his medications for several weeks?
    a. Diazepam
    b. Oxygen
    c. Midazoline
    d. Thiamine
20. The initial dose of diazepam for a patient with seizures would most likely be __________
    a. 2 mg.
    b. 5 mg.
    c. 8 mg.
    d. 12 mg.

See Answers to Review Questions at the back of this book.

References

1. Lloyd-Jones, D. M., Y. Hong, D. Labarthe, et al. "Defining and Setting National Goals for Cardiovascular Health Promotion and Disease Reduction: The American Heart Association's Strategic Impact Goal through 2020 and Beyond." *Circulation* 121 (2010): 586–613.
2. Epilepsy Foundation. 2011. http://www.epilepsyfoundation.org/about/statistics.cfm.
3. Parkinson's Disease Foundation 2016. Available at http://www.pdf.org/en/parkinson_statistics.
4. Brain Trauma Foundation. "Guidelines for the Prehospital Management of Traumatic Brain Injury, Second Edition." *Prehosp Emerg Care* 12 (2007): 1 (Supplement).
5. Jauch, E. C., B. Cucchiara, O. Adeoye, et al. "Part 11: Adult Stroke: 2010 American Heart Association Guidelines for Cardiopulmonary Resuscitation and Emergency Cardiovascular Care." *Circulation* 122 (2010): S818–S828.
6. Kidwell, C. S., J. L. Saver, G. B. Schubert, et al. "Design and Retrospective Analysis of the Los Angeles Prehospital Stroke Screen (LAPSS)." *Prehosp Emerg Care* 2(4) (1998): 267–273.
7. Kothari, R. U., A. Panicioli, T. Liu, et al. "Cincinnati Prehospital Stroke Scale: Reproducibility and Validity." *Ann Emerg Med* 33 (1999): 373–378.
8. Evenson, K. R., R. E. Foraker, D. L. Morris, and W. D. Rosamond. "A Comprehensive Review of Prehospital and In-Hospital Delay Times in Acute Stroke Care." *Int J Stroke* 4 (2009): 187–199.
9. Cucchiara, B. and M. Ross. "Transient IschemicAttack: Risk Stratification and Treatment." *Ann Emerg Med* 52 (2008): S27–S39.
10. De La Morandiere, K. P. and D. Walter. "Oxygen Therapy in Acute Stroke." *Emerg Med J* 20 (2003): 547.
11. Rønning, O. M. and B. Guldvog. "Should Stroke Victims Routinely Receive Supplemental Oxygen? A Quasi-Randomized Controlled Trial." *Stroke* 30 (1999): 2033–2037.
12. Michael, G. E. T. and R. E. O'Connor. "The Diagnosis and Management of Seizures and Status Epilepticus in the Prehospital Setting." *Emerg Med Clin North Am* 29 (2011): 29–39.
13. Friedman, B. W. and B. M. Grosberg. "Diagnosis and Management of the Primary Headache Disorders in the Emergency Department Setting." *Emerg Med Clin North Am* 27 (2009): 71–87.
14. Winters, M. E., P. Kleutz, and J. Zilbersten. "Back Pain Emergencies." *Med Clin North Am* 90 (2006): 503–523.

Further Reading

Brunner, L., et al. *Brunner and Suddarth's Textbook of Medical-Surgical Nursing.* 13th ed. Philadelphia: Lippincott Williams and Wilkins, 2013.

Fauci, A. S., et al. *Harrison's Principles of Internal Medicine.* 19th ed. New York: McGraw-Hill, 2013.

Guyton, A. C. and J. E. Hall. *Textbook of Medical Physiology.* 14th ed. Philadelphia: W. B. Saunders, 2013.

Limmer, D., M. F. O'Keefe, E. T. Dickinson, et al. *Emergency Care.* 12th ed. Fire Service Edition. Upper Saddle River, NJ: Pearson/Prentice Hall, 2011.

Martini, F. H., E. F. Bartholomew, and B. E. Bledsoe. *Anatomy and Physiology for Emergency Care.* 2nd ed. Upper Saddle River, NJ: Pearson/Prentice Hall, 2008.

Stone, C. K. and R. L. Humphries. *Current Emergency Diagnosis and Treatment.* 7th ed. New York: McGraw-Hill, 2011.

Tintanelli, J. E., et al. *Emergency Medicine: A Comprehensive Study Guide.* 7th ed. New York: McGraw-Hill, 2011.

2015 American Heart Association Guidelines for Cardiopulmonary Resuscitation and Emergency Care, *Circulation* 132 supp. 2) 2015, October 15, 2015. Available at http://circ.ahajournals.org/content/132/18_suppl_2/S444.full.

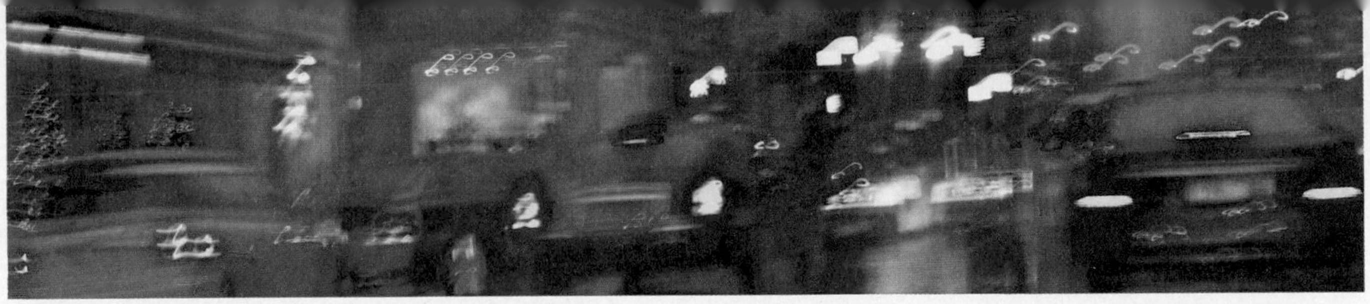

Chapter 4
Endocrinology

Bryan Bledsoe, DO, FACEP, FAAEM, EMT-P

STANDARD
Medicine (Endocrine Disorders)

COMPETENCY
Integrates assessment findings with principles of epidemiology and pathophysiology to formulate a field impression and implement a comprehensive treatment/disposition plan for a patient with a medical complaint.

Learning Objectives

Terminal Performance Objective: After reading this chapter, you should be able to integrate patient assessment findings, patient history, and knowledge of anatomy, physiology, pathophysiology, and basic and advanced life support interventions to recognize and manage patients with endocrine disorders.

Enabling Objectives: To accomplish the terminal performance objective, you should be able to:

1. Define key terms introduced in this chapter.
2. Review the anatomy and physiology of the endocrine system.
3. Explain the general pathophysiological changes of endocrine emergencies, and relate this to disturbances in normal endocrine physiology.
4. Adapt the scene size-up, primary assessment, history, secondary assessment, and use of monitoring technology to arrive at a field impression and differential diagnoses for endocrine emergencies.
5. Use a process of clinical reasoning to guide and interpret the patient assessment findings and develop a treatment plan for patients with endocrine disorders in the prehospital environment.
6. Given a variety of scenarios, describe the integration of assessment and management guidelines as they relate to endocrine emergencies.

KEY TERMS

Addison's disease, p. 257
Addisonian crisis, p. 258
anabolism, p. 248
autonomic nervous system, p. 240
catabolism, p. 248
Cushing's disease, p. 257
Cushing's syndrome, p. 257
diabetes insipidus, p. 243
diabetes mellitus, p. 247
diabetic ketoacidosis, p. 250
diuresis, p. 249
endocrine gland, p. 239
exocrine gland, p. 239
gluconeogenesis, p. 245
glycogenolysis, p. 245
glycosuria, p. 249
Graves' disease, p. 255
homeostasis, p. 239
hormone, p. 239
hyperglycemia, p. 248
hyperglycemic hyperosmolar nonketotic coma (HHNK), p. 252
hyperosmolar hyperglycemic state (HHS), p. 252
hyperthyroidism, p. 255
hypoglycemia, p. 248
hypoglycemic seizure, p. 255
hypothyroidism, p. 255
ketone bodies, p. 248
ketosis, p. 248
metabolism, p. 239
myxedema, p. 255
myxedema coma, p. 256
osmotic diuresis, p. 249
thyrotoxic crisis, p. 256
thyrotoxicosis, p. 255

Case Study

Shauna White and Steve Curran leave the hospital after the Quarterly Trauma Case Conference and notify dispatch that they are in service and en route to quarters. Within minutes, they receive a dispatch call for an unknown medical emergency in a nearby residential neighborhood. The response time is less than 3 minutes. They park the unit in front of the house and take Standard Precautions. As Steve removes the stretcher and jump kit from the back of the unit, a police cruiser pulls up to the curb. The officers intercept Steve and Shauna, explaining that they were dispatched after someone called 911 to report the sounds of a possible altercation in the home.

At that moment, a woman walks up and identifies herself as Mrs. Spencer, the 911 caller. She says that she was in her garden when she heard loud sounds suddenly coming from the McKenzies' house next door. She says she was alarmed because the noise lasted for only a short time, but it sounded like items were being thrown or broken. Moreover, she knows that Mr. McKenzie is traveling out of town. Mrs. McKenzie left the house about an hour before the noise occurred. At the moment, however, all is quiet.

The officers caution Steve, Shauna, and Mrs. Spencer to stand clear until they secure the scene. They approach the front door, identify themselves as police, and enter the house. In less than a minute, they call out "all clear," and summon the paramedics. Shauna and Steve quickly enter. In the living room, they see that the furniture in one corner has been overturned, and books and magazines are strewn about the floor. An officer crouches near an adolescent male who appears to be in his mid-teens. The boy is pale and diaphoretic. He looks confused as the officer speaks to him. His clothing is in disarray. Mrs. Spencer looks in from the open doorway and identifies the young man as Mark McKenzie.

Shauna's primary assessment reveals a 16-year-old male without airway compromise. He is breathing rapidly, but with good depth and volume. His carotid pulse is rapid and strong. Although the patient is conscious, he responds to Shauna with incoherent muttering. Steve quickly places a nonrebreather oxygen mask over the patient's face, and then he and Shauna move him onto the stretcher. His SpO_2 via pulse oximetry is 100 percent. One of the police officers says he will look around the scene for evidence of medications or illicit drugs.

Mark pulls the oxygen mask off and tries to get up and walk. Shauna replaces the mask and tries to reassure him. Finally, after he makes several more attempts to get up, Mark is gently restrained on the stretcher. Shauna begins a more detailed assessment while Steve looks for a vein to draw blood and start an intravenous line. He notes that Mark's skin is pale, cool, and clammy. Shauna observes no obvious injuries except a small bruise forming on the right cheek. In addition, she does not smell any unusual odors, such as alcohol or paint fumes. Mark is not wearing a MedicAlert tag. Shauna finds that Mark's blood pressure is 130/88 mmHg, his pulse is 120 beats per minute, and his respiratory rate is 28 breaths per minute. The oxygen saturation is 99 percent. No supplemental oxygen is then administered.

Prior to starting the IV line, Steve follows protocol, filling a red-top tube with blood and obtaining a sample for immediate determination of the blood glucose level. The portable glucose detection device reports the glucose level as "LOW." As Steve gives Shauna the information, the officer returns and tells them that he found a bottle of insulin in the refrigerator with Mark's name on the label.

Because hypoglycemia is potentially life threatening, Steve immediately administers 50 milliliters of 50 percent dextrose (25 grams) intravenously, per standing orders. Within minutes, Mark's skin becomes warm and dry, and he begins to speak more clearly. As Shauna prepares to contact medical direction prior to transporting Mark to the hospital for evaluation, his mother returns home. She says that Mark was diagnosed with diabetes at age 8 and it is usually well controlled, but his insulin dosage was recently changed. She thanks the team but says that she would prefer to contact Mark's physician, Dr. McGraw, directly rather than having Mark transported to the hospital. Shauna contacts medical direction and notifies them of the refusal of transport.

Steve aseptically discontinues Mark's IV while Shauna prepares the patient care report and transport refusal form for Mrs. McKenzie's signature. Before leaving the scene, Shauna reminds Mark and Mrs. McKenzie that they should not hesitate to call 911 again if they need help. She thanks the police officers for their assistance.

Introduction

The *endocrine system* is an important body system. Closely linked to the nervous system, it controls numerous physiologic processes. Unlike the nervous system, which exerts its control through nervous impulses, the endocrine system controls the body through specialized chemical messengers called **hormones**. The fundamental structural units of the endocrine system are the **endocrine glands**. Each endocrine gland produces one or more hormones. (An example of an endocrine gland is the pancreas. Specific endocrine glands will be described later. The endocrine glands are the chief focus of this chapter.)

Endocrine glands differ from other glands in that they are ductless. Instead of releasing hormones through ducts to a local site, they secrete their hormones directly into capillaries to circulate in the blood throughout the body. In contrast, the majority of glands are **exocrine glands**, which release their chemical products through ducts and tend to have a local effect. For example, the salivary glands are a type of exocrine gland. The salivary glands are located near the pharynx and secrete digestive enzymes, such as amylase, into the pharynx.

Keep in mind these important points about endocrine glands:

- In contrast to the exocrine glands, whose effects tend to be localized, endocrine glands tend to have widespread effects.
- The hormones released by endocrine glands typically act on distant tissues. They exert a very specific effect on their target tissues.
- Some hormones, such as insulin, have many target organs. Other hormones have only a few target organs.
- Through the release of hormones, the endocrine system plays an important role in regulating body function.

As noted, the principal product of an endocrine gland is a hormone. The term *hormone* comes from the Greek for "to set in motion," and hormones keep in motion, or regulate, numerous vital cell processes. For example, the hormones insulin and glucagon enable the body to maintain a stable blood glucose level, both after and between meals. This is an example of **homeostasis**, the natural tendency of the body to maintain an appropriate internal environment in the face of changing external conditions. Hormones such as growth hormone and thyroid hormone regulate **metabolism**. Metabolism encompasses all the cellular processes that produce the energy and molecules needed for growth or repair. In addition, hormones such as estrogen and testosterone regulate the sexual development of puberty and the subsequent reproductive function of adulthood.

Many people have endocrine disorders involving excessive or deficient hormone function. Some common conditions, such as hypothyroidism, are readily controlled by hormone replacement medication. Other hormonal disorders may have a more difficult course. You will find that the hormonal disorder diabetes mellitus is commonly involved in medical emergencies encountered in the prehospital setting.

Anatomy and Physiology

The eight major glands in the endocrine system are the hypothalamus, pituitary gland, thyroid gland, parathyroid glands, thymus, pancreas, adrenal glands, and gonads. The pineal gland is also an endocrine gland, but much of its function remains unclear. In addition to the endocrine glands, many body tissues have been found to have endocrine function. These include the kidneys, heart, placenta, and parts of the digestive tract.

CONTENT REVIEW

➤ Endocrine Glands
- Hypothalamus
- Pituitary
- Thyroid
- Parathyroid
- Thymus
- Pancreas
- Adrenals
- Gonads
- Pineal

The endocrine glands are located throughout the body (Figure 4-1). Although the figure shows an adult, remember that the thymus is active primarily during childhood, when it plays a role in maturation of the immune system. By adulthood, the thymus is so small that it is not visualized on chest X-rays. The hormones secreted by endocrine glands, their target tissues, and their effects are listed in Table 4-1.

Hypothalamus

The *hypothalamus* is located deep within the cerebrum of the brain. Hypothalamic cells act both as nerve cells, or neurons, and as gland cells. The hypothalamus is the junction, or connection, between the central nervous system and the endocrine system. As neurons, many hypothalamic cells receive messages from the **autonomic nervous system**—peripheral nerves that, among other functions, detect internal conditions such as blood pressure or blood glucose level and convey that information to the central nervous system through nerve impulses. Some hypothalamic cells respond by producing nerve impulses that travel to cells in the posterior pituitary gland. Other hypothalamic cells respond as gland cells by producing and releasing hormones into the stalk of tissue that connects the hypothalamus and the anterior pituitary gland (Figure 4-2).

In response to impulses from the autonomic nervous system, the hypothalamus—and other organs of the endocrine system—can release the hormones that promote homeostasis:

- Growth hormone releasing hormone
- Growth hormone inhibiting hormone
- Corticotropin releasing hormone
- Thyrotropin releasing hormone
- Gonadotropin releasing hormone
- Prolactin releasing hormone
- Prolactin inhibiting hormone

As shown in Table 4-1, most hypothalamic hormones, including thyrotropin releasing hormone (TRH) and growth hormone releasing hormone (GHRH), stimulate

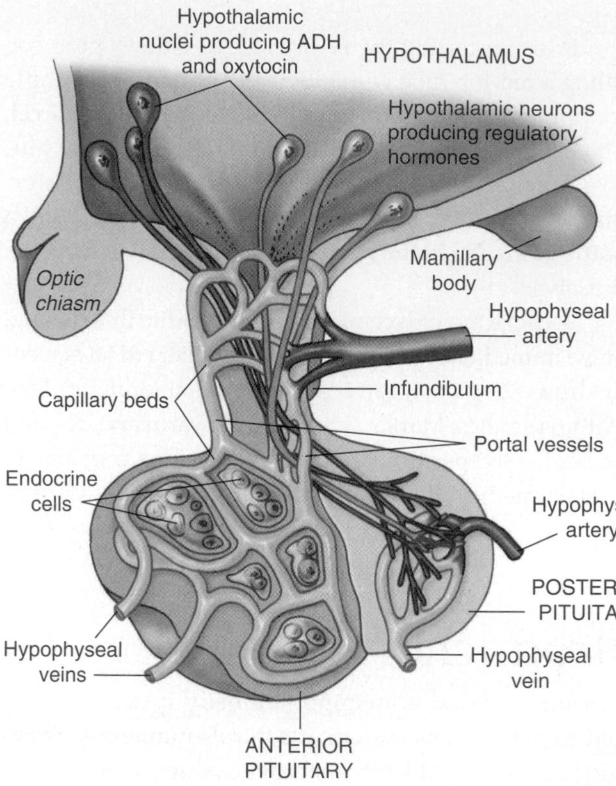

FIGURE 4-2 The hypophyseal portal system.

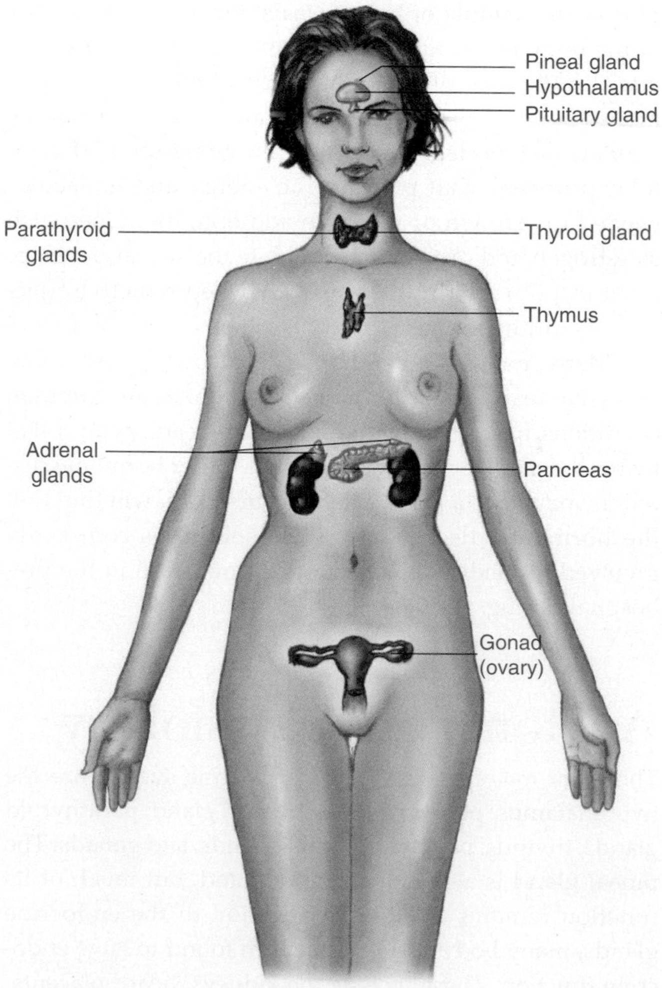

FIGURE 4-1 The major glands of the endocrine system.

Table 4-1 Endocrine System: Glands, Hormones, Target Tissues, Hormone Effects

Gland and Major Hormone(s)	Target Tissues	Major Hormone Effect(s)
Hypothalamus		
Growth hormone releasing hormone, GHRH	Anterior pituitary	Stimulates release of growth hormone
Growth hormone inhibiting hormone, GHIH (or somatostatin)	Anterior pituitary	Suppresses release of growth hormone
Corticotropin releasing hormone, CRH	Anterior pituitary	Stimulates release of adrenocorticotropin
Thyrotropin releasing hormone, TRH	Anterior pituitary	Stimulates release of thyroid stimulating hormone
Gonadotropin releasing hormone, GnRH	Anterior pituitary	Stimulates release of luteinizing hormone and follicle stimulating hormone
Prolactin releasing hormone, PRH	Anterior pituitary	Stimulates release of prolactin
Prolactin inhibiting hormone, PIH	Anterior pituitary	Suppresses release of prolactin
Posterior Pituitary Gland		
Antidiuretic hormone, ADH	Kidneys	Stimulates increased reabsorption of water into blood volume
Oxytocin	Uterus and breasts of females, kidneys	Stimulates uterine contractions and milk release
Anterior Pituitary Gland		
Growth hormone, GH	All cells, especially growing cells	Stimulates body growth in childhood; causes switch to fats as energy source
Adrenocorticotropic hormone, ACTH	Adrenal cortexes	Stimulates release of corticosteroidal hormones cortisol and aldosterone
Thyroid stimulating hormone, TSH	Thyroid	Stimulates release of thyroid hormones thyroxine and triiodothyronine
Follicle stimulating hormone, FSH	Ovaries or testes	FSH stimulates development of sex cells (ovum or sperm)
Luteinizing hormone, LH	Ovaries or testes	LH stimulates release of hormones (estrogen, progesterone, or testosterone)
Prolactin, PRL	Mammary glands	Stimulates production and release of milk
Thyroid Gland		
Thyroxine, T_4	All cells	Stimulates cell metabolism
Triiodothyronine, T_3	All cells	Stimulates cell metabolism
Calcitonin	Bone	Stimulates calcium uptake by bones, decreasing blood calcium level
Parathyroid Glands		
Parathyroid hormone, PTH	Bone, intestine, kidneys	Stimulates calcium release from bone, calcium uptake from GI tract, calcium reabsorption in kidney, all increasing blood calcium level
Thymus		
Thymosin	White blood cells, primarily T lymphocytes	Stimulates reproduction and functional development of T lymphocytes
Pancreas		
Glucagon	All cells, particularly in liver, muscle, and fat	Stimulates hepatic glycogenolysis and gluconeogenesis, increasing blood glucose level
Insulin	All cells, particularly in liver, muscle, and fat	Stimulates cellular uptake of glucose; increases rate of synthesis of glycogen, proteins, and fats; decreases blood glucose level
Somatostatin	Alpha and beta cells in the pancreas	Suppresses secretion of glucagon and insulin within islets of Langerhans

(*Continued*)

Table 4-1 Endocrine System: Glands, Hormones, Target Tissues, Hormone Effects (*Continued*)

Gland and Major Hormone(s)	Target Tissues	Major Hormone Effect(s)
Adrenal Medulla		
Epinephrine (or adrenaline)	Muscle, liver, cardiovascular system	Stimulates features of fight-or-flight response to stress
Norepinephrine	Muscle, liver, cardiovascular system	Stimulates vasoconstriction
Adrenal Cortex		
Glucocorticoids		
Cortisol	Most cells, particularly white blood cells (cells responsible for inflammatory and immune responses)	Stimulates glucagon-like effects; acts as anti-inflammatory and immunosuppressive agent
Mineralocorticoids		
Aldosterone	Kidneys, blood	Contributes to salt and fluid balance by stimulating kidneys to increase potassium excretion and decrease sodium excretion, increasing blood volume
Androgenic hormones		
Estrogen	Most cells	See effects under *Ovaries* and *Testes*
Progesterone	Uterus	
Testosterone	Most cells	
Ovaries		
Estrogen	Most cells, particularly those of female reproductive tract	Stimulates development of secondary sexual characteristics; plays role in maturation of egg prior to ovulation
Progesterone	Uterus	Stimulates uterine changes necessary for successful pregnancy
Testes		
Testosterone	Most cells, particularly those of male reproductive tract	Stimulates development of secondary sexual characteristics; plays role in development of sperm cells
Pineal Gland		
Melatonin	Exact action unknown	Released in response to light; may help determine daily, lunar, and reproductive cycles; may affect mood

secretion of pituitary hormones that rouse yet another endocrine gland or body tissue to increased activity. For example, in response to TRH, the anterior pituitary releases thyroid stimulating hormone, and thyroid stimulating hormone then acts on the thyroid gland to increase thyroid activity.

The pair of hypothalamic hormones—growth hormone releasing hormone (GHRH) and growth hormone inhibiting hormone (GHIH)—demonstrate a major trait of endocrine function: Many hormonal activities are driven not by one hormone, but by two hormones with opposing effects. GHRH stimulates secretion of growth hormone, and GHIH suppresses secretion of growth hormone. The actual amount of growth hormone secreted by the anterior pituitary depends on the net amount of stimulation (Figure 4-3).

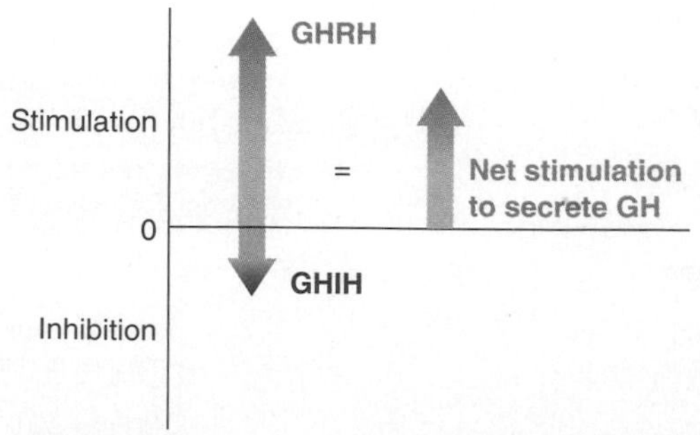

FIGURE 4-3 Regulation by hormone pairs. The net level of stimulation created by the opposing actions of growth hormone releasing hormone (GHRH) and growth hormone inhibiting hormone (GHIH) determines the amount of growth hormone (GH) secreted by the anterior pituitary.

Pituitary Gland

The *pituitary gland* is only about the size of a pea. It is divided into posterior and anterior pituitary lobes. These tissues have different embryonic origins and different functional relationships with the hypothalamus. The *posterior pituitary gland* responds to nerve impulses from the hypothalamus, whereas the *anterior pituitary gland* responds to hypothalamic hormones that travel down the stalk that connects the anterior pituitary and hypothalamus. As you look at the target tissues of the anterior pituitary in Table 4-1, you will understand why physiologists once thought of the pituitary gland as the "master gland." Its hormones have a direct impact on endocrine glands throughout the body. The term is used little today, because the dependence of the pituitary on the hypothalamus has been made clear.

As noted earlier, the pituitary gland has two lobes, the posterior and the anterior.

Posterior Pituitary

The posterior pituitary produces two hormones:

- ***Antidiuretic hormone (ADH)***—causes retention of body water
- ***Oxytocin***—causes uterine contraction and lactation

Antidiuretic hormone (ADH), also known as *vasopressin,* causes the kidneys to increase water reabsorption. This retention of water, or antidiuretic effect, results in increased circulating blood volume and decreased urine volume. Increased secretion of ADH is part of the homeostatic mechanism that can counteract losses of blood volume up to about 25 percent. Clinically, you will see increased ADH secretion in early shock states associated with dehydration or hemorrhage. Note that the opposite effect, decreased secretion of ADH, occurs after ingestion of alcohol and when there is a significant rise in circulating blood volume.

Although it is unlikely that a disorder in ADH secretion will present as a medical emergency, you should understand such endocrine dysfunction when patients discuss their medical histories. **Diabetes insipidus**, a disorder marked by large volumes of urine, is caused by inadequate ADH secretion relative to blood volume. The resultant reduction of blood volume, or diuretic effect, appears as excessive urine production. In a 24-hour period, the kidneys normally produce 1 to 1.5 liters of urine. In diabetes insipidus, it is not uncommon for urine output to increase to almost 20 liters per day. You can remember the characteristic urine presentation of diabetes insipidus by remembering that dilute urine has an insipid, or neutral, odor (and taste). Diabetes insipidus is often seen in conjunction with severe traumatic brain injuries.

Oxytocin, the natural form of the drug Pitocin, stimulates uterine contraction and lactation in women who have just delivered a baby. Oxytocin actually causes the "letdown" of milk by stimulating contractile cells within the mammary glands. An infant suckling at the breast stimulates receptors in the nipples that cause the release of oxytocin from the posterior pituitary. This, in turn, causes discharge of milk so the infant can feed. Following delivery, it is recommended that the infant be placed on the breast to suckle, thus stimulating the release of oxytocin. In addition to stimulating milk letdown, the oxytocin stimulates uterine contraction, which can help minimize postpartum bleeding.

In both sexes, oxytocin has a mild antidiuretic effect, which is similar to that of ADH due to their chemical similarity. The relationship between oxytocin and ADH has direct application to emergency medicine. Women in preterm labor are often given an IV fluid bolus in an attempt to suppress uterine contractions without the use of drugs. This works in the following way: The administration of an IV fluid bolus causes an increase in circulating blood volume, which is detected by autonomic nerves in the kidneys. An impulse is sent through the hypothalamus to the posterior pituitary, where it causes decreased secretion of ADH. This inhibition of ADH secretion, in turn, triggers decreased secretion of oxytocin, which contributes to the observed increase in urine production and, one hopes, the goal of suppression of preterm labor.

Anterior Pituitary

Because almost all of the anterior pituitary hormones regulate other endocrine glands, disorders directly involving the anterior pituitary are rarely a factor in endocrine emergencies. Table 4-1 lists the six hormones secreted by the anterior pituitary, as well as target tissues and hormone effects. As you can see, five of the six hormones regulate the activity of target glands, whereas the sixth affects almost all cells.

Five anterior pituitary hormones affect target glands:

- ***Adrenocorticotropic hormone (ACTH)***—targets the adrenal cortexes
- ***Thyroid stimulating hormone (TSH)***—targets the thyroid
- ***Follicle stimulating hormone (FSH)***—targets the gonads, or sex organs
- ***Luteinizing hormone (LH)***—also targets the gonads
- ***Prolactin (PRL)***—targets the mammary glands of women

The sixth anterior pituitary hormone has a broader effect:

- ***Growth hormone (GH)***—targets almost *all* body cells

GH has its most significant effects in children because it is the primary stimulant of skeletal growth. In adults, GH has several physiologic effects, but the most significant is metabolic. GH causes adipose cells to release their stored fats into the blood and causes body cells to switch from glucose to fats as the primary energy source. The net effect is that the body uses up fat stores and conserves its sugar stores.

Thyroid Gland

The two lobes of the *thyroid gland* are located in the neck anterior to and just below the cartilage of the larynx, with one lobe on either side of the midline. The two lobes are connected by a small isthmus, or band of tissue, that crosses the trachea at the level of the cricoid cartilage. The thyroid produces three hormones:

- ***Thyroxine (*** T_4 ***)***—stimulates cell metabolism
- ***Triiodothyronine (*** T_3 ***)***—stimulates cell metabolism
- ***Calcitonin***—lowers blood calcium levels

The thyroid is composed of tiny hollow sacs called *follicles*, which are filled with a thick fluid called *colloid*. The hormones *thyroxine* (T_4) and *triiodothyronine* (T_3) are produced within the colloid. When stimulated by the pituitary hormone TSH or by environmental conditions such as cold, the thyroid gland releases these hormones to increase the general rate of cell metabolism.

The thyroid gland also contains perifollicular cells called C cells that produce a different hormone, *calcitonin*. Calcitonin lowers blood calcium levels by increasing uptake of calcium by bones and inhibiting breakdown of bone tissue. Parathyroid hormone has the opposite, or antagonistic, effect on the blood calcium level, which is covered in the following discussion of the parathyroid glands.

Disorders of excessive or deficient production of thyroid hormones T_4 and T_3—called hyperthyroidism and hypothyroidism, respectively—are discussed later in this chapter.

Parathyroid Glands

Each *parathyroid gland* is very small, with a maximum diameter of 5 mm and weight of only 35 to 40 mg. Normally, four parathyroid glands are located on the posterior lateral surfaces of the thyroid, one pair above the other. Sometimes there are more than four parathyroid glands, but only rarely are there fewer. The parathyroid glands secrete:

- ***Parathyroid hormone (PTH)***—increases blood calcium levels

PTH increases blood calcium levels through actions on three different target tissues. In bone, the primary target, PTH causes release of calcium into the blood. In the intestines, PTH converts vitamin D into its active form, causing increased absorption of calcium. In the kidneys, PTH causes increased reabsorption of calcium. PTH is the antagonist of calcitonin, and the balance of PTH and calcitonin determines the level of blood calcium. The parathyroid glands rarely cause clinical problems. However, they can be accidentally damaged or removed during surgery or they may be damaged if the thyroid gland is irradiated. In either case, the loss of parathyroid function may result in hypocalcemia (low blood calcium levels).

Thymus Gland

The *thymus* is in the mediastinum just behind the sternum. It is fairly large in children but shrinks into a small remnant of fat and fibrous tissue in adults. Although the thymus is usually considered a lymphatic organ on the basis of its anatomy, its most important function is as an endocrine gland. During childhood, it secretes:

- ***Thymosin***—promotes maturation of T lymphocytes

Thymosin is critical to maturation of T lymphocytes, the cells responsible for cell-mediated immunity. The T of T lymphocyte stands for *thymus*.

Pancreas

The pancreas, located in the upper retroperitoneum behind the stomach and between the duodenum and spleen, is composed of both endocrine and exocrine tissues. The exocrine tissues, known as *acini*, secrete digestive enzymes—essential to digestion of fats and proteins—into a duct that empties into the small intestine.

The microscopic clusters of endocrine tissue found within the pancreas are known as the *islets of Langerhans*. Although 1 to 2 million islets are interspersed throughout the pancreas, they make up only about 2 percent of its total mass. The three most important types of endocrine cells in the islets of Langerhans are termed *alpha* (α), *beta* (β), and *delta* (δ) (Figure 4-4). Each type produces and secretes a different hormone. In addition, the islets contain a much

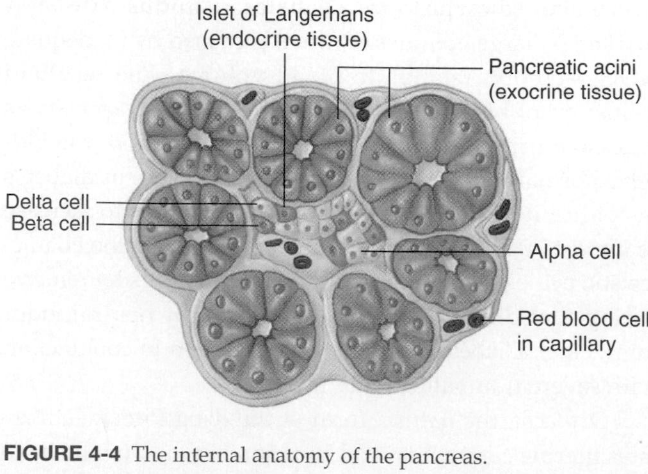

FIGURE 4-4 The internal anatomy of the pancreas.

smaller number of cells called *polypeptide cells*. These cells produce pancreatic polypeptide (PP), the function of which is still unclear.

The alpha and beta cells produce two hormones essential for homeostasis of blood glucose:

- *Glucagon*—increases blood glucose
- *Insulin*—decreases blood glucose

Approximately 25 percent of islet tissue is made up of alpha cells. Alpha cells produce the hormone *glucagon*. When the body's blood glucose level falls, alpha cells increase secretion of glucagon. Glucagon stimulates breakdown of glycogen, the complex carbohydrate that is the storage form of glucose, into individual glucose molecules that are released into the blood. This process, called **glycogenolysis**, takes place in more than one tissue, but activity in the liver is by far the most important in raising the blood glucose level.

The liver is the largest and heaviest of the internal organs, so it has many cells that can contain glycogen. In addition, liver cells have the greatest capacity to store glycogen—liver cells can store 5 to 8 percent of their weight as glycogen. (Compare this with the capacity of skeletal muscle (1 to 3 percent), another important storage tissue in the body.) In addition to stimulating glycogenolysis, the hormone glucagon also stimulates liver breakdown of body proteins and fats with subsequent chemical conversion to glucose. This second process, which produces glucose from nonsugar sources, is called **gluconeogenesis**. Both processes contribute to homeostasis by raising the blood glucose level.

Beta cells make up about 60 percent of islet tissue, and they produce the hormone *insulin*. Insulin is the antagonist of glucagon: Insulin lowers the blood glucose level by increasing the uptake of glucose by body cells. In addition, insulin promotes energy storage in the body by increasing the synthesis of glycogen, protein, and fat. Because the liver removes circulating insulin within 10 to 15 minutes of the time of secretion, it must be secreted constantly to sustain an appropriate balance of glucagon and insulin—a balance that results in a steady supply of glucose for immediate use as an energy source and for appropriate energy storage. Loss of functional beta cells leads to increased blood glucose levels, as seen in diabetes. The role of insulin deficiency in diabetes mellitus is discussed later in this chapter.

Delta cells, which make up about 10 percent of islet tissue, produce *somatostatin*. This hormone acts within islets to inhibit secretion of glucagon and insulin. Somatostatin also retards nutrient absorption from the intestines, although its mechanisms of action in the gut are poorly understood. As you look at Table 4-1, note that somatostatin is the same substance as growth hormone inhibiting hormone (GHIH).

Terminology Related to Glucose

You can remember terms related to glucose by performing some breakdown of your own. Look at the terms as they are listed below, where each word part is given along with its meaning and a sample sentence. Then you may want to reread the preceding discussion of glucagon and insulin, keeping the meanings of the word parts in mind as the terms appear. Also keep these meanings in mind when you read the discussion of diabetes mellitus later in the chapter.

Glucagon gluco = glucose, agon = to drive

The hormone glucagon drives an increase in blood glucose.

Glycogen glyco = sugar, gen = origin

The complex carbohydrate glycogen is the source for much of the blood glucose produced between meals.

Glycogenolysis *glycogen*, lysis = to loosen or unbind

Glycogenolysis breaks glycogen down into its component glucose molecules.

Gluconeogenesis *gluco = glucose, neo = new, genesis = origin*

New glucose molecules are synthesized from nonsugar sources through the process of gluconeogenesis.

Adrenal Glands

The paired *adrenal glands* are located on the superior surface of the kidneys. Each gland has two distinct anatomic divisions with different functions. The inner portion of the adrenal gland is called the *adrenal medulla*, and its cells behave both as nerve cells and as gland cells. The adrenal medulla is intimately related to the sympathetic component of the autonomic nervous system. When sympathetic nerves carry an impulse into the adrenal medulla, its cells respond by secreting the catecholamine hormones *epinephrine* (or adrenalin) and *norepinephrine* into the bloodstream. The outer portion of the adrenal gland is called the *adrenal cortex*, and it consists of endocrine tissue. The adrenal cortex secretes three classes of steroidal hormones that differ only slightly in chemical structure but have very distinct effects in the body:

- *Glucocorticoids*, of which *cortisol* is by far the most important, account for 95 percent of adrenocortical hormone production. Like glucagon, they increase the blood glucose level by promoting gluconeogenesis and decreasing glucose utilization as an energy source.

If you recall that cortisone is a commonly used medical glucocorticoid, you will realize that this class of hormones also inhibits inflammatory reactions and immune system responses, as well as potentiates the effects of catecholamines. The anterior pituitary hormone that promotes release, ACTH, is secreted in response to stress, trauma, or serious infection.

- *Mineralocorticoids,* of which *aldosterone* is the most important, contribute to salt and fluid balance in the body by regulating sodium and potassium excretion through the kidneys.
- *Androgenic hormones* have the same effects as those secreted by gonads; they will be covered in that discussion.

You may see disorders related to deficient or excessive secretion of adrenal hormones present as medical emergencies. They are discussed later in this chapter.

Gonads

Some differences in the gonads are obvious: Ovaries produce eggs, whereas testes produce sperm cells. However, the gonads of both sexes share one vital function: They are the endocrine glands chiefly responsible for the sexual maturation of puberty and any subsequent reproduction.

Ovaries

The ovaries, or female gonads, are paired organs about the size of an almond that are located in the pelvis on either side of the uterus. Under the regulation of the anterior pituitary hormones FSH and LH, the ovaries produce:

- *Estrogen*
- *Progesterone*

The hormone *estrogen* promotes the development and maintenance of secondary female sexual characteristics. Estrogen also plays a role in the egg development that precedes ovulation during each menstrual cycle. *Progesterone* is familiarly known as the "hormone of pregnancy" because it is necessary for implantation of the fertilized egg and maintenance of the uterine lining throughout pregnancy. Estrogen also serves to protect the female against heart disease. When estrogen levels fall at menopause, the female's risk of developing heart disease quickly increases to the male's level of risk. In addition, the ovaries produce small amounts of *testosterone,* which influences some body changes associated with puberty.

Testes

The male gonads, or *testes,* are located outside the abdominal cavity in the scrotum. Under the regulation of the anterior pituitary hormones FSH and LH, the testes produce:

- *Testosterone*

The hormone *testosterone* promotes the development and maintenance of secondary male sexual characteristics and plays a role in development of sperm.

Pineal Gland

The pineal gland is located in the roof of the thalamus in the brain. Its function has remained somewhat elusive. However, it has been shown that the pineal gland releases the hormone *melatonin* in response to changes in light. For example, melatonin production is lowest during daylight hours and highest in the dark of the night. Because of this, the pineal gland is felt to help determine day-length and lunar cycles and plays a role in controlling the reproductive "biological clock." Melatonin may affect a person's mood. The pineal gland has been implicated in "seasonal affective disorder" (SAD), which is characterized by severe depression during the winter months. Further research will help clarify the role of melatonin.

Patho Pearls

Anabolic and Catabolic Steroids. The term *steroid* refers to a variety of substances that have a similar chemical structure. There are two types of steroid medications: anabolic steroids and catabolic steroids.

The primary anabolic steroid hormones are the male sex hormones testosterone and dihydrotestosterone. These hormones increase protein synthesis and build muscle, bone, and body mass (thus, most men are bigger than most women). They also cause virilization (deepening of the voice, growth of the testicles, and body hair). There are numerous synthetic forms of anabolic steroids. They are sometimes used (nonmedically) to increase human physical performance and build body mass. Recent controversies about steroid use in professional sports are a testament to such nonmedical uses.

Catabolic steroids serve as anti-inflammatory medicines. These include such substances as hydrocortisone, prednisone, methylprednisolone, dexamethasone, and others. They are used in emergency medicine often and for many conditions. When they are administered as medications, the term *steroid* can be confusing or upsetting for some patients, who may associate steroids with the professional sports controversies. Therefore, it is best to refer to these substances by their proper names.

Other Organs with Endocrine Activity

We have discussed the principal glands of the endocrine system. Many tissues not considered part of the endocrine system have important endocrine functions. Certain organs in other systems secrete hormones directly into the blood. The placenta can be considered an endocrine gland because of its secretion of *human chorionic gonadotropin (hCG)* throughout gestation. It is the early secretion of hCG that is detected by at-home pregnancy tests. In the digestive tract, gastric and intestinal mucosa produce the hormones *gastrin* and *secretin,* both of which regulate digestive function.

Additionally, there are hormone-producing cells in the atrial walls of the heart. *Atrial natriuretic hormone (ANH)* and *brain natriuretic peptide (BNP)* are secreted by certain atrial cells in response to increased stretching of the atrial walls due to abnormally high blood volume or blood pressure. The hormone ANH is an antagonist to ADH and inhibits secretion of aldosterone, thus contributing to a homeostatic reduction in blood volume by increasing urine production.

The kidneys also have some endocrine function. Certain kidney cells will react to a decrease in blood volume or blood pressure by releasing the enzyme *renin.* Renin acts on *angiotensinogen,* converting it to *angiotensin I.* In the lungs, angiotensin I is converted to *angiotensin II* by *angiotensin-converting enzyme (ACE).* Angiotensin II stimulates the adrenal production of aldosterone, which causes water retention by the kidneys. This leads to increased blood volume and blood pressure. In addition to renin, the kidneys secrete the hormone *erythropoietin,* which stimulates the production of red blood cells by the bone marrow. (The role of erythropoietin is discussed in greater detail in the chapter "Hematology.")

Endocrine Disorders and Emergencies

The most common endocrine emergencies you should expect to treat will involve complications of diabetes mellitus. This section explains the pathophysiology of diabetes and its complications, including ketoacidosis and hypoglycemia, as a basis for discussion of field management. In addition, the section covers endocrine emergencies involving disorders of the thyroid and adrenal glands.

Disorders of the Pancreas

Diabetes Mellitus

The disease **diabetes mellitus** is marked by inadequate insulin activity in the body. As noted earlier, insulin is critical to maintaining normal blood glucose levels. Glucose is important for all cells, but it is especially important for brain cells. In fact, glucose is the *only* substance that brain cells can readily and efficiently use as an energy source. In addition, insulin enables the body to store energy as glycogen, protein, and fat.

Diabetes mellitus, or sugar diabetes, is not only a serious disease but also a common and ancient one. More than 29.1 million Americans (9.3 percent of the population) have been diagnosed with diabetes, and U.S. health experts believe that nearly the same number of Americans may be living with undiagnosed diabetes. The disease was named in ancient times by Greek physicians who noted that affected persons produced large volumes of urine that attracted bees and other insects; thus it was called diabetes (meaning "to siphon," or "to pass through") for excessive urine production and mellitus (meaning "honey sweet") for the presence of sugar in the urine. If you remember that *mellitus* means "sweet" and *insipidus* means "neutral," you will remember the common trait and the major distinctions in the presentations of untreated diabetes insipidus and diabetes mellitus.

Before presenting pathophysiology, we examine in detail the normal body's handling of glucose. The discussion of glucose metabolism focuses on events at the molecular and cellular levels, whereas the discussion on regulation of blood glucose focuses on events in the blood and in major target tissues such as the liver, fat cells, and kidneys.

Cultural Considerations

Who Is Most Affected by Diabetes? It has been estimated that 15.7 million individuals in the United States have diabetes. However, only two-thirds of them know that they have it. Each year, approximately 798,000 new cases of diabetes are diagnosed. Among individuals 20 years and older, approximately 11.3 million non-Latino whites (7.8 percent) have diabetes, compared with 2.3 million African Americans (10.8 percent) and 1.2 million Latinos (10.6 percent). These figures suggest that African Americans and Latinos are disproportionately affected by diabetes compared with non-Latino whites.

Diabetes is a particularly serious health problem among certain Latino groups. Type II diabetes is twice as prevalent among Latinos as among non-Latino whites. Approximately 24 percent of Mexican Americans in the United States and 26 percent of Puerto Ricans between 45 and 74 years of age have diabetes. In this same age group, about 16 percent of Cuban Americans have diabetes.

Additionally, diabetes-related complications affect Latinos at disproportionate rates. Lower-leg amputations, kidney disease, blindness, heart disease, and strokes resulting from diabetes occur at least twice as frequently among Latinos as among non-Latino whites. The disproportionate burden that this disease places on Latinos has been attributed to genetics and socioeconomic and environmental factors, among others. Whereas some researchers suggest that genetic factors play a prominent role in diabetes, other important factors must also be taken into account, including diet, sedentary lifestyles, cultural concepts of obesity or robustness, and access to care, information, and educational programs.

Paramedics who work in areas with large Latino populations may encounter more diabetic emergencies and more diabetic-related complications and should prepare accordingly.

GLUCOSE METABOLISM You learned in the chapter introduction that metabolism is the sum of the processes that produce the energy and molecules needed for cell growth or repair. The word *metabolism* comes from the Greek for "to change." Two kinds of change take place within a cell. One kind builds complex molecules from simpler ones. The synthesis of glycogen from glucose is an example. The other kind breaks down complex molecules into simpler ones. The breakdown of glucose into carbon dioxide, water, and energy (in the form of adenosine triphosphate, or ATP) is an example.

The building processes within a cell are collectively called **anabolism**. The prefix *ana-* comes from the Greek for "up," and anabolic pathways build molecules of higher complexity. Breakdown processes are collectively called **catabolism**. The prefix *cata-* comes from the Greek for "down," and catabolic pathways produce molecules of lower complexity. Anabolic pathways usually require energy to drive them, and catabolic pathways often release energy as part of the process. In other words, anabolic activity uses energy, whereas catabolic activity produces energy.

Look at the summary of effects of insulin and glucagon in Table 4-2. When materials are abundant after meals and blood glucose is high, insulin enables cells to use glucose directly and to store energy as glycogen, protein, and fat. Insulin stimulates anabolic pathways. In contrast, glucagon is the dominant hormone during periods of low blood glucose. It stimulates catabolic pathways to produce usable energy from the body's stores.

For anabolic pathways to proceed, insulin must first exert its stimulatory effects. Insulin acts by binding to receptors in the outer cell membrane. These receptors are proteins whose structure reacts specifically with insulin. When insulin is bound to a receptor, it changes the permeability of the membrane so glucose enters the cell far more readily. The rate at which glucose can be transported into cells can be increased tenfold or more by the action of insulin. Without insulin activity, the amount of glucose that can enter cells is far too small to meet average body energy demands. Note the two requirements for insulin effectiveness:

1. There must be sufficient insulin circulating in the bloodstream to satisfy cellular needs.
2. Insulin must be able to bind to body cells in such a way that adequate levels of stimulation occur.

The importance of these two requirements will become clear when you learn about the two types of diabetes mellitus.

Sometimes the body cannot use glucose as a primary energy source. In diabetes, this occurs when insufficient insulin activity exists for blood glucose to be taken in and used by cells. Other conditions, such as a high-fat, low-carbohydrate diet or starvation (which can occur in conjunction with some eating disorders), cause depletion of body stores of carbohydrate. Under any of these conditions, the body slowly switches from glucose to fat as the primary energy source. Adipose cells break down fats into their component free fatty acids, and the blood concentration of fatty acids rises considerably.

Most of the fatty acid is used directly by body cells as an energy source. Some is taken in by liver cells. In the liver, catabolism of fatty acids produces acetoacetic acid. When more acetoacetic acid is released from the liver than can be used by body cells, it accumulates in the blood along with two closely related substances, acetone and β-hydroxybutyric acid. These three substances are collectively called **ketone bodies**, and their presence in biologically significant quantity in the blood is called **ketosis**. This catabolic state is significant in the context of the emergency condition called diabetic ketoacidosis, or diabetic coma. (This condition will be discussed later in the chapter.)

REGULATION OF BLOOD GLUCOSE Homeostasis of blood glucose is remarkably effective. If you draw venous blood samples from a group of healthy people, you'll find that fasting blood glucose (generally done after an overnight fast) is usually between 80 to 90 mg glucose/dL blood. In the first hour or so after a meal, blood glucose may increase to about 120 to 140 mg/dL before falling toward the fasting, or baseline, level. The principal tissues involved in homeostasis are the alpha and beta tissues of the islets of Langerhans (producing glucagon and insulin, respectively) and the liver, as shown in Table 4-2. Liver disease, even in the presence of normal pancreatic function, can cause significant disturbances in glucose homeostasis.

A blood glucose level lower than baseline (often defined as less than 80 mg/dL) reflects **hypoglycemia**, or low blood sugar. Similarly, a blood glucose level higher than that expected shortly after a meal (often defined as greater than 140 mg/dL when drawn in a setting other than directly following a meal) reflects **hyperglycemia**, or

Table 4-2 Summary of Glucose Metabolism

Hormonal Effects of Insulin and Glucagon	
Insulin	**Glucagon**
Dominant hormone when blood glucose level is high	Dominant hormone when blood glucose level is low
Major Effects on Target Tissues	**Major Effects on Target Tissues**
All cells: ↑ uptake glucose Liver: ↑ production of glycogen, protein, fat Liver, fat: ↑ production of fats	Liver: ↑ glycogenolysis → glucose Liver: ↑ gluconeogenesis (protein, fat → glucose)

high blood sugar. Both terms indicate the blood glucose level only, not the cause of the abnormality.

The last factor to consider in discussing regulation of blood glucose is the role of the kidneys. When blood is filtered through the glomeruli of the kidneys, glucose—along with water and many other small molecules—passes from the blood into the proximal tubule. Water, glucose, and other useful materials are then reabsorbed, while waste products that are not reabsorbed become part of the urine, which will be excreted from the body. The amount of glucose that is reabsorbed depends on the blood level of glucose that already exists. Reabsorption of glucose is essentially complete at blood glucose levels up to about 180 mg/dL. Above that level, glucose begins to be lost in urine.

Glucose loss in urine can lead to dehydration, which has its physiologic basis in osmosis. Osmosis is the tendency of water molecules to migrate across a semipermeable membrane so that the concentrations of particles approach equivalence on both sides. Our example is the cell membranes that form the boundaries between the tubules of the kidney and the capillaries that surround them.

When glucose spills into urine, the osmotic pressure, or concentration of particulates, rises inside the kidney tubule to a level higher than that of the blood. Water follows glucose into urine to cause a marked water loss termed **osmotic diuresis**, which is the basis of the excessive urination characteristic of untreated diabetes. The term **diuresis** alone refers to increased formation and secretion of urine. The presence of glucose in urine, **glycosuria**, creates the sweet urine that added *mellitus* to *diabetes*.

Last, you should note that whenever the flow rate of fluid inside the kidney tubules rises, as in osmotic diuresis, an increase in excretion of potassium occurs. This leads to the potential for significant hypokalemia and its effects, including cardiac arrhythmias.

TYPE 1 DIABETES MELLITUS When we discussed the elements essential to normal insulin activity, the first was the presence of adequate amounts of insulin in the body. *Type 1 diabetes mellitus* is characterized by β-cell destruction with very low production of insulin by the pancreas. In many cases, no insulin is produced at all. Type 1 diabetes is commonly called juvenile onset diabetes because of the average age at diagnosis. The term *insulin-dependent diabetes mellitus (IDDM)* is also used because patients require regular insulin injections to maintain glucose homeostasis. This type of diabetes is less common than is type 2 diabetes, but it is more serious. Diabetes is regularly among the ten leading causes of death in the United States, and type 1 diabetes accounts for most diabetes-related deaths.

Heredity is an important factor in determining which persons will be predisposed to development of type 1 diabetes. The cause of type 1 diabetes is often unclear. However, viral infection, production of autoantibodies directed against beta cells (immune-related), and genetically determined early deterioration of beta cells are all possible. The immediate cause of the disease is destruction of beta cells.

CONTENT REVIEW

➤ Symptoms of Untreated Type 1 Diabetes Mellitus
- Polydipsia
- Polyuria
- Polyphagia
- Weakness
- Weight loss

In untreated type 1 diabetes, blood glucose levels rise because, without adequate insulin, cells cannot take up the circulating sugar. Hyperglycemia in the range of 300 to 500 mg/dL is not uncommon. As glucose spills into urine, large amounts of water are lost, too, through osmotic diuresis. Catabolism of fat becomes significant as the body switches to fatty acids as the primary energy source. Overall, this pathophysiology accounts for the constant thirst (polydipsia), excessive urination (polyuria), ravenous appetite (polyphagia), weakness, and weight loss associated with untreated type 1 diabetes. Ketosis can occur as the result of fat catabolism, and it may proceed to frank diabetic ketoacidosis, a medical emergency that you will encounter in the field and that will be discussed later in this chapter.

The treatment of type 1 diabetes almost always includes the periodic administration of insulin (Figure 4-5). Many patients take a morning and an evening dose of a moderate- to long-acting insulin. In addition, they monitor their glucose levels during the day and self-administer short-acting insulin on a sliding-scale system.

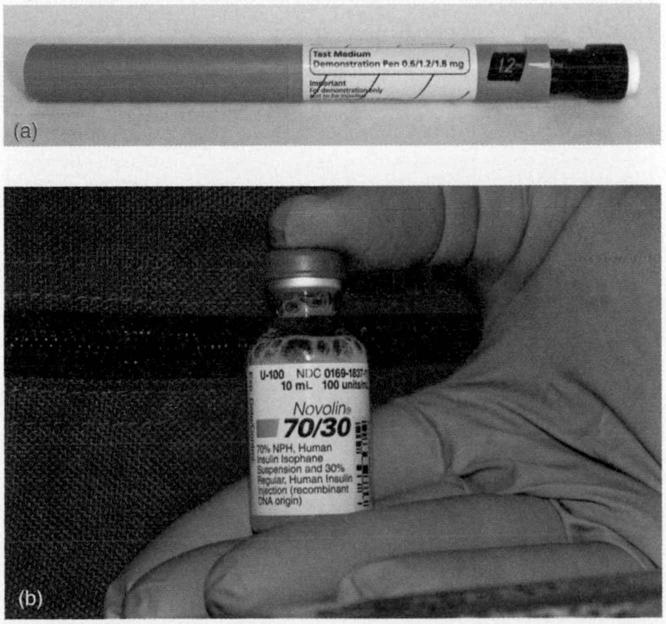

FIGURE 4-5 Insulin is the primary therapy for type 1 diabetes. (a) Syringe-style insulin. (b) Insulin vial.

(Photo a: © Dr. Bryan E. Bledsoe; Photo b: © Edward T. Dickinson, MD)

TYPE 2 DIABETES MELLITUS The second requirement for proper insulin activity is insulin binding so that adequate stimulation of cells occurs. Type 2 diabetes mellitus is associated with a moderate decline in insulin production accompanied by a markedly deficient response to the insulin that is present in the body (insulin resistance). Type 2 diabetes is also called *non-insulin-dependent diabetes mellitus (NIDDM)*, although some type 2 patients may also require insulin.

Heredity may play a role in predisposition. In addition, obese persons are more likely to develop type 2 diabetes, and obesity probably plays a role in development of the disease. Increased weight (and increased size of fat cells) causes a relative deficiency in the number of insulin receptors per cell, which makes fat cells less responsive to insulin. In fact, as obesity in children has become more prevalent, so has the occurrence of type 2 diabetes in children. Previously, type 2 diabetes was so uncommon in children that it was often called "adult onset diabetes," a descriptor that is, unfortunately, no longer appropriate.

Type 2 diabetes is far more common than type 1 diabetes, accounting for about 80 percent of cases of diabetes mellitus.

Untreated type 2 diabetes typically presents with a lower level of hyperglycemia and fewer major signs of metabolic disruption. For instance, glucose use is usually sufficient to keep the body from switching to fats as the primary energy source. Thus, diabetic ketoacidosis is uncommon in these patients. However, a complication called hyperosmolar hyperglycemic state (HHS) can occur, and you may see it as a medical emergency. It is discussed later in this chapter.

Medical treatment of type 2 diabetes is less intensive than that required for type 1 diabetes. Initial therapy often consists of dietary change and increased exercise in an attempt to improve body weight. If nonpharmacological therapy is insufficient to bring blood glucose levels down to the normal range, oral hypoglycemic agents may be prescribed. These drugs stimulate insulin secretion by beta cells and promote an increase in the number of insulin receptors per cell. In some cases, however, control may eventually require use of insulin.[1]

Diabetic Ketoacidosis (Diabetic Coma)

Diabetic ketoacidosis is a serious, potentially life-threatening complication associated with type 1 diabetes. It occurs when there is profound insulin deficiency coupled with increased glucagon activity. It may occur as the initial presentation of severe diabetes, as a result of patient noncompliance with insulin injections, or as the result of physiologic stress such as surgery or serious infection. Some of the major characteristics of diabetic ketoacidosis are listed in Tables 4-3 and 4-4.

PATHOPHYSIOLOGY Reread the discussion of ketosis in the preceding section, Glucose Metabolism. Diabetic ketoacidosis reflects amplification of the same physiologic mechanisms as ketosis.

In the initial phase of diabetic ketoacidosis, profound hyperglycemia exists because of lack of insulin. Body cells cannot take in glucose. The compensatory mechanism for low glucose levels within cells, gluconeogenesis, only contributes more blood glucose. The consequent loss of glucose in the urine, accompanied by loss of water through osmotic diuresis, produces significant dehydration (Figure 4-6).

Table 4-3 Diabetic Emergencies

Diabetic Ketoacidosis (DKA)	Hyperosmolar Hyperglycemic State (HHS)	Hypoglycemia
Common Causes	**Common Causes**	**Common Causes**
Cessation of insulin injections Physiologic stress (such as infection or surgery) that causes release of catecholamines, potentiating glucagon effects and blocking insulin effects	Physiologic stress (such as infection or stroke) producing hyperglycemia and a noncompensated diuresis, modulated by both insulin and glucagon activity	Excessive administration of insulin Excess insulin for dietary intake Overexertion, resulting in lowered blood glucose level
Signs and Symptoms	**Signs and Symptoms**	**Signs and Symptoms**
Polyuria, polydipsia, polyphagia Warm, dry skin and mucous membranes Nausea/vomiting Abdominal pain Tachycardia Deep, rapid respirations (Kussmaul's respirations) Fruity odor on breath Fever (if associated with infection) Decreased mental function or frank coma	Polyuria, polydipsia, polyphagia Warm, dry skin and mucous membranes Orthostatic hypotension Tachycardia Decreased mental function or frank coma	Weak, rapid pulse Cold, clammy skin Weakness, uncoordination Headache Irritable, agitated behavior Decreased mental function or bizarre behavior Coma (severe cases)
Management	**Management**	**Management**
Fluids, insulin as directed	Fluids, insulin as directed	Dextrose

Table 4-4 Diagnostic Signs by System for Diabetic Emergencies

System	Diabetic Emergency		
	Diabetic Ketoacidosis (DKA)	**HHS Coma**	**Hypoglycemia**
Cardiovascular			
Pulse	Rapid	Rapid	Normal
Blood pressure	Low	Normal to low (may be affected by position, or orthostatic)	Normal
Respiratory			
Respiration rate	Exaggerated air hunger	Normal, unlabored	Normal or shallow
Breath odor	Acetone (sweet, fruity)	None	None
Nervous			
Headache	Absent	None	Present
Mental state	Restlessness/unconsciousness	Lethargy/unconsciousness	Apathy, irritability/unconsciousness
Tremors	Absent	Absent	Present In late stages
Convulsions	None	Possible	
Gastrointestinal			
Mouth	Dry	Dry	Drooling
Thirst	Intense	Excessive	Absent
Vomiting	Common	Common	Uncommon
Abdominal pain	Frequent	Common	Absent
Ocular			
Vision	Dim	Normal	Double vision (diplopia)

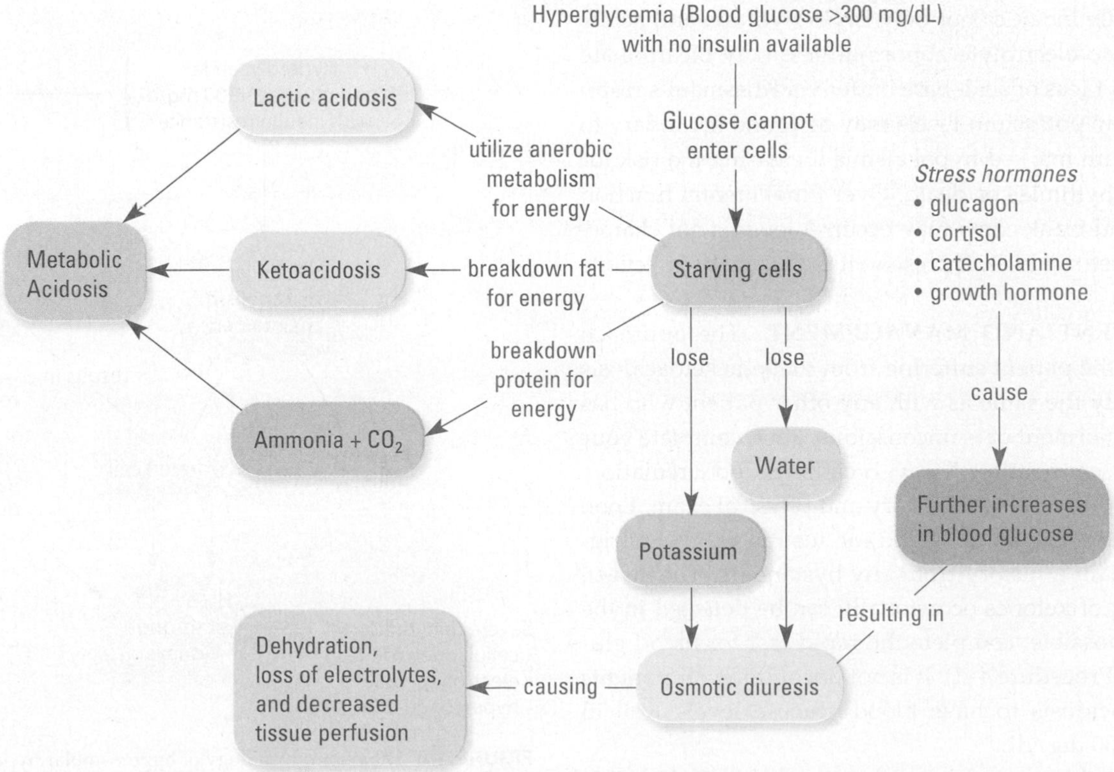

FIGURE 4-6 The pathophysiology of diabetic ketoacidosis.

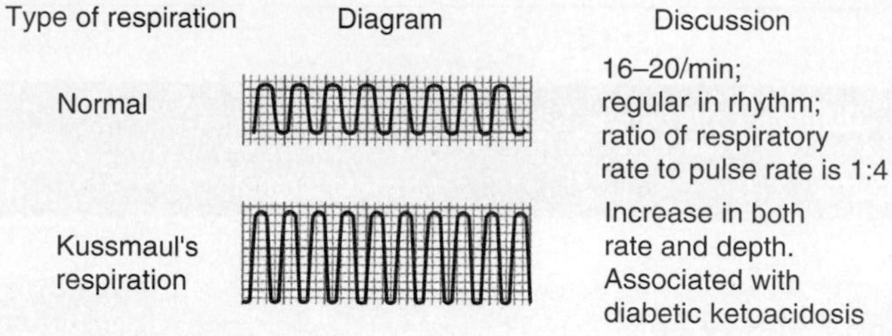

FIGURE 4-7 Kussmaul's respirations.

As the body switches to fat-based metabolism, the blood level of ketones rises. The ketone load accounts for the observed acidosis. By the time the characteristic decrease in pH from about 7.4 to about 6.9 has occurred, the patient is hours from death if left untreated.

SIGNS AND SYMPTOMS The onset of clinically obvious diabetic ketoacidosis is slow, lasting from 12 to 24 hours. In the initial phase, signs of diuresis appear, including increased urine production and dry, warm skin and mucous membranes. The individual often has excessive hunger and thirst, coupled with a progressive sense of general malaise. Volume depletion induces tachycardia and feelings of physical weakness.

As ketoacidosis develops, a major compensatory mechanism for acidosis appears: the rapid, deep breathing pattern termed *Kussmaul's respirations,* which helps expel carbon dioxide, CO_2, from the body (Figure 4-7). The breath itself may have a fruity or acetone-like smell, as some blood acetone is expelled through the lungs. The blood profile includes not only hyperglycemia and acidic pH, but also electrolyte abnormalities. Low bicarbonate levels reflect loss of acid–base buffer via Kussmaul's respirations. Low potassium levels may be found secondary to diuresis, with marked hypokalemia increasing the risk for cardiac arrhythmias or death. Over time, mental function declines and frank coma may occur. A fever is not characteristic of ketoacidosis. If present, it is a signal of infection.

ASSESSMENT AND MANAGEMENT The approach used with the patient suffering from diabetic ketoacidosis is essentially the same as with any other patient who has mental impairment or is unconscious. First, complete your primary assessment of airway, breathing, and circulation. Then complete a focused history and physical exam. Look for a MedicAlert bracelet and/or insulin in the refrigerator. Obtain a history from any bystanders. The sweet, fruity odor of ketones occasionally can be detected in the breath. If possible, complete the rapid test for blood glucose level (Procedure 4–1). It is not uncommon for patients with ketoacidosis to have blood glucose levels well in excess of 500 mg/dL.

Focus field management on maintenance of the ABCs and fluid resuscitation to counteract dehydration. In such cases, draw a red-top tube (or the tube specified by local protocols) of blood. Following blood sampling, administer 1 to 2 liters of normal saline per protocol. If transport time is lengthy, the medical direction physician may request intravenous or subcutaneous administration of regular insulin.

Expedite transport to an appropriate facility for definitive therapy.[2,3]

Hyperosmolar Hyperglycemic State (HHS)

Hyperosmolar hyperglycemic state (HHS), sometimes called **hyperglycemic hyperosmolar nonketotic coma (HHNK)**, is a serious complication associated with type 2 diabetes. Typically, both insulin and glucagon activity are present. HHS develops when two conditions occur: Sustained hyperglycemia causes osmotic diuresis sufficient to produce marked dehydration, and water intake is inadequate to replace lost fluids. Dialysis, high-osmolarity feeding supplements, infection, and certain drugs can also be associated with development of HHS. Some characteristics of HHS are listed in Tables 4-3 and 4-4.

PATHOPHYSIOLOGY As sustained hyperglycemia develops, glucose spills into the urine, causing osmotic diuresis and resultant dehydration (Figure 4-8). The level of hyperglycemia is often much higher than the levels seen in ketoacidosis (up to 1,000 mg/dL). However, insulin activity in patients with HHS coma prevents significant production of ketone bodies. Inadequate fluid replacement results in characteristic signs and symptoms.

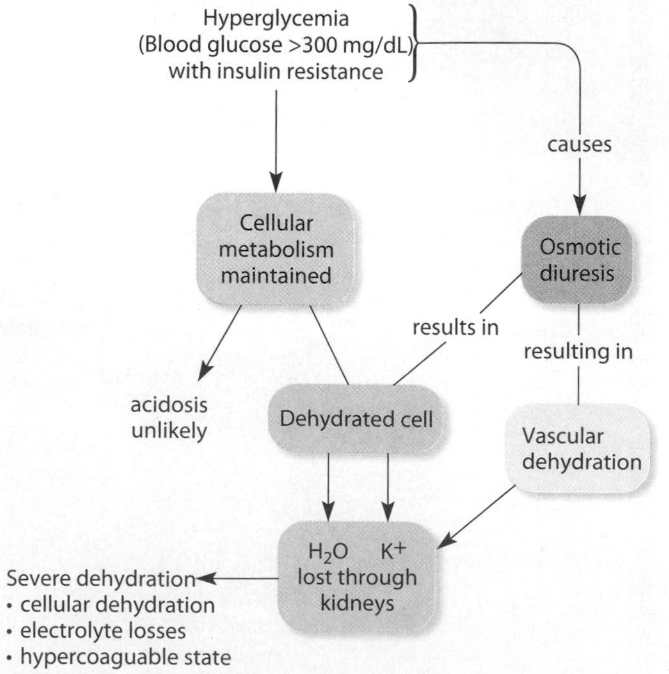

FIGURE 4-8 The pathophysiology of hyperosmolar hyperglycemic state (HHS)—also called hyperglycemic hyperosmolar nonketotic (HHNK) coma.

Procedure 4-1 Blood Glucose Determination

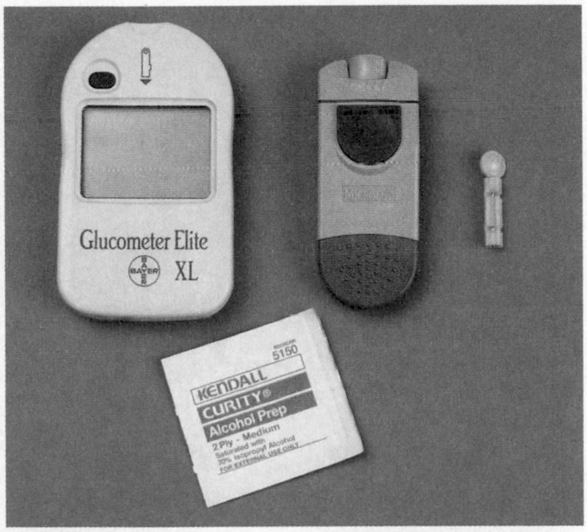

4-1a Prepare the equipment required for blood glucose measurement.

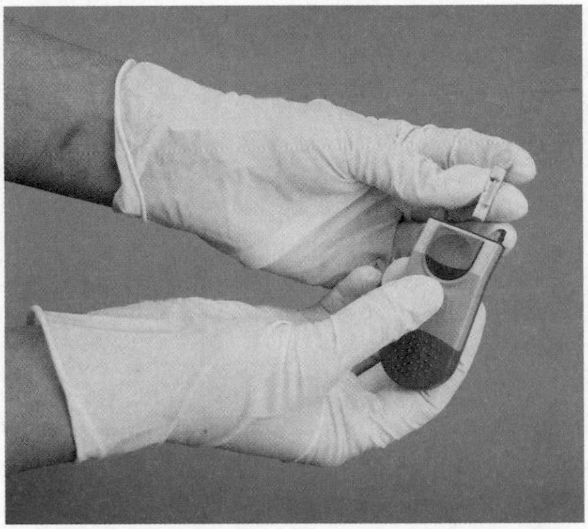

4-1b Insert the lancet into the adjustable lancing device.

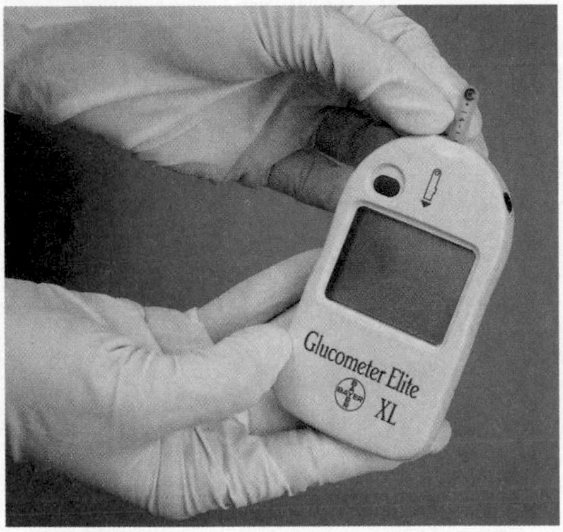

4-1c Remove the test strip and insert into the glucometer test slot.

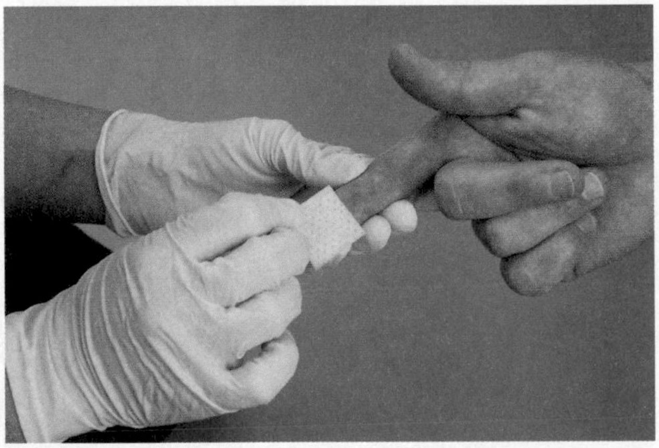

4-1d Cleanse the puncture site.

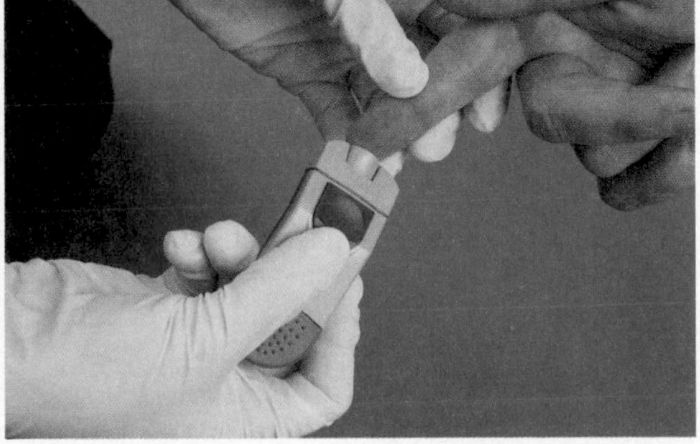

4-1e Perform the puncture.

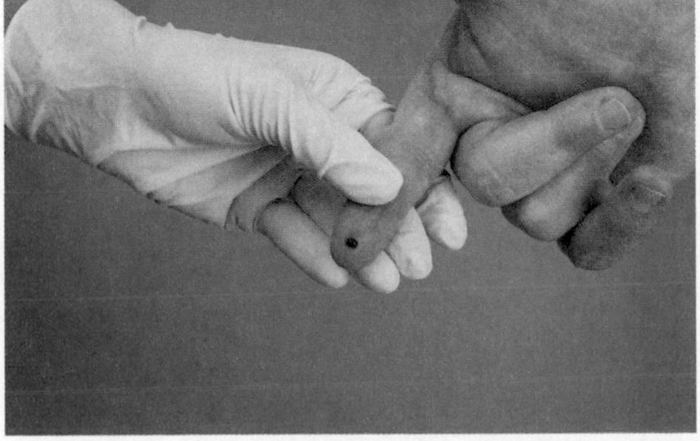

4-1f Obtain a drop of blood.

Procedure 4–1 *Continued*

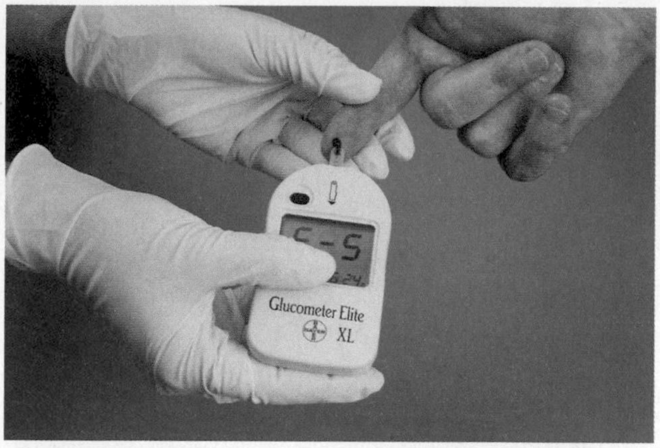

4-1g Apply the blood to the reagent strip in the glucose meter.

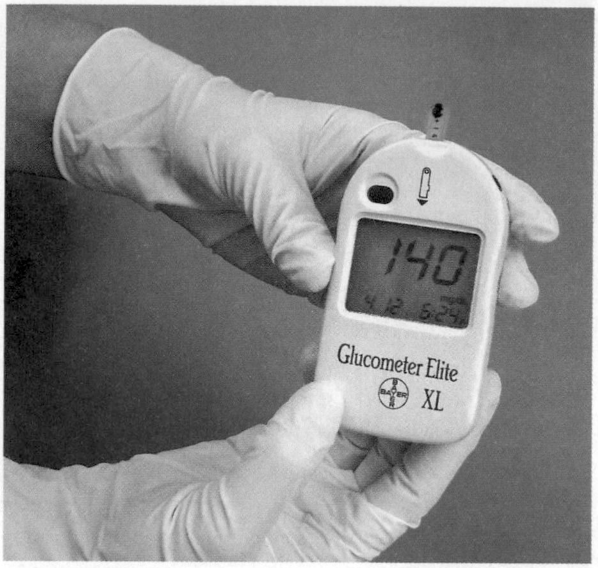

4-1h Read the blood glucose level.

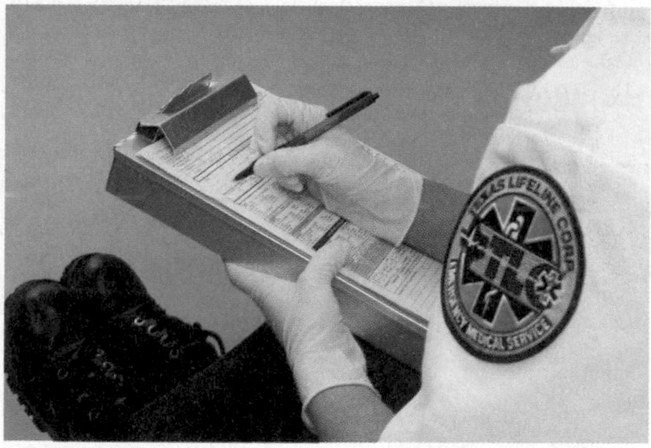

4-1i Record the results on the patient care report.

The mortality rate for HHS coma is higher than that for ketoacidosis, ranging from 40 to 70 percent. The higher mortality rate may be due to the lack of early signs and symptoms that bring patients with ketoacidosis to the attention of family or health care professionals. The mortality rate of HHS is also high because it primarily affects the elderly.

SIGNS AND SYMPTOMS The onset of HHS coma is even slower than that of ketoacidosis, with development often occurring over several days. Early signs include increased urination and increased thirst. Subsequent volume depletion can result in orthostatic hypotension when the patient gets out of bed, along with other signs such as dry skin and mucous membranes as well as tachycardia. The patient may become lethargic, confused, or enter frank coma. Kussmaul's respirations are rarely seen because of the lack of acidosis.

ASSESSMENT AND MANAGEMENT The approach used with the patient suffering from HHS coma is essentially the same as with any other patient who has mental impairment or is unconscious. It is often difficult in the field to distinguish diabetic ketoacidosis from HHS coma. Therefore, the prehospital treatment of both emergencies is identical (see earlier discussion of management of ketoacidosis) and transportation should be expedited.

Hypoglycemia (Insulin Shock)

Hypoglycemia, or low blood glucose, is a medical emergency. It can occur when a patient takes too much insulin, eats too little to match an insulin dose, or overexerts and uses almost all available blood glucose. As the period of hypoglycemia lengthens, the risk rises that brain cells will be permanently damaged or killed due to lack of glucose. You have learned that brain cells can adapt to use fats as an energy source. Note, however, that this adaptation requires hours to develop, and the switch to fat-based metabolism cannot correct any damage already incurred. This is why every second counts in treating hypoglycemia.

PATHOPHYSIOLOGY Hypoglycemia, or insulin shock, reflects high insulin and low blood glucose. Regardless of the reason for low blood sugar, insulin causes almost all remaining blood glucose to be taken up by cells. Because of the high level of insulin, glucagon may be ineffective in raising blood glucose levels. In prolonged fasts, almost half the glucose normally produced through gluconeogenesis is of renal origin. This activity is stimulated by epinephrine. Diabetic patients with kidney failure may be predisposed to hypoglycemia because of lack of renal gluconeogenesis.

SIGNS AND SYMPTOMS The signs and symptoms of hypoglycemia are many and varied. Altered mental status is the most important. Recall the case study that opened this chapter. Mark, who was hypoglycemic, was confused as the police officer spoke to him. In the earliest stages of hypoglycemia, the patient may appear restless or impatient or may complain of hunger. As blood glucose falls lower, he may display inappropriate anger (even rage) or display a bizarre behavior. Sometimes the patient may be placed in police custody for such behavior or be involved in an automobile crash.

Physical signs may include diaphoresis and tachycardia, both of which Mark showed. If blood glucose falls to a critically low level, the patient may have a **hypoglycemic seizure** or become comatose.

In contrast to diabetic ketoacidosis, hypoglycemia can develop quickly. A clear change in mental status can occur without warning. Always consider hypoglycemia when encountering a patient with bizarre behavior. Review Tables 4-3 and 4-4 for additional information.

ASSESSMENT AND MANAGEMENT In suspected cases of hypoglycemia, perform the initial assessment quickly. Look for a MedicAlert bracelet. If possible, determine the blood glucose level. Because of the urgency of this emergency, all paramedic units need to have the capability to perform this task or to rush a blood sample along with the patient.

If the blood glucose level is less than 60 mg/dL, draw a red-top tube of blood and start an IV of normal saline. Next, administer 50 to 100 mL (25 to 50 g) of 50 percent dextrose intravenously. If the patient is conscious and able to swallow, complete glucose administration with orange juice, sugared sodas, or commercially available glucose pastes. Some recent prehospital studies have shown 10 percent dextrose solutions to be just as effective as 50 percent dextrose, without the risks.[4]

If blood glucose cannot be obtained and the patient is unconscious, start an IV of normal saline and administer 50 to 100 mL (25 to 50 g) of 50 percent dextrose. Expedite transport to a medical facility. If you suspect alcoholism, also administer 100 mg of thiamine.

When an IV cannot be started, hypoglycemic patients may improve following the administration of glucagon. This is a much slower process and will work only if there are adequate stores of glycogen available. Glucagon must be reconstituted immediately prior to administration. A dose of 0.5 to 1.0 mg intramuscularly is usually adequate.

Disorders of the Thyroid Gland

You are more likely to see thyroid dysfunction as part of the medical history than as an emergency. However, you may see patients with acute complications of thyroid disorders.[5] The most common of these are:

- **Hyperthyroidism**—the presence of excess thyroid hormones in the blood
- **Thyrotoxicosis**—a condition that reflects prolonged exposure of body organs to excess thyroid hormones, with resultant changes in structure and function (Thyrotoxicosis is generally caused by Graves' disease.)
- **Hypothyroidism**—the presence of inadequate thyroid hormones in the blood
- **Myxedema**—a condition that reflects long-term exposure to inadequate levels of thyroid hormones, with resultant changes in structure and function

Graves' Disease

More than 95 percent of cases of thyrotoxicosis are due to **Graves' disease**. Roughly 15 percent of Graves' disease patients have a close relative with Graves', which suggests a strong hereditary role in predisposition to the disorder. In addition, Graves' disease is about six times more common in women than in men, with onset typically in young adulthood (20s and 30s).

PATHOPHYSIOLOGY Graves' disease has an autoimmune origin. Autoantibodies are generated that stimulate thyroid tissue to produce excessive amounts of thyroid hormones. The resultant changes in organ function are either responses to excess thyroid hormones or responses to the autoantibodies themselves.

SIGNS AND SYMPTOMS Signs and symptoms of Graves' disease include agitation, emotional changeability, insomnia, poor heat tolerance, weight loss despite increased appetite, weakness, dyspnea, and tachycardia

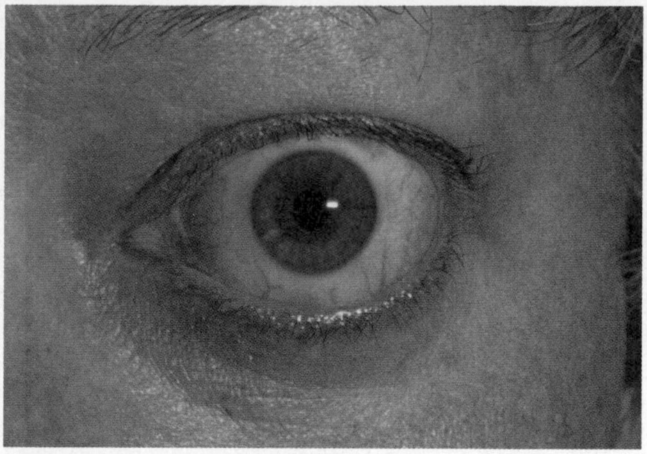

FIGURE 4-9 Exophthalmos.

(© Dr. P. Marazzi/Science Source)

or new-onset atrial fibrillation in the absence of a cardiac history. Nervous system symptoms tend to be more common in younger adults, whereas serious cardiovascular symptoms tend to predominate in older individuals. Prolonged reaction of orbital tissues with the pathological thyroid-stimulating autoantibodies can cause exophthalmos (protrusion of the eyeballs) (Figure 4-9), whereas interaction of autoantibodies with thyroid tissue often produces diffuse goiter (a generally enlarged thyroid gland) (Figure 4-10).

ASSESSMENT AND MANAGEMENT Cardiac dysfunction is probably the most likely context within which an emergency call may arise from thyrotoxicosis (usually caused by Graves' disease, as noted earlier). Use of β-adrenergic blockers such as propranolol may temporarily reduce cardiac stress, but make sure the patient does not have heart failure before considering use. Glucocorticoid therapy (namely, dexamethasone) is sometimes helpful in quickly reducing the level of circulating T_4.

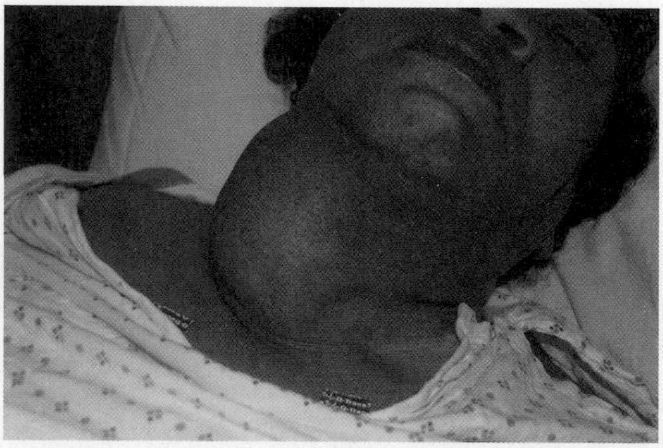

FIGURE 4-10 Generalized enlargement of the thyroid gland (goiter).

(© Edward T. Dickinson, MD)

Thyrotoxic Crisis (Thyroid Storm)

Thyrotoxic crisis, or *thyroid storm*, is a life-threatening emergency that can be fatal within as few as 48 hours if untreated. It is usually associated with severe physiologic stress (e.g., trauma, infection), less often with psychological stress. You may also encounter thyroid storm secondary to overdose of thyroid hormone in a hypothyroid individual.

PATHOPHYSIOLOGY The mechanisms underlying thyrotoxic crisis are poorly understood. An acute increase in the levels of thyroid hormones does not appear to be the cause. It is more likely that thyroid storm is caused by a shift of thyroid hormone in the blood from the protein-bound (biologically inactive) to the free (biologically active) state.

SIGNS AND SYMPTOMS The signs and symptoms associated with thyrotoxic crisis reflect the patient's extreme hypermetabolic state and increased activity of the sympathetic nervous system. The syndrome is characterized by high fever (106°F/41°C or higher), irritability, delirium or coma, tachycardia, hypotension, vomiting, and diarrhea. A less severe presentation may also occur, with slight fever and marked lethargy.

ASSESSMENT AND MANAGEMENT In the presence of the previously mentioned signs and symptoms of thyrotoxic crisis, field management is largely focused on supportive care: oxygenation, ventilatory assistance, fluid resuscitation, and cardiac monitoring. Glucocorticoids and β-adrenergic blockers may be helpful. Transport should be expedited for definitive therapy that blocks the high blood levels of thyroid hormones.

Hypothyroidism and Myxedema

Hypothyroidism can be congenital or acquired. Both sexes can be affected. The recent increase in incidence of hypothyroidism in middle-aged women may reflect better diagnostics, a true rise in incidence, or both. Advanced myxedema in middle-aged and elderly individuals is the condition you are most likely to see as part of a medical emergency, so we will focus most attention on myxedema and the uncommon complication of myxedema coma.

PATHOPHYSIOLOGY Hypothyroidism creates a low metabolic state, and early signs reflect poor organ function and poor response to challenges such as exercise or infection. Over time, untreated severe hypothyroidism causes the additional sign of myxedema: a thickening of connective tissue in the skin and other tissues, including the heart. Patients with myxedema may progress into a hypothermic, stuporous state called **myxedema coma**, which can be fatal if respiratory depression occurs. Triggers for progression include infection, trauma, a cold environment, or exposure

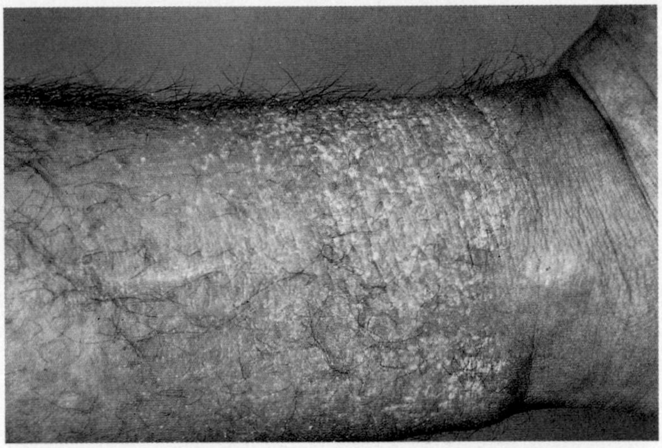

FIGURE 4-11 Doughy, edematous skin typical of myxedema.
(© Biophoto Associates/Science Source)

to central nervous system depressants such as alcohol or certain drugs.

SIGNS AND SYMPTOMS Early signs of hypothyroidism may be subtle. Symptoms may be as slight as fatigue and slowed mental function attributed falsely to aging. Typically, patients with hypothyroidism or myxedema show lethargy, cold intolerance, constipation, decreased mental function, or decreased appetite with increased weight. In addition, the relaxation stage of deep tendon reflexes (DTRs) is slowed. The classic appearance of myxedema is an unemotional, puffy face; thinned hair; enlarged tongue; and pale, cool skin that looks and feels like dough (Figure 4-11). Myxedema coma may be difficult to identify. Note whether the history is consistent with hypothyroidism, and look for the physical appearance of myxedema. Other signs include profound hypothermia (temperatures as low as 75°F/24°C are not uncommon), low-amplitude bradycardia, and carbon dioxide retention.

ASSESSMENT AND MANAGEMENT The presence of the described signs and symptoms may alert you to the possible presence of myxedema. Keep in mind that heart failure due to the combination of age, atherosclerosis, and myxedematous enlargement is not uncommon, so focus on maintenance of ABCs and close monitoring of cardiac and pulmonary status. Most patients with myxedema coma require intubation and ventilatory assistance. Active rewarming is contraindicated due to risk of cardiac arrhythmias and cardiovascular collapse secondary to vasodilation. Although IV access is important, limit fluids because fluid and electrolyte imbalance is common. Expedite transport to an appropriate facility for definitive treatment.

Disorders of the Adrenal Glands

Two disorders of the adrenal cortex can play a part in medical emergencies or complicate responses to trauma—hyperadrenalism and hypoadrenalism. Of these abnormalities, **Cushing's syndrome** and **Addison's disease** are the most commonly encountered. Cushing's syndrome is caused by excessive adrenocortical activity. In contrast, Addison's disease is caused by deficient adrenocortical activity. Reread the earlier section in which we discussed the anatomy and physiology of the adrenal glands to remind yourself how critical these hormones are to metabolic processes and to salt and water balance.[6]

Hyperadrenalism

Cushing's syndrome is a relatively common disorder of the adrenals and is caused by high levels of cortisol in the blood. It can be caused by medications (e.g., glucocorticoids, prednisone) or by tumors of the pituitary gland (adenomas). It usually affects middle-aged persons, with women affected more often than men. Check the patient's history to note any steroid treatment for nonendocrine conditions such as COPD, asthma, and cancer or rheumatologic disorders.

PATHOPHYSIOLOGY Cushing's syndrome is most commonly caused by long-term exposure to excess glucocorticoids, and it produces numerous changes. Metabolically, cortisol is an antagonist to insulin. Gluconeogenesis is prominent, with profound protein catabolism. The body's handling of fats is altered: Atherosclerosis and hypercholesterolemia are common. Over time, diabetes mellitus also may develop. Cortisol's mineralocorticoid activity causes sodium retention and increased blood volume. Increased vascular sensitivity to catecholamines occurs, which may also be a contributor to hypertension. Potassium loss through the kidneys may cause hypokalemia. Cortisol's anti-inflammatory and immunosuppressive properties predispose to infection.

Cushing's syndrome, when caused by pituitary tumors (adenomas), may be referred to as **Cushing's disease**. Outside of extrinsic steroid use, pituitary tumors account for approximately 70 percent of Cushing's syndrome cases.

SIGNS AND SYMPTOMS Regardless of the cause, the presenting signs and symptoms of Cushing's syndrome are the same. The earliest sign is weight gain, particularly through the trunk of the body, face, and neck. A "moon-faced" appearance often develops (Figure 4-12). The accumulation of fat on the upper back is occasionally referred to as a "buffalo hump." Skin changes are also common and may be an early clue to potential problems. These include thinning to an almost transparent appearance, a tendency to bruise easily, delayed healing from even minor wounds, and development of facial hair among women (hirsutism). Mood swings and impaired memory or concentration are also common.

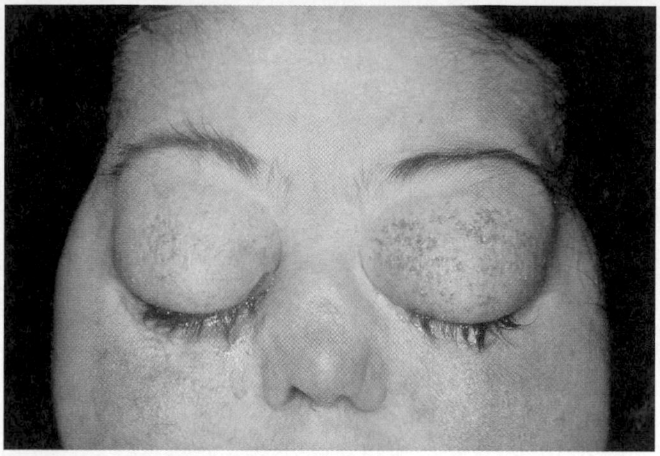

FIGURE 4-12 Facial features of Cushing's syndrome.
(© Biophoto Associates/Science Source)

ASSESSMENT AND MANAGEMENT Although it is unlikely that you will see a patient with acute hyperadrenal crisis, you are likely to encounter patients who exhibit signs and symptoms of Cushing's syndrome. Remember that these patients have a higher incidence of cardiovascular disease, including hypertension and stroke. Pay particular attention to skin preparation when starting IV lines because of skin fragility and susceptibility to infection. Observations indicative of Cushing's syndrome should be noted in your report and relayed to hospital staff.

Adrenal Insufficiency

Adrenal insufficiency, or Addison's disease, occurs when the adrenal glands fail to produce adequate amounts of the steroid hormones (primarily cortisol and aldosterone). Addison's disease is due to cortical destruction. Addison's has become less common as former leading causes of Addison's, such as tuberculosis, have come under control. Currently, more than 90 percent of Addison's disease cases are due to autoimmune disease. As with Graves' disease, another autoimmune disorder, heredity plays a prominent role in predisposition. In fact, patients with Addison's are more likely than average to have other autoimmune disorders, including Graves' disease. Persons with Addison's may be tipped into metabolic failure called **Addisonian crisis** by acute stresses such as infection or trauma. Be alert for this potentially life-threatening emergency.

Adrenal insufficiency can also result from other causes such as *congenital adrenal hyperplasia (CAH)* and *Waterhouse-Friderichsen syndrome (WFS)*. CAH can affect all adrenal hormones and can cause both hyperadrenalism and hypoadrenalism (depending on which hormones are affected). Hypoadrenalism occurs when mineralocorticoid production is reduced. WFS, also called *hemorrhagic adrenalitis*, occurs when an overwhelming bacterial infection (usually *Neisseria meningitides*) causes massive adrenal hemorrhage that reduces or shuts down hormone production by the glands.

PATHOPHYSIOLOGY Destruction of the adrenal cortex results in minimal production of all three classes of hormones: glucocorticoids, mineralocorticoids, and androgens. Low mineralocorticoid activity is key to the changes of Addison's disease: It causes major disturbances in water and electrolyte balance. Increased sodium excretion in urine causes low blood volume, and potassium retention can cause hyperkalemia and ECG changes. Note that many cases of adrenal insufficiency are due to therapy with steroids such as prednisone. Such therapy can completely suppress normal adrenal function, and sudden cessation of the drug may trigger symptoms of Addison's disease or even an Addisonian crisis, with cardiovascular collapse.

SIGNS AND SYMPTOMS Addison's disease is characterized by changes related to low corticosteroid activity: progressive weakness, fatigue, decreased appetite, and weight loss. Hyperpigmentation of the skin and mucous membranes, particularly in sun-exposed areas, is also characteristic.

Include Addisonian crisis in your list of possible causes of unexplained cardiovascular collapse, particularly if the history suggests primary Addison's or Addison's secondary to drug therapy. Many patients will have gastrointestinal problems such as vomiting or diarrhea, which will exacerbate electrolyte imbalances, low blood volume, and hypotension and increase the potential for cardiac arrhythmias.

ASSESSMENT AND MANAGEMENT The patient may reveal the presence of Addison's disease during the history, or the signs and symptoms just discussed may lead you to suspect the presence of Addison's. Focus emergency management on maintenance of the ABCs and close monitoring of cardiac and oxygenation status as well as blood glucose level. Hypoglycemia poses its own threat. Assess blood glucose levels and administer 25 to 50 g of 50 percent dextrose to patients with blood glucose levels less than 50 mg/dL or those with altered mental status. Obtain a baseline 12-lead ECG to check for arrhythmias related to electrolyte imbalance. Be aggressive in fluid resuscitation. Follow your local protocol or contact medical direction for specific orders based on your patient's presentation. Expedite transport to an appropriate facility for definitive treatment.

Summary

In conjunction with the nervous system, the endocrine system regulates body functions. The vast majority of endocrine emergencies you encounter will involve complications of diabetes mellitus, such as hypoglycemia or ketoacidosis. Other endocrine emergencies tend to be rare and will more likely be part of the patient history rather than the emergency itself.

In the field, always suspect diabetes when a patient presents with unexplained changes in mental status. A quick check with your glucometer will indicate the patient's glucose level.

A common diabetic emergency is a call to the home of a diabetic who has taken insulin but skipped a meal or, possibly, has vomited shortly after eating, thereby not taking in the sugar necessary to balance the insulin. Hypoglycemia, the most urgent diabetic emergency, must be quickly treated to prevent serious nervous system damage. When you cannot determine the exact type of diabetic emergency, treat for hypoglycemia.

Generally, when the patient's glucose level is low the skin becomes cool and clammy; when the glucose level is high, the skin generally is warm and dry. (A way to remember this is the rhyme, "When the skin is warm and dry, the sugar is high.") However, if you are unable to obtain a glucose level in a known diabetic who has an altered level of consciousness, treating the patient for hypoglycemia will not be detrimental, even if the patient is hyperglycemic, especially when compared to the consequences of withholding treatment of a hypoglycemic patient. A hyperglycemic patient, especially one in diabetic ketoacidosis (DKA), will need long-term treatment that will require hospitalization and constant monitoring.

Your primary responsibility for any diabetic emergency is to maintain a stable airway, oxygenate the patient, establish an IV line, and transport.

You Make the Call

It's a beautiful Sunday afternoon in spring. You and your partner are dispatched for an "unknown medical emergency" in a residential neighborhood. Within 4 minutes you are on scene with a 23-year-old woman who complains of extreme weakness and dizziness when she sits up or attempts to stand. She reports that over the past 48 hours she has had a fever (103°F) and abdominal pain, accompanied by nausea, vomiting, diarrhea, and loss of appetite. Blood pressure is 82/66 mmHg, pulse is 110 beats per minute, and respirations are 26 per minute and labored. Her skin is very pale but hot to the touch. Her mucous membranes are dry. Bilateral lung sounds are clear and equal. Pulse oximetry is 95 percent. ECG shows sinus tachycardia with peaked T waves and no ectopy. Glucometer reads "low" (<50 mg/dL).

When obtaining her history, you learn from her husband that she has had severe asthma since age 8 and is routinely managed with albuterol (Ventolin), cromolyn (Intal), and prednisone (Deltasone). She had not had any problems for several months, but over the past two weeks she was treated for bronchitis with antibiotics. She reports that she finished the antibiotics three days earlier. However, on further questioning you find out that she has not had any prednisone for four days. It seems that she ran out of prednisone but did not refill the prescription because she was feeling so much better. She intended to refill it tomorrow when she had a follow-up appointment with her doctor.

1. What is your first priority?
2. What additional intervention is needed?
3. What do you suspect is the likely cause of her signs and symptoms?
4. Should you transport this patient to the hospital or could her husband take her in their private vehicle?

See Suggested Responses at the back of this book.

Review Questions

1. The majority of the body's glands are of which type?
   a. Hormone
   b. Exocrine
   c. Endocrine
   d. Adrenal
2. The natural tendency of the body to maintain an appropriate internal environment despite changing external conditions is known as ____________
   a. hemostasis.
   b. metabolism.
   c. homeostasis.
   d. equilibrium.
3. Which endocrine gland is considered to be the "master gland" of the body?
   a. Pineal
   b. Adrenal
   c. Thymus
   d. Pituitary
4. ____________, the natural form of the drug Pitocin, stimulates uterine contraction and lactation in women who have just delivered a baby.
   a. Oxytocin
   b. Vasopressin
   c. Thyrotropin
   d. Antidiuretic hormone
5. The parathyroid glands secrete which hormone?
   a. TSH
   b. PTH
   c. FSH
   d. ACTH
6. The three most important types of endocrine cells in the islets of Langerhans include all of the following *except* ____________.
   a. beta cells.
   b. alpha cells.
   c. delta cells.
   d. gamma cells.
7. Which male hormone promotes the development and maintenance of secondary male sexual characteristics and plays a role in development of sperm?
   a. LH
   b. FSH
   c. Estrogen
   d. Testosterone
8. Which diabetic emergency will occur if a patient takes too much insulin, eats too little to match an insulin dose, or overexerts and uses almost all available blood glucose?
   a. HHNK
   b. Hyperglycemia
   c. Hypoglycemia
   d. Ketoacidosis
9. A condition that reflects long-term exposure to inadequate levels of thyroid hormones, which can result in an unresponsive patient, is known as ____________
   a. myxedema.
   b. thyrotoxicosis.
   c. hypothyroidism.
   d. hyperthyroidism.
10. The vast majority of endocrine emergencies seen in the prehospital environment involve complications of what pathology?
    a. Hyperthyroidism
    b. Hypoadrenalism
    c. Diabetes mellitus
    d. Hepatic failure

See Answers to Review Questions at the back of this book.

References

1. American Diabetes Association. "Diagnosis and Classification of Diabetes Mellitus." *Diabetes Care* 33 (2010) (Suppl 1): S62–S69.
2. Kitabchi, A. E. and E. A. Nyenwe. "Hyperglycemic Crisis in Diabetes Mellitus: Diabetic Ketoacidosis and Hyperglycemic Hyperosmolar State." *Endocrinol Metab Clin North Am* 35 (2006): 725–751.
3. Nugent, B. W. "Hyperosmolar Hyperglycemic State." *Emerg Med Clin North Am* 23 (2005): 629–648.
4. Noore, C. and M. Wollard. "Dextrose 10% or 50% in the Treatment of Hypoglycaemia Out of Hospital? A Randomized Trial." *Emerg Med J* 22 (2005): 512–515.
5. Sarlis, N. J. and L. Gourgiotis. "Thyroid Emergencies." *Rev Endocr Metab Disord* 4 (2003): 129–136.
6. Torrey, S. P. "Recognition and Management of Adrenal Emergencies." *Emerg Med Clin North Am* 23 (2005): 687–702.

Further Reading

Bledsoe, B. E. "No More Coma Cocktails: Using Science to Dispel and Improve Patient Care." *JEMS* 27(11) (2002): 54–60.

Gardner, D. and D. Shoback. *Greenspan's Basic & Clinical Endocrinology*. 9th ed. Philadelphia: McGraw-Hill, 2011.

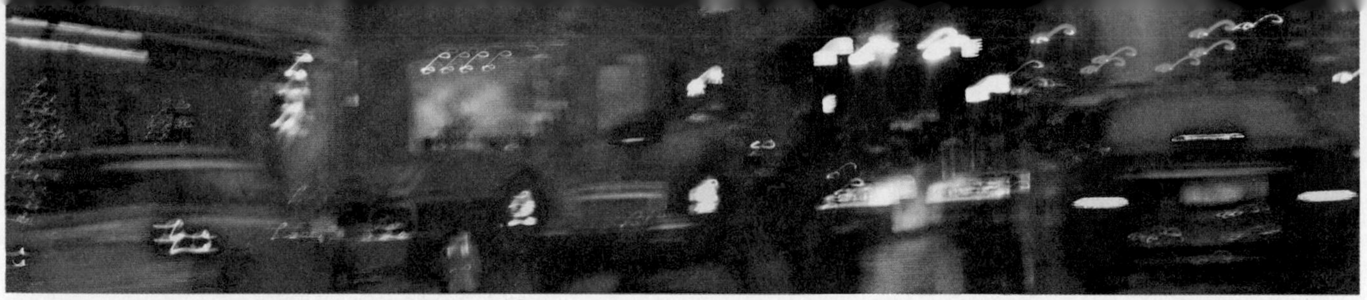

Chapter 5
Immunology

Bryan Bledsoe, DO, FACEP, FAAEM, EMT-P

STANDARD

Medicine (Immunology)

COMPETENCY

Integrates assessment findings with principles of epidemiology and pathophysiology to formulate a field impression and implement a comprehensive treatment/disposition plan for a patient with a medical complaint.

Learning Objectives

Terminal Performance Objective: After reading this chapter, you should be able to integrate patient assessment findings, patient history, and knowledge of anatomy, physiology, pathophysiology, and basic and advanced life support interventions to recognize and manage patients with allergic reactions and anaphylaxis.

Enabling Objectives: To accomplish the terminal performance objective, you should be able to:

1. Define key terms introduced in this chapter.
2. Review the anatomy and physiology of the immune system.
3. Explain the general pathophysiological changes of immunological emergencies, and relate this to disturbances in normal immune physiology.
4. Adapt the scene size-up, primary assessment, history, secondary assessment, and use of monitoring technology to arrive at a field impression and differentials for immunological emergencies.
5. Use a process of clinical reasoning to guide and interpret the patient assessment findings and develop a treatment plan for patients with immunological disorders in the prehospital environment.
6. Given a variety of scenarios, describe the integration of assessment and management guidelines as they relate to immunological emergencies.

KEY TERMS

acquired immunity, p. 264
active immunity, p. 264
allergen, p. 265
allergic reaction, p. 263
allergy, p. 264
anaphylaxis, p. 263
angioneurotic edema, p. 266
antibody, p. 263
antigen, p. 263
basophil, p. 265
cellular immunity, p. 263
delayed hypersensitivity, p. 265
histamine, p. 266
humoral immunity, p. 263
Hymenoptera, p. 263
hypersensitivity, p. 264
immediate hypersensitivity, p. 265
immune response, p. 263
immune system, p. 263
immunoglobulin (Ig), p. 263
induced active immunity, p. 264
mast cell, p. 265
natural immunity, p. 264
naturally acquired immunity, p. 264
passive immunity, p. 264
pathogen, p. 263
primary response, p. 264
secondary response, p. 264
sensitization, p. 264
slow-reacting substance of anaphylaxis (SRS-A), p. 266
toxin, p. 263
urticaria, p. 268

Case Study

Cherokee Nation EMS is dispatched to a clinic on the outskirts of town for a medical emergency. At the scene, clinic staff meet the paramedics and direct them to a treatment room. The nurse practitioner reports that a 39-year-old man received an immunization injection approximately 15 minutes earlier. Immediately after the injection, the man developed a red rash and generalized itching. This quickly progressed to obvious hives, wheezing, and associated dyspnea. As the reaction worsened, the patient became hoarse, more dyspneic, and hypotensive. A nurse was now administering supplemental oxygen while another clinic employee was setting up an intravenous infusion.

The primary assessment reveals an alert 39-year-old Native American man in marked distress. His airway is open, but there is marked stridor and audible wheezing. The carotid pulse is rapid and weak. Paramedics quickly remove the nasal cannula placed by the clinic staff and place a nonrebreather oxygen mask. The airway kit is opened in case rapid endotracheal intubation is required.

Steve Williams, the lead paramedic, begins a more detailed assessment while his partner, Beth White Cloud, begins to search for a vein to catheterize. The patient is diaphoretic and has urticarial lesions on the trunk and extremities. In addition, he is tachypneic, with a weak and thready pulse. The blood pressure is 108/50 mmHg, the pulse is 120 beats per minute, respirations are 32 breaths per minute, and oxygen saturation is 100 percent on the nonrebreather.

While Beth places the IV, Steve administers 0.5 milligrams of epinephrine 1:1,000 intramuscularly per system standing orders. Within approximately 2 minutes, the patient's stridor begins to improve and respirations slow. Beth completes placement of the IV and secures it with tape and tincture of benzoin because of the patient's marked diaphoresis. Beth administers 50 milligrams of diphenhydramine (Benadryl) intravenously. Steve prepares a prefill of epinephrine 1:10,000 for intravenous administration in case the patient does not improve.

Within 5 minutes, the paramedics note significant improvement. In fact, it appears that most of the urticarial lesions have cleared. The patient's respiratory rate is down to 22 breaths per minute, but the patient's heart rate is up to 136 beats per minute, which the paramedics attribute to the epinephrine. A repeat blood pressure reading is 100/74 mmHg. Steve opens the IV infusion and administers a 500-milliliter fluid bolus.

The patient continues to improve and is moved to the ambulance for transport to the emergency department. On arrival, the patient is assessed by Stephen Johnston, MD. Dr. Johnston orders the administration of an intravenous corticosteroid and additional IV fluids. The patient is observed for 2 hours and discharged, symptom free. A phone call to the clinic reveals that the patient received a tetanus immunization. In reviewing the case, Dr. Johnston learns from the patient that he had a similar reaction with a prior tetanus immunization but failed to relay this information to the clinic staff.

Introduction

An **allergic reaction** is an exaggerated response by the immune system to a foreign substance. Allergic reactions can range from mild skin rashes to severe, life-threatening reactions that involve virtually every body system. The most severe type of allergic reaction is called **anaphylaxis**. Anaphylaxis is a life-threatening emergency that requires prompt recognition and specific treatment by paramedics. The emergency treatment of anaphylaxis is one area of prehospital care in which advanced life support measures often mean the difference between life and death. Anaphylaxis can develop within seconds and cause death just minutes after exposure to the offending agent. Fortunately, several emergency medications are available to reverse the adverse effects of anaphylaxis.

The first complete description of anaphylaxis was reported in 1902 by Portier and Richet, French immunologists who were attempting to immunize dogs against the toxin of the deadly sea anemone (sea flower). They were injecting small, nonlethal quantities of the toxin into the animals in hopes of stimulating immunity to the toxin. However, when the animals received secondary injections of sublethal quantities of the toxin, at a time when it might be expected that they would be immune, the dogs developed shock and died. Richet called this dramatic and unexpected phenomenon *anaphylaxis*, which means the opposite of *phylaxis*, or protection.[1]

Anaphylaxis results from exposure to a particular substance that sets off a biochemical chain of events that can ultimately lead to shock and death. The exact incidence of anaphylaxis is unknown. However, an estimated 400 to 800 deaths annually in the United States are attributed to anaphylaxis. Injected penicillin and bee and wasp (**Hymenoptera**) stings are the two most common causes of fatal anaphylaxis. About 100 to 500 deaths per year are attributed to the parenteral administration of penicillin. Approximately 25 to 40 persons die each year from *Hymenoptera* stings. Fortunately, the incidence of anaphylaxis appears to be declining, presumably due to better recognition and treatment, as well as the availability of numerous potent antihistamines.

Pathophysiology

The immune system is the principal body system involved in allergic reactions. However, other body systems are also affected by an allergic reaction. These include the cardiovascular system, respiratory system, nervous system, and gastrointestinal system, among others. To fully appreciate the complexity of allergic and anaphylactic reactions, it is first necessary to review the anatomy and physiology of the immune system as it relates to the immune response.[2]

The Immune System

CONTENT REVIEW

- ➤ Allergic Reactions
  - Allergic reaction (exaggerated response by the immune system)
  - Anaphylaxis (the most severe form of allergic reaction)
- ➤ Anaphylaxis is often life-threatening

The **immune system** is a complicated body system responsible for combating infection. Components of the immune system can be found in the blood, bone marrow, and lymphatic system.

The **immune response** is a complex cascade of events that occurs following activation by an invading substance, or **pathogen**. The goal of the immune response is the destruction or inactivation of pathogens, abnormal cells, or foreign molecules such as **toxins**. The body can accomplish this through two mechanisms: cellular immunity and humoral immunity. **Cellular immunity** involves a direct attack of the foreign substance by specialized cells of the immune system. These cells physically engulf and deactivate or destroy the offending agent. **Humoral immunity**, on the other hand, is much more complicated. Humoral immunity is basically a chemical attack of the invading substance. The principal chemical agents of this attack are **antibodies**, also called **immunoglobulins (Igs)**. Antibodies are a unique class of chemicals that are manufactured by specialized cells of the immune system called *B cells*. There are five different classes of antibodies: IgA, IgD, IgE, IgG, and IgM.

The humoral immune response begins with exposure of the body to an antigen. An **antigen** is any substance capable of inducing an immune response (Table 5-1). Most antigens are proteins. Following exposure to an antigen, antibodies are released from cells of the immune system. These antibodies attach themselves to the invading substance to facilitate removal of that substance from the body by other cells of the immune system.

Table 5-1 Agents That May Cause Anaphylaxis

Antibiotics and other drugs
Foreign proteins (horse serum, streptokinase)
Foods (nuts, eggs, shrimp)
Allergen extracts (allergy shots)
Hymenoptera stings (bees, wasps)
Hormones (insulin)
Blood products
Aspirin
Nonsteroidal anti-inflammatory drugs (NSAIDs)
Preservatives (sulfiting agents)
X-ray contrast media
Dextran

If the body has never been exposed to a particular antigen, the response of the immune system is different than if it has been previously exposed to the particular antigen. The initial response to an antigen is called the **primary response**. Following exposure to a new antigen, several days are required before both the cellular and humoral components of the immune system respond. Generalized antibodies (IgG and IgM) are first released to help fight the antigen.

At the same time, other components of the immune system begin to develop antibodies specific for the antigen. These cells also develop a *memory* of the particular antigen. If the body is exposed to the same antigen again, the immune system responds much faster. This is called the **secondary response**. As a part of the secondary response, antibodies specific for the offending antigen are released. Antigen-specific antibodies are much more effective in facilitating removal of the offending antigen than the generalized antibodies released during the primary response.

Immunity may be either *natural* or *acquired*. **Natural immunity**, also called *innate immunity*, is genetically predetermined. It is present at birth and has no relation to previous exposure to a particular antigen. All humans are born with some innate immunity.

Acquired immunity develops over time and results from exposure to an antigen. Following exposure to a particular antigen, the immune system will produce antibodies specific for the antigen. This protects the organism, as subsequent exposure to the same antigen will result in a vigorous immune response. **Naturally acquired immunity** normally begins to develop after birth and is continually enhanced by exposure to new pathogens and antigens throughout life. For example, a child contracts chickenpox (varicella) at age 18 months. Following the infection, the child's immune system creates antibodies specific for the varicella virus. Repeated exposure to the varicella virus usually will not result in another infection. In fact, it is not unusual for a patient exposed to varicella to develop lifelong immunity to the infection.

Induced active immunity, also called *artificially acquired immunity*, is designed to provide protection from exposure to an antigen at some time in the future. This is achieved through vaccination and provides relative protection against serious infectious agents. In vaccination, an antigen is injected into the body to generate an immune response. This results in the development of antibodies specific for the antigen and provides protection against future infection. Most vaccines contain antigenic proteins from a particular virus or bacterium. Later, when the individual is actually exposed to the pathogen, the immune response will be vigorous and will often be enough to prevent the infection from developing.

An example of a vaccine commonly used is the DPT (diphtheria/pertussis/tetanus) vaccine. This vaccine contains antigenic proteins from the bacteria that cause diphtheria, whooping cough, and tetanus. The vaccine is administered at several intervals during the first five years of life. It provides protection against infection from these bacteria. Some vaccinations will impart lifelong immunity while others must be periodically followed with a "booster dose" to ensure continued protection.

Acquired immunity can be either *active* or *passive*. **Active immunity** occurs following exposure to an antigen and results in the production of antibodies specific for the antigen. Most vaccinations result in the development of active immunity, although it takes some time for a patient to develop specific antibodies. In certain cases, it is necessary to administer antibodies to provide protection until the active immunity can kick in. The administration of antibodies is referred to as **passive immunity**. There are two types of passive immunity. *Natural passive immunity* occurs when antibodies cross the placental barrier from the mother to the infant to provide protection against embryonic or fetal infections. *Induced passive immunity* is the administration of antibodies to an individual to help fight infection or prevent diseases.

An example of the clinical use of both active and passive immunity is the regimen used for the prevention of tetanus. Most persons who are from developed countries have typically received some form of tetanus vaccination during their lives. These people typically have some antibodies to tetanus and often need nothing more than a tetanus booster. However, some people have never received any sort of tetanus vaccination. When these people seek treatment for a tetanus-prone wound, they must receive prophylaxis for tetanus in addition to care for their wound. This is best achieved by the provision of both passive and active immunity. To provide immediate protection, the patient is administered antibodies specific for tetanus (tetanus immune globulin [TIG] Hypertet®). Then, they are administered a tetanus vaccination (Td or Dt). The tetanus immune globulin (TIG) provides passive immunity until such time as the body's immune system can respond to the tetanus vaccination with the development of antibodies specific for tetanus. This should be followed by periodic tetanus boosters until the patient's immunization program is complete.

Allergies

The initial exposure of an individual to an antigen is referred to as **sensitization**. Sensitization results in an immune response. Subsequent exposure induces a much stronger secondary response. Some individuals can become hypersensitive (overly sensitive) to a particular antigen. **Hypersensitivity** is an unexpected and exaggerated reaction to a particular antigen. In many instances, hypersensitivity is used synonymously with the term **allergy**. There are two types of hypersensitivity reactions, *delayed* and *immediate* (Table 5-2).

Table 5-2 Gell and Coombs Classification of Hypersensitivity Reactions

Type	Classification	Mediator	Examples
I	Immediate hypersensitivity reactions	Immunoglobulin E (IgE)	Common allergies Asthma
II	Cytotoxic hypersensitivity reactions	Immunoglobulin G (IgG) Immunoglobulin M (IgM)	Thrombocytopenia
III	Immune-complex reactions	Circulating antigen–antibody complexes	Serum sickness Systemic lupus erythematosus
IV	Delayed hypersensitivity reactions	Cell-mediated T cells	Poison ivy/oak Chronic transplant rejections

Delayed Hypersensitivity

Delayed hypersensitivity is a result of *cellular immunity* and therefore does not involve antibodies. Delayed hypersensitivity usually occurs in the hours and days following exposure and is the sort of allergy that occurs in normal people. Delayed hypersensitivity most commonly results in a skin rash and is often due to exposure to certain drugs and chemicals. The rash associated with poison ivy is an example of delayed hypersensitivity.

Immediate Hypersensitivity

When people use the term *allergy*, they are usually referring to **immediate hypersensitivity** reactions. Examples of immediate hypersensitivity reactions include hay fever, drug allergies, food allergies, eczema, and asthma. Some persons have an allergic tendency. This allergic tendency is usually genetic, meaning that it is passed from parent to child and is characterized by the presence of large quantities of IgE antibodies. An antigen that causes release of the IgE antibodies is referred to as an **allergen**. Common allergens include:

- Drugs
- Foods and food additives
- Animals
- Insects (*Hymenoptera* stings) and insect parts
- Fungi and molds
- Radiology contrast materials

Allergens can enter the body through various routes. These include oral ingestion, inhalation, topically, and through injection or envenomation (Figure 5-1). The vast majority of anaphylactic reactions result from injection or envenomation.

Parenteral penicillin injections are the most common cause of fatal anaphylactic reactions. Insect stings are the second most frequent cause of fatal anaphylactic reactions. Insects in the order *Hymenoptera* are the most frequent offending insects. There are three families in this order: fire ants (*Formicoidea*); wasps, yellow jackets, and hornets (*Vespidae*); and the honeybees (*Apoidea*). All produce a unique venom, although there are similar components in each. Honeybees often will leave their stinger embedded in the victim following a sting.

Following exposure to a particular allergen, large quantities of IgE antibodies are released. These antibodies attach to the membranes of **basophils** and **mast cells**—specialized cells of the immune system that contain chemicals that assist in the immune response. When the allergen binds to IgE attached to the basophils and mast cells, these cells release histamine, heparin, and other substances into

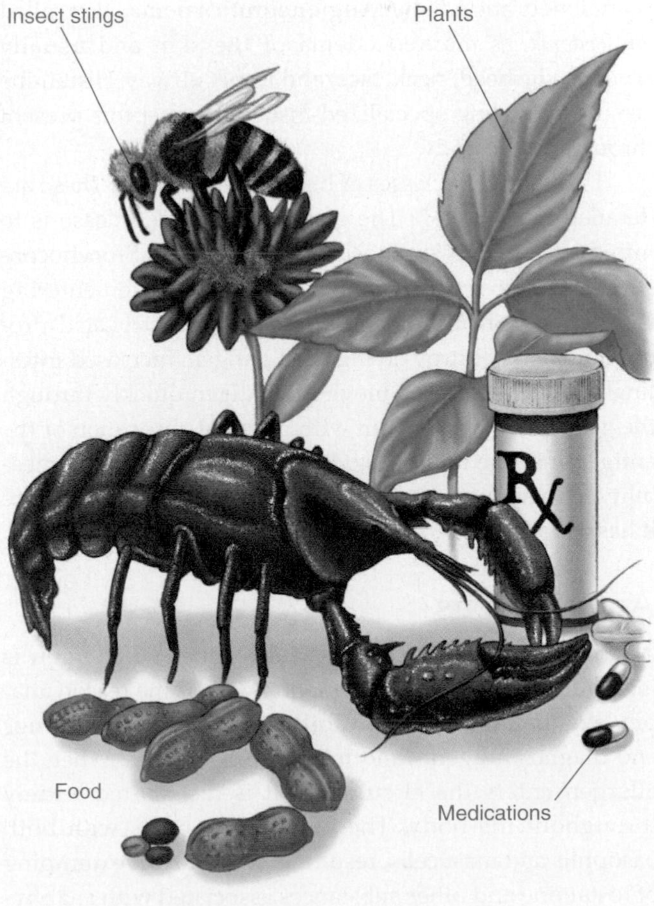

FIGURE 5-1 Anaphylactic reactions can result from a variety of causes.

Table 5-3 Histamine Receptor Types

Receptor Type	Major Tissue Locations	Major Biological Effects
H_1	Smooth muscle, endothelial cells	Acute allergic reactions
H_2	Gastric parietal cells	Secretion of gastric acid
H_3	Central nervous system	Modulation of neurotransmission
H_4	Mast cells, eosinophils, T cells	Regulate immune response

the surrounding tissues. Histamine and other substances are stored in *granules* found within the basophils and mast cells. In fact, because of this feature, basophils and mast cells are often called *granulocytes.* The process of releasing these substances from the cells is called *degranulation.* This release results in what people call an *allergic reaction*, which can be mild to severe.

The principal chemical mediator of an allergic reaction is histamine. **Histamine** is a potent substance that causes bronchoconstriction, increased intestinal motility, vasodilation, and increased vascular permeability. Increased vascular permeability causes the leakage of fluid from the circulatory system into the surrounding tissues. A common manifestation of severe allergic reactions and anaphylaxis is angioneurotic edema. **Angioneurotic edema**, also called *angioedema,* is marked edema of the skin and usually involves the head, neck, face, and upper airway. Histamine acts by activating specialized histamine receptors present throughout the body.

There are four classes of histamine receptors. These are detailed in Table 5-3. The goal of histamine release is to minimize the body's exposure to the antigen. Bronchoconstriction decreases the possibility of the antigen entering through the respiratory tract. Increased gastric acid production helps destroy an ingested antigen. Increased intestinal motility serves to move the antigen quickly through the gastrointestinal system with minimal absorption of the antigen into the body. Vasodilation and capillary permeability help remove the allergen from the circulation, where it has the potential to do the most harm (Figure 5-2).

Anaphylaxis

Anaphylaxis usually occurs when a specific allergen is injected directly into the circulation. This is the reason anaphylaxis is more common following injections of drugs and diagnostic agents and following bee stings. When the allergen enters the circulation, it is distributed widely throughout the body. The allergen interacts with both basophils and mast cells, resulting in the massive dumping of histamine and other substances associated with anaphylaxis. The principal body systems affected by anaphylaxis are the cardiovascular, respiratory, and gastrointestinal systems and the skin. Histamine causes widespread peripheral vasodilation, as well as increased permeability of the capillaries. Increased capillary permeability results in marked loss of plasma from the circulation. People sustaining anaphylaxis can actually die from circulatory shock.

Also released from the basophils and mast cells is a substance called **slow-reacting substance of anaphylaxis (SRS-A)**. This causes spasm of the bronchial smooth muscle, resulting in an asthmalike attack and, occasionally, asphyxia. SRS-A potentiates the effects of histamine, especially the effects on the respiratory system.

Patho Pearls

Allergic Responses: Some Are Lifesaving, Some Can Kill. The allergic response to an antigen is designed to rapidly eliminate the offending antigen from the body. In most people, this response is mild. However, in those previously sensitized to the antigen, the response can be massive, even life threatening.

The cascade of events following exposure to the antigen serves to remove the antigens from the body and to prevent additional ones from entering it. For example, shortly after exposure, persons previously sensitized to the antigen will develop bronchospasm and, in some cases, coughing with sputum. The bronchospasm serves to prevent additional antigens from entering the respiratory tract; the cough and increased sputum production help to remove any antigens there. Likewise, following exposure, histamine is released from mast cells and basophils. Histamine, in addition to causing bronchospasm, causes the capillaries to become leaky, allowing fluid to leave the intravascular space and enter the interstitial space. This can cause the antigen to be taken from the blood, where it is causing problems, and moved to the interstitial space, where it can eventually be removed by the lymphatic system and its components. Similarly, vomiting and diarrhea are common with severe allergic reactions. These help to remove any offending pathogens from the gastrointestinal tract.

Unfortunately, when the allergic response becomes severe (anaphylactic), it can lead to cardiovascular collapse, massive bronchospasm, and excessive fluid shifts. Because of this, paramedics may have to intervene with drugs such as epinephrine, diphenhydramine (Benadryl), and others discussed in this chapter, which will help counter some of the untoward effects described here.

Assessment Findings in Anaphylaxis

The signs and symptoms of anaphylaxis begin within 30 to 60 seconds following exposure to the offending allergen. In a small percentage of patients, the onset of signs and symptoms may be delayed by over an hour. The signs and symptoms of anaphylaxis (Table 5-4) can vary significantly. The severity of the reaction is often related to the speed of

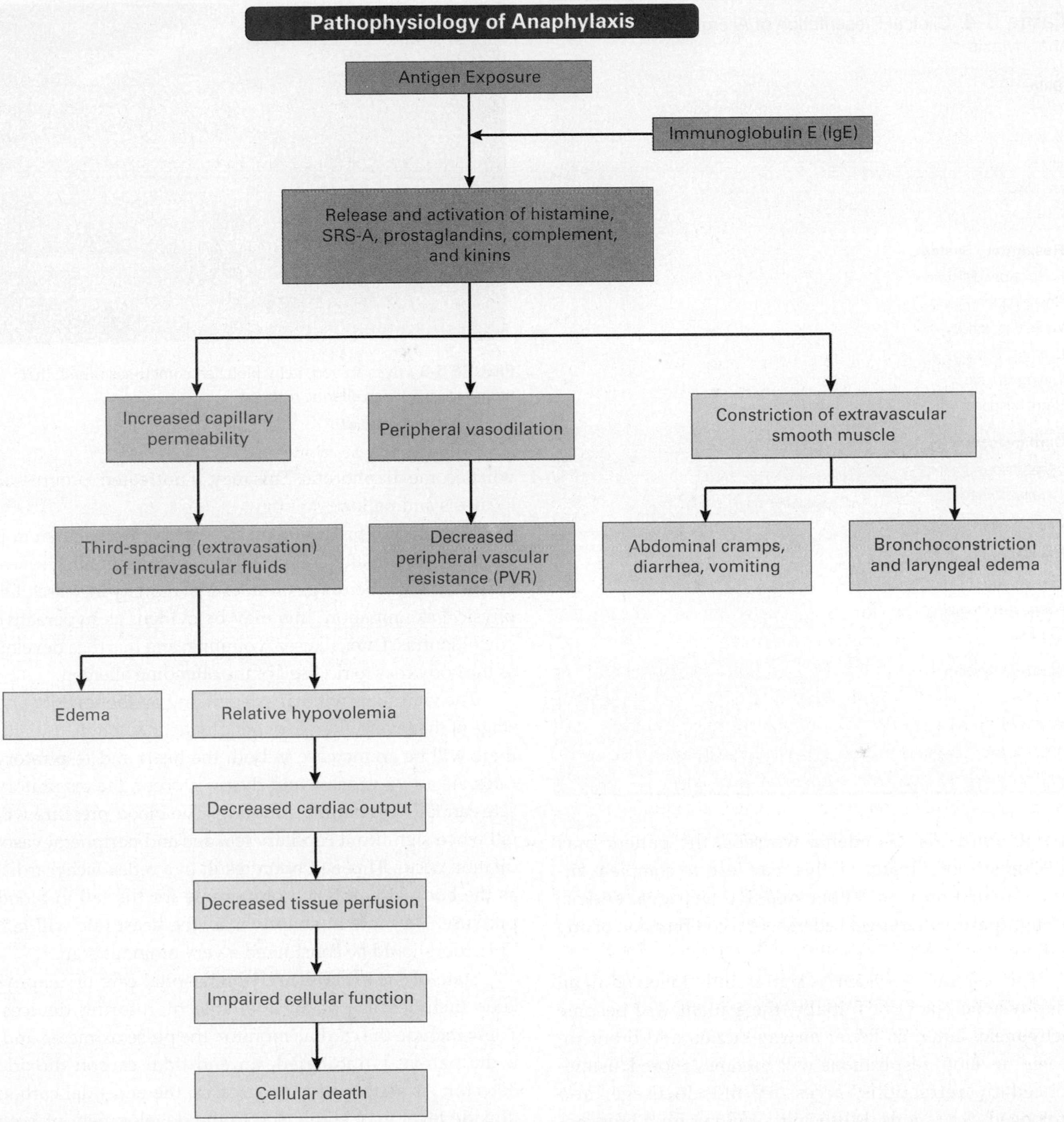

FIGURE 5-2 Pathophysiology of anaphylaxis.

onset. Reactions that develop very quickly tend to be much more severe.

A rapid and focused assessment is crucial to the early detection and treatment of anaphylaxis. Patients suffering an anaphylactic reaction often have a sense of impending doom. This sense of impending doom is often followed by development of additional signs and symptoms.

If the patient's condition permits, a brief history should be gathered, including previous allergen exposures and reactions. If possible, try to determine how quickly symptoms started and how severe they were.

Next, quickly evaluate the patient's level of consciousness. Upper airway problems, including laryngeal edema, may result in the patient being unable to speak. As the emergency progresses, the patient will become restless. As cardiovascular collapse continues, the patient will exhibit a decreased level of consciousness. If untreated, this may continue to unresponsiveness.

As noted earlier, a common manifestation of anaphylaxis is angioneurotic edema, involving the face and neck. Laryngeal edema is also a frequent complication and can threaten the airway. Initially, laryngeal edema will cause a

Table 5-4 Clinical Presentation of Allergies and Anaphylaxis

Skin
Flushing
Itching
Hives
Swelling
Cyanosis
Respiratory System
Respiratory difficulty
Sneezing, coughing
Wheezing, stridor
Laryngeal edema
Laryngospasm
Bronchospasm
Cardiovascular System
Vasodilation
Increased heart rate
Decreased blood pressure
Gastrointestinal System
Nausea and vomiting
Abdominal cramping
Diarrhea
Nervous System
Dizziness
Headache
Convulsions
Tearing

hoarse voice. As the edema worsens, the patient may develop stridor. Finally, all this may lead to complete airway obstruction from either massive laryngeal edema, laryngospasm, pharyngeal edema, or a combination of any of these.

The respiratory system is significantly involved in an anaphylactic reaction. Initially, the patient will become tachypneic. Later, as lower airway edema and bronchospasm develop, respirations will become labored, as evidenced by retractions, accessory muscle usage, and prolonged expirations. Wheezing, resulting from bronchospasm and edema of the smaller airways, is a common manifestation and may be so pronounced that it can be heard without the aid of a stethoscope. Ultimately, anaphylaxis can result in markedly diminished lung sounds, which reflect decreased air movement and hypoventilation.

The skin is typically involved early in severe allergic reactions and anaphylaxis. Generally, a fine red rash will appear diffusely on the body. As histamine is released, fluid will diffuse from leaky capillaries, resulting in urticaria. **Urticaria**, also called "hives," is a wheal and flare reaction characterized by red, raised bumps that may appear and disappear across the body (Figure 5-3). As cardiovascular collapse and dyspnea progress, the patient

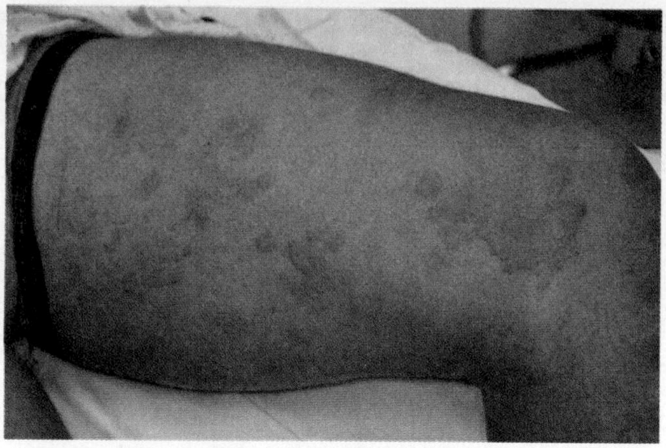

FIGURE 5-3 Hives are red, itchy blotches, sometimes raised, that often accompany an allergic reaction.

(© Edward T. Dickinson, MD)

will become diaphoretic. This may, if untreated, progress to cyanosis and pallor.

The effect of histamine on the gastrointestinal system is pronounced. Initially, the patient may note a rumbling sensation in the abdomen as gastrointestinal motility increases. On physical examination, this may be evident as hyperactive bowel sounds. Later, nausea, vomiting, and diarrhea develop as the body tries to rid itself of the offending allergen.

The vital signs will vary depending on the severity and stage of the severe allergic or anaphylactic reaction. Initially, there will be an increase in both the heart and respiratory rates. As airway edema and dyspnea occur, the respiratory rate can fall—an ominous finding. The blood pressure will fall when significant capillary leakage and peripheral vasodilation occur. This will often result in a reflex tachycardia, as the body attempts to compensate for the fall in blood pressure. Very late in anaphylaxis, the heart rate will fall. This, too, should be considered a very ominous sign.

State-of-the-art advanced prehospital care of anaphylaxis includes use of all available monitoring devices. These include the cardiac monitor, the pulse oximeter, and, if the patient is intubated, an end-tidal carbon dioxide detector. As anaphylaxis progresses, the end-tidal carbon dioxide level may climb due to the development of both respiratory and metabolic acidosis, which results in increased carbon dioxide elimination.

Management of Anaphylaxis

When responding to a patient with an anaphylactic reaction, first ensure that the scene is safe to approach. The presence of chemicals or patrolling bees can pose a risk to EMS personnel as well as to the patient and bystanders. If the patient is still in contact with the agent causing the reaction, he should be moved a safe distance away.

Honeybees often leave their stingers behind during a sting. If present, the stinger should be removed by scraping the skin with a fingernail or scalpel blade.

Always consider the possibility of trauma in anaphylaxis. If there is any suspicion of coincidental trauma, stabilize the cervical spine. It is not uncommon for people to fall or otherwise injure themselves as they try to escape from wasps and bees. The signs and symptoms of trauma may be masked by the signs and symptoms of anaphylaxis (Figure 5-4).

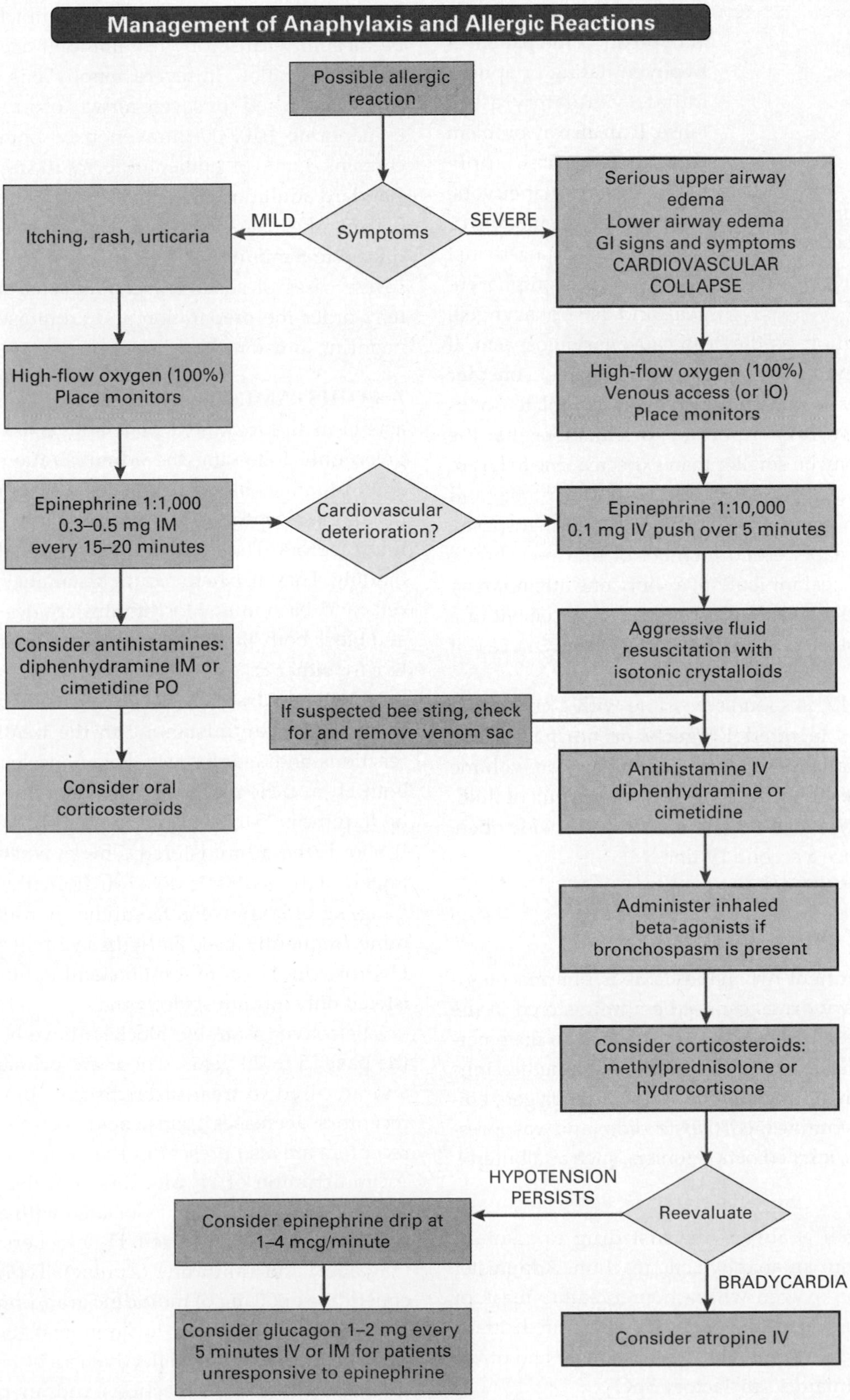

FIGURE 5-4 Management of anaphylaxis and allergic reactions.

CONTENT REVIEW

- Medications Used to Treat Anaphylaxis
  - Oxygen
  - Epinephrine
  - Antihistamines
  - Corticosteroids
  - Vasopressors
  - Beta-agonists
  - Other agents
  - Vasopressin
  - Atropine
  - Glucagon
- Epinephrine is the primary drug for management of anaphylaxis

Protect the Airway

Position the patient and protect the airway. Administer oxygen via a nonrebreather mask if the patient is hypoxic. If the patient is hypoventilating or apneic, initiate ventilatory assistance. If an airway problem is detected, first apply basic airway maneuvers, such as head positioning or the modified jaw-thrust maneuver. Use oropharyngeal and nasopharyngeal airways with caution, as they can cause laryngospasm. If the patient is having severe airway problems, consider early endotracheal intubation to prevent complete occlusion of the airway. It is important to remember that the glottic opening may be smaller than expected due to laryngeal edema. In addition, the larynx will be irritable and any manipulation of the airway may lead to laryngospasm. Ideally, the most experienced member of the crew should perform endotracheal intubation, as only one attempt may be possible. Have available equipment for placement of a surgical airway, such as a needle cricothyrotomy, in case it is needed.

Establish an IV as soon as possible with a crystalloid solution such as lactated Ringer's or normal saline. Remember that patients suffering anaphylaxis are volume depleted due to histamine-mediated third spacing of fluid. If the patient is hypotensive, administer fluids wide open. If time allows, place a second IV line.

Administer Medications

The primary treatment for anaphylaxis is pharmacological. If the necessary drugs cannot be administered in the field, then the patient should be transported to the emergency department immediately. Emergency medications used in the treatment of anaphylaxis include oxygen, epinephrine, antihistamines, corticosteroids, and vasopressors. Occasionally, inhaled beta-agonists, such as albuterol, may be required.

OXYGEN Oxygen is always the first drug to administer to a patient with an anaphylactic reaction. Administer high-concentration oxygen with a nonrebreather mask or similar device. If mechanical ventilation is required, attach supplemental oxygen. Apply the pulse oximeter and titrate the oxygen to maintain a satisfactory SpO_2.

EPINEPHRINE The primary drug for use in treatment of severe allergic reactions and anaphylaxis is epinephrine. Epinephrine is a sympathetic agonist. It causes an increase in heart rate, an increase in the strength of the cardiac contractile force, and peripheral vasoconstriction. It can also reverse some of the bronchospasm associated with anaphylaxis. Epinephrine also reverses much of the capillary permeability caused by histamine. It acts within minutes of administration. In severe anaphylaxis, characterized by hypotension and/or severe airway obstruction, administer epinephrine 1:10,000 intravenously. Epinephrine 1:10,000 contains 1 mg of epinephrine in 10 mL of solvent. The standard adult dose is 0.1 to 0.35 mg; the children's dose is 0.01 mg/kg. The effects of intravenous epinephrine wear off in 3 to 5 minutes, so repeat boluses may be required. In severe cases of sustained anaphylaxis, medical direction may order the preparation and administration of an epinephrine infusion.[3]

ANTIHISTAMINES Antihistamines are second-line agents in the treatment of anaphylaxis. They should be given only following the administration of epinephrine. Antihistamines block the effects of histamine by blocking histamine receptors. They do not displace histamine from the receptors. They only block additional histamine from binding. They also help reduce histamine release from mast cells and basophils. Most antihistamines are nonselective and block both H_1 and H_2 receptors. Others are more selective for either H_1 or H_2 receptors.

Diphenhydramine (Benadryl) is probably the most frequently used antihistamine in the treatment of allergic reactions and anaphylaxis. It is nonselective and acts on both H_1 and H_2 receptors. The standard dose of diphenhydramine is 25 to 50 mg intravenously or intramuscularly. It should be administered slowly when given intravenously. The pediatric dose of diphenhydramine is 1 to 2 mg/kg of body weight. Another nonselective antihistamine frequently used is hydroxyzine (Atarax, Vistaril). Hydroxyzine is a potent antihistamine, but it can be administered only intramuscularly.

Selective histamine blockers have been available for the past 15 to 20 years. These are primarily H_2 blockers and are used to treat ulcer disease. Blockage of the H_2 receptors decreases gastric acid secretion. However, H_2 receptors are also present in the peripheral blood vessels. Administration of H_2 blockers conceivably will reverse some of the vasodilation associated with anaphylaxis. The two most frequently used H_2 blockers are cimetidine (Tagamet) and ranitidine (Zantac). Typically, 300 mg of cimetidine or 50 mg of ranitidine are administered by slow intravenous push (over 3 to 5 minutes). (Some recent studies have questioned the effectiveness of H_2 blockers in the treatment of allergic reactions and anaphylaxis.) These agents are also considered more expensive than the nonselective antihistamines.[4]

CORTICOSTEROIDS Corticosteroids are important in the treatment and prevention of anaphylaxis. Although they are of little benefit in the initial stages of treatment, they help suppress the inflammatory response associated with these emergencies. Commonly used corticosteroids include methylprednisolone (Solu-Medrol), hydrocortisone (Solu-Cortef), and dexamethasone (Decadron).

VASOPRESSORS Severe and prolonged anaphylactic reactions may require the use of potent vasopressors to support blood pressure. Use these medications in conjunction with first-line therapy and adequate fluid resuscitation. Commonly used agents include dopamine, norepinephrine, and epinephrine. These medications are prepared as infusions and are administered continuously to support blood pressure and cardiac output.

BETA-AGONISTS Many patients with severe allergic reactions and anaphylaxis will develop bronchospasm, laryngeal edema, or both. In these cases, an inhaled beta-agonist can be useful. The most frequently used beta-agonist in prehospital care is albuterol (Ventolin, Proventil). Although usually used in the treatment of asthma, these agents will help reverse some of the bronchospasm and laryngeal edema associated with anaphylaxis. Give the adult patient 2.5 mg of albuterol via a handheld nebulizer. Children should receive 0.2 to 0.5 mL of albuterol based on their weight. Other beta-agonists, such as metaproterenol (Alupent) and levalbuterol (Xopenex), may be used instead of albuterol.

OTHER AGENTS Certain medications have been identified as potentially beneficial for anaphylaxis. These include vasopressin, atropine, and glucagon. There is some evidence that vasopressin may benefit hypotensive patients, whereas atropine may benefit those with bradycardia. Glucagon should be considered in patients unresponsive to epinephrine—especially those receiving beta-blockers.

Offer Psychological Support

A severe allergic or anaphylactic reaction is a harrowing experience for the patient. Although it is essential to work fast, prehospital crews should provide the patient with emotional support and explain the treatment regimen. Caution patients about the potential side effects of administered medications. For example, epinephrine will often cause a rapid heart rate, anxiety, and tremulousness. Likewise, the antihistamines may cause a dry mouth, thirst, and sedation. Careful explanation and emotional support will help allay patient anxiety and apprehension.

Table 5-5 Signs and Symptoms of Allergic and Anaphylactic Reactions

Mild Allergic Reaction	Severe Allergic Reaction or Anaphylaxis
Onset: Gradual	*Onset:* Sudden (30–60 seconds but can be more than an hour after exposure)
Skin/vascular system: Mild flushing, rash, or hives	*Skin/vascular system:* Severe flushing, rash, or hives; angioneurotic edema to the face and neck
Respiration: Mild bronchoconstriction	*Respiration:* Severe bronchoconstriction (wheezing), laryngospasm (stridor), breathing difficulty
GI system: Mild cramps, diarrhea	*GI system:* Severe cramps, abdominal rumbling, diarrhea, vomiting
Vital signs: Normal to slightly abnormal	Vital signs: Increased pulse early, may fall in late/severe case; increased respiratory rate early, falling respiratory rate late; falling blood pressure late
Mental status: Normal	*Mental status:* Anxiety, sense of impending doom, may decrease to confusion and to unconsciousness
	Other clues: Symptoms occur shortly after exposure to parenteral penicillin, *Hymenoptera* sting (fire ant, wasp, yellow jacket, hornet, bee), or ingestion of foods to which patient is allergic, such as nuts or shellfish
	Ominous signs: Respiratory distress, signs of shock, falling respiratory rate, falling pulse rate, falling blood pressure

Note: Not all signs and symptoms will be present in every case.

Assessment Findings in Allergic Reaction

Many patients you will be called to treat will be suffering from forms of allergic reaction less severe than anaphylaxis. An allergic reaction, as contrasted with an anaphylactic reaction, will have a more gradual onset, with milder signs and symptoms, and the patient will have a normal mental status (Table 5-5).

Management of Allergic Reactions

Common manifestations of mild (nonanaphylactic) allergic reactions include itching, rash, and urticaria. Patients with simple itching and nonurticarial rashes may be treated with antihistamines alone. In addition to antihistamines, epinephrine is often necessary for the treatment of urticaria.

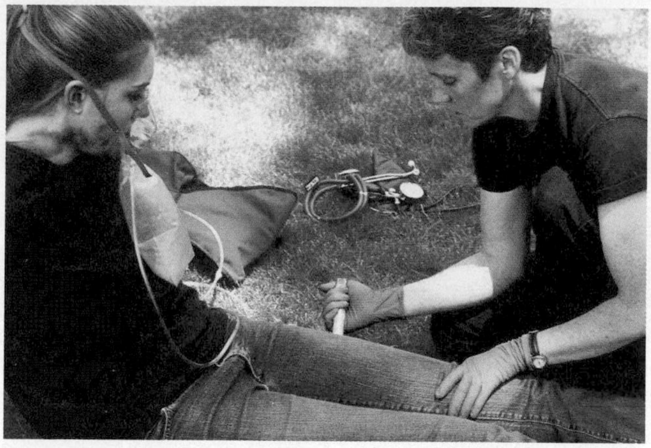

FIGURE 5-5 Epinephrine being administered using an autoinjector system.

Any patient suffering an allergic reaction who exhibits dyspnea or wheezing should receive supplemental oxygen if he is hypoxic. This should be followed by intramuscular epinephrine 1:1,000. Lesser allergic reactions that are not accompanied by hypotension or airway problems can be adequately treated with epinephrine 1:1,000 administered intramuscularly (Figure 5-5). Epinephrine 1:1,000 contains 1 mg of epinephrine in 1 mL of solvent. When administered into the muscle tissue, the drug is absorbed more slowly and the effect prolonged. The intramuscular dose is the same as the subcutaneous dose formerly used (0.3 to 0.5 mg). The intramuscular route should not be used in severe anaphylaxis, for which, as noted earlier, IV epinephrine should be administered.

Patient Education

Many severe allergic and anaphylactic reactions are preventable. People with a history of anaphylactic reactions should be educated about recognition and treatment. They should wear some sort of identification device, such as a MedicAlert bracelet, which will alert paramedics to their condition if they are unresponsive. In addition, many patients can initiate emergency anaphylactic treatment at home with epinephrine delivery systems such as the EpiPen.

The severity of an allergic reaction can be diminished in certain cases through a process called *desensitization.* In these cases, physicians begin therapy by administering an extremely small amount of the allergen that causes the patient's anaphylactic reaction. The quantity of the allergen present in the injection is gradually increased to a point at which the body's immune response to the allergen is blunted and anaphylactic reactions are averted.

Paramedics often keep reference cards for anaphylactic patients living in their service area so they can quickly identify them, their allergy, and their prehospital treatment history.[5]

Summary

Fortunately, severe allergies and anaphylaxis are uncommon. However, when they do occur, they can progress quickly and result in death in minutes. The central physiologic action in anaphylaxis is the massive release of histamine and other mediators. Histamine causes bronchospasm, airway edema, peripheral vasodilation, and increased capillary permeability. The prehospital treatment of anaphylaxis is intended to reverse the effects of these agents.

The primary, and most important, drug used in the treatment of anaphylaxis is epinephrine. Epinephrine helps reverse the effects of histamine. It also supports the blood pressure and reverses detrimental capillary leakage. Following the administration of epinephrine, potent antihistamines should be used to block the adverse effects of the massive histamine release. Inhaled beta-agonists are useful in cases of severe bronchospasm and airway involvement. Intravenous fluid replacement is crucial in preventing hypovolemia and hypotension.

The key to successful prehospital management of anaphylaxis is prompt recognition and treatment.

You Make the Call

You are assigned to a hospital-based EMS service that serves a beach town on the Gulf coast. At 1420 you are dispatched to an "injured person" on the beach just outside the Suntide III building. You and your partner are in a four-wheel-drive ambulance stationed only minutes from the call. You turn off Gulf Boulevard onto the beach access road and are able to pull up to a crowd of people on the beach.

You determine that the scene is safe and leave the ambulance with your jump kit and a monitor. The patient is a young man lying supine on the beach, moaning softly. He is in obvious distress. A rapid assessment reveals that the patient is breathing; has a rapid, thready pulse; and is alert but anxious and slightly agitated. He reports that he and his newlywed wife were taking a leisurely walk along the beach. He accidentally stepped on a dead "hardhead" saltwater catfish that a fisherman had discarded on the beach. The sharp dorsal fin had penetrated the patient's tennis shoe. He immediately developed a burning pain in his foot. Shortly thereafter, he became weak and dizzy and developed trouble breathing.

The patient is in moderate distress with audible wheezing. You and your partner notice the presence of hives on the patient's chest and back. A quick look at the dead fish confirms that it is a saltwater catfish, locally referred to as a "hardhead." You know that these fish have a toxin that can cause pain and burning. However, the reactions to such an injury are usually localized and this patient is certainly having a more generalized reaction.

1. What is the most likely explanation of the patient's emergency?
2. How would you treat this patient?
3. Should the local marine institute be advised of a potentially toxic strain of hardhead catfish?

See Suggested Responses at the back of this book.

Review Questions

1. Which body system is designed to combat infections?
   a. Immune
   b. Nervous
   c. Respiratory
   d. Cardiovascular
2. Innate immunity is also called ____________
   a. acquired immunity.
   b. natural immunity.
   c. naturally acquired immunity.
   d. induced active immunity.
3. The initial exposure of an individual to an antigen, precipitating a chain of events that leads to antibody formation, is referred to as ____________
   a. allergy.
   b. sensitization.
   c. hypersensitivity.
   d. active immunity.
4. What are the two leading causes of fatal anaphylactic reactions?
   a. Injected penicillin and insect stings
   b. Inhaled substances and bee stings
   c. Insect bites and ingested penicillin
   d. Injected penicillin and eating peanuts
5. A type of white blood cell that participates in allergic responses is a(n) ____________
   a. histamine.
   b. antibody.
   c. basophil.
   d. erythrocyte.
6. The type of shock (hypoperfusion) seen in an anaphylactic reaction most closely resembles what other type of shock?
   a. Septic
   b. Neurogenic
   c. Respiratory
   d. Circulatory
7. What is the primary drug for the management of anaphylaxis, which can help reverse the ongoing pathophysiological changes leading to death?
   a. Oxygen
   b. Decadron
   c. Proventil
   d. Epinephrine
8. Commonly used vasopressor agents include ____________
   a. dopamine.
   b. epinephrine.
   c. norepinephrine.
   d. all of the above.
9. A patient presents with urticaria, pruritus, exhalatory wheezing, a room air pulse oximetry reading of 95 percent, and anxiety. What type of allergic reaction would you classify this patient as having currently?
   a. None
   b. Mild
   c. Severe
   d. Near-fatal
10. Which of the following drug/dose combinations is *not* correct for a male patient with anaphylaxis?
    a. Epinephrine 1:1,000; 0.4 mg
    b. Albuterol; 2.5 mg
    c. Methylprednisone; 125 mg
    d. Norepinephrine infusion; 2 mcg/kg/min

See Answers to Review Questions at the back of this book.

References

1. Portier, P. and D. Richet. "De L'action Anphylactique de Certains Venins." *CR Soc Biol (Paris)* 6 (1902): 170.
2. Kemp, S. F. and R. F. Lockey. "Anaphylaxis: A Review of Causes and Mechanisms." *J Allergy Clin Immunol* 110 (2002): 341–348.
3. Simons, F. E. "Anaphylaxis." *J Allergy Clin Immunol* 125 (Suppl 2) (2010): S161–S181.
4. Winberry, S. L. and P. L. Lieberman. "Histamine and Antihistamines in Anaphylaxis." *Clin Allergy Immunol* 17 (2002): 287–317.
5. Liberman, D. B. and S. J. Teach. "Management of Anaphylaxis in Children." *Pediatr Emerg Care* 24 (2008): 861–866.

Further Reading

Bledsoe, B. E. and D. Clayden. *Prehospital Emergency Pharmacology.* 7th ed. Upper Saddle River, NJ: Pearson/Prentice Hall, 2012.

Salomone, J. A. "Anaphylaxis and Acute Allergic Reactions," in J. E. Tintinalli, et al., eds., *Emergency Medicine: A Comprehensive Study Guide.* 7th ed. New York: McGraw-Hill, 2011.

Chapter 6
Gastroenterology

Bryan Bledsoe, DO, FACEP, FAAEM, EMT-P

STANDARD
Medicine (Abdominal and Gastrointestinal Disorders)

COMPETENCY
Integrates assessment findings with principles of epidemiology and pathophysiology to formulate a field impression and implement a comprehensive treatment/disposition plan for a patient with a medical complaint.

Learning Objectives

Terminal Performance Objective: After reading this chapter, you should be able to integrate patient assessment findings, patient history, and knowledge of anatomy, physiology, pathophysiology, and basic and advanced life support interventions to recognize and manage patients with gastrointestinal disorders.

Enabling Objectives: To accomplish the terminal performance objective, you should be able to:

1. Define key terms introduced in this chapter.
2. Review the anatomy and physiology of the gastrointestinal system.
3. Describe the general pathophysiological changes of gastrointestinal emergencies, and relate this to disturbances in normal immune physiology.
4. Identify gastrointestinal problems as upper GI tract disorders, lower GI tract disorders, or GI accessory organ disorders.
5. Adapt the scene size-up, primary assessment, history, secondary assessment, and use of monitoring technology to arrive at a field impression and differential diagnoses for gastrointestinal emergencies.
6. Use a process of clinical reasoning to guide and interpret the patient assessment findings and develop a treatment plan for patients with gastrointestinal disorders in the prehospital environment.
7. Given a variety of scenarios, discuss the integration of assessment and management guidelines as they relate to gastrointestinal emergencies.

KEY TERMS

acute gastroenteritis, p. 283
adhesion, p. 292
appendicitis, p. 293
bowel obstruction, p. 292
cholecystitis, p. 294
chronic gastroenteritis, p. 285
cirrhosis, p. 283
colic, p. 288
Crohn's disease, p. 289
Cullen's sign, p. 280
cyclical vomiting syndrome (CVS), p. 286
diverticula, p. 290
diverticulitis, p. 290
diverticulosis, p. 290
esophageal varix, p. 282
Grey Turner's sign, p. 280
hematemesis, p. 282
hematochezia, p. 284
hemorrhoid, p. 291
hepatitis, p. 296
hernia, p. 292
infarction, p. 292
intussusception, p. 292
irritable bowel syndrome (IBS), p. 291
ligament of Treitz, p. 281
lower gastrointestinal bleeding, p. 287
Mallory-Weiss syndrome, p. 281
McBurney's point, p. 294
melena, p. 282
mesenteric ischemia, p. 293
Murphy's sign, p. 295
pancolitis, p. 288
pancreatitis, p. 295
peptic ulcer, p. 285
peritonitis, p. 277
portal, p. 282
proctitis, p. 288
referred pain, p. 278
somatic pain, p. 278
ulcerative colitis, p. 288
upper gastrointestinal bleeding, p. 281
visceral pain, p. 277
volvulus, p. 292
Zollinger-Ellison syndrome, p. 286

Case Study

George Kastner and his partner, Stephanie Emrick, are working a 12-hour shift on Sunday morning when they are dispatched Code 3 to an "unknown medical emergency" in an affluent section of the city. They arrive on scene within 5 to 6 minutes.

The house is well off the road, hidden by a row of large pine trees. As George and Stephanie are transferring their equipment from the truck to the cot, a woman runs from the house, panic stricken. She screams, "I think he's dead! There's blood all over the bathroom!" The woman identifies herself only as the victim's wife and begins to cry uncontrollably. Because George and Stephanie do not know the circumstances, they decide that it will be safer to have police officers enter the house first. Stephanie radios dispatch, requesting the police and an additional advanced life support unit.

Deputy Sheriff Marcus Eliot arrives within a few moments. Almost immediately after entering the house, he screams for George and Stephanie to hurry inside.

In the house, they find their patient lying face down in a pool of blood. With Standard Precautions already in place, Stephanie and George logroll the victim onto his back. Their primary assessment reveals a middle-aged man who has shallow, gurgling respirations. His radial pulse is extremely rapid, weak, and barely palpable. They find no external hemorrhages to account for the pool of blood.

George and Stephanie's first concern is the patient's compromised airway. They size an oropharyngeal airway and attempt to insert it with the help of a tongue depressor. Their patient still has a gag reflex and begins to vomit. Stephanie has the suction ready, and George begins to suction copious amounts of bright red blood. When the patient takes a shallow breath, they fear that he will aspirate the blood. Unable to control the hemorrhage, they decide to intubate to control the patient's airway and prevent aspiration.

The second crew arrives and paramedic Nicia Logan begins to search for a vein for intravenous access. Her partner, Anthony Rivera, readies the cot for removal.

The patient's intact gag reflex inhibits George's initial attempts at intubation, so he decides to perform rapid sequence intubation. He administers etomidate and succinylcholine (Anectine) and successfully intubates the patient with a 7.5-mm tube. Nicia and Anthony administer a 500-mL fluid bolus of 0.9 percent NaCl.

His airway secured, they move the patient to the truck and begin rapid transport to the hospital. En route, George reassesses the patient: respirations are 18, assisted with 100 percent oxygen via a bag-valve unit; breath sounds are diminished, with crackles in the bases. The cardiac monitor reveals sinus tachycardia at 124 beats per minute without ectopy. Blood pressure is 78/42 mmHg. Stephanie radios ahead to the hospital, giving a full report on the patient and the seriousness of his status.

The emergency department staff readies the resuscitation bay with the rapid transfuser and pages the surgical resident on call. When George and Stephanie wheel the patient through the door, the emergency department team immediately recognizes the patient as someone they see regularly. He has been diagnosed with severe portal hypertension from alcoholic-induced hepatic failure. They begin resuscitation as the surgical resident performs an upper endoscopic examination, which reveals a bleeding esophageal varix at the junction of the patient's esophagus and his stomach. The emergency physician places a central line for hemodynamic monitoring and volume fluid resuscitation. Then the staff hurries the patient to the operating room for emergency surgery.

After George and Stephanie complete their charting and restock the unit, they stop at the emergency desk to chat with the attending physician. She tells them that increased portal pressure and forceful retching probably caused the varix to tear. She explains the injury's pathophysiology and assures George and Stephanie that their actions probably saved the patient's life.

Introduction

Gastrointestinal emergencies account for more than 500,000 emergency visits and hospitalizations every year—approximately 5 percent of all visits to the emergency department. Of that number, more than 300,000 are due to gastrointestinal bleeding. These figures will probably increase as more and more people treat themselves with over-the-counter medications and delay seeing a physician until their symptoms become severe. Perhaps more important, the numbers will rise as the general population ages. In the past few years, the number of patients over 60 years of age included in these statistics has risen from approximately 3 percent to more than 45 percent.

General Pathophysiology, Assessment, and Treatment

Gastrointestinal (GI) emergencies usually result from an underlying pathological process that can be predicted by evaluating numerous risk factors. These risk factors are commonly known to physicians; most are self-induced by patients. They include excessive alcohol consumption, excessive smoking, increased stress, ingestion of caustic substances, and poor bowel habits. The wide variety of risk factors and potential causes requires the emergency care provider to complete a thorough secondary assessment before making a field diagnosis, along with assessing the seriousness of the emergency and the need for any prevention strategy to minimize organ damage.

CONTENT REVIEW

- Gastrointestinal Disease Risk Factors
  - Excessive alcohol consumption
  - Excessive smoking
  - Increased stress
  - Ingestion of caustic substances
  - Poor bowel habits

General Pathophysiology

CONTENT REVIEW

- Types of Gastrointestinal Pain
  - Visceral
  - Somatic
  - Referred
- Pain from hollow organs tends to be vague and nondescript, whereas pain from solid organs tends to be localized.

Pain is the hallmark of the acute abdominal emergency. The three main classifications of abdominal pain are visceral, somatic, and referred. **Visceral pain** originates in the walls of hollow organs such as the gallbladder or appendix, in the capsules of solid organs such as the kidney or liver, or in the visceral peritoneum. Three separate mechanisms can produce this pain: inflammation, distention (being stretched out or inflated), and ischemia (inadequate blood flow). Because these processes progress at varying rates, they likewise can cause varying intensities, characteristics, and locations of pain.

Inflammation, distention, and ischemia all transmit a pain signal from visceral afferent neural fibers back to the spinal column. Because the nerves enter the spinal column at various levels, visceral pain usually is not localized to any one specific area. Instead, it is often described as vague or poorly localized, dull, or crampy. The body most often responds to this vague pain with sympathetic stimulation that causes nausea and vomiting, diaphoresis, and tachycardia.

Organs that consist of hollow viscera—for example, the gallbladder (cholecystitis) and the small and large intestines—can frequently cause visceral pain. Many hollow organs first cause visceral pain when they become distended and then cause a different, more specific type of pain (somatic pain, described next) when they rupture or tear. For example, appendicitis initially presents with vague periumbilical abdominal pain that is classified as visceral. If the appendix ruptures, it can spill its contents into the peritoneal cavity, causing bacterial **peritonitis** and generating somatic pain. Various microbes associated with pelvic inflammatory diseases can also cause bacterial peritonitis.

Somatic pain, as contrasted to visceral pain, is a sharp type of pain that travels along definite neural routes (determined by the dermatomes, or tissue blocks, present during embryonic development) to the spinal column. Because these routes are clearly defined, the pain can be localized to a particular region or area. As previously noted, bacterial and chemical irritations of the abdomen commonly cause somatic pain. Bacterial irritation can originate from a perforated or ruptured appendix or gallbladder. Chemical irritation of the abdomen can result from leakage of acidic juices from a perforated ulcer or from an inflamed pancreas. Whether the cause is bacterial or chemical, the resulting peritonitis can lead to sepsis and even death. The degree of pain is initially proportional to the spread of the irritant through the abdominal cavity. Somatic pain allows the examiner to locate the specific area of irritation, providing valuable information.

The third type of pain, referred pain, is not a true pain-producing mechanism. As its name implies, **referred pain** originates in a region other than where it is felt (Figure 6-1). Many neural pathways from various organs pass through or over regions where the organ was formed during embryonic development. For example, the afferent neural pathways that originate in the diaphragm enter the spinal column at the cervical enlargement at the fourth cervical vertebra. Therefore, patients who have an inflammation or injury of the diaphragm often feel pain in their necks or shoulders. One of the most significant hemorrhagic emergencies, the dissecting abdominal aortic artery, produces referred pain felt between the shoulder blades. Some common nonhemorrhagic emergencies are associated with referred-pain patterns, too. Appendicitis often presents with periumbilical pain, whereas pneumonia can cause pain below the lower margin of the rib cage.

General Assessment

Your assessment of a patient who complains of abdominal discomfort or whom you suspect of having an abdominal pathology is similar to a trauma assessment with an expanded history. Do not approach the patient until you and your partner have determined the scene to be free and clear of any apparent dangers. Always take Standard Precautions, including gloves, eyewear, mask, and disposable body gown, to prevent contamination. As you approach the patient, survey the scene for potential evidence of your patient's problem. Medication bottles, alcohol containers, ashtrays, and buckets with emesis or sputum, for instance, can provide valuable information.

Scene Size-Up and Primary Assessment

As you approach, look for mechanisms of injury to help determine whether the call is medical or trauma. If you suspect trauma, always immobilize the cervical spine as you assess the adequacy of the patient's airway and his

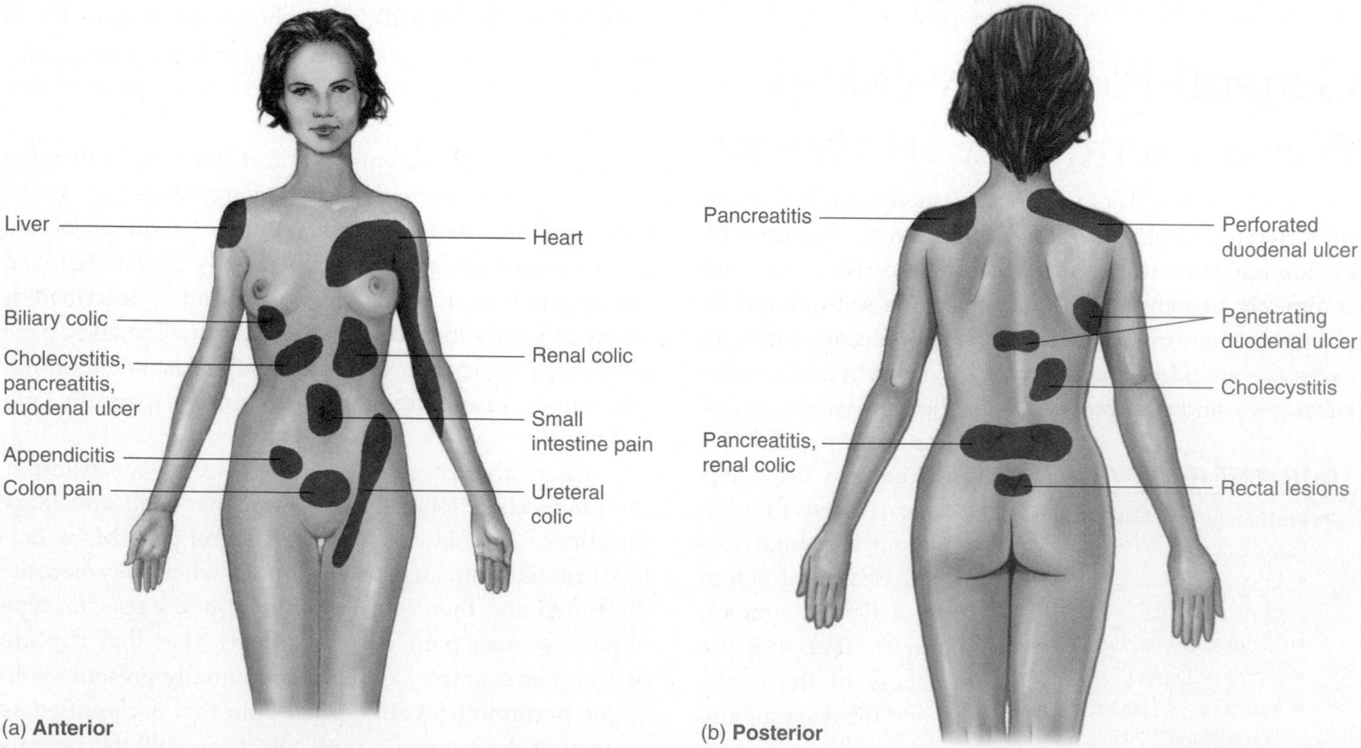

FIGURE 6-1 Referred pain patterns: (a) anterior, (b) posterior.

level of responsiveness. In the vast majority of medical patients, you can check responsiveness and airway patency by asking the patient his name and chief complaint (why he called the ambulance today) and noting the answers. You can further evaluate the rate, depth, and quality of the patient's respirations fairly rapidly and without great difficulty. As you evaluate the respiratory functions, quickly palpate a pulse and check skin color, temperature, and circulation, including signs of bleeding and capillary refill. If you discover a life-threatening condition during the primary assessment, treat it and then rapidly continue the assessment to identify any other life threats.

Secondary Assessment

Once you have completed the primary assessment and dealt with any life threats, conduct the secondary assessment. Your ability to obtain a history from the patient will depend on his level of responsiveness. In some cases, you may detect deterioration of the patient's mental status over time as you take the history.

HISTORY An accurate and thorough history can provide invaluable information. After you conduct the SAMPLE history (symptoms, *a*llergies, *m*edications, *p*ast medical history, *l*ast oral intake, and *e*vents), you can take a more thorough history, exploring the chief complaint, the history of the present illness, the past medical history, and the current health status. The history of the present illness and the past medical history will be especially helpful in sorting the multitude of signs and symptoms and piecing together a clear picture of the underlying pathophysiology.

History of the Present Illness Your OPQRST-ASPN history for gastrointestinal patients should address the following specific concerns:

- ***Onset.*** When did the pain first start? Was the onset sudden or gradual? Sudden onsets of abdominal pain are generally caused by perforations of abdominal organs or capsules. Gradual onset of pain usually is associated with the blockage of hollow organs.
- ***Provocation/palliation.*** What makes the pain worse? What makes the pain better? If the pain lessens when the patient draws his legs up to his chest or lies on his side, it usually indicates peritoneal inflammation, which is often of GI origin. If walking relieves the pain, the cause may be in the GI or urinary systems—perhaps an obstruction of the gallbladder or a stone caught in the renal pelvis or ureter.
- ***Quality.*** How would you describe the pain: dull, sharp, constant, intermittent? Localized, tearing pain is usually associated with the rupture of an organ. Dull, steadily increasing pain may indicate a bowel obstruction. Sharp pain, particularly in the flank, may indicate a kidney stone.
- ***Region/radiation.*** Does the pain travel to any other part of your body? Radiated pain, or pain that seems to change location, is common because it involves the same neural routes as referred pain. Pain referred to the shoulder or neck is usually associated with an irritation of the diaphragm, as happens with cholecystitis.
- ***Severity.*** On a scale of 1 to 10, with 10 representing the worst pain possible, how would you rate the pain you are feeling now? The severity of pain usually worsens as the pathology (ischemia, inflammation, or stretching) of the organ advances.
- ***Time.*** When did the pain first start? Estimation of the pain's time of onset is important to determine its possible causes. Any abdominal pain lasting more than 6 hours is considered a surgical emergency and needs to be evaluated in the emergency department.
- ***Associated symptoms.*** Have you experienced any associated nausea and/or vomiting with the discomfort? If yes, try to determine the content, color, and smell of the vomitus. Ask if the vomitus contained any bright red blood, "coffee grounds," or clots. Determining whether your patient has an active gastrointestinal bleed is imperative.

  Have you experienced any changes in bowel habits—constipation or diarrhea—associated with this discomfort/pain? Question the patient further to determine if there have been any changes in feces such as a tarry, foul-smelling stool. Changes in bowel morphology, color, or smell can be the only indication of such conditions as a lower GI hemorrhage, gastritis, or bleeding diverticula.
- Have you had an associated loss of appetite or weight loss? Patients who have an acute abdomen usually have an associated loss of appetite.
- ***Pertinent negatives.*** The absence of symptoms associated with GI function or the presence of symptoms related to urinary function may mean the problem originates in the urinary system. Pain in the lowest part of the abdomen, the pelvis, can be due to problems in the reproductive system. Last, remember that an inferior myocardial infarction (MI) can irritate the diaphragm and generate its referred-pain pattern. Be sure to check for cardiovascular history when this pain pattern (pain in shoulder and/or neck area) is present.

Keep in mind the information that your SAMPLE history provides about your patient's last oral intake. It can help you to differentiate the possible causes of your patient's pain if the problem is in the GI system.

Not all abdominal emergencies result in abdominal pain. Some may cause chest pain. This, typically, is referred pain. Common gastrointestinal emergencies that can cause chest pain include gastroesophageal reflux, gastric ulcers, duodenal ulcers, and, in some cases, gallbladder disease. When confronted by a patient with chest pain, always consider the GI system as a possible cause.

Past Medical History Have you ever experienced this same type of pain or discomfort before? If the patient answers yes, then investigate whether he saw a physician for the problem and how it was diagnosed. Commonly, patients have been treated for the complaint in the past and the pain is a flareup of an old problem.

PHYSICAL EXAMINATION While you are conducting the history, you can also begin the physical examination. Your patient's general appearance and posture strongly suggest his apparent state of health and the severity of his complaint. Usually patients with severe abdominal pathology lie as still as possible, often in the fetal position. They do not writhe around on the floor or cry out, because doing so increases the pain. You also should continually monitor the patient's level of consciousness for any subtle changes that indicate early signs of shock.

Take a complete set of vital signs to establish a baseline for further evaluation and treatment. These include pulse, respiratory rate, blood pressure, and pulse oximetry. You can also ascertain additional important information such as body temperature.

Visually inspect the abdomen before palpating it, auscultating it, or moving the patient. Remove the patient's clothing as necessary to freely visualize the entire abdomen. Distention of the abdomen may be an ominous sign. It can be caused by a buildup of free air due to an obstruction of the bowel. If the distention is caused by hemorrhage, the patient has lost a large amount of his circulating volume, for the abdomen can hold from 4 to 6 L of fluid before any noticeable change in abdominal girth occurs. Other signs of fluid loss include periumbilical ecchymosis (**Cullen's sign**) and ecchymosis in the flank (**Grey Turner's sign**).

Auscultating the abdomen usually provides little helpful information because bowel sounds are heard throughout this area. If you auscultate the abdomen, you must do so before palpating it. Listen for at least 2 minutes in each quadrant, beginning with the quadrant farthest from the affected area and auscultating the affected area last. Like auscultation, percussion requires a quiet environment and an experienced clinician. It, too, provides little or no useful information and, therefore, is not routinely performed in the field.

Palpating the abdomen, on the other hand, can give you a plethora of information. It can define the area of pain and identify the associated organs. Before palpating, ask the patient to point to where he is experiencing the most discomfort. Then work in reverse order, palpating that area last. Palpate the abdomen with a gentle pressure, feeling for muscle tension or its absence, as well as for masses, pulsations, and tenderness beneath the muscle. If you identify a pulsating mass, stop palpating at once; the increase in pressure may cause the affected blood vessel or organ to rupture.

General Treatment

Once you have completed the primary assessment and the secondary assessment, you can address treatment and transport. Your highest priority when treating a patient with abdominal pain is to secure and maintain his airway, breathing, and circulation. Be prepared to suction the airway of vomitus and blood. Supplemental oxygen and aggressive airway management may be indicated, depending on your patient's status. Monitor circulation by placing the patient on a cardiac monitor and frequently assessing his blood pressure. Measurement of the hematocrit will give an indirect measure of blood loss.

Establish a large-bore IV line in patients who complain of abdominal discomfort for use if emergency blood transfusion becomes necessary. You can use the IV for pharmacological intervention or to replace volume lost to hemorrhage or dehydration. In general, the need to avoid masking any abdominal pain for further evaluation will limit your pharmacological interventions to palliative agents such as antiemetics. Place the patient in a comfortable position and provide emotional reassurance based on your field assessment, any conversation with hospital staff or family, and knowledge of estimated transport time. Keep your voice and actions quiet and collected. Calm, as well as anxiety, are transmitted easily to patients and family. How you transport the patient will depend on his physiologic status. Normally, gentle but rapid transport is sufficient. Remember that persistent abdominal pain lasting longer than 6 hours is classified as a surgical emergency and always requires transport. In all cases, be sure to maintain monitoring of mental status and vital signs and to give nothing by mouth. Bring vomitus to the emergency department for evaluation.

Specific Illnesses

The gastrointestinal tract is essentially one long tube, divided structurally and functionally into different parts (Figure 6-2). Three other organs—the liver, gallbladder, and pancreas—are intimately associated with it, as is the

CONTENT REVIEW

➤ The Gastrointestinal System
- GI tract
- Liver
- Gallbladder
- Pancreas
- Appendix

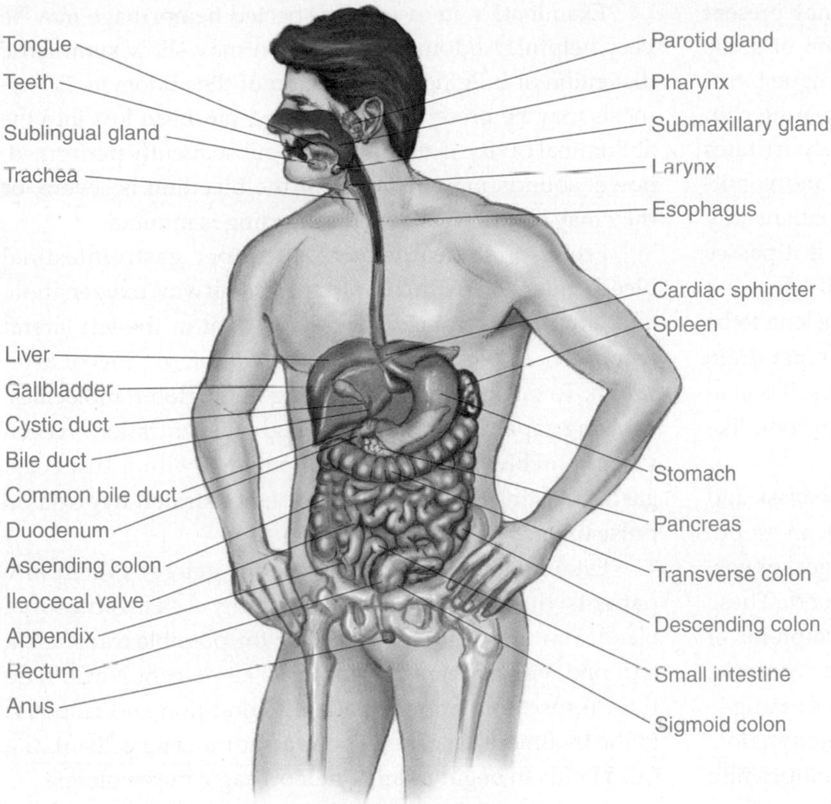

FIGURE 6-2 The gastrointestinal tract is one long tube divided structurally and functionally into different parts.

small structure called the vermiform appendix, which protrudes from the first portion of the large intestine. Collectively, these organs are called the GI, or digestive, system. The GI system converts food into nutrient molecules that individual cells can use, and it excretes solid wastes from the body.

Upper Gastrointestinal Diseases

For convenience, clinicians often divide the GI tract broadly into the upper and lower GI tracts. The upper GI tract consists of the mouth, esophagus, stomach, and duodenum, the latter being the first part of the small intestine. Physical digestion of food and some chemical digestion take place here. As food passes through the lower GI tract, consisting of the remainder of the small intestine and the large intestine, nutrients are absorbed into the blood and solid wastes are formed and excreted.

CONTENT REVIEW

➤ The Upper GI Tract
- Mouth
- Esophagus
- Stomach
- Duodenum

Upper GI Bleeding

Upper gastrointestinal bleeding can be defined as bleeding within the gastrointestinal tract proximal to the **ligament of Treitz**, which supports the duodenojejunal junction, the point where the first two sections of the small intestine (the duodenum and the jejunum) meet.

CONTENT REVIEW

➤ Major Causes of Upper GI Hemorrhage
- Peptic ulcer disease
- Gastritis
- Varix rupture
- Mallory-Weiss syndrome
- Esophagitis
- Duodenitis

Upper gastrointestinal bleeds account for more than 300,000 hospitalizations per year. The mortality rate has remained fairly steady, at approximately 10 percent, over the past few years. Many factors contribute to this high mortality. First, the number of patients who treat their symptoms with home remedies and over-the-counter medications is increasing rapidly. Many of these patients come under medical care only when their disease has caused significant damage, such as large-scale hemorrhage from an ulcerated lesion. Second, the overall age of the population is increasing. The infirmities of age and its greater likelihood of coexisting illnesses, such as hypertension, atherosclerosis, diabetes, and substance abuse (including abuse of medications), make this older population more vulnerable to the effects of upper gastrointestinal bleeds. The mortality rate is highest in those over 60 years of age. One prevention strategy for the field is to check for such coexisting problems, especially in elderly patients, and to treat accordingly. In particular, look at the history and physical for evidence of tobacco or alcohol use, or both.

The six major identifiable causes of upper GI hemorrhage, in descending order of frequency, are peptic ulcer disease, gastritis, variceal rupture, **Mallory-Weiss syndrome** (esophageal laceration, usually secondary to vomiting), esophagitis, and duodenitis. Peptic ulcer disease accounts for approximately 50 percent of upper GI bleeds, with gastritis accounting for an additional 25 percent. Overall, irritation or erosion of the gastric lining of the stomach causes more than 75 percent of upper GI bleeds. Most cases of upper GI bleeding are chronic irritations or inflammations that cause minimal discomfort and minor hemorrhage. Physicians can manage these conditions on an outpatient basis; however, if a peptic ulcer erodes through the gastric mucosa, if the esophagus is lacerated in Mallory-Weiss syndrome, or if varices (often secondary to alcoholic liver damage) rupture, an acute-onset, life-threatening, and difficult-to-control hemorrhage can result.

Upper GI bleeds may be obvious, or they may present quite subtly. Most often patients will complain of some type of abdominal discomfort ranging from a vague burning sensation to an upset stomach, gas pain, or tearing pain in the upper quadrants. Because blood severely irritates the GI system, most cases present with nausea and vomiting. If the bleeding is in the upper GI tract, the patient may experience **hematemesis** (bloody vomitus) or, if it passes through the lower GI tract, **melena**. The partially digested blood will turn the stool black and tarry. For melena to be recognizable, approximately 150 mL of blood must drain into the GI tract and remain there for 5 to 8 hours. Blood in emesis may be bright red (new, fresh blood) or look like coffee grounds (old, partially digested blood).

Upper GI bleeding may be light or it may be brisk and life threatening. Patients who suffer a rupture of an esophageal varix or a tear or disruption in the esophageal or gastric lining may vomit copious amounts of blood. These hemorrhages can cause the classic signs and symptoms of shock, including alteration in mental status, tachycardia, peripheral vasoconstriction, diaphoresis (sweating—producing pale, cool, clammy skin), and hemodynamic instability. Besides shock, the vomitus itself can compromise the airway, resulting in impaired respirations, aspiration, and ultimately respiratory arrest.

A frequently employed clinical indicator is the tilt test, which indicates whether the patient has orthostatic hypotension (a 10-mmHg change in blood pressure or a 20-bpm change in heart rate when the patient rises from supine to standing). Hypotension suggests a decreased circulating volume. The human body can compensate for a circulating volume deficit of approximately 15 percent before clinical indicators such as the tilt test show positive results. Thus, patients whose systolic blood pressure drops 10 mmHg or whose heart rate increases 20 bpm or more need aggressive fluid resuscitation.

When evaluating the patient and his laboratory values, remember that the hematocrit might be within normal ranges when the patient is in the early phase of an acute hemorrhage. The key prevention strategy is to identify subtle indicators and treat the condition before it worsens. More general complaints include malaise, weakness, syncopal (fainting) and near-syncopal (lightheadedness) spells, tachycardia, and indigestion.

Your patient's general appearance may be the best indicator of his condition's severity. Because the hemorrhage is internal and histories are often misleading, you must perform a thorough physical examination. The patient may present doubled over in pain or lying very still. The latter is usually an ominous sign that any movement causes extreme pain. If you place the patient supine, be alert to the possibility of vomitus compromising the airway. Patients with a history of GI problems may have scars from past surgeries.

Examination in cases of suspected hemorrhage may be very helpful. Abdominal inspection may show symmetric distention or bulging in one region of the abdomen. Ecchymosis may be present if much blood has been lost into the abdominal cavity. If auscultation is subsequently performed, bowel sounds may be absent if the bleeding is severe, or they may be hyperactive if the bleeding is minimal.

Prehospital treatment of an upper gastrointestinal bleed centers on maintaining a patent airway, oxygenation, and circulatory status. Place the patient in the left lateral recumbent or high semi-Fowler's position to prevent aspiration. To maximize the remaining hemoglobin molecules' carrying capability, administer high-concentration oxygen via a nonrebreather mask to all patients with a suspected gastrointestinal bleed who have demonstrated hypoxia on pulse oximetry.

Establish two large-bore (14–16 gauge) IVs in any patient whom you suspect of having a gastrointestinal bleed. Start one with blood tubing for possible transfusion and one with volume-replacement 0.9 percent NaCl. Base fluid resuscitation on the patient's condition and response to the treatment. In general you can administer a 20 mL/kg fluid bolus to begin treating hemorrhagic hypovolemia.

Once the patient reaches the emergency department, treatment may include gastric decompression and lavage with a nasogastric tube, further fluid/blood resuscitation, endoscopy, antacid and histamine-antagonist administration, proton-pump inhibitors, or immediate surgery.[1]

Esophageal Varices

An **esophageal varix** is a swollen vein of the esophagus. Often these varices rupture and hemorrhage. When they do, the mortality rate is over 35 percent.

The cause of esophageal varices usually is an increase in **portal** pressure (portal hypertension). The blood flows from the abdominal organs, through the portal vein, and into the liver, where nutrients are absorbed into liver tissue and numerous compounds are detoxified and returned to the blood. From the liver, blood courses directly into the inferior vena cava through the hepatic veins. Blood flow through the liver ordinarily encounters little, if any, resistance. Damage to that organ, however, can impede circulation, causing blood to back up into the left gastric vein and, from there, into the esophageal veins. The dramatically higher pressure in these normally low-pressure pathways causes the esophageal veins to dilate and emerge from their sheaths (to evaginate, or "outpocket"). These small evaginations are called esophageal varices (Figure 6-3). As they become engorged, the varices continue to dilate outward

CONTENT REVIEW

➤ Upper GI Diseases
- Esophageal varices
- Acute gastroenteritis
- Gastroenteritis (chronic)
- Peptic ulcers
- Cyclical vomiting syndrome

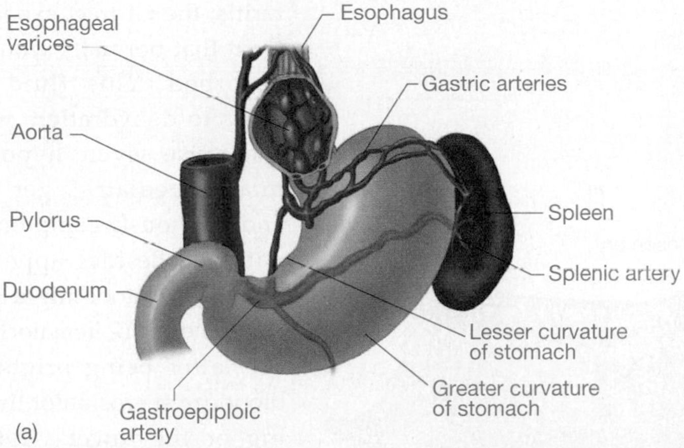

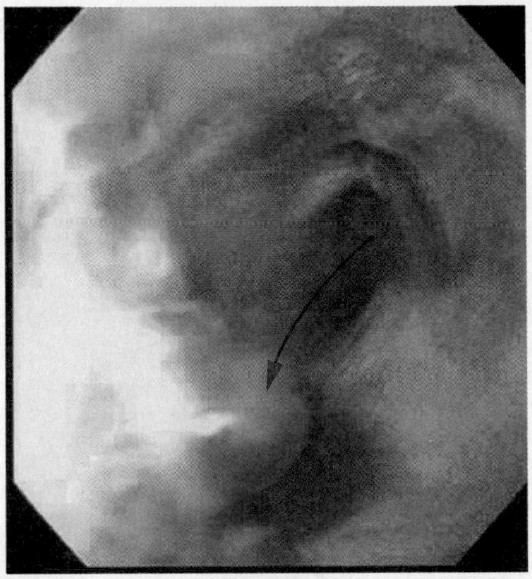

FIGURE 6-3 (a) Esophageal varices occur when the esophageal veins dilate and emerge from their sheaths. (b) Endoscopic view of an esophageal varix.

(Photo: © Dr. Bryan E. Bledsoe)

under extreme pressure until they rupture, causing massive hemorrhage. They may also erode through the submucosal layer and directly into the esophagus.

The primary causes of esophageal varices are the consumption of alcohol and the ingestion of caustic substances. Alcoholic liver cirrhosis accounts for two-thirds of cases of esophageal varices. Over time, alcohol consumption can cause a degenerative process known as **cirrhosis** of the liver. Cirrhosis results in fatty deposits and fibrosis in the liver parenchymal tissue (key functional tissues of the liver), thus obstructing portal blood flow. Consequently, esophageal varices are common in the United States and the Western Hemisphere in general, where the alcohol consumption rate is high. In fact, cirrhosis is one of the leading causes of death in the Western Hemisphere. Caustic substances such as battery acid or drain cleaners can erode the esophagus from the inside out, causing hemorrhage of a vessel. Caustic ingestion, along with variceal formation due to viral hepatitis and erosive esophagitis, accounts for the remaining one-third of cases of esophageal varices.

Patients suffering from leaking or ruptured esophageal varices often present initially with painless bleeding and signs of hemodynamic instability. They may complain of hematemesis with bright red blood, dysphagia (difficulty swallowing), and a burning or tearing sensation as the varices continue to bleed, irritating the lining of the esophagus. The hematemesis can be forceful and copious if the hemorrhage is large. Clotting time increases because the high portal pressure backs up blood into the spleen, destroying platelets. In addition, many of the clotting elements (e.g., prothrombin) are manufactured in the liver, and the inability of the liver to make these elements decreases with liver failure and cirrhosis. The patient may exhibit the classic signs of shock, including an increased pulse, increased respirations, and cool, clammy, diaphoretic skin, possibly associated with an altered level of consciousness and hypotension.

Because paramedics cannot tamponade the bleeding in the prehospital setting, your care should focus on aggressive airway management, intravenous fluid resuscitation, and rapid transport to the emergency department. Airway management is a top priority. You may need to suction emesis frequently and diligently from the airway. Endotracheal intubation also may be needed to maintain airway patency. To maximize oxygenation, administer high-concentration oxygen via a nonrebreather mask if the patient is hypoxic. If the patient shows signs and symptoms of shock, place him in the shock position and begin fluid resuscitation. The drug octreotide is the drug of choice for acute variceal bleeding. It is an analog of the peptide somatostatin and works by inhibiting the release of vasodilatory hormones such as glucagon. It indirectly causes vasoconstriction of the viscera and decreased portal vein flow. If the patient continues to hemorrhage, management in the emergency department might include endoscopic cauterization or sclerotherapy (injection of a thrombus-forming drug into the vein itself).[2]

Acute Gastroenteritis

Acute gastroenteritis is defined as inflammation of the stomach and intestines with associated sudden onset of vomiting and/or diarrhea. It affects from 3 to 5 million people yearly worldwide and affects approximately 20 percent of all hospitalized patients. The pathological inflammation causes hemorrhage and erosion of the

Layers of the Small Intestine (Jejunum)

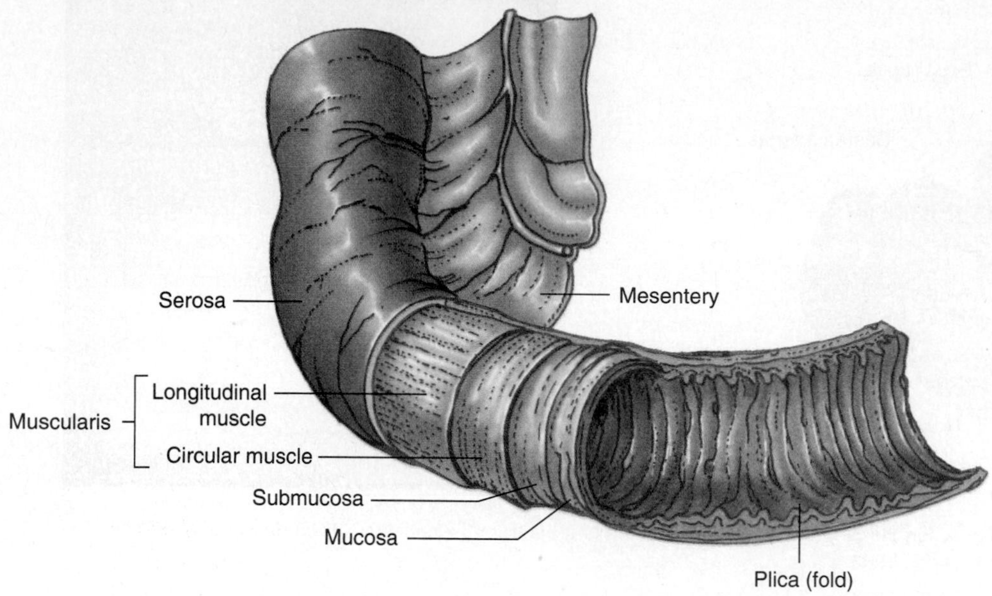

FIGURE 6-4 Mucosal surfaces of GI tract (small intestine).

mucosal and submucosal layers of the gastrointestinal tract (Figure 6-4). This inflammation and erosion can, in turn, damage the villi inside the intestine, which absorb water and nutrients. The water that healthy villi normally would absorb now moves through the bowel at an increased rate. Dehydration secondary to diarrhea is a common cause of death in developing nations but is seen far less frequently in the United States. Adequate volume replacement is your major prehospital prevention strategy to minimize the likelihood of hypovolemia, or even possible hypovolemic shock.

Individuals who abuse alcohol and tobacco are at high risk for gastritis (inflammation of the stomach) and gastroenteritis (inflammation of the stomach and intestines). A wide variety of chemical agents and incidents can lead to acute gastritis. One of the most common is the use of nonsteroidal anti-inflammatory drugs (NSAIDs) such as aspirin, which break down the mucosal surfaces of the stomach and GI tract. Other causes include excessive alcohol intake and tobacco use; alcohol and nicotine have the same irritating effect on the mucosa as NSAIDs. Stress, chemotherapeutic agents, and the ingestion of acidic or alkalotic agents can also cause acute gastroenteritis. Both systemic infection (e.g., salmonellosis) and infection from ingested pathogens (e.g., staphylococcus) can cause infectious acute gastroenteritis.

As the name implies, the onset of acute gastroenteritis is rapid and usually severe. The swift movement of fluid through the gastrointestinal tract causes multiple problems. First, and most obvious, diarrhea is almost always associated with this condition. Approximately 7 to 9 L of fluid (secretions and ingested fluids) normally move through the GI tract every 24 hours. Of that, less than 2 percent, or approximately 100 mL, is lost in the stool. With acute gastroenteritis, the GI tract expels the fluid that normally would be absorbed. This fluid loss leads to dehydration, which can cause severe hypovolemia in pediatric, geriatric, and previously compromised patients. Besides appearing watery, the stool might show either melena or **hematochezia**, the latter being bright red blood from erosion of the lining of the lower GI tract. Along with the changes in stool, patients may have bouts of hematemesis, fever, nausea and vomiting, and general malaise. Due to dehydration and hemorrhage, the patient can be hemodynamically unstable; the exam may show hypotension, tachycardia, and pale, cool, and clammy skin. The patient may appear restless or show decreased mental status. If dehydration is severe, he can develop chest pain and cardiac arrhythmias from electrolyte disturbances. The patient may complain of widespread and diffuse abdominal pain that is not specific to any one region. Visible distention is relatively unlikely unless significant gas has built up within the intestines; palpation will probably reveal tenderness throughout the abdomen.

Treatment for acute gastroenteritis is mainly supportive and palliative. Keep the patient positioned with head forward or face to the side to minimize the likelihood of aspiration should vomiting occur. Be prepared to clear the airway of vomit or secretions. Maintaining adequate oxygenation is also a high priority. When there is no significant blood loss, the circulatory system's oxygen-carrying capabilities remain intact. Administer supplemental oxygen to correct hypoxia. Avoid hyperoxia. Rehydration is the next step in treating your patient. If he is conscious and alert, oral fluid rehydration may be appropriate. The easiest and quickest route, however, is IV fluid administration. In the prehospital setting, the fluid of choice is either 0.9 percent NaCl or lactated Ringer's solution to replace the patient's circulating volume. Pharmacological treatment can involve antiemetics such as ondansetron (Zofran), prochlorperazine (Compazine), or similar agents. Additional replacement of electrolytes such as potassium may be needed. Offer emotional support during transport. Exercise extreme caution and use Standard Precautions throughout patient contact to prevent any spread of infectious disease.

Chronic Gastroenteritis

Chronic gastroenteritis is inflammation of gastrointestinal mucosa marked by long-term mucosal changes or permanent mucosal damage. Unlike acute gastroenteritis, chronic gastroenteritis is due primarily to microbial infection. The most prevalent pathogen in the United States is the *Helicobacter pylori* bacillus. Other bacteria that can cause chronic gastroenteritis include *Escherichia coli, Klebsiella pneumoniae, Enterobacter, Campylobacter jejuni, Vibrio cholerae, Shigella,* and *Salmonella.* Many of these bacteria can be found as part of normal enteric flora, and effective vaccination against pathogenic strains has not been possible. *Shigella* and *Salmonella* are not part of the normal spectrum of intestinal flora. Viral pathogens include the norovirus and rotavirus. Among the parasitic causes are the protozoa *Giardia lamblia, Cryptosporidium parvum,* and *Cyclosporidium cayetenis.*

All these microbes and their associated gastric disorders are far more common in underdeveloped countries. They are transmitted via the fecal–oral route or through infected food or water. Fecal–oral transmission can occur when people practice poor personal hygiene or food-handling techniques. Local water supplies can become contaminated during natural disasters that disrupt normal water distribution and sewage treatment practices. In such instances, people from outside the endemic area may be more vulnerable to infection than is the local population. *Cyclosporidium* infection reportedly can be contracted by swimming in contaminated water.

Gastroenteritis patients commonly present with nausea and vomiting, fever, diarrhea, abdominal pain, cramping, anorexia (loss of appetite), lethargy, and, in severe cases, shock. Usually the intensity of signs and symptoms reflects the degree of microbial contamination. On the other hand, infection with *H. pylori,* the most common infectious gastroenteritis in the United States, often presents with common signs such as heartburn, abdominal pain, and, on endoscopic examination, gastric ulcers.

When in contaminated conditions, be sure to decontaminate the drinking water or use a different water source; when in doubt about the reliability of the water, drink only beverages that have been briskly boiled or disinfected. Make sure proper sanitation and preparation of foods are maintained. Standard Precautions will protect most EMS providers and prevent transmitting the organism further. To avoid transmitting the disease to patients, health care providers should not work when they are ill.

Prehospital treatment involves protecting yourself and the patient from further contamination, monitoring the ABCs, and transport. Medical treatment of infectious gastroenteritis will require identification of the offending organism. Some of the causative microorganisms are sensitive to antibiotics, but in most cases the patient will be supported while the disease takes its natural path.

Peptic Ulcers

Peptic ulcers are erosions caused by gastric acid (Figure 6-5a). They can occur anywhere in the gastrointestinal tract; terminology is based on the portion of the GI tract affected. Duodenal ulcers (Figure 6-5b) occur most frequently in the proximal portion of the duodenum; gastric ulcers occur exclusively in the stomach. Overall, peptic ulcers occur in males four times more frequently than in females, and duodenal ulcers occur from two to three times more frequently than do gastric ulcers. Current statistics place the number of peptic ulcers at 4 to 5 million, with approximately 500,000 new cases diagnosed yearly. Patients who are more likely to have gastric ulcers are over 50 years old

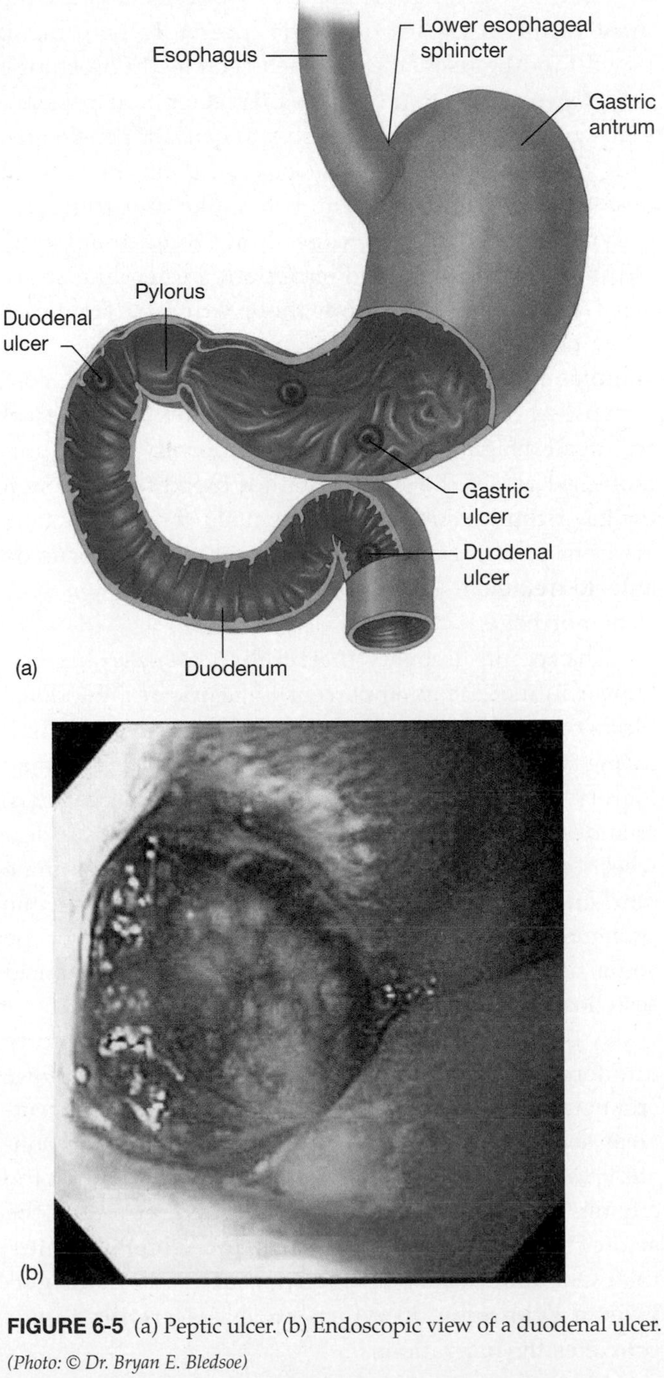

FIGURE 6-5 (a) Peptic ulcer. (b) Endoscopic view of a duodenal ulcer.
(Photo: © Dr. Bryan E. Bledsoe)

and work in jobs requiring physical activity. Their pain usually increases after eating or with a full stomach and they usually have no pain at night. Duodenal ulcers are more common in patients from 25 to 50 years old who are executives or leaders under high stress. There is also some familial tendency toward duodenal ulcers, suggesting a genetic predisposition. Patients with duodenal ulcers commonly have pain at night or when their stomach is empty. Thus, it is important in taking the focused history to get family history and a reliable estimate of the patient's last oral intake. Measurement of hematocrit may substantiate any suspicions of chronic or acute hemorrhage.

Nonsteroidal anti-inflammatory medications (aspirin, ibuprofen, naproxen), acid-stimulating products (alcohol, nicotine), or *Helicobacter pylori* bacteria are the most common causes of peptic ulcers. To help break down food boluses, the stomach secretes hydrochloric acid. One enzyme that controls this secretion is pepsinogen. The hydrochloric acid helps to convert pepsinogen into its active form, pepsin. Between them, the pepsin and the hydrochloric acid can make the digestive enzymes very irritating to the GI tract's mucosal lining. Ordinarily, mucous gland secretions protect the stomach's mucosal barrier from these irritants. However, when nonsteroidal anti-inflammatory medications, acid stimulators, or *H. pylori* damage the barrier, the mucosa is exposed to the highly acidic fluid, and peptic ulcers result. Prostaglandin, an important locally acting hormone, decreases the stimulation for blood flow through the gastric mucosa, thus allowing its further destruction. Treatment strategies in the prehospital setting focus on antacid treatment and support of any complications such as hemorrhage.

The recent discovery that *Helicobacter pylori* bacteria appear in more than 80 percent of gastric and duodenal ulcers has enabled physicians to treat the disease by eliminating its cause with antacids and antibiotics, rather than merely treating its symptoms. Definitive treatment includes tamponade of any bleed, possibly by surgical resection, and antibiotic therapy, along with histamine blockers and antacids. If medical therapy fails and the problem persists, it may require surgical resection of the vagus nerve (vagotomy) to reduce the stimulation for acid secretion.[3]

A blocked pancreatic duct can also contribute to duodenal ulcers. As chyme passes through the pyloric sphincter from the stomach into the duodenum, the pancreas secretes an alkalotic solution laden with bicarbonate ions that neutralize the acidic hydrogen ions in the chyme. If the pancreatic duct is blocked, however, the acidic chyme can cause ulcerations throughout the intestine. One other cause of duodenal ulcers is **Zollinger-Ellison syndrome**, in which an acid-secreting tumor provokes the ulcerations.

Findings on clinical examination of a patient with peptic ulcer can vary. Chronic ulcers can cause a slow bleed, with resulting anemia. Visual inspection of the abdomen is usually helpful only if significant hemorrhage has occurred, in which case the same signs of ecchymosis and distention are found, as in other causes of upper GI bleeding. On palpation, pain may be localized or diffuse. These patients often have relief of pain after eating or coating their GI tract with a liquid such as milk.

Acute, severe pain is probably due to a rupture of the ulcer into the peritoneal cavity, causing hemorrhage. Depending on the ulcer's location, the patient may have hematemesis or may have melena-colored stool. Bouts of nausea and vomiting due to the irritation of the mucosa are common. If the ulcer has eroded through a highly vascular area, massive hemorrhage can occur. Along with the signs of hemorrhage on visual inspection, these patients will appear very ill and have signs of hemodynamic instability, such as pale, cool, and clammy skin, tachycardia, decreased blood pressure, and, possibly, altered mental status. Most patients will lie still to decrease the pain. They may have surgical scars from previous ulcer repair. Bowel sounds will usually be absent.

Treatment for peptic ulcers depends on the severity of the patient's pain. Patients who have abdominal pain or hemodynamic instability may require comfortable positioning and psychological support; high-concentration oxygen (if hypoxia is present); IV access for fluid resuscitation and pharmacological administration; and rapid transport. Common medications to reduce the mucosal irritation include histamine blockers such as ranitidine and famotidine, proton-pump inhibitors such as omeprazole and esomeprazole, and antacids such as sucralfate.

Cyclical Vomiting Syndrome

Cyclical vomiting syndrome (CVS) is an increasingly common disorder characterized by repeated sudden attacks, called episodes, of severe nausea, vomiting, and physical exhaustion without apparent cause. The episodes often last from several hours to several days. They can be variable in severity, sometimes leaving the patient unable to work or even to get out of bed. The syndrome can occur over an extended period of time with recurrent events.

There appear to be four distinct cycles of CVS:

- *Prodrome phase.* During the prodrome phase, the person feels that nausea and vomiting are about to begin. This is often accompanied by intense sweating and may last for minutes to hours.
- *Vomiting phase.* During this phase, the patient has intense nausea, vomiting, and retching. These episodes tend to last 20 to 30 minutes at a time and are

often associated with severe abdominal pain. This phase can last from hours to days.

- *Recovery phase.* During the recovery phase, the vomiting and retching stop and eventually the nausea subsides. The patient is able to eat and return to the normal activities of daily living.
- *Well phase.* During this phase, the patient is asymptomatic.

CVS can result in dehydration, esophagitis, tearing of the upper GI tract, and decay and damage from the frequent and excessive exposure to gastric acids.

The exact cause of CVS is unknown, but it is known to be more common with the following conditions:

- Emotional stress (e.g., anxiety)
- Unrelated infections (e.g., sinusitis, upper respiratory infections)
- Menstruation
- Motion sickness
- Exposure to certain foods (e.g., chocolate, caffeine)
- Chronic marijuana usage
- Hot weather
- Physical exhaustion and/or increased exercise
- Dietary changes, including overeating, fasting, or eating immediately before bed

CVS appears to be more common in children than adults. It is also more common in people who are prone to migraine headaches.

Treatment of CVS can be challenging. Often, the patient has already taken the common antinausea/antiemetic medications. IV hydration is typically indicated and the patients may require pain medication. Is often worthwhile to try a different antiemetic from the one that the patient typically takes. Prevention is often the best treatment, and it may be possible to prevent an occurance of cyclical vomiting if the patient can identify and avoid or modify a factor, such as any of those just listed, that seems to occur before or in conjunction with CVS episodes.

Lower Gastrointestinal Diseases

The lower GI tract consists of the jejunum and ileum of the small intestine and the entire large intestine, rectum, and anus. As digestive fluid moves through the small intestine (which is approximately 6 meters long), nutrients are absorbed into the blood. Water is absorbed and solid wastes form in the large intestine, also called the large bowel or colon, which is roughly 1.5 meters long (review Figure 6-2).

CONTENT REVIEW

- Lower GI Tract
  - Jejunum
  - Ileum
  - Large intestine
  - Rectum
  - Anus

Lower GI Bleeding

Lower gastrointestinal bleeding occurs in the GI tract distal to the ligament of Treitz. Lower GI hemorrhages occur most frequently in conjunction with chronic disorders and anatomic changes associated with advanced age. The most common cause is diverticulosis, which is most prevalent in elderly people. Other causes are colon lesions (cancer or benign polyps), rectal lesions (hemorrhoids, anal fissures, anal fistulas), and inflammatory bowel disorders such as ulcerative colitis and Crohn's disease. These chronic disorders and diverticulosis rarely result in a massive hemorrhage such as that which can occur in the esophagus or stomach.

CONTENT REVIEW

- Major Causes of Lower GI Hemorrhage
  - Diverticulosis
  - Colon lesions
  - Rectal lesions
  - Inflammatory bowel disorder
- Lower gastrointestinal bleeding is usually chronic and rarely results in exsanguinating hemorrhage.

Your assessment of patients with suspected lower GI bleeds will be identical to your assessment of those with suspected upper GI bleeds. After you complete your primary assessment and treat all life-threatening conditions, you can conduct your secondary assessment. First, ask the patient whether this is a new complaint or a chronic problem. If a chronic problem, check the abdomen visually for scars from previous surgery. Frequent complaints with lower GI bleeding include cramping pain that may be described as like a muscle cramp or like gas pain, nausea and vomiting, and changes in stool. Melenic stool usually indicates a slow GI bleed. If the stool contains bright red blood, the hemorrhage either is very large (thus passing through the intestines before melenic change can occur) or has occurred in the distal colon. In the latter case, hemorrhoids or rectal fissures are possible causes. The abdominal exam will show findings similar to those for a bleeding peptic ulcer. If the abdomen has the distention or ecchymosis characteristic of significant hemorrhage, check for signs of early shock, such as pale, cool, and clammy skin; tachycardia; decreased blood pressure; and, possibly, altered mental status. Because most patients with lower GI bleeds have not lost significant amounts of blood, they will present with hemodynamic stability, including warm dry skin, on physical exam.

How you manage the patient with a lower GI bleed will depend on his physiologic status. Watch his airway and oxygenation status closely. If hypoventilation or inadequate respirations develop, administer high-concentration oxygenation via a nonrebreather mask or positive pressure ventilation. Establish IV access and fluid resuscitation based on your patient's hemodynamic status. If you find a drop in hematocrit along with other signs of significant

CONTENT REVIEW

➤ Lower GI Diseases
- Ulcerative colitis
- Crohn's disease
- Diverticulitis
- Hemorrhoids
- Irritable bowel syndrome
- Bowel obstruction

blood loss, be especially sure that one IV line is of sufficiently large bore for emergency transfusion. Place the patient in a comfortable position, offer psychological support, and transport him for further examination.

Ulcerative Colitis

Ulcerative colitis is classified as an idiopathic inflammatory bowel disorder (IBD)—that is, one of unknown origin. The inflammatory (ulcerative) process creates a continuous length of chronic ulcers in the mucosal layer of the colon; extension of the ulcers into the submucosal layer is uncommon. As ulcers heal, granular tissue replaces the ulcerations, thickening the mucosa (Figure 6-6). Approximately 75 percent of all ulcerative colitis involves the rectum or rectosigmoid portion of the large intestine. The inflammatory process usually starts in the rectum and then extends proximally into the colon, sometimes affecting the entire large intestine. If it spreads throughout the entire colon it is called **pancolitis**; if limited to the rectum, it is called **proctitis**.

Although ulcerative colitis is relatively unusual in Africa or Asia, its occurrence in the Western Hemisphere is increasing rapidly. In the United States, more than 10,000 new cases are diagnosed each year. It most frequently strikes people between the ages of 20 and 40 years.

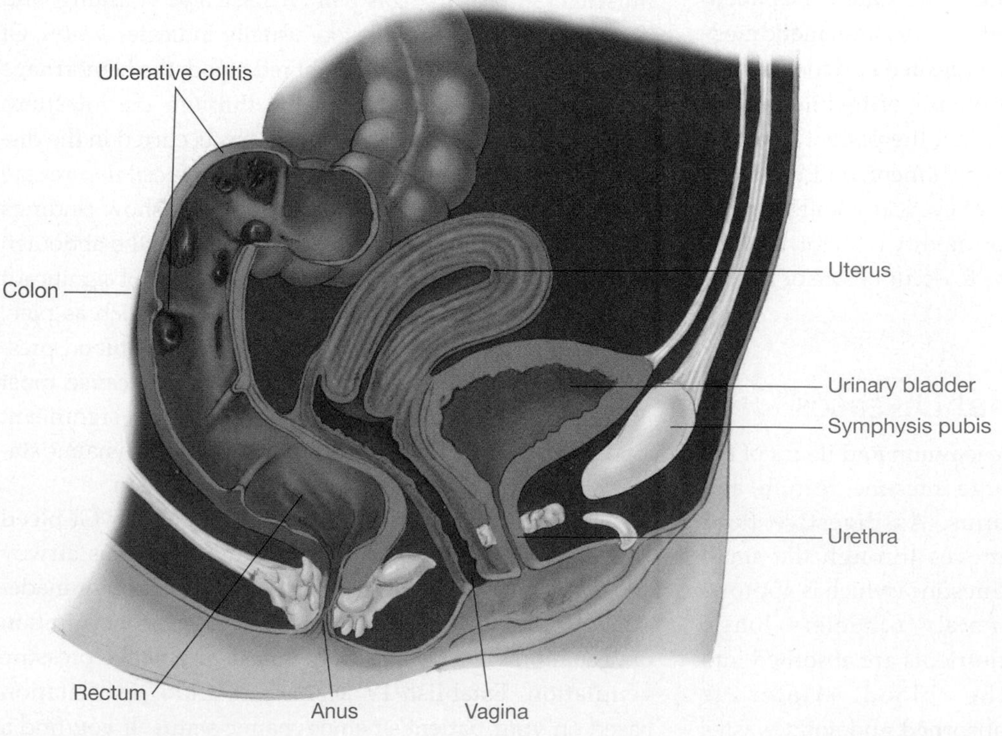

FIGURE 6-6 Ulcerative colitis.

Although researchers have not found a specific pathogen or cause of ulcerative colitis, they have determined many different contributing factors—psychological, allergic, toxic, environmental, immunologic, and infectious. Current research has found that the release of cytokines can cause an overwhelming inflammatory response in the submucosa much like the release of histamines during anaphylaxis.

Acute ulcerative colitis is difficult to differentiate from other causes of lower GI bleeding. Because of its insidious presentation, diagnosing, tracking, and treating ulcerative colitis may require hematocrit and hemoglobin results, guaiac analyses of the stool, and endoscopic examinations. The severity of ulcerative colitis's signs and symptoms is usually related directly to the extent and severity of current inflammation in the colon. In patients with mild signs and symptoms, the disease often is isolated in one distal segment of the GI tract. Severe presentations, on the other hand, normally involve the entire colon.

Typically, ulcerative colitis presents as a recurrent disorder with occasional bloody diarrhea or stool-containing mucus. Accompanying the stool abnormalities are **colic** (acute abdominal pain with cramping or spasms), nausea and vomiting, and occasionally, fever (suggesting infection) or weight loss (suggesting severe or longer-term colonic dysfunction). The cramping is usually limited to the lower quadrants, depending on the extent of colonic involvement, and it occurs when hypertrophic muscles lying beneath the submucosa prevent the colon from stretching in response to pressure from its contents. These patients will typically appear restless due to abdominal discomfort but will not show signs of hemodynamic instability (that is, skin will be warm and dry rather than cool and clammy).

More severe cases may present with bloody diarrhea and intense colicky abdominal pain, electrolyte derangements due to fluid loss through the colon, ischemic damage to the colon itself, or, eventually, perforation of the bowel. Often, these patients present with signs and symptoms of hypovolemic shock such as pale, cool, clammy skin; hypotension; and tachycardia. Such patients with advanced disease and ongoing hemorrhage may have distention or ecchymosis on the skin and may show guarding of the lower quadrants during the physical examination. Significant hemorrhage is common in patients with ulcerative colitis.

Your management of the patient with ulcerative colitis will depend on his physiologic status. If he presents with signs and symptoms of hypovolemic shock, administer high-concentration oxygen (if the patient is hypoxic) and circulatory support, including intravenous access and fluid resuscitation. If your patient has bouts of nausea and vomiting, you must diligently manage his airway to prevent aspiration of vomitus. Additional management may include antiemetics and antispasmodic medications. Transport any patient who presents with lower GI bleeding or colicky pain to the emergency department for diagnostic evaluation.[4]

Crohn's Disease

Crohn's disease, along with ulcerative colitis, is the other idiopathic inflammatory bowel disorder in humans. It is more common in the Western Hemisphere, with from 20,000 to 30,000 new cases reported annually in the United States. This disease, which strongly tends to run in families, is most prevalent among white females, those under frequent stress, and in the Jewish population.

Unlike ulcerative colitis, which affects the large intestine, Crohn's disease can occur anywhere from the mouth to the rectum. Between 35 and 45 percent of less severe cases involve the small intestine only; approximately 40 percent involve the colon itself. Severe cases of Crohn's disease may involve any portion of the GI tract, causing a variety of problems ranging from diarrhea to intestinal and perianal abscesses and fistulas (the latter, abnormal passages connecting two internal organs or different lengths of intestine). Complete intestinal obstruction, a surgical emergency, can also occur. Significant lower GI bleeding, on the other hand, is rare with Crohn's disease.

As the pathological inflammation begins, it damages the innermost layer of tissue, the mucosa. Granulomas then form and further break down the mucosal and submucosal layers. The affected section of intestinal wall eventually becomes rubbery and nondistensible due to hypertrophy and fibrosis of the muscles underlying the submucosa (Figure 6-7). The patchwork-quilt formation of granulomas, fibrosis, and hypertrophy also decreases the intestine's internal diameter, resulting in fissures (incomplete tears) in the mucosa and possibly deeper into the submucosa as food boluses pass through. If a tear extends into the blood vessels in the submucosal layer, small bleeds result. The same pathological pattern of ulceration and scarring can lead to creation of fistulas, most commonly between lengths of small intestine, or to obstruction of the small bowel. Increased suppressor T lymphocyte activity suggests an immune-mediated role in the inflammatory process.

Crohn's patients' clinical presentations can vary drastically as the disease progresses, and prehospital diagnosis is difficult or next to impossible. Common signs and symptoms include GI bleeding, recent weight loss, intermittent abdominal cramping/pain, nausea and vomiting, diarrhea, and fever. Onset of a flareup in disease activity is usually rapid, often requiring a visit to the emergency department or physician's office. Abdominal pain cannot be localized to any specific quadrant because the disease can affect any portion of the small intestine and often affects more than one. The physical exam is also nonspecific and nonlocalized, with diffuse tenderness the most commonly found sign. Absence of bowel sounds in a patient with Crohn's disease strongly suggests intestinal obstruction, a surgical emergency.

Because the vast majority of patients with Crohn's disease are hemodynamically stable, prehospital treatment is largely palliative. Your management depends on the patient's physiologic status. If he has bouts of nausea and vomiting, you must diligently manage the airway to

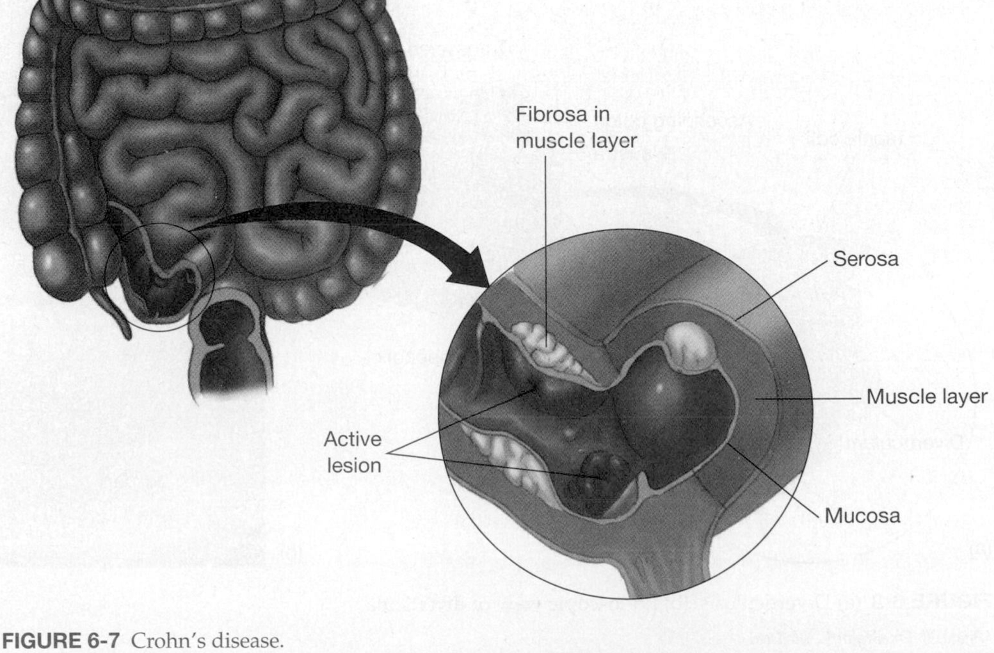

FIGURE 6-7 Crohn's disease.

prevent aspiration of vomitus. Additional management may include antiemetics and antispasmodic medications. Particularly if the patient presents with signs and symptoms of obstruction or significant hemorrhage, administer high-concentration oxygenation (if the patient is hypoxic) and circulatory support, including intravenous access and fluid resuscitation. As always, calmly and quietly inform the patient of all measures taken and offer psychological support en route to the emergency facility.

Diverticulitis

Diverticulitis is a relatively common complication of diverticulosis. **Diverticulosis** is a condition characterized by the presence in the intestine of **diverticula**, small outpouchings of mucosal and submucosal tissue that push through the outermost layer of the intestine, the muscle. Colonic diverticula are far more common in developed countries such as the United States and increase markedly in prevalence with increased age. They are present in more than half of patients over 60 years of age. Diverticulitis is an inflammation of diverticula secondary to infection. Unlike diverticulosis, it is symptomatic: Patients will complain of lower left-sided pain (because most diverticula are in the sigmoid colon); exam and testing will show fever and an increased white blood cell count.

The pathogenesis of an acquired diverticulum is twofold. First, stool passes sluggishly through the colon, a condition associated with the relatively low-fiber diets common in developed countries. The colon responds with muscle spasms that increase bulk movement by raising the pressure on the contents inside the colon and pushing the fecal material forward. Second, the outermost layer of colon tissue is made up of fibrous bands of muscle wrapped around one another. Among them are muscles called the *teniae coli*. Nerves and blood vessels enter the colon through small openings within the teniae coli. These openings become weakened with age, and the increased pressure of muscle spasms can cause the inner layers of tissue, the mucosa and submucosa, to herniate through the openings, forming diverticula (Figure 6-8).

These diverticula commonly trap small amounts of fecal material, including sunflower seeds, popcorn fragments, okra seeds, sesame seeds, and others. The entrapped feces may allow bacteria other than the normal flora to grow and cause an infection. The problem is compounded when the diverticula become inflamed, causing diverticulitis. Complications secondary to diverticulitis include possible hemorrhage or larger perforations of the colon wall through which the infected fecal contents can spill into the peritoneal cavity and cause peritonitis.

The most common presentation of diverticulitis is colicky pain associated with a low-grade fever, nausea and vomiting, and tenderness on palpation. The pain is usually localized to the lower left side because the sigmoid colon is involved in 95 percent of reported cases. Thus, diverticulitis is often called left-sided appendicitis. If the diverticula begin to bleed significantly, the usual signs and symptoms associated with severe lower GI bleeding may be present: cool, clammy skin; tachycardia; and diaphoresis. Bleeding diverticula can also result in bright red and bloody feces (hematochezia) because of their close proximity to the rectum. Patients may additionally complain of the perception that they cannot empty their rectums, even after defecation.

Prehospital treatment for diverticulitis is mainly supportive. Measures to counter hypovolemic shock will be needed only when significant hemorrhage has occurred.

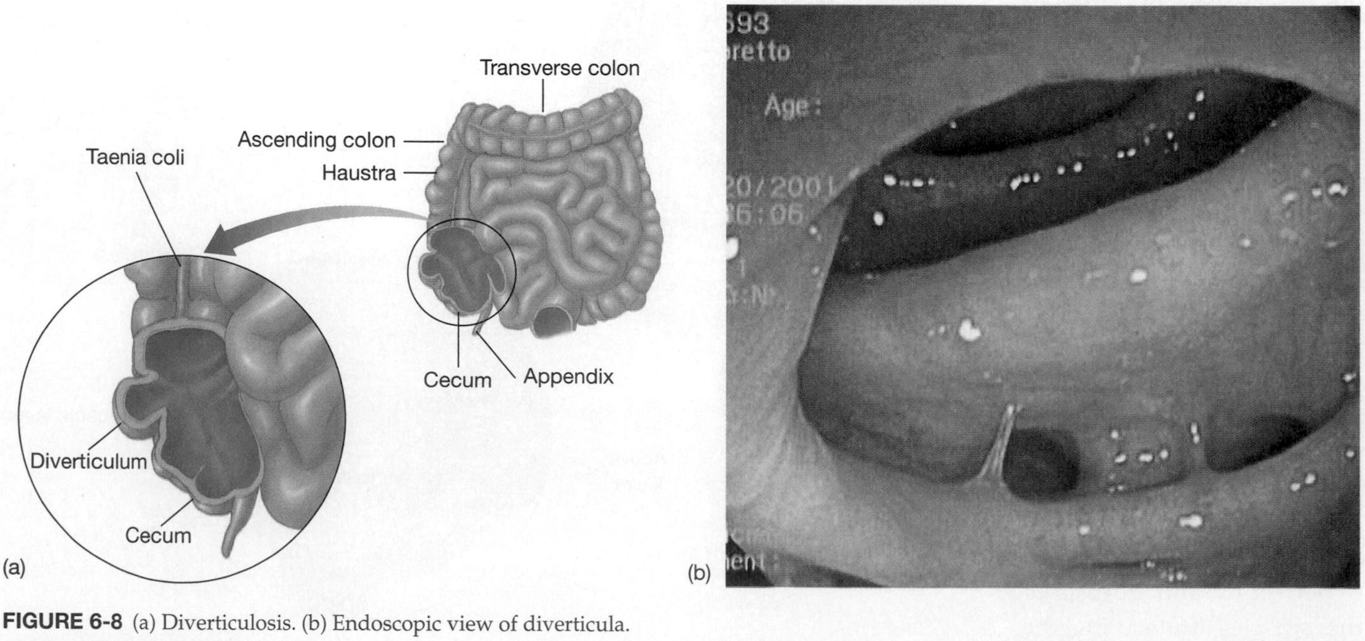

FIGURE 6-8 (a) Diverticulosis. (b) Endoscopic view of diverticula.

(Photo: © Dr. Bryan E. Bledsoe)

Monitor the patient's airway and oxygenation and provide supplemental oxygen if the patient is hypoxic. Establish intravenous access and begin fluid resuscitation if the patient is hemodynamically unstable. Antiemetics (ondansetron) may comfort the patient. Treatment in the hospital includes antibiotic therapy, endoscopy, and radiologic tests to locate the diverticula. Long-term treatment includes implementing a high-fiber diet to stimulate daily bowel movements.

Hemorrhoids

Hemorrhoids are small masses of swollen veins that occur in the anus (external) or rectum (internal) (Figure 6-9). They frequently develop during the fourth decade of life. Most hemorrhoids are idiopathic (of unknown cause), although they can result from pregnancy or portal hypertension. External hemorrhoids often result from lifting a heavy object. Other causes of hemorrhoids include straining at defecation and a diet low in fiber. Overall, hemorrhoids are common, particularly in persons over the age of 50 years. Their morbidity is low in most cases; one marked exception is in alcoholic patients with cirrhosis of the liver.

Internal hemorrhoids most often involve the inferior hemorrhoidal plexus and vasculature. They commonly bleed during the process of defecation because of straining and then thrombose into a closed state again. External hemorrhoids result from thrombosis of a vein, often following lifting or straining, causing bright red bleeding with a bowel movement. The increased venous pressure sometimes causes the vessels to erode and bleed spontaneously, which increases the risk of infection. Rarely do hemorrhoids cause a significant hemorrhage.

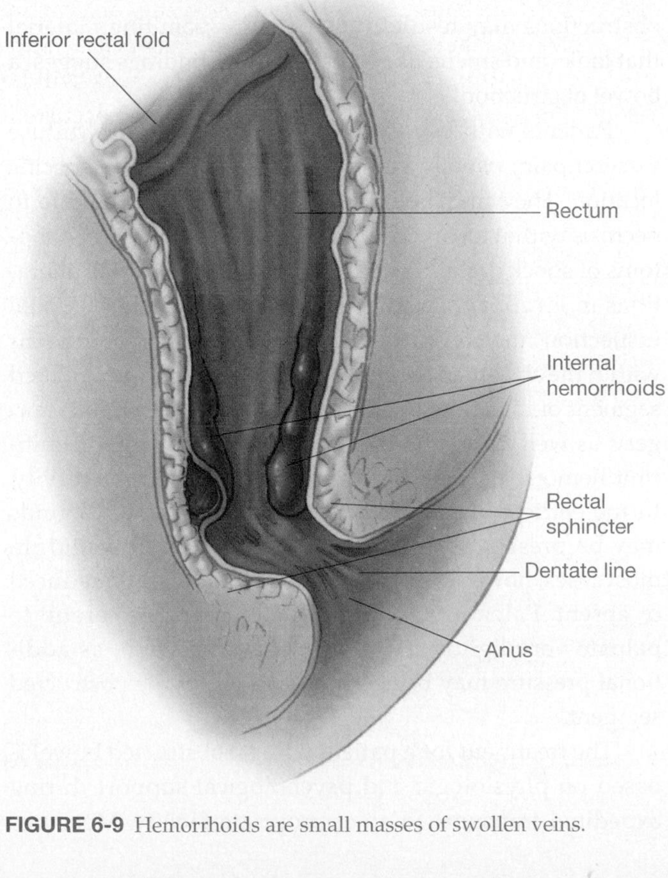

FIGURE 6-9 Hemorrhoids are small masses of swollen veins.

Patients with hemorrhoids commonly call for emergency care because of bright red bleeding and pain on defecation. Physical assessment usually reveals a hemodynamically stable patient with relatively normal appearance (warm, dry skin, perhaps with slight tachycardia consistent with anxiety) who bleeds with defecation. Visual examination of the stool may reveal gross bleeding. Treatment for hemorrhoids depends on the patient's condition. Most frequently, emotional reassurance and transport are all that is needed; however, you should remain alert to the possibility that the bleeding could be from a lower GI bleed, potentially resulting in uncontrolled hemorrhage. Either significant hemorrhage or bleeding hemorrhoids in an alcoholic patient warrant closer monitoring and transport for immediate follow-up.

Irritable Bowel Syndrome

Irritable bowel syndrome (IBS), sometimes called *spastic colon*, is a gastrointestinal system disorder that is characterized by the presence of common signs and symptoms that include:

- Abdominal pain
- Cramping
- Increased gas
- Altered bowel habits
- Food intolerance
- Abdominal distention (bloating)

IBS is defined as a functional issue rather than a structural problem. It can occur in both adults and children. The exact cause is uncertain but may be due to various factors, including food sensitivities, hypersensitivity to the pain that occurs with gaseous distention, abnormal peristalsis, hormonal imbalances, hereditary factors, and psychological conditions such as depression and/or anxiety. There is no defined cure for IBS, but treatment is available. In a prehospital setting, IBS should be treated as any other abdominal complaint.

Rectal Foreign Body

Some patients will present with a foreign body in the rectum. In most cases, the foreign body was inserted into the rectum with the patient's knowledge for various reasons, including sexual gratification or psychosis. However, foreign bodies (e.g., gallstones, fecaliths) can also pass into the lower GI tract from upper GI structures or swallowing. Most swallowed foreign bodies pass readily, but others may not. Most patients will report rectal pain or pressure. Some may show signs of infection or even frank shock.

Prehospital treatment is supportive, and analgesia may be required. The situation can be quite embarrassing for some patients and should be addressed with empathy and concern.

Bowel Obstruction

Bowel obstructions are blockages of the hollow space, or lumen, within the small and large intestines. Obstructions can be either partial or complete. An obstructed bowel segment can be catastrophic if not rapidly diagnosed and treated. Of this malady's varied causes, **hernias** (Figure 6-10), **intussusception** (Figure 6-11), **volvulus** (Figure 6-12), and **adhesions** (Figure 6-13) are the four most frequent, accounting for more than 70 percent of all reported cases. Other common causes are foreign bodies, gallstones, tumors, adhesions from previous abdominal surgery, and bowel **infarction**. The most common location for obstructions is the small intestine, due to its smaller diameter and greater length, flexibility, and mobility.

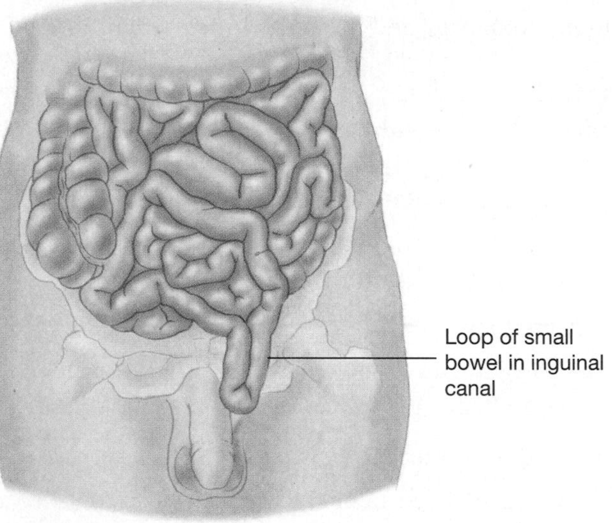

FIGURE 6-10 Inguinal hernia.

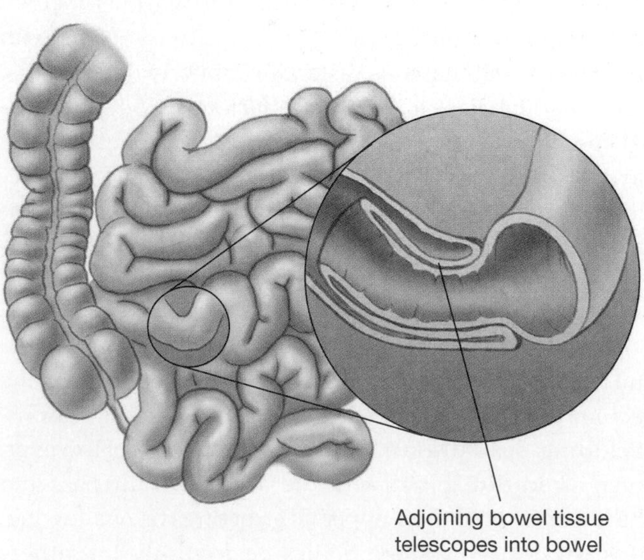

FIGURE 6-11 Intestinal intussusception.

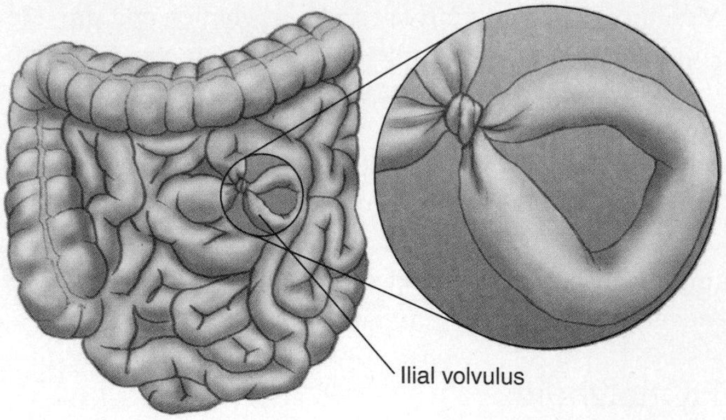

FIGURE 6-12 Intestinal volvulus.

The obstruction may be chronic, as with tumor growth or adhesion progression, or its onset may be sudden and acute, as with obstruction by a foreign body. Chronic obstruction usually results in a decreased appetite, fever, malaise, nausea and vomiting, weight loss, or, if rupture occurs, peritonitis. Acute-onset pain may follow ingestion of a foreign body. Pain might also be due to a strangulated hernia, one that has rotated through the muscle wall of the abdomen such that blood flow is suddenly cut off (the herniated tissue has been "strangulated") and ischemia, or even infarction, of tissue occurs. Patients with bowel obstruction will frequently vomit, with the vomitus often containing a significant amount of bile. Severe bowel obstructions may result in the patient's vomiting material that looks and smells like feces. All these findings suggest a bowel obstruction.

Patients with bowel obstruction present with diffuse visceral pain, usually poorly localized to any one specific location. They may be hemodynamically unstable due to necrosis within an organ, and you may see signs and symptoms of shock (pale, cool, clammy skin; tachycardia; alterations in level of consciousness; and hypotension). Visual inspection may reveal distention, peritonitis, or free air within the abdomen secondary to rupture of a strangulated segment of intestine. Look for scars left from previous surgery, as well as for the ecchymosis indicating that significant hemorrhage has occurred into the abdominal cavity. In the earliest phase of acute obstruction, bowel sounds may be present as a high-pitched obstruction sound. In most cases, however, bowel sounds will be greatly reduced or absent. Palpation will reveal tenderness. Be careful to palpate very lightly if you suspect obstruction, as additional pressure may bring about rupture of the obstructed segment.

The treatment for a patient with an obstructed bowel is based on physiologic and psychological support during expedited transport to an appropriate facility. Measures

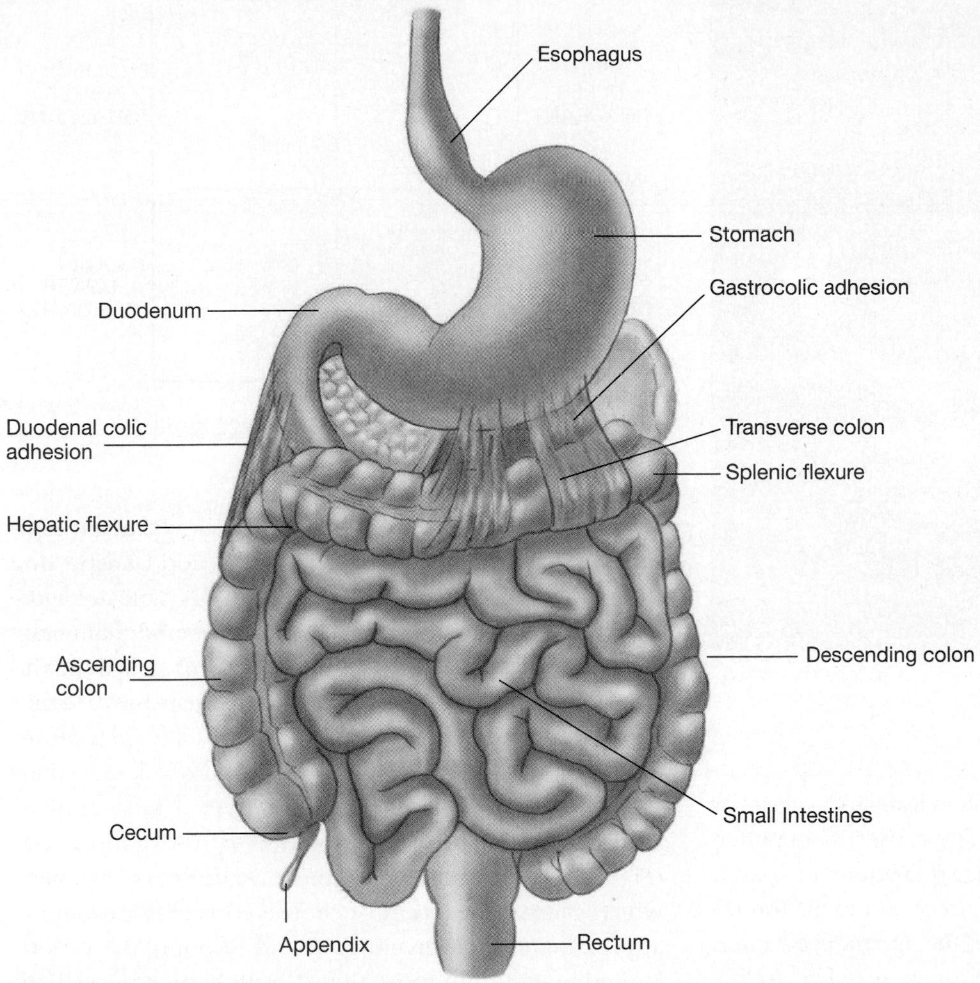

FIGURE 6-13 Intestinal adhesion.

include airway management, supplemental oxygenation (if the patient is hypoxic), position of comfort or shock position, and fluid resuscitation to prevent shock.

Mesenteric Ischemia

Mesenteric ischemia occurs when one of the mesenteric arteries becomes narrowed or occluded. There are two mesenteric arteries:

- Superior mesenteric artery (SMA). The SMA supplies the intestine from the lower part of the duodenum through two-thirds of the transverse colon, as well as the pancreas.
- Inferior mesenteric artery (IMA). The IMA supplies the large intestine from the splenic flexure to the upper part of the rectum, which includes the descending colon, the sigmoid colon, and part of the rectum.

When blood flow through either of these vessels is reduced or stopped, abdominal pain occurs. Nausea, vomiting, and diarrhea are common. Over time, if untreated, the bowel will become ischemic and die, causing infection. Mesenteric ischemia usually occurs in people older than age 60. It is more common in smokers and those with elevated cholesterol levels. Mesenteric ischemia can be either chronic or acute. Chronic mesenteric ischemia can progress without warning to acute mesenteric ischemia—sometimes very quickly. Prehospital treatment should include hydration, pain control, and antiemetics. The treatment is usually surgical.

Accessory Organ Diseases

As you learned earlier in this chapter, the GI tract has three closely associated organs—the liver, gallbladder, and pancreas—as well as the small structure called the vermiform appendix. Accessory organ emergencies can arise in all four locations.

Appendicitis

Appendicitis is an inflammation of the vermiform appendix, located at the junction of the large and small intestines (the ileocecal junction) (Figure 6-14). Appendicitis occurs in approximately 10 to 20 percent of the population in the United States, and it is most common in young adults. Acute appendicitis is the most common surgical emergency you will encounter in the field, mostly in older children and young adults. There are no particular risk factors.

The appendix has no known anatomic or physiologic function; most of its tissue is lymphoid in type. It lies just inferior to the ileocecal valve and the first section of the ascending colon. Depending on the individual patient, it may be in the retroperitoneal, pelvic, or abdominal cavity. The appendix can become inflamed, and if left untreated it can rupture, spilling its contents into the peritoneal cavity and setting up peritonitis.

The pathogenesis of appendicitis is most often due to obstruction of the appendiceal lumen by fecal material. The shape and location of the appendix make it particularly vulnerable to obstruction by feces or other material, such as food particles or tumors. This

CONTENT REVIEW

- ➤ Accessory Organ Diseases
  - Appendicitis
  - Cholecystitis
  - Pancreatitis
  - Hepatitis

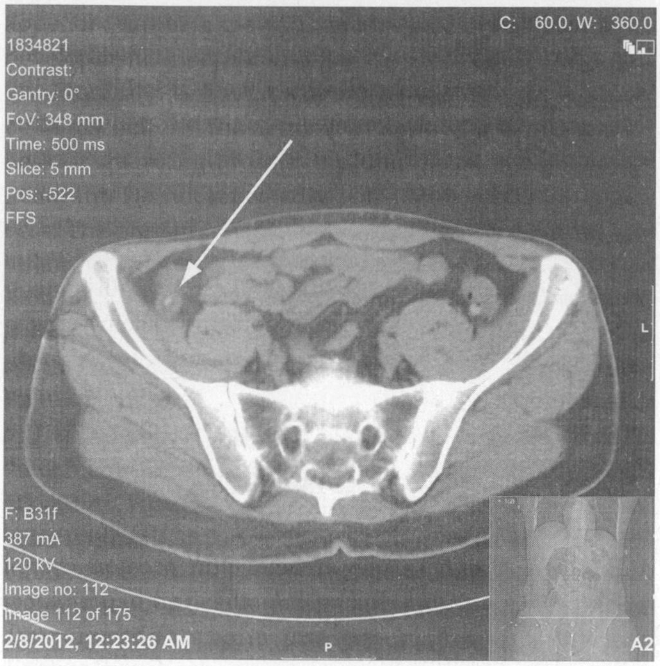

FIGURE 6-14 Acute appendicitis.

(© Dr. Bryan E. Bledsoe)

inflames the lymphoid tissue and often leads to bacterial or viral infection that ulcerates the mucosa. The inflammation also causes the appendix's internal diameter to expand, which can block the appendicular artery and cause thrombosis. With its blood supply cut off, the appendix becomes ischemic, and infarction and necrosis of tissue follow. At this point, the vessel walls often weaken to the point of rupture, spilling the appendiceal contents into the peritoneal cavity.

Appendicitis was often frequently misdiagnosed due to the wide variety of signs and symptoms that can accompany it. Now, with advanced computer tomography (CT) imaging, appendicitis can be diagnosed reliably.[5] Mild or early appendicitis causes diffuse, colicky pain often associated with nausea and vomiting and sometimes a low-grade fever. Often, the pain is initially located in the periumbilical region. Because of the appendiceal blockage, the patient usually loses his appetite. As the appendix continues to dilate, the pain will localize in the right lower quadrant. A common site of pain is **McBurney's point**, 1 to 2 inches above the anterior iliac crest along a direct line from the anterior crest to the umbilicus (Figure 6-15). Once the appendix ruptures the pain will become diffuse, owing to development of peritonitis.

Physical assessment will find a patient who appears to be in discomfort. The abdominal exam will reveal tenderness or guarding around the umbilicus or right lower quadrant. Do not repeatedly palpate for rebound tenderness. The pressure that this procedure exerts can cause an inflamed appendix to rupture.

Prehospital care for appendicitis includes placing the patient in a position of comfort, giving psychological support, diligently managing the airway to prevent aspiration, establishing intravenous access, and transporting the patient. In most cases, the appendix will not have ruptured, and the patient will remain hemodynamically stable. Monitor as you would for bowel obstruction, and treat any complications such as tachycardia or other signs of shock as they arise.

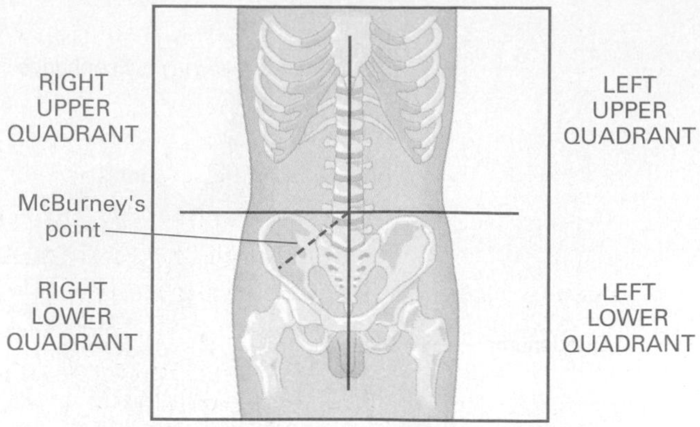

FIGURE 6-15 McBurney's point is a common site of pain in appendicitis.

Cholecystitis

Cholecystitis is an inflammation of the gallbladder (Figure 6-16). Cholelithiasis (the formation of gallstones), which causes 90 percent of cholecystitis cases, occurs in approximately 15 percent of the adult population in the United States, with more than 1 million new cases diagnosed annually. The two types of gallstones are cholesterol based and bilirubin based. Cholesterol-based stones are far more common and are associated with a

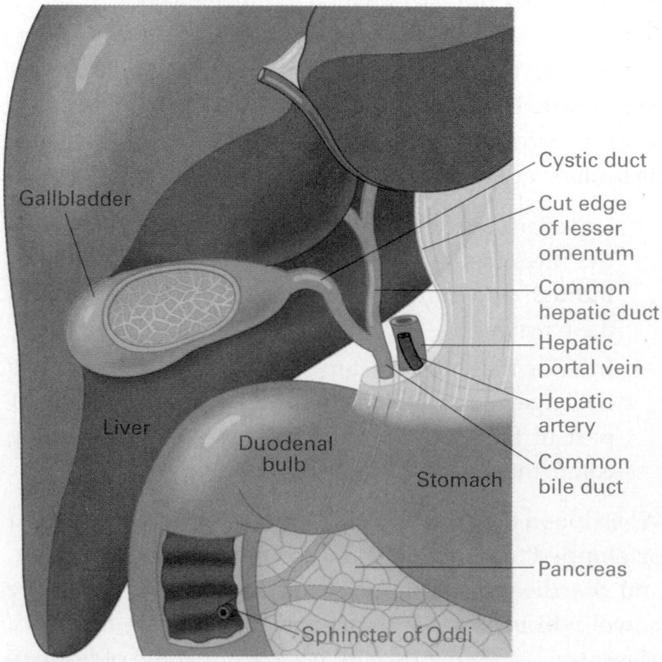

FIGURE 6-16 The gallbladder is located below the liver.

CONTENT REVIEW

- Causes of Acute Pancreatitis
  - Alcohol abuse
  - Gallstones
  - Elevated serum lipids (cholesterol and triglycerides)
  - Drug induced

specific risk profile: obese, middle-aged women with more than one biological child.

Definitive treatment of acute cholecystitis includes antibiotic therapy, laparoscopic surgery, lithotripsy (ultrasound treatment to break up the stones), and surgery if the other, less invasive, therapies fail. With the advent of laparoscopic surgery, mortality has fallen to less than 1 percent, with an overall morbidity of approximately 6 percent.

Cholecystitis caused by gallstones can be chronic or acute. The liver produces bile, the primary vehicle for removing cholesterol from the body. The bile travels down the common bile duct to empty into the small intestine at the sphincter of Oddi. The sphincter of Oddi opens when chyme exits the stomach through the pyloric sphincter. When the sphincter of Oddi closes, the flow of bile backs up into the gallbladder via the cystic duct. The bile remains in the gallbladder until the sphincter of Oddi opens again.

The bile can become supersaturated and calculi—stonelike masses based on bilirubin, cholesterol, or both—form. These calculi travel down the cystic duct, frequently lodging in the common bile duct. When they obstruct the flow of bile, gallbladder inflammation and irritation result. The bile salts subsequently attack the mucosal membrane lining the gallbladder, leaving the underlying epithelial tissue without protection. Prostaglandins are also released, further irritating the epithelial wall. As irritation continues, the inflammation grows, increasing intraluminal pressure and ultimately reducing blood flow to the epithelium.

Other causes of cholecystitis include acalculus cholecystitis (cholecystitis without associated stones) and chronic inflammation caused by bacterial infection. Acalculus cholecystitis usually results from burns, sepsis, diabetes, or multiple organ failure. Chronic cholecystitis resulting from a bacterial infection (*Escherichia coli* and enterococci) presents with an inflammatory process similar to cholelithiasis.

An inflamed gallbladder usually causes an acute attack of upper right quadrant abdominal pain. The inflammation can cause an irritation of the diaphragm with referred pain in the right shoulder. If the gallstones are lodged in the cystic duct, the pain may be colicky, due to expansion and contraction of the duct. Often, the pain occurs after a meal that is high in fat content because of the secondary release of bile from the gallbladder. The right subcostal region may be tender because of abdominal muscle spasms. Patients may experience extreme pain as the epithelium in the gallbladder erodes away. Sympathetic stimulation because of the pain may cause pale, cool, clammy skin. If peritonitis occurs, the skin may be warm due to increased blood flow to the inflamed peritoneum. Nausea and vomiting are common, due to cystic duct spasm.

Visual inspection may reveal scars from previous gallstone surgeries, but distention and ecchymosis are rarely seen. Palpation may reveal either diffuse right-sided tenderness or point tenderness under the right costal margin, a positive **Murphy's sign**.

Prehospital treatment of the patient with acute cholecystitis is mainly palliative. Place the patient in the position of comfort; maintain his ABCs, ensuring adequate oxygenation; and, finally, establish intravenous access. Pain medications commonly used include hydromorphone (Dilaudid) and fentanyl (Sublimaze). Morphine has historically been contraindicated because it was believed to cause spasms of the cystic duct.

Cultural Considerations

Race and Sex as Risk Factors. Although patients should never be stereotyped based on race or sex, both appear to be risk factors for several gastroenterologic problems. Because of this, you should consider racial and gender differences as they may affect various disease states. For example, acute pancreatitis affects males more commonly than females. In addition, the hospitalization rate for acute pancreatitis per 100,000 patients is three times higher in black patients compared with their white counterparts.

Cholecystitis also seems to have racial and gender predilections. Pima Indians and Scandinavians have the highest risk for gallstones and, subsequently, cholecystitis. In the United States, whites have a higher incidence of cholecystitis than blacks. Asians and sub-Saharan Africans have an extremely low risk of cholecystitis. Cholecystitis is two to three times more frequent in females than in males.

Thus, always consider race and gender factors as part of the total picture when trying to determine the possible cause of a gastroenterologic emergency.

Pancreatitis

Pancreatitis is an inflammation of the pancreas. Its four main categories, based on cause, are metabolic, mechanical, vascular, and infectious. Metabolic causes—specifically, alcoholism—account for approximately 80 percent of all cases; consequently, pancreatitis is widespread in the United States, owing to the high incidence of alcoholism. Mechanical obstructions caused by gallstones or elevated serum lipids account for another 9 percent. Vascular injuries caused by thromboembolisms or shock, along with infectious diseases, account for the remaining 11 percent. Overall mortality in acute pancreatitis is relatively high, approximately 30 to 40 percent, mainly due to accompanying sepsis and shock, which lead to multisystem organ failure. In acute pancreatitis, the rate of serious morbidity and mortality has been found to be 14 percent in patients with fewer than three positive findings. The mortality rate exceeded 95 percent, however, when there were three or more positive findings.

The vast bulk of the pancreas's tissue is arranged in glandular structures called *acini* (singular, *acinus*). These cells produce digestive enzymes that empty into the duodenum at the ampulla of Vater, near the junction with the stomach. The other function of the pancreas is endocrine: A small amount of tissue located in isolated islets of tissue secretes the hormones insulin and glucagon. Frequently, gallstones leaving the common bile duct become lodged at the ampulla of Vater and obstruct the pancreatic duct (Figure 6-17). These obstructions back up pancreatic digestive enzymes into the pancreatic duct and the pancreas itself. The digestive enzymes inflame the pancreas and cause edema, which reduces blood flow, as in the pathogenesis of acute appendicitis. In turn, the decreased blood flow causes ischemia and, finally, acinar destruction. This is often called *acute pancreatitis* based on rapidity of onset.

Acinar tissue destruction causes a second form of pancreatitis, chronic pancreatitis. Acinar tissue destruction commonly occurs due to chronic alcohol intake, drug toxicity, ischemia, or infectious diseases. Alcohol ingestion results in the deposit of platelet plugs in the acinar tissue. The plugs disrupt enzyme flow from the pancreas. When digestive juices back up into the pancreas from the ampulla of Vater, the digestive enzymes can become activated and begin to digest the pancreas itself. Morphologically, this autodigestion appears as lesions and fatty tissue changes on the pancreas.

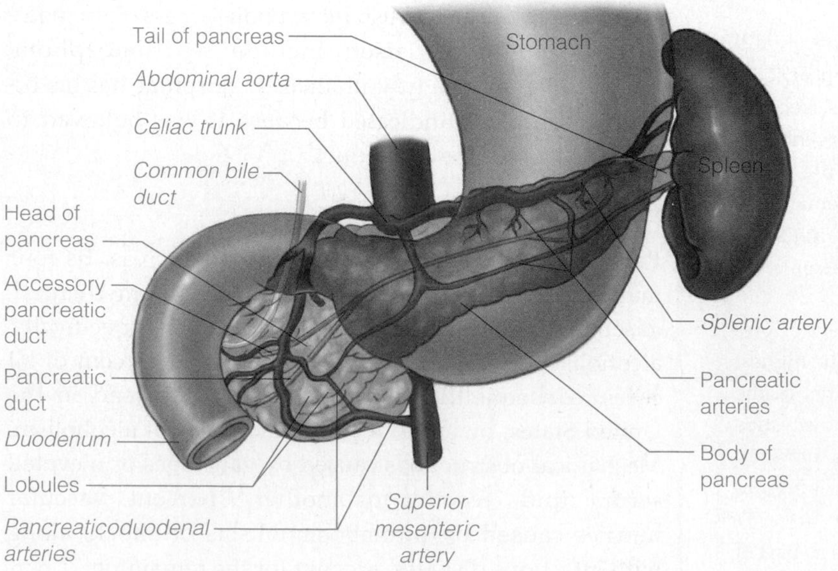

FIGURE 6-17 Anatomy of the pancreas and surrounding structures.

As tissue digestion continues, the lesion can erode and begin to hemorrhage. This acute exacerbation of pancreatitis causes intense abdominal pain. Its intensity reflects the number of lesions affected or the degree of acinar tissue death. The pain can be localized to the left upper quadrant or may radiate to the back or the epigastric region. Most patients experience nausea followed by uncontrolled vomiting and retching that can further aggravate the hemorrhage. Visual inspection may reveal previous surgical scars for lesion removal; ecchymosis and swelling of the left upper quadrant may also be present due to hemorrhage or significant organ edema. The patient will appear acutely ill with diaphoresis, tachycardia, and possible hypotension if massive hemorrhaging is involved.

CONTENT REVIEW

➤ Severe Pancreatitis Signs and Symptoms
- Acute abdominal pain to left upper quadrant or radiating to back or epigastric region
- Nausea/vomiting/retching
- Possible ecchymosis and swelling of left upper quadrant
- Patient appears acutely ill with diaphoresis and tachycardia
- Hypotension if massive hemorrhaging is involved

Prehospital treatment is supportive and aimed at maintaining the ABCs by providing high-concentration oxygen (if the patient is hypoxic) and establishing intravenous access. Fluid resuscitation with crystalloid may be warranted if the patient appears hemodynamically unstable. Definitive treatment involves gastric intubation and suctioning for emesis control, diagnostic peritoneal lavage, antibiotic therapy, fluid resuscitation, and surgery to remove the blockage.[6]

Hepatitis

Hepatitis involves any injury to hepatocytes (liver cells) associated with an inflammation or infection. Because of its wide range of potential causes, hepatitis has a high mortality rate. Six viruses—hepatitis types A, B, C, D, E, and G—are the disease's most common causes, resulting in six different kinds of hepatitis that together account for 60 to 70 percent of all cases. Hepatitis F virus (HFV) has been proposed as a cause of hepatitis, but was never substantiated. Alcoholic hepatitis, which arises from alcoholic cirrhosis (Figure 6-18), rather than an infectious agent, is responsible for another 20 to 30 percent of cases. Trauma and other diseases account for the remaining 10 percent. Factors that increase the risk of contracting

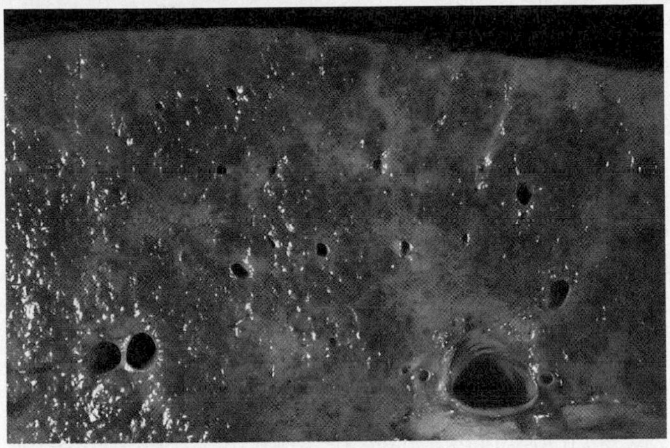

FIGURE 6-18 Liver cirrhosis.

(© Centers for Disease Control and Prevention/Dr. Edwin P. Ewing, Jr.)

hepatitis include crowded and unsanitary living conditions, poor personal hygiene that invites oral–fecal transmission, exposure to bloodborne pathogens, and chronic alcohol intake. (Specific risk factors are associated with the different types of hepatitis.)

The liver is in the upper right abdominal quadrant. A highly vascular organ, it filters and detoxifies blood returning from the abdomen and certain abdominal organs. Its other important functions include synthesizing fatty acids, converting glucose to glycogen, and helping to remove toxic products such as ammonia from the body. Any of the viral pathogens, alcoholic exposure, or trauma can injure the hepatocytes, causing inflammation and, possibly, chronic liver disease. Whatever its cause, the results are usually similar. The changes in the liver include enlargement and hypertrophy, fatty changes, loss of architecture, and appearance of lesions and spontaneous hemorrhages. The symptoms' severity can range from mild to complete liver failure and death.

Of the six types of viral hepatitis, hepatitis A (HAV) is probably the best known. Commonly referred to as infectious hepatitis, HAV spreads by the oral–fecal route. The disease is self-limiting, usually lasting between two and eight weeks. It rarely causes severe hepatic injury and, thus, has a very low mortality rate. Hepatitis B (HBV), known as "serum hepatitis," is transmitted as a bloodborne pathogen that can stay active in bodily fluids outside the body for days. With well over 310 million carriers worldwide, HBV is an epidemic. Its effects may be only minimal, but they can also range to severe liver ischemia and necrosis. Hepatitis C (HCV) is caused by the pathogen most commonly responsible for spreading hepatitis through blood transfusions. Hepatitis C is marked by chronic and often debilitating damage to the liver. Hepatitis D (HDV) is a less common disorder because its pathogen is dormant until activated by HBV. Hepatitis E (HEV) is a waterborne infection that has caused epidemics in Africa, Mexico, and other third-world nations. Its mortality rate for pregnant women is high. Hepatitis G (HGV) has been reported in persons who developed hepatitis after a transfusion. Infection with HGV can lead to chronic infection in 15 to 30 percent of adults. The long-term outcomes of the infection are not yet known. People with hepatitis A, B, or C can be super-infected with HGV.

CONTENT REVIEW

➤ Severe Hepatitis Signs and Symptoms
- Abdominal tenderness to upper right quadrant or radiating to right shoulder
- Loss of appetite/weight loss
- Clay-colored stool
- Jaundice/yellowing of skin and whites of eyes
- Nausea/vomiting
- Possible fever
- Pharyngitis, coughing
- General malaise, photophobia

Patients with hepatitis commonly present with symptoms relative to the severity of their disease. Usually they complain of upper right quadrant abdominal tenderness, not relieved by antacids, food, or positioning. They may lose their appetite and become anorexic, usually losing weight. The decrease in bile production changes their stool to a clay color, and increased bilirubin retention causes jaundice, a yellow coloring of the skin, and scleral icterus, a yellowing of the whites of the eyes. Other signs and symptoms include severe nausea and vomiting, general malaise, photophobia, pharyngitis, and coughing.

Physical examination will reveal a sick patient, possibly with a jaundiced appearance. Depending on the patient's severity, his positioning can range from standing up and walking around to lying in a fetal position with his knees drawn to his chest. Pain may present in the right upper quadrant or the right shoulder (referred from diaphragmatic irritation). Fever may be secondary to infection or to tissue necrosis. Inspection may yield nonspecific findings. Palpation may reveal an enlarged liver. Skin color and temperature can range from warm and dry (due to the infection) to cool, clammy, and diaphoretic if a hepatic lesion has ruptured and begun to bleed.

Prehospital treatment is mainly palliative. Secure the ABCs and establish intravenous access for fluid resuscitation or antiemetic administration. You must carefully consider any pharmacological administration because the liver breaks down many active drug metabolites. Definitive treatment involves antiviral and anti-inflammatory medications and symptomatic treatment. Vaccinations are available for hepatitis A and B.

Summary

Abdominal pain can originate from a wide variety of causes, either from the abdominal organs or from areas outside the abdominal cavity. Generally, the patient's description of the pain (sharp, dull, burning, tearing, cramping) may help narrow the differential diagnosis; however, prehospital management priorities for the abdominal patient are to establish and maintain the patient's airway, breathing, and circulation. The differential diagnosis can include a multitude of causes that usually cannot be identified without laboratory and radiographic analysis. Correction of the most life-threatening conditions generally requires surgical intervention.

Airway management is of paramount importance, as patients frequently suffer from severe bouts of nausea and vomiting. Be prepared to turn the patient onto his side, if necessary, to clear large amounts of vomitus from the airway. Fluid loss, hemorrhage, or sepsis may compromise the circulatory status. Initiate fluid resuscitation for the hemodynamically unstable patient in the field, but never delay transport. Patients who have abdominal pain lasting more than 6 hours should always be evaluated by a physician. The key to successful treatment of gastrointestinal ailments is prompt recognition, treatment, and rapid transport to the hospital.

You Make the Call

You are working your third straight day. The tones in the ambulance bay go off and the call comes through: "Medic 22 respond to 727 McCluer Road for a man down." You and your partner find the road on the GPS and leave the station.

When you arrive on the scene, it appears to be free of danger. At the door a woman meets you. She says she found her husband slumped over in the bathroom. You enter the bathroom and find an approximately 30-year-old male patient, extremely pale and diaphoretic, sitting on the toilet. As you begin your assessment, the patient tells you he feels lightheaded and then passes out.

1. What are your first steps in caring for this patient?
2. What are possible causes for the patient's condition?
3. What information would you attempt to ascertain from the patient's wife?
4. What physical clues might you identify in this situation?

See Suggested Responses at the back of this book.

Review Questions

1. What is the hallmark finding for a patient with an acute abdominal emergency?
   a. Pain
   b. Fever
   c. Nausea
   d. Vomiting
2. What type of pain is characterized as sharp and travels along definite neural routes to the spinal column?
   a. Tearing
   b. Somatic
   c. Referred
   d. Visceral
3. How many liters of fluid can the abdomen hold before any noticeable change in abdominal girth occurs?
   a. 4 to 6 pints
   b. 6 to 10 pints
   c. 4 to 6 liters
   d. 6 to 10 liters
4. Persistent abdominal pain lasting longer than ____________ hours is classified as a surgical emergency and always requires transport.
   a. 2
   b. 4
   c. 5
   d. 6
5. What is the bolus amount of an isotonic crystalloid used when treating hemorrhagic hypovolemia from a gastrointestinal bleed?
   a. 10 mL/kg
   b. 20 mL/kg
   c. 600–1,000 mL
   d. 800–1,000 mL
6. What is the most common cause of lower GI hemorrhages?
   a. Benign polyps
   b. Crohn's disease
   c. Diverticulosis
   d. Ulcerative colitis

7. What is the most common surgical emergency the paramedic will encounter in the field, mostly in older children and young adults?
   a. Gastritis
   b. Appendicitis
   c. Cholecystitis
   d. Diverticulitis
8. An inflamed gallbladder usually causes an acute attack of pain in which abdominal quadrant?
   a. Upper left
   b. Lower left
   c. Upper right
   d. Lower right
9. You are treating a patient with a positive Murphy's sign, nausea, and point tenderness. If you desired to administer an analgesic, you would _______
   a. use diazepam.
   b. use fentanyl.
   c. use nitroglycerin.
   d. use none of these, as analgesics are not warranted for this patient.
10. Which type of hepatitis is a waterborne infection that has caused epidemics in Africa, Mexico, and other third-world nations?
   a. Hepatitis A
   b. Hepatitis C
   c. Hepatitis D
   d. Hepatitis E

See Answers to Review Questions at the back of this book.

References

1. Chen, Z. J. and M. L. Freeman. "Management of Upper Gastrointestinal Bleeding Emergencies: Evidence-Based Medicine and Practical Considerations." *World J Emerg Med* 2 (2011): 5–12.
2. Smith, M. N. "Emergency: Variceal Hemorrhage from Esophageal Varices Associated with Alcoholic Liver Disease." *Am J Nurs* 110 (2010): 32–39.
3. Malfertheiner, P., F. Megraud, C. O'Morain, et al. "Current Concepts in the Management of *Helicobacter pylori* Infection: The Maastricht III Consensus Report." *Gut* 56 (2007): 772–781.
4. Caprilli, R., A. Viscido, and G. Latella. "Current Management of Severe Ulcerative Colitis." *Nat Clin Pract Gastroenterol Hepatol* 4 (2007): 92–101.
5. Pritchett, C. V., N. C. Levinsky, Y. P. Ha, A. E. Dembe, and S. M. Steinberg. "Management of Acute Appendicitis: The Impact of CT Scanning on the Bottom Line." *J Am Coll Surg* 210 (2010): 699–705, 705–707.
6. Thompson, D. R. "Narcotic Analgesic Effects on the Sphincter of Oddi: A Review of the Data and Therapeutic Implications in Treating Pancreatitis." *Am J Gastroenterol* 96 (2001): 1266–1272.

Further Reading

Hall, J. *Guyton and Hall Textbook of Medical Physiology*. 13th ed. Philadelphia: W. B. Saunders, 2015.

Kuma, V., A. Abbas, and J. Aster. *Robbins and Cotran Pathological Basis of Disease*. 9th ed. Philadelphia: W. B. Saunders, 2014.

Marx, J., R. Hockberger, and R. Walls. *Emergency Medicine: Concepts and Clinical Practice*. 8th ed. St. Louis: Mosby, 2013.

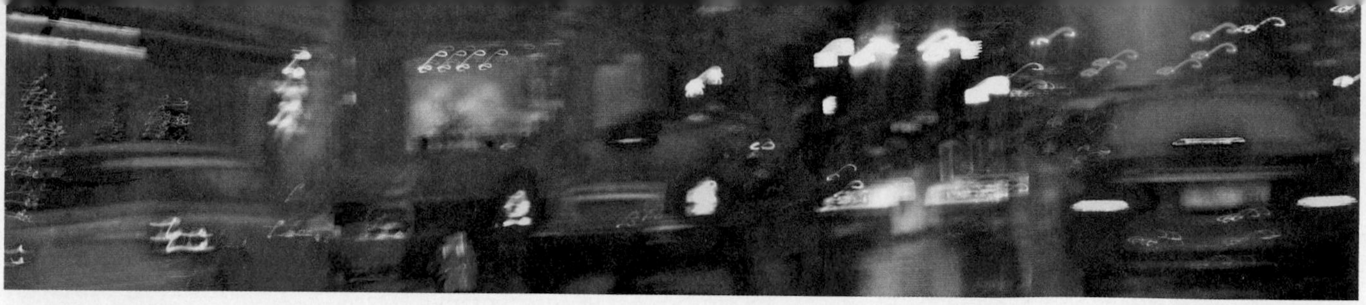

Chapter 7
Urology and Nephrology

Bryan Bledsoe, DO, FACEP, FAAEM, EMT-P

STANDARD
Medicine (Genitourinary/Renal)

COMPETENCY
Integrates assessment findings with principles of epidemiology and pathophysiology to formulate a field impression and implement a comprehensive treatment/disposition plan for a patient with a medical complaint.

Learning Objectives

Terminal Performance Objective: After reading this chapter, you should be able to integrate patient assessment findings, patient history, and knowledge of anatomy, physiology, pathophysiology, and basic and advanced life support interventions to recognize and manage patients with urologic and renal disorders.

Enabling Objectives: To accomplish the terminal performance objective, you should be able to:

1. Define key terms introduced in this chapter.
2. Review the anatomy and physiology of the urinary system.
3. Describe the general pathophysiological changes of urologic and renal emergencies, and relate this to disturbances in normal renal physiology.
4. Adapt the scene size-up, primary assessment, history, secondary assessment, and use of monitoring technology to arrive at a field impression and differential diagnoses for renal emergencies.
5. Use a process of clinical reasoning to guide and interpret the patient assessment findings and develop a treatment plan for patients with urologic and renal disorders in the prehospital environment.
6. Given a variety of scenarios, discuss the integration of assessment and management guidelines as they relate to urologic and renal emergencies.

KEY TERMS

active transport, p. 305
acute kidney injury (AKI), p. 311
acute tubular necrosis, p. 312
antidiuresis, p. 305
anuria, p. 311
ascending loop of Henle, p. 304
benign prostatic hypertrophy, p. 303
Bowman's capsule, p. 304
chronic ambulatory peritoneal dialysis (CAPD), p. 317
chronic kidney disease (CKD), p. 314
chronic renal failure (CRF), p. 314
circumcision, p. 307
collecting duct, p. 304
community-acquired infection, p. 321
cortex, p. 303
creatinine, p. 306
cystitis, p. 321
descending loop of Henle, p. 304
dialysate, p. 317
distal tubule, p. 304
diuresis, p. 305
end-stage renal failure (ESRF), p. 314
end-stage kidney disease (ESKD), p. 314
epididymis, p. 307
erythropoietin, p. 306
facilitated diffusion, p. 305
filtrate, p. 304
flanks, p. 303
genitourinary system, p. 302
glomerular filtration, p. 304
glomerular filtration rate (GFR), p. 304
glomerulus, p. 304
glucose intolerance, p. 315
hemodialysis, p. 317
hilum, p. 303
hyperosmolar, p. 305
hypo-osmolar, p. 305
interstitial nephritis, p. 312
intrarenal abscess, p. 321
isosthenuria, p. 315
kidney, p. 303
medulla, p. 303
microangiopathy, p. 312
nephrology, p. 302
nephron, p. 303
nosocomial infection, p. 321
oliguria, p. 311
osmolarity, p. 305
osmosis, p. 304
osmotic diuresis, p. 306
papilla, p. 303
penis, p. 307
perinephric abscess, p. 321
peritoneal dialysis, p. 317
postrenal AKI, p. 313
prerenal AKI, p. 312
preventive strategy, p. 303
priapism, p. 320
prostate gland, p. 307
prostatitis, p. 321
proximal tubule, p. 304
pyelonephritis, p. 321
pyramids, p. 303
reabsorption, p. 304
reduced nephron mass, p. 314
reduced renal mass, p. 315
referred pain, p. 308
renal, p. 302
renal AKI, p. 312
renal calculi, p. 303
renal dialysis, p. 316
renal pelvis, p. 303
renin, p. 306
scrotum, p. 307
secretion, p. 304
semen, p. 307
simple diffusion, p. 304
sperm cell, p. 307
testes, p. 307
testicular torsion, p. 320
urea, p. 302
uremia, p. 315
ureter, p. 306
urethra, p. 306
urethritis, p. 321
urinary bladder, p. 306
urinary stasis , p. 320
urinary system, p. 302
urinary tract infection (UTI), p. 320
urine, p. 302
urology, p. 302
vas deferens, p. 307
visceral pain, p. 308

Case Study

Shortly after midnight, Rachel Gutierrez and Jack White receive a call that a man has fallen in his bathroom and cannot get up. As they arrive at the house, a young woman meets them and identifies herself as Amy Jackson, the patient's wife and the person who called 911 for help. She says she woke up hearing her husband, David, yelling from the bathroom that he needed help. As the three go up the steps, they can hear a man calling, "Hurry up. This pain is awful."

Rachel and Jack see an athletic-looking man in pajamas lying in the bathroom and moaning. He is pale, sweating profusely, and restlessly moving over the floor.

When Rachel asks about the pain, he says, "It's in my lower back. On the right. I can't move, it's so bad. And I have to pee. Help me." Rachel gets a urine bottle while Jack introduces himself quietly to David and begins the assessment. Jack helps David to void and then checks the bottle. The urine is reddish yellow. Jack looks for a vein to start an IV line, and Rachel asks David about the pain. He answers that the same spot in his back hurt a bit after dinner, but he was in a lot of pain when he woke up and tried to go to the bathroom. David says his brother had a kidney stone last year. "Could this be one? Am I going to die?" Rachel answers that it might be a kidney stone and that they will take care of him and get him to a hospital. Then she asks more questions quietly, trying to find out if his urination pattern had been normal before he got up, and whether he has ever had bloody urine or been told he had any kind of urinary system trouble before. Jack completes the physical exam, and Rachel reports vital signs of blood pressure 140/90 mmHg, pulse 150, respirations 36/min, and SpO_2 of 99 percent on room air. After an IV line is established, Rachel and Jack help the patient onto the stretcher and out to the ambulance. Following standing orders, the paramedics administer 4 milligrams of ondansetron (Zofran) and 50 mcg of fentanyl. Within minutes of administration, the patient is much more comfortable.

David stays in the emergency department for almost 24 hours, medicated with additional fentanyl to relieve pain and with an IV drip to keep him well hydrated and move fluid through his kidneys. An IVP (intravenous pyelogram, an X-ray test) shows complete obstruction midway down the right ureter with what appears to be a radiopaque stone. His urine is intermittently bloody, and all samples are screened for stones. Finally, David passes a visible stone, and with his pain easing back to an ache, he sleeps a bit before going home.

Introduction

The **urinary system** performs a number of vital functions. It maintains blood volume and the proper balance of water, electrolytes, and pH (acid–base balance). It ensures that key substances such as glucose remain in the bloodstream, yet it also removes a variety of toxic wastes from the blood. It plays a major role in arterial blood pressure regulation. In addition, the urinary system controls development of red blood cells, or erythrocytes.

The body eliminates water and other substances removed from blood in the form of the fluid **urine**. The kidneys' regulation of water and other important substances in blood is an example of homeostasis, the body's ability to maintain an appropriate internal environment despite changing conditions. Metabolism, the intracellular processes that generate the energy and materials necessary for cell growth and repair, also creates many waste products. For example, significant amounts of ammonia form in the liver when amino acids are broken down in gluconeogenesis, a process that produces glucose between meals. Ammonia is highly toxic to body cells, particularly brain cells. Liver cells convert the ammonia into **urea**, a less toxic compound. The kidneys remove urea efficiently from the blood and pass it into the urine. Moreover, the urinary system eliminates many foreign chemicals such as drug metabolites.

The urinary system in women is physically distinct from the reproductive system: They share no structures. (The chapters "Gynecology" and "Obstetrics" discuss medical emergencies related to the female reproductive system.) In contrast, the urinary system in men shares some structures with the reproductive system. For instance, both urine and the male reproductive fluid are eliminated from the body through the opening at the tip of the penis. Consequently, the term **genitourinary system** is often used with men. The urinary and reproductive systems' proximity in women and their shared structures in men are due to the common embryonic origin of their tissues.

The most significant medical disorders involving the urinary system affect the kidneys and kidney function. **Nephrology** (from the Greek *nephros,* kidney) is the medical specialty devoted to kidney disorders. **Urology** is the surgical specialty devoted to care of the entire urinary system in women and the genitourinary system in men. We will use nephrology and nephrologic (or the preferred adjective, **renal**, from the Latin *renes,* kidneys) to refer to conditions primarily affecting the kidneys. We will use *urology* and *urologic* to refer to conditions that significantly affect other parts of the urinary or genitourinary systems.

Renal and urologic disorders are common, affecting about 20 million Americans. Many disorders are very serious. More than 50,000 Americans die annually from kidney disease. More than 250,000 Americans suffer from the most severe form of long-term kidney failure, end-stage renal failure. They require either dialysis, a process that artificially performs the most important kidney functions, or kidney transplantation, implantation of a kidney from another person, to survive. The leading causes of end-stage renal failure are poorly controlled diabetes mellitus (both type 1 and type 2) and uncontrolled or inadequately controlled hypertension.

Among acute, or sudden-onset, disorders, **renal calculi**, or kidney stones, are very common. More than 500,000 Americans are treated for kidney stones each year. Infections are also common, and they may have different causes in women and men. A woman complaining of burning pain on urination probably has an infection in the urinary system. Men with the same chief complaint may have an infection that arose in the urinary system or as a sexually transmitted disease. Noncancerous enlargement of the prostate gland, or **benign prostatic hypertrophy**, affects about 60 percent of men by age 50 and about 80 percent by age 80. If prostatic hypertrophy obstructs urine flow, a medical emergency involving sharp pain and inability to urinate may result.

All of these conditions, as well as others described later, are sufficiently common that you will see them in the field. Whenever existing kidney function may be jeopardized, prehospital care includes **preventive strategies**, or steps to minimize the likelihood of any further loss of function. Our discussion of assessment and management will cover these procedures.

Anatomy and Physiology

The urinary system contains four major structures, the kidneys, ureters, urinary bladder, and urethra (Figure 7-1). First we will discuss the structures and functions of the urinary system, focusing on the kidneys. Then we will cover the additional structures of the male genitourinary system.

Kidneys

The left kidney lies in the upper abdomen behind the spleen, and the right kidney lies behind the liver. These locations correspond to the left and right areas of the small of the back, or the **flanks**. A healthy **kidney** in a young adult is about the size of a fist and contains about 1 million **nephrons**, the microscopic structures that produce urine. With aging comes a normal loss of nephrons—10 percent per decade of life after age 40—so always be alert to the possibility of compromised kidney function in elderly patients.

Gross and Microscopic Anatomy of the Kidney

The renal artery and vein, as well as nerves, lymphatic vessels, and the ureter, pass into the kidney through the notched region called the **hilum**. The tissue of the kidney itself is visibly divided into an outer region, the **cortex**, and an inner region, the **medulla**. Medullary tissue is divided into fan-shaped regions, or **pyramids**. Each pyramid ends in a portion of tissue called the **papilla**, which projects into the hollow space of the **renal pelvis** (Figure 7-2). The spaces of the pelvis come together at the origin of the ureter. Urine forms in the cortical and medullary tissue of the kidney and leaves the kidney through the renal pelvis and ureter.

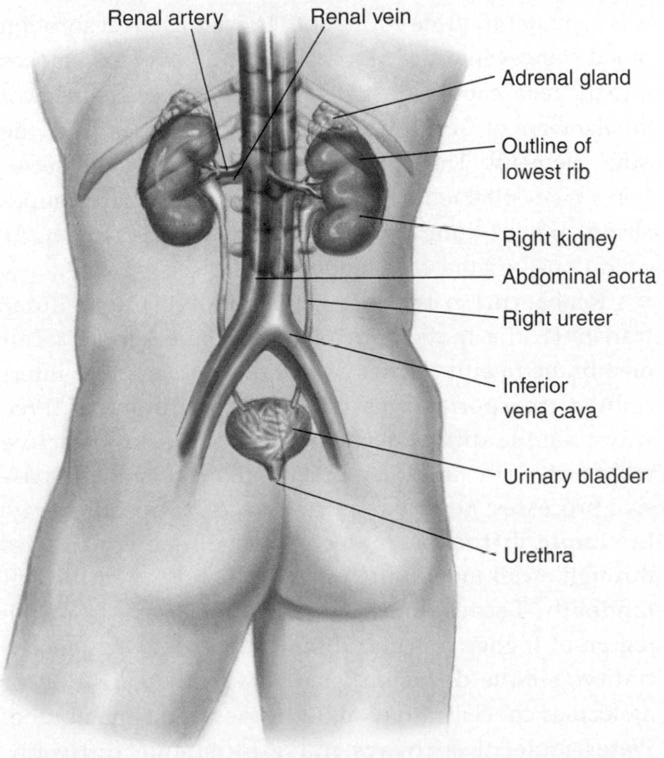

FIGURE 7-1 Anatomy of the urinary system, posterior view.

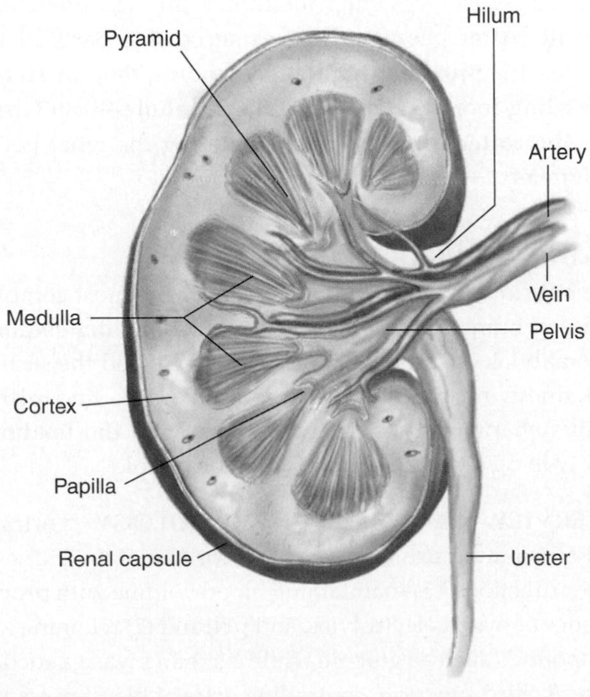

FIGURE 7-2 Cross section of the kidney.

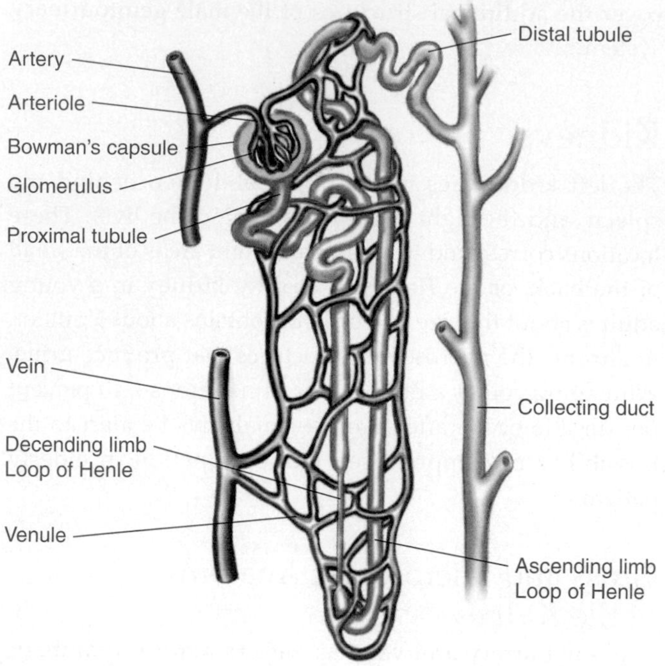

FIGURE 7-3 Anatomy of the nephron.

The functional unit of the kidney, the nephron, forms urine (Figure 7-3). Each nephron consists of a tubule divided into structurally different portions and capillaries that form a complex net of vessels covering the surface of the tubule. Blood that has entered the kidney through the renal artery flows through successively smaller vessels until it reaches a **glomerulus**, a cluster of capillaries surrounded by **Bowman's capsule**, the cup-shaped, hollow structure that is the first part of the nephron. Water and chemical substances enter the tubule through Bowman's capsule. After passage through successive parts of the tubule—the **proximal tubule**, **descending loop of Henle**, **ascending loop of Henle**, and **distal tubule**—urine drips into the **collecting duct** before entering the renal pelvis and ureter.

Kidney Physiology

The physiology of the kidneys is one of the most complex topics in human physiology. Its explanation often requires several book chapters. You may wish to reread the section on kidneys in your physiology book before reading further in this chapter, or you may wish to keep the textbook handy in case you need more detail on a topic.

OVERVIEW OF NEPHRON PHYSIOLOGY Forming and eliminating urine are the basis for two of the kidneys' major functions: (1) maintaining blood volume with proper balance of water, electrolytes, and pH, and (2) retaining key compounds such as glucose while excreting wastes such as urea. A third function, controlling arterial blood pressure, relies both on urine formation and on a second mechanism (the renin–angiotensin system) that does not involve urine production. Last, kidney cells regulate erythrocyte development, but this process does not involve urine formation in any way.

Urine is produced through the interactions among capillary blood flowing over the nephron tubule, the fluid flowing inside the tubule, and the capillary and tubular cells themselves. Three general processes are involved in formation of urine: **glomerular filtration**, **reabsorption** of substances from the renal tubule into blood, and **secretion** of substances from blood into the renal tubule.

The first step in urine formation is filtration of blood. As blood flows through the capillaries of the glomerulus, water and numerous chemical materials are filtered out of the blood and into Bowman's capsule. Normally, the only blood elements that are not freely filtered into the capsule are blood cells and the plasma proteins, all of which are too large to pass through the pores formed by cell junctions in the capillary walls. Consequently, the fluid formed in the capsule—the **filtrate**—roughly resembles blood plasma except for the absence of proteins.

The rate at which blood is filtered, the **glomerular filtration rate (GFR)**, averages 180 L/day, the equivalent of 60 complete passages of blood plasma through the glomerular filters. This remarkable efficiency underlies the kidneys' ability to excrete toxic or foreign substances such as urea or drug metabolites so quickly that the substances do not accumulate in the blood.

Filtration is a nonselective process based primarily on molecular size (electrical charge is a secondary factor), and it is essential to urine formation. In contrast, reabsorption of substances into the blood and secretion of substances into the renal tubule are highly selective processes. Almost all elements of filtrate are handled independently of the other elements. The processes of reabsorption and secretion are essential to forming urine with the correct composition and volume to compensate for current body conditions—that is, to maintain homeostasis.

Reabsorption and secretion involve intercellular transport, the movement of a molecule across a cell membrane to either enter or exit a cell. Like other intercellular transport processes, they occur in one of three ways: simple diffusion, facilitated diffusion, or active transport. Both simple and facilitated diffusion are passive processes: neither requires the cell to spend energy. In **simple diffusion**, molecules small enough to pass through a cell membrane move into and out of the cell randomly. Because net movement is always from the region of higher concentration to that of lower concentration, simple diffusion leads toward equalization of molecular concentration on both sides of the membrane. Water molecules always move by simple diffusion. **Osmosis** is the process in which water molecules move so that the concentrations of particles dissolved in water (or **osmolarity**) approach equivalence on both sides of a membrane. A solution with a higher concentration than another solution is **hyperosmolar** to the other; a solution with a lower, more dilute concentration is **hypo-osmolar** to the other.

In **facilitated diffusion**, molecules still move from the region of higher concentration to that of lower concentration. However, a molecule-specific carrier in the membrane acts as a tunnel and speeds the molecules' movement through the membrane. The body cells' normal handling of glucose is an example of this process. When insulin binds to a glucose-specific carrier in the cell membrane, glucose can pass into the cell ten times faster than when insulin is not bound to the carrier.

Active transport is the only process that can produce a net movement of molecules from a region of lower concentration to one of higher concentration. This uphill movement against the concentration gradient is possible because energy is spent to drive the action of the molecule-specific carrier in the membrane. Active transport processes are vital to renal tubular physiology because they allow for the precise balance of reabsorption and secretion that results in independent, homeostatic handling of electrolytes and other substances such as glucose.

TUBULAR HANDLING OF WATER AND ELECTROLYTES Tubular handling of water and electrolytes, including sodium (Na^+), potassium (K^+), hydrogen (H^+), and chloride (Cl^-), is the basis for control of blood volume and maintenance of electrolyte balance, including pH. As you recall, Na^+ is the dominant cation in the body's extracellular fluids, including blood, whereas K^+ is the dominant cation in intracellular fluid. Appropriate retention of Na^+ in the body, along with osmotic retention of water, is key to maintaining blood volume. Selective retention of K^+ and H^+, along with anions such as Cl^-, maintains the balance of blood electrolytes and blood pH.

Filtrate formed in Bowman's capsule enters the proximal tubule (review Figure 7-3). The cells of the proximal tubule have an extensive brush border that maximizes contact between cell membrane and filtrate. They also have high concentrations of molecule-specific carriers in their membranes and maintain a high level of metabolic activity, producing energy that can support active transport. Under normal conditions, about 65 percent of filtered Na^+ and Cl^- is reabsorbed in the proximal tubule, along with osmotic reabsorption of about the same percentage of filtered water. Reabsorption takes place by both passive and active transport processes. Much of the active Na^+ reabsorption is coupled with secretion of H^+ into the tubule; H^+ secretion raises the pH of the arterial-derived blood flowing in capillaries surrounding the tubule. Further handling of H^+ as the filtrate moves through the tubule determines the pH both of the venous blood leaving the kidneys and of the urine excreted from the body.

As filtrate moves through the next part of the nephron, the loop of Henle, its volume and composition change further. Simple diffusion is the dominant process in the first part of the loop. By the time filtrate has moved through the descending limb of the loop, roughly another 20 percent of the filtrate's original water load has been reabsorbed. The cells of the second, ascending, limb of the loop of Henle are normally virtually impermeable to water; however, passive and active reabsorption of significant amounts of electrolytes occurs in the same part of the tubule. This reabsorption of electrolytes without reabsorption of water produces a relatively dilute fluid that may exit the collecting duct as dilute urine. Healthy kidneys can produce urine with an osmolarity as low as one-sixth the osmolar concentration of blood plasma, an action termed **diuresis**. A number of hormones alter tubular handling of water and electrolytes (Table 7-1). Some increase the permeability of the distal tubule, collecting duct, or both, so that far more water is reabsorbed. **Antidiuresis**, the result of this hormonal activity, can form a very

Table 7-1 Hormones That Affect Tubular Handling of Water and Key Electrolytes

Hormone	Target Tissue	Effect(s)
Aldosterone	Distal tubule, collecting duct	Increase in reabsorption of Na^+, Cl^-, and water Increase in secretion of K^+
Angiotensin II	Proximal tubule	Increase in reabsorption of Na^+, Cl^-, and water Increase in secretion of H^+
Antidiuretic hormone (ADH)	Distal tubule, collecting duct	Increase in reabsorption of water
Atrial natriuretic hormone (ANH)	Distal tubule, collecting duct	Decrease in reabsorption of Na^+ and Cl^-

Note: *Aldosterone, ADH, and ANH are discussed in detail in the chapter "Endocrinology"; angiotensin II is discussed in the chapter "Cardiology."*

Table derived from Arthur C. Guyton and John E. Hall, Textbook of Medical Physiology, *9th ed. Philadelphia: W.B. Saunders Company, 1996.*

concentrated urine with an osmolarity as high as four times that of plasma.

The ability of healthy kidneys to handle significant swings in water and electrolyte intake is remarkably large. Studies have shown that an individual can increase his sodium intake to ten times the average amount or decrease it to roughly one-tenth the average, and the kidneys will still compensate properly. Blood volume and sodium content will change only modestly from their baseline, normal levels.

TUBULAR HANDLING OF GLUCOSE AND UREA Glucose and urea represent substances that the kidneys handle in opposite fashion. Critical substances such as glucose are retained in the body, and wastes such as urea are excreted.

Glucose is freely filtered into Bowman's capsule as an element of filtrate. Normally, glucose is completely reabsorbed through an active transport process by the time filtrate leaves the proximal tubule. The body's absolute retention of glucose is usually maintained until the blood glucose level reaches about 180 mg/dL; above that level, glucose begins to be lost in urine. This pattern, in which glucose is completely reabsorbed until a ceiling, or threshold level, of blood glucose is reached, is due to saturation of the active transport process responsible for reabsorption of glucose. At excessively high blood glucose levels, so much glucose enters the filtrate that the proximal tubule's transport capacity to reabsorb it is insufficient. When this occurs, as in uncontrolled type 1 diabetes mellitus, the body loses not only glucose but also large amounts of water through **osmotic diuresis**.

Urea, a waste product, is also freely filtered into Bowman's capsule. However, tubular handling of this small molecule is very different from that of glucose. Urea is passively reabsorbed throughout most of the tubule, and about half of the filtered load will remain in urine. Thus, the kidneys' ability to excrete urea efficiently depends on the glomerular filtration rate, or GFR. If blood passes through the glomerular capillaries at an adequate rate, the net result of filtration and passive reabsorption will keep the blood level from rising toward a toxic level. The blood urea nitrogen test, or BUN, directly measures blood concentration of urea and is an indirect indicator of GFR. **Creatinine**, another waste product of metabolism, has larger molecules than urea and is not reabsorbed. Because all the filtered creatinine will be eliminated in urine, the blood concentration of creatinine is a direct indicator of GFR.

CONTROL OF ARTERIAL BLOOD PRESSURE The kidneys regulate systemic arterial blood pressure in several ways. Over the long term, they control the body's balance of water and electrolytes, thus maintaining blood volume at a healthy level. In addition, juxtaglomerular cells—specialized cells adjacent to glomerular capillary cells—respond to low blood pressure by releasing an enzyme called **renin**. Within seconds of its release, renin produces significant amounts of the active hormone angiotensin I. As angiotensin I flows through the lungs, angiotensin converting enzyme (ACE) produces angiotensin II, the powerful vasoconstrictor that immediately raises arterial blood pressure. Angiotensin II acts both on kidney tubular cells (Table 7-1) and on adrenal cells, causing the latter to secrete aldosterone. The renin–angiotensin system's maintenance of blood pressure, as well as its role in hypertension, is covered in detail in the chapters "Pathophysiology" and "Emergency Pharmacology."

CONTROL OF ERYTHROCYTE DEVELOPMENT The kidneys produce 90 percent of the body's **erythropoietin**, a hormone that regulates the rate at which erythrocytes mature in bone marrow. The exact mechanism that produces erythropoietin is unclear. The impact of renal tissue death, however, is clear and profound; the nonkidney sources of erythropoietin can produce only about one-third to one-half the red cell mass (measured as hematocrit) needed by the body.

Ureters

Urine drains from the renal pelvis into the **ureter**, the long duct that runs from the kidney to the urinary bladder (Figure 7-1). Each ureter is about 25 cm long and, like the kidney, is located in the retroperitoneum of the abdomen. A thin muscular layer in the ureters' walls limits their ability to distend in response to internal pressure. The ureters' nerves derive from renal, gonadal, or hypogastric nerve trunks. The microscopic structure of the ureters and the nature of their nerve supply are important in understanding the symptoms caused by kidney stones caught in a ureter.

Urinary Bladder

The **urinary bladder**, the anteriormost organ in the pelvis of both men and women, stores urine. The muscular bladder usually contains at least a small amount of urine, which produces its roughly spherical shape. The bladder neck, through which urine passes during urination, is held in place by ligaments. In women, connective tissue loosely attaches the bladder's posterior wall to the anterior vaginal wall. In men, the bladder wall is structurally continuous with the prostate gland (Figure 7-4).

Urethra

The **urethra** is the duct that carries urine from the bladder to the exterior of the body. In women, the urethra is only

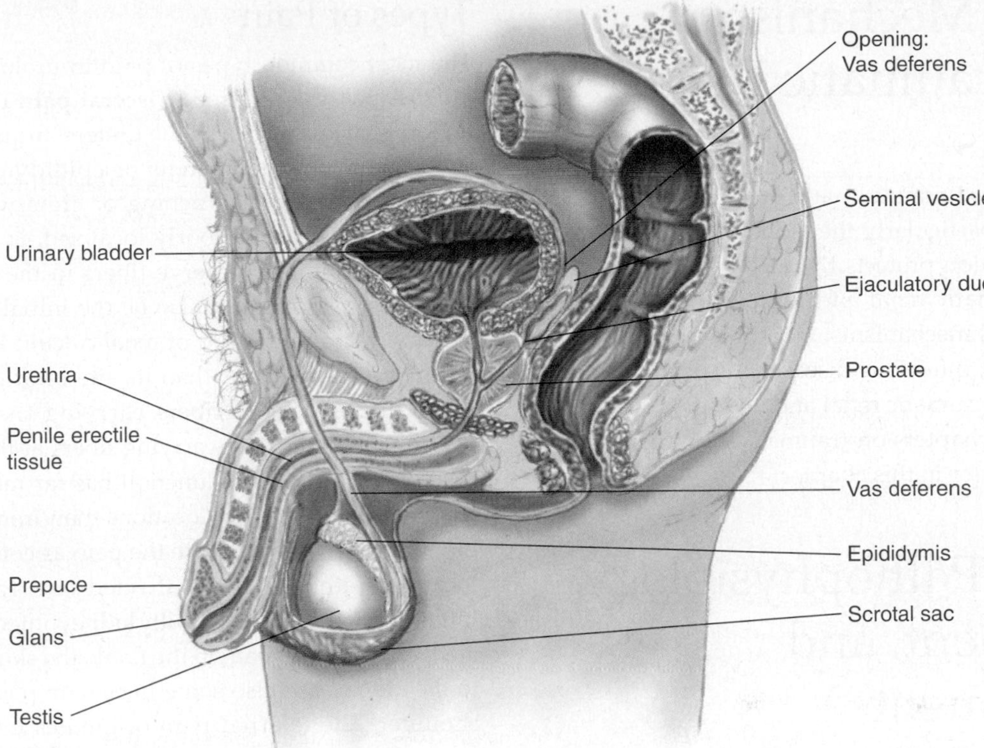

FIGURE 7-4 Anatomy of the male genitourinary system.

about 3 to 4 cm long and opens to the external environment via a small orifice just anterior to that of the vagina. In men, the urethra is about 20 cm long and ends at the tip of the penis. The female urethra's shortness is probably one reason the female urinary system is more vulnerable to bacterial infection from environmental (largely skin) sources. Because the male urethra carries both urine and male reproductive fluid, it can be a point of entry for sexually transmitted diseases.

Testes

The **testes** (singular, *testis*), are the primary male reproductive organs. They produce both the hormones responsible for sexual maturation and **sperm cells**, male sex cells. The testes lie outside the abdomen in a muscular sac called the **scrotum**. Normal scrotal temperature is about 2°C to 3°C lower than the abdominal temperature, which is critical for development of sperm.

Epididymis and Vas Deferens

Sperm cells pass from the testis into the **epididymis**, a small sac where they are stored. Each testis, with its paired epididymis, is palpable inside the scrotum (Figure 7-4). Sperm are channeled from the epididymis into the **vas deferens**, a muscular duct that carries them into the pelvis and through the substance of the prostate gland to its opening into the urethra. Sperm cells mix with special fluid before passing into the urethra for ejaculation—elimination from the body.

Prostate Gland

The **prostate gland** surrounds the male urinary bladder neck, and the first part of the urethra runs through its tissue. The prostate gland is a major source of the fluid that combines with sperm to form **semen**, the ejaculated male reproductive fluid. In emergency care, the prostate is probably most important in its role as part of the urinary system. Because the first part of the urethra passes through the prostate, any enlargement of the prostate that narrows or obstructs the urethra can block urine flow and create a possible medical emergency.

Penis

The **penis** is the male organ of copulation. Its spongy internal tissues fill with blood to produce penile erection. The skin covering the end of the penis, the foreskin, is often surgically removed in infancy through **circumcision**; the difference in appearance will be noticeable after you have treated a number of male patients.

CONTENT REVIEW

- Mechanisms of Nontraumatic Urologic Disorders
  - Inflammatory or immune-mediated disease
  - Infectious disease
  - Physical obstruction
  - Hemorrhage

General Mechanisms of Nontraumatic Tissue Problems

Both traumatic and nontraumatic problems can affect the urinary system, particularly the kidneys. The kidneys' retroperitoneal location protects them relatively well against injury. Nontraumatic renal and urologic disorders result from four general mechanisms: inflammatory or immune-mediated disease, infectious disease, physical obstruction, or hemorrhage. Traumatic renal and urologic disorders are discussed in the chapters on trauma. We discuss nontraumatic disorders later in this chapter.

General Pathophysiology, Assessment, and Management

As you learned in the "Gastroenterology" chapter, emergencies are common. Because of the similar presentations of both gastrointestinal (GI) and urologic emergencies, you may have difficulty determining the source of an abdominal problem when pain is the sole complaint. You can often find clues to the eventual diagnosis when you take a focused history and perform the focused physical exam. Before reading further, you may want to review the discussion of GI pathophysiology, assessment, and management in the chapter "Gastroenterology."

Pathophysiologic Basis of Pain

The nerve fibers that carry pain messages to the brain are triggered by different stimuli. Some are triggered when damage to the epithelial lining of an organ exposes the underlying tissue layer, where the nerve endings are located. Others respond to stretching forces generated when an organ is inflamed or enlarged by internal hemorrhage or obstruction.

Causes of Pain

Bacterial infection damages the epithelial tissue that lines structures such as the urethra and urinary bladder. This damage causes pain that often worsens when urine flows over the affected tissue during urination. Bacteria normally found on the skin can cause infections in women. In men, the same symptom, pain on voiding, is often due to a sexually transmitted disease such as gonorrhea. Distention of a ureter by a renal calculus (kidney stone) causes a sharp pain that may ease or worsen when the stone shifts position inside the ureter.

Types of Pain

The most common types of pain in urologic emergencies are visceral and referred. **Visceral pain** usually arises in hollow structures such as the ureters, urinary bladder, and urethra, or the vas deferens or epididymis in males. Its chief characteristic, an aching or crampy pain felt deep within the body and poorly localized, is due to the relatively low number of nerve fibers in the involved structures. Visceral pain can also be the initial presentation of urinary tract infection or of renal calculi. **Referred pain** is felt in a location other than its site of origin. This occurs when afferent nerve fibers carrying the pain message merge with other pain-carrying fibers at the junction with the spinal cord. If that junction has far more nerve fibers from one or more other locations than from the site of origin, the brain may perceive the pain as coming from those locations rather than the affected one. Pyelonephritis—inflammation associated with kidney infection—is associated not only with pain in the flank, the skin surface closest to the kidney, but also sometimes with pain in the neck or shoulder. The referred pain originates in diaphragmatic irritation due to kidney inflammation, but the brain perceives the pain as coming from the area of the neck or shoulder.

Assessment and Management

The assessment steps are the same for all abdominal emergencies. Do not try to pinpoint the cause of abdominal pain in the field; diagnosis is often difficult even in the hospital setting. However, you do need to do an assessment to detect and manage life-threatening conditions such as shock and to provide historical and physical information that will be helpful in the hospital.

Scene Size-Up

During scene size-up, look for evidence of a traumatic versus medical cause and for signs of a life-threatening situation, perhaps an observer performing CPR or the presence of blood. Remember to employ personal protective equipment and proper handling.

Primary and Secondary Assessments

Primary assessment of the patient concentrates on the ABCs of airway, breathing, and circulation, as well as on patient disability (for example, signs of agitation and confused mental state). If the patient is conscious and responsive, ask for the chief complaint. Secondary assessment includes the history, physical exam, and vital signs.

History

INFORMATION ABOUT PAIN When the chief complaint is pain or involves pain, initial questions should elicit information about the timing, character, and associated symptoms of the pain. The OPQRST template is useful for beginning your questions:

- ***Onset.*** When did the pain start, and what were you doing at the time? Visceral pain often arises gradually, with the patient first aware of vague discomfort and only later aware of pain.
- ***Provocation/palliation.*** What makes the pain worse or better? Increased pain on urination, particularly in light of a fever or history of fever, suggests a urinary/genitourinary tract infection. Pain associated with the inability to urinate, particularly in elderly men, points toward urethral obstruction due to prostatic enlargement. Improvement with knees drawn up to the chest points toward peritonitis, whereas improvement with walking may indicate a kidney stone that has moved into a less painful position.
- ***Quality.*** What is the pain like? Visceral pain is frequently described as dull or crampy; because many urinary system structures are hollow, visceral pain is common in these emergencies. Vague discomfort followed by a change to sharp pain localized in the flank, for instance, may indicate ureteral obstruction due to a kidney stone that has moved.
- ***Region/radiation.*** Where is the pain located, or do you feel pain in several places? Does the pain seem to move from one part of your body to another? Listen for patterns of referred pain such as pain in the lower back and the neck or shoulder, as well as changes in perception of pain on movement of a limb or the whole body. In postpubertal women, be sure to ask for menstrual history, particularly if menstrual-like cramps are described or blood is present in the perineal area. (See more in the chapters "Gynecology" and "Obstetrics.")
- ***Severity.*** Where is the pain on a scale of one to ten? Has the intensity changed over time, and, if so, how? Sudden changes to sharp pain, particularly when associated with decreased responsiveness and early signs of shock, may indicate rupture of an internal organ such as the appendix in appendicitis or the fallopian tube in an ectopic pregnancy. Most urologic problems will not show this pattern of abrupt and significant shift in severity and type of pain.
- ***Time.*** How long ago did the pain start? Is it constant or does it come and go? Remember that any case of abdominal pain lasting about 6 hours or longer is considered a surgical emergency until proven otherwise, and the patient should be transported to an appropriate facility. Pelvic visceral pain of long duration and unchanging intensity, particularly if associated with signs suggesting urinary tract origin such as fever and increased pain on urination, suggests a medical case rather than a surgical one, but you still may need to transport the patient to the hospital. When confronted with an acute abdomen (sudden onset of severe abdominal pain), always err on the side of considering it a potential surgical emergency.
- ***Previous history of similar event.*** Some urologic emergencies such as renal calculus and infection may recur. This makes it especially important to elicit any history of a similar event, the diagnosis at the time, and the treatment given. Because increased risk for renal calculi is genetic in some cases, listen for a history of family members similarly affected.
- ***Nausea/vomiting.*** As you learned in the "Gastroenterology" chapter, severe pain is often associated with autonomic nervous system discharge producing the signs of nausea, possibly with vomiting, along with profuse sweating, clammy skin, and rapid heart rate. Remember that such a presentation does not necessarily indicate that the problem is in the GI system. For instance, the severe pain of a kidney stone can cause this presentation.
- ***Changes in bowel habits and stool.*** Frequent stools, especially if they are diarrheal or contain signs of blood (either melena or hematochezia), suggest a problem in the GI system. Recent constipation may not be relevant except in the context of physical findings.
- ***Weight loss.*** Significant weight loss over a very short period (hours or days) almost always reflects water loss, and signs of dehydration will be evident. Longer-term weight loss may suggest chronic illness or GI dysfunction. Be sure to ask about conditions including diabetes, cardiovascular disease, and cancer, as well as medications and medication changes.
- ***Last oral intake.*** The timing and content of the last meal may indicate an acute, progressive problem (a normal appetite, normal meal) or exacerbation of a long-standing one (poor appetite, small meal). Ask explicitly about fluid intake, because patients may not consider beverages to be food. The timing of the last oral intake is also important if the patient will be undergoing general anesthesia for a surgical procedure.
- ***Chest pain.*** Chest pain, particularly left sided, does not necessarily indicate a myocardial infarction (MI). Assess whether the pain pattern suggests angina (for example, chest pain associated with radiation to jaw and left arm). Also remember that patients with long-standing or severe diabetes may not show the typical pain pattern of an MI due to diabetic neuropathy (nerve damage), but signs of ischemia may appear on an ECG.

Physical Examination

For the patient with abdominal pain, the physical examination includes forming an overall impression as well as examining the abdomen. Remember that you will not be able to diagnose most cases of abdominal pain in the field. Your job is to gather the historical and physical evidence that can be used in the hospital and to make sure that the patient is supported before and during transport.

APPEARANCE In general, any person with significant pain, particularly pain of some duration, will appear uncomfortable. A patient may show discomfort by rigidly maintaining the position of least pain or by constantly pacing if walking helps ease the pain.

POSTURE Lying with knees drawn to chest suggests peritonitis, which is often of GI origin. Relief with walking suggests visceral pain; kidney stones may shift position during walking, easing the sharp pain. Check visually if the patient who is walking is upright or favoring one side. Someone who looks feverish and walks hunched up, leaning to one side, and complaining of back pain may have a pyelonephritis (kidney infection).

LEVEL OF CONSCIOUSNESS In the absence of fever, acute-onset decreases in responsiveness often suggest hemorrhage and evolution of hypovolemic shock. Hemorrhage is far more often tied to GI or reproductive (namely, obstetric) emergencies than to urinary system problems. You may see a decreased level of consciousness in sick patients who are undergoing dialysis, the artificial technique that replaces some vital kidney functions, including maintenance of electrolyte balance and removal of wastes. Try to determine whether the change in responsiveness is acute or chronic, which may suggest a new problem or an aggravation of preexistent problems.

APPARENT STATE OF HEALTH Patients with chronic illness, whether or not it originates in the urinary system, often look ill even without an acute problem. Extreme thinness, pale skin or mucous membranes, or the presence of home health equipment such as a bedside toilet, dialysis machine, or an oxygen tank, all suggest chronic problems. In significant emergency states, the patient will usually not be tidy and neatly dressed. If he is, this may suggest that the emergency occurred suddenly, as with a hemorrhage or painful passage of a stone.

SKIN COLOR Pale, dry, cool skin and mucous membranes may suggest chronic anemia, such as that found in persons with chronic renal failure. Pale, clammy skin suggests severe pain or shock, whereas flushed, dry skin may accompany fever.

EXAMINATION OF THE ABDOMEN The four components of the abdominal exam are inspection, auscultation, percussion, and palpation.

Always inspect the abdomen first. Note any ecchymotic discoloration or distention, as well as any surgical or traumatic scars. Most nephrologic and urologic emergencies will not show acute abnormalities on exam, whereas a number of GI emergencies will. Auscultation rarely produces a positive finding because bowel sounds are almost always present. Absence of bowel sounds, however, is important and suggests a GI emergency such as bowel obstruction.

Percussion and palpation may be more useful in the field. Percussion of the abdomen or other involved areas may produce clues to the origin of a urologic problem. Pain induced by percussion of the flanks, especially when accompanied by fever, strongly suggests pyelonephritis, or kidney infection. Pain on percussion just above the pelvic rim of the abdomen, especially when accompanied by fever and an increased urge to void, suggests cystitis—bladder infection. Constant, sharp pain increased by percussion of the affected flank may indicate where a kidney stone has lodged in a ureter.

In postpubescent girls and women, abdominal palpation may reveal pregnancy if you feel the firm, muscular mass of the gravid uterus above the pelvic rim. A ruptured ectopic pregnancy is possible when palpation increases pain in the lower quadrant, particularly when accompanied by evidence of hemorrhage or early shock. A vaginal exam is rarely indicated in the field; however, you should check for blood or other discharge at the urethral or vaginal openings. In all cases, ask the patient for the date of her last menstrual period.

Palpation of the lower abdomen may help diagnose acute urinary obstruction in older men due to prostatic enlargement. If enough urine has been retained, you will feel a large (up to roughly the size of a 2-liter bottle), painful, fluctuant mass above the pelvic rim of the abdomen. This represents the distended bladder. The male abdominal exam should also include inspection of the penis and scrotum. Purulent discharge from the penis may indicate a sexually transmitted disease (STD). Palpation of the scrotum may detect a testicular mass (remember that testicular cancer is far more common in younger men—the opposite of the age risk for prostatic cancer). Palpable nontesticular masses may be painful (infectious epididymitis) or nonpainful (varicocele, a noninfectious swelling of the epididymis). Tenderness of the testicle can result from testicular torsion. This usually involves only one side and often is associated with the testicle being high in the scrotum. Ask relevant questions, such as whether swelling has been present for some time (as occurs with a varicocele) or is of recent onset (epididymitis).

ASSESSMENT TOOLS A hematocrit may detect significant or chronic bleeding. If blood is present in underwear or on the perineum itself, consider obtaining a small amount of material from the rectum or penile opening or opening of the vagina to be checked for visible blood or occult bleeding. The latter may help to localize the affected system.

Vital Signs

Temperature is important because fever suggests an infectious process. If you found high blood pressure, increased heart rate, or both during the ABC assessment, put those findings into context with other impressions from the exam. For instance, both heart rate and blood pressure commonly increase in someone with severe pain. On the other hand, it is also important to find out the patient's usual readings, if either he or a bystander can tell you. Uncontrolled chronic hypertension is one of the two most common causes of nephron damage and chronic renal failure (with the other cause being diabetes mellitus).

Management and Treatment Plans

Management of the patient with abdominal pain includes general and case-specific elements.

AIRWAY, BREATHING, CIRCULATION Field management always starts with the ABCs—airway, breathing, and circulation. Be sure to assess oxygenation. If the patient is hypoxic, provide enough supplemental oxygen to correct hypoxia. Avoid hyperoxia. Be prepared for vomiting in any patient with severe pain, whether or not it is likely of genitourinary origin. Circulatory support is also vital, especially when there is any indication of hemorrhage, dehydration, or shock or the patient appears to have any compromise of renal function. Monitor blood pressure closely, and monitor cardiac status with ECG per local protocol or discussion with medical direction.

PHARMACOLOGICAL INTERVENTIONS Consider placing a large-bore IV line for volume replacement or drug administration. When possible, use a needle of sufficiently large bore for any emergency blood transfusion. In almost all cases involving abdominal pain, the question of analgesics (pain-relieving medications) will arise. Nausea is common and should be treated with antiemetics such as ondansetron (Zofran) or prochlorperazine (Compazine). Pain should be treated—preferably with an opiate (e.g., hydromorphone, fentanyl).

NONPHARMACOLOGICAL INTERVENTIONS Remember that patients with an acute abdominal problem are possible surgical cases. Thus, nothing should be given by mouth. Administer fluid or medication only by IV or IM routes. Monitor vital signs closely and look for any change in level of consciousness. Be sure the patient is in a position of relative comfort, but also ensure that the position minimizes risk of aspiration if vomiting occurs.

CONTENT REVIEW

- Patients Most at Risk for Significant Kidney Problems
  - Older patients
  - Patients with diabetes
  - Patients with chronic hypertension
  - Patients with more than one risk factor

TRANSPORT CONSIDERATIONS Each patient with abdominal pain of greater than 6 hours is considered a surgical emergency until hospital evaluation proves otherwise. Rapidly, yet gently, transport all such patients. During transportation, talk quietly to the patient, both to calm him and to keep him informed of time until arrival or other pertinent matters. All of your actions, both with the patient and any family or friends in the ambulance, should reflect caring and competence.

Renal and Urologic Emergencies

You must know how to respond properly and quickly to each major type of urinary or genitourinary emergency. Prevention strategies—procedures that minimize further loss of any existing kidney function—are vital. Most of this discussion focuses on renal emergencies, those affecting the kidneys. The leading causes of kidney failure are diabetes mellitus (both types) and uncontrolled or inadequately controlled hypertension. Add to that profile the fact that nephron number decreases with age, and you have the general profiles of patients most at risk for significant problems affecting kidney function: older patients, those with diabetes or chronic hypertension, or those with more than one risk factor.

We will discuss three renal emergencies—acute kidney injury, chronic kidney disease, and renal calculi (kidney stones). We will also discuss one urologic disorder, urinary tract infection, which can affect any or all parts of the urinary/genitourinary system.

Acute Kidney Injury

Acute kidney injury (AKI), also called acute renal failure (ARF), is a sudden (often over a period of days) drop in urine output to less than 400 to 500 mL per day, a condition called **oliguria**. Output may literally fall to zero, a condition called **anuria**. AKI is not uncommon among severely ill, hospitalized patients. It is less common in the field. Noting AKI in the prehospital

CONTENT REVIEW

- Common Renal and Urologic Emergencies
  - Acute kidney injury
  - Chronic kidney disease
  - Renal calculi
  - Urinary tract infection

CONTENT REVIEW

- Types of AKI
  - Prerenal
  - Renal
  - Postrenal

setting is vital because the condition may be reversible, dependent on the cause and extent of damage associated with the disorder. Overall mortality is roughly 50 percent, in part because the condition usually appears in significantly injured or ill persons.

Pathophysiology

The three types of AKI are prerenal, renal, and postrenal. The distinct initial pathophysiology of each type determines both the severity of AKI and the likelihood for reversal and preserving renal function. The common point among the three types is their clinical presentation: sudden-onset oliguria or anuria. You may wish to reread the summary of kidney physiology before reading about the pathophysiology for each type of AKI.

PRERENAL AKI **Prerenal AKI** begins with dysfunction before the level of the kidney; that is, with insufficient blood supply to the kidneys, or hypoperfusion. Prerenal AKI not only accounts for the highest proportion of AKI cases—40 to 80 percent—but also is often reversible through restoration of proper perfusion. These factors make it extremely important to know conditions associated with increased risk of renal hypoperfusion and to treat the patient quickly and properly. Problems that can trigger prerenal AKI include some common field conditions: hemorrhage, heart failure (MI or CHF), sepsis, and shock (Table 7-2). These triggers decrease renal blood supply through a drop in blood volume, blood pressure, or both. In addition, any anomaly directly affecting blood flow into the kidneys (such as thrombosis of a renal artery or vein) can trigger prerenal AKI through an increase in renal vascular resistance. When renal vascular resistance becomes higher in the renal vessels than in systemic vessels, blood is effectively shunted away from the kidneys.

Normally, the kidneys receive about 20 to 25 percent of cardiac output. This high level of perfusion is essential to sustaining a GFR sufficient to maintain blood volume and composition and to clear wastes such as urea and creatinine from the bloodstream. As GFR drops, less urine forms, and the bloodstream retains water, electrolytes, and wastes such as urea and creatinine. Because the retained electrolytes include H^+ and K^+, metabolic acidosis and hyperkalemia may appear.

If hypoperfusion is prolonged or worsens in degree, two things happen. First, GFR decreases still further, and less filtrate means still less urine formation. Second, the nephron tubular cells become ischemic and active reabsorption and secretion decrease or cease. All these metabolic effects of decreased nephron function further stress the body, particularly the cardiovascular system, and increase the likelihood that tubular ischemia will advance toward tubular cell death. At this point, the process is renal AKI, not prerenal.

RENAL AKI In **renal AKI**, the pathological process is within the kidney tissue, or renal parenchyma, itself. Three different processes cause renal AKI. The first is injury to small blood vessels (or **microangiopathy**) or glomerular capillaries; the second is injury to tubular cells; the third is inflammation or infection in the interstitial tissue surrounding nephrons (Table 7-2).

Microangiopathy and glomerular injury both result in obstruction of these minute vessels that are a vital part of the blood vessel–tubule structure of the nephron; consequently, nephron function is lost. Microangiopathy and glomerular injury are often immune mediated and may be associated with systemic immune-mediated diseases such as type 1 diabetes mellitus and systemic lupus erythematosus. In these cases, AKI involves both preexistent and ongoing (that is, chronic and acute) nephron destruction.

Tubular cell death, or **acute tubular necrosis**, can follow prerenal AKI or can develop directly due to toxin deposition. Along with heavy metals and miscellaneous inorganic and organic compounds, a number of medications (including some antibiotics and cisplatin, an anticancer agent) can cause acute tubular necrosis.

Interstitial nephritis, a chronic inflammatory process also commonly due to toxic compounds including drugs (antibiotics, nonsteroidal anti-inflammatory drugs, diuretics), can also result in renal AKI.

Table 7-2 Causes of Prerenal, Renal, and Postrenal Acute Kidney Injury (AKI)

Prerenal AKI	Renal AKI	Postrenal AKI
Hypovolemia (hemorrhage, dehydration, burns)	Small vessel/glomerular damage (vasculitis—often immune mediated, acute glomerulonephritis, malignant hypertension)	Abrupt obstruction of both ureters (secondary to large stones, blood clots, tumor)
Cardiac failure (myocardial infarction, congestive heart failure, valvular disease)	Tubular cell damage (acute tubular necrosis—either ischemic or secondary to toxins)	Abrupt obstruction of the bladder neck (secondary to benign prostatic hypertrophy, stones, tumor, clots)
Cardiovascular collapse (shock, sepsis)	Interstitial damage (acute pyelonephritis, acute allergic interstitial reactions)	Abrupt obstruction of the urethra (secondary to inflammation, infection, stones, foreign body)
Renal vascular anomalies (renal artery stenosis, or thrombosis, embolism of renal vein)		

Note: *AKI secondary to transplant rejection is considered an immune-mediated form of renal AKI.*

POSTRENAL AKI The third form of AKI, **postrenal AKI,** originates in a structure distal to the kidney—the ureters, bladder, or urethra. In its earliest phase (before urine has backed up into the kidneys, shutting down further urine formation), postrenal AKI is reversible simply by removing the obstruction that is preventing elimination of urine. Urinary tract obstruction causes fewer than 5 percent of AKI cases, but, like prerenal AKI, it is important to identify because the odds of reversal are good. If the obstruction is not cleared, renal AKI may develop secondary to nephron and interstitial injury caused by renovascular obstruction.

Because both ureters must be blocked simultaneously for postrenal AKI to develop (assuming two kidneys are present), it is probably the least likely cause of the cases you will see. Far more common will be obstruction of the bladder neck or of the urethra.

Regardless of probable cause, treat AKI aggressively in the field so the patient will have the best chance for recovery.

Assessment

The focused history will often provide clues to the severity and duration of AKI. For instance, if the patient complains of inability to void for a number of hours associated with a feeling of painful bladder fullness, the cause may simply be acute obstruction at the bladder neck or urethra. In contrast, a patient with poor mentation may be unable to give a coherent history, and a family member will tell you that the patient has felt increasingly ill for several days and has not urinated at all within the past 12 hours or so. Questions likely to provide useful information include the following:

- *When was the decrease or absence of urine first noticed, and has there been any observed change in output since the problem was first noted? What was the patient's previous output?* The last question may be useful because patients with chronic kidney disease due to inadequate renal function can develop AKI as a complication.
- *Has the patient noted development of edema (swelling) in the face, hands, feet, or torso? How about feelings of heart palpitations or irregular rhythm? Has a family member or friend noticed decreased mental function, lethargy, or overt coma?* If the patient continued to consume fluids after AKI developed, retention of water and Na^+ can lead to visible edema in a relatively short time. Retention of K^+ can lead to hyperkalemia, a condition that can be lethal, especially in a person with previously compromised heart function. Increasingly poor mentation can be a sign of metabolic acidosis.

The focused physical examination may be helpful in assessing the degree of AKI present, the antecedent condition, and any immediate threats to life. Impaired mentation or clear decreases in consciousness in a person with previously good mental function suggest severe AKI and a potential threat to life. In a patient without evidence of shock, cardiovascular findings may include hypertension due to fluid retention, tachycardia, and ECG evidence of hyperkalemia (Figure 7-5). If shock triggered the AKI or has developed more recently, profound hypotension may be present, accompanied by tachycardia and hyperkalemia.

General visual inspection will usually show pale, cool, moist skin; if shock is not present, these findings may still represent homeostatic shunting of blood to the internal organs, including the kidneys. Look for edema in the patient's face, hands, and feet (Figure 7-6). Examination of the abdomen will reveal very different findings, depending on the cause of AKI. As with any abdominal complaint, look for scars, ecchymosis, and distention. If the abdomen is distended, note whether the swelling is symmetric. Palpate for pulsating masses, which may indicate an abdominal aortic aneurysm. Auscultation is rarely helpful in renal

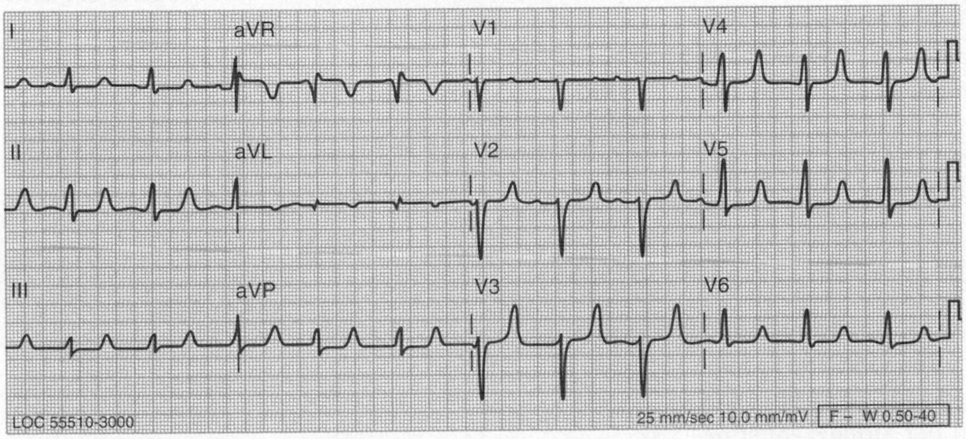

FIGURE 7-5 ECG with signs of hyperkalemia.

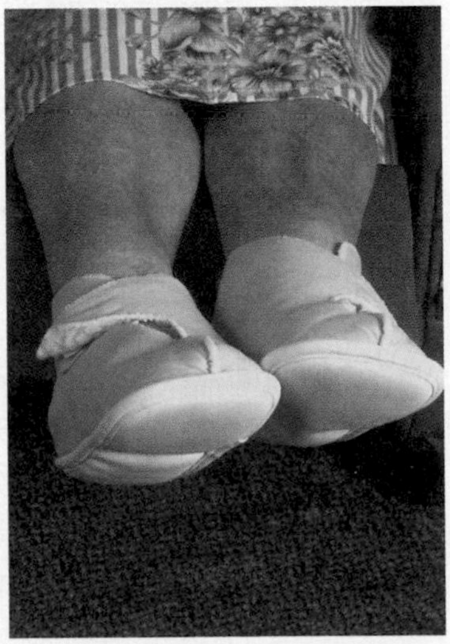

FIGURE 7-6 Edema of the feet consistent with fluid retention in acute kidney injury.

and urologic emergencies, and bowel sounds may be muffled if ascites (fluid within the abdomen) is present. Percussion and palpation findings will depend on the trigger condition.

A hematocrit may be useful if either acute hemorrhage or chronic anemia is suspected (the latter is common in patients with cancer or chronic renal failure). Urinalysis can offer useful information very quickly. Proteinuria and glycosuria (urinary protein and glucose, respectively) suggest renal dysfunction. In some infections, notably pyelonephritis, the urine may contain so many white blood cells that they form a visible sediment in the specimen.

Renal function is clinically evaluated by laboratory analysis of the blood. Two frequently used indicators of renal function are the blood urea nitrogen (BUN) level and the serum creatinine. An elevation in either of these two values points toward renal insufficiency or failure. Usually, the ratio of BUN to creatinine (BUN/creatinine ratio) should be 20. A BUN/creatinine ratio greater than 20 indicates prerenal or postrenal problems, whereas a BUN/creatinine ratio of less than 20 indicates a renal problem.

Management

Because AKI can lead to life-threatening metabolic derangements, monitoring and supporting the ABCs is vital. Use supplemental oxygen if the patient is hypoxic. Provide only enough to correct hypoxia. Avoid hyperoxia. Initial fluid resuscitation may be required if hypovolemia is present. Monitor ECG readings closely and adjust supports per local protocol or discussion with medical direction.

The chief prevention strategies are protecting fluid volume and cardiovascular function, as indicated by some of the steps previously noted, and eliminating or reducing exposure to any nephrotoxic agents or medications. If you are unsure whether an antibiotic, analgesic, or other drug is nephrotoxic and you are not in a position to check, discontinue the medication until the patient is at the appropriate care facility.

During transportation, be sure to talk quietly to the patient, both to calm him and to keep him informed of time until arrival or other pertinent matters. As always, your actions should reflect caring competence. Even if the patient is confused or comatose, you should still address him respectfully as you perform procedures and avoid saying anything you do not want him to hear.

Chronic Kidney Disease

Chronic kidney disease (CKD), also called **chronic renal failure (CRF)**, is inadequate kidney function due to permanent loss of nephrons. Usually, at least 70 percent of the nephrons (healthy norm, 1 million per kidney) must be lost before significant clinical problems develop and the diagnosis is made. Metabolic instability does not occur until about 80 percent or more of nephrons are destroyed. When this point of dysfunction is reached, an individual is said to have developed **end-stage renal failure (ESRF)** or **end-stage kidney disease (ESKD)**, and must have either dialysis or a kidney transplant to survive. Anuria is not necessarily present in either CKD or end-stage renal failure.

Together, diabetes mellitus and hypertension cause more than half of all cases of end-stage renal failure. The death toll from CKD is high: More than 250,000 Americans have end-stage renal failure, and more than 50,000 die yearly from kidney disease. Roughly 30,000 new cases of CKD are diagnosed each year. The number of donor kidneys available in recent years has been sufficient for only about one-third of the persons on the waiting list to receive a kidney.

Pathophysiology

The three pathological processes that initiate the nephron damage of CKD are the same as those underlying renal AKI: microangiopathy or glomerular capillary injury, tubular cell injury, and inflammation or infection in interstitial tissue (Table 7-3). Although the cause of initial nephron destruction is different for each of the three pathological processes, the same cycle of ongoing nephron damage becomes established: Functional nephrons adapt primarily by increasing glomerular filtration (through decreased vascular resistance in glomerular vessels and hypertrophy of capillary vessels) and secondarily by increasing tubular reabsorption and secretion (through cellular hypertrophy and functional adaptation of tubular cells). After a time, the compensatory changes damage these nephrons, leading to their destruction and initiating adaptive changes in additional, functional nephrons. Most of the damage seems to affect the glomeruli. Under the microscope, surviving nephrons often show dilated, abnormal glomeruli, and nonfunctional nephrons have heavily scarred glomeruli or no visible glomeruli, only sclerotic tissue.

This characteristic loss of nephrons, or **reduced nephron mass**, is also visible at the level of gross anatomy

Table 7-3 Causes of Chronic Kidney Disease (CKD)

Type of Tissue Injury	Examples
Microangiopathy, glomerular injury	Systemic hypertension, diabetes mellitus, atherosclerosis, glomerulonephritis, systemic lupus erythematosus
Tubular cell injury	Nephrotoxins including analgesics and heavy metals, stones, obstruction at bladder neck or urethra
Interstitial injury	Infections including pyelonephritis, tuberculosis

Note: *Congenital disorders resulting in CKD include polycystic disease and renal hypoplasia.*

as shrunken, scarred kidneys, or **reduced renal mass**. Physiologically, each of the kidney's four major functions is highly disturbed or absent, depending on the degree of renal failure:

- ***Maintenance of blood volume with proper balance of water, electrolytes, and pH.*** In CKD, active transport in the tubules decreases significantly or ceases. Filtrate simply passes through the tubules, leading to characteristic **isosthenuria**, the inability to concentrate or dilute urine. As overall GFR falls over time, retention of Na^+ and water increases, causing a high-volume stress on the cardiovascular system. Retention of K^+ can lead to dangerous hyperkalemia, and retention of H^+ can lead to equally dangerous metabolic acidosis. Hypocalcemia is also common. It results from several causes, including renal retention of phosphate ions (with higher levels of serum phosphate facilitating Ca^{++} absorption into bone) and lack of renal production of vitamin D.
- ***Retention of key compounds such as glucose with excretion of wastes such as urea.*** Glucose and other substances that normally are actively reabsorbed are also lost in urine as filtrate flows passively through the nephron. Any hypoglycemic effect is overshadowed, however, by the significant hyperglycemic effect (**glucose intolerance**) in most patients due to cellular resistance to insulin. The wastes urea and creatinine accumulate in blood almost in direct proportion to the number of nephrons lost. In fact, the general syndrome of signs and symptoms caused by severe CKD is termed **uremia**, for this characteristic buildup of blood urea.
- ***Control of arterial blood pressure.*** The renin–angiotensin loop is disrupted; even small amounts of renin can lead to severe hypertension. Hypertension may also develop due to retention of Na^+ and water. Cardiac decompensation, with hypotension and tachycardia, can develop suddenly, especially if cardiac function has been independently impaired.
- ***Regulation of erythrocyte development.*** Because erythropoietin is no longer produced in normal quantities (or at all, in some end-stage patients), chronic anemia develops. Anemia is another cardiac stressor, and it can contribute to cardiac failure.

Assessment

During the focused history and physical exam, you will probably find many characteristics of uremia in patients with CKD and end-stage disease. Table 7-4 lists some of these signs and symptoms, which affect nearly every organ system. Many of the listed problems can precipitate shock or other major physiologic instability; this is one reason you must always be alert when dealing with patients with CKD or end-stage disease, even when they initially appear stable. In addition, this list is by no means exhaustive. Kidney failure affects almost every organ and major function in the body.

The focused history will typically show GI symptoms such as anorexia and nausea, sometimes with vomiting. The patient's mentation as he speaks is an important clue to CNS impairment. Signs may be as subtle as anxiety or mood swings or as immediately serious as seizures or coma.

Your general impression before the focused physical exam is likely to note marked abnormalities. Skin will typically be pale, moist, and cool. Scratches and ecchymoses are common skin changes associated with CKD. Mucous membranes may also be very pale, dependent on the degree of anemia. Jaundice may be present, dependent on the degree of retention of urea and other pigmented metabolic wastes. A skin condition called *uremic frost* appears when excessive amounts of urea are eliminated through sweat. As the sweat dries, a white "frosty" dust of urea may appear on the skin.

The major organ systems often show significant abnormalities on direct examination (Table 7-4). Because of the failure of vital urinary system functions, cardiovascular stress can be enormous. Either hypertension or hypotension may occur, dependent on the degree of fluid retention (retention detectable as peripheral edema or pulmonary edema) and the level of cardiac function; tachycardia is common with both presentations. ECG findings may include an arrhythmia secondary to hyperkalemia. Metabolic acidosis, when present, compounds the effects of hyperkalemia. Pericarditis is also common, and a rub may be heard on chest auscultation. Neuromuscular abnormalities, in addition to impaired mentation, include muscle cramps and "restless legs syndrome," as well as muscle twitching or tonic–clonic or other forms of seizure.

Your abdominal exam will reveal many abnormalities. The challenge is to begin separating (by exam and history) chronic findings from those of recent onset or aggravated by the emergency that led to your call. For instance, you know that ecchymoses on the abdomen or flank may suggest acute hemorrhage. You may find a patient with ecchymoses scattered over the body surface. Look for evidence of new abdominal ecchymoses versus older bruises or a clear history of recent onset as signs of a current problem. Be sure to note abdominal contour, including the presence of symmetric distention or localized bulges, scars, and ecchymoses before the exam and to clearly document the pre-exam appearance. Findings on auscultation, percussion, and palpation will depend on the presenting problem.

The hematocrit and urinalysis generally have less value in CKD than in AKI. A hematocrit is useful only if you know the patient's baseline value, and recent changes in the amount of urinary output may be more significant than the content. The exceptions are blood (red blood cells)

Table 7-4 Common Elements of Uremic Syndrome

System	Pathophysiology	Clinical Sign/Symptom
Fluid/electrolyte	Water/Na^+ retention	Edema, arterial hypertension[1]
	H^+ retention	Metabolic acidosis
	HPO_4^{2-} retention	Hyperphosphatemia/hypocalcemia[1]
Cardiovascular/pulmonary	Fluid volume overload	Ascites, pulmonary edema
	Arterial hypertension	Congestive heart failure, accelerated atherosclerosis
	Dysfunctional fat metabolism; retention of urea, other wastes	Pericarditis
Neuromuscular		
Central nervous system	Retention of urea, other wastes	Headache, sleep disorders, impaired mentation, lethargy, coma, seizures
Skeletal muscle	Retention of urea, other wastes; hypocalcemia	Muscular irritability and cramps, muscle twitching
Gastrointestinal (GI)	Retention of urea, other wastes	Anorexia, nausea, vomiting
	Impaired hemostasis	Peptic ulcer, GI bleeding
Endocrine/metabolic	Low vitamin D, other factors	Osteodystrophy
	Cellular resistance to insulin	Glucose intolerance
	Mechanisms unclear	Poor growth and development, delayed sexual maturation[2]
Dermatologic	Chronic anemia	Pale skin, mucous membranes
	Retention urea, pigments	Jaundice, uremic frost
	Clotting disorders	Ecchymoses, easy bleeding
	Secondary hyperparathyroidism	Pruritus, scratches
Hematologic	Lack of renal erythropoietin	Chronic anemia
	Impaired platelet function and prothrombin consumption	Impaired hemostasis with easy bleeding, bruising; splenomegaly
Immunologic	Lymphopenia, general leukopenia	Vulnerability to infection

[1]Although relatively uncommon, fluctuations to the other extreme (example, hypokalemia) may occur if oral intake is poor over a prolonged period or during or after dialysis treatment.

[2]Primarily seen in children, adolescents, and young adults.

in urine, which is always a significant finding on dipstick analysis, and visible amounts of white blood cells, which suggest significant infection.

Management

IMMEDIATE MANAGEMENT As with AKI, CKD can lead to life-threatening complications, so monitoring and supporting the ABCs is vital. Provide supplemental oxygen if the patient is hypoxic. Consider a small IV bolus for fluid resuscitation if hypovolemia is evident. Monitor the ECG readings closely and adjust supports according to your local protocol or discussion with medical direction.

The chief prevention strategies are regulation of fluid volume and cardiovascular function and major electrolyte disturbances (for example, use of a vasopressor in hypotension and administration of bicarbonate for partial correction of acidosis, respectively) and elimination or reduction of exposure to any nephrotoxic agents or medications. Although uncommon, severe swings in electrolyte levels may occur during and after dialysis, so be cautious about replacement measures in the field in these patients. Err on the side of conservative treatment except for clearly life-threatening complications. If you are unsure whether a drug is nephrotoxic and you are not in a position to check, discontinue it until the patient is at the emergency department.

Expedite transportation to an appropriate facility in the same manner appropriate for patients with AKI. Be sure to talk quietly to the patient, both to calm him and to keep him informed of the time until arrival or other pertinent matters. If the patient is confused, ask short orientation questions periodically to assess lucidity and level of consciousness.

LONG-TERM MANAGEMENT **Renal dialysis**, the artificial replacement of some of the kidney's most critical functions, is a fact of life for most patients with CKD and end-stage disease (Figure 7-7). Although dialysis is necessary

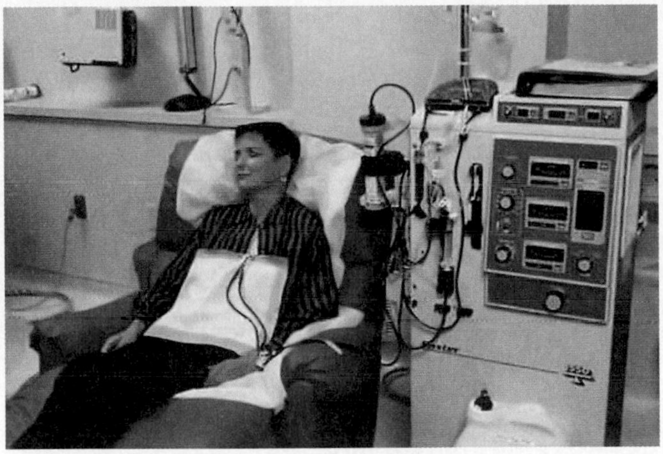

FIGURE 7-7 Hemodialysis has allowed many renal failure patients to live a relatively normal life.

(© Michal Heron)

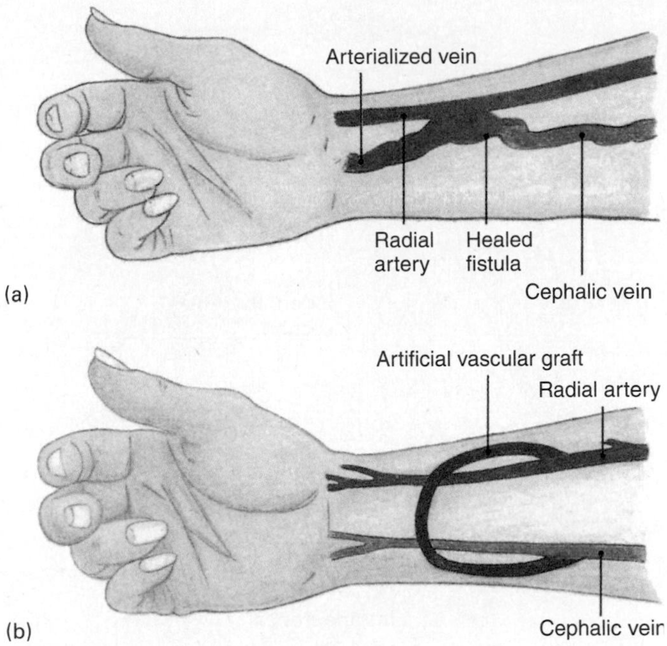

FIGURE 7-8 Vascular access for hemodialysis. (a) Arteriovenous fistula; (b) artificial graft between artery and vein.

for survival, it is not without risk. One risk that you have already learned about is the possibility of physiologically destabilizing shifts in blood volume and composition and arterial blood pressure.

Dialysis was first developed about 30 years ago. Since then, two different technologies, hemodialysis and **peritoneal dialysis**, have been refined. Both rely on the same physiologic principles: osmosis and equalization of osmolarity across a semipermeable membrane such as that of the renal nephron. (You may wish to reread the explanation of osmosis in this chapter's physiology section before reading further.) In dialysis, the patient's blood flows past a semipermeable membrane that has a special cleansing fluid on the other side that is hypo-osmolar to blood for a number of impurities (such as urea, creatinine) and critical substances (such as Na^+, K^+, and H^+). As the blood flows over the membrane, these substances in blood move into the hypo-osmolar solution, called the **dialysate**, and their concentrations in blood are thus reduced. The effect of dialysis is to temporarily lessen or eliminate volume overload and toxically high blood concentrations of electrolytes, urea, and other substances.

In **hemodialysis** (*hemo* = blood, *dia* = across, *lysis* = separation), the patient's blood is passed through a machine that contains an artificial membrane and the dialysate solution. Vascular access is required to achieve the necessary blood flow of 300 to 400 mL/minute. Often, a superficial, internal fistula is created surgically by anastomosing an artery and vein in the lower forearm. If the required healthy artery and vein are not available, surgeons can insert a special vascular graft made of artificial material between an artery and vein (Figure 7-8). If creating such a fistula is not possible, an indwelling catheter may need to be placed in the internal jugular vein. Because hemodialysis can be performed in settings including outpatient clinics and at home, you may see patients both between and during hemodialysis sessions. The three most common complications relate to vascular access. Two of the three complications are bleeding from the needle puncture site and local infection. The third is the narrowing or closing of the internal fistula. Under normal flow conditions, the internal fistula will have a palpable thrill (vibration), or bruit, due to the relatively high-volume turbulent flow from artery into vein. If the fistula narrows significantly or closes, however, this vibration is lost. The leading complications that require hospitalization are thrombosis, infection, and aneurysm development. They are particularly common in patients with grafts of artificial material.

CONTENT REVIEW

- Types of Renal Dialysis
  - Hemodialysis
  - Peritoneal dialysis
- Peritoneal dialysis is also known as chronic ambulatory peritoneal dialysis (CAPD)

Chronic ambulatory peritoneal dialysis (CAPD) uses the peritoneal membrane within the patient's abdomen as the semipermeable dialysis membrane, and dialysate solution is introduced and removed from the abdominal cavity via an indwelling catheter (Figure 7-9). This simpler technique, which used to be significantly less effective than hemodialysis, has been improved greatly in recent years. Currently, many patients practice either chronic peritoneal lavage (intermittent cycles in which dialysate is introduced, allowed to remain for an extended period, and then removed) or CPAD (in which dialysate is introduced via a closed system that allows the patient to remain ambulatory during dialysis). Peritoneal dialysis avoids some of the risk of fluid and electrolyte shifts seen during hemodialysis,

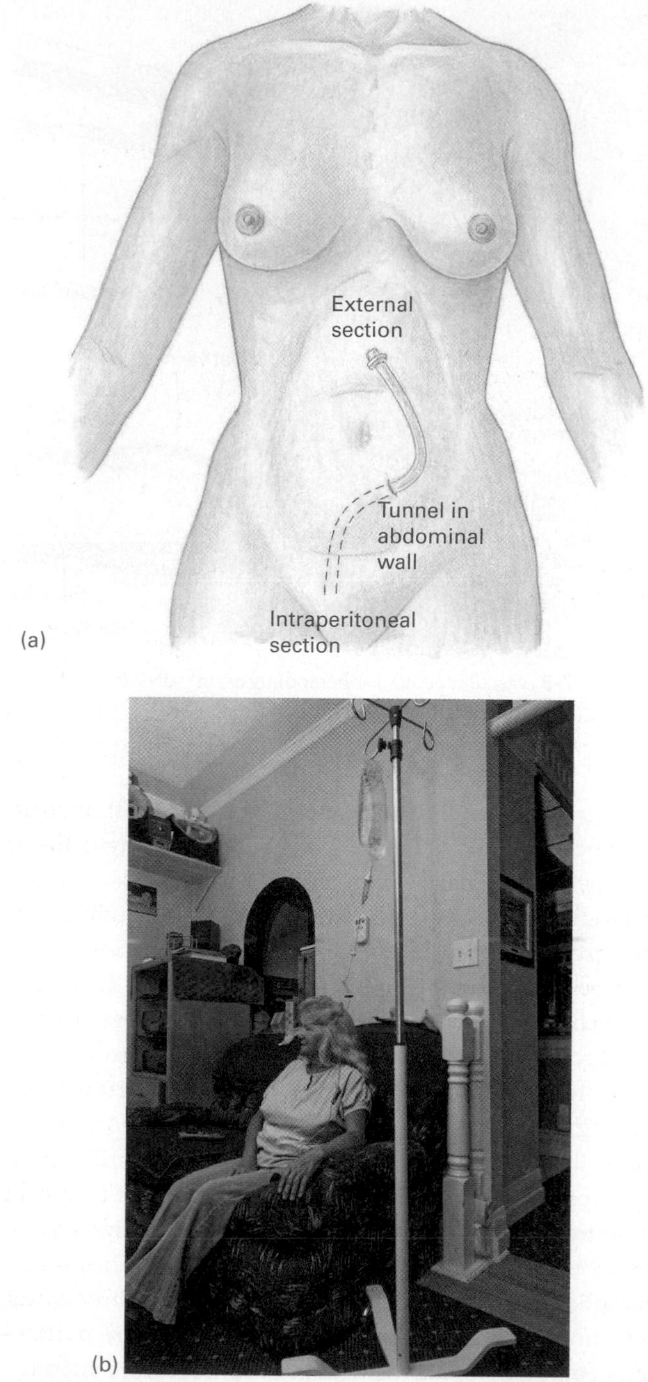

FIGURE 7-9 Peritoneal dialysis. (a) A catheter is placed into the patient's peritoneal space. (b) Patients will dialyze at home three to four times a day.

but its success requires additional physical characteristics (such as healthy vasculature around the peritoneum). The most common complication is infection in the catheter, the abdominal tunnel containing the catheter, or the peritoneum itself. The incidence of peritonitis is about one episode per year, so you may find its signs in these patients.

Both forms of dialysis have complications in common that are not related to vascular access. They include hypotension, shortness of breath, chest pain, and neurologic abnormalities ranging from headache to seizure or coma. If the patient is hypotensive, check for dehydration, hemorrhage, or infection. Shortness of breath and chest pain may reflect cardiac arrhythmias (often secondary to hyperkalemia) or may be without identifiable cause. Be aware that these patients, many of whom have cardiac compromise, are at higher risk for ischemia or MI during these periods. Neurologic abnormalities may occur before, during, or after treatment. In most cases they represent neurotoxicity of accumulated blood urea; in some cases, rapid removal of urea from blood causes an osmotic diuresis from brain tissue with a resulting increase in intracranial pressure. Benzodiazepines may be useful in patients who develop seizures.

Renal Calculi

Kidney stones, or *renal calculi* (singular, *calculus*), represent crystal aggregation in the kidney's collecting system (Figure 7-10). This condition is also called *nephrolithiasis* (from the Greek *lithos,* stone). Kidney stones affect about 500,000 persons each year. Brief hospitalization is common due to the severity of pain as a stone travels from the renal pelvis, through the ureter, to the bladder, and is eliminated in urine. If necessary, additional inpatient treatment may include shockwave lithotripsy, a procedure that uses sound waves to break large stones into smaller ones. Overall morbidity and mortality are low, however, unless a complication such as hemorrhage or urinary tract obstruction results. Stones form more commonly in men than women, although the ratio varies for types of stones with different

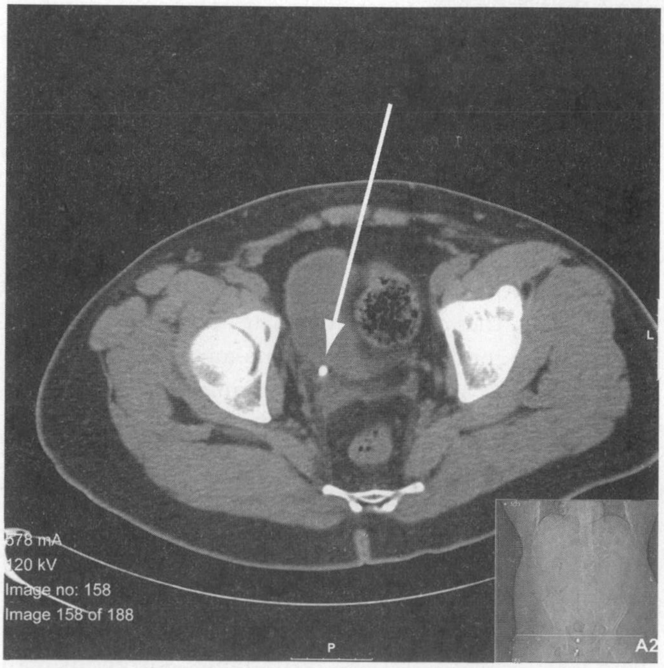

FIGURE 7-10 CT scan of abdomen. Arrow points to kidney stone.
(© *Dr. Bryan E. Bledsoe*)

compositions. Certain stones also occur in familial patterns, suggesting hereditary factors. Another risk factor for calculus formation is immobilization due to surgery or injury, with the latter including immobilization secondary to paraplegia or other paralysis syndromes that involve the absence of motor impulses, sensation, or both. Last, the use of certain medications, including anesthetics, opiates, and psychotropic drugs, increases the risk for stones.

Patho Pearls

About Kidney Stones. Kidney stones are more common in the warmer months—usually summer and fall. Kidney stones also tend to be more common in the southern United States, from Texas and New Mexico to the Carolinas. This region is often referred to as "the kidney stone belt."

The exact reasons that kidney stones occur more frequently in this region and at this time of year are unclear, but there are several theories. First, the South may have more of the inorganic salts of which kidney stones are made. Second, this region of the country is considerably warmer than the others, and the fluid intake of its people may often be too low to prevent kidney stone formation. Other theories include dietary and cultural considerations. In the warmer months in the South, iced tea is often the drink of choice on long, hot days. Tea contains a large amount of tannic acid, which contributes to kidney stone formation. It has also been suggested that the Southern diet is high in green, leafy plants (spinach, turnip greens, mustard greens), and these plants contain salts and other compounds that contribute to kidney stone formation.

The best prevention for kidney stone development is to stay well hydrated with water. Drinking large quantities of water (not tea, coffee, or sodas) during the summer months helps to maintain fluid movement through the kidneys and inhibits kidney stone formation. Once you have suffered a kidney stone, you will go to great lengths to avoid a second occurrence.

Pathophysiology

Stones may form in metabolic disorders such as gout and primary hyperparathyroidism, which produce excessive amounts of uric acid and calcium, respectively. More often, they occur when the general balance between water conservation and dissolution of relatively insoluble substances, such as mineral ions and uric acid, is lost and excessive amounts of the insolubles aggregate into stones. The problem boils down to "too much insoluble stuff" and urine "too concentrated," a situation that may more likely arise with change in diet, climate, or physical activity.

Stones consisting of calcium salts (namely, calcium oxalate and calcium phosphate) are by far the most common. These compounds are found in 75 to 85 percent of all stones. Calcium stones are from two to three times more common in men than in women, and the average age at onset is between 20 and 30 years. Their formation frequently runs in families, and anyone who has had a calcium stone is at fairly high risk to form another within two to three years.

Struvite stones (chemically denoted $MgNH_4PO_4$) are also common, representing about 10 to 15 percent of all stones. The pathophysiology of struvite stones differs from that of calcium stones. Their formation is associated with chronic urinary tract infection (UTI) or frequent bladder catheterization. The association with bacterial UTI makes struvite stones much more common in women than in men. These stones can grow to fill the renal pelvis, producing a characteristic "staghorn" appearance on X-rays.

Far less common are stones made of uric acid or cystine. Uric acid stones form more often in men than in women and tend to occur in families; about half of all patients with uric acid stones have gout. Cystine stones are the least common. They are associated with excess levels of cystine in filtrate and are probably due at least in part to hereditary factors, as they often run in families.

Assessment

The focused history almost always centers on pain. (Kidney stones are generally conceded to be among the most painful of human medical conditions.) Typically, the patient first notes discomfort as a vague, visceral pain in one flank. Within 30 to 60 minutes it progresses to an extremely sharp pain that may remain in the flank or migrate downward and anteriorly toward the groin. Migrating pain indicates that the stone has passed into the lowest third of the ureter. Stones that lodge in the lowest part of the ureter, within the bladder wall, often cause characteristic bladder symptoms such as frequency of urination during the day or during the night (nocturia), urgency, and painful urination. Because these three symptoms far more frequently suggest bladder infection, making the probable diagnosis may be difficult, particularly in women. Visible hematuria is not uncommon in urine specimens taken during passage of a stone. Fever, however, is not typical unless infection is present. When kidney stones are suspected, be sure to get the patient's personal medical history and family history, because both will often provide useful information.

The physical exam will almost always reveal someone who is very uncomfortable. The patient may be agitated or physically restless; walking sometimes reduces the pain. Vital signs will vary with level of discomfort, with highest blood pressure and heart rate associated with greatest pain. Skin will typically be pale, cool, and clammy. Abdominal examination may be difficult, depending on the patient's ability to remain still. First inspect the abdomen for contour and symmetry. Auscultation and percussion are generally useful only in ruling out GI conditions. Palpation results will vary and may depend, in part, on whether pain is so great that muscle guarding is present, making palpation of underlying structures impossible.

Management

As always, management begins with the ABCs. Positioning should center on comfort, but be prepared for vomiting due to the severe pain, especially if the patient's last meal was within several hours. Consider analgesia en route to the hospital, according to your local protocol and your perception of the patient's condition. Medications such as hydromorphone, morphine, or fentanyl can be effective. There are some studies that show that ketorolac (Toradol), an injectable nonsteroidal anti-inflammatory drug, is effective in renal colic—especially if used with an opiate such as morphine.[1] If the pain is in the initial, intermittent, colicky phase, consider coaching pain management through breathing techniques similar to those used for women in labor. An IV line is useful for volume replacement or drug administration. Nausea and vomiting are common and antiemetics should be provided. The usual prevention strategy, if kidney function is adequate, is IV fluid to promote urine formation and movement through the system. Transport is the same as that for other abdominal conditions—that is, position of comfort and supportive care.

Priapism

Priapism is a painful and prolonged erection of the penis. Priapism affects only the *corpora cavernosa*. The *corpora spongiosum* remains flaccid. Although in many instances the cause is unclear, priapism has been associated with certain disease processes. The most common cause of nontraumatic priapism is sickle cell disease, in which sickling of erythrocytes prevents normal venous drainage of the penis. Other causes of priapism include leukemia, multiple myeloma, tumors, spinal cord injury, spinal anesthesia, carbon monoxide poisoning, malaria, and black widow spider bites. Priapism has also been associated with use of the following drugs: psychotropic omeprazole, hydroxyzine, prazosin, calcium channel blockers, anticoagulants, cocaine, marijuana, ethanol, and MDMA (ecstasy). Some of the erectile dysfunction drugs, especially vardenafil (Levitra), have been associated with priapism.

A priapism is a medical emergency and requires prompt intervention by a urologist to prevent permanent damage and penile dysfunction.[2]

Testicular Torsion

Testicular torsion is the twisting of the spermatic cord, which cuts off the blood supply to the testicle and surrounding structures within the scrotum. This results in severe testicular pain and associated abdominal pain. Certain men are predisposed to testicular torsion as a result of inadequate connective tissue within the scrotum (bell-clapper deformity). However, it can also result from trauma to the scrotum—particularly if significant swelling occurs. It can also occur after strenuous exercise or may not have an obvious cause. Testicular torsion is more common during infancy and at the beginning of adolescence, although it can occur at any age.

The signs and symptoms of testicular torsion include the sudden onset of severe testicular pain (usually limited to one testicle). The testicle is exquisitely tender and swollen. The testicle is often high in the scrotum (when compared to the other testicle) because of shortening of the spermatic cord due to twisting. Nausea, vomiting, and dizziness are common. The patient may also report blood in the semen. The cremasteric reflex is typically absent on the affected side.

Prehospital treatment includes identification of the condition and pain control. Paramedics should maintain a high index of suspicion for this condition and report it to the emergency department staff. Intravenous analgesics and antiemetics are often required. In the emergency department, testicular torsion is diagnosed by physical exam and testicular ultrasound (which shows blood flow to the testicles). Prompt (<6 hours) treatment is necessary if the affected testicle is to be salvaged. The chances of saving the testicle diminish over time. On occasion, the affected testicle can be manually detorsed (derotated). However, in most cases, the patient will require surgery, in which the affected testicle is detorsed. Following detorsion, the testicle is surgically fixed (pexed) in the scrotum so that the torsion will not occur again. Typically, the opposite testicle is pexed as well.

Urinary Tract Infection

Urinary tract infection (UTI) affects the urethra, bladder, or kidney, as well as the prostate gland in men. UTIs are extremely common, accounting for more than 6 million office visits yearly. Almost all UTIs start with pathogenic colonization of the bladder by bacteria that enter through the urethra. Thus, females in general are at higher risk because of their relatively short urethra. Other groups at risk for UTI are paraplegic patients or patients with nerve disruption to the bladder, including some diabetic persons. Any condition that promotes **urinary stasis** (incomplete urination with urine remaining in the bladder that may serve as nutrition for pathogens) places a person at higher risk. Pregnant women often have urinary stasis due to pressure from the gravid uterus. People with neurologic impairment (some patients with spina bifida or with diabetic neuropathy, for example) also tend to have urinary stasis, which predisposes them to infection. The use of instrumentation in patients who require bladder catheterization places them at even higher risk of UTIs.

Morbidities such as scarring, abscesses, or eventual development of CRF are most likely in persons with anatomic abnormalities of the urinary system or chronic calculi (the latter acting as a focus for continuing infection and inflammation), those who are immunocompromised, or those who have renal disease due to diabetes mellitus or another condition.

Pathophysiology

UTIs are generally divided into those of the lower urinary tract—namely, urethritis (urethra), cystitis (bladder), and prostatitis (prostate gland)—and those of the upper urinary tract, pyelonephritis (kidney).

Lower UTIs are far more common than upper UTIs, for two reasons. First, seeding of infection via the bloodstream is rare. Second, asymptomatic bacterial colonization of the urethra, especially in females, is very common, and can predispose a person to infection by other, pathogenic bacteria.

In females, infection may begin when gram-negative bacteria normally found in the bowel (that is, the enteric flora) colonize the urethra and bladder. Symptomatic **urethritis**, inflammation secondary to urethral infection, is very uncommon. More often you will see joint symptomatic infection of the urethra and bladder (urethritis and **cystitis**, respectively). Sexually active females are at higher risk, which may be attributed to use of contraceptive devices or agents, to the introduction of enteric flora during intercourse, or both. Recently, homosexually active men who engage in anal sex have also been found to be at higher risk for bacterial cystitis, possibly due to introduction of enteric bacterial flora during intercourse. In any case, sexually active persons who suffer from urinary stasis are at even higher risk for infection. Persons who urinate after intercourse might lower their risk because voiding eliminates some bacteria. The pathophysiology for persons using bladder catheterization probably differs only in that pathogenic bacteria are introduced directly into the bladder via the catheter. In general, the likelihood that active cystitis will develop, that antibiotic treatment will clear such infections, and that reinfection will occur are all determined by the interplay of the pathogen's virulence, the size of its colony, its sensitivity to antibiotic treatment, and the strength of the host's local and systemic immune functions.

Prostatitis, inflammation of the prostate gland, in our context, denotes inflammation secondary to bacterial infection, as well as any general inflammatory condition. Men with acute bacterial prostatitis, the closest parallel to acute cystitis in women, also tend to show evidence of joint urethritis, and the same bowel flora tend to be involved. The major difference between acute bacterial prostatitis and acute cystitis is the much lower incidence of prostatitis among men who do not require bladder catheterization.

Upper UTIs usually evolve from infection that spreads upward into the kidney. **Pyelonephritis** is an infectious inflammation of the renal parenchyma: nephrons, interstitial tissue, or both. Acute pyelonephritis is ten times more common in women than in men. Its incidence is highest in pregnancy and during periods of sexual activity, reflecting the epidemiology of lower UTIs. If the infection of pyelonephritis persists, intrarenal or perinephric abscesses may occur, but these complications are uncommon. **Intrarenal abscesses** form within the renal parenchyma. If they rupture and spill their contents into the adjacent fatty tissue, **perinephric abscesses** may result. From 20 to 60 percent of patients who develop perinephric abscesses have a clear predisposing factor, such as renal calculi, anatomic abnormalities of the kidney, history of urologic surgery or injury, or diabetic renal disease.

Urinary tract infections may be community acquired or nosocomial. Among **community-acquired infections**, Gram-negative enteric bacteria predominate. In fact, *E. coli* accounts for roughly 80 percent of infections in persons without the complicating factors of bladder catheterization, renal calculi, or anatomic abnormalities. In **nosocomial infections**, cases acquired in an inpatient setting or related to catheterization, *Proteus*, *Klebsiella*, and *Pseudomonas* are commonly identified. Less common, but still important, are sexually transmitted pathogens (among women and men) such as *Chlamydia* and *N. gonorrhoeae*. Fungi such as *Candida* are rarely seen except in catheterized or immunocompromised patients or patients with diabetes mellitus.

Assessment

The focused history of lower UTI typically centers on three symptoms: painful urination, frequent urge to urinate, and difficulty in beginning and continuing to void. Pain often begins as visceral discomfort that progresses to severe, burning pain, particularly during and just after urination. The evolution of pain corresponds roughly to the degree of epithelial damage caused by the pathogen. In both men and women, pain is often localized to the pelvis and perceived as being in the bladder (in women) or bladder and prostate (in men). The patient may complain of a strong or foul odor in the urine. Many women will give a history of similar episodes, which may or may not have been diagnosed or treated. Patients with pyelonephritis are more likely to feel generally ill or feverish. They typically complain of constant, moderately severe, or severe pain in a flank or lower back (just under the rib cage). Pain may be referred to the shoulder or neck. The triad of urgency, pain, and difficulty may be present or included in the past history.

On physical exam, patients with UTI appear restless and uncomfortable. Typically, patients with pyelonephritis appear more ill and are far more likely to have a fever. Skin will often be pale, cool, and moist (in lower UTI) or warm and dry (in febrile upper UTI). Vital signs will vary with the degree of illness and pain, but in an otherwise healthy individual they should not be far from the norms. Inspect and auscultate the abdomen to document findings, but neither procedure is likely to be very useful, as visible appearance and bowel sounds are usually within normal limits. Percussion and palpation will probably reveal painful tenderness over the pubis in lower UTI and at the flank in upper UTI. Lloyd's sign—tenderness to percussion of the lower back at the costovertebral angle (CVA)—indicates pyelonephritis.

Management

UTI management should center on the ABCs and circulatory support. If pain is severe, help the patient to a comfortable position, but consider the risk of aspiration during vomiting. Analgesics should be considered, as with renal calculi; they will probably be needed only for severely painful cases of pyelonephritis. Consider nonpharmacological pain management, with breathing and relaxation techniques. The best prevention technique is hydration to increase blood flow through the kidneys and to produce a more dilute urine. In many cases, this is better accomplished by IV administration, which eliminates the risk of vomiting and satisfies the guidelines for possible surgical cases. Expedite transport to an appropriate facility.

Summary

The urinary system (1) maintains blood volume and the proper balance of water, electrolytes, and pH; (2) enables the blood to retain key substances, such as glucose, and removes a variety of toxic wastes from the blood; (3) plays a major role in regulation of arterial blood pressure; and (4) controls maturation of red blood cells. Kidney nephrons produce urine. Homeostasis through urine production is responsible for the first two functions and assists in the third (regulating blood pressure) by producing renin, the enzyme through which blood pressure is controlled. Other kidney cells produce erythropoietin, the hormone that stimulates red blood cell maturation.

Renal and urologic emergencies typically present as an acute abdomen. The most common are acute kidney injury (AKI), chronic kidney disease (CKD), and renal calculi. Both AKI and CKD may present with life-threatening complications and impaired function of other systems. Be prepared for apparently stable patients to acutely develop destabilizing complications (often, cardiovascular). Urinary tract infections (UTIs) are divided into those of the lower urinary tract (urethra, bladder, and prostate in men) and those of the upper urinary tract (kidney). Both types of infection can present with considerable pain, but pyelonephritis is the more serious, with fever likely and complications including abscesses possible.

Because renal function is often lowered in the elderly and in persons with hypertension or diabetes, consider it potentially impaired in all these patients. The best prevention strategies are to minimize the likelihood of prerenal failure by protecting blood volume and blood pressure and to investigate possible postrenal urinary tract obstruction.

You Make the Call

Shortly after dinner, you are called to an "unknown medical" case in a nearby apartment complex. You are met by a middle-aged woman who introduces herself as the person who called in the emergency. She tells you she is worried about her neighbor, whom she describes as an elderly gentleman who has been on his own since his wife died. She is concerned tonight that he seemed very shaky on his feet when she brought dinner for him and his speech did not make sense when she asked if he was all right. She says he normally speaks "like an educated gentleman."

A thin, elderly man opens the door. He is neatly dressed in shirt and pants but is pale and shaky. As he says he is fine and starts to close the door, you introduce yourselves and ask if you may come in and check to be sure he is all right. He reluctantly agrees. When you ask about his health, he says the doctor told him he had the flu and he was supposed to take it easy. He seems worried about your approval and repeats that he is fine. He cannot tell you the day of the week or his apartment number, and he sits down, trembling slightly. You note that his skin is cool and dry, and the inside of his mouth seems dry when he speaks. While your partner takes his vital signs, you ask about his problems with the flu. He says he had diarrhea for a few days but it is better. When you ask if he has eaten, he says he cannot remember but he knows he made tea to take his pills. He shows you a bottle of antibiotic capsules and one of a diuretic. He thinks there might be some other bottles in the kitchen. He mentions he might stop taking the water pills because he is not making water anymore. When you ask him about that, he says he slept all day and did not need to go to the bathroom. Your partner reports blood pressure of 80/60 mmHg, heart rate of 130 beats per minute, and labored respirations of 28 per minute. He also notes that the heartbeat seems somewhat irregular.

The patient says he will go to the hospital, but only if he can "finish dressing" and have his neighbor drive him.

1. What is your first management priority?
2. What risk factors, if any, might the patient have for a renal complication to his condition? Which renal complication, if any?
3. Should you agree to the neighbor's driving the patient to the hospital after he finishes dressing? If not, why?

See Suggested Responses at the back of this book.

Review Questions

1. What is the name of the medical specialty devoted to care of the entire urinary system in women and the genitourinary system in men?
   a. Urology
   b. Neurology
   c. Nephrology
   d. Renology
2. What is the functional unit of the kidney, which forms urine?
   a. Hilum
   b. Papilla
   c. Nephron
   d. Renal pelvis
3. What is the name of the structure that transports urine from the kidneys to the urinary bladder?
   a. Hilum
   b. Ureters
   c. Urethra
   d. Retroperitoneum
4. The general profiles of patients most at risk for significant problems affecting kidney function include __________
   a. older patients with cardiovascular disease.
   b. patients with chronic hypertension.
   c. patients with diabetes mellitus.
   d. all of the above.
5. You are transporting a patient between hospitals. While reading the patient's medical charts, you see that his daily output of urine has been 200 to 300 mL/day. Producing this amount of urine is called __________
   a. anuria.
   b. oliguria.
   c. dysuria.
   d. polyuria.
6. What is the name of the condition that is a chronic inflammatory process commonly due to toxic compounds, which can result in renal AKI?
   a. Cystitis
   b. Postrenal AKI
   c. Interstitial nephritis
   d. Chronic renal failure
7. Patients who require hemodialysis three times a week are prone to which complication(s) requiring hospitalization?
   a. Infection
   b. Thrombosis
   c. Cellulitis
   d. Infection and thrombosis
8. Kidney stones most commonly consist of __________
   a. cystine.
   b. struvite.
   c. uric acid.
   d. calcium salts.

9. ____________ is an infectious inflammation of the renal parenchyma: nephrons, interstitial tissue, or both.
   a. Cystitis
   b. Urethritis
   c. Pyelonephritis
   d. Prostatitis

10. Types of AKI include ____________
   a. renal.
   b. prerenal.
   c. postrenal.
   d. all of the above.

11. If a patient has sepsis and hypoperfusion, this will likely lead to which type of AKI?
   a. Prerenal
   b. Nephrotoxic
   c. Postrenal
   d. Intrarenal

See Answers to Review Questions at the back of this book.

References

1. Ghuman, J. and R. Vadera. "Ketorolac and Morphine for Analgesia in Acute Renal Colic: Is This Combination More Effective than Monotherapy?" *CJEM* 10 (2008): 66–68.
2. Rosenstein, D. and J. W. McAninch. "Urologic Emergencies." *Med Clin North Am* 88 (2004): 495–518.

Further Reading

Mumtaz, F., C. R. Woodhouse, J. W. McAninch, and D. L. Cochlin. *Management of Urological Emergencies*. London, UK: Informal Healthcare, 2004.

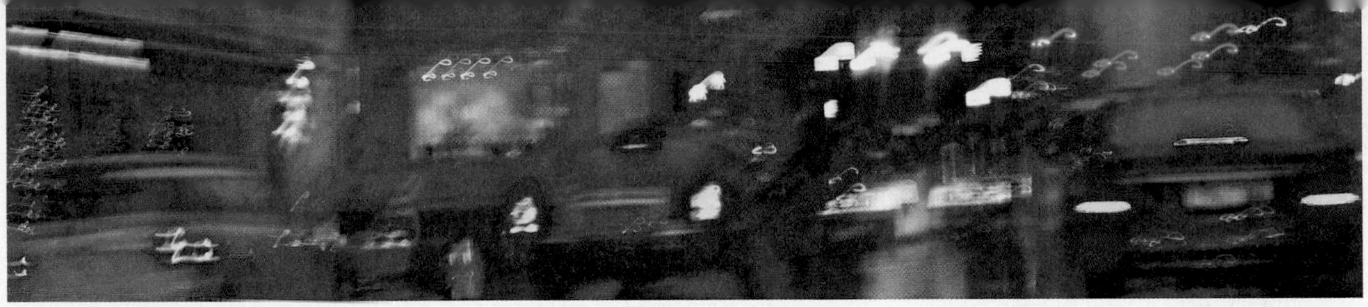

Chapter 8

Toxicology and Substance Abuse

Bryan Bledsoe, DO, FACEP, FAAEM, EMT-P

STANDARD

Medicine (Toxicology)

COMPETENCY

Integrates assessment findings with principles of epidemiology and pathophysiology to formulate a field impression and implement a comprehensive treatment/disposition plan for a patient with a medical complaint.

Learning Objectives

Terminal Performance Objective: After reading this chapter, you should be able to integrate patient assessment findings, patient history, and knowledge of anatomy, physiology, pathophysiology, and basic and advanced life support interventions to recognize and manage patients with toxicologic emergencies and substance abuse disorders.

Enabling Objectives: To accomplish the terminal performance objective, you should be able to:

1. Define key terms introduced in this chapter.
2. Review the epidemiology of toxicologic disorders and substance abuse.
3. Describe the role of poison control centers in surveillance and management of toxicologic emergencies.
4. Identify the routes by which toxins can enter the body, and the fundamental management when a toxin enters by each route.
5. Adapt the scene size-up, primary assessment, history, secondary assessment, and use of monitoring technology to arrive at a field impression and differentials for toxicologic emergencies.
6. Describe the pathophysiology and consistent assessment findings that would be present in specific toxins or toxidromes as seen prehospitally.
7. Use a process of clinical reasoning to guide and interpret the patient assessment findings and develop a treatment plan for patients displaying a toxicologic emergency in the prehospital environment.
8. Given a variety of scenarios, discuss the integration of assessment and management guidelines as they relate to toxicologic and substance abuse emergencies.

KEY TERMS

acid, p. 344
activated charcoal, p. 330
addiction, p. 359
alkali, p. 344
antidote, p. 330
decontamination, p. 329
delirium tremens (DTs), p. 363
drug overdose, p. 360
enterotoxin, p. 351
exotoxin, p. 351
gastric lavage, p. 330
ingestion, p. 328
inhalation, p. 328
injection, p. 328
organophosphates, p. 328
substance abuse, p. 359
surface absorption, p. 328
therapeutic index, p. 346
tolerance, p. 359
toxicology, p. 326
toxidrome, p. 333
toxin, p. 326
whole bowel irrigation, p. 330
withdrawal, p. 359

Case Study

Paramedics rush to their vehicle as a call comes in to Rescue 190. Rescue 190 is staffed by paramedics John Osborn, Stephen Johnson, and Tony Greenway. Dispatch reports an unconscious person at 1301 North 7th Street. The address seems very familiar. As the paramedics turn the corner and approach the residence, they immediately remember this location. They have been called here many times in the past to attend to a chronically depressed young woman who has trouble coping with stressful situations. Stephen reports that the crew from another shift was there four days ago.

Inside they find the young woman unresponsive and lying on the floor beside the sofa. She was found like this by her boyfriend, who states that she called him at work 2 hours earlier, crying that "she just couldn't take it anymore." On the floor beside her are an empty bottle of acetaminophen (Tylenol) and an empty bottle of nortriptyline (Pamelor), a tricyclic antidepressant. There is a pharmacy receipt on the floor showing that the bottles were just purchased today. Because of this, the paramedics have to assume that the bottles were full. The smell of alcohol pervades the air. A quick look around the scene reveals several empty bottles of an expensive wine on the sofa table.

Primary assessment shows that the young woman is unresponsive but alive. Respirations are slow and shallow. She is tachycardic with weak pulses. The paramedics intubate her and begin mechanical ventilation. They then establish an IV and place the various monitors. A focused history from the patient's boyfriend provides no additional information. The police arrive and start to interrogate the boyfriend in an adjacent room. Tony and John complete a rapid medical assessment. The only noteworthy findings are multiple shallow scars across both wrists.

The paramedics quickly transport the patient to the hospital, remembering to bring all bottles of medicines (full and empty) found at the scene. The patient does not seem to improve while en route. Shortly after arrival at the emergency department, the patient has a grand mal seizure that requires intravenous diazepam for treatment. The patient continues to deteriorate despite aggressive medical intervention. She does not regain consciousness and is eventually transferred to the ICU. She dies in the ICU 48 hours later from cardiac arrhythmias and hepatic failure. Her physicians hope to learn the cause of death from an autopsy performed by the hospital's pathologist. Results should be known in several weeks.

Introduction

Toxicology is the study of **toxins** (drugs and poisons) and their antidotes, and their effects on living organisms. Toxicologic emergencies result from the ingestion, inhalation, surface absorption, or injection of toxic substances that then exert their adverse effects on the body's tissues and metabolic mechanisms. Theoretically, all toxicologic emergencies can be classified as poisoning. However, in this discussion, the term *poisoning* will be used to describe exposure to nonpharmacological substances. The term *overdose* will be used to describe exposure to pharmacological substances, whether the overdose is accidental or intentional. Substance abuse, although technically a form of poisoning, will be addressed separately.

In this chapter, we discuss various aspects of toxicologic emergencies as they apply to prehospital care. We will establish general treatment guidelines for each type of toxic exposure, then address the specific issues surrounding some of the more common substances involved. Because the field of toxicology is rapidly changing, it is virtually impossible for a paramedic to remain up to date on treatment guidelines for each type of toxic exposure. Specific treatment should be supervised by medical direction in association with a poison control center. This plan ensures that the patient receives the most current level of care available.

Epidemiology

Over the years, the occurrence of toxicologic emergencies has continued to increase in number and severity.[1] The following figures reveal the high potential for toxic substance involvement on an EMS call:

- The American Association of Poison Control Centers estimates that more than 3.1 million poisonings occur annually.
- Ten percent of all emergency department visits and EMS responses involve toxic exposures.
- Fifty percent of accidental poisonings occur in children under the age of 6 years.
- A child who has experienced an accidental ingestion has a 25 percent chance of another, similar ingestion within one year.
- Eighty percent of all attempted suicides involve a drug overdose.

Although over half of all poisonings occur in children aged 1 through 5, they are generally accidental and relatively mild, accounting for only 10 percent of hospital admissions for poisoning and only 5 percent of the fatalities. EMS personnel must be aware that more serious poisonings, especially in children older than 5 years, may represent intentional poisoning by parents or caretakers (Figure 8-1). Unfortunately, poisoning due to drug experimentation and suicide attempts are also becoming a common consideration in older children.

Adult poisonings and overdoses, although less frequent, account for 90 percent of hospital admissions for toxic substance exposure. They also account for 95 percent of the fatalities in this category. Most adult poisonings and overdoses are intentional. Intentional poisonings and overdoses can be due to illicit drug use, alcohol abuse, attempted suicide, and "suicidal gesturing," in which the patient is making a cry for help but may miscalculate and take a type or amount of toxin that does actually cause injury. More rarely, intentional poisoning can result from attempted homicide or chemical warfare. Accidental poisonings are increasingly caused by exposure to chemicals and toxins on the farm or in the industrial workplace. More often, they are the result of idiosyncratic (individual hypersensitivity) reactions or dosage errors when taking prescribed medications, but these usually do not require medical attention.

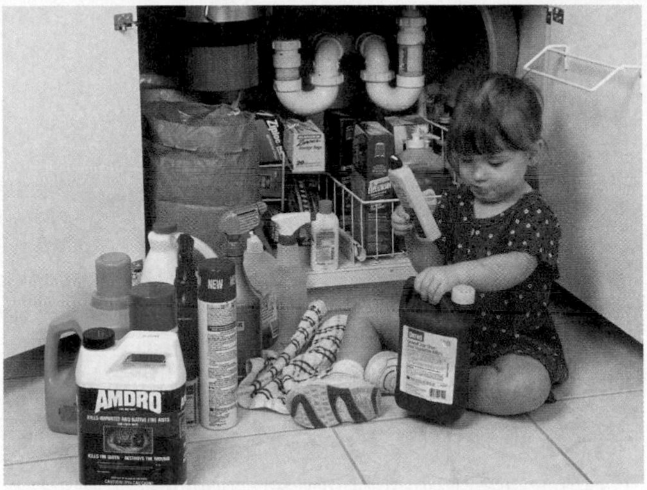

FIGURE 8-1 The suspected accidental pediatric poisoning is among the more common EMS calls.

Poison Control Centers

Poison control centers have been set up across the United States and Canada to assist in the treatment of poison victims and to provide information on new products and new treatment recommendations. They are usually based in major medical centers and teaching hospitals and serve a large population. Almost all poison control centers now have computer systems to access information rapidly.

Poison control centers are usually staffed by physicians, toxicologists, pharmacists, nurses, or paramedics with special training in toxicology. These experts provide information to callers 24 hours a day, 7 days a week. They update information regularly and offer the most current treatment guidelines.

Memorize the number of the nearest poison control center and access it routinely. There are several advantages to this. First, the poison control center can help you immediately determine potential toxicity based on the type of agent, amount and time of exposure, and physical condition of the patient. Second, the most current, definitive treatment can sometimes be started in the field. The poison control center also can notify the receiving hospital of current treatment and recommendations even before arrival of the patient.

Routes of Toxic Exposure

To have a destructive effect, poisons must gain entrance into the body. The four portals of entry are *ingestion, inhalation, surface absorption,* and *injection.* It is important to

CONTENT REVIEW

- Routes of Toxic Exposure
  - Ingestion
  - Inhalation
  - Surface absorption
  - Injection
- It is important to remember that toxic substances have both immediate and delayed effects.

note that, regardless of the portal of entry, toxic substances have both immediate and delayed effects.

Ingestion

Ingestion is the most common route of entry for toxic exposure. Frequently ingested poisons include:

- Cleaning agents (alkalis and soaps)
- Cosmetics
- Drugs (prescription, nonprescription, illicit)
- Foods
- Household products
- Petroleum-based agents (gasoline, paint)
- Plants

Immediate toxic effects of ingestion of corrosive substances, such as strong acids or alkalis, can involve burns to the lips, tongue, throat, and esophagus. Delayed effects result from absorption of the poison from the gastrointestinal tract. Most absorption occurs in the small intestine, with only a small amount being absorbed from the stomach. Some poisons may remain in the stomach for up to several hours, because the intake of a large bolus of poison can retard absorption. Aspirin ingestion is a classic example of this. When a patient ingests a large number of aspirin tablets, the tablets can bind together to form a large bolus that is difficult to remove or break down.

Inhalation

Inhalation of a poison results in rapid absorption of the toxic agent through the alveolar–capillary membrane in the lungs. Inhaled toxins can irritate pulmonary passages, causing extensive edema and destroying tissue. When these toxins are absorbed, wider systemic effects can occur. Causative agents can appear as gases, vapors, fumes, or aerosols. Common inhaled poisons include:

- Ammonia
- Carbon monoxide
- Carbon tetrachloride
- Chlorine
- Cyanide
- Freon
- Methyl chloride
- Mustard gas
- Nitrous oxide
- Tear gas
- Toxic gases
- Toxic vapors, fumes, or aerosols

Surface Absorption

Surface absorption is the entry of a toxic substance through the skin or mucous membranes. This most frequently occurs from contact with poisonous plants such as poison ivy, poison sumac, and poison oak. Many toxic chemicals may also be absorbed through the skin. **Organophosphates**, often used as pesticides, are easily absorbed through dermal contact (Figure 8-2).

Injection

Injection of a toxic agent under the skin, into muscle, or into a blood vessel results in both immediate and delayed effects. The immediate reaction is usually localized to the site of the injection and appears as red, irritated, edematous skin. An allergic or anaphylactic reaction can also appear (see the "Immunology" chapter). Later, as the toxin is distributed throughout the body by the circulatory system, delayed systemic reactions can occur.

Other than intentional injection of illicit drugs, most poisonings by injection result from the bites and stings of insects and animals. Most insects that can sting and bite belong to the class *Hymenoptera,* which includes honeybees, hornets, yellow jackets, wasps, and fire ants. Only the females in this group can sting. In addition, spiders, ticks, and other arachnids, such as scorpions, are notorious for causing poisonings by injection. Higher animals that bite and sting include snakes and certain marine animals. Marine animals with venomous stings include jellyfish (especially the Portuguese man-of-war), stingrays, anemones, coral, hydras, and certain spiny fish.

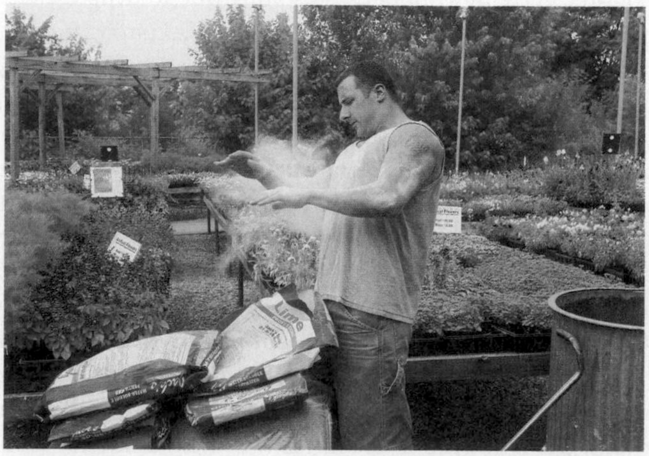

FIGURE 8-2 Significant toxic exposures can result from surface absorption of agricultural products.

General Principles of Toxicologic Assessment and Management

Although specific protocols for managing toxicologic emergencies may vary, certain basic principles apply to most situations. Keep in mind the importance of recognizing the poisoning promptly. Have a high index of suspicion if circumstances suggest involvement of a toxin in the emergency.

Scene Size-Up

Always begin assessment with a thorough evaluation of the scene. Take note of where you are and who is around you. Be alert for any potential danger to you, the rescuer. Remember, despite your natural urge to immediately assess and treat the patient, if you are incapacitated you will not be able to help anyone and you will become a patient yourself. In toxicologic emergencies, there are specific hazards to keep in mind:

- Patients who are suicidal may have the potential for violence. They are often intoxicated, may act irrationally, and will not always be cooperative or happy to see you. Therefore, look for signs of overdose such as empty pill bottles and used needles or other drug paraphernalia. Never put your hand blindly into a patient's pocket, as it may contain used needles.
- Chemical spills and hazardous material emergencies can quickly incapacitate any individuals who are nearby. Make sure you have the proper clothing and equipment needed for the particular emergency. Distribute this gear to rescuers who have been trained in their use.

Primary Assessment

After the scene size-up, perform the standard primary assessment. Form a general impression and quickly assess mental status. Assessment of the ABCs is critical in toxicologic emergencies because airway and respiratory compromise are common complications. This can be due to direct airway injury, pulmonary injury, profuse secretions, or decreased respiratory effort secondary to altered mental status. After assessing the ABCs, set a transport priority for the patient.

Secondary Assessment

For responsive patients, start by obtaining a history. It is important to find out not only what toxin the patient was exposed to but when the exposure took place, because toxic effects develop over time. Then proceed to a physical exam with full vital signs. With unresponsive patients, start with a rapid head-to-toe exam. Be alert for signs of trauma inconsistent with the suspected intoxication. Then proceed to obtain a history from relatives or other bystanders. Relay this information to the local poison control center. The center will advise you on the most current protocol for treatment. Be aware of your local policy, which will outline whether you can initiate this protocol or whether you must first contact on-line medical direction. Never delay supportive measures or immediate transport to the hospital based on a delay in contacting or obtaining information from the poison control center.

CONTENT REVIEW

➤ Standard Toxicologic Emergency Procedures
- Recognize a poisoning promptly (have a high index of suspicion).
- Assess the patient thoroughly to identify the toxin and measures required to control it.
- Initiate standard treatment procedures for all toxicologic emergencies:
  - Protect rescuer safety.
  - Remove the patient from the toxic environment.
  - Support ABCs.
  - Decontaminate the patient.
  - Administer an antidote if one exists.
- Rescuer safety takes particular priority during scene size-up for a toxicologic emergency.

A detailed physical exam can be performed en route if time and the patient's condition permit. Ongoing assessment is essential for these patients. Poisoned patients can deteriorate suddenly and quickly. Repeat the primary assessment and vitals and reevaluate every 5 minutes for critical/unstable patients and every 15 minutes for stable patients.

Treatment

Decontamination

Once you have initiated supportive treatment (airway control, breathing assistance, and IV fluids), proceed to a mode of treatment that is specific to toxicologic emergencies: decontamination. **Decontamination** is the process of minimizing toxicity by reducing the amount of toxin absorbed into the body. There are three steps to decontamination:

1. ***Reduce intake of toxin.*** This means that you must remove a person from an environment where he is inhaling toxic fumes, or you must properly remove a stinger and sac from someone stung by a bee. A classic example involves a person who has had organophosphates spilled on him. The patient's clothes

CONTENT REVIEW

➤ Principles of Decontamination
- Reduce intake
- Reduce absorption
- Enhance elimination

must be removed and his skin cleaned with soap and water to reduce absorption of the toxins.

2. ***Reduce absorption of toxin once in the body.*** This usually applies to ingested toxins, which wait in the stomach and intestines while the body absorbs them into the bloodstream.

   In the past, syrup of ipecac was used to induce vomiting in order to empty the stomach. *Use of syrup of ipecac is no longer recommended.*[2]

   Gastric lavage ("pumping the stomach") has also been found to be of limited use. This process involves passing a tube into the stomach and repeatedly filling and emptying the stomach with water or saline in hopes of removing the ingested poison. Most studies have shown that gastric lavage removes almost no poisons from the stomach unless it is initiated within 1 hour of the ingestion. Possible complications, such as aspiration or perforation, make this procedure a risk without much benefit. Except in limited situations with ingestions of highly toxic substances that do not bind to charcoal and for which there is no antidote, gastric lavage has become an uncommon decontamination procedure.

   The most effective and widely used method of reducing absorption of toxins is **activated charcoal**. Because of its extremely large surface area, it can adsorb, or bind, molecules from the offending toxin and prevent their absorption into the bloodstream.

3. ***Enhance elimination of toxin.*** Cathartics, such as sorbitol (often mixed with activated charcoal), increase gastric motility, thereby shortening the amount of time toxins stay in the gastrointestinal tract to be absorbed. Cathartics must be used cautiously, as there is controversy regarding their effectiveness. Cathartics should not be used in pediatric patients because of the potential to cause severe electrolyte derangements.

   Whole bowel irrigation is another method of enhancing elimination. Using a gastric tube, polyethylene glycol electrolyte solution is administered continuously at 1 to 2 L/hr until the rectal effluent is clear or objects recovered. This technique seems effective with few complications and is therefore gaining popularity. Its availability, however, is limited to a few centers.

Antidotes

Finally, if indicated, the appropriate antidote should be administered. An **antidote** is a substance that will neutralize a specific toxin or counteract its effect on the body. There are not many antidotes (Table 8–1), and they will rarely be 100 percent effective. Most poisonings will not require the administration of an antidote.

Table 8–1 Antidotes for Toxicologic Emergencies

Toxin	Antidote	Adult Dosage
Acetaminophen	N-Acetylcysteine	Initial: 140 mg/kg
Arsenic	*see Mercury, arsenic, gold*	
Atropine	Physostigmine	Initial: 0.5–2 mg IV
Benzodiazepines	Flumazenil	Initial: 0.2 mg q 1 min to total of 1–3 mg
Carbon monoxide	Oxygen	
Cyanide	Hydroxocobalamin	Reconstitute a 5 g vial with 200 mL of normal saline, mix, and administer IV over 15 minutes. A repeat 5 g dose may be required.
Ethylene glycol	Fomepizole (or as methyl alcohol)	Initial: 15 mg/kg IV
Gold	*see Mercury, arsenic, gold*	
Iron	Defreoxamine	Initial: 10–15 mg/kg/hr IV
Lead	Edetate calcium disodium or Dimercaptosuccinic acid (DMSA)	1 amp/250 mL D_5W over 1 hr 250 mg PO
Mercury, arsenic, gold	BAL (British anti-Lewisite) DMSA	5 mg/kg IM 250 mg PO
Methyl alcohol	Ethyl alcohol ± dialysis	1 mL/kg of 100% ethanol IV
Nitrates	Methylene blue	0.2 mL/kg of 1% solution IV over 5 min
Opiates	Naloxone	0.4–2.0 mg IV
Organophosphates	Atropine Pralidoxime (Protopam)	Initial: 2–5 mg IV Initial: 1 g IV

The specific actions you take when dealing with toxicologic emergencies will be dictated by consultation with medical direction, by protocols obtained from the poison control center, and by your local policy and procedures on initiating these protocols.

Suicidal Patients and Protective Custody

Before leaving a suicidal patient who claims to have been "just kidding," consider the legal ramifications. You may be charged later with patient abandonment. At the same time, be aware of protective custody laws in your state. Always involve law enforcement personnel in these cases and involve them early. Only law enforcement personnel can place a patient in protective custody and ultimately consent to treatment.

Ingested Toxins

Poisoning by ingestion is the most common route of poisoning you will encounter in prehospital care. It is essential to initiate the following principles of assessment and treatment promptly.

Assessment

It takes time for an ingested toxin to make its way from the gastrointestinal system into the circulatory system. Therefore, you need to find out not only what was ingested, but also when it was ingested. Following are some general guidelines for managing patients who have ingested toxins, as well as information about specific substances.

HISTORY Begin your history by trying to find out the type of toxin ingested, the quantity of the toxin, the time elapsed since ingestion, and whether the patient took any alcohol or other potentiating substance. Also ask the patient about drug habituation or abuse and underlying medical illnesses and allergies. Remember that in cases of poisoning, inaccuracies creep into nearly half the histories because of drug-induced confusion, patient misinformation, or deliberate patient attempts at deception.

The following questions will help you to develop a relevant history:

- What did you ingest? (Obtain pill containers and any remaining contents, samples of the ingested substance, or samples of vomitus. Bring them with the patient to the emergency department.)
- When did you ingest the substance? (Time is critical for decisions regarding lab tests and the use of gastric lavage and/or antidotes.)
- How much did you ingest?
- Did you drink any alcohol?
- Have you attempted to treat yourself (including inducing vomiting)?
- Have you been under psychiatric care? If so, why? (Answers may indicate a potential for suicide.)
- What is your weight?

PHYSICAL EXAMINATION Because the history can be unreliable, the physical examination is extremely important. It has two purposes: (1) to provide physical evidence of intoxication and (2) to find any underlying illnesses that may account for the patient's symptoms or that may affect the outcome of the poisoning. As you complete the primary assessment and rapid physical exam, pay attention to the following patient features:

- ***Skin.*** Is there evidence of cyanosis, pallor, wasting, or needle marks? Flushing of the skin may indicate poisoning with an anticholinergic substance. Staining of the skin may occur from chronic exposure to mercuric chloride, bromine, or similar chemicals.
- ***Eyes.*** Constriction or dilation of the pupils can occur with various types of poisons (e.g., marijuana, methamphetamines, narcotics). Ask about impaired vision, blurring of vision, or coloration of vision.
- ***Mouth.*** Look for signs of caustic ingestion, presence of the gag reflex, the amount of salivation, any breath odor, or the presence of vomitus.
- ***Chest.*** Breath sounds may reveal evidence of aspiration, atelectasis, or excessive pulmonary secretions.
- ***Circulation.*** Cardiac examination may give clues as to the type of toxin ingested. For example, the presence of tachyarrhythmias (e.g., from methamphetamine) or bradyarrhythmias (e.g., from organophosphates) may suggest specific toxins.
- ***Abdomen.*** Abdominal pain may result from poisoning by salicylates, methyl alcohol, caustics, or botulism toxin.

You can frequently expect to encounter patients who have ingested more than one toxin. This may be the result of a suicide attempt or of experimentation with illicit drugs. Such multiple ingestions present a diagnostic and therapeutic dilemma. Signs and symptoms may be inconsistent with a single diagnosis, and attempted treatment may produce unexpected results. A common example of this is the "speedball" (heroin mixed with cocaine). If the narcotic overdose is treated, the rescuer is often presented with a patient who is now in a cocaine-induced catecholamine crisis (tachycardia, hypertension, seizures). In such cases, or if you cannot identify what the patient has ingested, consult medical direction and/or the poison control center according to your local protocols.

Management

PREVENT ASPIRATION As previously discussed, initiation of supportive measures (maintaining airway, breathing, and circulation) is the top priority in the treatment of the poisoned patient. Aspiration is a frequent complication of poisoning, resulting from an altered level of consciousness and a decreased gag reflex. Preventing aspiration must be one of your major objectives. If insertion of an endotracheal tube is necessary, nasotracheal intubation is preferred in patients who have a gag reflex.

Poisoning is a situation in which rapid sequence intubation (RSI) may be required (see the chapter "Airway Management and Ventilation"). It is not uncommon to encounter a patient with altered mental status who is vomiting. The prevention of aspiration is a primary concern, but attempts at endotracheal intubation fail because the patient will "clamp down" his teeth. In these situations, it is often prudent to use RSI to quickly control and maintain the airway. This is far superior to waiting for the patient to deteriorate to the point at which an endotracheal tube can be placed without the aid of neuromuscular blockers. Remember, most poisoning patients will have compromised respiration or circulation, so routinely provide supplemental oxygen if the patient is hypoxic.

ADMINISTER FLUIDS AND DRUGS Once you have ensured the ABCs, establish intravenous access. An IV of lactated Ringer's or normal saline at a to-keep-open rate is recommended for all potentially dangerous ingestions. In addition to volume replacement with a crystalloid solution, conduct cardiac monitoring and repeat assessments, including frequent monitoring of vital signs.

Many EMS systems still use an empiric therapeutic regimen for comatose patients, consisting of $D_{50}W$, naloxone (Narcan), and thiamine (vitamin B_1). This so-called coma cocktail should not be used. Instead, treatment should be guided by objective patient information obtained on scene. If immediate determination of blood glucose levels is available (glucometer and chemstrips), withhold the administration of $D_{50}W$ until determination of hypoglycemia is made. If indicated, use 25 to 50 g of $D_{50}W$ IV push. If narcotic intoxication is suspected (respiratory depression or pinpoint pupils), give 1 to 2 mg of naloxone IV push. Naloxone reverses the effects of narcotic intoxication. If chronic alcoholism is suspected, consider administration of 100 mg of thiamine IV to address possible encephalopathy. Do not give these medications empirically!

Follow these supportive measures with the decontamination procedures outlined earlier. Often, decontamination is performed in the emergency department rather than on scene or during transport. This also applies to the use of most antidotes. There are exceptions, of course, and each case needs to be treated individually. Consult the poison control center and medical direction according to local protocols.

DO NOT INDUCE VOMITING As mentioned earlier, induction of vomiting is no longer an accepted routine intervention for patients who have ingested toxins. It is still important to contact the poison control center about this, because, in rare cases of pediatric ingestion, induction of vomiting may play some role. However, for the overwhelming majority of cases, induction of vomiting is not required and may even be contraindicated.

Inhaled Toxins

Toxic inhalations can be self-induced or the result of accidental exposure from such sources as house fires or industrial accidents. Commonly abused inhaled toxins include paint (and other hydrocarbons), Freon, propellants, glue, amyl nitrite, butyl nitrite, and nitrous oxide. The general guidelines for assessment and management of toxicologic emergencies apply to inhaled toxins, but the following sections provide some specifics.

Assessment

Inhaled toxic substances produce signs and symptoms primarily in the respiratory system. These symptoms are particularly severe in patients who have inhaled chemicals and propellants concentrated in paper or plastic bags. Patients who inhale paint or propellants are often referred to as "huffers." Look for the presence of paint on the upper or lower lip. (Huffers, who report it to be more potent, often prefer gold paint.) The presence of paint on the upper or lower lips should alert you to the possibility of inhalant abuse. The sniffing of paint, propellants, or hydrocarbons has become an epidemic problem in many developing countries. This is particularly true in the lower socioeconomic groups, most notably the legions of street children in Latin and South America. Huffing can lead to serious, irreversible brain damage. As the toxins are inhaled, oxygen is gradually displaced from the respiratory system, producing a relative hypoxia. Signs and symptoms of aerosol inhalation include:

- ***Central nervous system:*** dizziness, headache, confusion, seizures, hallucinations, coma
- ***Respiratory:*** tachypnea, cough, hoarseness, stridor, dyspnea, retractions, wheezing, chest pain or tightness, crackles (rales) or rhonchi
- ***Cardiac:*** arrhythmias

Management

Your first priority in the case of toxin inhalation is to remove the patient from the source as soon as it is safe to do so. Then follow these guidelines:

- Safely remove the patient from the poisonous environment. In doing so, take the following essential precautions:
    - Wear protective clothing.
    - Use appropriate respiratory protection.
    - Remove the patient's contaminated clothing.

- Perform the primary assessment, history, and physical exam.
- Initiate supportive measures.
- Contact the poison control center and medical direction according to local protocols.

Surface-Absorbed Toxins

Many poisons, including organophosphates, cyanide, and other toxins, can be absorbed through the skin and mucous membranes.

Assessment and Management

Signs and symptoms of absorbed poisons can vary, depending on the toxin involved. See the discussion of specific toxins in the sections that follow. When you suspect absorption of a toxin (especially cyanide or organophosphates), take the following steps:

- Safely remove the patient from the poisonous environment. It is essential that you follow these guidelines:
  - Wear protective clothing.
  - Use appropriate respiratory protection.
  - Remove the patient's contaminated clothing.
- Perform the primary assessment, history, and physical exam.
- Initiate supportive measures.
- Contact the poison control center and medical direction according to local protocols.

Specific Ingested, Inhaled, and Absorbed Toxins

CONTENT REVIEW

- ➤ Toxidromes
  - Anticholinergic
  - Acetylcholinesterase inhibition
  - Cholinergic
  - Extrapyramidal
  - Hemoglobinopathies
  - Metal fume fever
  - Narcotic
  - Sympathomimetic
  - Withdrawal
- ➤ Similar toxins with similar signs and symptoms are organized into toxidromes, which make remembering the details of their effects much simpler.

To recognize and implement the proper procedure in a given poisoning, you must be familiar with the signs and symptoms that a particular toxin will trigger. Often, you may not be able to identify the exact toxin a patient has been exposed to, but usually a group of toxins will have similar manifestations and effects and will require similar interventions. Similar toxins with similar signs and symptoms are organized into **toxidromes** (toxic syndromes), which make remembering the details of their effects much simpler. Study the toxidromes listed in Table 8–2.

The following sections address specific toxins commonly encountered. Although the standard toxicologic emergency procedures, discussed earlier, apply to all these toxins, pay close attention to variations in treatment. Variations include specific procedures you must perform in a particular case or a poisoning in which an antidote is available or immediately necessary. Management of injected toxins, drug overdose, and substance abuse will be covered later in the chapter.

CONTENT REVIEW

- ➤ Specific Toxins Commonly Encountered
  - Carbon monoxide
  - Cyanide
  - Cardiac medications
  - Caustic substances
  - Hydrofluoric acid
  - Alcohol
  - Hydrocarbons
  - Tricyclic antidepressants
  - MAO inhibitors
  - Newer antidepressants
  - Lithium
  - Acetaminophen
  - Other nonprescription pain medications
  - Theophylline
  - Metals
  - Contaminated food
  - Poisonous plants and mushrooms

Carbon Monoxide

Carbon monoxide is the number-one cause of poisoning in industrialized countries. Carbon monoxide (CO) is an odorless, tasteless gas that is often the byproduct of incomplete combustion of carbon-containing compounds. The CO molecule consists of one carbon atom and one oxygen atom joined by a triple bond. CO is an extremely stable molecule.

Although CO is often associated with fossil fuels, it is important to remember that it also results from the incomplete combustion of wood and charcoal. CO is a major source of poisoning in many third-world countries, where much of the cooking is done with wood-fired stoves and ovens. It is also prevalent when wood-fired heaters are used to warm a structure (Figure 8-3).[3]

Sources

Sources of CO fall into three primary classes: endogenous, exogenous, and the hydrocarbon methylene chloride.

Small amounts of CO are routinely produced through endogenous sources. The primary source is a normal breakdown of hemoglobin in a process called *heme catabolism*. In certain disease states, the breakdown of hemoglobin is increased. These conditions include the hemolytic anemias and, in some instances, sepsis.

Certainly, most CO exposure is related to exogenous causes. Among these are house fires, automobile exhaust fumes, fumes from propane-powered vehicles (e.g., forklifts), heaters, indoor stoves, camp stoves, boat exhaust

Table 8–2 Toxic Syndromes

Toxidromes	Toxin/Substances	Signs and Symptoms
Anticholinergic	1. Anticholinergic antiparkinson drugs (including benzotropine, orphenadrine) 2. Antihistamines (including diphenhydramine, chlorpheniramine) 3. Gastroinestinal antispasmodics (including dicyclomine, isopropamide) 4. Urinary tract antispasmodics (including oxybutynin, fesoterodine) 5. Opthalmic anticholinergics/cycloplegics (including homatropine, tropicamide) 6. Belladonna alkaloids (including belladonna tincture, atropine sulfate) 7. Tricyclic antidepressants (including amitriptyline, doxepin) 8. Other anticholinergic drugs (including ipratropium bromide, dipheniodol, piprenzepine) 9. Plants (including *Atropa belladonna*, deadly nightshade, jimson weed, angel's trumpet, datura, *Amanita muscaria, Amanita pantherina*)	Dry skin and mucous membranes, dry mouth, flushing, erythema, dilated pupils, blurred vision, mild hypertension, tachycardia, nausea, vomiting, hyperthermia, urinary retention, decreased bowel sounds, constipation, somnolence, confusion to restlessness, excitement, agitation, delirium, hallucinations, seizures, arrhythmias, respiratory failure
Cholinergic	1. Cholinergic agonists (including acetylcholine, choline, pilocarpine, carbachol, bethanechol, methacholine, muscarine) 2. Pesticides (including organophosphates and carbamates) 3. Plants (including *Areca catechu*—betel nuts)	Salivation, sweating, sedation, lacrimation, urination, diarrhea, vomiting, bronchorrhea, constricted pupils, fasiculations, paralysis, early hypertension-late hypotension, early tachycardia-late bradyarrhythmias), seizures, coma
Sympathomimetic	1. Direct-acting beta-agonist sympathomimetics (including epinephrine, norepinephrine) 2. Direct-acting alpha-agonist sympathomimetics (including phenylephrine) 3. Indirect-acting sympathomimetics (including amphetamines, cocaine, "bath salts") 4. Mixed-acting sympathomimetics (including ephedrine, phenylpropanolamine)	Tachycardia, hypertension, dilated pupils, hyperthermia, agitation, tremors, seizures
Sedative-Hypnotics	1. Barbiturates (including phenobarbital, butalbital) 2. Benzodiazepines (including diazepam, lorazepam) 3. Ethanol (including vodka, wine)	Hypotension, bradycardia, respiratory depression, hypothermia, ataxia, hyporeflexia, central nervous system depression, agitation
Opioids	1. Synthetic (including tramadol, diphenoxylate, propoxyphene, fentanyl) 2. Semisynthetic (including dextromethorphan, hydrocodone, oxycodone) 3. Natural (including codeine, morphine, paregoric)	Euphoria, pinpoint pupils, hypotension, bradycardia, respiratory depression, hypothermia, hyporeflexia, central nervous system depression, constipation, coma
Atypical Antipsychotics	1. Aripiprazole 2. Asenapine maleate 3. Clozapine 4. Iloperidone 5. Lurasidone 6. Olanzapine 7. Paliperidone 8. Quetiapine 9. Risperidone 10. Ziprasidone	Central nervous system depression, dizziness, some anticholinergic symptoms such as sinus tachycardia and urinary retention, hypotension, seizures, extrapyramidal symptoms, neuroleptic malignant syndrome. Some agents (such as quetiapine and risperidone) may cause QTC prolongation. Clozapine can cause agranulocytosis.
Extrapyramidal Symptoms	1. Phenothizanes (including chlorpromazine, acetophenazine, perphenazine) 2. Butyprophenones (including haloperidol, droperidol) 3. Atypical antipsychotics (including risperidone, olanzapine)	Dystonic reactions (including protruding tongue, twisted neck, deviated gaze, abdominal rigidity), akathisia (unpleasant sensations of inner restlessness that may manifest as an inability to sit still), pseudoparkinsonism
Hemoglobinopathies	1. Carbon monoxide 2. Methemoglobin (inducers including butyl nitrites, nitrotoluene, aniline, aminophenol)	Headache, nausea, dizziness, vomiting, weakness, confusion, seizures, coma, cardiac arrhythmias, death

Table 8–2 Toxic Syndromes (*Continued*)

Toxidromes	Toxin/Substances	Signs and Symptoms
Metal Fume Fever	Inhalation of metal oxide fumes from welding various metals including brass, cadmium, arsenic, zinc, antimony, manganese, nickel, copper, magnesium, cobalt, tin, lead, silver, chromium, iron	Fever, chills, nausea, vomiting, abdominal pain, respiratory symptoms, fatigue, joint pain, muscle aches, metallic taste. Symptoms usually self-limiting and resolve within 2 days.
Opioid Withdrawal		Tachycardia, hypertension, anxiety, dilated pupils, sweating, vomiting, rhinorrhea, piloerection, diarrhea, yawning
Ethanol Withdrawal		Tachycardia, hypertension, increased respirations, hyperthermia, agitation, disorientation, hallucinations, tremor, seizures

Source: Deutsch, C.M., Bronstein, A.C., Rocky Mountain Poison Center, Denver Health, Denver, CO. Used by permission.

fumes, cigarette smoke, and smoke from charcoal-fired cookstoves and ovens. Essentially, any combustible item should be considered a possible source of CO.

Methylene chloride is an organic hydrocarbon consisting of two hydrogen ions and two chloride ions bound to a carbon molecule. It is often used as an industrial solvent, particularly as a paint remover and adhesive remover. Methylene chloride is converted to CO in the liver after inhalation. Persons exposed to high levels of methylene chloride can develop *carboxyhemoglobinemia* and the signs and symptoms of CO toxicity.

Pathophysiology

CO competes with oxygen for the oxygen-binding sites on hemoglobin. Each hemoglobin molecule contains four oxygen-binding sites. These binding sites contain iron and form a complex referred to as *heme*. The heme structure is, in turn, connected to the protein segments of hemoglobin. Because of its molecular structure, CO will bind to hemoglobin with an affinity that is approximately 200 to 250 times that of oxygen. The binding of CO to hemoglobin results in the formation of a compound called *carboxyhemoglobin (COHb)*. As CO levels increase in the blood, oxygen molecules will be displaced from hemoglobin, causing a premature release of the remaining oxygen in the tissues. Furthermore, CO will prevent oxygen molecules from binding to hemoglobin. Carboxyhemoglobin cannot carry oxygen. As CO poisoning increases, and carboxyhemoglobin levels rise, the amount of hemoglobin that is saturated with oxygen, called *oxyhemoglobin*, is increasingly diminished. This ultimately affects organ systems that are highly dependent on aerobic metabolism and, thus, oxygen.

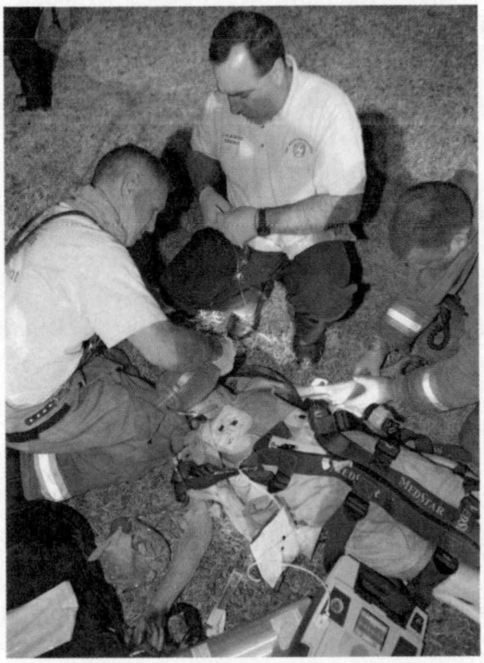

FIGURE 8-3 Carbon monoxide poisoning is the number-one cause of poisoning in industrialized countries.

(© Glen E. Ellman/FortWorthFire.com)

Once CO binds to hemoglobin and forms carboxyhemoglobin, it can only be removed slowly or via degradation of carboxyhemoglobin. That is, carboxyhemoglobin is ultimately removed from the circulation and destroyed. The normal half-life of carboxyhemoglobin, when the patient is breathing room air, is 240 to 360 minutes (4–6 hours). The half-life of CO can be decreased to 80 minutes with the administration of 100 percent oxygen. The administration of oxygen under pressure, termed *hyperbaric oxygen (HBO) therapy*, further reduces the half-life of carboxyhemoglobin to approximately 22 minutes.

Besides binding to hemoglobin, CO also binds to other iron-containing proteins. These include *myoglobin* and *cytochrome*, among others. The effects of CO on myoglobin are particularly important. Myoglobin is an iron-containing protein similar to hemoglobin. It is found in selected tissues, particularly muscles, and serves as a storage site for oxygen. Myoglobin is especially important in the heart. A reduction in functional myoglobin results in decreased oxygen levels in the heart. This could lead to cardiac ischemia, arrhythmias, and other types of cardiac dysfunction.

One mechanism of action of CO has only recently been understood. CO causes an increase in the circulating levels of *nitric oxide (NO)*. Nitric oxide is a highly reactive gas that is essential in many biochemical processes. Nitric oxide relaxes the smooth muscle in the walls of the arterioles, causing vasodilation. Following contraction of the heart (systole), the endothelial cells lining the interior of the arterioles will release small amounts of NO that promote vasodilation, allowing the pulsatile blood to readily pass through the vessel. CO causes an increase in the circulating levels of NO. This results in both cerebral and peripheral vasodilation and plays a major role in causing the syncope and headache associated with CO toxicity. Increased NO levels result in the formation of oxygen-free radicals—especially following periods of ischemia. These are thought to cause oxidative damage to the brain and are the probable cause of delayed neurologic sequelae (DNS). Nitric oxide oxidizes hemoglobin, forming *methemoglobin*. As methemoglobin levels increase, the oxygen-carrying capacity of the blood falls.[4]

Some levels of carboxyhemoglobin are normally present in the blood—either from environmental exposure or from endogenous sources. These levels are, of course, higher in tobacco smokers. Endogenous CO production usually results in carboxyhemoglobin (COHb) levels between 0.4 and 0.7 percent. Persons who smoke one pack of cigarettes per day will often have COHb levels ranging from 5 to 6 percent. Persons who smoke two to three packs per day will often have levels ranging from 7 to 9 percent (or even higher), depending on the cigarette type and filter. CO production from cigar smoking varies significantly. COHb levels of up to 20 percent have been reported with cigar smoking. However, these levels are extremely variable, depending on whether or not the smoker inhales the cigar smoke and the duration of exposure. COHb levels are higher in urban commuters. Interestingly, CO toxicity is a particular concern for persons working in tollbooths—particularly in urban areas where cars idle. COHb following methylene chloride exposure (100 ppm for 8 hours) can result in levels of 3 to 5 percent.

The impact of CO poisoning on major body systems is quite varied. Body systems that are highly reliant on aerobic metabolism are particularly vulnerable to the effects of CO. Of these, the central nervous system and the cardiovascular system are most frequently affected.

As a rule, the impact of CO on the central nervous system causes nervous system depression. This results in impairment manifesting as headache, dizziness, confusion, seizures, and ultimately coma. It has been well documented that there are long-term complications associated with CO exposure. These are primarily cognitive and psychiatric problems.

CO also adversely affects the cardiovascular system. This usually manifests as depressed myocardial function and results in several signs and symptoms. These may include chest pain, hypotension with tachycardia, cardiac arrhythmias, myocardial ischemia, and ultimately ventricular fibrillation. Most deaths from CO poisoning are due to ventricular fibrillation. It has been shown that CO has adverse long-term effects on the cardiovascular system. For example, the risks of a premature cardiac death are higher in patients who sustain a myocardial injury during the initial CO insult.

In addition to affecting the central nervous system and cardiovascular system, CO poisoning adversely affects other body systems. For example, metabolic derangements are common following CO exposure. Initially, respiratory alkalosis occurs primarily from hyperventilation. Later, and with severe exposures, metabolic acidosis is noted.

CO also adversely affects the respiratory system. In approximately 10 to 30 percent of patients with CO poisoning, pulmonary edema will occur. This can result from the direct effect of CO on the alveolar membrane. It can also occur with left ventricular failure that is secondary to myocardial depression. Because CO is often associated with nausea and vomiting, the possibility of aspiration as a cause of acute pulmonary edema must also be considered. In addition, because of the effects of CO on the central nervous system, neurogenic pulmonary edema must also be considered.

Ultimately, *multiple organ dysfunction syndrome (MODS)* can result, especially with significant exposures. MODS occurs when two or more organ systems fail to maintain their essential functions. The mortality rate with MODS is quite high.

In summary, the pathophysiologic effects of CO can be detailed as follows:

- ***Limits oxygen transport***—CO binds more readily to hemoglobin than does oxygen, forming carboxyhemoglobin, which cannot transport oxygen.
- ***Inhibits oxygen transfer***—CO changes the structure of hemoglobin, thus causing the premature release of oxygen into the tissues.
- ***Causes tissue inflammation***—Poor and inadequate tissue perfusion initiates and maintains an inflammatory response. This response may, at times, further injure body cells and tissues.
- ***Causes reduced cardiac function***—CO is a myocardial depressant and adversely affects myocardial function. This can lead to arrhythmias, myocardial ischemia, and even myocardial infarction. Long-term cardiac effects, including an increased risk of premature cardiac death, have been documented.
- ***Increases activation of nitric oxide***—Nitric oxide levels are increased following CO exposure, resulting in cerebral and systemic vasodilation. This can result in

headache and syncope. In addition, increased nitric oxide levels induce an inflammatory response that can harm delicate tissues.

- *Causes vasodilation*—Vasodilation, as just noted, can cause syncope and worsen tissue perfusion. This vasodilation is mediated primarily through the increased release of gaseous nitric oxide. Nitric oxide oxidizes hemoglobin, forming methemoglobin. As methemoglobin levels increase, the oxygen-carrying capacity of the blood falls.
- *Induces free-radical formation*—The increase in nitric oxide levels following CO exposure results in the increased formation of free radical compounds. These free radicals can cause injury to the inner lining of blood vessels and oxidative brain damage.

Several patient populations are at increased risk for significant CO poisoning. Persons at the extremes of age—the very young and the elderly—are at increased risk of developing toxic effects from CO due to the special characteristics of their physiology. In addition, persons with heart disease are more vulnerable to the ill effects of CO. They are already having problems related to poor or inadequate myocardial oxygenation. The added effects of CO for these patients can be problematic—or even fatal. Pregnant women, for reasons previously detailed, are at risk for the adverse effects of CO. CO affects the fetus more than the mother, because fetal hemoglobin has a higher affinity for CO than it does for oxygen. Patients with a decreased oxygen-carrying capacity, such as those with anemia (iron-deficiency, sickle cell), are also at increased risk for developing toxic effects from CO because of the already limited oxygen-carrying capacity of their blood. Finally, patients with chronic respiratory disease (asthma, COPD, cystic fibrosis) are at increased risk because their respiratory system is already compromised and inefficient in hemoglobin oxygenation. Any decline in oxygen levels from CO exposure will exacerbate the situation.[5]

Signs and Symptoms

The signs and symptoms of carbon monoxide poisoning are vague and nonspecific and closely resemble those of other diseases. Thus, CO poisoning is often called "the great imitator." It is for this reason that CO poisoning is often misdiagnosed. CO poisoning is often diagnosed as a viral illness (influenza), acute coronary syndrome, or even migraine.

CO poisoning is typically classified as either *acute* or *chronic*. Acute carbon monoxide poisoning results from short exposure to a relatively high level of carbon monoxide. Chronic CO exposure, by contrast, results from long or recurrent exposures to relatively low levels of carbon monoxide.

Table 8–3 Signs and Symptoms of Acute CO Poisoning

Malaise	Agitation	Seizures
Flu-like symptoms	Nausea	Fecal incontinence
Fatigue	Vomiting	Urinary incontinence
Dyspnea on exertion	Diarrhea	Memory disturbances
Chest pain	Abdominal pain	Gait disturbances
Palpitations	Headache	Bizarre neurologic symptoms
Lethargy	Drowsiness	Coma
Confusion	Dizziness	Death
Depression	Weakness	
Impulsiveness	Confusion	
Hallucinations	Visual disturbances	
Confabulation	Syncope	

The signs and symptoms of acute CO poisoning are diverse. Some patients will develop certain signs and symptoms, whereas others will not. Table 8–3 lists signs and symptoms associated with acute CO poisoning.

The signs and symptoms of chronic CO poisoning are essentially the same as those of acute CO poisoning. However, their onset and severity may be extremely varied.

As a rule, the signs and symptoms of acute CO poisoning worsen with increasing levels of COHb. Table 8–4 illustrates the signs and symptoms of CO poisoning and the associated classifications. It is important to point out that COHb levels do not always correlate with signs and symptoms, nor do they predict sequelae. Interestingly, the cherry-red skin color so often associated with CO poisoning is actually an unreliable finding. When present, it is usually associated with a significant CO exposure.

Table 8–4 Signs and Symptoms of CO Poisoning Classified by Severity

COHb	Severity	Signs and Symptoms
<15–20%	Mild	Headache, nausea, vomiting, dizziness, blurred vision
21–40%	Moderate	Confusion, syncope, chest pain, dyspnea, tachycardia, tachypnea, weakness
41–59%	Severe	Arrhythmias, hypotension, cardiac ischemia, palpitations, respiratory arrest, pulmonary edema, seizures, coma, cardiac arrest
>60%	Fatal	Death

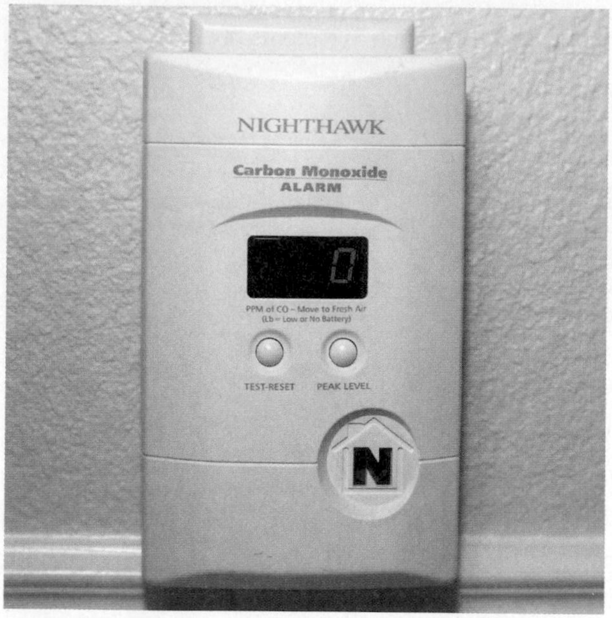

FIGURE 8-4 Household carbon monoxide detectors are effective and can reduce the incidence of carbon monoxide deaths.

(© Dr. Bryan E. Bledsoe)

CO Detection

Carbon monoxide detectors have been widely available for more than a decade. However, even today, they remain vastly underutilized. Numerous models of very inexpensive CO detectors are available for the home. It is important to point out that in 1998 Underwriters Laboratories (UL) revised the guidelines for CO detectors. Thus, units made before 1998 should not be used (Figure 8-4).

Handheld CO detectors have been available for some time. Noncommercial detectors will detect only CO. Commercial detectors, such as those used by most fire departments, measure several gases. The most commonly measured gases are CO, oxygen, hydrogen sulfide, and combustible gases (Figure 8-5).

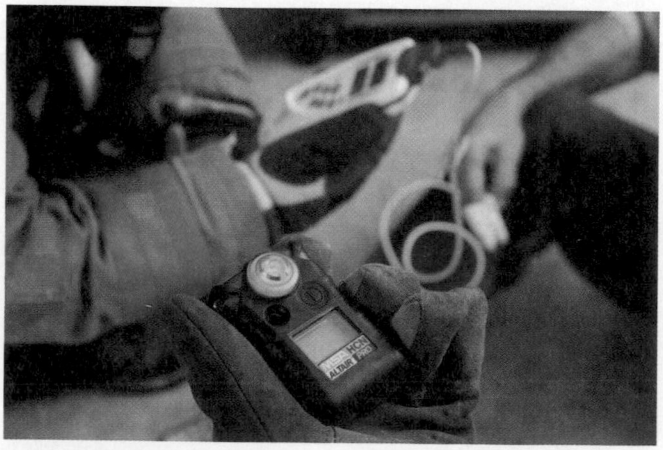

FIGURE 8-5 Handheld carbon monoxide (and poisonous gas) detectors can detect the presence of poisonous gases in the environment.

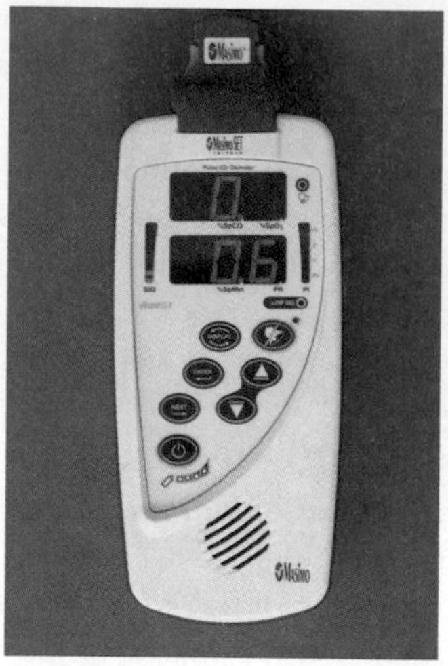

FIGURE 8-6 A CO-oximeter allows for the rapid detection of carbon monoxide poisoning through the noninvasive measurement of carboxyhemoglobin levels.

(© Dr. Bryan E. Bledsoe)

Until recently, biological detection of CO required hospital-based arterial blood gas sampling or venous blood analysis. Now, technologies developed to detect biological carboxyhemoglobin levels in the prehospital and emergency department setting are available. This technology, referred to as *CO-oximetry*, functions in a fashion similar to that of pulse oximetry. However, unlike pulse oximetry, CO-oximetry can detect deoxyhemoglobin (Hb), oxyhemoglobin (O_2Hb), carboxyhemoglobin (COHb), and methemoglobin (MetHb). The CO-oximeter can provide the following values: oxygen saturation (SpO_2), carboxyhemoglobin percentage (SpCO), methemoglobin percentage (SpMet), and pulse rate. CO-oximetry uses a finger probe similar to that for pulse oximetry, but instead of measuring only two wavelengths of light, the CO-oximeter is able to measure eight wavelengths. Research has demonstrated that carboxyhemoglobin levels as measured by CO-oximetry correlate favorably to those measured with hospital-based technologies (Figure 8-6).

Because the signs and symptoms of CO poisoning are so vague and nonspecific, CO exposure and poisoning are easy to miss. Failing to detect and diagnose CO poisoning can result in the patient being allowed to return to the contaminated environment, with devastating outcomes. Missed CO poisonings are a particular area of legal liability for fire and emergency personnel. Because of the associated risk and the insidious nature of CO poisoning, CO-oximetry should be routine for all fire service and EMS personnel (Procedure 8–1).

Management

It is important to maintain a low threshold of suspicion for treating victims of CO exposure. The Centers for Disease Control and Prevention (CDC) has established diagnostic

Procedure 8–1 Pulse CO-oximeter Use

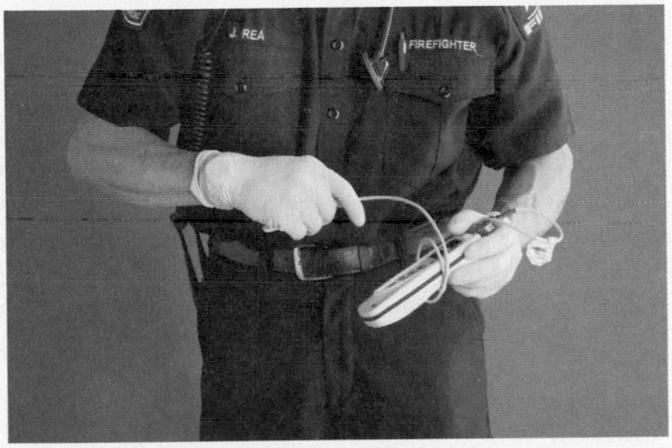

8-1a Prepare the pulse CO-oximeter.

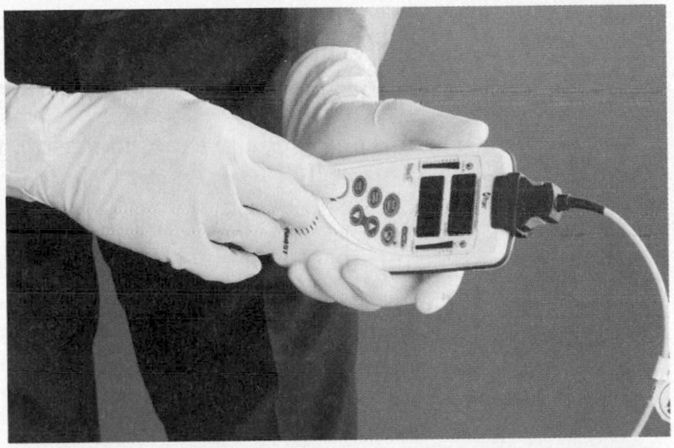

8-1b Turn on the pulse CO-oximeter and allow it to complete the startup routine.

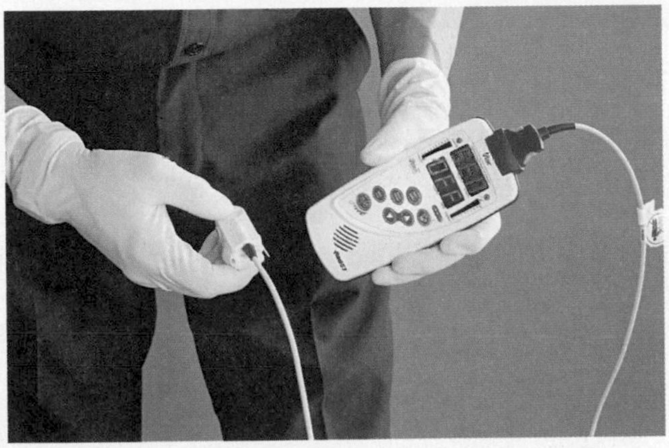

8-1c The pulse CO-oximeter will complete the startup. Prepare the sensor for placement.

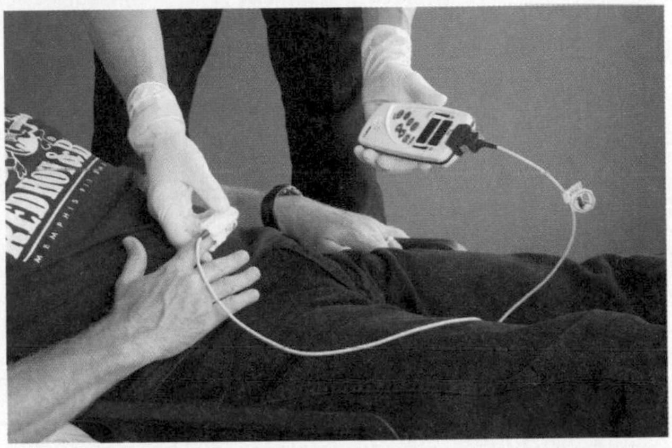

8-1d Place the sensor on the patient's finger. Be sure the sensor is properly placed.

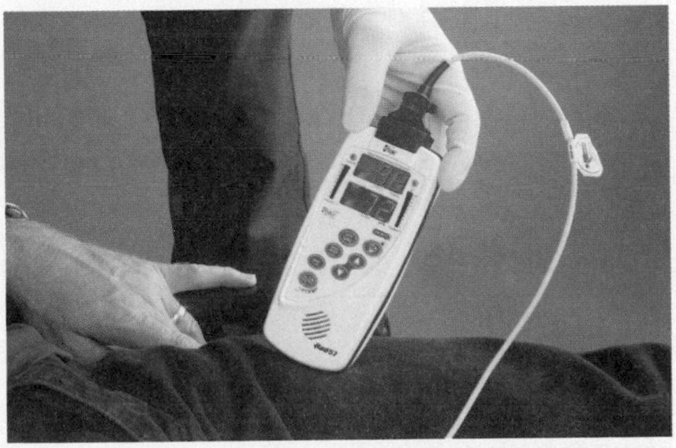

8-1e First, measure the SpO_2 and pulse rate as with any oximeter.

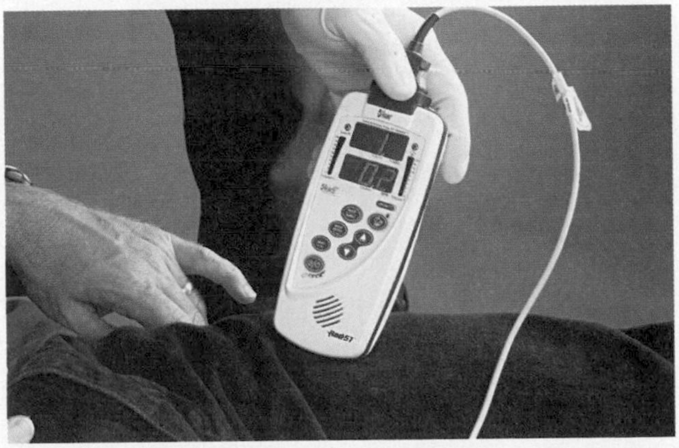

8-1f Then press the SpCO button and measure the SpCO and SpMet (if the unit has a methemoglobin module).

criteria for CO poisoning. CO poisoning can be diagnosed through biological testing when carboxyhemoglobin levels (SpCO) exceed 5 percent in nonsmokers and 10 percent in smokers. At present, there is no environmental test for confirmation of CO poisoning. In addition, the CDC has established diagnostic categories for CO poisoning. These are:

- *Suspected*—There is a potentially exposed person, yet no credible threat.
- *Probable*—There is a clinically compatible case in which a credible threat exists.
- *Confirmed*—There is a clinically compatible case in which biological tests have confirmed exposure.

The treatment of CO poisoning should be based on the severity of symptoms. As a rule, treatment is indicated when the SpCO exceeds 10 to 12 percent. It is important to always be prepared to treat the complications of CO poisoning, such as seizures, cardiac arrhythmias, and cardiac ischemia (Figure 8-7).

After the patient has been removed to a safe area, it is important to begin the administration of high-concentration oxygen. Consider the use of CPAP. This will serve to maximize hemoglobin oxygen saturation. As oxygen levels in the blood increase, some carbon monoxide molecules will be displaced from hemoglobin. Further, studies have shown an improvement in neurologic outcome and cardiac

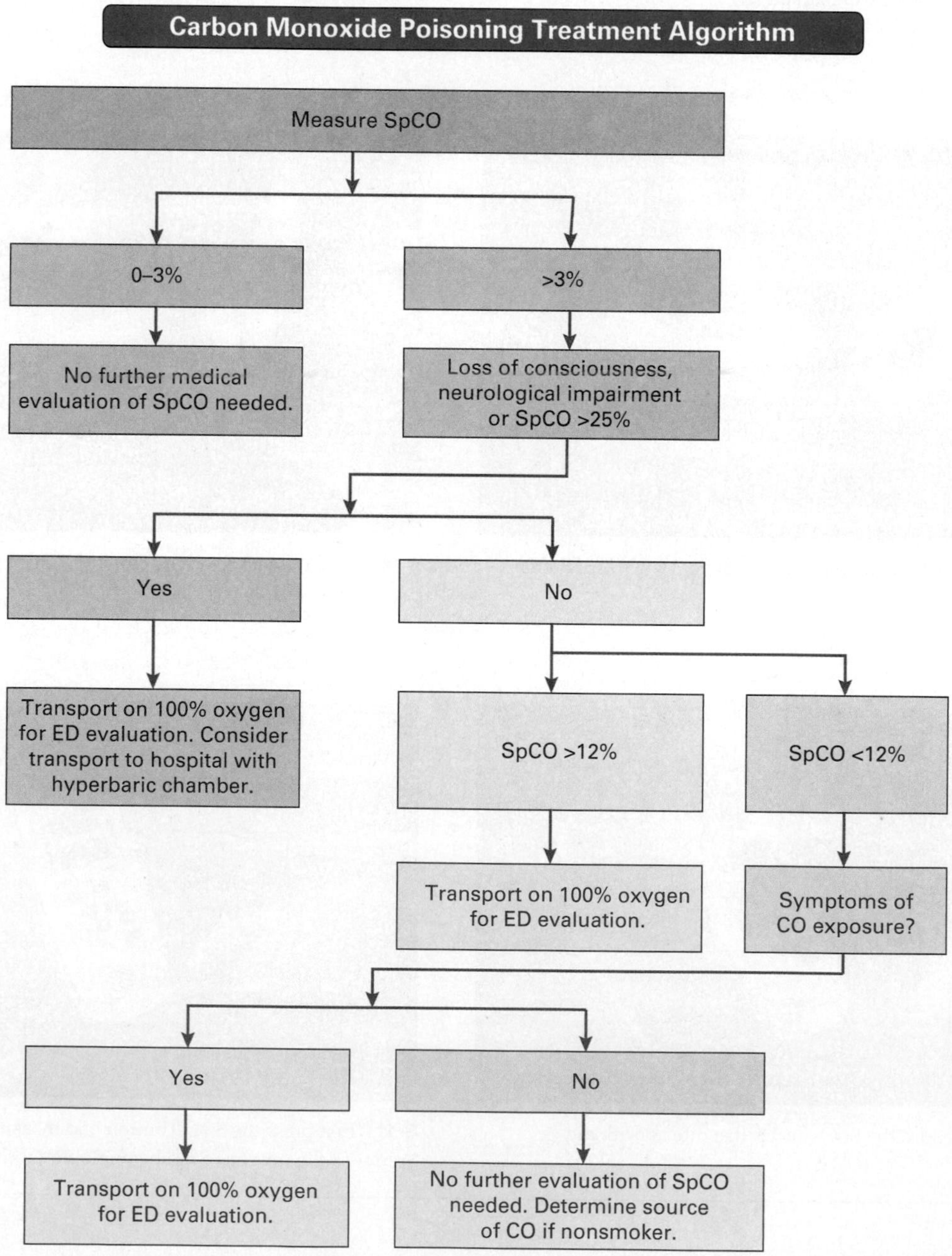

FIGURE 8-7 Diagnosis and treatment algorithm for carbon monoxide poisoning.

complications following early administration of high concentrations of oxygen.

It has been common practice to place patients with moderate to severe CO poisoning in a hyperbaric oxygen (HBO) therapy chamber. This increases the atmospheric pressure around the patient and serves to drive oxygen into the tissues and to fully saturate remaining hemoglobin oxygen-binding sites. There is no significant body of research, however, that demonstrates that patient outcomes are better following HBO therapy.[6] Regardless, it is still commonly used. The benefits of HBO therapy include the alleviation of tissue hypoxia and a reduction in the half-life of carboxyhemoglobin. Normally, the half-life of carboxyhemoglobin is 4 to 6 hours. Through HBO therapy, the effective half-life of carboxyhemoglobin can be decreased to 22 minutes. HBO therapy should be considered for patients who have altered mental status, coma, or focal neurologic deficits; patients who are pregnant and have a carboxyhemoglobin level greater than 15 percent; and patients with a history of a loss of consciousness. HBO therapy should be less strongly considered for patients who exhibit signs or symptoms of cardiovascular compromise or metabolic acidosis, or patients who are at the extremes of age (Figure 8-8).

Treatment and monitoring of the patient with CO exposure should continue on scene and en route to the hospital. It is important to continuously monitor SpO_2 and SpCO levels. ALS providers should obtain a 12-lead ECG and monitor the ECG en route. Always document your findings and plot any trends. It is important to remember that older, first-generation pulse oximeters may give falsely elevated SpO_2 readings in the presence of carbon monoxide poisoning.

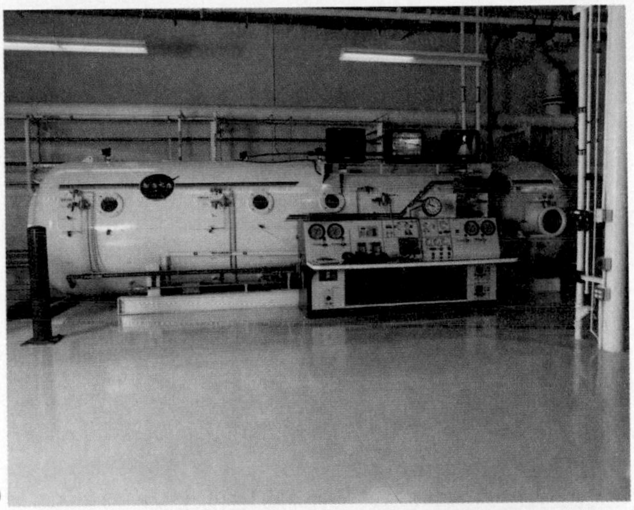

(a)

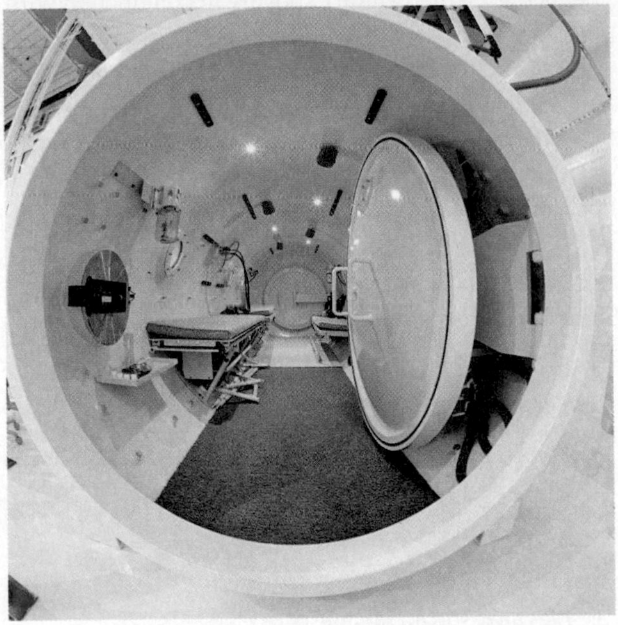

(b)

FIGURE 8-8 Hyperbaric oxygen (HBO) therapy was commonly used for carbon monoxide poisoning although the scientific literature documenting the effectiveness is lacking. Large HBO chambers (a) can be used for multiple patients. Large chambers (b) allow the patient to rest comfortably.

(Both photos: NASA/Johnson Space Center)

Cyanide

Cyanide is a colorless gas that has a faint, bitter-almond smell. However, approximately 40 percent of the population cannot smell cyanide. The cyanide molecule consists of one atom of carbon and one atom of nitrogen held together by a triple bond. The cyanide anion is extremely toxic. Cyanide-containing products are routinely used in some manufacturing processes. However, in these uses cyanide is present as a salt—usually as sodium cyanide or potassium cyanide. Both are white powders.

Hydrogen cyanide is a gaseous product of combustion. High levels of cyanide are found during the combustion of plastics, wool, silk, synthetic rubber, polyurethane, and asphalt. Many of these products are frequently encountered during structural firefighting. The toxicity of cyanide varies by its chemical form. The OSHA permissible level of cyanide is 10 ppm as an 8-hour, time-weighted average. Cyanide can be either ingested or inhaled. Most accidental cyanide exposures result from inhalation of cyanide gas. The ingestion of a cyanide powder is more common with suicide and homicide attempts.

Cyanide is a cellular toxin. It inhibits an enzyme called cytochrome c oxidase (aa_3) that is found in the fourth complex of the electron transport chain. The electron transport chain is found on the shelves (cristae) of the mitochondria in the cells. The mitochondria are organelles primarily responsible for energy production in the cell. The inhibition of cytochrome c oxidase effectively stops energy production (ATP) by the cell. This causes the cell to shift from aerobic metabolism to anaerobic metabolism. When this occurs, energy production by the cell is markedly reduced. The tissues that are most affected by this interruption of electron transport are those that are highly dependent on aerobic metabolism, such as the heart and the central nervous system.[7]

Cyanide can enter the body by a variety of routes. It is present in many commercial and household items that can be either ingested or absorbed—rodenticides, silver polish, and fruit pits and seeds (such as those of apricots, cherries, pears). It also can be inhaled, especially in fires that release cyanide from products containing nitrogen. A roomful of burning plastics, silks, or synthetic carpeting can also be a roomful of cyanide-filled smoke. Cyanide also forms in patients on long-term sodium nitroprusside therapy. Suicidal patients have been known to take cyanide salt. Regardless of the entry route, cyanide is an extremely fast-acting toxin.

Cyanide and Carbon Monoxide

The incidence of cyanide exposure in conjunction with CO poisoning is higher than once thought. Cyanide, like CO, results from the combustion of selected materials. Unfortunately, the effects of CO and cyanide are cumulative. Many times the symptoms of cyanide toxicity are often attributed to CO poisoning because rescuers and medical personnel lack a high index of suspicion for cyanide poisoning.

Signs and Symptoms

Signs and symptoms of cyanide poisoning include:

- Burning sensation in the mouth and throat
- Headache, confusion, combative behavior
- Hypertension and tachycardia followed by hypotension and further arrhythmias
- Seizures and coma
- Pulmonary edema
- Elevated serum lactate

Management

First, safely remove the patient from the source of exposure. To prevent inhalation, always wear breathing equipment when entering the scene of a fire. Initiate supportive measures immediately. For many years, the standard treatment for cyanide poisoning was the Lilly or Pasadena cyanide antidote kit (Figure 8-9). This kit contains amyl nitrite ampules, a sodium nitrite solution, and a sodium thiosulfate solution. The nitrites induce the formation of methemoglobin (MetHb). Cyanide has a greater affinity for methemoglobin than it does for cytochrome oxidase. Thus, the binding of cyanide to methemoglobin frees cytochrome oxidase so that cellular energy production resumes. Amyl nitrite is a volatile gas that can be immediately inhaled while intravenous access is obtained. It should be followed as soon as possible by intravenous sodium nitrite. Finally, sodium thiosulfate should be administered. Sodium thiosulfate binds cyanide, forming thiocyanate. Thiocyanate is considerably less toxic than cyanide and can be excreted through the kidneys.

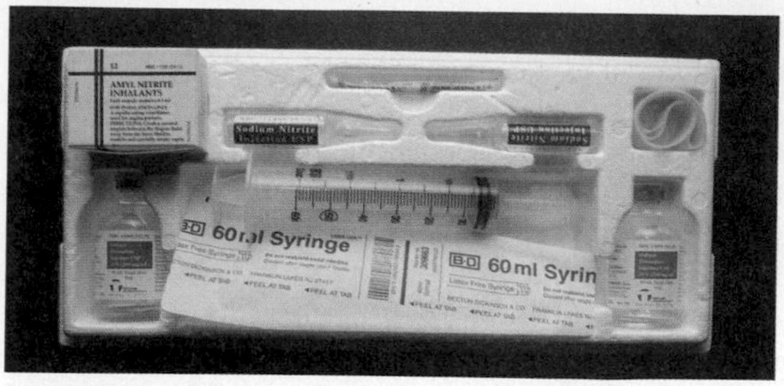

FIGURE 8-9 Cyanide antidote kit.
(© Jeff Forster)

There are, however, several problems associated with the administration of nitrites in CO poisoning. First, and most important, methemoglobin cannot transport oxygen. This occurs because the conversion of hemoglobin to methemoglobin changes the state of the iron on the heme molecule where oxygen binds. Methemoglobin contains iron in the *ferric* (Fe^{3+}) state, whereas hemoglobin contains iron in the *ferrous* (Fe^{2+}) state. Oxygen can bind only to heme that is in the Fe^{2+} state. Thus, concomitant CO poisoning and cyanide poisoning can significantly decrease the oxygen-carrying capacity of the blood when nitrites are administered. The induction of methemoglobinemia by the nitrites, along with the presence of carboxyhemoglobin, can lead to a functional anemia. Children are at particular risk for methemoglobinemia. The signs and symptoms of methemoglobinemia are detailed in Table 8–5. Because of this, sodium nitrite should be avoided in combination CO/cyanide poisonings when the SpCO is greater than 10 percent.

The second antidote available for cyanide poisoning is *hydroxocobalamin*. Hydroxocobalamin is a precursor to cyanocobalamin (vitamin B_{12}). Hydroxocobalamin combines with the cyanide ion (chelates from cytochrome oxidase) to form cyanocobalamin. Vitamin B_{12} is harmless and eliminated through the kidney. Hydroxocobalamin has been used for many years in France as an antidote for cyanide poisoning. In December 2006, it received FDA approval for use in the United States. It is commercially marketed under the name Cyanokit (Figure 8-10).[8]

Because cyanide and CO come from similar combustion sources, firefighters are at particular risk for concomitant

Table 8–5 Signs and Symptoms of Methemoglobinemia

SpMET	Symptoms
1–3%	Normal, asymptomatic
3–15%	Slight grayish-blue skin discoloration
15–20%	Asymptomatic, but cyanotic
20–50%	Headache, dyspnea, confusion, weakness, chest pain
50–70%	Altered mental status, delirium

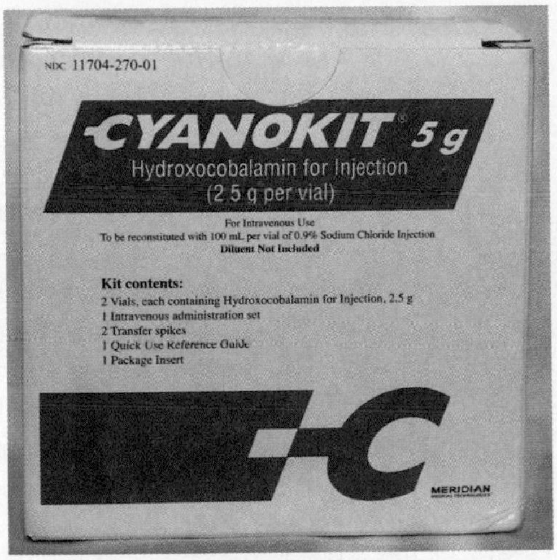

FIGURE 8-10 Cyanokit containing hydroxocobalamin.
(© Dr. Bryan E. Bledsoe)

CO and cyanide poisoning. If dual CO/cyanide poisoning is suspected, hydroxocobalamin should be the preferred antidote. The induction of methemoglobinemia by the nitrites may complicate the already elevated carboxyhemoglobin levels resulting from the CO poisoning. These two factors increase the patient's chances of developing both short-term and long-term complications.

Cardiac Medications

The list of cardiac medications grows almost daily. Many classes of these drugs exist, including antiarrhythmics, beta-blockers, calcium channel blockers, glycosides, and ACE inhibitors. Generally, these medications regulate heart function by decreasing heart rate, suppressing automaticity, and/or reducing vascular tone. Overdoses of these drugs can be intentional but are more often due to errors in dosage.

Signs and Symptoms

In overdose quantities, signs and symptoms of cardiac medication poisoning include:

- Nausea and vomiting
- Headache, dizziness, confusion
- Profound hypotension
- Cardiac arrhythmias (usually bradycardia)
- Heart conduction blocks
- Bronchospasm and pulmonary edema (especially with beta-blockers)

Management

Initiate standard toxicologic emergency assessment and treatment immediately. Be aware that severe bradycardia may not respond well to atropine; therefore, you may need to use an external pacing device. Some cardiac medications do have antidotes that may help with severe adverse effects. These include calcium for calcium channel blockers, glucagon for beta-blockers, and digoxin-specific Fab (Digibind) for digoxin. Contact medical direction before giving these antidotes. The American Association of Poison Control Centers has issued out-of-hospital treatment guidelines for calcium channel blocker poisonings (Figure 8-11) and beta-blocker poisonings (Figure 8-12).[9,10]

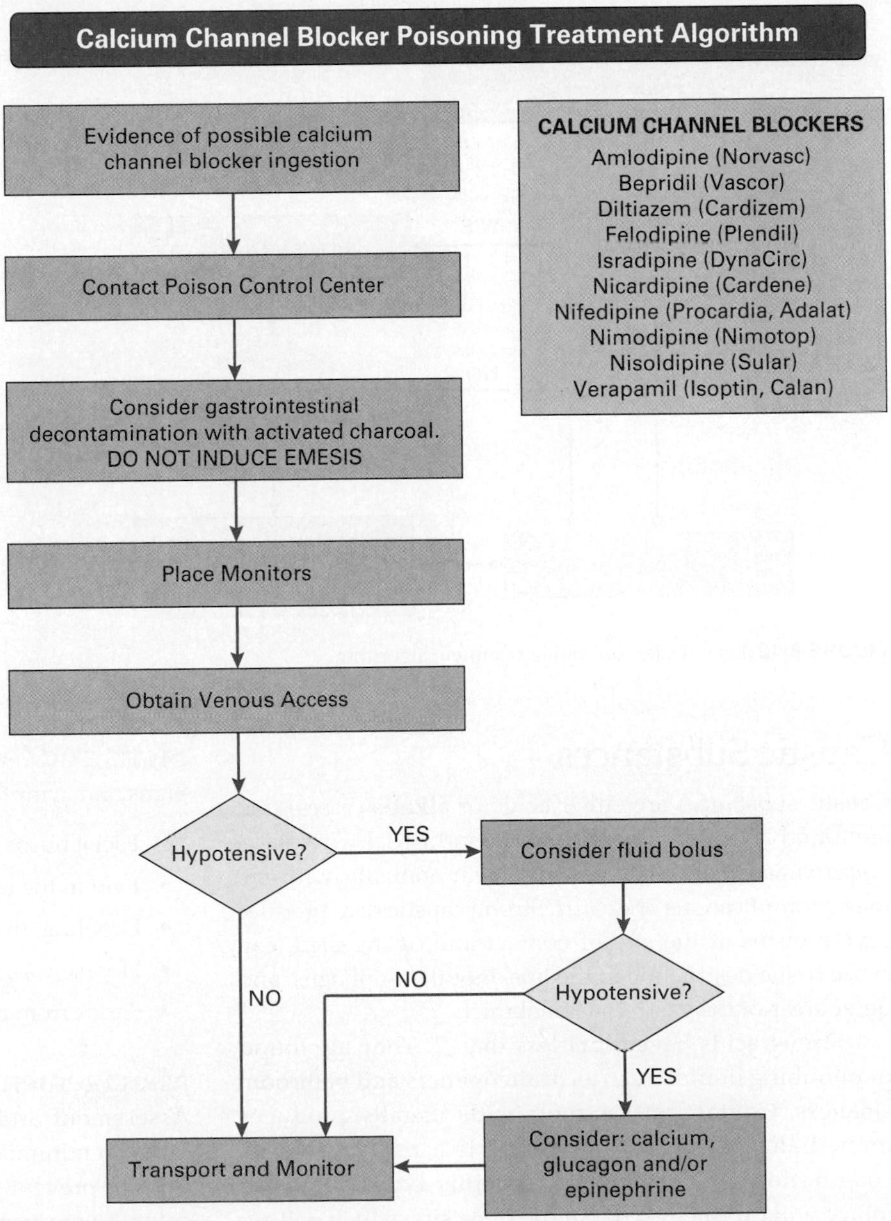

FIGURE 8-11 Calcium channel blocker poisoning treatment algorithm.

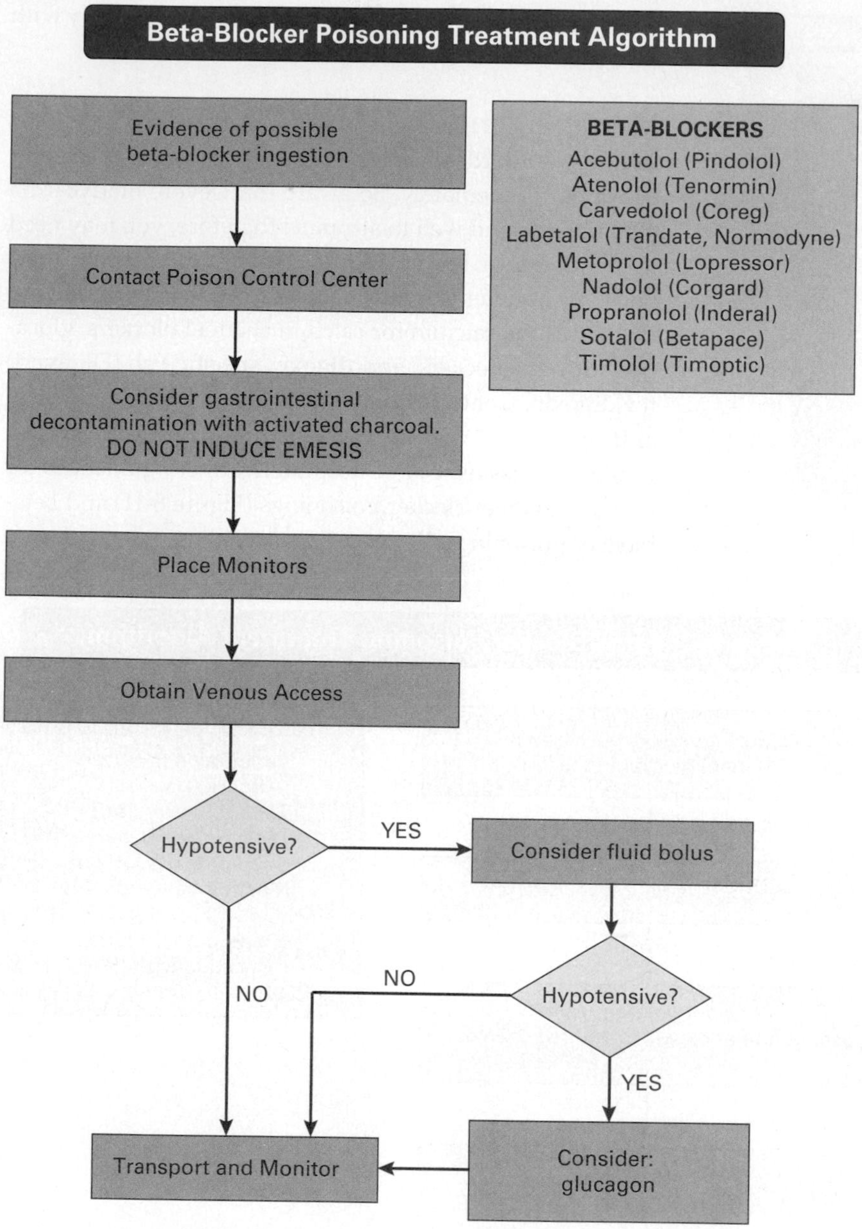

FIGURE 8-12 Beta-blocker poisoning treatment algorithm.

Caustic Substances

Caustic substances are either **acids** or **alkalis** (bases) that are found in both the home and the industrial workplace. Approximately 12,000 exposures occur annually, with 150 major complications or deaths. Strong caustics can produce severe burns at the site of contact and, if ingested, can cause tissue destruction at the lips, mouth, esophagus, and other areas of the gastrointestinal tract.

Strong acids have a pH less than 2. They are found in plumbing liquids such as drain openers and bathroom cleaners. Contact with strong acids usually produces immediate and severe pain. This is a result of tissue coagulation and necrosis. Often this type of contact injury will produce eschar at the burn site, which will act like a shield and prevent further penetration or damage to deeper tissues. If ingested, acids will cause local burns to the mouth and throat. Because of the rapid transit through the esophagus, the esophagus is not usually damaged. More likely, the stomach lining will be injured. Immediate or delayed hemorrhage can occur and may be associated with perforation. Pain is severe and usually due to direct injury and spasm from irritation. Absorption of acids into the vascular system will occur quite readily, causing a significant acidemia, which will need to be managed along with the direct local effects.

Strong alkaline agents typically have a pH greater than 12.5. They can be in solid or liquid form (such as in Drano or Liquid-Plumr) and are routinely found around the house. These agents cause injury by inducing liquefaction necrosis. Pain is often delayed, which allows for longer tissue contact and deeper tissue injury before the exposure is even recognized. Solid alkaline agents can stick to the oropharynx or esophagus. This can cause perforation, bleeding, and inflammation of central chest structures. Liquid alkalis are more likely to injure the stomach because they pass quickly through the esophagus. Within 2 to 3 days of exposure, complete loss of the protective mucosal tissue can occur, followed by either gradual healing and recovery or further bleeding, necrosis, and stricture formation.

Signs and Symptoms

Signs and symptoms of caustic injury include:

- Facial burns
- Pain in the lips, tongue, throat, or gums
- Drooling, trouble swallowing
- Hoarseness, stridor, or shortness of breath
- Shock from bleeding, vomiting

Management

Assessment and intervention must be aggressive and rapid to minimize morbidity and mortality. Take precautions to prevent injury to rescuers. Initiate standard toxicologic emergency assessment and treatment, but pay particular attention to establishing an airway. Injury to the oropharynx and larynx may make airway control and ventilation difficult and may even require cricothyrotomy. Because caustics will not adsorb to activated charcoal, there is no indication to administer it. In the past, rescuers often gave water or milk to dilute any ingested caustics, but there is controversy as to whether this is beneficial. Rapid transport to the emergency department is essential.

Hydrofluoric Acid

Hydrofluoric acid (HF) deserves special attention because it is extremely toxic and can be lethal despite the appearance of only moderate burns on skin contact. HF penetrates deeply into tissues and is inactivated only when it comes in contact with cations such as calcium ion (Ca^{++}). Calcium fluoride is formed by this inactivation and settles in the tissue as a salt. The removal of calcium from cells causes a total disruption of cell functioning and can even cause bone destruction as calcium is leached out of the bones. Death has been reported from exposure of <2.5 percent body surface area to a highly concentrated solution.

Signs and Symptoms

Signs and symptoms of HF acid exposure include:

- Burning at site of contact (Figure 8-13)
- Trouble breathing
- Confusion
- Palpitations
- Muscle cramps

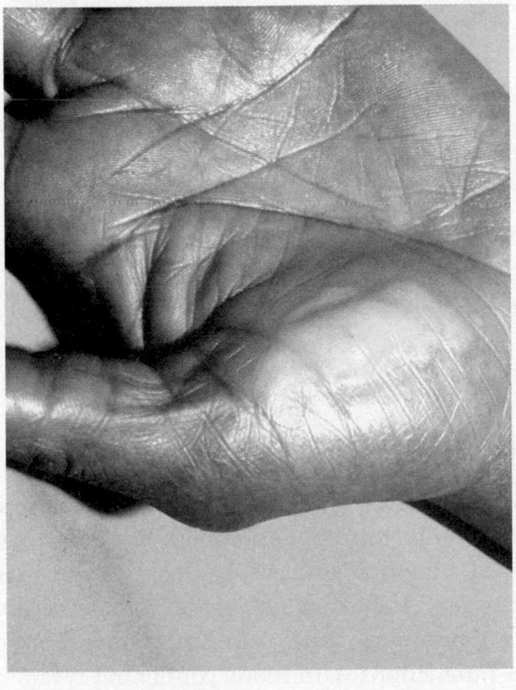

FIGURE 8-13 Hydrofluoric acid burn to left palm. Note green swelling. *(© David Effron, MD)*

Management

Management includes:

- Ensure the safety of rescue personnel.
- Initiate supportive measures.
- Remove exposed clothing.
- Thoroughly irrigate the affected area with water.
- Immerse the affected limb in iced water with magnesium sulfate, calcium salts, or benzethonium chloride.
- Transport immediately for definitive care.

Alcohol

See the section on Alcohol Abuse later in this chapter.

Hydrocarbons

Hydrocarbons are organic compounds of mostly carbon and hydrogen. They include such common recognizable names as kerosene, naphtha, turpentine, mineral oil, chloroform, toluene, and benzene. These chemicals are found in common household products such as lighter fluid, paint, glue, lubricants, solvents, and aerosol propellants. Toxicity from hydrocarbons can occur through any route, including ingestion, inhalation, or surface absorption.

Signs and Symptoms

Signs and symptoms of hydrocarbon poisoning will vary with the type and route of exposure but may include:

- Burns due to local contact
- Wheezing, dyspnea, hypoxia, and pneumonitis from aspiration/inhalation
- Headache, dizziness, slurred speech, ataxia (irregular and difficult-to-control movements), and obtundation (dulled reflexes)
- Foot and wrist drop with numbness and tingling
- Cardiac arrhythmias

Management

Recent studies have shown that very few poisonings with hydrocarbons are serious, and fewer than 1 percent require physician intervention. If you know the exact chemical that the patient has been exposed to and the patient is asymptomatic, medical direction may suggest that the patient can be left at home. On the other hand, a few hydrocarbon poisonings can be very serious. Any patient who is symptomatic, does not know what he has taken, or who has taken a hydrocarbon that requires gastrointestinal decontamination (halogenated or aromatic hydrocarbons) must be treated using standard toxicologic emergency procedures. Because charcoal will not bind hydrocarbons, this may be one of the few cases in which gastric lavage can be useful.

Tricyclic Antidepressants

Tricyclic antidepressants were once commonly used to treat depression. Close monitoring was required because these medications have a narrow **therapeutic index**, meaning that a relatively small increase in dose can quickly lead to toxic effects. The very nature of their use, treating depression, presents a dilemma because the patients most seriously in need of treatment may also be the most likely to attempt to take an overdose. Deaths due to antidepressant overdose have dropped significantly in recent years since the development and rapid acceptance of safer agents unrelated to tricyclics. However, tricyclic antidepressants are still used for various clinical problems, such as chronic pain or migraine prophylaxis, and may still be responsible for more deaths due to intentional overdose than any other medication. Common agents include amitriptyline (Elavil), amoxapine, clomipramine, doxepin, imipramine, and nortriptyline.

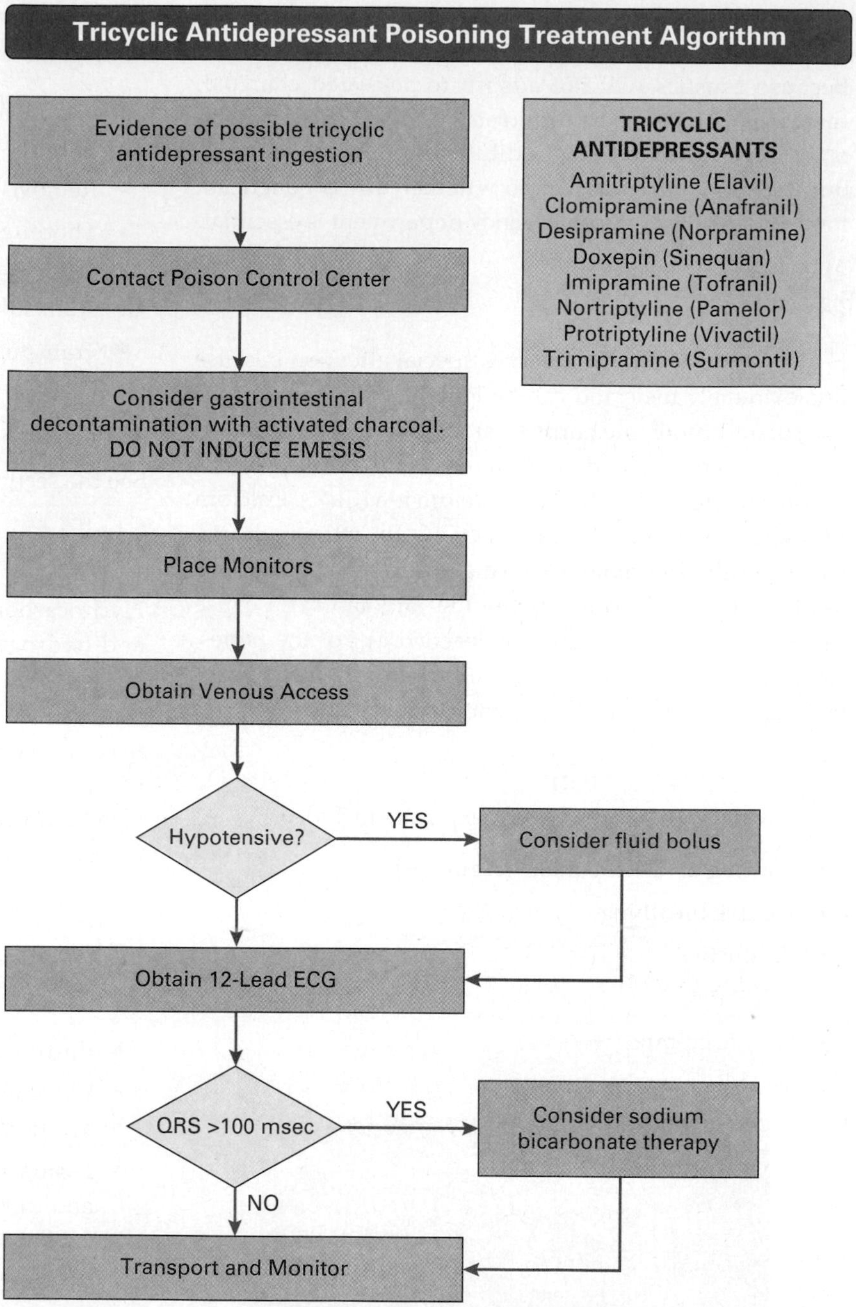

FIGURE 8-14 Tricyclic antidepressant poisoning treatment algorithm.

Signs and Symptoms

Signs and symptoms of tricyclic antidepressant toxicity include:

- Dry mouth
- Blurred vision
- Urinary retention
- Constipation

Late into an overdose, more severe toxicity may produce:

- Confusion, hallucinations
- Hyperthermia
- Respiratory depression
- Seizures
- Tachycardia and hypotension
- Cardiac arrhythmias (heart block, wide QRS, *torsades de pointes*)

Management

Toxicity from tricyclic antidepressants requires immediate initiation of standard toxicologic emergency procedures. Cardiac monitoring is critical, as arrhythmias are the most common cause of death. If you suspect a mixed overdose with benzodiazepines, do *not* use Flumazenil, because it may precipitate seizures. If significant cardiac toxicity occurs, sodium bicarbonate can be used as an additional therapy. Contact medical direction as necessary (Figure 8-14).[11]

MAO Inhibitors

Monoamine oxidase inhibitors (MAOIs) have been used, although rarely, to treat depression. Recently they have been used, on a limited basis, to treat obsessive-compulsive disorders. They are relatively unpopular because of a narrow therapeutic index, multiple-drug interactions, serious interactions with foods containing tyramine (for example, certain red wines and cheeses), and high morbidity and mortality when taken in overdose. These drugs inhibit the breakdown of neurotransmitters such as norepinephrine and dopamine while increasing the availability of the components needed to make even more neurotransmitters. When taken in overdose, MAOIs can be extremely dangerous, although symptoms may not appear for up to 6 hours.

Signs and Symptoms

Signs and symptoms of MAOI overdose include:

- Headache, agitation, restlessness, tremor
- Nausea
- Palpitations
- Tachycardia
- Severe hypertension
- Hyperthermia
- Eventually, bradycardia, hypotension, coma, and death

New MAOIs have recently entered the marketplace. These next-generation drugs are reversible, less toxic, and do not have the same reactions with food as the older MAOIs. Data are not yet available on the outcome of patients overdosing with these newer agents.

Management

No antidote exists for MAOI overdose because the inhibition is not reversible, except with newer drugs. Therefore, institute standard toxicologic emergency procedures as soon as possible. If necessary, give symptomatic support for seizures and hyperthermia using benzodiazepines. If vasopressors are needed, use norepinephrine.

Newer Antidepressants

In recent years, several new agents have been developed to treat depression. Because of their high safety profile in therapeutic and overdose amounts, these drugs have been widely accepted and have virtually replaced tricyclic antidepressants.

Recently introduced drugs include trazodone (Desyrel), bupropion (Wellbutrin), and the large group of popular selective serotonin reuptake inhibitors, or SSRIs (Prozac, Luvox, Paxil, Zoloft). SSRIs prevent the reuptake of serotonin in the brain, theoretically making it more available for brain functions. The true mechanism by which these drugs treat depression is unclear.

Signs and Symptoms

When the newer antidepressants are taken in overdose, the signs and symptoms are usually mild. Occasionally, trazodone and bupropion will cause CNS depression and seizures, but deaths are rare and have been reported only in mixed overdoses with multiple ingestions. More commonly, signs and symptoms of overdose with the newer antidepressant agents include:

- Drowsiness
- Tremor
- Nausea and vomiting
- Sinus tachycardia

Serotonin Syndrome

Overdose of SSRIs can sometimes result in *serotonin syndrome*. Serotonin syndrome is a clinical syndrome that manifests as autonomic instability, altered mental status, seizures, extrapyramidal syndrome including muscle rigidity, hyperthermia, and, rarely, death. The onset of serotonin syndrome is usually within 6 hours of ingestion, with an increasing severity of clinical findings. Serotonin syndrome appears to be due, in large part, to excessive stimulation of the serotonin receptors in the nervous system. Drug interactions are also commonly implicated in serotonin syndrome. Although not exclusively related to interactions with SSRIs, drugs that can interact with SSRIs to cause serotonin syndrome include monoamine oxidase inhibitors, meperidine (Demerol), dextromethorphan, lithium, clonazepam, methylenedioxymethamphetamine (MDMA, Ecstasy), and the dietary supplements tryptophan and St. John's wort.

The signs and symptoms of serotonin syndrome can develop rapidly, often occurring within minutes after ingestion or a change in medication. The symptoms of serotonin syndrome are diverse.

- *Mild symptoms of serotonin syndrome* may include tachycardia, shivering, diaphoresis, mydriasis, intermittent tremor or myoclonus, and overactive or hyperactive reflexes.
- *Moderate symptoms of serotonin syndrome* include abnormalities such as hypertension and hyperthermia; a temperature greater than 40°C (104°F) is common in moderate intoxication. In addition to the mild symptoms, other symptoms may include hyperactive bowel sounds. The hyperactive reflexes and clonus in moderate cases may be greater in the lower limbs than in the upper limbs. Mental status changes include hypervigilance and agitation.
- *Severe symptoms of serotonin syndrome* include severe hypertension and tachycardia that may eventually lead to shock. With severe cases, agitated (excited) delirium, as well as muscular rigidity and high muscular tension, may be seen. Other abnormalities include metabolic acidosis, rhabdomyolysis, seizures, renal failure, and disseminated intravascular coagulation.

The symptoms of serotonin syndrome are often described as a clinical triad of abnormalities:

- *Cognitive effects:* confusion, hypomania, hallucinations, agitation, headache, coma
- *Autonomic effects:* shivering, sweating, fever, hypertension, tachycardia, nausea, diarrhea
- *Somatic effects:* myoclonus/clonus (muscle twitching), hyperreflexia, tremor

Management

Overdose with these new antidepressants is not as life threatening as with previous agents, unless other drugs or alcohol are taken simultaneously. Consequently, treat overdoses with the standard toxicologic emergency procedures. Also have the patient discontinue all serotonergic drugs and implement supportive measures. Benzodiazepines occasionally are used to improve patient comfort, but these are rarely given in the field. Beware of serotonin syndrome and prepare to treat accordingly (Figure 8-15).[12]

Lithium

In the treatment of bipolar (manic-depressive) disorder, no other drug has been proven to be more effective than lithium. It is unclear how lithium exerts its therapeutic effect. However, like tricyclic antidepressants, lithium has a narrow therapeutic index that results in toxicity during normal use and in overdose situations.

Signs and Symptoms

Signs and symptoms of lithium toxicity include:

- Thirst, dry mouth
- Tremor, muscle twitching, increased reflexes
- Confusion, stupor, seizures, coma
- Nausea, vomiting, diarrhea
- Bradycardia, arrhythmias

Management

Treat lithium overdose with mostly supportive measures. Use the standard toxicologic emergency procedures, but remember that activated charcoal will not bind lithium and need not be given. Alkalinizing the urine with sodium bicarbonate and osmotic diuresis using mannitol may increase elimination of lithium, but severe toxic cases require hemodialysis.

Salicylates

Salicylates are some of the more common drugs taken in overdose, largely due to the fact that they are readily available over the counter. The most recognizable forms are aspirin, oil of wintergreen, and some prescription combination medications.

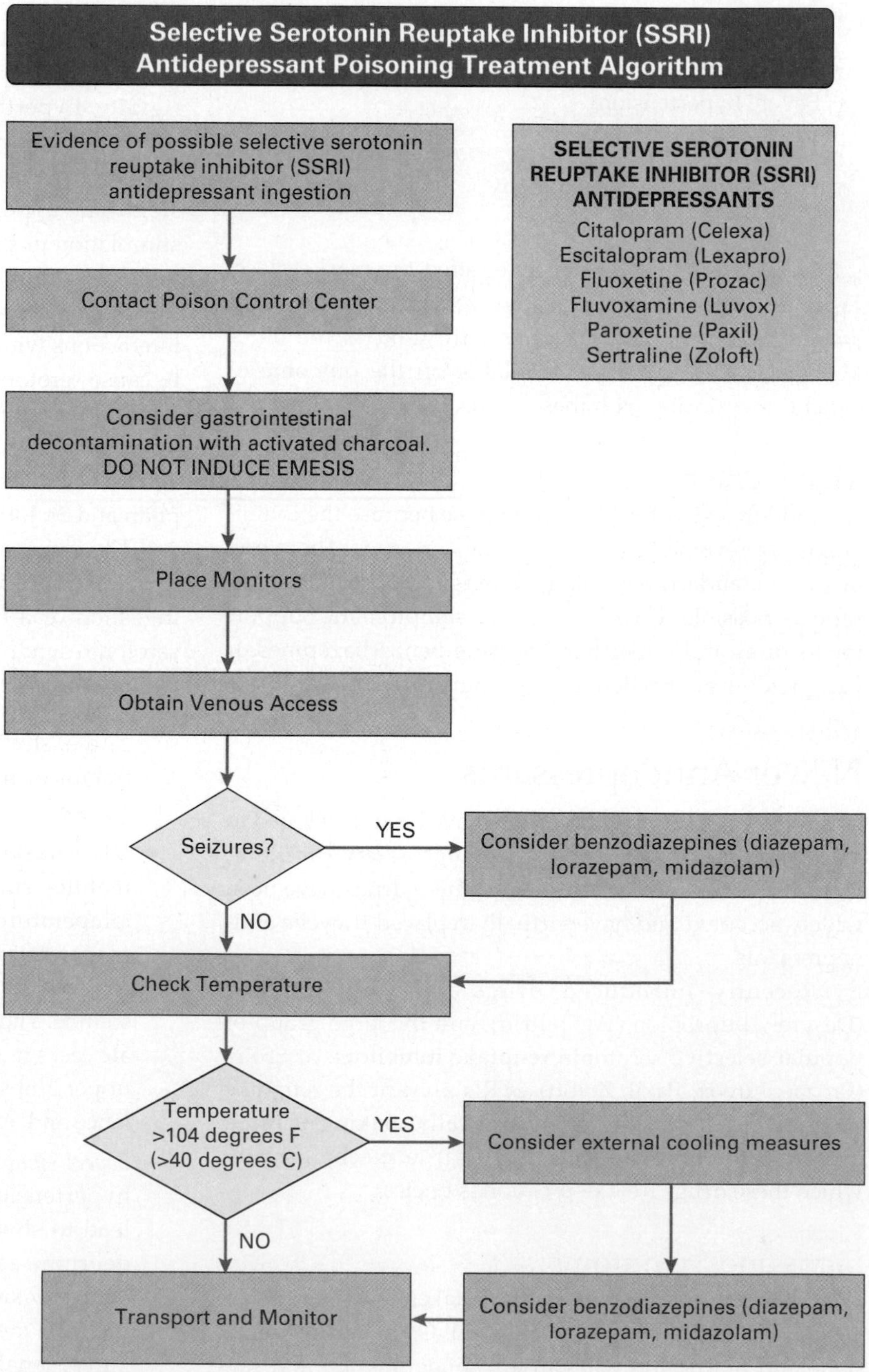

FIGURE 8-15 Selective serotonin reuptake inhibitor (SSRI) poisoning treatment algorithm.

Aspirin in large doses can cause serious consequences. About 300 mg/kg is required to cause toxicity. In such amounts, salicylates inhibit normal energy production and acid buffering in the body. This results in a metabolic acidosis, which further injures other organ systems.

Signs and Symptoms

Signs and symptoms of salicylate overdose include:

- Rapid respirations
- Hyperthermia
- Confusion, lethargy, coma
- Cardiac failure, arrhythmias
- Abdominal pain, vomiting, hematemesis
- Pulmonary edema, adult respiratory distress syndrome (ARDS)

Chronic overdose symptoms are somewhat less severe and do not tend to include abdominal complaints. It is difficult to distinguish chronic overdose from very early acute overdose or early overdose that has progressed past the abdominal irritation stage.

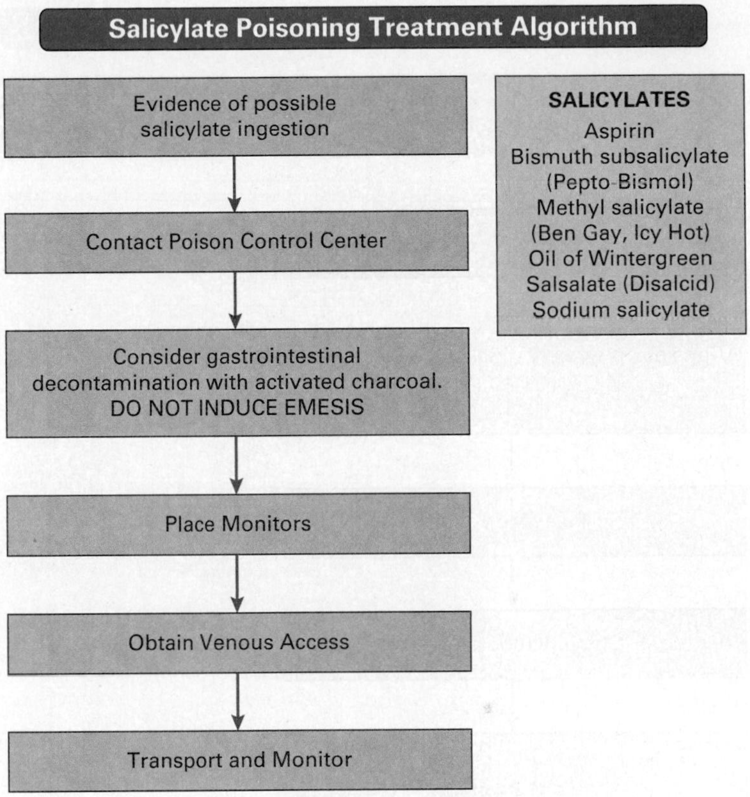

FIGURE 8-16 Salicylate poisoning treatment algorithm.

Management

In all cases, salicylate poisoning should be treated using standard toxicologic emergency procedures. Activated charcoal definitely reduces drug absorption and should be used. If possible, find out the time of ingestion, as blood levels measured at the right time can indicate the expected degree of injury. Most symptomatic patients will require generous IV fluids. Severe cases may require dialysis (Figure 8-16).[13]

Acetaminophen

Because of its few side effects in normal dosages, acetaminophen (e.g., paracetamol, Tylenol) is one of the most common drugs in use today. It is used to treat fever and/or pain and is a common ingredient in hundreds of over-the-counter preparations. It also can be obtained by prescription in combination with various other drugs.

In large doses, however, acetaminophen can be very dangerous. A dose of 150 mg/kg is considered toxic and may result in death due to injury to the liver. A highly reactive byproduct of acetaminophen metabolism is responsible for most adverse effects, but this is usually avoided by the body's detoxification system. When large amounts of acetaminophen enter the system, the detoxification system is overwhelmed and gradually depleted, leaving the toxic metabolite in the circulation to cause hepatic necrosis.

Signs and Symptoms

Signs and symptoms of acetaminophen toxicity appear in four stages.

Stage 1	½ hour to 24 hours	Nausea, vomiting, weakness, fatigue
Stage 2	24 to 48 hours	Abdominal pain, decreased urine, elevated liver enzymes
Stage 3	72 to 96 hours	Liver function disruption
Stage 4	4 to 14 days	Gradual recovery or progressive liver failure

Management

Treat acetaminophen overdose with standard toxicologic emergency procedures. Find out the time of ingestion, as blood levels taken at the right time can predict the potential for injury. An antidote called N-acetylcysteine (NAC, Mucomyst) is available and highly effective. However, NAC is usually administered based on clinical and laboratory studies and is rarely given in the prehospital setting. Cimetidine (Tagamet) has been proposed as an antidote for acetaminophen toxicity, although the literature on the effectiveness is inconclusive (Figure 8-17).[14]

Other Nonprescription Pain Medications

Nonsteroidal anti-inflammatory drugs (NSAIDs) are another group of medications that are readily available and

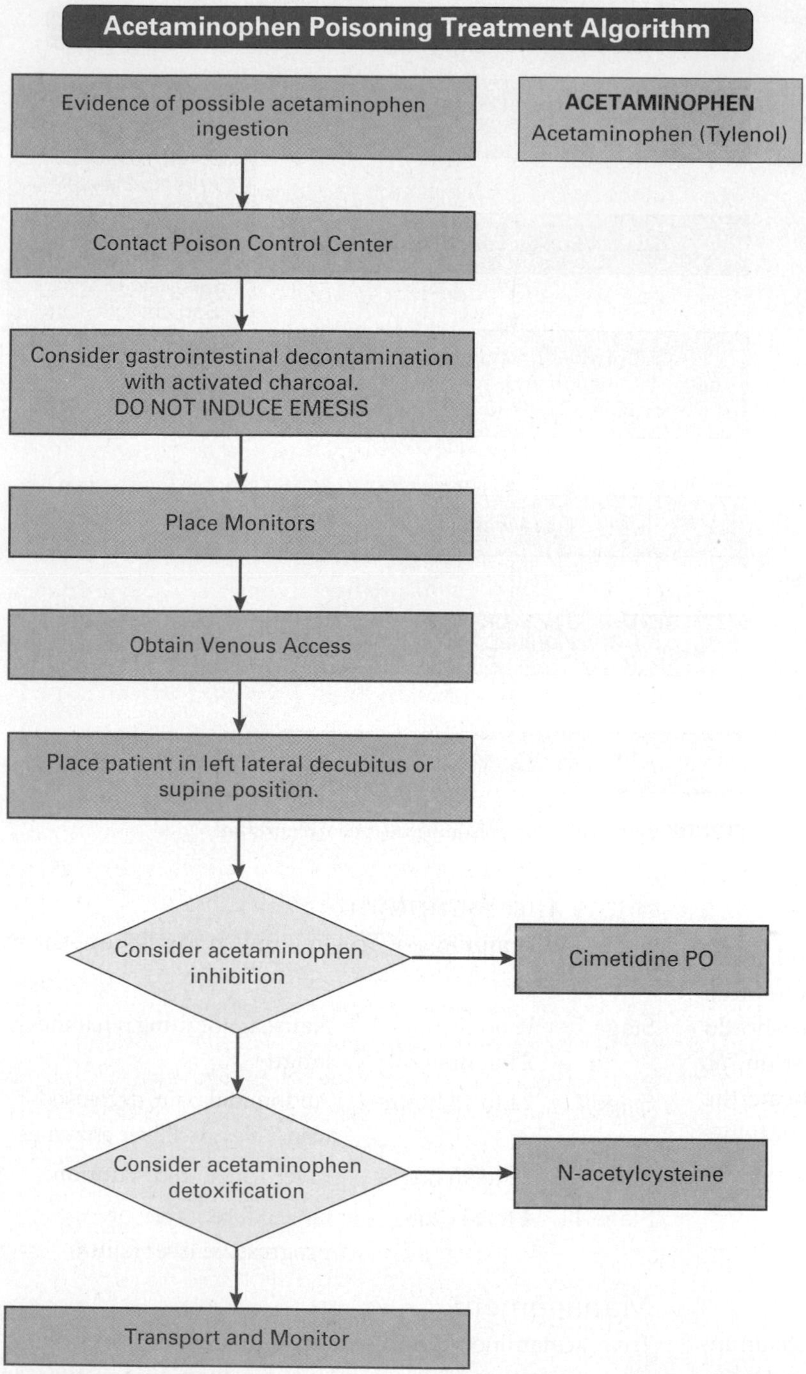

FIGURE 8-17 Acetaminophen poisoning treatment algorithm.

are often overdosed. Common examples include naproxen sodium, indomethacin, ibuprofen, and ketorolac (Toradol).

Signs and Symptoms

The presentation of toxicity caused by NSAIDs varies greatly, but can include:

- Headache
- Ringing in the ears (tinnitus)
- Nausea, vomiting, abdominal pain
- Swelling of the extremities
- Mild drowsiness
- Dyspnea, wheezing, pulmonary edema
- Rash, itching

Management

There is no specific antidote for NSAID toxicity. Use general overdose procedures, including supportive care, as soon as possible and transport the patient to the emergency department for observation and any necessary symptomatic treatment.

Theophylline

Theophylline belongs to a group of medications called *xanthines*. It is occasionally used for patients with asthma or COPD because of its moderate bronchodilation and mild anti-inflammatory effects. Like other drugs with a narrow therapeutic index and high toxicity, theophylline has become less popular recently and therefore is not implicated in as many overdose injuries as in the past.

Signs and Symptoms

Symptoms of theophylline toxicity include:

- Agitation
- Tremors
- Seizures
- Cardiac arrhythmias
- Nausea and vomiting

Management

Theophylline can cause significant morbidity and mortality. In overdose situations, it is essential that you institute toxicologic emergency procedures immediately. In fact, theophylline is on the small list of drugs that have significant *enterohepatic circulation*. This means that multiple doses of activated charcoal over time will continuously remove more and more of the drug from the body. Treat any arrhythmias according to ACLS procedures.

Metals

With the exception of iron, overdose of heavy metals is a rare occurrence. Other possible involved metals include lead, arsenic, and mercury. All metals affect numerous enzyme systems within the body and therefore present with a variety of symptoms. Some also have direct local effects when ingested and when accumulated in various organs.

Iron

The body requires only small amounts of iron on a daily basis to maintain a sufficient store for enzyme and hemoglobin production. Excess amounts are easily obtained from nonprescription supplements and multivitamins. Children have a tendency to accidentally overdose on iron by taking too many candy-flavored chewable vitamins containing iron. To determine the amount of iron ingested, calculate the amount of elemental iron present in the type of pill ingested. Symptoms occur when more than 20 mg/kg of elemental iron are ingested.

SIGNS AND SYMPTOMS Excess iron will cause gastrointestinal injury and possible shock from hemorrhage, especially if it forms *concretions* (lumps of iron formed when tablets fuse together after being swallowed). Patients with significant iron ingestions will often have visible tablets or concretions in the stomach or small intestine on X-ray. Other signs and symptoms of iron ingestion include:

- Vomiting (often hematemesis), diarrhea
- Abdominal pain, shock
- Liver failure
- Metabolic acidosis with tachypnea
- Eventual bowel scarring and possible obstruction

MANAGEMENT It is essential to initiate standard toxicologic emergency procedures immediately. Because iron tends to inhibit gastrointestinal motility, pills sit longer in the stomach and may possibly be easier to remove through gastric lavage. Because activated charcoal will not bind iron (or any metals), it should not be used. Deferoxamine, a chelating agent, may be used in iron overdose as an antidote, as it binds to iron so that less is moved into cells and tissues to cause damage.[15]

Lead and Mercury

Both lead and mercury are heavy metals found in varying amounts in the environment. Lead was often used in glazes and paints before the toxic potential of such exposure became apparent. Mercury is a contaminant from industrial processing but is also found in thermometers and temperature-control switches in most homes. Chronic and acute exposures are possible with both metals.

SIGNS AND SYMPTOMS Signs and symptoms of heavy metal toxicity include:

- Headache, irritability, confusion, coma
- Memory disturbance
- Tremor, weakness, agitation
- Abdominal pain

MANAGEMENT Chronic poisoning can cause permanent neurologic injury, which makes it imperative that the proper agencies monitor heavy metal levels in the environment of a patient who has presented with toxicity. Learn to recognize the signs of heavy metal toxicity and institute standard toxicologic emergency procedures as needed. Activated charcoal will not bind heavy metals, but various chelating agents (DMSA, BAL, CDE) are available and may be used in definitive management in the hospital.

Contaminated Food

Food poisoning is caused by a spectrum of different factors. For example, bacteria, viruses, and toxic chemicals notoriously produce varying levels of gastrointestinal distress. The patient may present with nausea, vomiting, diarrhea, and diffuse abdominal pain.

Bacterial food poisonings range in severity. Bacterial **exotoxins** (secreted by bacteria) or **enterotoxins** (exotoxins associated with gastrointestinal diseases, including food poisoning) cause the adverse GI complaints noted previously. Food contaminated with other bacteria, such as *Shigella, Salmonella,* or *E. coli*, can produce even more severe gastrointestinal reactions, often leading to electrolyte imbalance and hypovolemia. *Clostridium botulinum,* the world's most toxic poison, presents as severe respiratory distress or arrest. The incubation of this toxin can range from 4 hours to 8 days. Fortunately, botulism rarely occurs, except in cases of improper food storage methods such as canning.

A variety of seafood poisonings are a result of specific toxins found in dinoflagellate-contaminated shellfish such as clams, mussels, oysters, and scallops and can produce a syndrome referred to as *paralytic shellfish poisoning.* This condition can lead to respiratory arrest in addition to standard gastrointestinal symptoms.

Increased fish consumption by North Americans has also increased the number of cases of poisonings from toxins found in many commonly eaten fish. *Ciguatera (bony fish) poisoning* most frequently turns up in fish caught in the Pacific Ocean or along the tropical reefs of Florida and the West Indies. Ciguatera normally takes 2 to 6 hours to incubate and may produce myalgia and paresthesia. *Scombroid (histamine) poisoning* results from bacterial contamination of mackerel, tuna, bonitos, and albacore. Both types of poisoning cause the common gastrointestinal symptoms. Scombroid poisoning will present with an immediate facial flushing, as histamines cause vasodilation.

Signs and Symptoms

As mentioned, signs and symptoms of food poisoning may include:

- Nausea, vomiting, diarrhea, abdominal pain
- Facial flushing, respiratory distress (with some seafood poisonings)

Management

Except for botulism, food poisoning is rarely life threatening. Treatment, therefore, is largely supportive. In suspected cases of food poisoning, contact poison control and medical direction, and take the following steps:

- Perform the necessary assessment.
- Collect samples of the suspected contaminated food source.
- Perform the following management actions:
  - Establish and maintain the airway.
  - Administer high-concentration oxygen initially.
  - Intubate and assist ventilations, if appropriate.
  - Establish venous access.
- Consider the administration of antihistamines (especially in seafood poisonings) and antiemetics.

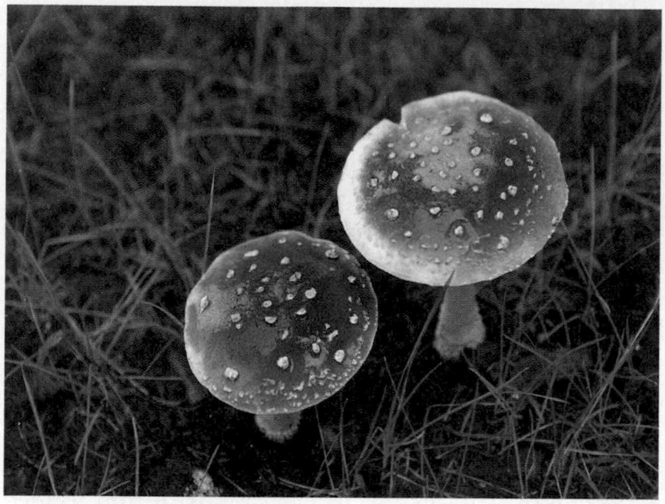

FIGURE 8-18 Poisonous *Amanita* mushrooms.
(Steve Hillebrand/U.S. Fish and Wildlife Service)

Poisonous Plants and Mushrooms

Plants, trees, and mushrooms contribute heavily to the number of accidental toxic ingestions. Although the vast majority of plants are nontoxic, many of the popular decorative houseplants can present a danger to children, who frequently ingest nonfood items. Most poison control centers distribute pamphlets that identify toxic household plants. (These pamphlets will help "poison proof" the home.)

It is impossible to cover all the toxic plants and mushrooms. Few rescuers are trained as botanists, and they find it difficult to identify the offending material. Mushrooms are particularly difficult to identify from small pieces. Additionally, most people recognize mushrooms and other plants by common names rather than by the nomenclature of scientific species. A general approach is to obtain a sample of the plant, if possible. Try to find a full leaf, stem, and any flowers.

Because many ornamental plants contain irritating chemicals or crystals, examine the patient's mouth and throat for redness, blistering, or edema. Identify other abnormal signs during the physical exam.

Mushroom poisonings generally fall into two categories: people seeking edible mushrooms and accidental ingestions by children. Fortunately, few of the many mushroom species possess extremely dangerous toxins. Toxic mushrooms fall into seven classes. *Amanita* and *Galerina* belong to the deadly cyclopeptide group. *Amanita* accounts for more than 90 percent of all deaths (Figure 8-18). These mushrooms produce a poison that is extremely toxic to the liver, with a mortality rate of about 50 percent.

Signs and Symptoms

Signs and symptoms of poisonous plant ingestion include:

- Excessive salivation, lacrimation (secretion of tears), diaphoresis
- Abdominal cramps, nausea, vomiting, diarrhea
- Decreasing levels of consciousness, eventually progressing to coma

Management

For guidance on the treatment of plant poisonings, call the poison control center. If contact cannot be made, use the procedures outlined for treatment of food poisoning.

Injected Toxins

Although we generally think of intentional or accidental drug overdoses as sources of injected poisons, the most common source for these poisonings is the animal kingdom. Bites and stings from a variety of insects, reptiles, and animals are among the most common injuries sustained by humans. Further injury can result from bacterial contamination or from a reaction produced by an injected substance.

General Principles of Management

The general principles of field management for bites and stings include the following:

- Protect rescue personnel—the offending organism may still be around.
- Remove the patient from danger of repeated injection, especially in the case of yellow jackets, wasps, or hornets.
- If possible, identify the insect, reptile, or animal that caused the injury and bring it to the emergency department along with the patient (if it can be done safely).

CONTENT REVIEW

- ➤ Bites and Stings
  - Insect stings
  - Africanized honeybees
  - Brown recluse spider bites
  - Black widow spider bites
  - Scorpion stings

- Perform a primary assessment and rapid physical exam.
- Prevent or delay further absorption of the poison.
- Initiate supportive measures as indicated.
- Watch for anaphylactic reaction (see the chapter "Immunology").
- Transport the patient as rapidly as possible.
- Contact the poison control center and medical direction according to local protocols.

Bites and Stings

Insect Stings

Many people die from allergic reactions to the stings from an order of insects known as *Hymenoptera.* As mentioned earlier, *Hymenoptera* includes wasps, bees, hornets, and ants. Only the common honeybee leaves a stinger. Wasps, yellow jackets, hornets, and fire ants sting repeatedly until they are removed from contact.

In most cases of insect bite, local treatment is all that is necessary. Unless an allergic reaction occurs, most patients will tolerate the isolated *Hymenoptera* sting.

SIGNS AND SYMPTOMS Signs and symptoms include:

- Localized pain
- Redness
- Swelling
- Skin wheals

Idiosyncratic reactions to the toxin may occur, resulting in a progressing localized swelling and edema. This is not an allergic reaction, however, if it responds well to an antihistamine such as diphenhydramine hydrochloride. The major problem resulting from a *Hymenoptera* sting is an allergic reaction or anaphylaxis. Signs and symptoms of allergic reaction include the following:

- Localized pain, redness, swelling, and a skin wheal
- Itching or flushing of the skin, rash
- Tachycardia, hypotension, bronchospasm, or laryngeal edema
- Facial edema, uvular swelling

MANAGEMENT For *Hymenoptera* stings, take the following supportive measures:

- Wash the area.
- Gently remove the stinger, if present, by scraping without squeezing the venom sac.
- Apply cool compresses to the injection site.
- Observe for and treat allergic reactions and/or anaphylaxis (see the chapter "Immunology").

Africanized Honeybees

Africanized honeybees (AHBs), also referred to as "Africanized bees" or "killer bees," are descendants of southern African bees imported in 1956 by Brazilian scientists attempting to breed a honeybee better adapted to the South American tropics. Some of these bees escaped quarantine in 1957 and began breeding with local Brazilian honeybees. The resultant bees multiplied quickly and extended their range throughout South and Central America at a rate greater than 200 miles per year. In the past decade, AHBs began invading North America, primarily through south Texas. The bees have spread across the southwestern United States and into California (Figure 8-19).

Africanized bees acquired the name "killer bees" because they will viciously attack people and animals that unwittingly stray into their territory, often resulting in serious injury or death. Only a minimal disturbance is necessary to cause an AHB attack. Although all honeybees respond to threats to their colonies, AHBs respond more quickly and in much greater numbers than do European honeybees. In comparison to European honeybees, greater numbers of AHBs will pursue intruders for much greater

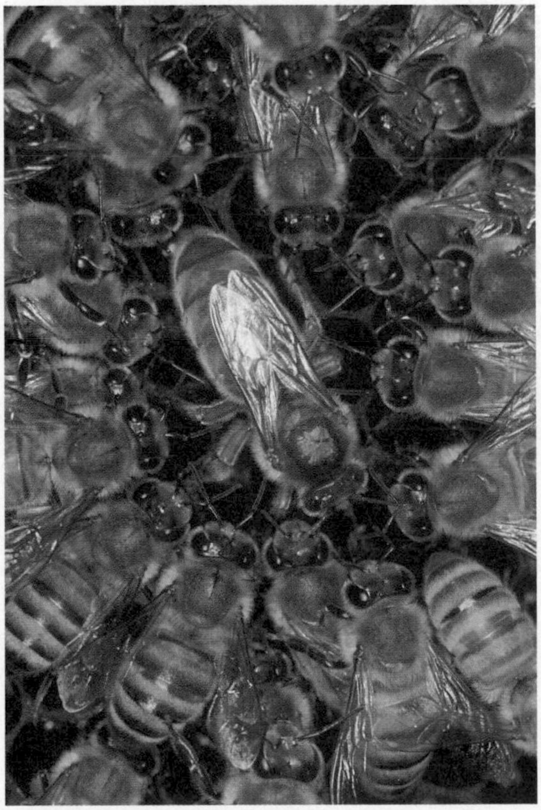

FIGURE 8-19 Africanized honeybees *(Apis mellifera).*

(USDA photo by Scott Bauer)

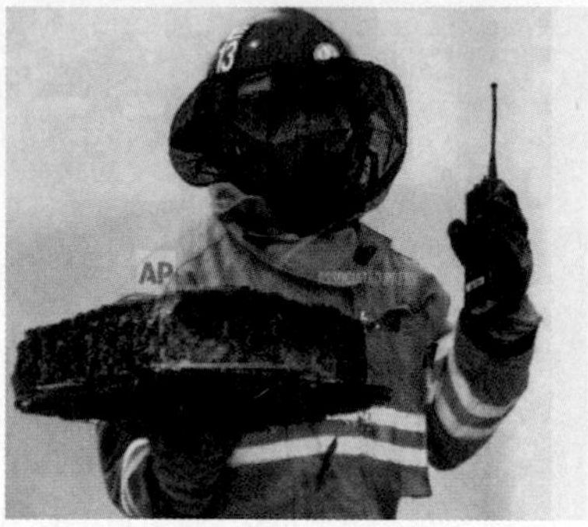

FIGURE 8-20 Firefighting foam as a repellant for Africanized honeybees.

(© Chris Richards—Arizona Daily Star/AP Images)

distances. Recent research reported that three to four times as many AHBs responded and left eight to ten times more stings than their European counterparts.

AHBs pose a particular risk for firefighters and EMS personnel. Heavy turnout gear can provide good protection as long as a properly fitting bee veil is also used. Hazardous material suits can also be used. AHBs can be immobilized and killed with wetting agents (surfactants), including commercial dishwashing detergents (Figure 8-20).[16]

Brown Recluse Spider Bites

The brown recluse spider lives in the southern and midwestern states. It is found in large numbers in Tennessee, Arkansas, Oklahoma, and Texas. It has also been reported in Hawaii and California.

The brown recluse is about 15 mm in length. It generally lives in dark, dry locations and can often be found in and around the house. There is a characteristic violin-shaped marking on the back, giving the spider its nickname, "fiddleback spider" (Figure 8-21). Another identifying feature is the presence of six eyes (three pairs in a semicircle), instead of the eight eyes common to most spiders.

SIGNS AND SYMPTOMS Brown recluse spider bites are usually painless. Not uncommonly, bites occur at night while the patient sleeps. Most victims are unaware that they have been bitten until the local reaction starts. Initially, a small erythematous macule surrounded by a white ring forms at the site (Figure 8-22). This usually appears within a few minutes of the bite. Over the next 8 hours, localized pain, redness, and swelling develop. Tissue necrosis at the site occurs over days to weeks (Figure 8-23). Other symptoms include chills, fever, nausea and vomiting, joint pain, and, in severe situations, bleeding disorders (disseminated intravascular coagulation).

MANAGEMENT Treatment is mostly supportive. Because there is no antivenin, the emergency department treatment consists of antihistamines to reduce systemic reactions and possible surgical excision of necrotic tissue.[17]

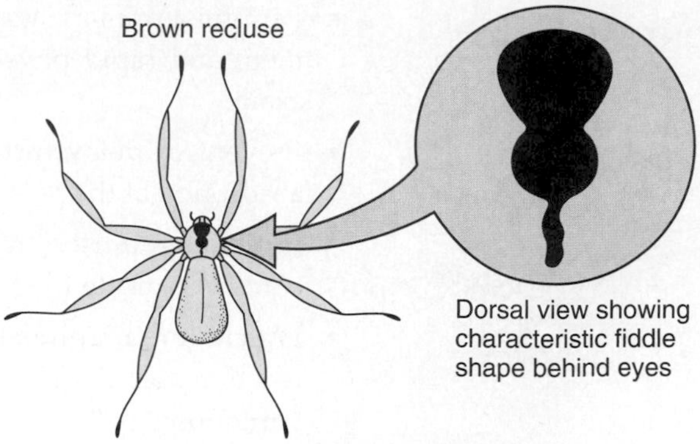

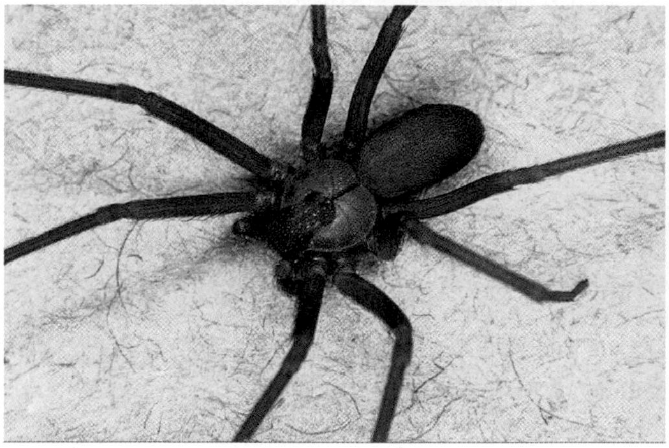

FIGURE 8-21 Brown recluse spider.

(Photo: Centers for Disease Control and Prevention)

Black Widow Spider Bites

Black widow spiders live in all parts of the continental United States. They are usually found in woodpiles or brush. The female spider is responsible for bites and can be

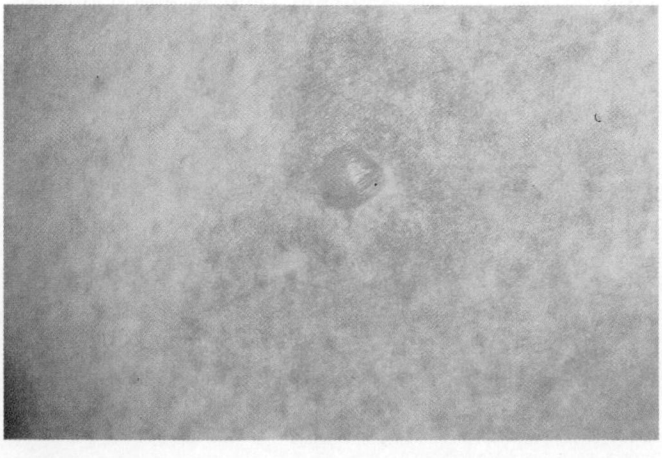

FIGURE 8-22 Brown recluse spider bite 24 hours after bite. Note the bleb and surrounding white halo.

(Courtesy of Baylor Scott and White Health Care)

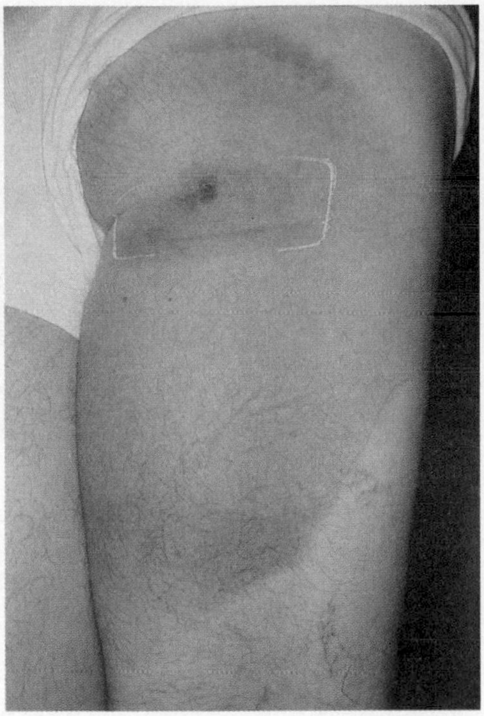

FIGURE 8-23 Brown recluse spider bite four days after the bite. Note the spread of erythema and early necrosis.

(Courtesy of Baylor Scott and White Health Care)

easily identified by the characteristic orange hourglass marking on her black abdomen (Figure 8-24). The venom of the legendary black widow is very potent, causing excessive neurotransmitter release at the synaptic junctions.

SIGNS AND SYMPTOMS Signs and symptoms of black widow spider bites start as immediate localized pain, redness, and swelling. Progressive muscle spasms of all large muscle groups can occur and are usually associated with severe pain. Other systemic symptoms include nausea, vomiting, sweating, seizures, paralysis, and decreased level of consciousness.

MANAGEMENT Prehospital treatment is mostly supportive. It is important to reassure the patient. IV muscle relaxants may be necessary for severe spasms. With physician order, you may use diazepam (2.5 to 10 mg IV) or calcium gluconate (0.1 to 0.2 mg/kg of 10 percent solution IV). Calcium chloride is not effective and should not be used. Because hypertensive crisis is possible, monitor blood pressure carefully. Antivenin is available, so transfer the patient to the emergency department as soon as possible.[18]

Scorpion Stings

There are many species of scorpion in the United States (Figure 8-25). All can sting, causing localized pain, but only one, the bark scorpion, has caused fatalities. These arthropods live mostly in Arizona and adjacent areas of California, Nevada, New Mexico, and Texas. There have been no deaths in Arizona from scorpion stings since 1970.

Scorpions move mostly at night, hiding in the day under debris and buildings. The venom they inject is stored in a bulb at the end of the tail. If provoked, the scorpion will sting with its tail, injecting only a small amount of poison.

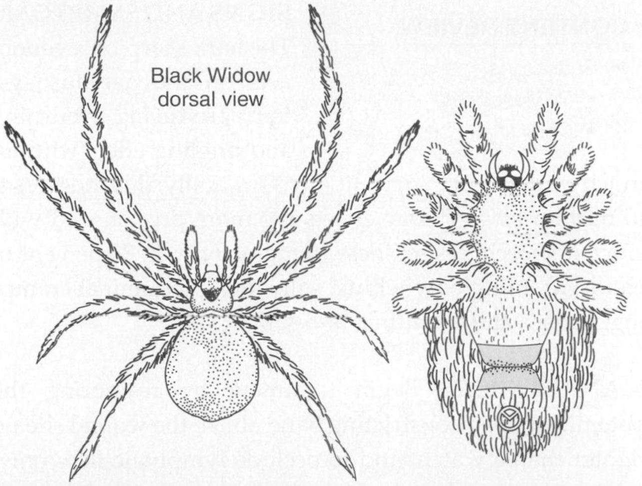

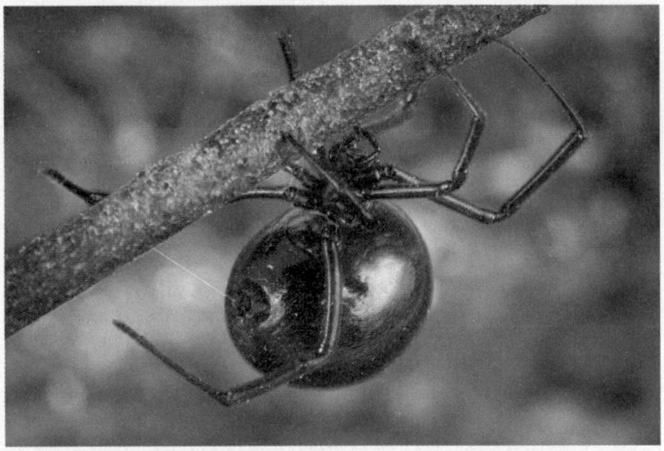

FIGURE 8-24 Black widow spider.

(Photo: Centers for Disease Control and Prevention/Paula Smith)

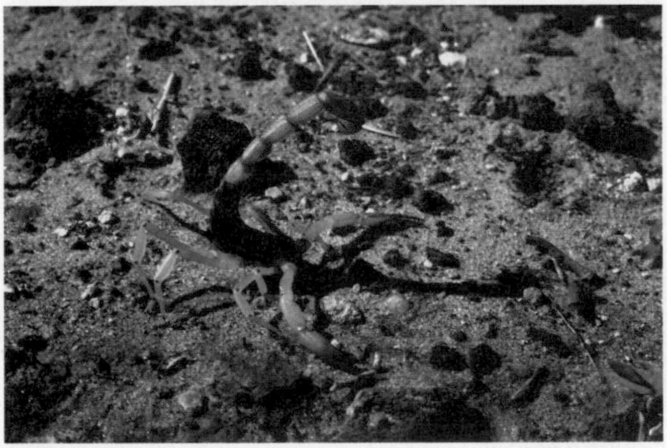

FIGURE 8-25 Scorpion.

(U.S. Fish and Wildlife Service/Gary M. Stolz)

CONTENT REVIEW

- ➤ Snakebites
  - Pit viper bites
  - Coral snake bites

SIGNS AND SYMPTOMS The bark scorpion's venom acts on the nervous system, producing a burning and tingling effect without much evidence of injury initially. Gradually, this progresses to numbness. Systemic effects are more pronounced with slurred speech, restlessness (hyperactivity in 80 percent of children), muscle twitching, salivation, abdominal cramping, nausea and vomiting, and seizures.

MANAGEMENT Begin treatment by reassuring the patient. Apply a constricting band above the wound site no tighter than a watchband to occlude lymphatic flow only. Avoid the use of analgesics, which may increase toxicity and potentiate the venom's effect on airway control. Transport the patient to the emergency department if systemic symptoms develop. Antivenin is available but should be used only in severe cases.[19]

Snakebites

There are several thousand snakebites each year in the United States. Fortunately, these bites result in very few deaths. The signs and symptoms of snakebite depend on the snake, the location of the bite, and the type and amount of venom injected.

Two families of poisonous snakes are native to the United States. One family (*Crotalidae*) includes the pit vipers. Common pit vipers are cottonmouths (water moccasins) (Figure 8-26), rattlesnakes (Figure 8-27), and copperheads (Figure 8-28). Pit vipers are so named because of the distinctive pit between the eye and the nostril on each side of the head. These snakes have elliptical pupils, two well-developed fangs, and a triangular-shaped head. Only the rattlesnake, the most common pit viper, has rattles on the end of its tail.

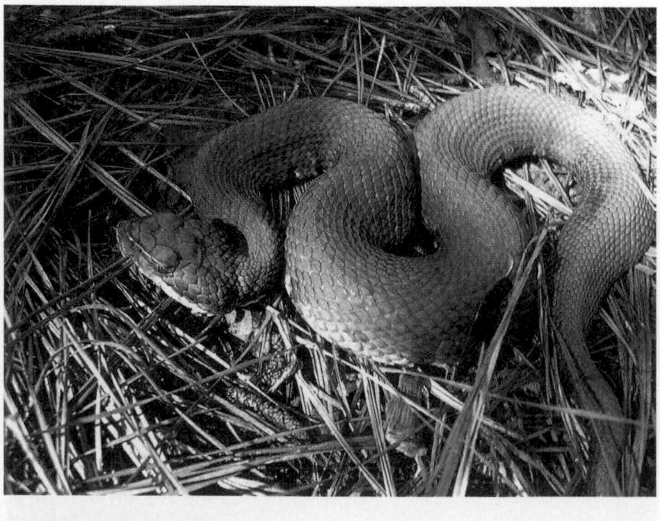

FIGURE 8-26 Cottonmouth.

(Centers for Disease Control and Prevention/Edward J. Wozniak, DVM, PhD, Michael Smith)

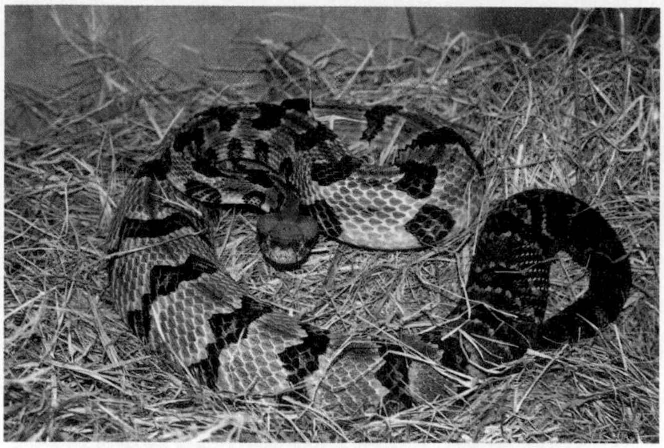

FIGURE 8-27 Rattlesnake.

(Centers for Disease Control and Prevention/Edward J. Wozniak, DVM, PhD, Michael Smith)

The second family of poisonous snakes is the *Elapidae*, or coral snake, which is a distant relative of the cobra. Several varieties of coral snakes are found in the United States, primarily in the Southwest. Because it is a small snake and has small fangs, the coral snake cannot readily attach itself to a large surface, such as an arm or leg. The coral snake has round eyes, a narrow head, and no pit. It has characteristic yellow-banded red and black rings around its body. Several nonpoisonous snakes, such as the king snake, mimic this coloration pattern. Keep in mind a helpful mnemonic: "red touch yellow, kill a fellow; red touch black, venom lack." This rhyme indicates the distinctive pattern of the coral snake—a pattern that signals danger (Figure 8-29).

Pit Viper Bites

Pit viper venom contains hydrolytic enzymes that are capable of destroying proteins and most other tissue

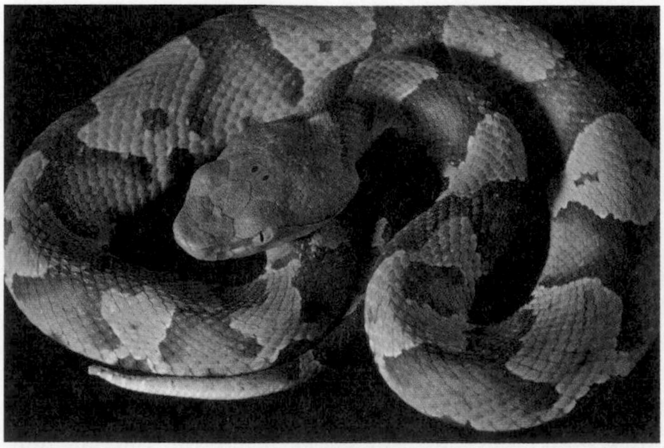

FIGURE 8-28 Copperhead.

(Centers for Disease Control and Prevention/James Gathany)

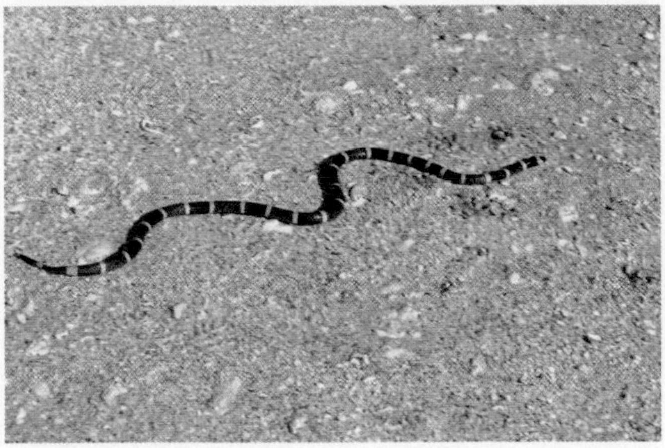

FIGURE 8-29 Coral snake.

(U.S. Fish and Wildlife Service/Luther C. Goldman)

components. These enzymes may produce destruction of red blood cells and other tissue components and may affect the body's blood clotting system within the blood vessels. This will produce infarction and tissue necrosis, especially at the site of the bite.

A severe pit viper bite can result in death from shock within 30 minutes. However, most deaths from pit viper bites occur from 6 to 30 hours after the bite, with 90 percent occurring within the first 48 hours.

SIGNS AND SYMPTOMS Signs and symptoms of pit viper bite include:

- Fang marks (often little more than a scratch mark or abrasion)
- Swelling and pain at the wound site
- Continued oozing at the wound site
- Weakness, dizziness, or faintness
- Sweating and/or chills
- Thirst
- Nausea and vomiting
- Diarrhea
- Tachycardia and hypotension
- Bloody urine and gastrointestinal hemorrhage (late)
- Ecchymosis
- Necrosis
- Shallow respirations, progressing to respiratory failure
- Numbness and tingling around face and head (classic)

MANAGEMENT In treating a person who has been bitten by a pit viper, the primary goal is to slow absorption of the venom. Remember, about 25 percent of all rattlesnake bites are "dry" and no venom is injected. The amount of venom a pit viper injects varies significantly. It is helpful to try to classify the degree of envenomation:

Degree of Envenomation	Signs and Symptoms
None	None (either local or systemic)
Minimal	Swelling Pain No systemic symptoms
Moderate	Progressive swelling Mild systemic symptoms • Paresthesias • Nausea and vomiting • Unusual tastes • Mild hypotension • Mild tachycardia • Tachypnea
Severe	Swelling (spreading rapidly) Severe pain Systemic symptoms • Altered mental status • Nausea and vomiting • Hypotension (systolic <80) • Severe tachycardia • Severe respiratory distress Blood oozes freely from puncture wounds

Antivenin is available for the various common pit vipers found in the United States (Figure 8-30). However, antivenin should be considered only for severe cases when there is marked envenomation, as evidenced by severe systemic symptoms. In 2000, a safer antivenin, Crotalidae Polyvalent Immune Fab (Ovine) (FabAV), was approved for the management of patients with minimal to moderate North

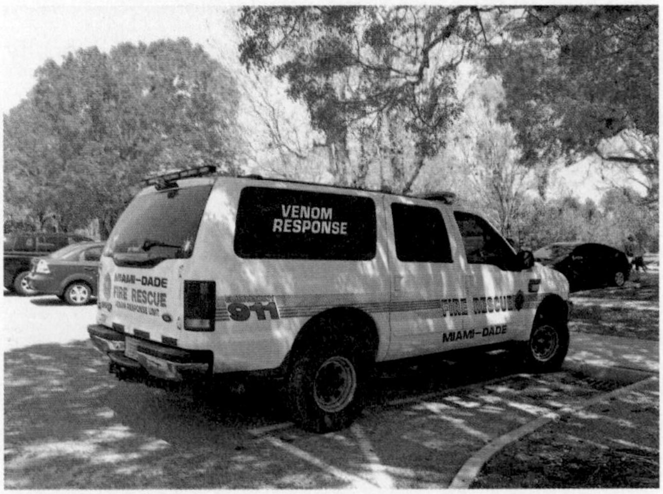

FIGURE 8-30 Antivenin is available for the various common pit vipers found in the United States.

(© Caroline Bennet/www.LotsaFunMaps.com)

American *Crotalid* envenomation. It has been found to be safer and better tolerated than older antivenins and is now the only one available in the United States.[20] Routine emergency treatment of pit viper bites includes the following steps:

- Keep the patient supine.
- Immobilize the limb with a splint.
- Maintain the extremity in a neutral position. Do not apply constricting bands.
- Initiate supportive care using the following guidelines:
  - Provide supplemental oxygen if the patient is hypoxic.
  - Start IV with crystalloid fluid.
  - Transport the patient to the emergency department for management, which may include the administration of antivenin in the ED.
  - *Do not* apply ice, cold pack, or Freon spray to the wound.
  - *Do not* apply an arterial tourniquet.
  - *Do not* apply electrical stimulation from any device in an attempt to retard or reverse venom spread.

Coral Snake Bites

The venom of the coral snake contains some of the enzymes found in pit viper venom. However, because of the presence of neurotoxin, coral snake venom affects primarily nervous tissue. The classic, severe coral snake bite will result in respiratory and skeletal muscle paralysis.[21]

SIGNS AND SYMPTOMS After the bite of a coral snake, there may be no local manifestations or even any systemic effects for as long as 12 to 24 hours. Signs and symptoms of a coral snake bite include:

- Localized numbness, weakness, and drowsiness
- Ataxia
- Slurred speech and excessive salivation
- Paralysis of the tongue and larynx (produces difficulty breathing and swallowing)
- Drooping of eyelids, double vision, dilated pupils
- Abdominal pain
- Nausea and vomiting
- Loss of consciousness
- Seizures
- Respiratory failure
- Hypotension

MANAGEMENT Treatment in cases of suspected coral snake bites includes the following steps:

- Wash the wound with copious amounts of water.
- Apply a compression bandage and keep the extremity at the level of the heart.
- Immobilize the limb with a splint.
- Start an IV using crystalloid fluid.
- Transport the patient to the emergency department for administration of antivenin.
- *Do not* apply ice, cold pack, or Freon sprays to the wound.
- *Do not* incise the wound.
- *Do not* apply electrical stimulation from any device in an attempt to retard or reverse venom spread.

Marine Animal Injection

Although most dangerous marine life prefer warm, tropical waters, some can be found in more northern waters. With the large number of people who flock to beaches and coastal recreation areas every year, the number of injuries from marine life has increased moderately. The most common encounters occur while the person is walking on the beach, but they can also happen while wading in shallow waters or scuba diving in deeper waters. Injection of toxins from marine life can result from stings of jellyfish and corals or from punctures by the bony spines of animals such as sea urchins and stingrays. All venoms of marine animals contain substances that produce pain out of proportion to the size of the injury. These poisonous toxins are unstable and heat sensitive. Heat will relieve pain and inactivate the venom.

Both freshwater and saltwater contain considerable bacterial and viral pollution. Therefore, secondary infection is always a possibility in injuries from marine animals. Particularly severe and life-threatening infections can be inflicted by a number of organisms. In all cases of marine-acquired infections, *Vibrio* species must be considered.

SIGNS AND SYMPTOMS Signs and symptoms of marine animal injection include:

- Intense local pain and swelling
- Weakness
- Nausea and vomiting
- Dyspnea
- Tachycardia
- Hypotension or shock (severe cases)

MANAGEMENT In suspected cases of marine animal injection, take the following steps:

- Establish and maintain the airway.
- Apply a constricting band between the wound and the heart no tighter than a watchband to occlude lymphatic flow only.
- Apply heat or hot water (110°F–113°F).[22]
- Inactivate or remove any stingers.

CONTENT REVIEW

➤ Marine Poisonings
- Marine animal injection
- Ciguatera poisoning

Ciguatera Poisoning

Ciguatera fish poisoning (or ciguatera) is an illness caused by eating fish that contain toxins produced by marine microalgae called *Gambierdiscus toxicus*. Thus, ciguatera poisoning occurs primarily from predator reef fish species near the top of the food chain in tropical waters, such as barracuda, moray eel, parrotfish, grouper, and amberjack. Barracuda are most frequently associated with ciguatoxin poisoning.

Ciguatera fish poisoning generally begins with a gastrointestinal syndrome consisting of nausea, vomiting, diarrhea, and abdominal pain, with onset ranging from 2 to 30 hours after ingestion. However, symptoms most commonly begin within 2 to 6 hours. Within approximately 3 hours of eating contaminated fish, neurologic symptoms can occur and include profound weakness, paresthesias (tingling), severe pruritus, tooth pain or the feeling that teeth are loose, pain on urination, and blurred vision. Hot–cold temperature sensation reversal is characteristic, although not always present. Ciguatera often is associated with signs of cardiovascular dysfunction, such as hypotension, bradycardia (slowed heartbeat), or arrhythmia (irregular heartbeat), which typically occur one to three days after eating contaminated fish. Complete recovery usually occurs within a few weeks, but neurologic symptoms can recur periodically. No diagnostic tests for ciguatera fish poisoning exist; diagnosis is based on the presence of characteristic symptoms in a patient with a recent history of fish ingestion. The diagnosis can be confirmed through laboratory testing indicating the presence of ciguatoxin in fish samples saved from a meal; the level of ciguatoxin in fish that causes human illness varies. In addition, no proven screening test exists for detecting ciguatoxin in fish before they are distributed and eaten. Ciguatoxins are odorless, colorless, and tasteless and cannot be eliminated or reduced by cooking or freezing.

Ciguatera has no cure. Some studies have demonstrated a benefit with administration of mannitol. Symptoms usually go away in days or weeks but can last for years. People who have ciguatera can be treated for their symptoms.[23]

Substance Abuse and Overdose

Substance abuse, the use of a pharmacological substance for purposes other than medically defined reasons, is a very serious problem in our nation. Drugs are abused because they stimulate a feeling of euphoria in the abuser. Eventually, abusers begin to crave the feeling the drug gives them and therefore develop a dependence on the drug, also called **addiction**. An addiction exists when a person repeatedly uses and feels an overwhelming need to obtain and continue using a particular drug. Becoming accustomed to the use of the drug is called *habituation*. Physiologic dependence is the resulting condition if removal of the drug causes adverse physical reactions. There can also be psychological dependence, in which use of the drug is required to prevent or relieve tension or emotional stress. With continued use, **tolerance** develops, which means that the abuser must use increasingly larger doses to get the same effect.

Patho Pearls

Addiction, Tolerance, and Withdrawal. Prolonged exposure to many drugs can result in addiction to and tolerance of the drug in question. *Addiction* is the continued use of the drug despite the fact that it may be harmful and serves no medical purpose. *Tolerance* is the need for an increased amount of the drug to obtain effects previously obtained from a lower dose of the same drug. Addiction can be psychological, physical, or both. With addiction and the development of tolerance, patients will often use larger and larger quantities of the drug to get the euphoria they seek.

As they become physically addicted, patients will begin to suffer physical manifestations when the drug levels fall. This phenomenon is referred to as *withdrawal*. Most drug withdrawals are very uncomfortable for the patient but are rarely life threatening. However, with alcohol and the benzodiazepines, withdrawal can be potentially fatal and may be complicated by seizures and similar problems.

The symptoms of drug withdrawal vary depending on the drug involved. As a rule, however, withdrawal symptoms are the physiologic opposite of those caused by the drug. For example, alcohol is a central nervous system depressant. Withdrawal from alcohol is characterized by CNS stimulation that causes anxiety, tremulousness, difficulty sleeping, hallucinations, and possibly seizures. Patients addicted to amphetamines, a CNS stimulant, have withdrawal symptoms that include a loss of energy, excessive sleepiness, slowed mentation, and similar symptoms. Thus, it is not necessary to memorize the various withdrawal syndromes—simply remember the physiologic effects of the drug in question and remember that patients withdrawing from those drugs often manifest symptoms that are exactly the opposite of those caused by the drugs.

Attempts to stop the drug can trigger a psychological or physical reaction known as **withdrawal**. Withdrawal reactions can be quite unpleasant and severe. In some cases (especially with alcohol and benzodiazepines), withdrawal can be severe enough to cause death. These reactions further strengthen the victim's dependence on the drug. At this point, the abuser may begin to withdraw from regular activities. He may have conflicts with family, friends, and coworkers as his personality and priorities change. Often, the abuser will be involved in criminal activities to support the habit. The abuser has formed an addiction at the point when the substance abuse begins to affect some part of his life. This includes affecting the abuser's health, work, or relationships. Also, the abuser begins to seek out the drug he abuses.

The National Institute on Drug Abuse performed a survey to estimate national use and exposure to illicit drugs. The results were astounding:

- 28 million Americans used illicit drugs at least once.
- 14.5 million use illicit drugs regularly.
- 20 million Americans have tried cocaine.
- 860,000 people use cocaine weekly.
- 11.6 million use marijuana regularly.
- 770,000 people use hallucinogens such as PCP or LSD regularly.
- 2.5 million have used heroin.

The use of illicit drugs has fluctuated in recent years. Most recently, heroin has regained popularity, especially among middle- to upper-class teenagers and young adults. Beyond hurting themselves, substance abusers are 18 times more likely to be involved in criminal activities. These include violent crimes as well as theft to support drug habits. (The Secretary of Health and Human Services has estimated that cocaine is a $65 billion-per-year industry.)

In general terms, **drug overdose** refers to poisoning from a pharmacological substance, either legal or illegal. This can occur by accident, miscalculation, changes in the strength of a drug, suicide, polydrug use, or recreational drug use. Many overdose emergencies seen in the field occur in the habitual drug abuser. It is most difficult to obtain a good history in these cases. However, if the paramedic is familiar with street-drug slang, a more accurate history may be obtained. It is imperative that the paramedic maintains a nonjudgmental attitude in these cases, even though this may be difficult.

The presentation of the drug overdose will vary based on the substance used. Management should be the same as for any ingested, inhaled, or injected poison. Poison control should be contacted for additional direction.

CONTENT REVIEW

➤ Drugs Commonly Abused
- Alcohol
- Barbiturates
- Cocaine
- Narcotics
- Marijuana
- Amphetamines
- Hallucinogens
- Sedatives
- Benzodiazepines

Commonly Abused Drugs

Drugs of abuse are both common and dangerous. These drugs all have various signs and symptoms and require supportive treatment and general toxicologic emergency management. Refer to Table 8–6 for further details on what you may find on assessment and the interventions required.

Remember these specific guidelines for patients who have taken the following drugs:

- ***Alcohol***—May require thiamine and $D_{50}W$ for hypoglycemia.
- ***Amphetamines/stimulants***—Use benzodiazepines (diazepam) for seizures and in combination with haloperidol for hyperactivity.
- ***Barbiturates***—Forced diuresis and alkalization of the urine improve elimination of barbiturates from the body.
- ***Benzodiazepines***—Use flumazenil to counteract adverse effects. Be careful not to trigger a withdrawal syndrome with seizures.
- ***Cocaine***—Benzodiazepines (diazepam) may be needed for sedation and to treat seizures. Beta-blockers are absolutely contraindicated because unopposed alpha-receptor stimulation can cause cardiac ischemia, hypertension, and hyperthermia.
- ***Hallucinogens***—Use benzodiazepines for seizures and in combination with haloperidol for hyperactivity.
- ***Narcotics/opiates***—Naloxone is effective in reversing respiratory depression and sedation, but be careful, as it may trigger a withdrawal reaction in chronic opiate abusers.

Drugs Used for Sexual Purposes

There are a number of drugs that deserve mention as a separate category. These drugs are used to stimulate and enhance the sexual experience, but without medically approved indications for such use. *Ecstasy*, also called *MDMA*, is one such drug. Ecstasy is a modified form of methamphetamines and has similar, although milder, effects. It is very popular in today's university and nightclub environments.

Use of Ecstasy initially causes anxiety, nausea, tachycardia, and elevated blood pressure, followed by relaxation, euphoria, and feelings of enhanced emotional insight. No definitive data exist as to whether the experience of sexual intercourse is improved. Studies show that prolonged use may cause brain damage. Some deaths from MDMA ingestion have been reported. These cases present with confusion, agitation, tremor, high temperature, and diarrhea. No specific treatment exists. Standard supportive measures should be initiated.

Rohypnol (flunitrazepam) is another drug abused for sexual purposes. Illegal in the United States, it is commonly called the "date rape drug," because it can be slipped secretly into a woman's drink. This drug is a strong benzodiazepine like diazepam, lorazepam, and midazolam. The resulting sedation and amnesia allows the

Table 8–6 Common Drugs of Abuse

Drug	Signs and Symptoms	Routes	Prehospital Management
Alcohol Boor Whiskey Gin Vodka Wine Tequila	CNS depression Slurred speech Disordered thought Impaired judgment Diuresis Stumbling gait Stupor Coma	Oral	ABCs Respiratory support Oxygenate, if hypoxic Establish IV access Administer 100 mg thiamine IV ECG monitor Check glucose level Administer $D_{50}W$, if hypoglycemic
Barbiturates Thiopental Phenobarbital Primidone Butalbital	Lethargy Emotional lability Incoordination Slurred speech Nystagmus Coma Hypotension Respiratory depression	Oral IV	ABCs Respiratory support Oxygenate, if hypoxic Establish IV access ECG monitor Contact poison control—may order bicarbonate
Cocaine Crack Rock	Euphoria Hyperactivity Dilated pupils Psychosis Twitching Anxiety Hypertension Tachycardia Arrhythmias Seizures Chest pain	Snorting Injection Smoking (freebasing)	ABCs Respiratory support Oxygenate, if hypoxic ECG monitor Establish IV access Treat life-threatening arrhythmias Seizure precautions: diazepam 5–10 mg
Narcotics Heroin Codeine Meperidine Morphine Fentanyl Hydromorphone Pentazocine Methadone Desomorphine (Krokodil)	CNS depression Constricted pupils Respiratory depression Hypotension Bradycardia Pulmonary edema Coma Death	Oral Injection	ABCs Respiratory support Oxygenate, if hypoxic Establish IV access *Administer 1–2 mg naloxone IV or endotracheally as ordered by medical direction until respirations improve. Larger than average doses (2–5 mg) have been used in the management of overdose of synthetic opiates and alcoholic coma ECG monitor
Marijuana Grass Weed Hashish Synthetic cannabis	Euphoria Dry mouth Dilated pupils Altered sensation	Smoked Oral	ABCs Reassure the patient Speak in a quiet voice ECG monitor if indicated
Amphetamines Benzedrine Dexadrine Ritalin Methamphetamine Synthetic cathinones (bath salts)	Exhilaration Hyperactivity Dilated pupils Hypertension Psychosis Tremors Seizures	Oral Injection	ABCs Oxygenate, if hypoxic ECG monitor Establish IV access Treat life-threatening arrhythmias Seizure precautions: diazepam 5–10 mg

(*Continued*)

Table 8–6 Common Drugs of Abuse (*Continued*)

Drug	Signs and Symptoms	Routes	Prehospital Management
Hallucinogens	Psychosis	Oral	ABCs
LSD	Nausea	Smoked	Reassure the patient
DMT	Dilated pupils		"Talk down" the "high" patient
MDMA	Rambling speech		Protect the patient from injury
Mescaline	Headache		Provide a dark, quiet environment
Peyote	Dizziness		Speak in a soft, quiet voice
Psilocybin	Suggestibility		Seizure precautions: diazepam 5–10 mg
Ayahuasca	Distortion of sensory perceptions		Hallucinations
PCP**			
Sedatives	Altered mental status	Oral	ABCs
Seconal	Hypotension		Respiratory support
Valium	Slurred speech		Oxygenate, if hypoxic
Librium	Respiratory depression		Establish IV access
Xanax	Shock		ECG monitor
Ativan	Bradycardia		Medical direction may order naloxone
Restoril	Seizures		
Ambien			
Phenobarbital			
Ketamine			
GHB			
Benzodiazepines***	Altered mental status	Oral	ABCs
Valium	Slurred speech		Respiratory support
Librium	Arrhythmias		Oxygenate, if hypoxic
Xanax	Coma		Activated charcoal as ordered by medical direction
Halcion			Establish IV access
Restoril			ECG monitor
Dalmane			Contact poison control
Centrax			
Ativan			
Serax			

*With the advent of the opiate antagonist naloxone, narcotic overdosage has become easier to manage. It is possible to titrate this effective medication to increase respirations to normal levels without fully awakening the patient. In the case of narcotic addicts, this prevents hostile and confrontational episodes.

**PCP was originally an animal tranquilizer, but it manifests hallucinogenic properties when used by humans. In addition to bizarre delusions, it can cause violent and dangerous outbursts of aggressive behavior. The rescuer is advised to remain safe when attempting to treat this type of overdose. PCP patients have been known to have almost superhuman strength and high pain tolerance.

***Deaths due to pure benzodiazepine ingestion are very rare. Minor toxicity ranges are 500–1,500 mg. A benzodiazepine antagonist (Romazicon) is available. IV dosage is 1–10 mg, or an infusion of 0.5 mg/hr. It may cause seizures in a benzodiazepine-dependent patient.

perpetrator to rape the victim. Treatment is the same as for any benzodiazepine, but consequences of the sexual assault require attention as well.

Alcohol Abuse

Alcohol is the most common substance of abuse in the United States and most of the world. Almost 75 percent of Americans have at least one drink per year. The average American consumes 2.5 gallons of pure ethanol every year. Alcohol has been linked to 5 percent of deaths in the United States. Alcoholism costs more than $100 billion per year due to lost work time and medical costs to treat complications and injuries. Alcoholism progresses in much the same way as drug dependence, discussed earlier.

Physiologic Effects

Alcohol (ethyl alcohol, or ethanol) depresses the central nervous system, potentially to the point of stupor, coma, and death. In patients with severe liver disease, metabolism of alcohol may become impaired, which increases the course and severity of intoxication. At low doses, alcohol has excitatory and stimulating effects, thus depressing inhibitions. At higher doses, alcohol's depressive effect is more obvious. Abuse of and dependence on alcohol is called *alcoholism*. It is a major problem in our society, contributing to many highway traffic fatalities, drownings, burns, trauma, and drug overdoses.

Alcohol is completely absorbed from the stomach and intestinal tract approximately 30 to 120 minutes after ingestion. Once absorbed, alcohol is distributed to all body tissues and fluids, with concentrations of alcohol in the brain rapidly approaching the alcohol level in the blood.

Some alcoholics will drink methanol (wood alcohol) or ethylene glycol (a component of antifreeze) if ethanol is unavailable. Both are readily available and, when ingested, will be absorbed quickly from the gastrointestinal tract. Ingestion of these chemicals can cause blindness or death.

In addition, alcohol causes a peripheral vasodilator effect on the cardiovascular system, resulting in flushing and a feeling of warmth. In cold conditions, alcohol's dilation of the blood vessels results in an increased loss of body heat. The diuretic effect seen when large amounts of alcohol are ingested is due to the inhibition of *vasopressin*, which is the hormone responsible for the conservation of body fluids. Without vasopressin, an increase in urine flow occurs. The "dry mouth syndrome" experienced after alcohol consumption may be the result of alcohol-induced cellular dehydration.

In addition, methanol will also cause visual disturbances, abdominal pain, and nausea and vomiting even at low doses. In fact, death has been reported after ingestion of only 15 mL of a 40 percent solution. Occasionally patients will complain of headache or dizziness and may even present with seizures and obtundation. Ethylene glycol ingestion has similar symptoms, but the CNS effects such as hallucinations, coma, and seizures are more pronounced in the early stages.

General Alcoholic Profile

The classic alcoholic portrayed in movies is an unkempt, continually intoxicated street person who is completely nonfunctional. Although alcoholics of this type exist, it would be a grave error to consider this the typical picture of someone dependent on alcohol. More commonly, alcoholism is characterized by impaired control over drinking, preoccupation with the drug ethanol, use of ethanol despite adverse consequences, and distortions in thinking, such as denial. This is the definition used by the National Council on Alcoholism and Drug Dependence. Obviously, this definition applies to many people, including many functional people at all levels of society who have masked their addiction well. Take note of these warning signs, which may indicate alcohol abuse:

- Drinking early in the day
- Prone to drink alone and secretly
- Periodic binges (may last for several days)
- Partial or total loss of memory ("blackouts") during period of drinking
- Unexplained history of gastrointestinal problems (especially bleeding)
- "Green tongue syndrome" (using chlorophyll-containing substances to disguise the odor of alcohol on the breath)
- Cigarette burns on clothing
- Chronically flushed face and palms
- Tremulousness
- Odor of alcohol on breath under inappropriate conditions

Consequences of Chronic Alcohol Ingestion

Alcohol has many deleterious effects on the body. Chronic abuse can be devastating, affecting every organ system, as shown in Figure 8-31. Some of the more common effects include:

- Poor nutrition
- Alcohol hepatitis
- Liver cirrhosis with subsequent esophageal varices
- Loss of sensation in hands and feet
- Loss of cerebellar function (balance and coordination)
- Pancreatitis
- Upper gastrointestinal hemorrhage (often fatal)
- Hypoglycemia
- Subdural hematoma (due to falls)
- Rib and extremity fractures (due to falls)

Keep in mind that conditions such as subdural hematomas, sepsis, and other life-threatening disease processes may mimic the signs and symptoms of alcohol intoxication. For example, diabetic ketoacidosis produces a breath odor that can easily be confused with the odor of alcohol.

Alcohol Withdrawal Syndrome

The alcoholic may suffer a withdrawal reaction from either abrupt discontinuation of ingestion after prolonged use or from a rapid fall in blood alcohol level after acute intoxication. Alcohol withdrawal can be potentially fatal. Withdrawal symptoms can occur several hours after sudden abstinence and can last up to five to seven days. Seizures (sometimes called "rum fits") may occur within the first 24 to 36 hours of abstinence. **Delirium tremens (DTs)** usually develops on the second or third day of the withdrawal. Delirium tremens is characterized by a decreased level of consciousness during which the patient hallucinates and

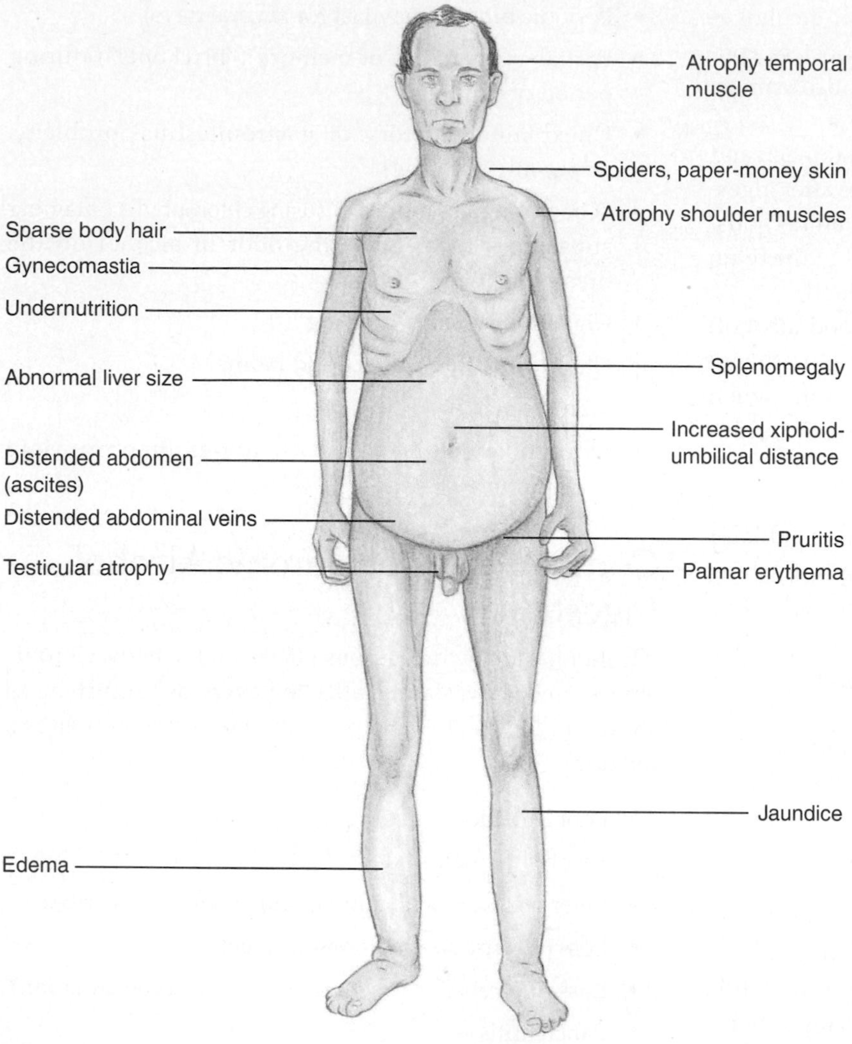

FIGURE 8-31 The chronic alcoholic.

misinterprets nearby events. Seizures and delirium tremens are ominous signs. There is a significant mortality from delirium tremens. Benzodiazepines (e.g., diazepam, lorazepam) are an effective treatment and can prevent seizures in severe cases.[24]

SIGNS AND SYMPTOMS Signs and symptoms of withdrawal syndrome include:

- Coarse tremor of hands, tongue, and eyelids
- Nausea and vomiting
- General weakness
- Increased sympathetic tone
- Tachycardia
- Sweating
- Hypertension
- Orthostatic hypotension
- Anxiety
- Irritability or a depressed mood
- Hallucinations
- Poor sleep

MANAGEMENT Alcohol intoxication, whether acute or chronic, should not be underestimated as a toxic emergency problem. In cases of suspected alcohol abuse, take the following steps:

- Establish and maintain the airway.
- Determine whether other drugs are involved.
- Start an IV using lactated Ringer's or normal saline.
- Chemstrip and administer 25 g of $D_{50}W$ if hypoglycemic.
- Consider benzodiazepines.
- Maintain a sympathetic attitude and reassure the patient of help.
- Transport to the emergency department for further care.

Summary

Toxicologic emergencies are a broad spectrum of emergencies that range from common alcohol ingestion to something as severe, and extremely rare, as contact with a military-grade biological chemical. No matter what scenario you find yourself in, keeping in mind a few simple rules will help you to effectively manage these situations:

- ***Recognize and identify the poisoning promptly.*** In other words, you must have a high index of suspicion when circumstances suggest that a toxin may be involved. Do your best to identify the specific poison, and retrieve the container if at all possible and if you can do it safely.

- ***Be thorough in your primary assessment and evaluation of the patient.*** This will facilitate your efforts to identify the toxin and the measures needed to control the situation. Treatment is largely based on symptoms and the type and route of the toxin.
- ***Initiate the standard treatment procedures required for all toxicologic emergencies.*** Beyond the usual concern for rescuer safety and rapid implementation of ABCs and supportive measures, consider the methods needed to minimize any further exposure to the toxin. One of the most important treatments you can perform is to decontaminate the patient as best you can. When the toxin is on the surface of the skin and clothes, decontamination is usually done by removing the clothes and flushing the skin with copious amounts of water. (The solution to pollution is dilution.)
- ***Contact poison control and/or medical direction for toxin-specific treatment instructions.*** You will get the best advice if you can identify the specific toxin; state the amount that was ingested, absorbed, inhaled, or injected; and obtain the container.
- ***Administer an antidote if one exists for the particular toxin.***

These few simple steps are the necessary early response to all toxicologic emergencies. The majority of such emergencies will require simple ALS procedures, including establishing an airway, maintaining oxygenation, IV therapy, supportive care, and transport to the emergency department. Some cases may require you to treat symptoms of the poisoning, such as seizures, brady/tachycardia, respiratory arrest, or burns, to name just a few. Basic airway care should always be at the top of your list.

You Make the Call

It is a beautiful sunny day in south Oshawa, where you and your partner, Amit Shaw, are polishing up your truck, Medic 24. A call comes in from central dispatch, sending you to 1502 Tom Sawyer Lane, the home of local pest-control guru Robert Walsh and his wife, Leslie. As you pull into the driveway, Leslie is standing in front of the garage and motions you to come quickly. She informs you that her husband is very ill. He was packaging some of the new chemicals for work when he dropped the bottle onto the floor of the garage, spilling it everywhere.

When you look into the garage, you see Rob sitting on a chair looking sweaty and weak and he is having some difficulty breathing. He has vomited twice. There is a strong, vaguely familiar odor (like the last time you sprayed your lawn for bugs) emanating from a big puddle in the back of the garage. As you complete your scene size-up, it becomes clear that quick intervention is needed. You spring into action.

1. What class of toxin are you dealing with?
2. What toxidrome (including signs and symptoms) will you expect to find when you make a further assessment of the patient?
3. What are your priorities in managing this situation?
4. Beyond standard supportive measures, what other intervention will help treat this patient?

See Suggested Responses at the back of this book.

Review Questions

1. The American Association of Poison Control Centers estimates that more than ____________ poisonings occur annually.
   a. 2 million
   b. 3 million
   c. 2 thousand
   d. 3 thousand
2. What is the most common route of entry into the body for toxic exposures?
   a. Injection
   b. Inhalation
   c. Ingestion
   d. Surface absorption

3. Which of the following is a common inhaled poison?
   a. Nitrous oxide
   b. Carbon tetrachloride
   c. Methyltrihydrochloride
   d. Triazide

4. The use of which of the following is the most effective and widely used method of reducing absorption of toxins?
   a. Gastric lavage
   b. Activated charcoal
   c. Syrup of ipecac
   d. Whole bowel irrigation

5. Amitriptyline, amoxapine, clomipramine, doxepin, imipramine, and nortriptyline are common agents called ____________
   a. hydrocarbons.
   b. antiemetics.
   c. tricyclic antidepressants.
   d. calcium channel blockers.

6. Which medication will likely be used by a patient diagnosed with bipolar disorder?
   a. Lithium
   b. Codeine
   c. Valium
   d. Dextromethorphan

7. Which is the most common pit viper?
   a. Copperhead
   b. Rattlesnake
   c. Water moccasin
   d. Coral snake

8. Because of the presence of neurotoxin, coral snake venom primarily affects which type of tissue?
   a. Cardiac
   b. Nervous
   c. Muscle
   d. Skeletal

9. What is the most common substance of abuse in the United States and most of the world?
   a. Cocaine
   b. Alcohol
   c. Amphetamines
   d. Narcotics/opiates

10. In cases of poisoning, patient histories are often unreliable because of ____________
    a. deliberate deception.
    b. patient misinformation.
    c. drug-induced confusion.
    d. all of the above.

11. Which of the following toxic/abuse situations is *incorrectly* paired with its prehospital management?
    a. Alcohol: thiamine
    b. Cocaine: diazepam
    c. Opiates: naloxone
    d. TCAs: flumazenil

See Answers to Review Questions at the back of this book.

References

1. Bronstein, A. C., D. A. Spyker, L. R. Cantilena, Jr., et al. "2009 Annual Report of the American Association of Poison Control Centers' National Poison Data Systems (NPDS): 27th Annual Report." *Clin Tox* 48 (2010): 979–1178.
2. Manoguerra, A. S. and D. J. Cobaugh. "Guidelines for the Management of Poisoning Consensus Panel. Guideline on the Use of Ipecac Syrup in the Out-of-Hospital Management of Ingested Poisons." *Clin Toxicol (Phila)* 43 (2005): 1–10.
3. Alarie, Y. "Toxicity of Fire Smoke." *Crit Rev Toxicol* 32 (2002): 259–289.
4. Thom, S. R., V. M. Bhopale, S. T. Han, J. M. Clark, and K. R. Hardy. "Intravascular Neutrophil Activation Due to Carbon Monoxide Poisoning." *Am J Respir Crit Care Med* 174 (2006): 1239–1248.
5. Satran, D., C. R. Henry, C. Adkinson, C. I. Nicholson, Y. Bracha, and T. D. Henry. "Cardiovascular Manifestations of Moderate to Severe Carbon Monoxide Poisoning." *J Am Coll Cardiol* 45 (2005): 1513–1516.
6. Buckley, N. A., D. N. Juurlink, G. Isbister, M. H. Bennett, and E. J. Lavonas. "Hyperbaric Oxygen for Carbon Monoxide Poisoning." *Cochrane Database Syst Rev* 4 (2011): CD002041.
7. Baud, F. J. "Cyanide: Critical Issues in Diagnosis and Treatment." *Hum Exp Toxicol* 26 (2007): 191–201.
8. Shepherd, G. and L. I. Velez. "Role of Hydroxocobalamin in Acute Cyanide Poisoning." *Ann Pharmacother* 42 (2008): 661–669.
9. Olson, K. R., A. R. Erdman, A. D. Woolf, et al. "Calcium Channel Blocker Ingestion: An Evidence-Based Consensus Guideline for Out-of-Hospital Management." *Clin Toxicol* 43 (2005): 797–822.
10. Christianson, G., A. Woolf, and K. R. Olson. "β-Blocker Ingestion: An Evidence-Based Consensus Guideline for Out-of-Hospital Management." *Clin Toxicol* 43 (2005): 131–146.
11. Woolf, A. D., A. R. Erdman, L. S. Nelson, et al. "Tricyclic Antidepressant Poisoning: An Evidence-Based Consensus Guideline for Out-of-Hospital Management." *Clin Toxicol (Phila)* 45 (2007): 203–233.
12. Nelson, L. S., A. R. Erdman, L. L. Booze, et al. "Selective Serotonin Reuptake Inhibitor Poisoning: An Evidence-Based Consensus Guideline for Out-of-Hospital Management." *Clin Toxicol (Phila)* 45 (2007): 315–332.
13. Chyka, P. A., A. R. Erdman, G. Christianson, et al. "Salicylate Poisoning: An Evidence-Based Consensus Guideline for Out-of-Hospital Management." *Clin Toxicol (Phila)* 45 (2007): 95–131.
14. Dart, R. C., A. R. Erdman, K. R. Olson, et al. "Acetaminophen Poisoning: An Evidence-Based Consensus Guideline for Out-of-Hospital Management." *Clin Toxicol* 44 (2006): 1–18.
15. Manoguerra, A. S., A. R. Erdman, L. L. Booze, et al. "Iron Ingestion: An Evidence-Based Consensus Guideline for Out-of-Hospital Management." *Clin Toxicol (Phila)* 43 (2005): 553–570.
16. Vetter, R. S., P. K. Visscher, and S. Camazine. "Mass Envenomations by Honey Bees and Wasps." *West J Med* 170 (1999): 223–227.
17. de Roodt, A. R., J. Estevez-Ramírez, S. Litwin, P. Magaña, A. Olvera, and A. Alagón. "Toxicity of Two North American Loxosceles (Brown Recluse Spiders) Venoms and Their Neutralization by Antivenoms." *Clin Toxicol (Phila)* 45 (2007): 678–687.
18. Diaz, J. H. and K. E. Leblanc. "Common Spider Bites." *Am Fam Physician* 15 (2007): 869–873.

19. White, J. "Venomous Animals: Clinical Toxicology." *EXS* 100 (2010): 233–291.
20. Lavonas, E. J., T. H. Schaeffer, J. Kokko, S. L. Mlynarchek, and G. M. Bogdan. "Crotaline Fab Antivenom Appears to Be Effective in Cases of Severe North American Pit Viper Envenomation: An Integrative Review." *BMC Emerg Med* 9 (2009): 13.
21. Weinstein, S., R. Dart, A. Staples, and J. White. "Envenomations: An Overview of Clinical Toxinology for the Primary Care Physician." *Am Fam Physician* 80 (2009): 793–802.
22. Atkinson, P. R., A. Boyle, D. Hartin, and D. McAuley. "Is Hot Water Immersion an Effective Treatment for Marine Envenomation?" *Emerg Med J* 23 (2006): 503–508.
23. Friedman, M. A., L. E. Fleming, M. Fernandez, et al. "Ciguatera Fish Poisoning: Treatment, Prevention and Management." *Mar Drugs* 6 (2008): 456–479.
24. Amato, L., S. Minozzi, S. Vecchi, and M. Davoli. "Benzodiazepines for Alcohol Withdrawal (Review)." *Cochrane Database Syst Rev* 2010: CDC005063.

Further Reading

Auerbach, P. S., ed. *Wilderness Medicine.* 6th ed. St. Louis: Mosby Year Book, 2012.

Bledsoe, B. E. and D. E. Clayden. *Prehospital Emergency Pharmacology.* 7th ed. Upper Saddle River, NJ: Pearson/Prentice Hall, 2012.

Hoffman, R. et al. *Goldfrank's Toxicologic Emergencies.* 10th ed. New York: McGraw-Hill, 2014.

Tintinalli, J. E., et al., eds. *Emergency Medicine: A Comprehensive Study Guide.* 7th ed. New York: McGraw-Hill, 2013.

Chapter 9
Hematology

Bryan Bledsoe, DO, FACEP, FAAEM, EMT-P

STANDARD

Medicine (Hematology)

COMPETENCY

Integrates assessment findings with principles of epidemiology and pathophysiology to formulate a field impression and implement a comprehensive treatment/disposition plan for a patient with a medical complaint.

Learning Objectives

Terminal Performance Objective: After reading this chapter, you should be able to integrate patient assessment findings, patient history, and knowledge of anatomy, physiology, pathophysiology, and basic and advanced life support interventions to recognize and manage patients with hematologic disorders.

Enabling Objectives: To accomplish the terminal performance objective, you should be able to:

1. Define key terms introduced in this chapter.
2. Explain the demographics and the role of heredity in the risk factors for hematologic disorders.
3. Review the anatomy and physiology of the hematologic system.
4. Adapt the scene size-up, primary assessment, history, secondary assessment, and use of monitoring technology to arrive at a field impression and differentials for hematologic emergencies.
5. Describe the pathophysiology and consistent assessment findings that would be present in a patient experiencing a hematologic emergency.
6. Use a process of clinical reasoning to guide and interpret the patient assessment findings and develop a treatment plan for patients displaying a hematologic emergency in the prehospital environment.
7. Given a variety of scenarios, discuss the integration of assessment and management guidelines as they relate to hematologic emergencies.

KEY TERMS

2,3-bisphosphoglycerate (2,3-BPG), p. 372
anemia, p. 383
antigen, p. 377
autoimmune disease, p. 375
Bohr effect, p. 372
chemotaxis, p. 373
disseminated intravascular coagulation (DIC), p. 388
erythrocyte, p. 371
erythropoiesis, p. 372
erythropoietin, p. 370
fibrinolysis, p. 377
hematocrit, p. 372
hematology, p. 369
hematopoiesis, p. 370
hemoglobin, p. 371
hemolysis, p. 372
hemophilia, p. 387
hemostasis, p. 376
inflammatory process, p. 375
leukemia, p. 386
leukocyte, p. 373
leukocytosis, p. 385
leukopenia, p. 385
leukopoiesis, p. 373
lymphoma, p. 386
major basic protein (MBP), p. 374
multiple myeloma, p. 388
neutropenia, p. 374
phagocytosis, p. 373
plasma, p. 370
pluripotent stem cell, p. 370
polycythemia, p. 383
sequestration, p. 372
sickle cell disease, p. 384
thrombocyte, p. 375
thrombocytopenia, p. 387
thrombocytosis, p. 387
thrombosis, p. 377
von Willebrand's disease, p. 388

Case Study

Medic 102 responds to the scene of what appears to be a minor fall down three steps at a local shopping mall. The patient, a 36-year-old man, is at the base of the stairs, complaining of pain and swelling of the right knee and right flank. It is difficult to get a clear history from the patient and he appears somewhat confused.

The primary assessment reveals a very thin patient who states his name is C.J. He is alert to name only and is confused as to how he came to be on the floor. He is tachypneic and tachycardic, with a weakly palpable radial pulse and obvious profuse diaphoresis. As C.J. appears shocky and complains of back pain, Christian and Victoria, the responding paramedics, immediately place him supine and logroll him onto a backboard. While they are log-rolling C.J., Christian and Victoria note a large area of ecchymosis on his right flank. They initiate an IV of normal saline and administer a fluid bolus.

After they quickly place C.J. in the ambulance, Christian initiates rapid transport while Victoria performs a more complete assessment. Additional findings include a large joint effusion of the right knee and a Medic-Alert tag on a wrist bracelet that reads Hemophilia A. C.J. is responding to the fluid bolus and is becoming less confused. Vital signs reflect a blood pressure of 90/60 mmHg, a pulse of 120, and respirations of 24. SpO_2 is 96 percent. Victoria applies a splint to C.J.'s right knee and calls in to medical direction at Southside Medical Center. She alerts them that they are transporting a patient with hemophilia A and a probable hemarthrosis and retroperitoneal hematoma from a fall. In anticipation of the patient's arrival, the emergency physician alerts the hospital pharmacy to send factor VIII to the department. In addition, he alerts the trauma team. The transport is uneventful and the paramedics of Medic 102 turn C.J. over to the emergency department team. It seems that C.J. is well known to the emergency department staff because of his illness. They quickly begin therapy with factor VIII and administer intravenous fluids and packed red blood cells. The emergency physician performs an arthrocentesis of the right knee, primarily to help with pain. He removes 160 mL of blood from the knee. The patient is stabilized in the emergency department and then admitted to the medical floor for additional therapy.

Introduction

Hematology is the study of the blood and the blood-forming organs. It exemplifies the way that multiple organ systems interact to maintain homeostasis, the normal balance of body functions. Hematologic disorders are common and include red blood cell disorders, white blood cell disorders, platelet disorders, and coagulation problems. Although these disorders are common, they rarely are the primary cause of a medical emergency. They usually accompany other ongoing disease processes. Some hematologic diseases are genetic in origin. Hemophilia A is a classic example. It is a sex-linked disease that causes abnormally low levels of an essential blood clotting protein (factor VIII). It affects approximately 1 or 2 persons per 10,000 in the United States. Some hematologic diseases are more common in certain ethnic groups. For example, among the population as a whole, sickle cell anemia is relatively uncommon. However, among African Americans specifically, 8 percent of the population has the sickle cell trait. In addition to their primary effects, hematologic disorders may predispose patients to infection and intolerance to exercise, hypoxia, acidosis, and blood loss.

Patients with hematologic problems often complain of signs and symptoms that do not point directly to a specific disease process. Careful examination and history taking may be necessary to further clarify the diagnosis. Often, however, laboratory findings will be needed to confirm the diagnosis. Thus, the final diagnosis of patients for whom you provide prehospital care is often not immediately apparent. You must use your assessment skills to recognize and treat injuries, pain, and instabilities, while formulating a field impression that enables you to anticipate further complications and thus enhance patient outcome and survivability. Because of this, it is essential that you have a good understanding of the basic pathophysiologic processes of your patients' diseases, including hematologic disorders.

Anatomy, Physiology, and Pathophysiology

The hematopoietic system consists of blood (both cells and plasma), bone marrow, the liver, the spleen, and the kidneys. The cellular components of blood are formed by the differentiation of a **pluripotent stem cell** in a process termed **hematopoiesis**. In the fetus, hematopoiesis occurs first outside the bone marrow (*extramedullary hematopoiesis*) in the liver, spleen, lymph nodes, and thymus. By the fourth month, the developing bone marrow begins to produce blood cells (*intramedullary hematopoiesis*). After birth, the bone marrow is the primary site of blood cell production and extramedullary hematopoiesis greatly diminishes, occurring mostly in the liver and spleen. By adulthood, hematopoiesis occurs exclusively in the bone marrow unless a pathological state exists.

CONTENT REVIEW

- Hematopoietic System Components
  - Blood
  - Bone marrow
  - Liver
  - Spleen
  - Kidneys

In hematopoiesis, the stem cell reproduces to maintain a constant population of cells. Some stem cells then further differentiate into myeloid multipotent stem cells that, in turn, differentiate into unipotent progenitors. These unipotent progenitors ultimately mature into basophils, eosinophils, neutrophils, monocytes (types of white blood cells), erythrocytes (red blood cells), and thrombocytes (platelets). Pluripotent stem cells may also differentiate into common lymphoid stem cells that ultimately mature into lymphocytes (another type of white cell). The kidney, and to a lesser extent the liver, produce **erythropoietin**, the hormone responsible for red blood cell production. The liver also removes toxins from the blood and produces many of the clotting factors and proteins in plasma. The spleen, an important part of the immune system, has cells that scavenge abnormal blood cells and bacteria.

Blood volume normally remains relatively constant at about 6 percent of total body weight. With an average of 80 to 85 mL of blood per kilogram of body weight, a person who weighs 75 kg has approximately 6 L of blood. The body can easily handle up to about 0.5 L of lost blood or fluid. An example is routine blood donations, in which healthy donors tolerate the blood loss without complication.

The major determinants of the blood volume are red cell mass and plasma volume. Red blood cells remain confined to the intravascular compartment. If their destruction remains constant, then only changes in the rate of production can alter the size of the circulating red cell mass. The plasma volume, on the other hand, can rapidly change due to fluid shifts between the intravascular and extravascular space. These fluid shifts help to preserve circulating blood volume in the event of acute hemorrhage. Other compensatory mechanisms include vasoconstriction, tachycardia, and increased cardiac contractility to maintain adequate tissue perfusion until significant losses overwhelm these measures. When these compensatory measures fail, the patient enters decompensated shock. Fortunately, young healthy individuals' bodies can compensate for loss of as much as 25 to 30 percent of blood volume.

Components of Blood

Blood consists of liquid, or plasma, and formed elements—red blood cells, white blood cells, and platelets.

Plasma

Plasma is a thick, pale yellow fluid that is 90 to 92 percent water and 6 to 7 percent proteins. Fats, carbohydrates, electrolytes, gases, and certain chemical messengers compose the remaining 2 to 3 percent. Plasma transports the cellular components of blood and dissolved nutrients throughout the body and, at the same time,

CONTENT REVIEW

- Components of Blood
  - Plasma
  - Formed elements
  - Red blood cells
  - White blood cells
  - Platelets

transports waste products from cellular metabolism to the liver, kidneys, and lungs, where they can be removed from the body.

Most plasma components can move back and forth across the capillary membranes to the interstitial fluid. However, plasma proteins, such as albumin, are large molecules and have great difficulty diffusing across the membranes. This is fortunate, as they remain in the plasma to help retain water in the capillaries. This is known as *osmotic pull*, or *oncotic pressure*. Plasma proteins perform many other functions, including clotting of blood, dismantling of clots, buffering of the blood's acid–base balance, transporting hormones and regulating their effects, and providing a source of energy.

Electrolytes are also found in the plasma. These are chemical substances that dissociate into charged particles in water. They are essential for nerve conduction, muscle contraction, and water balance. They can easily diffuse across capillary membranes, based on their concentration gradients. Carbohydrates in plasma are generally in the form of glucose, the primary energy source for all body tissues. Glucose is especially important to brain cells, which cannot obtain energy from fat metabolism. (As you learned in the "Endocrinology" chapter, glucose cannot diffuse across most cell membranes without assistance from the hormone insulin.) Plasma also performs a role in gas transport. In addition to being carried by red blood cells, carbon dioxide and oxygen are dissolved and transported in plasma.

Red Blood Cells

The primary function of blood is to transport oxygen from the lungs to the tissues. At rest, the body consumes about 4 mL of oxygen per kilogram of body weight every minute. Because it stores little oxygen, the body would quickly succumb to anoxia without the continued transport provided by the blood.

The red blood cell (RBC), or **erythrocyte**, is a biconcave disk that does not have a nucleus when mature (Figure 9-1). It contains **hemoglobin** molecules that transport oxygen. Hemoglobin comprises four subunits of *globin*, each bonded to a *heme* (iron-containing) molecule. Each globin subunit can bind with one oxygen molecule; thus, each complete hemoglobin molecule can carry up to four oxygen molecules. When all four subunits are carrying an oxygen molecule, the hemoglobin is 100 percent saturated. When fully saturated, each gram of hemoglobin can transport 1.34 mL of oxygen.

OXYGEN TRANSPORT The effectiveness of oxygen transport depends on many factors. Red blood cell mass (the number of red blood cells present) is obviously a factor in oxygen transport. The greater the number of red blood cells, the greater will be the potential oxygen-carrying

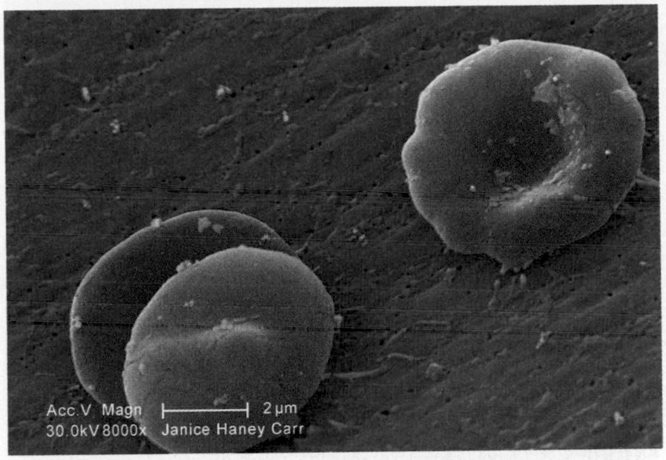

FIGURE 9-1 Scanning electron photomicrograph of red blood cells moving through a blood vessel.

(Centers for Disease Control and Prevention/Janice Haney Carr)

capacity. The percentage of oxygen bound to hemoglobin increases as the PO_2 increases. This is illustrated in the oxygen-hemoglobin dissociation curve (Figure 9-2). Normal PO_2 is approximately 95 to 100 mmHg. Based on this, the oxygen-hemoglobin dissociation curve indicates that normal oxygen saturation is about 97 percent. Hemoglobin's affinity for oxygen is also a factor in oxygen transport. Several factors affect oxygen affinity, including pH, PCO_2, concentration of 2,3-bisphosphoglycerate (2,3-BPG), and temperature.

The lower the pH (that is, the more acidic the blood), the more readily hemoglobin will release oxygen. This shifts the oxygen-hemoglobin dissociation curve to the right. In contrast, alkalosis makes hemoglobin bind to oxygen more tightly. This shifts the oxygen-hemoglobin dissociation curve to the left (Figure 9-3). The PCO_2 is directly related to the pH. Thus, in the lungs, as PCO_2 decreases with diffusion of CO_2 into the alveoli, the quantity of oxygen that binds with the hemoglobin increases. The opposite effect occurs when the blood reaches the tissues. There,

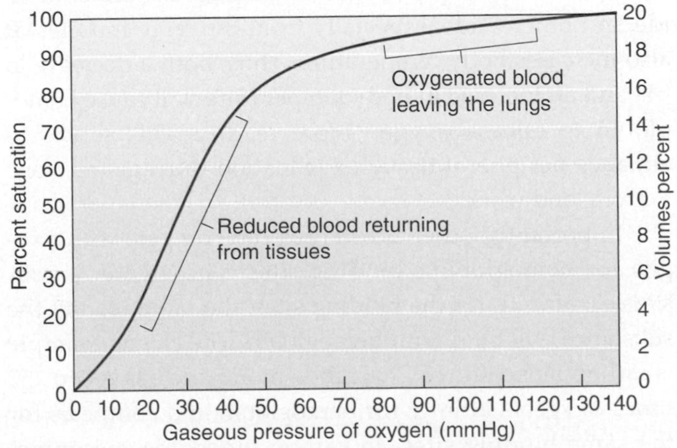

FIGURE 9-2 The oxygen–hemoglobin dissociation curve.

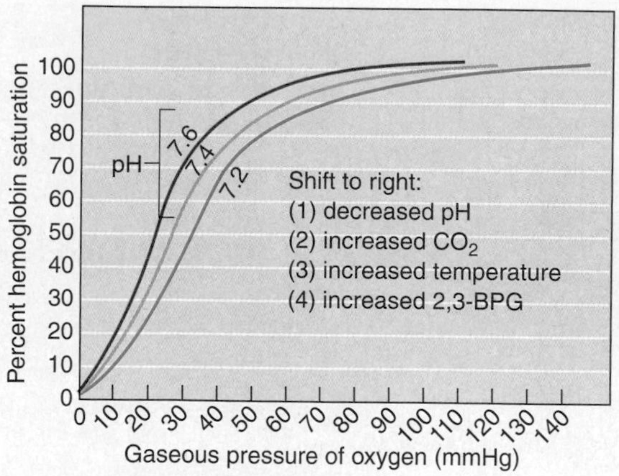

FIGURE 9-3 Effects of pH, increased carbon dioxide, temperature, and 2,3-BPG on the oxygen–hemoglobin dissociation curve.

waste CO_2 from the tissues diffuses into the blood, causing the hemoglobin to give up more oxygen to the tissues. This is called the **Bohr effect**.

Except for hemoglobin, the most abundant chemical in red blood cells is **2,3-bisphosphoglycerate (2,3-BPG)** [formerly called 2,3-diphosphoglycerate (2,3-DPG)]. During prolonged periods of hypoxia, the level of 2,3-BPG increases. This shifts the oxygen-hemoglobin dissociation curve to the right and can increase the PO_2 in the plasma as much as 10 percent more than it otherwise would have been. However, the increased 2,3-BPG makes it more difficult for oxygen to combine with hemoglobin in the lungs. This effect casts doubt on whether 2,3-BPG's effect in hypoxia is as beneficial as was once thought.

An elevation in the body temperature causes a shift of the oxygen–hemoglobin dissociation curve to the right and a decrease in hemoglobin's affinity for oxygen. Conversely, a fall in body temperature causes hemoglobin to bind oxygen more tightly. During periods of hyperthermia and pyrexia (fever), hemoglobin's decreased affinity for oxygen enhances oxygenation of the peripheral tissues and end organs.

Exercise has several effects on oxygen affinity. First, exercise causes the production and release of carbon dioxide and other acids, especially from the large muscles. It also increases body temperature. Thus, both a decrease in pH and an increase in body temperature will cause hemoglobin to release oxygen more readily. This serves to enhance peripheral tissue oxygenation during strenuous exercise and work.

Importantly, other substances can compete with oxygen for hemoglobin's binding sites. The greater a substance's affinity for the binding sites, the more readily the substance will bind with hemoglobin. The classic example is carbon monoxide (CO). Carbon monoxide has 200 to 250 times oxygen's affinity for hemoglobin and competes for the same binding sites. In carbon monoxide poisoning, when CO binds to one of the hemoglobin molecule's four binding sites, the hemoglobin molecule is altered so that the remaining three oxygen molecules are held more tightly. This inhibits oxygen release in the peripheral tissues, contributing to hypoxia, acidosis, and, eventually, shock.

RED BLOOD CELL PRODUCTION Red blood cell (RBC) production is termed **erythropoiesis**. Erythropoietin, a hormone produced primarily by the kidney, stimulates the bone marrow's production of erythrocytes. Erythropoietin is secreted when the renal cells sense hypoxia. This, in turn, stimulates the bone marrow to increase RBC production, resulting in increased red cell mass. Although it is a relatively slow process, this effectively increases the oxygen-carrying capacity of blood, thereby increasing oxygen delivery to the tissues.

The red blood cell lives approximately 120 days. Hemorrhage, **hemolysis** (destruction of the RBC), or **sequestration** of the RBCs by the liver or spleen may significantly reduce its life span. Hemorrhage may occur outside the body or be hidden within a body cavity, such as the peritoneum, retroperitoneum, or GI tract. Hemolysis may occur within the circulatory system in sickle cell disease and in rare autoimmune anemias. The spleen and liver contain specialized scavenger cells called *macrophages* (a type of white blood cell) that can remove damaged or abnormal red blood cells from the circulation.

LABORATORY EVALUATION OF RED BLOOD CELLS AND HEMOGLOBIN Red blood cells are quantified or measured and reported in two ways: red blood cell count and hematocrit. The red blood cell count is the total number of RBCs reported in millions per cubic millimeter (mm^3) of blood. Normal values vary with age and sex but in general run between 4.2 and 6.0 million/mm^3. The **hematocrit** is the packed cell volume of red blood cells per unit of blood (Figure 9-4). This measurement is obtained by placing a sample of blood in a centrifuge and spinning it at high speed so the cellular elements separate from the plasma.

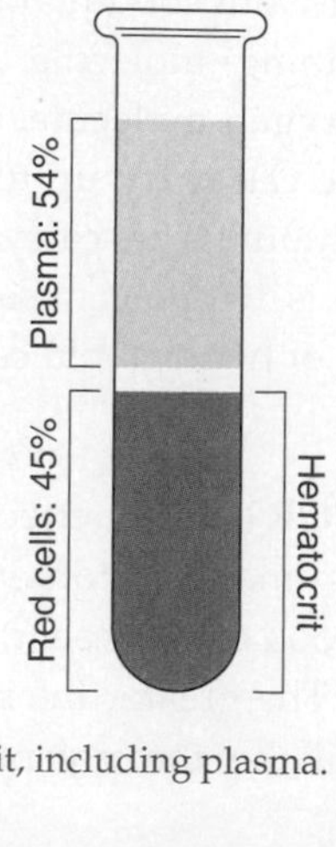

FIGURE 9-4 Hematocrit, including plasma.

The red blood cells are the heaviest blood component because they carry the iron-containing pigment hemoglobin. They are forced to the bottom of the tube. Above the red blood cells are the white blood cells. On the top of the specimen is the plasma, which consists primarily of water. The RBCs' column height is divided by the blood's total column height (cellular component plus plasma) and reported as a percentage. Normal values range between 40 and 52 percent, with females generally running a few percentage points below males.

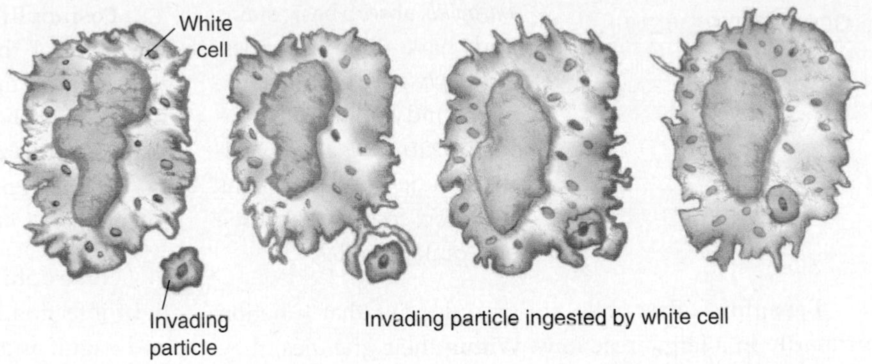

FIGURE 9-5 White blood cells engulfing and destroying an invader in the process called phagocytosis.

Another way to determine the status of the red blood cell is to measure the concentration of hemoglobin present. This is typically expressed as the number of grams of hemoglobin present per deciliter of whole blood. The hemoglobin concentration will decrease in two ways. First, when the number of red blood cells present is below normal, the hemoglobin will also be below normal. In some cases, the red blood cell volume can be normal, but the amount of hemoglobin present may be decreased. In emergency medicine, it is commonplace to measure the hemoglobin in addition to the hematocrit (H&H). Both values indicate red blood cell volume and capability. The normal hemoglobin in a man is 12.0 to 15.0 g/dL; for females, it is 10.5 to 14.0 g/dL.

White Blood Cells

White blood cells (WBCs), called **leukocytes** or white corpuscles, circulate through the bloodstream and tissues, providing protection from foreign invasion. White blood cells are extremely mobile, traveling through the bloodstream to wherever they are needed to fight infection. A large population of leukocytes does not move freely within the bloodstream, but instead is attached to the blood vessels' walls. These *marginated* leukocytes may quickly return to the circulating pool in response to stress, corticosteroids, seizures, epinephrine, and exercise. This process is called *demargination.* Marginated leukocytes that attach more firmly to the vascular lining through adhesion may then leave the blood vessels by diapedesis. This enables the leukocytes to squeeze between the cells lining the blood vessels and to follow chemical signals (**chemotaxis**) to the infection site. There, they may engulf and destroy an invader by **phagocytosis** (Figure 9-5). Others stimulate either chemical or immune responses to fight infection.

CONTENT REVIEW

➤ White Blood Cell Blasts
- Myeloblasts
- Monoblasts
- Lymphoblasts

Healthy people have from 5,000 to 9,000 white blood cells per microliter of blood. An infection can increase that number to more than 16,000 white blood cells. An increase in the white blood cell number is a classic sign of bacterial infection. White blood cells originate in the bone marrow from undifferentiated stem cells. Through a process termed **leukopoiesis**, these stem cells respond to specific growth factors that allow them to differentiate into three main blasts (immature forms): *myeloblasts, monoblasts,* and *lymphoblasts.*

CONTENT REVIEW

➤ White Blood Cell Categories
- Granulocytes
- Monocytes
- Lymphocytes

White blood cells are categorized as *granulocytes, monocytes,* or *lymphocytes* (Figure 9-6).

GRANULOCYTES Granulocytic white blood cells, so named for the granules they contain, form from stem cells that differentiate in the bone marrow in response to hormonal stimulation. These cells mature through several stages from myeloblast to promyelocyte, myelocyte, metamyelocyte, band form, and mature form (Figure 9-7). Their mature forms are classified by the type of stain they absorb.

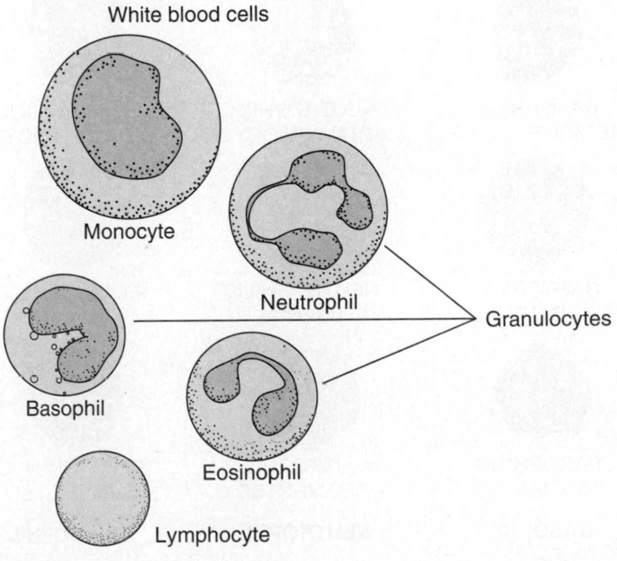

FIGURE 9-6 Types of white blood cells.

CONTENT REVIEW

➤ Granulocyte Classifications
- Basophils
- Eosinophils
- Neutrophils

Basophils absorb basic stains and have blue granules. *Eosinophils* absorb acidic stains and contain red granules. *Neutrophils* absorb neither acidic nor basic stains well and contain pale blue and pink granules.

Basophils Basophils are granulocytes that function primarily in allergic reactions. Within their granules, they store all the histamine in the circulating blood. In response to an allergic stimulus, the cells degranulate, releasing histamines that cause vasodilation, bronchoconstriction, rhinorrhea, increased vascular permeability, and increased neutrophil and eosinophil chemotaxis. Basophils also contain heparin, which breaks down blood clots.

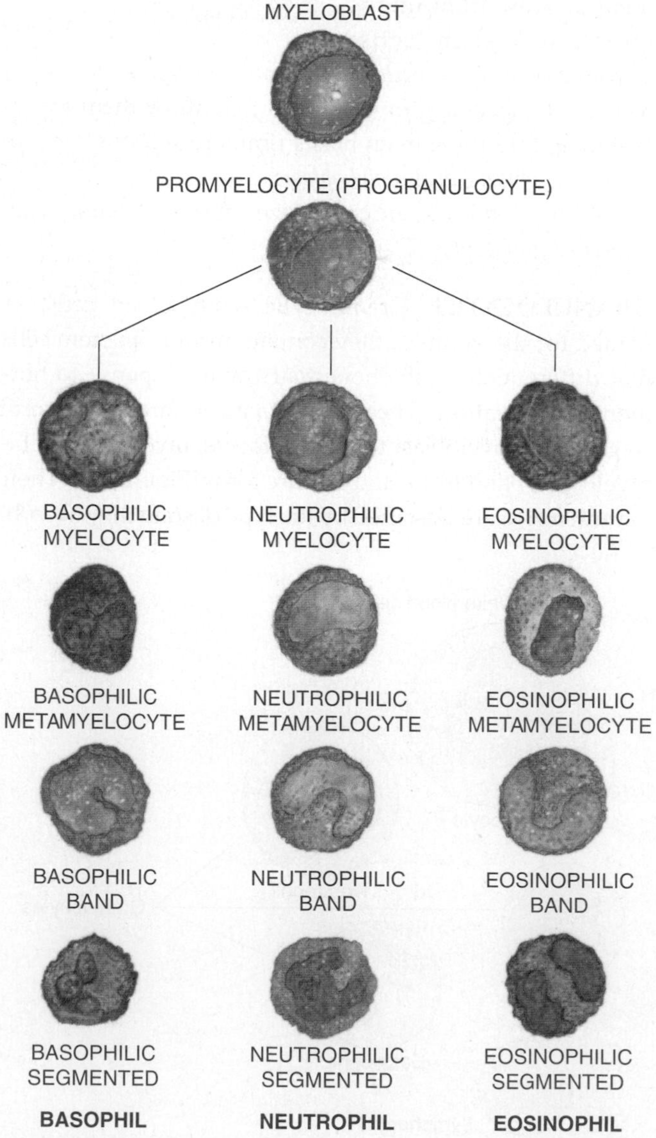

FIGURE 9-7 Granulocyte maturation.

Eosinophils Eosinophils are highly specialized members of the granulocytic series. They can inactivate the chemical mediators of acute allergic reactions, thereby modulating the anaphylactic response. They also contain **major basic protein (MBP)**, which they release in conjunction with an antibody response shown to fight parasitic infections.

Neutrophils The neutrophils' primary function is to fight infection. They leave the bloodstream by diapedesis and engulf and kill microorganisms that have invaded the body. Once they have phagocytized the microorganism, primary and secondary granules within the neutrophil fuse with the phagosome, and the organism is killed and digested. In severe infections the total neutrophil count may rise rapidly, with immature (band) forms apparent on the peripheral blood smear under microscopic examination. If the neutrophil count is low (**neutropenia**), the body cannot mount an appropriate response to infection, and the infection may overwhelm the body's defenses and kill the individual. Neutropenia may result from primary bone marrow disorders that decrease production; from overwhelming infection, viral syndrome, autoimmune disease, or drugs; and from nutritional deficiencies.

MONOCYTES Monocytes are unique in that after their initial phase of maturation they are released into the circulation and can remain there as circulating monocytes or migrate to distant sites to further mature into free or fixed tissue macrophages. Macrophages, the "garbage collectors" of the immune system, engulf both foreign invaders and dead neutrophils. They also can attack tumor cells and participate in tissue repair. Monocytes and macrophages also secrete growth factors to stimulate production of granulocytes and red blood cells. Some macrophages are fixed within tissues, residing in the liver, spleen, lungs, and lymphatic system. These cells are part of the reticuloendothelial system. They remove foreign matter, cellular debris, and proteins from the blood. After engulfing foreign proteins or infectious agents, these fixed macrophages of the reticuloendothelial system can stimulate lymphocyte production in an immune response against these agents.

LYMPHOCYTES Lymphocytes are the primary cells involved in the body's immune response. They are located throughout the body in the circulating blood, as well as in other tissues such as lymph nodes, circulating in lymph fluid, bone marrow, spleen, liver, lungs, intestine, and skin. Lymphocytes are characteristically small, round, white blood cells containing no granules on staining. However similar they may appear, though, these cells are highly specialized. They contain surface receptor sites specific to a single antigen (foreign protein) and stand ready to initiate the immune response to rid the body of that particular substance or infectious agent.

IMMUNITY The two basic subpopulations of lymphocytes are T cells and B cells. T cells mature in the thymus gland, located in the mediastinum, and then migrate throughout the body. They are responsible for developing *cell-mediated,* or *cellular, immunity.* Once an antigen activates them, they generate other cells called *effector cells* that are responsible for delayed-type hypersensitivity reactions, tumor suppression, graft rejection (organ transplant rejections), and defense against intracellular organisms. B cells produce antibodies to combat infection, which is termed *humoral immunity.* B cells originate in the bone marrow and then migrate to peripheral lymphatic tissues. There, they can be exposed to antigens from invading organisms and respond by producing the specific antibodies necessary to defend against them. Some of these B cells' lines are maintained and give the body a "memory" of the previous infection. When the body is subsequently exposed to the same antigen or infection, it generates a rapid response to quickly overwhelm the infection (see the chapter "Immunology").

AUTOIMMUNE DISEASE **Autoimmune disease** occurs when the body makes antibodies against its own tissues. These antibodies may be limited to specific organs, such as the thyroid, as occurs in Hashimoto's thyroiditis, or they may involve virtually every tissue type, as in the antinuclear antibodies of systemic lupus erythematosus (SLE) that attack the body's cell nuclei. Several anemias result from autoimmunity and will be discussed later in this chapter. Mechanisms for the development of autoimmune disease include genetic factors and viral infections.

ALTERATIONS IN IMMUNE RESPONSE Several factors can alter the body's immune response. For example, patients who receive an organ transplant must take drugs that inhibit cellular immunity and prevent graft rejection. If they do not, the T cells will recognize the new organ as "not self" and begin the process of attacking it. This is called *rejection.* Unfortunately, immunosuppressed organ recipient patients are at risk for infections from many different organisms, including bacteria, viruses, fungi, and protozoa. Human immunodeficiency virus (HIV) effectively destroys cell-mediated immunity by selectively attacking, and ultimately killing, T cells. This also leaves the patient at risk for opportunistic infections against which the body cannot defend itself, ultimately causing death. Patients who have cancer are often immunocompromised by the disease itself or by chemotherapy agents that also attack the bone marrow. These agents decrease leukocyte production to extremely low levels, leaving the body defenseless against infection. As a paramedic, you must protect your immunosuppressed patients from undue exposure to infection by good hand-washing technique, correct IV technique, and proper wound care. If you have an infection, you must take precautions not to transmit it to your patients. If the infection is highly contagious, as in influenza or chickenpox, you may have to work in a non-patient care setting.

INFLAMMATORY PROCESS The **inflammatory process** is a nonspecific defense mechanism that wards off damage from microorganisms or trauma. It attempts to localize the damage while destroying the source, at the same time facilitating repair of the tissues. Causes of the inflammatory process may be an infectious agent, trauma, chemical, or immunologic. After local tissue injury occurs, the damaged tissues release chemical messengers that attract white blood cells (chemotaxis), increase capillary permeability, and cause vasodilation. If bacteria are present, responding neutrophils or macrophages will phagocytize them and tissue repair will begin. The greater capillary permeability and vasodilation allow increased blood flow to the area and enable fluid to leak out of the capillaries. The process of local inflammation results in redness, warmth, swelling, and usually pain. The pain serves as a reminder against overuse, allowing time for rest and repair. Systemic inflammation is an inflammatory reaction, often in response to a bacterial infection. Fever is a common symptom and likely occurs in response to chemical mediators that macrophages release in response to the infectious agent. These chemical mediators act on the brain and lead to stimulation of the sympathetic nervous system, which causes vasoconstriction, heat conservation, and fever. The macrophages also release factors that stimulate the release of leukocytes from the bone marrow, leading to an elevated white blood cell count.

Platelets

Platelets, or **thrombocytes**, are small fragments of large cells called *megakaryocytes.* Like the other blood cells described so far, megakaryocytes come from an undifferentiated stem cell in the bone marrow. The hormone *thrombopoietin* stimulates these stem cells to differentiate through several stages into megakaryocytes, which then mature and break up into platelets—small fragments without nuclei. The normal number of platelets ranges from 150,000 to 450,000 per microliter of blood. As they function to form a plug at an initial bleeding site and also secrete factors important in clot formation, too few platelets, a condition called *thrombocytopenia,* can lead to bleeding problems and blood loss. Too many platelets, *thrombocytosis,* may cause abnormal clotting, plugs in vessels, and emboli that may travel to the extremities, heart, lungs, or brain. Platelets survive from 7 to 10 days and are removed from circulation by the spleen.

Platelets are activated when they contact injured tissue. This contact stimulates an enzyme within the platelet, causing the surface to become "sticky," which, in turn, leads the platelets to aggregate and form a plug. Platelets also adhere to the damaged tissue to keep the plug in place.

As the platelets aggregate, they release chemical messengers that also activate the blood clotting system.

Hemostasis

Hemostasis—from *hemo* (blood) and *stasis* (standing still)—is the term used to describe the combined three mechanisms that work to prevent or control blood loss. These mechanisms are:

- Vascular spasms
- Platelet plugs
- Stable fibrin blood clots (coagulation)

When a blood vessel tears, the smooth muscle fibers (tunica media) in the vessel walls contract. This causes vasoconstriction and reduces the size of the tear. Less blood flows through the constricted area, effectively limiting blood loss, and the smaller tear makes it easier for a platelet plug to develop and stop blood loss (Figure 9-8). At any tear in a blood vessel, platelets aggregate and adhere to collagen, a connective tissue that supports the blood vessels. This forms a platelet plug, which acts much like bubble gum stuck into a hole. The plug is unstable, however, and would permit the vessel to bleed again if not for the formation of a stable fibrin clot. This process, blood coagulation, is initiated in part by the platelet plug (Figure 9-9).

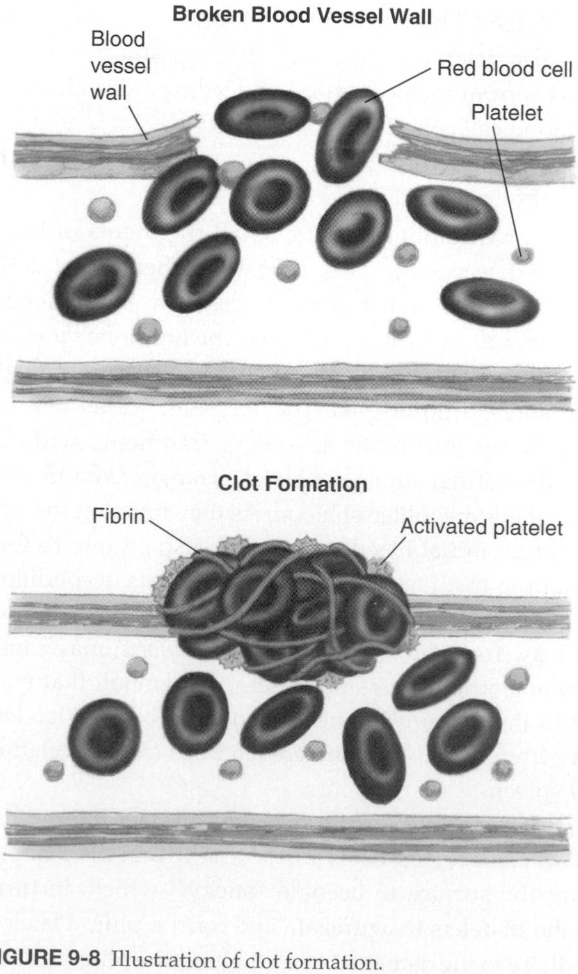

FIGURE 9-8 Illustration of clot formation.

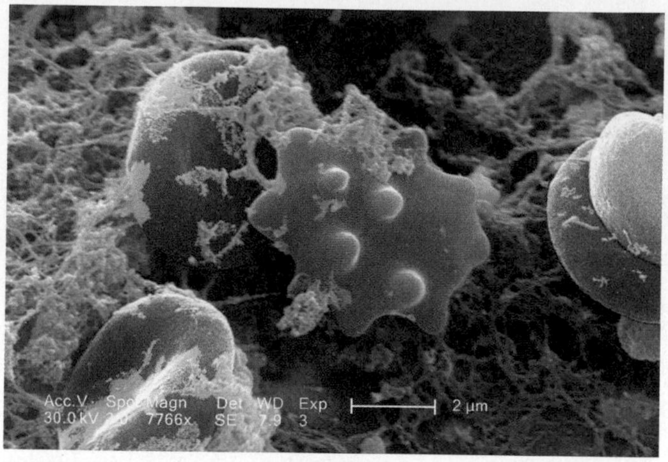

FIGURE 9-9 Scanning electron photomicrograph of clot formation. *(Centers for Disease Control and Prevention/Janice Haney Carr)*

Because of the smoothness of the tunica intima, the blood vessels' innermost lining, blood normally flows through the vessels without frictional damage to cells or platelets. Damage to cells or to the vessel lining, however, starts the coagulation cascade. This cascade, or sequence of events, can be activated either by damage to vessels (extrinsic pathway) or by trauma to blood from turbulence (intrinsic pathway). Either results in the cascade's progression to a clot. Most clotting proteins are produced in the liver and circulate in an inactive state. The best known of these are *prothrombin* and *fibrinogen*. The damaged cells send out a chemical message that activates a specific clotting factor. This activates each protein in turn, until a stable fibrin clot forms. To completely stop the bleeding, the coagulation cascade relies on the platelet plug and the clotting factors to interact. Once the bleeding stops, the inflammatory and healing processes can begin. The coagulation cascade can be summarized thus (Figure 9-10):

1. A. ***Intrinsic pathway.*** Platelets release substances that lead to the formation of prothrombin activator

   or

   B. ***Extrinsic pathway.*** Tissue damage causes platelet aggregation and the formation of prothrombin activator.
2. ***Common pathway.*** The prothrombin activator, in the presence of calcium, converts prothrombin to thrombin.
3. ***Thrombin.*** In the presence of calcium, thrombin converts fibrinogen to stable fibrin, which then traps blood cells and more platelets to form a clot.

The development of a clot does not end the coagulation cascade. What the body can do, it usually can undo, given sufficient time. Once a fibrin clot is formed, it releases a chemical called *plasminogen*. Plasminogen is converted to

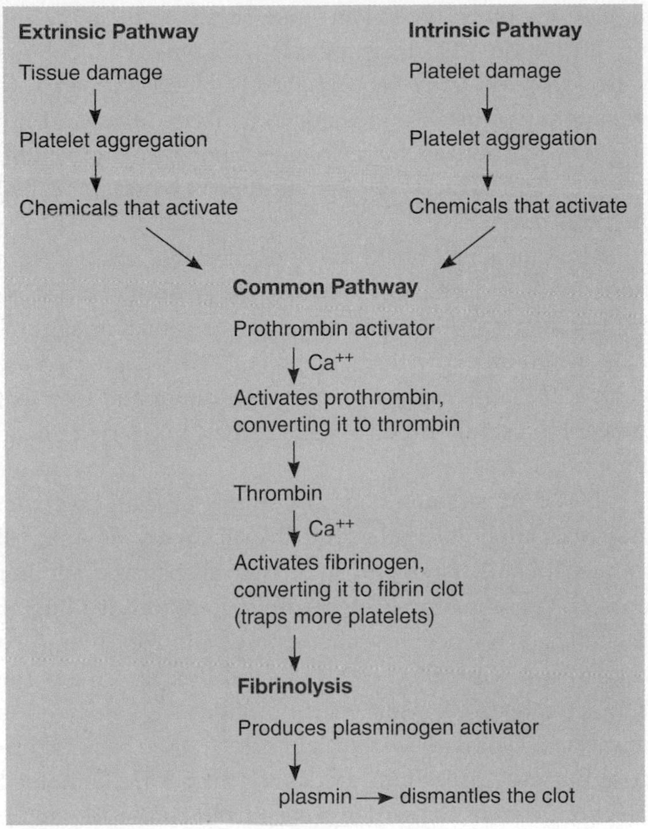

FIGURE 9-10 The coagulation cascade.

plasmin and is then capable of dismantling, or lysing, a clot through the process of **fibrinolysis**. A clot's dismantling generally takes from hours to days. By that time, scarring has begun.

Thrombosis (clot formation), when it occurs in coronary arteries or cerebral vasculature, may lead to heart attack and stroke. To stimulate or speed fibrinolysis and thus break down clots, medical researchers have developed several fibrinolytic agents. These agents may help reestablish blood flow to these vital organs, limiting or preventing tissue death, and thus help to prevent the patient's disability or death. Fibrinolytics are effective only against blockages whose components include a fibrin clot.

Patients who lack certain clotting factors can have bleeding disorders that may complicate their assessment and treatment. Other patients take medications that decrease the effectiveness of platelets or the coagulation cascade. Recall that an enzyme on a platelet membrane makes the membrane sticky. Certain medications such as aspirin, dipyridamole (Persantine), and ticlopidine (Ticlid) irreversibly alter the enzyme, thus decreasing the platelets' ability to aggregate and initiate the coagulation cascade. Other medications, such as heparin and warfarin (Coumadin), cause changes within the clotting cascade that prevent clot formation. Heparin, in conjunction with antithrombin III (a naturally occurring thrombin inactivator), rapidly inactivates thrombin, which then prevents formation of the fibrin clot. Warfarin blocks vitamin K activity necessary to generate the activated forms of clotting factors II, VII, IX, and X, effectively interrupting the clotting cascade.

Glycoprotein IIb-IIIa receptors are present on the platelet membrane and are the major platelet surface receptor involved in the final common pathway of platelet aggregation. When platelets become activated, the glycoprotein IIb/IIIa receptor undergoes a conformational change and becomes able to crosslink fibrinogen, thereby serving as the final common pathway resulting in platelet aggregation. Glycoprotein IIb/IIIa inhibitors are medications used in the treatment of acute coronary syndrome, often in combination with angioplasty with or without stent placement. These agents are frequently given in combination with heparin or aspirin to prevent clotting before and during invasive heart procedures. Glycoprotein IIb/IIIa inhibitors are classified as potent platelet inhibitors. The following are specific glycoprotein IIb/IIIa inhibitors and their brand names:

- Abciximab (ReoPro)
- Eptifibatide (Integrilin)
- Tirofiban (Aggrastat)

Vitamin K (AquaMEPHYTON) enhances clotting. Certain byproducts of tobacco smoking (especially in women on birth control pills) also enhance clotting. Relative or complete immobility, trauma, polycythemia (high red blood cell count), and cancer may also lead to increased clotting, as blood becomes relatively stagnant. The stagnation of blood allows platelet activation to begin, which leads to clotting. To counteract the effects of decreased activity, many patients take aspirin or other antiplatelet inhibitors and wear compressive stockings to facilitate venous drainage from the lower extremities.

Blood Products and Blood Typing

A blood transfusion is the transplantation of blood or a component of blood from one person to another. It is accomplished by IV infusion (Figure 9-11). Various types of transfusions are given for various purposes (Table 9-1).

In the 1800s, when patients received blood from others, some had a reaction that led to multiple organ failure and death. Karl Landsteiner discovered the reason for this was reaction **antigens**, proteins on the surface of the donor's red blood cells that the patient's body recognized

CONTENT REVIEW

➤ Blood Types
- A
- B
- AB
- O

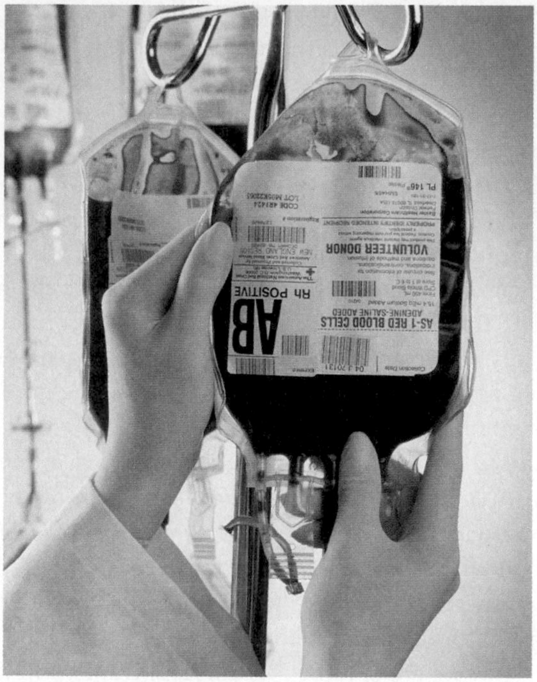

FIGURE 9-11 Blood transfusion.

(Steve Dunwell/The Image Bank/Getty Images)

as "not self." Following transfusion, antibodies in the patient's own blood attacked the foreign antigens present in the transfused blood. Landsteiner named the antigens A and B and the opposing antibodies anti-A and anti-B. Someone with A antigen on his red blood cells would have anti-B antibodies. His blood type would be A. Someone with B antigens on the red blood cell surface would have anti-A antibodies; his type would be B. Some people's red blood cells have both antigens on their surface but neither antibody. Their blood type is AB. Others have neither antigen but both antibodies; their blood type is O (for zero antigens, but pronounced "Oh"). Blood type is an inherited trait. Approximately 45 percent of the U.S. population has type O, 39 percent type A, 11 percent type B, and 5 percent type AB.

Because only the antibodies recognize and attack foreign tissue, a person with no antibodies (type AB) can receive any blood type in an emergency, and the body will not attack the cells. Thus, people with type AB blood are called *universal recipients.* Conversely, blood with no antigens to any other blood group type (type O) would not trigger a reaction, as the recipient's blood recognizes nothing "foreign." Thus, people with type O blood are called *universal donors.*

Crossmatching blood involves checking samples from both donor and recipient to ensure the greatest compatibility. If a donor's blood does not clump together, or agglutinate, when mixed with the recipient's blood, the two are compatible. Reliance on the universal donor and recipient concept is useful only in an emergency, when there is no time to check samples.

Blood transfusion is not as simple as that, however. Approximately 40 years after the discovery of A and B antigens, Landsteiner and A. S. Weiner observed another antigen present on red blood cells. Research leading to this antigen's discovery used rhesus monkey blood, so the antigen was called the Rh factor. If a person has the Rh factor, he is Rh positive; if not, he is Rh negative. As many as 500 other lesser antigens have since been identified, but they usually do not cause the severe hemolytic reaction seen in the patients sensitized to the Rh factor. *Erythroblastosis fetalis,* more commonly called hemolytic disease of the newborn, can lead to a fatal hemolytic reaction in neonates. In this disease, the mother who is Rh^- is sensitized by previous exposure to the Rh antigen during a previous pregnancy with an Rh^+ child or from a previous blood transfusion. Therefore, if she subsequently becomes pregnant with an Rh^+ child, the mother produces antibodies that attack the fetus's red blood cells, leading to a severe—and often fatal—hemolytic reaction. Fortunately, the incidence of hemolytic disease of newborns has been declining due to the administration of Rh immune globulin (RhoGAM) to mothers. This inhibits formation of anti-Rh antibodies. Additionally, transfusions *in utero* or fetal exchange transfusions immediately after birth can diminish or eliminate the likelihood of infant death.

Table 9-1 Types of Transfusions

Type of Transfusion	Contents	Use
Whole blood	All cells, platelets, clotting factors, and plasma	Replace blood loss from hemorrhage
Packed red blood cells (PRBCs)	Red blood cells and some plasma	Replace red blood cells in anemic patients
Platelets	Thrombocytes and some plasma	Replace platelets in a patient with thrombocytopenia
Fresh frozen plasma (FFP)	Plasma, a combination of fluids, clotting factors, and proteins	Replace volume in a burn patient or in hypovolemia secondary to low oncotic pressure
Clotting factors	Specific clotting factors needed for coagulation	Replace factors missing due to inadequate production, as in hemophilia

Transfusion Reactions

There are many types of transfusion reactions. One, hemolytic transfusion reaction, occurs when a donor's and recipient's blood are not compatible. Antigens on the donor's red blood cells trigger a response from the antibodies in the recipient's blood. The antibodies attach to the red blood cells, which are then *hemolyzed*, or taken up by the fixed macrophages of the spleen's reticuloendothelial system.

Signs and symptoms of a hemolytic transfusion reaction may include facial flushing, hyperventilation, tachycardia, and a sense of dread. Hives may appear on the skin, and the patient may develop chest pain, wheezing, fever, chills, and cyanosis. Flank pain may occur as small clots begin to clog the microvasculature of the kidneys, which can lead to kidney failure requiring dialysis. The damage can be permanent.

If you are caring for a patient receiving a blood transfusion and he develops what you believe to be a hemolytic reaction, stop the transfusion immediately. Change all associated IV tubing and initiate IV therapy with normal saline or lactated Ringer's solution. Administer a bolus as necessary to maintain good perfusion and blood pressure. Furosemide (Lasix) is often administered to promote diuresis. Low dose dopamine (2–5 mcg/kg/minute) should be considered along with the IV fluid to help maintain adequate renal perfusion. If you observe evidence of an allergic reaction, you can give diphenhydramine (Benadryl) 25 to 50 mg IV to help with some of the histamine-mediated effects such as itching or hives. In extreme cases of anaphylactic reaction, you may need to administer IV epinephrine if the patient is hypotensive or demonstrates severe bronchospasm.

The most common transfusion reaction is the febrile nonhemolytic reaction. It is caused by sensitization to antigens on the white blood cells, platelets, or plasma proteins. Signs and symptoms include headache, fever, and chills. As with any other transfusion reaction, always stop the transfusion before attempting to treat it. After stopping the blood product, change all tubing and initiate normal saline IV. Patients are often given diphenhydramine (Benadryl) and an antipyretic (e.g., ibuprofen, acetaminophen) for the fever. No further treatment may be necessary, as this reaction rarely progresses to more serious complications. However, close observation is required to exclude development of a hemolytic reaction. In the event of any transfusion reaction, return all blood bags, tubing, and filters to the blood bank for analysis. Medical direction may order you to take blood and urine samples.

Because blood transfusion adds fluid to the system, a patient may experience signs and symptoms of circulatory overload. In fact, signs and symptoms are the same as those for left ventricular failure and may include pulmonary edema, dyspnea, and chest pain. Hypotension is not usually a problem, and you may treat the patient successfully by slowing the heart rate and administering diuretics.[1]

General Assessment and Management

In general, patients with disorders of the hematopoietic system may present with a variety of complaints and physical findings. Patients with infection, white blood cell abnormalities (immunocompromised and prone to infection), or transfusion reactions may present with febrile symptoms. Subsequently, these patients may develop hemodynamic instability as infection progresses to sepsis or as the transfusion reaction leads to a hemolytic reaction, renal failure, and disseminated intravascular coagulation (DIC). Acute hemodynamic compromise can also be found in patients with anemia secondary to acute blood loss, coagulation defects, or autoimmune disease. These disease processes may not be easily differentiated in the field and often require significant laboratory testing to confirm the diagnosis. In most cases, however, if you obtain a careful history, you will have a good working diagnosis.

Most hematopoietic disorders are chronic conditions that present with acute exacerbation when the patient is exposed to an additional stress such as infection or trauma. Treatment of patients with disorders of the hematopoietic system, in most cases, is supportive. Some patients may have hemodynamic instability from blood or fluid loss. These patients may require intravenous fluids to support end-organ perfusion and prevent shock. In addition, they should receive oxygen therapy to prevent hypoxia from poor perfusion and diminished oxygen-carrying capacity of the blood. It is important to recognize the need for rapid transport in patients with hemodynamic instability who may require transfusion or other definitive care measures. Always contact medical direction for questions or problems.

Scene Size-Up

Assessment of the patient with a possible hematopoietic abnormality begins the same as for any other patient. Perform a scene size-up and take standard precautions. During your approach, form a general impression of the patient. Is the patient a trauma or medical patient? In how much distress is the patient?

Primary Assessment

Complete a primary assessment for life threats. Determine responsiveness and assess the airway, breathing, and circulation. Alterations in the hematopoietic system may present as life-threatening bleeds or overwhelming infections with septic shock. Do not spend time obtaining a complete set of vital signs during the primary assessment. Check the ABCs and quickly determine your priority for transport. Critical or unstable patients should be considered candidates for expeditious transport.

Secondary Assessment

Next, complete a secondary assessment. Use your general impression to choose a format for a responsive or unresponsive medical patient or trauma patient with significant or nonsignificant mechanism of injury. Each format follows a sequence of history gathering and physical examination designed to meet the needs of that particular patient. Trauma patients and unresponsive medical patients often present life-threatening problems that you will have noted in your primary assessment.

History

For a responsive medical patient, obtain a SAMPLE history and perform a physical exam. Obtain a set of vital signs and place the pulse oximeter. Keep in mind that an anemic patient will have increased heart and respiratory rates as his body attempts to compensate for less oxygen reaching the tissues. Ask for the chief complaint—why did the patient call for assistance? What *s*igns or *s*ymptoms (*S*AMPLE) accompanied or preceded the complaint? Pay attention to generalized complaints such as fatigue, lethargy, malaise, apprehension, or confusion. These may indicate inadequate oxygen delivery to the tissues. Have there been any unusual skin changes, such as coloring or bruising? Does the patient complain of itching? Inquire about lymph node enlargement (swollen glands), sore throat, or pain upon swallowing. These may indicate infection.

Any change in the blood's ability to deliver oxygen to the body will appear in the cardiovascular and respiratory systems. Note dyspnea, palpitations, and dizziness with changes in the patient's position. Patients with hematologic problems may suffer syncope. Did the patient have a syncopal episode, or is he just weak? Syncope can be due to several factors but is often related to a sudden change in position in a patient who has a marked anemia. Bleeding abnormalities may be disguised as gastrointestinal upset. Ask about overt bleeding with vomiting or diarrhea, but do not overlook complaints of nausea or anorexia, vomiting of "coffee ground" material, or having black tarry or cranberry, sticky, odoriferous stools. Many patients will notice bleeding of the gums when they brush their teeth. This can, on occasion, be hard to control. Atraumatic bleeding of the gums almost always points to an underlying hematologic abnormality. Ask about changes in urination, hematuria (blood in the urine), and alterations in the usual menstrual pattern in females. Keep in mind that hematologic disorders are often diagnosed when the patient seeks assistance for another medical condition.

Determine any *a*llergies (S*A*MPLE). Be sure to ask about use of prescription or over-the-counter *m*edications (SA*M*PLE). Make note of the patient's medication, dose, and the condition for which he takes the medication. Also, if time allows, note the dosing schedule of the medications. Ask about compliance. Does the patient take medication as prescribed? When was the last dose taken? Medications that may indicate an alteration in the hematologic system, or that might make the patient more susceptible to an alteration in the system, include pain relievers, antibiotics, anticoagulants, hormones, and medications for heart disease, arthritis, and seizures.

When asking about *p*ast medical history (SAM*P*LE), make note of surgeries such as a splenectomy, heart-valve replacement, or placement of long-term venous access devices. Ask about bloodborne infections such as HIV or hepatitis B or C. Make note of liver or bone marrow disease or cancers. Include questions about family history such as hemophilia, sickle cell disease, cancer, or death at an early age that was not trauma related. Inquire also about social habits such as smoking, alcohol consumption, IV drug use, or long-term exposure to chemicals or radiation.

If you find a significant history, ask about the last episode of an incident or last use of a medication. Remember to include the usual questions about *l*ast oral intake (SAMP*L*E). Also, inquire about any unusual *e*vents (SAMPL*E*) that preceded the onset of the complaint, such as the start of a new medication, recent transfusion, fall, or injury.

Physical Examination

When performing the physical exam, evaluate each system methodically as you would in any other patient. If the history suggests a hematopoietic problem, look for potential pathology during the physical exam that may confirm your working diagnosis and be a clue to developing complications.

- ***Nervous system***—Always evaluate the nervous system in any patient with a suspected hematologic problem. First, note the patient's level of consciousness using the AVPU system. Be alert for other nervous system disorders. Many patients with hematologic problems will complain of being "weak and dizzy." Try to clarify this further. Is the patient fatigued, weak all over, or does he have focal weakness? Is he dizzy, or is he suffering true vertigo? Both can be associated with hematologic problems such as anemia. Ask if the patient has any numbness or motor deficits. Pernicious anemia can cause sensory deficits that are often unilateral. Try to determine whether the patient had a syncopal episode. What were the patient's condition and position immediately prior to the syncopal episode? Many of the

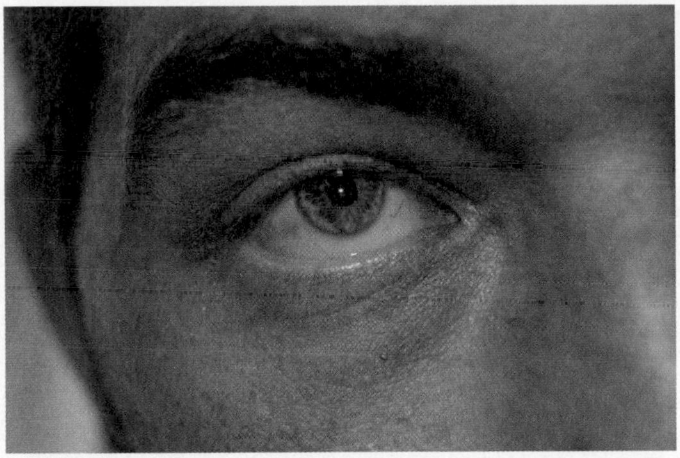

FIGURE 9-12 Jaundice.
(© Edward T. Dickinson, MD)

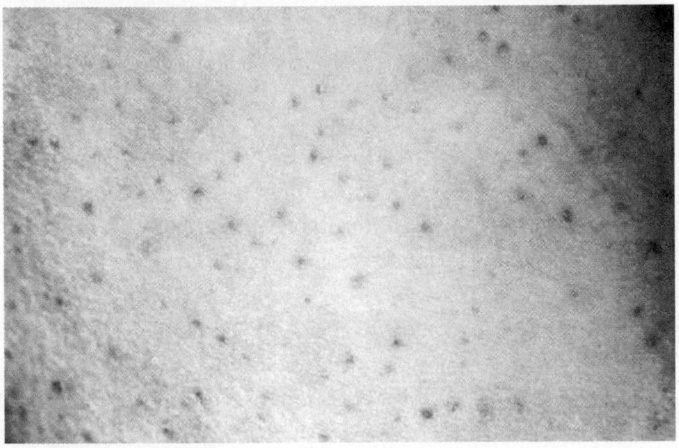

FIGURE 9-13 Petechiae.
(Centers for Disease Control and Prevention)

hematologic diseases, especially the autoimmune diseases, will affect the eye. Always examine the eyes for abnormalities. Question the patient about any visual disturbances or visual loss. In addition to the autoimmune diseases, sickle cell anemia is notorious for causing eye problems.

- *Skin*—Note the patient's skin color (Figure 9-12). Jaundice (yellow skin) may indicate liver disease or hemolysis of red blood cells, whereas a florid (reddish) appearance is often associated with polycythemia. Patients with anemia typically exhibit pallor. Observe for petechiae (tiny red dots in the skin) (Figure 9-13), purpura (large purplish blotches related to multiple hemorrhages into the skin), and bruising. (Figure 9-14 compares the appearance of petechiae and purpura.) Inquire about pruritus (itching). Patients with hematologic disorders often develop pruritus. Some hematologic problems, such as sickle cell anemia, cause the destruction of red blood cells. This results in hemoglobin's spilling into the circulatory system. Macrophages then break down the hemoglobin. The iron is removed and transported to the bones or liver. The porphyrin portion of the hemoglobin is subsequently converted into bilirubin, which is taken up by the liver. An excess of bilirubin, either from liver disease or from the breakdown of hemoglobin associated with the hemolytic anemias, can cause pruritus. Often, patients will develop itching over a bruise. As the hemoglobin breaks down within the bruise, the localized accumulation of bilirubin causes the itching. This is most common one to two weeks after the bruise occurs. When examining the skin, be alert for any evidence of prolonged bleeding. The patient may have several bandages over relatively minor wounds where he could not stop the bleeding.
- *Lymphatic*—The lymphatic system is affected early in hematopoietic diseases, especially those of the immune system. During your physical exam, pay particular attention to the lymph nodes. Palpate the lymph nodes of the neck, clavicle, axilla, and groin. Note any enlargement. Compare sides. Splenomegaly (an enlarged spleen) is also often present, but this can be hard to examine in the field.
- *Gastrointestinal*—The gastrointestinal effects of hematologic problems can be quite varied. Epistaxis (nosebleed) is common. The nasal mucosa is quite vascular, as it warms and humidifies the inhaled air. A slight crack in the nasal mucosa can result in brisk bleeding. This is a particular problem in people with blood clotting abnormalities, as stopping the bleeding is very difficult for them. These patients may swallow a great deal of blood and may become nauseated. Also, blood acts as a cathartic (laxative). Patients who swallow even moderate amounts of blood will often report loose bowel movements. These are often dark (melena). Blood present in emesis may be bright red or appear like coffee grounds.

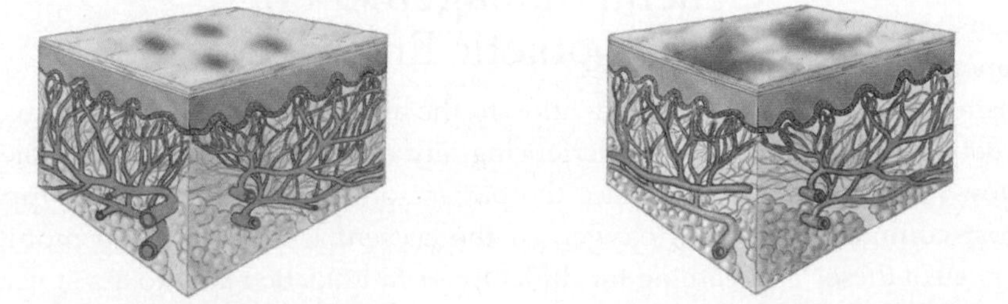

(a) *Petechiae* – Reddish-purple spots, diameter less than 0.5 cm

(b) *Purpura* – Reddish-purple blotches, diameter more than 0.5 cm

FIGURE 9-14 (a) Petechiae; (b) purpura.

- *Musculoskeletal*—Many hematopoietic problems are autoimmune in nature. That is, a problem develops in which the immune system has trouble determining which tissues are self and which are nonself. Autoimmune diseases such as rheumatoid arthritis result from the body's immune system attacking various tissues in the joints. This can cause arthralgia (pain and swelling of the joints). Autoimmune diseases tend to affect more than one joint, whereas infectious processes tend to affect only a single joint. Patients with blood clotting disorders such as hemophilia will often develop hemarthrosis (bleeding into a joint) with only minor trauma. This can result in an extremely swollen, discolored, and painful joint. Always inquire about joint pain and examine the major joints in any patient suspected of having hematopoietic disease.
- *Cardiorespiratory*—The effects of hematopoietic problems on the cardiorespiratory system are varied. Patients with anemia will often develop dyspnea, tachycardia, and chest pain from the increased cardiac work caused by the anemia. In severe cases, patients can develop high-output heart failure, in which the heart works excessively hard to compensate for a profound anemia. If untreated, heart failure and pulmonary edema can result. Patients with bleeding disorders may report expectorating blood with coughing. This can be due to small tears in the respiratory mucosa from the coughing. Normally, these heal quickly. Patients with bleeding disorders, however, will continue to bleed, resulting in potential airway obstruction and, in severe cases, shock. Always auscultate for breath sounds. Note crackles or rhonchi indicative of heart problems or infection.
- *Genitourinary*—The genitourinary effects of hematopoietic problems are typically due to bleeding disorders or infection. Bleeding disorders can cause hematuria (blood in the urine) and blood in the scrotal sac in males. A woman who still has her uterus may develop menorrhagia (heavy menstrual bleeding) or frank vaginal bleeding (dysfunctional uterine bleeding). Immunocompromised patients are at increased risk for developing genitourinary infections. These can range from recurrent urinary tract infections to severe sexually transmitted diseases. Sickle cell anemia, especially in the later stages, can cause priapism. This is a prolonged, painful erection due to obstruction of the blood vessels that drain the penis and allow for detumescence. Sickle cell disease is the most common cause of priapism in the emergency setting. All of these require additional evaluation in the emergency department. Detailed evaluation of the genitourinary system is not appropriate for field settings.

Bleeding of the gums is one of the earliest findings of hematologic problems. Patients with blood clotting abnormalities and low platelet levels will often develop atraumatic bleeding of the gums. Any patient with bleeding gums requires a detailed investigation for a possible hematologic disorder. Gingivitis (infection of the gums) can be due to poor hygiene, disease, or both. However, chronic gingivitis should cause increased suspicion of a hematologic disorder, especially one involving the immune system. In addition, gingivitis increases a patient's risk of developing sepsis. Slight trauma, such as brushing the teeth, can cause the bacteria to enter the circulatory system, resulting in generalized sepsis. Always note the presence of gingivitis when examining for bleeding gums. Ulcerations of the gums and oral mucosa are typically due to viral diseases. These infections are more common in immunosuppressed patients. Thrush (yeast infection in the mouth) in adults is almost always associated with AIDS. (Thrush in children is common and not a reason for concern.)

The liver plays a major role in manufacturing many of the substances required for blood clotting. Liver disease can slow blood clotting. This is most evident in a prolonged prothrombin (PT) time. Also, as the liver fails, the bilirubin level will increase, resulting in jaundice. Thus, any patient with jaundice should be evaluated for liver disease.

Abdominal pain is not uncommon in persons with hematologic disease. Two of the major organs associated with the hematopoietic system, the liver and spleen, are in the abdomen. Problems with the spleen, the liver, or both can lead to abdominal pain. Splenomegaly is common in hematologic problems, as the spleen is active in the removal of abnormal or aged red cells. In some of the anemias, especially the hemolytic anemias, the spleen can become markedly enlarged. Patients with sickle cell anemia will often develop splenic infarcts as sickled cells accumulate and block blood supply to parts of the spleen. By the time children with sickle cell disease are 5 years of age, they are virtually asplenic (without a spleen), as the disease has completely infarcted their spleen. Because the spleen is not functional, these patients are placed at increased risk of infection, especially by encapsulated bacteria.

General Management of Hematopoietic Emergencies

Pay close attention to the airway and ventilation status of patients experiencing any alteration in the hematopoietic system. Place the patient on high-concentration supplemental oxygen (if the patient is hypoxic) and monitor breathing for difficulty or fatigue. Be ready to assist ventilations with a bag-valve mask.

Assess the circulatory system. Consider fluid volume replacement, but remember that crystalloid solutions cannot carry oxygen. Too much fluid can "dilute" the blood and reduce its capacity per unit volume to carry oxygen. Be alert for arrhythmias and treat accordingly. Based on your assessment and evaluation, create the optimum environment for the blood to perform its tasks of oxygen delivery and waste product removal. Creating such an environment may include giving the patient aspirin to inhibit platelet aggregation or ventilating the patient to compensate for acidosis and to allow oxygen to unload from hemoglobin at the tissues.

Transport the patient to the appropriate facility, provide comfort measures including analgesia, and provide psychological support to both the patient and his family.

Managing Specific Hematopoietic Disorders

The rest of this chapter will detail the more common hematopoietic diseases that you might encounter in prehospital care. Again, it is important to remember that many hematologic problems occur in conjunction with other illnesses. For example, someone with a cancer or significant renal disease quite commonly will have a coexisting anemia. In the following sections, we first examine diseases of the red blood cells. These are the most common hematologic problems encountered. Second, we look at the white blood cell diseases. These include the leukemias, lymphomas, and similar illnesses. Finally, we present diseases of the platelets and blood coagulation disorders.

Diseases of the Red Blood Cells

Red blood cell diseases result in too many red blood cells, too few red blood cells, or improperly functioning red blood cells. An excess of red blood cells is called **polycythemia**. Although uncommon, several conditions can cause polycythemia. An inadequate number of red blood cells or inadequate hemoglobin within the red blood cells is called **anemia**. Anemia is common, and several types are frequently encountered. Finally, red blood cell function can be impaired. Most commonly, this is due to problems with either hemoglobin structure and function or the red blood cell membrane. Problems with red blood cell function include the thalassemias and sickle cell anemia.

CONTENT REVIEW

- ➤ Diseases of the Red Blood Cells
  - Anemia
  - Sickle cell disease
  - Polycythemia

Anemias

The most common diseases of the red blood cells are the anemias. Anemia is typically classified as a hematocrit of less than 37 percent in women or less than 40 percent in men. Most patients with anemia will remain asymptomatic until the hematocrit drops below 30 percent. The decreased hematocrit in anemia is due to a reduction in the number of red blood cells or in the amount or quality of hemoglobin in the red blood cells. Anemia is actually a sign of an underlying disease process that is either destroying red blood cells and hemoglobin or decreasing the production of red blood cells and hemoglobin. Blood loss, either acute or chronic, also can cause anemia. Anemia can be a self-limiting disease or it can be a lifelong illness requiring periodic transfusions. Anemias that result from the destruction of red blood cells are called *hemolytic anemias*. These can be hereditary or acquired. Examples of hereditary hemolytic anemias include sickle cell anemia, thalassemia, and glucose-6-phosphate dehydrogenase deficiency (G6PD). Acquired hemolytic anemias can result from immune system disorders, drug effects, or environmental effects. Anemias caused by inadequate red blood cell production include such problems as iron deficiency anemia, pernicious anemia, and anemia of chronic disease. Table 9-2 shows the numerous types of anemia, all of which must be confirmed by laboratory diagnosis.

Table 9-2 Types of Anemia

Cause	Type	Pathophysiology
Inadequate production of red blood cells	Aplastic	Failure to produce red blood cells
	Iron deficiency	Iron is primary component of hemoglobin
	Pernicious	Vitamin B_{12} is necessary for correct red blood cell division during its development
	Sickle cell	Genetic alteration causes production of a hemoglobin that changes the shape of a red blood cell to a *C*, or sickle, in low-oxygen states
Increased red blood cell destruction	Hemolytic	Body destroys red blood cells at greater rate than production; red blood cell parts interfere with blood flow
Blood cell loss or dilution	Chronic disease	Hemorrhage leads to cell loss, whereas excessive fluid leads to a dilution of red blood cell concentration

Anemia is a sign, not a disease process in itself. Because the red blood cells' primary purpose is to transport oxygen, anemia results in hypoxia. The signs and symptoms of anemia vary, depending on the rapidity of its onset and the patient's age and underlying general health. A mild anemia may not exhibit signs or symptoms until the body is stressed, as during exercise. Then a mild dyspnea, fatigue, palpitations, and syncope may be present. Chronic anemias may present signs or symptoms of pica (the craving of unusual substances such as clay or ice), headache, dizziness, ringing in the ears, irritability or difficulty concentrating, pallor, and tachycardia. Angina pectoris can be an important indicator.

If anemia develops rapidly, the body does not have time to compensate for the change. Signs and symptoms of shock may be present, including postural hypotension and decreased cardiac output, resulting in a shunting of blood away from the periphery to the heart, lungs, and brain. Compensatory mechanisms can cause diaphoresis, pallor, cool skin, anxiety, thirst, and air hunger. If the onset of anemia is slower, the body can adjust to the reduced availability of oxygen with a right shift of the oxyhemoglobin dissociation curve and an increase in plasma volume.

Prehospital treatment of anemia is primarily symptomatic. Treat hypoxia with supplemental oxygen. Avoid hyperoxia. Transport to a medical facility for treatment of the cause. Start volume replacement if there is evidence of dehydration.

Sickle Cell Disease

Sickle cell disease, often termed "sickle cell anemia," is a disorder of red blood cell production. Normal hemoglobin is very flexible, and the red blood cell can pass easily through the tiny capillaries. Sickle hemoglobin has an abnormal chemical sequence that gives red blood cells a C, or sickle, shape when oxygen levels are low (Figure 9-15). Patients with sickle cell disease will have a chronic anemia that results from destruction of abnormal red blood cells (hemolytic anemia). The average life span of sickled red blood cells is 10 to 20 days, compared to 120 days for normal red blood cells. In addition, sickled red blood cells increase the blood's viscosity, leading to sludging and obstruction of the capillaries and small blood vessels. Blockage of blood flow to various tissues and organs is common and usually occurs following a period of stress. This process, called a *vasoocclusive crisis*, is characteristic of sickle cell anemia. Because of the vasoocclusive crisis, tissues and organs are eventually damaged. Adult sickle cell patients often have multiple organ problems, including cardiopulmonary disease, renal disease, and neurologic disorders.

Sickle cell disease is inherited. It primarily affects African Americans, although other ethnic groups can be affected. These include Puerto Ricans and people of Spanish, French, Italian, Greek, and Turkish heritage. If both parents carry a gene for sickle cell anemia, the chances are 1 in 4 that the child will have normal hemoglobin. The chances are 2 in 4 that he will have both normal hemoglobin and sickle hemoglobin, which is referred to as *sickle cell trait.* The chances are 1 in 4 that he will have only sickle hemoglobin (no normal hemoglobin). This condition is referred to as *sickle cell disease.*

CONTENT REVIEW

➤ Sickle Cell Crises
- Vasoocclusive
- Hematologic
- Infectious

Patients with sickle cell disease will develop three types of problems. *Vasoocclusive crises* cause musculoskeletal pain, abdominal pain, priapism, pulmonary problems, renal crises (renal infarctions), and central nervous system crises (cerebral infarctions). In addition, they will develop *hematologic crises* that consist of a fall in the hemoglobin level, sequestration of red blood cells in the spleen, and problems with bone marrow function. In severe cases, the bone marrow can shut down, causing an aplastic crisis. These are usually self-limited. Finally, sickle cell patients often develop *infectious crises.* They are functionally immunosuppressed, and the loss of splenic function makes them particularly vulnerable to encapsulated bacteria. Infections become common and are often the cause of death in sickle cell anemia.

Prehospital care for patients in sickle cell crisis is primarily supportive. Begin high-concentration oxygen (if hypoxic) to saturate as much hemoglobin as possible.

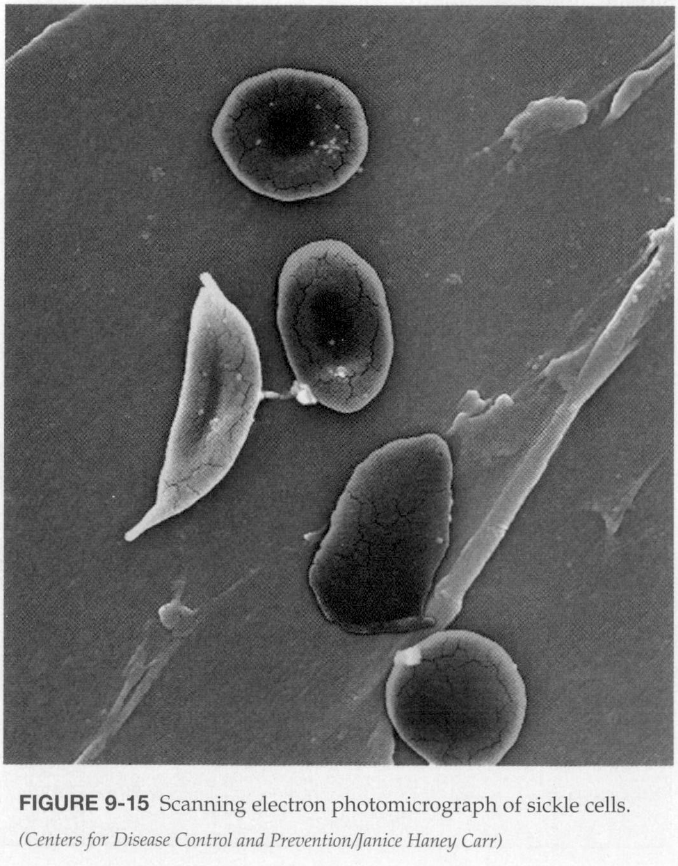

FIGURE 9-15 Scanning electron photomicrograph of sickle cells.
(Centers for Disease Control and Prevention/Janice Haney Carr)

Initiate IV therapy with an isotonic crystalloid solution. These patients are often dehydrated, and hydration will sometimes help with the vasoocclusive process. Venous access is sometimes difficult in older patients with sickle cell disease because of the large number of IV starts they have required in their lifetime. Placing a central line is occasionally necessary. Vasoocclusive crises can be extremely painful. Start analgesic therapy in the field, if possible. Often, these patients will require large amounts of narcotics for pain control. Always consult medical direction if there is a question regarding management. Transport is indicated.[2,3]

Polycythemia

Polycythemia is an abnormally high hematocrit. It is due to excess production of red blood cells. Polycythemia is a relatively rare disorder and typically occurs in patients 50 years of age or older. It can occur secondarily to dehydration. The increased red blood cell load increases the patient's risk of thrombosis. Most deaths from polycythemia are due to thrombosis.

Polycythemia's signs and symptoms vary. The principal finding is a hematocrit of 50 percent or greater. The patient will usually have an increased number of white blood cells and platelets. However, the large number of red blood cells may cause a platelet dysfunction. This can result in bleeding abnormalities such as epistaxis, spontaneous bruising, and gastrointestinal bleeding. Patients with polycythemia may complain of headache, dizziness, blurred vision, itching, and gastrointestinal disease. Severe cases can result in congestive heart failure.

The prehospital treatment of polycythemia is supportive. Ensure that the airway and breathing are adequate. Administer supplemental oxygen if hypoxic. Initiate an IV with an isotonic crystalloid solution. The principal treatment is phlebotomy, which removes excess red blood cells.

Cultural Considerations

Racial Bias and Analgesia. Unfortunately, racial and ethnic bias is still present in medicine. Several recent studies have shown that minority patients are less apt to receive adequate analgesia when compared to nonminority patients. Sickle cell anemia is the most common of the hereditary disorders and almost exclusively affects African Americans. In patients with sickle cell disease, the abnormal blood cells can obstruct blood flow to a region of the body, resulting in a very painful vasoocclusive event (called sickle cell crisis). Many patients in sickle cell crisis require large amounts of narcotic analgesics for relief; the more chronic the disease, the greater the required amounts of narcotic analgesics tend to be. There has been a documented racial/ethnic bias and stereotyping when it comes to pain management in sickle cell crisis. Many in medicine have attempted to address this problem by establishing pain management protocols for sickle cell crisis and ongoing quality assurance programs.

EMS has, historically, done a poor job of treating pain in the prehospital setting. If your system has a large African American community, then consider asking your medical director for a treatment protocol that addresses sickle cell crisis and affords adequate pain relief. This will help to alleviate any treatment bias—whether real or perceived.

CONTENT REVIEW

- Diseases of the White Blood Cells
  - Leukopenia/neutropenia
  - Leukocytosis
  - Leukemia
  - Lymphoma

Diseases of the White Blood Cells

The white blood cells are the body's principal defense system. Problems with white blood cells typically result from too few white blood cells (**leukopenia**), too many white blood cells (**leukocytosis**), or improper white blood cell function. The neutrophil is the main blood component protecting against a bacterial or fungal infection. A reduction in the number of neutrophils (neutropenia) predisposes the patient to bacterial and fungal infections.

Leukopenia/Neutropenia

The status of the white blood cells is easily determined by obtaining a complete blood count. A normal white blood cell count ranges from 5,000 to 9,000 per cubic millimeter of blood. A decrease in the number of white blood cells indicates a problem with white blood cell production in the marrow or destruction of white blood cells. Because bacterial infections pose a major risk to humans, an absolute neutrophil count is a better indicator of the immune system's status. The prehospital treatment of leukopenia or neutropenia is supportive. Pay special attention to preventing infection in the patient, as his immune system is overstressed or may be functioning inadequately.

Leukocytosis

Leukocytosis is an increase in the number of circulating white blood cells. This occurs when the body is exposed to an infectious agent or is particularly stressed. Following exposure, the immune system is stimulated and the marrow and spleen start releasing white blood cells to help the body fight infection. A white blood cell count between 10,800 and 23,000 per cubic millimeter of blood is characteristic of a bacterial infection. During periods of stress, immature neutrophils may be released into the circulation. These differ from mature neutrophils in that they have a segmented nucleus. These cells are referred to as "bands" or "segs." An increase in the number of bands is indicative of a significant bacterial infection. Causes of leukocytosis include bacterial infection, rheumatoid arthritis, DKA, leukemia, pain, and exercise. Viral infections tend to have little effect on the white blood cell count or, in some cases, actually cause a decrease in the white blood cell count. A white blood cell count greater than 30,000 per cubic millimeter is called a *leukemoid reaction.* A white blood cell count this high indicates a problem with excess white blood cell production. Any patient with a significantly elevated white blood cell count should be evaluated for possible leukemia.

Leukemia

Leukemias are cancers of hematopoietic cells. Precursors of white blood cells in the bone marrow begin to replicate abnormally. The cells proliferate initially in the bone marrow and then spread to the peripheral blood. Leukemias affect approximately 13 in 100,000 persons. They are classified by the type of cell or cells involved. The most common types of leukemia are:

- Acute lymphocytic leukemia (ALL)
- Acute myelogenous leukemia (AML)
- Chronic lymphocytic leukemia (CLL)
- Chronic myelogenous leukemia (CML)
- Hairy cell leukemia

Discussion of the pathology of the various leukemias is not within the scope of this text. ALL is primarily a disease of children and young adults. CML occurs in both children and adults. AML, CLL, and hairy cell leukemia tend to occur in the sixth and seventh decades of life. Medicine has made significant advances in the treatment of leukemia. Treatments such as chemotherapy, radiation therapy, and bone marrow transplantation have resulted in cures of certain types of leukemias. The treatment of pediatric leukemia is one of the great successes of modern medicine. More than 50 percent of pediatric patients with ALL live a normal life with the disease in remission or cured. Infections are a common complication of leukemia, primarily due to the low number of circulating neutrophils. Deaths from leukemias are typically secondary to infection or bleeding.

The signs and symptoms of leukemia vary. Most patients will have a moderate to severe anemia, as the cancerous cell production overwhelms the bone marrow. Thrombocytopenia (an abnormal decrease in platelets) is common for the same reason. Many leukemia patients will present with bleeding, usually due to the thrombocytopenia. With the initial presentation, leukemia patients will appear acutely ill. They will be febrile and weak, usually due to a secondary infection. Various lymph nodes may be enlarged. Patients often have a history of weight loss and anorexia. In addition, liver and spleen enlargement are typical, resulting in a sensation of abdominal fullness or abdominal pain. The sternum may be tender, secondary to the increased bone marrow activity. Fatigue is a common complaint.

The prehospital treatment of the patient with leukemia is primarily supportive. Place the patient in a position of comfort. Administer supplemental oxygen if hypoxic. Initiate an IV with an isotonic crystalloid solution such as lactated Ringer's or normal saline. Consider a fluid bolus if the patient is dehydrated. If the patient is having pain secondary to the leukemia, consider administration of an analgesic. Remember, leukemia patients are at increased risk of developing infection. Employ proper isolation techniques.

Lymphomas

Lymphomas are cancers of the lymphatic system. Malignant lymphoma is typically classified as follows:

- Hodgkin's lymphoma
- Non-Hodgkin's lymphoma

Malignant lymphoma is classified by the cell type involved, which indicates the stem cell from which the malignancy arises. In the United States, each year, approximately 40,000 persons are diagnosed with non-Hodgkin's lymphoma, and 7,500 are diagnosed with Hodgkin's lymphoma. The long-term survival rate is much better with Hodgkin's lymphoma. In fact, many patients with Hodgkin's lymphoma who have been treated with radiation, chemotherapy, or both are considered cured.

The most common presenting sign of non-Hodgkin's lymphoma is painless swelling of the lymph nodes. The majority of patients with Hodgkin's lymphoma typically have no related symptoms. Patients with lymphoma may report fever, night sweats, anorexia, weight loss, fatigue, and pruritus. Treat patients with lymphomas symptomatically. Place the patient in a position of comfort. Administer supplemental oxygen if the patient is hypoxic. Initiate an IV with an isotonic crystalloid solution such as lactated Ringer's or normal saline. Consider a fluid bolus if the patient is dehydrated. If the patient is having pain secondary to the lymphoma, consider administration of an analgesic. As with leukemia patients, lymphoma patients are at increased risk of developing infection. Employ proper isolation techniques.[4]

Diseases of the Platelets/Blood Clotting Abnormalities

Various disorders can affect the platelets or the body's blood clotting system. Some of these are hereditary, whereas others may be acquired. Examples of platelet abnormalities include thrombocytosis (increased platelets) and thrombocytopenia (reduced platelets). Various disorders can affect the coagulation system, including hemophilia A and hemophilia B (Christmas disease). Von Willebrand's disease involves problems of both platelet formation and coagulation.

CONTENT REVIEW

- Platelet Abnormalities
  - Thrombocytosis
  - Thrombocytopenia
  - Hemophilia
  - von Willebrand's disease

Thrombocytosis

Thrombocytosis is an increase in the number of platelets, usually due to increased platelet production (essential thrombocytosis). It is also seen in polycythemia vera, in which both red blood cells and platelets are increased. Thrombocytosis often complicates chronic myelogenous leukemia. Thrombocytosis can be secondary to other disorders, such as malignant diseases, hemolytic anemias, acute hemorrhage, and autoinflammatory diseases. Most patients with thrombocytosis are asymptomatic. Prehospital treatment is supportive.

Thrombocytopenia

Thrombocytopenia is an abnormal decrease in the number of platelets. It is due to decreased platelet production, sequestration of platelets in the spleen, destruction of platelets, or any combination of the three. Many drugs can induce thrombocytopenia. *Acute idiopathic thrombocytopenia purpura (ITP)* results from destruction of platelets by the immune system. It is most commonly seen in children following a viral infection. ITP is characterized by easy bruising, bleeding, and a falling platelet count. Chronic ITP usually occurs in adult women and is often associated with autoimmune disease. Prehospital treatment is supportive.[5]

Hemophilia

Hemophilia is a blood disorder in which one of the proteins necessary for blood clotting is missing or defective. A deficiency of factor VIII is called hemophilia A. A deficiency of factor IX is known as hemophilia B (Christmas disease). Hemophilia A is the most common inherited disorder of hemostasis. The severity of the disease is directly related to the amount of circulating factor VIII available. Patients are classified as mild, moderate, or severe, based on the amount of circulating factor VIII. Hemophilia B is more rare, but also more severe, than hemophilia A.

When a person with hemophilia is injured, the bleeding will take longer to stop because the body cannot form stable fibrin clots. Simple trauma, such as nosebleeds or tooth extractions, can lead to prolonged, occasionally life-threatening bleeds. In extensive trauma such as pelvic fractures, blood loss can be overwhelming. A common problem with hemophilia is hemarthrosis (bleeding into the joint space). This can result from even the most minor trauma. Eventually, repeated bleeding episodes will lead to permanent joint damage.

Hemophilia is a sex-linked, inherited bleeding disorder (Figure 9-16). The gene with the defective information is carried on the X chromosome. Females have two X chromosomes, one from their mother and one from their father. If one chromosome has the defective gene and the other does not, the disease is not expressed. Females who have one X chromosome containing the defective gene are referred to as carriers. Males, however, have an X chromosome from their mother and a Y chromosome from their father. If that X chromosome carries the defective gene, males will express the disease. Hemophilia A affects approximately 1 in 10,000 males. A female, on the other hand, can inherit hemophilia only if she receives two X chromosomes that express the disease. That is, she must be the offspring of a carrier mother and a father with hemophilia.

MOTHER		FATHER	
X (healthy)	x (hemophilia gene-carrier)	X (healthy)	Y (healthy)
DAUGHTER XX (both healthy)	DAUGHTER Xx (carrier of trait-no disease)	SON XY no disease	SON xY hemophilia

FIGURE 9-16 Familial (sex-linked) characteristics of hemophilia.

The signs and symptoms of hemophilia include numerous bruises, deep muscle bleeding characterized as pain or a "pulled muscle," and the joint bleeding called *hemarthrosis*. Most patients will be aware of their diagnosis and will tell you. Some may wear MedicAlert bracelets or similar devices.

Hemophiliacs can be treated in the hospital with infusions of factor VIII. In addition to factor VIII, some hemophiliacs will require blood transfusions due to bleeding from trauma. Unfortunately, before blood and blood products were routinely tested, transfusions infected many hemophiliacs with the human immunodeficiency virus, hepatitis B, and/or hepatitis C.

Prehospital treatment of the patient with hemophilia should be comprehensive. The normal hemostatic mechanisms of vasoconstriction and platelet aggregation will still occur, but the platelet plug will not be stable, due to the deficiency of factor VIII. Thus, you should be attentive to prolonged bleeding or possible rebleeds. The hemophiliac is at risk of both. Administer supplemental oxygen if the patient is hypoxic and initiate IV therapy with an isotonic crystalloid such as normal saline. Be careful to help prevent additional trauma, which can result in further hemorrhage. If the patient sustained a joint injury with resultant hemarthrosis, splinting the extremity will sometimes help control pain. Occasionally, analgesics will be required.

Von Willebrand's Disease

Factor VIII actually consists of several components. One of these components is factor VIII:vWF, also called von Willebrand's factor. In **von Willebrand's disease**, this component of factor VIII is deficient. It is produced by the endothelial cells and is necessary for normal platelet adhesion. Thus, in addition to the clotting problem, platelet function is abnormal in patients with von Willebrand's disease. Although the disease is inherited, it is not sex linked, equally affecting both females and males. A sign of this disease is excessive bleeding, primarily after surgery or injury. It is not associated with the deep muscle or joint bleeding of hemophilia, nor is it usually as serious, although nosebleeds, excessive menstruation, and gastrointestinal bleeds can occur. Prehospital treatment is supportive. Aspirin is generally contraindicated, as it further inhibits platelet aggregation, thus exacerbating the disease. Definitive treatment is the administration of von Willebrand's factor.

Other Hematopoietic Disorders

Other hematopoietic disorders that you may encounter in the prehospital setting include disseminated intravascular coagulation and multiple myeloma.

Disseminated Intravascular Coagulation

Disseminated intravascular coagulation (DIC), also called consumption coagulopathy, is a disorder of coagulation caused by systemic activation of the coagulation cascade. Normally, inhibitory mechanisms localize coagulation to the affected area. A combination of protein inhibitors, rapid blood flow, and absorption of the fibrin clot restricts circulating free thrombin to the site of coagulation. In DIC, circulating thrombin cleaves fibrinogen to form fibrin clots throughout the circulation. This can cause widespread thrombosis and, occasionally, end-organ ischemia. Bleeding is the most frequent sign of DIC and is due to the reduced fibrinogen level, consumption of coagulation factors, and thrombocytopenia. DIC most commonly results from sepsis, hypotension, obstetric complications, severe tissue injury, brain injury, cancer, and major hemolytic transfusion reactions. The disease is quite grave. Its signs include oozing blood at venipuncture and wound sites. The patient may exhibit a purpuric rash, often over the chest and abdomen. Minute hemorrhages may be noted just under the skin. Prehospital care is symptomatic. The patient with DIC may be hemodynamically unstable and may require intravenous fluids. Definitive treatment includes the administration of fresh frozen plasma and platelets.[6]

Multiple Myeloma

Multiple myeloma is a cancerous disorder of plasma cells. Plasma cells are a type of B cell responsible for producing immunoglobulins (antibodies). The disease is rarely found in persons under the age of 40. Approximately 14,000 new cases are diagnosed each year. Usually, multiple myeloma begins with a change or mutation in a plasma cell in the bone marrow. These cancerous plasma cells crowd out healthy cells and lead to a reduction in blood cell production. The patient then becomes anemic and prone to infection.

The first sign of multiple myeloma often is pain in the back or ribs. The diseased marrow weakens the bones and pathological fractures (those occurring with minimal or no trauma) may occur. The resulting anemia leads to fatigue, and reduced platelet production places the patient at risk for bleeding. Laboratory evaluation will reveal an elevation in the level of a circulating antibody or part of an antibody (light chain), due to the proliferation of plasma cells. Despite this, the patient is at increased risk of infection, as the plasma cells do not secrete specific antibodies in response to infection. In addition, the calcium level is often elevated in multiple myeloma due to bone destruction. This can lead to renal failure.

Treatment of multiple myeloma includes chemotherapy, radiation, and bone marrow transplants. Prehospital care is supportive. Establish an IV of isotonic crystalloid solution. Consider a fluid bolus if there are symptoms of dehydration. Multiple myeloma can be very painful because of the proliferation of the plasma cells and destruction of the marrow. Consider analgesics if pain is severe. It is not uncommon for EMS to be summoned following a pathological fracture in a patient with multiple myeloma. Again, these are very painful, and you should start analgesic therapy if so indicated.

Summary

Hematology is the study of blood and blood-forming organs. Blood consists of a liquid portion, or plasma, and the formed elements—red blood cells, white blood cells, and platelets. Each component of blood has various functions that are intrinsic to sustaining homeostasis. Plasma draws water into the capillaries, and it assists in clotting blood, dismantling clots, buffering the blood's acid–base balance, transporting hormones and regulating their effects, and providing a source of energy. Red blood cells contain hemoglobin and transport oxygen to the body tissues and remove wastes. White blood cells protect the body from foreign invasion through the processes of chemotaxis and phagocytosis. Platelets travel to the site of damaged tissue and help to prevent blood loss.

Hemostasis is the body's way of preventing or controlling blood loss. The three phases of hemostasis are vascular spasm, development of the platelet plug, and formation of a stable fibrin clot (blood coagulation). Some diseases interfere with parts of the processes of hemostasis, and people who have these diseases may incur life-threatening hemorrhages from minor injuries.

Numerous conditions and diseases affect the hematologic system, with varying and sometimes disastrous outcomes. As a paramedic, you must understand hematology because breakdowns in the hematologic system can complicate patient assessment and care.

You Make the Call

Your crew is just starting a Sunday afternoon barbecue lunch when the call comes in to respond to a patient who is hemorrhaging following a lawn mower accident. The accident occurred at 2424 Eighth Avenue, which is just around the corner from your location, and you arrive within minutes. As you approach the scene, you see that the lawn mower has been turned off and a middle-aged man is calling for you to come quickly. The man's 17-year-old son, Jim, was walking through the yard when a sharp stone was kicked out from the blades and struck him in the arm. He has a nasty laceration to his left upper arm, which is spurting blood with each pulse beat. Jim is trying vainly to stem the bleeding.

Applying pressure during the primary assessment, your EMT partner, Tina, obtains a set of vital signs. The pulse is 110 and regular; the respiratory rate is 22 and nonlabored; the blood pressure is 112/84 mmHg.

After you transport the patient to the hospital, the hospital staff closes the patient's wound, but they are concerned about a possible infection at the wound site.

1. What hemostatic responses will seek to control this blood loss?
2. Why are the heart rate and respiratory rate elevated?
3. What will the body do to replace red blood cells?
4. What body mechanisms will fight off an infection?

See Suggested Responses at the back of this book.

Review Questions

1. The kidney—and, to a lesser extent the liver—produces which hormone that is responsible for red blood cell production?
   a. Oxytocin
   b. Thyrotoxin
   c. Testosterone
   d. Erythropoietin
2. Young, healthy individuals' bodies can compensate for loss of as much as ___________ percent of blood volume.
   a. 25–30
   b. 30–35
   c. 35–40
   d. 40–45
3. Carbohydrates in plasma are generally in which form, which is the primary energy source for all body tissues?
   a. Oxygen
   b. Glucose
   c. Estrogen
   d. Hemoglobin
4. What is the name of the specialized scavenger cells in the spleen and liver?
   a. Leukophages
   b. Neutrophages
   c. Macrophages
   d. Hematophages

5. What are the primary cells involved in the body's immune response?
   a. Monocytes
   b. Erythrocytes
   c. Lymphocytes
   d. Granulocytes
6. Most clotting proteins are produced in which organ and circulate in an inactive state?
   a. Femur
   b. Liver
   c. Spleen
   d. Sternum
7. A person with type ____________ blood is called a universal recipient.
   a. O
   b. A
   c. AB
   d. B
8. What is typically classified as a hematocrit of less than 37 percent in women or less than 40 percent in men?
   a. Anemia
   b. Leukemia
   c. Polycythemia
   d. Thrombocytopenia
9. Many leukemia patients will present with bleeding, usually due to ____________
   a. anemia.
   b. infection.
   c. hypoxemia.
   d. thrombocytopenia.
10. What is the most frequent sign of disseminated intravascular coagulation (DIC) and is due to the reduced fibrinogen level, consumption of coagulation factors, and thrombocytopenia?
    a. Fever
    b. Bleeding
    c. Purpuric rash
    d. Oozing blood at wound sites
11. The majority of prehospital treatment of hematologic emergencies is ______
    a. symptomatic in nature.
    b. the infusion of large quantities of IV fluid.
    c. geared toward creating a state of hyperoxia.
    d. irrelevant and unnecessary.

See Answers to Review Questions at the back of this book.

References

1. Davenport, R. D. "Pathophysiology of Hemolytic Transfusion Reactions." *Semin Hematol* 42 (2005): 165–168.
2. Ellison, A. M. and K. Shaw. "Management of Vasoocclusive Pain Events in Sickle Cell Disease." *Pediatr Emerg Care* 23 (2007): 832–838.
3. Hick, J. L., S. C. Nelson, K. Hick, and M. O. Nwaneri. "Emergency Management of Sickle Cell Disease Complications: Review and Practice Guidelines." *Minn Med* 89 (2006): 42–44.
4. Behl, D., A. W. Hendrickson, and T. J. Moynihan. "Oncologic Emergencies." *Crit Care Clin* 26(1) (2010): 181–205.
5. Neunert, C., W. Lim, A. Crowther, et al. "The American Society of Hematology 2011 Evidence-Based Practice Guideline for Immune Thrombocytopenia." *Blood* 117 (2011): 4190–4207.
6. Kitchens, C. S. "Thrombocytopenia and Thrombosis in Disseminated Intravascular Coagulation (DIC)." *Hematology Am Soc Hematol Educ Program* (2009): 240–246.

Further Reading

Hall, J. *Guyton and Hall Textbook of Medical Physiology*. 13th ed. Philadelphia: W. B. Saunders, 2015.

Martini, F. H., E. F. Bartholomew, and B. E. Bledsoe. *Anatomy and Physiology for Emergency Care*. 2nd ed. Upper Saddle River, NJ: Pearson/Prentice Hall, 2008.

Tintanelli, J. E., et al. *Emergency Medicine: A Comprehensive Study Guide*. 7th ed. New York: McGraw-Hill, 2013.

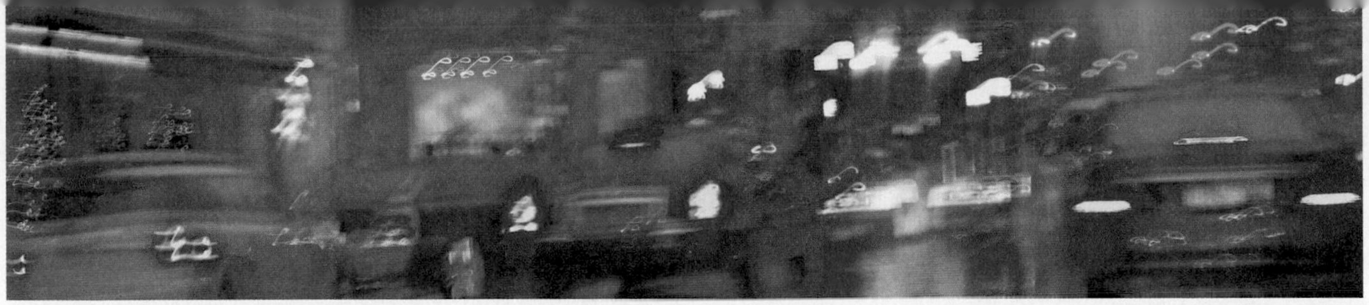

Chapter 10
Infectious Diseases and Sepsis

Bryan Bledsoe, DO, FACEP, FAAEM, EMT-P
Brad Buck, NRP, CEMT-P

STANDARD
Medicine (Infectious Diseases)

COMPETENCY
Integrates assessment findings with principles of epidemiology and pathophysiology to formulate a field impression and implement a comprehensive treatment/disposition plan for a patient with a medical complaint.

Learning Objectives

Terminal Performance Objective: After reading this chapter, you should be able to integrate patient assessment findings, patient history, and knowledge of anatomy, physiology, pathophysiology, and basic and advanced life support interventions to recognize and manage patients with infectious diseases and sepsis.

Enabling Objectives: To accomplish the terminal performance objective, you should be able to:

1. Define key terms introduced in this chapter.
2. Explain public health principles related to infectious diseases, and the roles of local, state, and federal agencies involved in infectious disease surveillance and outbreaks.
3. Differentiate among the characteristics of bacteria, viruses, prions, fungi, protozoa, and parasites as causes of infectious diseases.
4. Describe the interactions of the agent, host, and environment as determining factors in disease transmission.
5. Describe the phases of the infectious process and the body's normal defenses against disease.
6. Explain the principles and practices of infection control in prehospital care, including your responsibilities and your rights under the Ryan White Act.
7. Adapt the scene size-up, primary assessment, history, secondary assessment, and use of monitoring technology to arrive at a field impression for patients with infectious disease emergencies.
8. Describe the pathophysiology of infectious diseases of immediate concern to EMS providers.
9. Use a process of clinical reasoning to guide and interpret the patient assessment findings and develop a treatment plan for

patients displaying an infectious disease emergency.

10. Describe the actions to take if you are exposed to an infectious disease.
11. Discuss EMS providers' roles in patient education and preventing disease transmission.
12. Explain the pathophysiology, risk factors, assessment, and prehospital management of sepsis/systemic inflammatory response syndrome (SIRS).
13. Given a variety of scenarios, discuss the integration of assessment and management guidelines as they relate to infectious disease emergencies.

KEY TERMS

active immunity, p. 401
airborne, p. 397
antibody, p. 399
antigen, p. 399
autoimmunity, p. 400
B lymphocytes, p. 400
bacteria, p. 395
bactericidal, p. 396
bacteriostatic, p. 396
bloodborne, p. 397
Brudzinski's sign, p. 422
cell-mediated immunity, p. 400
chancroid, p. 436
chickenpox, p. 420
Chikungunya virus disease, p. 420
chlamydia, p. 435
communicable, p. 398
communicable period, p. 399
contamination, p. 398
croup, p. 427
decontaminate, p. 407
disease period, p. 399
disinfection, p. 407
Ebola virus disease (EVD), p. 419
encephalitis, p. 429
endotoxin, p. 395
epiglottitis, p. 427
exotoxin, p. 395
fecal–oral route, p. 397
food poisoning, p. 429
fungus, p. 396
gastroenteritis, p. 428
genital warts, p. 434
German measles, p. 425
gonorrhea, p. 433
Gram stain, p. 395
hantavirus, p. 428
hepatitis, p. 412
herpes simplex virus, p. 426
hookworm, p. 397
human immunodeficiency virus (HIV), p. 410
humoral immunity, p. 400
immune system, p. 399
immunoglobulin, p. 400
impetigo, p. 436
incubation period, p. 399
index case, p. 394
infection, p. 398
infectious disease, p. 393
infestation, p. 436
influenza, p. 422
Kernig's sign, p. 422
latent period, p. 399
leukocyte, p. 399
lice, p. 436
Lyme disease, p. 432
lymph, p. 400
lymphatic system, p. 400
lymphocyte, p. 400
macrophage, p. 400
mask, p. 416
measles, p. 424
meningitis, p. 421
Middle East respiratory syndrome (MERS), p. 418
mononucleosis, p. 426
mumps, p. 424
neutrophil, p. 399
normal flora, p. 395
nosocomial, p. 438
obligate intracellular parasite, p. 396
opportunistic pathogen, p. 395
parasite, p. 397
passive immunity, p. 401
pathogen, p. 395
pertussis, p. 425
phagocytosis, p. 400
pharyngitis, p. 427
pinworm, p. 397
pneumonia, p. 417
PPD, p. 402
prions, p. 396
protozoan, p. 396
rabies, p. 430
reservoir, p. 397
resistance, p. 399
respirator, p. 416
respiratory syncytial virus (RSV), p. 425
reticuloendothelial system (RES), p. 399
rubella (German measles), p. 425
Ryan White Act, p. 408
scabies, p. 437
sepsis, p. 439
septicemia, p. 439
seroconversion, p. 399

severe acute respiratory syndrome (SARS), p. 418
sexually transmitted disease (STD), p. 433
sinusitis, p. 428
sterilization, p. 408
syphilis, p. 433
systemic inflammatory response syndrome (SIRS), p. 439
T lymphocytes, p. 400
tetanus, p. 431
trichinosis, p. 397
trichomoniasis, p. 436
tuberculosis (TB), p. 414
varicella, p. 420
virulence, p. 398
virus, p. 396
window phase, p. 399
Zika virus disease (ZVD), p. 419

Case Study

Elizabeth Fletcher and her partner, Stuart Pratt, are performing routine duties at the station one cool spring evening when the call comes in. They are dispatched to a local residence for a patient complaining of difficulty breathing.

Elizabeth and Stuart arrive to find a 52-year-old man sitting on the edge of his bed, complaining of shortness of breath. The patient's wife reports that his symptoms began as a cough and congestion. Over the past two weeks, the symptoms have gradually worsened.

While Stuart gathers the history and records the patient's vital signs, Elizabeth begins the physical exam. The patient is an undernourished man who appears much older than his 52 years. His vital signs are blood pressure, 156/96 mmHg; pulse, 118; respirations, 30 and slightly labored; and temperature, 99.4°F via a tympanic thermometer. The patient's electrocardiogram shows a sinus tachycardia with occasional unifocal premature ventricular contractions. His skin is pale and dry. Oxygen saturation is 90 percent on room air and improves to 95 percent after several minutes of oxygen by mask. Auscultation of the patient's chest reveals scattered dry crackles bilaterally. He coughs occasionally, but it is nonproductive. He is a one-pack-per-day smoker with a 20-pack/year history. There is no history of obstructive lung disease. Before this episode, he has never experienced any difficulty breathing.

When Stuart questions him further, the patient admits to night sweats and loss of 15 pounds of body weight over the past month. He has coughed up blood on at least three occasions during the past several days. Based on these examination findings, Stuart and Elizabeth suspect tuberculosis (TB) as a possible cause of the patient's signs and symptoms and ensure that airborne PPE is being used.

Elizabeth and Stuart establish an IV of normal saline at a to-keep-open rate. While they transport the patient to the emergency department, he remains stable and his shortness of breath (breathing difficulty) improves. On arrival, the emergency physician diagnoses the patient with possible tuberculosis based on the history and chest X-ray findings. An infectious disease specialist admits the patient to an isolation room on a medical floor for treatment and subsequent evaluation.

The EMS system is notified about the possible exposure. Cultures for the bacterium that causes tuberculosis can take up to six weeks to complete. The paramedics involved in the call are informed about the possible exposure, and postexposure protective measures are started. Cultures later confirm the diagnosis of tuberculosis. Fortunately, neither of the paramedics has been infected.

Introduction

Infectious diseases are illnesses caused by infestation of the body by biological organisms such as bacteria, viruses, fungi, protozoans, and helminths (worms). Most infectious disease states are not life threatening and the patient recovers completely. Some types of infection, however, such as human immunodeficiency virus (HIV), hepatitis B virus (HBV), hepatitis C virus (HCV), and acute bacterial meningitis, are particularly dangerous and may result in death or permanent disability.

All health care professionals must maintain a strong working knowledge of public health principles and infectious diseases. This is especially true for paramedics, who are often the first to encounter patients with communicable diseases. Early recognition and management of these patients may make a difference in how the patient is treated and may also ensure that care providers take necessary precautions to prevent the spread of the disease to others.

This chapter discusses infectious diseases, including the types of disease-causing organisms, functions of the immune system, and general pathophysiology of infectious diseases. It emphasizes the specific diseases, discussing those that you may encounter during interhospital transports or out-of-hospital care, especially those that you are most likely to encounter in the field.

Public Health Principles

Paramedics should be alert to specific illness patterns related to infectious diseases. Patients presenting with clinical findings such as those listed throughout this chapter should cause paramedics to have a heightened sense of awareness that this might not be an isolated incident. It is the early detection of a possible outbreak that can make it possible to contain the threat to the community.

When dealing with infectious diseases, you must consider the impact of the disease process on the community as well as on the infected patient. An infectious agent is a "hazardous material" that can affect large numbers of people.

Epidemiologists—health professionals who study how infectious diseases affect populations—attempt to describe and predict how diseases move from individuals to populations. Through various clinically based studies and statistical techniques, they try to determine how effectively an infectious agent can travel through a population. Using the population of infected individuals as a standard, they attempt to predict those individuals in the larger population who may be most at risk for contracting the infectious agent. Recognizing that risk may be predictable, and not just random, is important. The characteristics of the host, the infectious agent, and the environment may yield clues as to how the infectious agent is transmitted and reveal individuals or populations susceptible to infection.

How a population is identified is important. It may be defined by such parameters as geographic boundary, workplace, school, correctional institution, age group, income level, or ethnic group. All the characteristics of a certain population are known as its *demographics*. The population's tendency to expand, decline, or move is important as well. Besides stimulating social and economic progress, the movement of people and animals within and among other societies also provides a vehicle for infectious agents.

To track the progress of infection within a population, epidemiologists work backward through the chain of infection to determine the **index case**, the individual who first introduced the infectious agent to the population. From the index case, they then retrace the chain forward to verify their reconstruction of the infection's pattern.

To gauge a disease's potential impact on the community, paramedics must evaluate the host (patient), what they believe to be the infectious agent, and the environment. Based on that assessment, they may use more aggressive personal protective equipment. They must also consider the patient, those in the patient's immediate environment, and those in the environment where the patient is being transported all to be at risk for infection. On a more personal level, paramedics must appreciate that they and their families could also be at risk.

Legal Considerations

Reporting Contagious Diseases. All states have provisions for reporting contagious diseases without fear of violating the patient's privacy or confidentiality issues. Even the Health Insurance Portability and Accountability Act (HIPAA) has provisions in place for reporting contagious disease without violating provisions of the act. More than 60 diseases in the United States are reportable at a national level. In addition, there are state-reportable diseases that vary from state to state. Some illnesses, including anthrax, brucellosis, diphtheria, pertussis, plague, and others, must be reported immediately. Others, including AIDS, gonorrhea, leprosy, and syphilis, must be reported within one week. Some require reporting of individual cases and others require reporting of numbers only.

It is usually not the role of EMS personnel to report infectious diseases to the various health departments unless the paramedic is also functioning in a public health or industrial health role. However, any information about or suspicions of infectious diseases should be reported to emergency department staff for subsequent investigation. Of course, if a communicable disease is suspected, always wear the appropriate personal protective equipment.

Public Health Agencies

Local agencies are the first line of defense in disease surveillance and outbreak. Municipal, city, and county agencies, including fire departments, ambulance services, and health departments, must cooperate to monitor and report the incidence and prevalence of disease.

At the state level, a designated agency (health department or board of health, for instance) generally monitors infectious diseases. These agencies may set policies requiring vaccinations and regulate or implement control programs in vector and animal control, food preparation, water, sewer, and other sanitation control programs. State and local laws sometimes require these agencies to meet or exceed federal guidelines and recommendations.

A number of federal agencies are involved in tracking the morbidity and mortality of infectious diseases. The U.S. Department of Health and Human Services (DHHS) Centers for Disease Control and Prevention (CDC) in Atlanta, Georgia, is the most visible federal agency. The CDC monitors national disease data and freely disseminates this information to all health care providers. It sends personnel nationally and internationally to assist with studying, characterizing, and managing serious disease outbreaks. The CDC is also involved in researching infectious diseases. The National Institute for Occupational Safety and Health (NIOSH), also under the aegis of DHHS, works with the U.S. Department of Labor's Occupational

Safety and Health Administration (OSHA) in setting standards and guidelines for workplace and worker controls to prevent infectious diseases in the workplace. This level of federal government involvement would not be possible without the leadership of the U.S. Congress in establishing national health policies and in drafting the federal budget.

Other organizations and governmental agencies that might serve as resources for your organization include the Federal Emergency Management Agency (FEMA), the National Fire Protection Association (NFPA), the United States Fire Protection Administration (USFPA), and the International Association of Firefighters (IAFF). These groups develop helpful blueprints for incorporating OSHA, NIOSH, and other standards and guidelines into daily operations.

Microorganisms

The vast majority of disease-causing organisms are microscopic (visible only under a microscope). These microorganisms surround us. They are on our skin and in the air we breathe, and they colonize virtually every orifice of our bodies. Some can even live in the highly acidic environment of our stomachs, which destroys other disease-producing microorganisms or deactivates their toxic products. Microorganisms that reside in our bodies without ordinarily causing disease are part of the *host defenses* known as **normal flora**. Normal flora help keep us disease free by creating environmental conditions that are not conducive to disease-producing microorganisms, or **pathogens**. Competition between colonies of normal flora and pathogens also discourages the survival of pathogens. Common bacterial pathogens include *Staphylococci, Streptococci,* and *Enterobacteriaceae.* Certain viruses, rickettsiae, fungi, and protozoans are also pathogenic.

Opportunistic pathogens are ordinarily nonharmful bacteria that cause disease only under unusual circumstances. Most opportunistic pathogens are normal flora. Patients who have a weakened immune system or who are under unusual stress become susceptible to diseases caused by opportunistic organisms. For example, the fungus *Pneumocystis jiroveci* is usually harmless but can cause a deadly form of pneumonia in patients with HIV. The fungus overwhelms the weakened immune system and begins to reproduce rapidly in the lungs. Left untreated, *P. jiroveci* pneumonia may be fatal. Organ transplant recipients are also at increased risk for infectious diseases because they must take immunosuppressant medications to prevent organ rejection. A more common (and less harmful) opportunistic infection is thrush (oral candidiasis), often seen in patients who take broad-spectrum antibiotics. As the antibiotic kills normal bacterial flora in the mouth, the fungus *Candida albicans* grows almost uninhibited on the tongue and in the pharynx, producing a white coating on the mucosa.

Bacteria

Bacteria are microscopic single-celled organisms that range in length from 1 to 20 micrometers. These living cells are classified as *prokaryotes* because they do not have a distinct nuclear membrane and possess only one chromosome in the cytoplasm. Bacteria reproduce independently, but they require a host to supply food and a supportive environment. Some common diseases caused by pathogenic bacteria include sinusitis, otitis media, bacterial pneumonia, pharyngitis (strep throat), tuberculosis, and most urinary tract infections.

Most bacteria are easily identifiable with stains or by their appearance under a microscope. Similar colorfastness indicates similarities in cell wall structure and other anatomic features. The **Gram stain** is the most common method of differentiating bacteria. Bacteria that turn purple by this process are Gram-positive; those that turn red are Gram-negative. Because of the similarities in their cell walls, bacteria that stain alike may respond to similar treatments.

Bacteria are further categorized into groups based on their general appearance: Cocci or spheres (*Staphylococci, Streptococci*) are round; rods (*Enterobacter* sp., *E. coli*) are elongated; and spirals (spirochetes, vibrio) are coiled. *Enterobacter* sp. and *E. coli* are Gram-negative rods. *Staphylococci* and *Streptococci* are Gram-positive cocci. Regardless of how bacteria stain or appear under a microscope, the specific tissues and organs that are infected chiefly determine the patient's signs and symptoms.

Pathogenic bacteria may harm their human hosts in a number of ways. Heavy colonization may result in direct damage to tissues as the bacteria feed. Bacteria may also cause indirect damage by releasing toxic chemicals that can have localized or systemic effects. The two general categories of toxins are exotoxins and endotoxins. This classification is no longer based primarily on where they originate, as their names imply, but rather by their chemical structures. **Exotoxins** are poisonous proteins shed by bacteria during bacterial growth. They stimulate the immune system to form antibodies to these proteins, and chemicals, light, or heat may also deactivate them. Exotoxins are more toxic than endotoxins. For example, the infectious agent of toxic shock syndrome, *Staphylococcus aureus,* releases an exotoxin, as does anthrax, which can be delivered as a biological weapon of mass destruction.

Endotoxins consist of proteins, polysaccharides (large sugar molecules), and lipids. The immune system cannot form antibodies specific to a particular endotoxin unless both the protein and polysaccharide portions are present. Endotoxins come from the bacterial cell wall and are released when the bacterial cell is destroyed.

CONTENT REVIEW

➤ Types of Bacteria
- Spheres (cocci)
- Rods
- Spirals

They are more stable in heat than exotoxins. Only Gram-negative bacteria make endotoxins. The skin lesions of meningococcemia and the signs of shock that sometimes accompany it are due to large amounts of endotoxin released by the infectious agent, *Neisseria meningitidis.*

Most bacterial infections respond to treatment with antibiotics that are either **bactericidal** (kill bacteria) or **bacteriostatic** (inhibit bacterial growth or reproduction). Antibiotics are prescribed based on bacterial sensitivity; different antibiotics are required to treat different bacteria. Their administration usually decreases bacterial presence and reduces symptoms. Some types of bacterial infections respond quickly to antibiotics; others take longer. In recent years, a number of bacterial strains have developed resistance to antibiotic therapy, making treatment more difficult. The more a type of bacterium is exposed to an antibiotic, the greater the likelihood of its developing resistance. The overuse of antibiotics in both medical and veterinary settings has contributed to this serious problem. Resistant forms of tuberculosis (mycobacterium) and *S. aureus* are of particular concern. Antibiotics may now be ineffective against these diseases, and the mortality rate is high. The willingness of some physicians and other practitioners to prescribe the newest antibiotics for relatively minor infections and the widespread addition of antibiotics to animal feed have only added to the problem.

Antimicrobial treatment alters the normal flora of the skin, mouth, mucosa, and gastrointestinal tract and often results in colonization of those areas by new microorganisms that resist antibiotics. In some cases, an antibiotic may kill normal flora and allow more virulent and dangerous opportunistic pathogens to multiply freely. This can lead to a secondary infection that is more severe than the original infection being treated. For all these reasons, antibiotics should be prescribed cautiously.

Viruses

Viruses are much smaller than bacteria and can be seen only with an electron microscope. Viruses cannot reproduce and carry on metabolism by themselves. Therefore, they are considered to be neither prokaryotes nor eukaryotes. Instead, viruses are **obligate intracellularparasites**; that is, they can grow and reproduce only within a host cell. Once inside, the virus takes control of the host cell's protein synthesis mechanism and directs it to begin reproducing the virus. The cell then releases new virus particles, which infect nearby cells.

Because viruses "hide" inside the host's cells, they resist antibiotic treatment. Once a virus enters a host cell, it becomes part of that host cell, making selective eradication of the virus virtually impossible, as any treatment capable of killing the virus will generally kill the host cell as well. This is the major obstacle facing researchers as they work to find cures for HIV and other viruses.

Approximately 400 types of viruses have been identified. One frequently encountered viral disorder, the common cold, is caused by a number of different viruses (nearly 200) that all produce similar symptoms. Fortunately, most viral diseases are mild and self-limiting. They run their course until the patient's immune system eventually fights them off. A host is generally susceptible to any particular virus only once. Once a person's immune system develops active immunity against a particular type of virus, it becomes attuned to similar attacking viruses and will destroy them.

Other Microorganisms

Prions are a new classification of disease-producing agents that microbiologists used to refer to as "slow viruses." They are neither prokaryotes nor eukaryotes but particles of protein, folded in such a way that proteases (enzymes that break down proteins) cannot act on them. These protein particles accumulate in nervous system and brain tissue, destroying them and giving them a spongy appearance on gross examination. Prions are known to cause progressive, untreatable dementia in kuru, Creutzfeldt-Jakob disease, mad cow disease, and fatal familial insomnia. Although EMS providers will rarely respond to patients with diseases caused by prions, a general discussion of infectious agents must acknowledge their existence.

Fungi are plantlike microorganisms, most of which are not pathogenic. Yeasts, molds, and mushrooms are types of fungi. Some fungi have a capsule around the cell wall that provides additional protection against phagocytes. Fungi compose a large part of the body's normal flora, but they may become pathogenic in patients with compromised immune function, such as those with HIV. Fungi may also lead to disease states in patients taking broad-spectrum antibiotics. As the antibiotics kill off bacteria, the fungi are able to grow uninhibited. Fungi are a common cause of vaginal infections and often cause pneumonia in patients with weakened immune systems.

Protozoa are single-celled parasitic organisms with flexible membranes and the ability to move. Most protozoa live in the soil and ingest decaying organic matter. Although rarely a cause of disease in humans, they are considered opportunistic pathogens in patients with compromised immune function. These organisms may enter the body by the fecal–oral route or through a mosquito bite. Common diseases caused by protozoa include malaria and forms of gastroenteritis. Protozoa also cause vaginal infections (trichomoniasis) in women with normal immune function.

Parasites are common causes of disease where sanitation is poor (generally in developing countries). Occasional cases are seen in this country. Roundworms (ascarides) live in the intestinal mucosa and may reach 30–50 cm in length. Symptoms include abdominal cramping, fever, and cough. Diagnosis usually depends on finding eggs in the patient's stool.

Pinworms (*Enterobius vermicularis*) are common in the United States and in other civilized countries. It is estimated that 20 percent of children living in temperate climates harbor this disease. These tiny worms (3–10 mm long) live in the distal colon and crawl onto the anal mucosa to lay their eggs, usually when the host is asleep. Although the disease may remain asymptomatic, it is a common cause of anal pruritus (itching) and infection and is easily spread among children, especially in day care centers. Children may carry the disease home and infect their entire family. This disease is often endemic among institutionalized children. Treatment involves a single dose of an antibiotic (mebendazole); all family members must be treated simultaneously to avoid reinfection.

Hookworms (*Ancylostoma duodenale, Necator americanus*) are found in warm, moist climates. This **parasite** infects an estimated 25 percent of the world's population, although it is relatively rare in the United States. The larvae are passed in the stool of infected animals. The disease is most commonly contracted when a barefoot child walks in a contaminated area. The larvae enter through the skin and migrate to the intestines, where they grip and irritate the intestinal wall and feed on blood. Epigastric pain and anemia are possible. Prevention involves wearing shoes; treatment is similar to that for pinworms.

Trichinosis (*Trichinella spiralis*) may be contracted by eating raw or inadequately cooked pork products, most commonly sausage. Females burrow into the intestinal wall and produce thousands of living larvae that migrate to skeletal muscle, where each forms a cyst and remains. Symptoms include gastrointestinal disturbances, edema (especially of the eyelids), fever, and a variety of other diffuse and secondary symptoms. If the worms invade the heart, lungs, or brain in large numbers, death may result. Diagnosis is made by finding encysted worms during examination of muscle biopsy. Mebendazole is the antibiotic of choice.

Other types of worms, such as tapeworms and flukes, are rarely encountered in the United States.

Contraction, Transmission, and Stages of Disease

As a paramedic, you must understand the relationship between the pathophysiology and the assessment and management of patients with infections or diseases resulting from infections. This knowledge will prepare you for leadership in recognizing infectious diseases and curbing their transmission.

The interactions among host, infectious agent, and environment are the elements of disease transmission. Studying each of these factors individually and then looking for relationships among them often reveals how an infectious agent has been effectively transmitted. Infectious agents exist in all types of **reservoirs**—animals, humans, insects, and the environment. While inhabiting animal or insect reservoirs, they do not cause disease. Their presence at any time in a given environment is affected by their life cycle, by the presence of stressors that may force them outside their normal reservoirs, and by the climate. The initiation of therapy can sometimes disrupt the life cycle of the infectious agent and may eradicate the infection. When a host and infectious agent come together at the right time and under the right conditions, disease transmission takes place.

Infectious agents may invade hosts through one of two basic mechanisms. The more common is direct transmission from person to person through a cough, sneeze, kiss, or sexual contact. The other mechanism, indirect transmission, can spread organisms in a number of ways. Infected persons often shed organisms into the environment. These organisms come to rest on doorknobs, handrails, computer keyboards, and so on. Other people who contact those surfaces are at risk for contracting the disease. Similarly, microorganisms may be transmitted via food products, water, or even through the soil.

Bloodborne diseases are transmitted by contact with the blood or body fluids of an infected person. They include AIDS; hepatitis B, C, and D; Ebola virus disease (EVD); and syphilis. The risk of transmission of bloodborne diseases increases if a patient has open wounds, active bleeding, or increased secretions. Assume that every patient has an infectious bloodborne disease and take precautions to avoid contact with blood and other body fluids.

Some infectious diseases may be transmitted through the air on droplets expelled during a productive cough or sneeze. They include tuberculosis, meningitis, mumps, measles, rubella, and chickenpox (varicella). Other, more common diseases such as the common cold, influenza, and respiratory syncytial virus (RSV) may also be transmitted by the **airborne** route.

Some infectious diseases are transmitted orally (primarily by eating) or by the **fecal–oral route**, in which enteric microorganisms (normally found in the GI system and the feces) are transmitted between potential hosts, as in shaking hands or other social customs, and then having the recipient somehow introduce the infectious agent into his mouth by scratching or eating with his hands. Fecal–oral diseases are prevalent in third-world countries and in areas with unsanitary conditions. Hepatitis A and E and other viruses can be transmitted by the fecal–oral route. Foodborne illnesses include food poisoning, certain parasitic infections, and trichinosis.

The risk of infection is considered *theoretical* if transmission is acknowledged to be possible but has not actually

Table 10-1 Modes of Transmission of Infectious Diseases

Disease	Bloodborne	Airborne	Sexual	Indirect	Opportunist	Fecal–Oral
Hepatitis A						✓
Hepatitis B	✓					
Hepatitis C	✓		✓			
HIV	✓		✓			
Influenza		✓	✓	✓		
Syphilis			✓			
Gonorrhea			✓			
Measles		✓				
Mumps		✓				
Strep throat		✓			✓	
Herpes virus	✓		✓	✓		
Food poisoning		✓		✓		✓
Lyme disease	✓					
Pneumonia		✓			✓	
Ebola	✓		✓	✓		✓

been reported. It is considered *measurable* if factors in the infectious agent's transmission and their associated risks have been identified or deduced from reported data. Generally, the risk of disease transmission rises if a patient has open wounds, increased secretions, active coughing, or any ongoing invasive treatment in which exposure to an infectious body fluid is likely (Table 10-1). In the prehospital setting, the unpredictable environment and behavior of patients increase the risk of exposure. For example, a patient with a closed head injury and multiple lacerations may be combative, thereby contaminating EMS personnel with blood or other body fluids. Broken windshield glass contaminated with blood may easily penetrate examination gloves and skin. Patients who are violent and aggressive may deliberately bite, scratch, or spit at rescuers. Many EMS patient care activities occur in a closed, poorly ventilated environment, such as the back of an ambulance. Thus, you must have available, and routinely use, protective clothing and other barrier devices, as indicated. Regular cleaning and sanitization of the ambulance and equipment will also help to reduce exposure and create a cleaner, safer working environment.

CONTENT REVIEW

➤ Factors Affecting Disease Transmission
- Mode of entry
- Virulence
- Number of organisms transmitted
- Host resistance

Not all exposures to microorganisms from body fluids or infected patients will result in transmission of those agents. Nor are all infectious agents and diseases **communicable** (capable of being transmitted to another host). Communicability depends on several factors. Exposure to an infectious agent may just result in **contamination**, in which the agent exists only on the surface of the host without penetrating it. Penetration of the host implies that **infection** has occurred, but infection should never be equated with disease. Factors that affect the likelihood that an exposed individual will become infected and then actually develop disease include:

- ***Correct mode of entry.*** Certain external barriers in hosts, particularly the skin, make it impossible for infectious agents to establish themselves. Mucous membranes, however, often present an effective point of entry.
- ***Virulence.*** **Virulence** is an organism's strength or ability to infect or overcome the body's defenses. Some organisms, such as the hepatitis B virus (HBV), are highly virulent and can remain infectious on a surface for weeks. Others, such as HIV and syphilis, die when exposed to air and light. Some bacteria (*Clostridium*) may remain dormant in the soil for months and be capable of causing disease if contracted. Infection generally occurs either when a highly virulent

microorganism interacts with a normal, intact host or when a less virulent microorganism enters a host with impaired defenses (immunosuppression).

- *Number of organisms transmitted (dose).* For most diseases, a minimum number of organisms must enter the host to cause infection. As a rule, the higher the number, the greater the likelihood of contracting the disease.
- *Host resistance.* **Resistance** is the host's ability to fight off infection. Several factors affect the host's resistance. They include general health and fitness, genetic predisposition or resistance to infection, nutrition status, recent exposure to stressors, hygiene, and the presence of underlying disease processes. Persons with decreased immune function are at significantly increased risk for contracting infectious diseases. Cigarette smokers and those regularly exposed to secondhand cigarette smoke are also at increased risk.
- *Other host factors.* The tendency of the host to travel or be in contact with other potential hosts, the age and socioeconomic status of the host, and the characteristics of other hosts within the population of which the infected host is a member all affect the likelihood of contracting disease.

Phases of the Infectious Process

Disease progression varies greatly, depending on the infectious agent and the host. Conditions can manifest themselves in various ways. Once infected with an infectious agent, the host goes through a **latent period** when he cannot transmit the agent to someone else. Following the latent period is a **communicable period**, when the host may exhibit signs of clinical disease and can transmit the infectious agent to another host.

The appearance of symptoms often lags after exposure to an infectious disease. The time between exposure and presentation, known as the **incubation period**, may range from a few days, as in the common cold, to months or years, as in HIV/AIDS or hepatitis. Thus, prehospital personnel must be notified if any patient for whom they provide care subsequently develops a life-threatening infectious disease.

Most viruses and bacteria have surface proteins, or **antigens**, that stimulate the body to produce **antibodies**. These antibodies react to or unite with the antigens. The antibodies' presence in the blood indicates exposure to the disease that they fight. Although testing for the presence of a specific disease antigen is difficult, laboratory tests can often spot antibodies that are specific for the disease or antigen. For example, they detect the human immunodeficiency virus (HIV) through the presence of antibodies specific to HIV. When a person develops antibodies after exposure to a disease, his previously negative test will be positive and **seroconversion** has occurred. The time between exposure to disease and seroconversion is referred to as the **window phase**. A person in the window phase may test negative even though he is infected. From the standpoint of the immune system response, the window phase is the period when antigen is present but antibody production has not reached detectable levels. The **disease period** is the duration from the onset of signs and symptoms until the resolution of symptoms or death occurs. Keep in mind that the resolution of symptoms does not necessarily imply that the infectious agent has been eradicated.

The Body's Defenses Against Disease

The body protects itself from disease in many ways. At the basic level, skin defends against invading infection and pathogens. Parts of the respiratory system assist by creating turbulent airflow and capturing foreign bodies with nasal hair. Mucus can trap and kill foreign materials, transport them to the mouth and nose via the mucociliary escalator, and expel them as sputum. (Nicotine from cigarette smoke paralyzes the individual cilia of the escalator, making the expulsion of lower airway mucus, sometimes referred to as phlegm, difficult.) The urinary and gastrointestinal systems work cooperatively to eliminate pathogens via feces and urine. Three body systems that specifically protect against disease are the immune system, the complement system, and the lymphatic system.

The Immune System

As you learned in the chapters "Pathophysiology" and "Immunology," the human body has a sophisticated **immune system**. The various cells involved in the immune response are sometimes collectively referred to as the **reticuloendothelial system (RES)** because their locations are so widely scattered throughout the body. (*Reticulo* means "network"; *endothelial* refers to certain cells that line blood vessels, the heart, and various body cavities.)

The immune system fights disease by protecting the body from foreign invaders. It must be able to differentiate "self" from "nonself." The immune system can recognize the antigens of most bacteria and viruses as foreign, or nonself. Once the immune system identifies a material as nonself, it starts a series of actions intended to eliminate the foreign material. This series of mechanisms is initiated by the inflammatory response, which results from local tissue injury. Although this discussion focuses on infection, the initial injury may also be physical, chemical, or thermal.

The inflammatory response involves selected **leukocytes** (white blood cells), the functional units of blood in the immune response. The two types of white cells, **neutrophils**

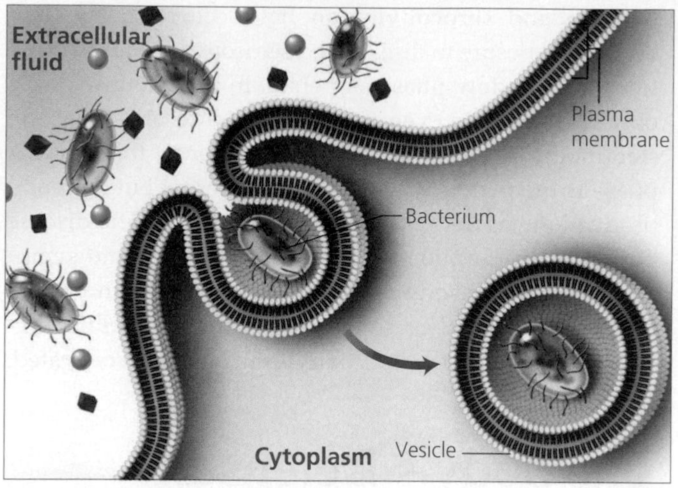

FIGURE 10-1 Phagocytosis occurs when cells engulf infectious agents.

and **macrophages**, both attack the infectious agent by a combination of digestive enzymes and ingesting it in a process called **phagocytosis** (Figure 10-1). Neutrophils act first and are followed 12 to 24 hours later by the macrophages. Once phagocytosis occurs, the macrophages release chemicals called *chemotactic factors*, which trigger additional immune system responses.

Two types of immune system response are **cell-mediated immunity** and **humoral immunity**. Both are time-consuming processes that involve the actions of **lymphocytes**, which are another type of leukocyte. Cell-mediated immunity does not result in the formation of antibodies against the foreign antigens; humoral immunity does. The antibodies remain in the blood, ready to attack the same antigen upon any future reexposure.

Cell-mediated immunity generates various forms of **T lymphocytes** that react against specific antigens. Helper T cells, suppressor T cells, killer T cells, and inflammatory T cells work together against bacteria such as *Mycobacterium tuberculosis,* the causative agent of tuberculosis, and viruses that have been taken up by host cells. This defense mechanism also responds to the presence of cancer cells and transplanted tissue. Humoral immunity, by contrast, results from the action of antibodies formed from mature **B lymphocytes** (plasma cells) in the lymph nodes and bone marrow. It aims primarily at toxins and pathogens not yet ingested by phagocytes. Humoral immunity is responsible for the immune system's properties of *memory* and *specificity.* These properties mean that a particular antigen is "remembered" when it enters the body again and, as a result, plasma cells produce antibodies that work specifically against that antigen. In this way, antibodies (also called **immunoglobulins**) protect against most infectious agents to which the body is repeatedly exposed.

CONTENT REVIEW

➤ Classes of Human Antibodies
- IgG
- IgM
- IgA
- IgD
- IgE

Other classes of white blood cells, monocytes, eosinophils, basophils, and natural killer (NK) cells, also participate in the general immune system response. The five classes of human antibodies are:

- *IgG* remembers an antigen and recognizes any repeated invasions. It is the principal immunoglobulin in human serum and is the major class of immunoglobulin in the immune response. It crosses the placental barrier from mother to fetus and is important in producing immunity prior to birth.
- *IgM* is formed early in most immune responses.
- *IgA* is the main immunoglobulin in exocrine secretions (milk, respiratory, saliva, and tears).
- *IgD* is present on the surface of B lymphocytes and acts as an antigen receptor.
- *IgE* attaches to mast cells in the respiratory and intestinal tracts. It plays a major role in allergic reactions. Patients with allergies generally have increased levels of this immunoglobulin.

An unfortunate occasional aspect of humoral immunity is **autoimmunity**, the body's formation of antibodies against itself (autoantibodies). We do not completely understand autoimmunity, but it may be due in part to antigens that chemically "look like" the body's own tissues.

The Complement System

Because cell-mediated and humoral immunity are time-consuming processes, the complement system provides an alternate pathway to react more quickly to foreign bodies. This system of at least 20 proteins works with antibody formation and the inflammatory reaction to combat infection. It responds by recognizing surface complex molecules (endotoxins) from Gram-negative bacteria. Originally named because it "complemented" the action of antibodies so foreign cell lysis could occur, complement is now known to start a cascade of biochemical events triggered by tissue injury. The number of reactions and products in this cascade increases almost exponentially. The net result is that complement is involved with the acute inflammatory response, helping phagocytosis, and the outright killing of certain bacteria such as *Neisseria* species.

The Lymphatic System

The **lymphatic system** is a secondary circulatory system. It comprises the spleen, thymus, lymph nodes, and lymphatic ducts—a separate set of small, thin-walled vessels that collect overflow fluid from the tissue spaces and return it to the circulatory system. This fluid, known as **lymph**, has the same composition as normal interstitial fluid.

The lymphatic system is important in disease prevention. The lymph nodes filter the lymph before returning it to the circulatory system. They are lined with reticuloendothelial cells that attach to and destroy particulate matter, including microorganisms, through phagocytosis. The leftovers, usually amino acids and other cell fragments, return to the circulatory system to be used as building blocks in cellular metabolism.

An essential organ in the lymphatic system is the spleen, a solid organ in the left upper abdominal quadrant. The spleen essentially functions as two separate organs. The white pulp of the spleen generates antibodies and produces B and T lymphocytes. The red pulp removes unwanted particulate matter, such as old or damaged red blood cells and other blood elements. Blood loss from the spleen, which is vulnerable to abdominal trauma, can be massive and rapidly fatal.

Individual Host Immunity

The interaction of cell-mediated immunity, humoral immunity, complement, the lymphatic system, the leukocytes, and all the cells of the RES result in *resistance,* the host's defense against present and future infection. An individual is said to have acquired **passive immunity** if he has received antibodies from the maternal circulation via the placenta (transplacental transmission) or from inoculation (injection). Passive immunity generally lasts from days to months. An individual who develops antibodies in response to inoculation by a killed or modified form of an infectious agent in an attenuated vaccine or its parts is said to have acquired **active immunity**. Active immunity is humoral immunity and generally lasts for years or the lifetime of the individual. After immunization or natural exposure to an antigen, an individual should *seroconvert* (show evidence of antibody response). The *assay,* or laboratory measure of the amount of antibodies against a particular antigen, is the *titer.* The measure of a particular vaccine's effectiveness is reported as the antibody titer. The titer most familiar to health care workers is the one reported after the hepatitis B vaccination series.

The immune system's ability to develop antibodies is also used to classify microorganisms into serotypes. A serotype is determined by exposing a microorganism to known antibody solutions. When a reaction indicates the formation of an antigen–antibody complex, the antigens associated with that microorganism are then known, and the microorganism is thereafter designated as a certain serotype. The designation may be in letters, numbers, or alphanumerics and often depends on how the antigens are identified.

Immunizing against tetanus is common practice in emergency medicine. Tetanus is a rare, but frequently fatal, disease that results from a wound infected with the bacterium *Clostridium tetani.* This bacterium releases an exotoxin called *tetanospasmin* that causes the clinical signs and symptoms of the disease. Thus, the infection can be localized, but the patient will experience generalized symptoms because of the presence of the exotoxin in the circulation. Generalized tetanus causes pain and stiffness in the jaw muscles (hence the common name "lockjaw") and stiffness in the trunk muscles. This progresses to reflex convulsive spasms and tonic contractions of muscle groups. These are accompanied by autonomic nervous system dysfunction, laryngospasm, and other problems. As a rule, people in developed countries receive several doses of tetanus vaccine during their childhood. Periodic boosters follow every 5 to 10 years.

CONTENT REVIEW

- ➤ Phases of Prehospital Infection Control
  - Preparation for response
  - Response
  - Patient contact
  - Recovery
- ➤ Infection control begins long before an emergency call.

Occasionally, patients who have never received any form of tetanus vaccination will present with a tetanus-prone wound. This is a particular problem along the United States–Mexico border. In these cases, patients require passive antibodies until their immune system can begin to manufacture specific antibodies in response to the tetanus vaccine. Passive immunity is provided by injection of tetanus immune globulin (TIG) (Hypertet). This provides antibodies for immediate protection. Because the patient did not manufacture them, they are considered passive immunity. At the same time, the patient will receive a dose of tetanus toxoid. This will cause the patient's immune system to manufacture antibodies against tetanus, providing a form of active immunity. Because there is no specific treatment for tetanus, the best approach is to prevent it by aggressive immunization.

Infection Control in Prehospital Care

To supplement the body's natural defenses against disease, EMS providers must protect themselves from infectious exposures (Figure 10-2). The four phases of infection control in prehospital care are preparation for response, response, patient contact, and recovery.

Preparation for Response

Infection control begins long before an emergency call. To ensure proper protection, the EMS agency should implement the following procedures:

- Establish and maintain written standard operating procedures (SOPs) for infection control, and monitor employee compliance.
- Prepare an infection control plan that includes a schedule of when and how to implement OSHA, NIOSH, and CDC pathogen standards and guidelines.

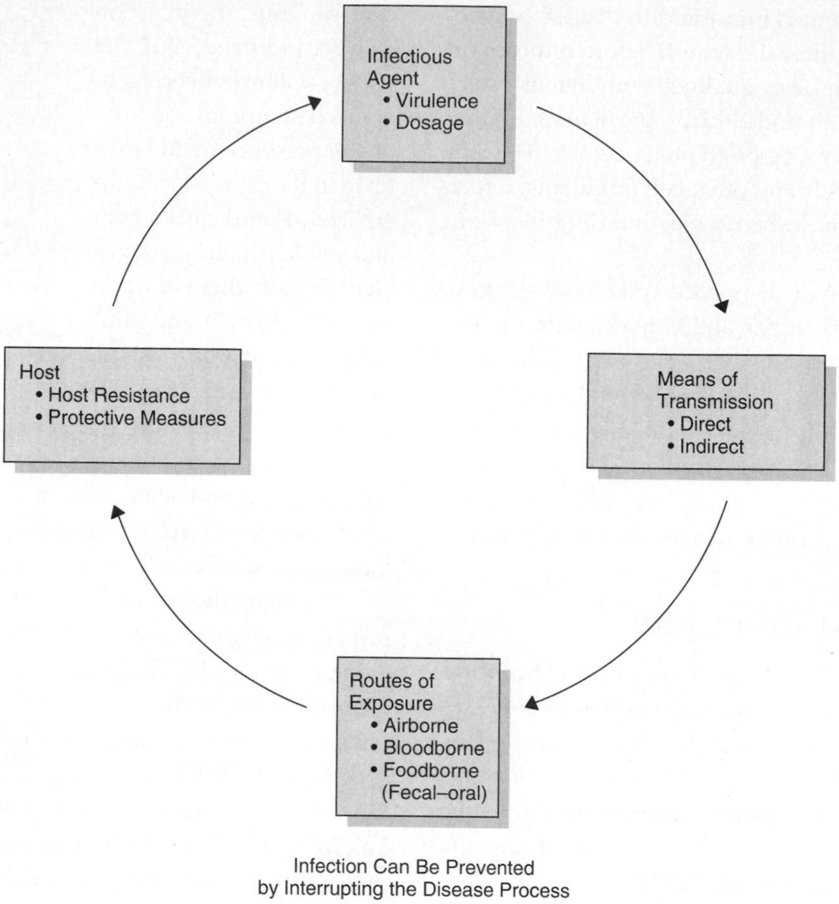

FIGURE 10-2 Interruption of infectious disease transmission is a role of prehospital personnel.

- Provide adequate original and ongoing infection control training to all personnel, including engineering and work practice controls.
- Ensure that all employees are provided with personal protective equipment (PPE) and that it is fitted appropriately, checked regularly, maintained properly, and can be located easily.
- Ensure that all EMS personnel treat and bandage all personal wounds (e.g., open sores, cuts, or skin breaks) before any emergency response.
- Use disposable supplies and equipment when possible. The risk of transmitting disease is generally much lower than when reusing items, even though they have been cleaned or disinfected.
- Ensure that all EMS personnel have access to the facilities and supplies needed to maintain a high level of personal hygiene.
- Do not allow EMS personnel to deliver patient care if they exhibit signs or symptoms of an infectious disease.
- Monitor all EMS personnel for compliance with vaccinations and appropriate diagnostic tests (e.g., **PPD**, antibody titers).
- Appoint a designated infectious disease control officer (IDCO) to serve as a contact person for personnel exposed to an infectious disease and monitor the infection control program.
- Identify specific job classifications and work processes in which the possibility of exposure exists.
- Provide hazmat (hazardous materials) education for employees, including how to locate and interpret safety data sheets (SDS) regarding chemicals or chemical mixtures with information on the associated health hazards.

Do not assume that your EMS agency can protect you from exposure to all infectious agents. Your attitude toward protecting yourself against infectious agents is one measure of your professionalism.

Response

When responding to an EMS call, take the following infection control measures:

- Obtain as much information as possible from dispatch regarding the nature of the patient's illness or injury.

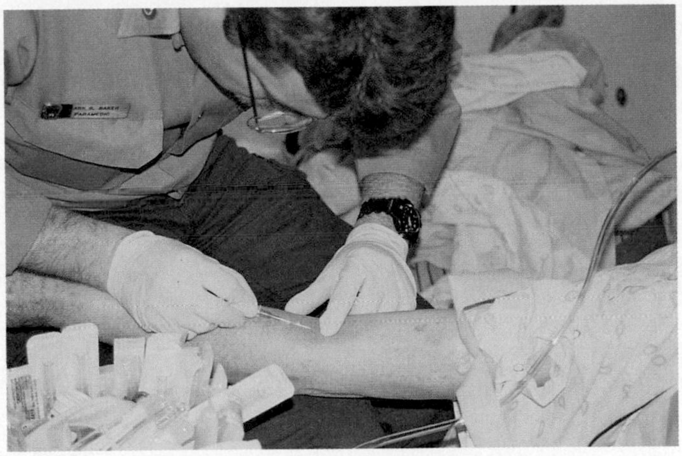

FIGURE 10-3 Always use the personal protection recommended for the degree of exposure anticipated.

- Prepare for patient contact. Put on gloves and don eye and face protection before patient contact when practical.
- Prepare mentally for the call. Think *infection control!*

Patient Contact

Your contact with a patient, especially at an emergency scene, poses your highest risk for acquiring an infectious disease. Have all personal protective equipment with you before leaving the emergency vehicle, and follow these guidelines:

- Isolate all body substances and avoid any contact with them.
- Take Standard Precautions. Wear appropriate personal protective equipment such as gowns, gloves, face shields, masks, protective eyewear, aprons, and similar items (Figure 10-3).
- Allow only necessary personnel to make patient contact. Limit the risk to as few people as possible, thus minimizing exposure.
- Use airway adjuncts such as a pocket mask or bag-valve-mask unit to minimize exposure. Disposable items are preferable.
- Properly dispose of biohazardous waste.
- Use extreme caution with sharp instruments. Use retractable IV needles and needleless injection systems when possible. *Never* bend, recap, or remove contaminated needles. Dispose of all contaminated sharps in properly labeled puncture-resistant containers (Figure 10-4).
- Never smoke, eat, or drink in the patient compartment of the ambulance. Each service should have strict guidelines regarding the presence of food and drink in the driver compartment during down times. Strictly adhere to OSHA guidelines.
- Do not apply cosmetics or lip balm, or handle contact lenses, when a likelihood of exposure exists.

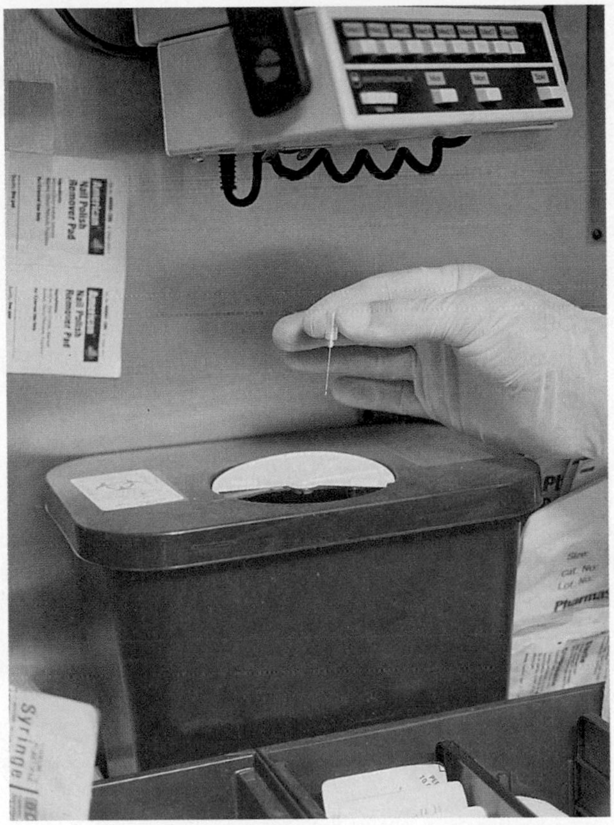

FIGURE 10-4 Dispose of needles and other sharp objects properly.

Table 10-2 details specific measures for protection against HIV (human immunodeficiency virus) and HBV (hepatitis B virus) infections.

Standard Precautions

The CDC, OSHA, and NIOSH recommend Standard Precautions for health care workers at increased risk for exposure to HIV and other bloodborne pathogens. Because it is impossible to reliably determine which patients have bloodborne infections, the following precautions are recommended for all patients:

- All health care workers should routinely use appropriate barrier precautions to prevent exposure of the skin and mucous membranes to any contact with blood, or other body fluids, from any patient. Wear disposable gloves whenever touching blood and body fluids, mucous membranes, or broken skin; handling items or surfaces soiled with blood or body fluids; and performing venipuncture or other vascular access procedures. Change and discard gloves after contact with each patient. To prevent exposure of the mucous membranes of the mouth, nose, and eyes, wear masks and protective eyewear or protective face shields during procedures likely to aerosolize blood or other body fluids. If a glove is torn or a needle stick occurs, remove the glove and replace it as soon as possible. Discard

Table 10-2 Guidelines for Prevention of Transmission of HIV and HBV to Prehospital Personnel

Protective Task or Activity	Disposable Gloves	Gown	Mask	Protective Eyewear
Bleeding control with active bleeding	Yes	Yes	Yes	Yes
Bleeding control with minimal bleeding	Yes	No	No	No
Emergency childbirth	Yes	Yes	Yes	Yes
Blood drawing	Yes	No	No	No
IV insertion	Yes	No	No	No
Endotracheal intubation	Yes	No	Yes	Yes
EOA insertion	Yes	No	Yes	Yes
Oral/nasal suctioning; manually clearing airway	Yes	Yes	Yes	Yes
Handling/cleaning instruments with possible contamination	Yes	Yes	Yes	Yes
Measuring blood pressure	Yes	No	No	No
Giving an injection	Yes	No	No	No
Measuring temperature	Yes	No	No	No
Rescuing from a building fire	Yes	No	No	No
Cleaning back of ambulance after a medical call	Yes	No	No	No

the needle or instrument and obtain another. Wear gowns or aprons during any procedure likely to generate splashes of blood or other body fluids.

- Wash your hands (including the webs between your fingers) and other skin surfaces thoroughly with soap and warm water after removal of gloves and especially after contamination with blood or other body fluids. (Use of a hand-sanitizing agent is an acceptable alternative when soap and water are not available.)
- Take precautions to prevent injuries caused by needles, scalpels, or other sharp instruments or devices when performing procedures, cleaning instruments, or disposing of instruments. To prevent needle stick injuries, needles should not be recapped, purposely bent, broken by hand, removed from disposable syringes, or otherwise manipulated by hand. Position puncture-resistant containers as close as possible to work areas and place disposable syringes and needles, scalpel blades, and other sharp items in them for disposal.
- Although saliva has not been directly implicated in HIV transmission, use mouthpieces with one-way valves or filters, bag-valve-mask devices, and other ventilation devices to avoid mouth-to-mouth contact. Place these resuscitation items where the need for resuscitation is predictable.
- Do not put gloved hands close to your mouth, and avoid wiping your face with your forearms or the backs of your gloved hands. Use clean towels to deal with perspiration.
- If you have exudative or weeping skin lesions, refrain from direct patient care and from handling patient care equipment until the condition resolves.
- Pregnant health care workers are not believed to be at greater risk of HIV infection than health care workers who are not pregnant. If a health care worker develops HIV infection during pregnancy, however, the infant is at risk for transplacental transmission. Therefore, pregnant health care workers should be especially familiar with, and strictly adhere to, precautions to minimize the risk of HIV transmission.
- Disinfection of diagnostic or therapeutic equipment and supplies is mandatory.

Enhanced Precautions

The occurrence of Ebola virus disease (EVD) in 2014 in the United States resulted in the Centers for Disease Control and Prevention issuing recommendations for enhanced protection of EMS personnel when exposure to EVD or a similar highly contagious disease was possible. When state and local EMS authorities determine that there is an increased risk (based on information provided by local, state, and federal public health authorities, including the city or county health department, state health department, and/or the CDC), they may direct EMS providers to modify their practices as described here:

- *Patient assessment*:
  - To minimize potential exposure, only one EMS provider should approach the patient and should

perform the initial screening from at least three feet away from the patient. Based on the initial screening, if the EMS provider suspects that the patient could have EVD, then PPE should be donned before coming into close contact with the patient. Keep other emergency responders farther away, while ensuring that they are still able to support the provider with primary assessment duties.

- No one should have direct contact with a patient who may have EVD without wearing appropriate PPE.
- During patient assessment and management, EMS personnel should consider the signs, symptoms, and risk factors of EVD. A relevant exposure history should include the following:
  - Residence in, or travel to, a country or area with widespread EVD or cases in urban settings with uncertain control measures.
  - Contact with blood or body fluids (including but not limited to urine, saliva, vomit, sweat, and diarrhea) of a patient under investigation or patient with confirmed EVD.
- Patients who meet the criteria should be further questioned regarding the presence of signs or symptoms of EVD such as fever, severe headache, muscle pain, weakness, fatigue, diarrhea, vomiting, abdominal pain, diarrhea, and unexplained hemorrhage.

- *Safety and PPE:*
  - If 911 call takers advise the patient is suspected of having EVD, EMS personnel should put on the PPE appropriate for patients under investigation before entering the scene. PPE options are described in local protocols.
  - To minimize potential exposure, only one EMS provider should approach the patient and should perform the initial screening from at least three feet away from the patient. If, based on the initial screening, the EMS provider suspects that the patient might have EVD, then PPE should be put on before coming into close contact with the patient. Keep the other emergency responders farther away, while ensuring they are still able to support the provider with primary assessment duties.
  - No one should have direct contact with a patient who may have EVD without wearing appropriate PPE. Based on the clinical presentation of the patient, there are two PPE options:
    - If the patient is *not* exhibiting obvious bleeding, vomiting, or diarrhea and there is no concern for bleeding, vomiting, or diarrhea, EMS personnel should follow the PPE guidelines for clinically stable patients under investigation.

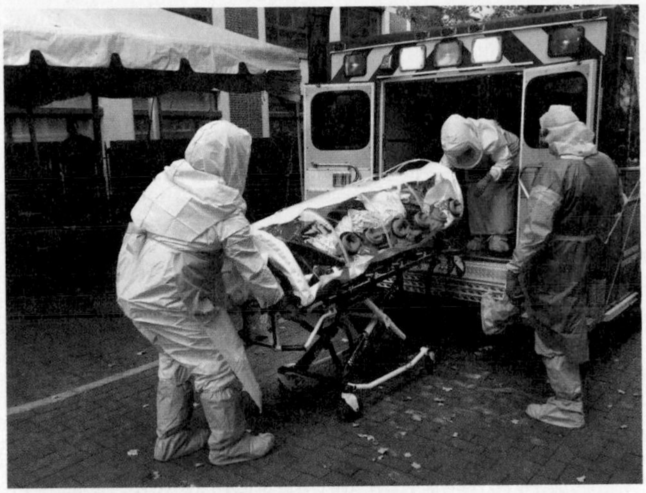

FIGURE 10-5 Enhanced PPE for patients under investigation for Ebola virus disease (EVD).
(Edward T. Dickinson, MD)

    - If the patient is exhibiting obvious bleeding, vomiting, or diarrhea or there is concern for potential bleeding, vomiting, or diarrhea, then EMS personnel should wear recommended PPE equipment for EVD. PPE should be put on before entering a scene with a patient under investigation and continue to be worn until providers no longer are in contact with the patient. PPE should be carefully put on and taken off under the supervision of a trained observer (Figure 10-5).
  - If the patient exhibits obvious bleeding, vomiting, copious diarrhea, or a clinical condition that warrants invasive or aerosol-generating procedures (such as intubation, suctioning, active resuscitation), then use PPE as designated for the care of hospitalized patients.
  - If blood, body fluids, secretions, or excretions from a patient under investigation come into direct contact with the EMS provider's unprotected skin or mucous membranes, then the EMS provider should immediately stop working. The exposed provider should wash the affected skin surfaces with a cleansing or antiseptic solution, and mucous membranes (e.g., conjunctiva) should be irrigated with a large amount of water or eyewash solution, according to the usual protocols. All waste should be placed in a biohazard bag. EMS providers should report exposure to an occupational health provider, supervisor, or designated infection control officer for immediate care.

- *Patient Management:*
  - No one should have direct contact with a patient under investigation without wearing appropriate PPE.

- Use caution when approaching a patient under investigation. On rare occasions, illness can cause delirium, with erratic behavior, such as flailing or staggering. This type of behavior can place EMS providers at additional risk of exposure.
- Keep the patient separated from others as much as possible.
- Limit the number of providers who care for a patient under investigation. All EMS personnel having direct contact with a patient under investigation must wear PPE.
- Limit the use of needles and other sharps as much as possible. Needles and sharps should be handled with extreme care and disposed in puncture-proof, sealed containers specific to the care of this patient. Do not dispose of used needles and sharps in containers that have sharps from other patients in them.
- Consider giving the patient oral medicine to reduce nausea, per EMS protocols and consistent with scope of practice.
- If the patient is vomiting, give the patient a large red biohazard bag to contain any emesis.
- If patient has profuse diarrhea, consider wrapping the patient in an impermeable sheet to reduce contamination of other surfaces.
- Prehospital resuscitation procedures such as endotracheal intubation, open suctioning of airways, and cardiopulmonary resuscitation frequently result in a large amount of body fluids, such as saliva and vomit. Performing these procedures in a less controlled environment (for example, a moving vehicle) increases EMS providers' risk of exposure to infectious pathogens. Perform these procedures under safer circumstances (when the vehicle has stopped, upon arrival at the hospital destination) and wear the PPE recommended by the CDC to use during aerosol-generating procedures.

- *Prehospital care considerations:*
  - Prehospital patient care is frequently provided in an uncontrolled environment with unique operational challenges. EMS systems must design their procedures to accommodate their local operational challenges while still following the principles of the CDC's PPE guidance.
  - Procedures designed by an EMS system may be as simple as having one provider put on PPE and manage the patient while the other provider does not engage in patient care but serves in the role of trained observer.
  - There may be situations in which a patient must be carried and multiple providers are required to put on PPE. EMS providers wearing PPE who have cared for the patient must remain in the back of the ambulance; none of these should serve as the driver.
  - EMS agencies may consider sending additional resources to eliminate the need for putting on PPE (field-donning) by additional providers. For example, a dedicated driver for the EMS unit may not need to wear PPE if the patient compartment is isolated from the cab.
  - Doffing of PPE must be performed with meticulous care to prevent self-contamination. See guidance on PPE doffing and ensure that training emphasizes adherence to a standardized protocol.

- *Additional Considerations:*
  - Prepare and use safe procedures to treat and transport the patient to the hospital.
  - The EMS provider driving the ambulance should contact the receiving hospital and follow local or regional protocols for transporting this kind of patient to the receiving hospital.
  - Remove and keep nonessential equipment away from the patient on the scene and in the ambulance. This will eliminate or minimize contamination.
  - Avoid contamination of reusable porous surfaces not designated for single use. Cover the stretcher with an impermeable material.
  - Conduct appropriate patient assessment according to established protocols, using minimal equipment.

Recovery

Infection control does not end when you deliver the patient to the emergency department. Decontaminating the ambulance and equipment is essential. Take the following steps at the completion of each response:

- Wash hands immediately after patient contact (Figure 10-6). Ample data substantiate that *effective, vigorous* hand washing is superior to some disinfectants. On scene, you can wipe your hands with a waterless hand-cleansing solution. However, this provides for only partial cleansing because it cannot grossly remove the particles to which microorganisms adhere. Only soap and water can do that. On returning to quarters, or at the earliest opportunity, thoroughly wash your hands with soap and warm water, paying attention to the webs between fingers. Overlooking this important habit may result in the inadvertent contamination of personal clothing or anything else that you contact. Such oversight can result in transmitting the disease to family and friends.

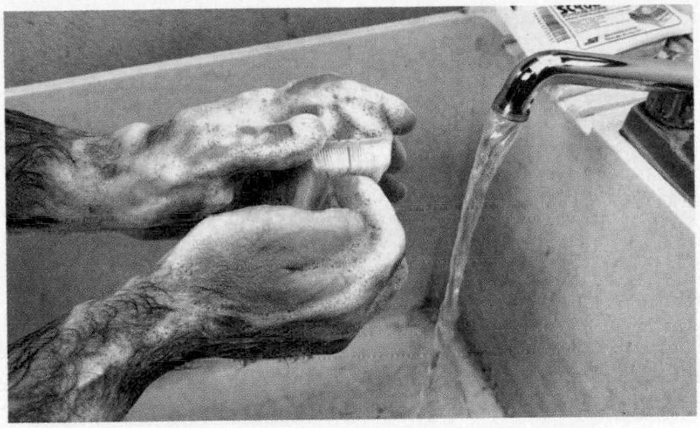

FIGURE 10-6 Handwashing is one of the most effective methods of preventing disease transmission.

- If you sustain a wound and are exposed to the body fluids of others, vigorously wash the wound with soap and warm water immediately, *before* contacting your employer or IDCO.
- Dispose of all biohazardous wastes in accordance with local laws and regulations.
- Place potentially infectious wastes in leakproof biohazard bags. Bag any soiled linen and label for laundry personnel (Figure 10-7).
- Decontaminate all contaminated clothing and reusable equipment.
- Handle uniforms in accordance with the agency's standard procedures for personal protective equipment.

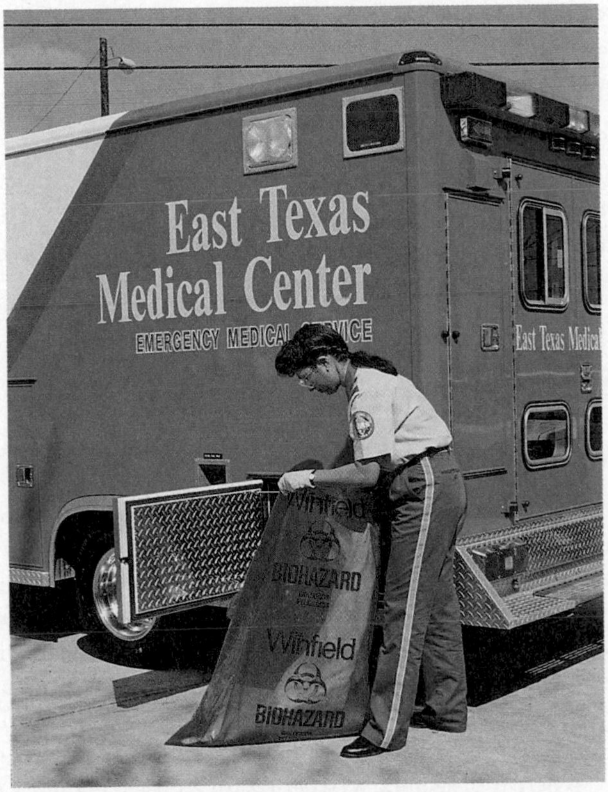

FIGURE 10-7 Bag all linens and label them infectious.

Decontamination Methods and Procedures

CONTENT REVIEW

➤ Decontamination Levels
- Low-level disinfection
- Intermediate-level disinfection
- High-level disinfection
- Sterilization

Decontaminate infected equipment according to local protocol and SOPs established by the EMS agency. Perform decontamination in a designated area that is properly marked and secured. The room should have a suitable ventilation system and adequate drainage. Be sure to wear gloves, gowns, boots, protective eyewear, and a face mask. To begin decontamination, remove surface dirt and debris with soap and water. Then disinfect and, if required, sterilize all items. The four levels of decontamination are low-level disinfection, intermediate-level disinfection, high-level disinfection, and sterilization.

LOW-LEVEL DISINFECTION Low-level **disinfection** destroys most bacteria and some viruses and fungi. It does not destroy *Mycobacterium tuberculosis* or bacterial spores. Use low-level disinfection for routine housekeeping and cleaning (Figure 10-8), as well as for removing visible body fluids. All EPA-registered disinfectants are suitable for low-level disinfection.

INTERMEDIATE-LEVEL DISINFECTION Intermediate-level disinfection destroys *Mycobacterium tuberculosis* and most viruses and fungi. It does not, however, destroy bacterial spores. Use it for all equipment that has come into contact with intact skin such as stethoscopes, splints, and blood pressure cuffs. A 1:10 to 1:100 dilution of water and chlorine bleach is acceptable for intermediate-level disinfection. Hard-surface germicides and EPA-registered disinfectants/chemical germicides are also effective.

HIGH-LEVEL DISINFECTION High-level disinfection destroys all forms of microorganisms except certain

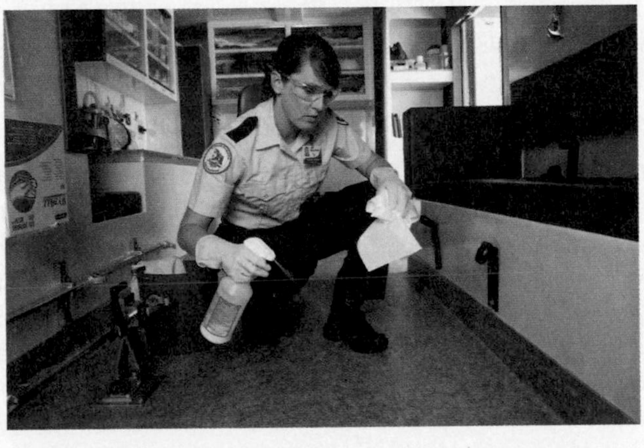

FIGURE 10-8 Complete routine cleaning and other housekeeping chores after each patient encounter.

bacterial spores. High-level disinfection is required for all reusable devices that have come into contact with mucous membranes, including laryngoscopes, Magill forceps, and airway adjuncts. For high-level disinfection, immerse objects in an EPA-approved chemical-sterilizing agent for 10 to 45 seconds (depending on the manufacturer's instructions). Alternatively, immerse the device in hot water (176°F–212°F) for 30 minutes.

STERILIZATION **Sterilization** destroys all microorganisms and is required for all contaminated invasive instruments. An autoclave that uses pressurized steam or ethylene-oxide gas effectively sterilizes equipment. These methods, however, are rarely available outside of a hospital setting. Alternatively, prolonged immersion (6–10 hours, depending on the manufacturer's instructions) in an EPA-approved chemical-sterilizing agent is usually adequate. When possible, use disposable instruments for invasive procedures.

Infectious Disease Exposures

Infectious disease exposures occur during all hours of a workshift. Because you may not always be able to contact an agency administrator, you need a working knowledge of your agency's standard operating procedures, as well as the laws and regulations applicable to exposures. The following recommendations will help to ensure that exposure management will protect you, other emergency responders and health care professionals, the agency, and confidentiality of patient information.

REPORTING AN INFECTIOUS DISEASE EXPOSURE Immediately report exposures of EMS personnel to the designated IDCO, according to local protocol. Report all exposures to blood, blood products, or any potentially infectious material, regardless of their perceived severity. This will permit immediate medical follow-up, including counseling for the EMS provider and identification of the infectious agent. It also enables the IDCO to evaluate the circumstances of the exposure and implement changes to prevent future exposures, if needed. Finally, it facilitates follow-up testing if the source individual consents.

THE RYAN WHITE ACT The **Ryan White Act** is a federal law, originally passed in 1990, that outlines the rights and responsibilities of agencies and health care workers when an infectious disease exposure occurs. In 2009, Congress passed the Ryan White HIV/AIDS Treatment Extension Act, which continued the rights and responsibilities that were part of the original act. Under the provisions of this law, the exposed employee has the right to ask the source patient's infection status, but neither the agency nor the employee can force the source individual to be tested. Employers must also tell their employees what to do if an exposure occurs.

Federal law further mandates that each agency designate an IDCO to whom exposures are reported. This officer coordinates implementation of the exposure control plan and follows local reporting requirements.

POSTEXPOSURE Employers are required to provide a medical evaluation and treatment for any paramedic or other EMS provider exposed to an infectious disease. The nature of the exposure is assessed based on the route, dose, and nature of the infectious agent. As part of the medical evaluation, employees are entitled to receive counseling about alternatives for treatment, the risks of treatment, signs, symptoms, the possibility of developing disease, and preventing further spread of the potential infection. This includes the available medications, their potential side effects, and their contraindications. Treatment must be in line with current U.S. Public Health Service recommendations.

After a paramedic is exposed to an infectious disease, he has the option to submit a blood sample for baseline testing. If the employee does not consent to having his blood screened for specific diseases, the blood samples are normally maintained for 90 days in the event that he changes his mind.

The IDCO or other health care professional who specializes in occupational infectious diseases should counsel the exposed employee and obtain informed consent for postexposure prophylaxis (PEP) based on CDC guidelines. All records related to employee counseling and PEP are forwarded to the IDCO. Vaccines may be made available to the employee if deemed appropriate by an occupational medicine physician.

CONFIDENTIALITY The IDCO will maintain records of all exposures as required by law. All these exposure records (like any medical records) are confidential. They must not be released to anyone without express written permission from the employee.

Assessment of the Patient with Infectious Disease

When assessing a patient, always maintain a high index of suspicion that an infectious agent may be involved. Consider the dispatch information, evaluate the environment for its suitability for transmitting infectious agents, and maintain appropriate Standard Precautions. Gloves are the mandatory minimum level of personal protective equipment (PPE) required on every patient contact. Consider eye protection.

When approaching a patient with a possible infectious disease, look for general indicators of infection such as unusual skin signs, fever, weakness, profuse sweating, malaise, anorexia, and unexplained worsening of existing disease states. If an infection is localized, signs of inflammation may include redness, swelling, tenderness to palpation, capillary streaking, and warmth in the affected area. A rash or other diagnostic skin signs may make identifying an infectious disease much easier.

Past Medical History

The patient's past medical history (PMH) may provide valuable clues to his illness. Patients who have AIDS or are taking immunosuppressant medications such as steroids are particularly susceptible to infection. COPD patients, patients with autoimmune diseases, and transplant recipients frequently take steroids and immunosuppressants. Persons with diabetes and other endocrine disorders are also more likely to get infections due to additional stressors on their immune systems. Other conditions that increase the risk for developing infectious diseases include alcoholism, malnutrition, IV drug abuse, malignancy (cancer), and splenectomy (removal of the spleen), as well as artificial heart valves (aortic or mitral) or joints (hip or knee). Any significant increase in emotional stress may also increase a person's risk of significant illness, including infectious diseases.

A patient with a PMH of numerous untreated throat infections who suddenly develops a heart murmur, fever, and malaise may have rheumatic fever, a streptococcal infection that can affect the heart. Such patients are often found in medically underserved areas where access to primary care is difficult or nonexistent. Patients with cancer are at increased risk for acquiring numerous opportunistic infectious diseases. A recently transmitted sexual disease may precede systemic infection. Recent unfinished antibiotic treatment may lead to the proliferation of drug-resistant infectious agents, causing recurrent, persistent bacterial infections or development of other opportunistic infections.

In addition to determining past or current illnesses or diseases, thoroughly investigate the patient's chief complaint and any history of the present illness, including:

- When did signs and symptoms begin?
- Is fever present? How has the temperature changed over time?
- Has the patient taken any medications—including aspirin, ibuprofen, or acetaminophen—that treat fever?
- Does the patient have any neck pain or stiffness when his head is moved, especially during flexion?
- Has the patient had any difficulty swallowing?
- Has the patient had any previous symptoms or illnesses similar to this one?

The Physical Examination

Physical examination of the patient whom you suspect of having an infectious disease follows the standard format for assessing a medical patient. Determine the patient's level of consciousness and vital signs early on. Increased temperature commonly indicates infection. Significant increases in pulse may occur due to the infection and as a result of elevated body temperature. As a consequence, metabolic needs will increase. The patient will require more oxygen and more nutrients to maintain normal physiologic function. This may be a serious problem for elderly, very young, or debilitated patients with concurrent illnesses that limit their cardiovascular and respiratory reserve.

Hypotension in the patient with an infectious disease may result from dehydration, vasodilation, or both, as seen in sepsis or septic shock. In rare cases, infections of the heart muscle (endocarditis) may result in decreased cardiac output (cardiogenic shock). In any case, assess the cause of the hypotension and treat it promptly. If the lungs are clear, the judicious use of fluids may be beneficial; if fluid status is not a problem, vasopressors such as dopamine may be necessary.

Dehydration is a common consequence of infectious diseases. Increased body temperature is often accompanied by increased respiratory rate and concomitant fluid loss, of which the patient is often unaware (insensible fluid loss). Vomiting or diarrhea can quickly cause life-threatening dehydration, especially in pediatric patients who have large body surface areas relative to their volume. Electrolyte imbalances often occur with fluid loss. Advances in technology that may soon make the prehospital evaluation of electrolytes cost effective may be indicated in the setting of significant dehydration. Clinically significant dehydration will usually cause tachycardia and hypotension, but be vigilant for more subtle signs that include thirst, poor skin turgor, and a shrunken and furrowed tongue. A history of decreased fluid intake, fever, vomiting, and/or diarrhea should trigger a thorough assessment of fluid status. While performing a physical exam similar to that for any patient with a medical emergency, assess the following:

- Skin for temperature, hydration, color, or rash
- Sclera (white of eye) for icterus (jaundice)
- Reaction to neck flexion (Is nuchal rigidity [neck stiffness] present?)
- Lymph nodes for swelling or tenderness (lymphadenopathy)
- Breath sounds (for adventitious sounds and evidence of consolidation)
- Hepatomegaly (enlargement of the liver)
- Purulent (pus-filled) lesions

Specific Infectious Diseases

The following section profiles infectious diseases that either may be encountered in the prehospital setting or are commonly known by emergency health care practitioners. The first major category includes diseases of immediate concern to EMS. General profiles of other diseases follow. You should be familiar with the terminology of these profiles and realize which diseases you will more commonly encounter in your patients. Always employ Standard Precautions.

Diseases of Immediate Concern to EMS Providers

The diseases of immediate concern to EMS providers include HIV, hepatitis, tuberculosis, pneumonia, chickenpox, pandemic outbreaks such as avian flu, bacterial meningitis, and Ebola virus disease. They are infectious diseases that have gained notoriety, pose a high risk for communicability and debilitating disease, or are relevant to direct patient care. Although most attention focuses on reducing transmission from patient to health care worker, the profiles also consider reverse transmission, because responsible health care workers protect both themselves and their patients. The inclusion of chickenpox may surprise some EMS personnel, but the disease is highly communicable and poses a serious occupational risk for unvaccinated or previously unexposed health care workers.

Human Immunodeficiency Virus/AIDS

The **human immunodeficiency virus (HIV)** was the most discussed and feared infectious agent of the modern era, especially of the past three decades. The clinical condition that it causes, acquired immunodeficiency syndrome (AIDS), is not a disease per se, but a collection of signs and symptoms that share common anatomic, physiologic, and biochemical derangements in the immune system. Like other viruses, HIV uses the host cell's reproductive apparatus to copy itself. HIV is a retrovirus; that is, it normally carries its genetic material in RNA (instead of DNA) and uses an enzyme called *reverse transcriptase* (hence the designation "*retro*virus") to use RNA to synthesize DNA. This is the reverse of the usual process of transcription of DNA into RNA. The action of reverse transcriptase enables genetic material from a retrovirus to become permanently incorporated into the DNA of an infected cell. Two types of HIV have been identified, HIV-1 and HIV-2. Most research targets the HIV-1 variant, which has proven much more pathogenic than HIV-2.

CONTENT REVIEW

- Diseases of Immediate Concern to EMS Providers
  - HIV
  - Hepatitis
  - Tuberculosis
  - Pneumonia
  - SARS
  - Chickenpox
  - Meningitis

The emergence of HIV and AIDS, more than any other infectious process, has increased emergency and health care workers' awareness of the dangers of infectious disease. The worldwide research and educational activities resulting from concern about HIV and AIDS are effective models for teaching health care workers and lay persons about how other infectious diseases are transmitted and for providing personal and community action plans to prevent the spread of infectious agents. Although it is a worldwide epidemic, with an especially high mortality rate in sub-Saharan Africa, AIDS poses a significantly lower *occupational* risk to health care workers in developed countries than other infectious agents.

PATHOGENESIS In the past 20 years, we have learned about the dynamics of HIV infection and the development of AIDS. It was first assumed that the virus caused a cellular immune system response and then remained in a dormant phase. The humoral response was known to produce antibodies within one to three months after infection, with clinical disease developing in one to ten years. For unexplained reasons, the virus would become active, and the worsening clinical signs were attributed to an increasing viral population. The extent of immune cell activity during the incubation phase, reported to be from months to ten years, was not immediately understood.

Research in the mid-1980s and early 1990s determined that HIV specifically targets T lymphocytes with the CD4 marker, a surface molecule that attaches the virus to the cell, and a better understanding of the cellular immune response and CD4 markers emerged. A reasonably reliable correlation between disease progression and the decrease in CD4 T lymphocyte count was developed. Physicians could predict the development of specific clinical events as the CD4 count decreased. For example, *Pneumocystis jiroveci* (formerly *Pneumocystis carinii)* pneumonia [PJP], an opportunistic AIDS infection, frequently develops when CD4 counts drop to a certain level. The CD4 count thus became a guide to treatment. Its usefulness, however, was limited because it only reflected the immune system's destruction.

Recent advances in molecular biology and more reliable and cost-effective assays of proteins and other biochemical molecules have revealed a tremendous increase in virus production immediately after infection and have shown that the immune system increases its activity to counter it. Eventually the number of immune system cells (T lymphocytes) offsets the viral load, reflected by the HIV RNA. This equilibrium, or set point, may take years to establish. Even during the dynamic phase, when the equilibrium has not yet been set, measurement of viral load is still the best available indicator of response to therapy and long-term clinical outcome.

AIDS, once a disease that was almost always fatal, can now be treated, allowing infected patients to live a relatively normal life and have a relatively normal life span. Numerous medications, including antiretroviral agents, have changed the face of AIDS. Although the number of new HIV infections has remained relatively constant, the number of patients who are living with HIV infection and AIDS has increased significantly and AIDS diagnosis and deaths have decreased significantly. (Treatment is controlling HIV infection, thus avoiding AIDS in many cases.) Most people with AIDS do not transmit the disease to others.[1]

RISK TO THE GENERAL PUBLIC HIV is transmitted through contact with blood, blood products, and body fluids. The virus has been noted in blood, semen, vaginal secretions, and breast milk.

The virus can enter the body through breaks in the skin, mucous membranes, the eyes, or by placental transmission. Mother-to-child transmission of HIV can occur through pregnancy, labor and delivery, and breastfeeding. The incidence of mother-to-child HIV transmission is highest in Africa (approximately 90 percent of cases).[2] The virus is most commonly contracted through sexual contact or sharing contaminated needles. Before the initiation of stringent controls in screening donor blood and blood products, hemophiliacs and individuals needing frequent blood transfusions were at increased risk of HIV infection. Persons at high risk for HIV exposure in the United States include:

- Men who have sex with men
- African Americans
- Urban dwellers

Recovery from AIDS has been extremely rare, although, as already noted, current medication regimens now allow most AIDS patients a relatively normal life span. Postexposure prophylaxis has been demonstrated to reduce the transmission of AIDS. This typically involves the administration of antiretroviral drugs. Even with the tremendous advances in AIDS treatment, it remains a major cause of death in Africa.

RISK TO HEALTH CARE WORKERS Although contact with contaminated blood or body secretions potentially places health care workers at risk, infection from HIV-positive patients has been exceedingly rare. This has been attributed to use of Standard Precautions, immediate washing of hands and other skin surfaces after body substance exposure, and careful handling of sharp instruments after use. Accidental needle-stick injuries are the most frequent source of infection in health care workers. Through December 2001, there were 57 documented cases of occupational HIV transmission to health care workers in the United States; only one reported case has been confirmed since 2001.[3]

The risk for effective transmission of HIV to health care workers initially depends on whether the exposure to HIV was percutaneous, mucosal, or cutaneous (to intact skin). Within each of those categories, the risk depends on fluid type. Blood is the most dangerous, followed by fluids that may or may not contain blood: semen, vaginal secretions, and cerebrospinal, synovial, pleural, peritoneal, pericardial, and amniotic fluid. Urine and saliva, unlikely to contain blood, pose a very low risk. Source patients (those possibly infecting health care workers) who are HIV positive or die within two months after the health care worker's exposure, are considered to increase the risk. The highest risk exposure involves a large volume of blood, high antibody titer against a retrovirus in the source patient, deep percutaneous injury, or actual intramuscular injection.

CLINICAL PRESENTATION The CDC first established the case definition of what constituted AIDS in 1982. Since then, it has expanded the definition of the syndrome to include other diseases such as extrapulmonary and pulmonary tuberculosis, recurrent pneumonia, wasting syndrome, HIV dementia, and sensory neuropathy. The AIDS patient may first develop a mononucleosis-like syndrome with nonspecific signs and symptoms such as fatigue, fever, sore throat, lymphadenopathy (lymph node disease), splenomegaly (enlarged spleen), rash, and diarrhea. Because not all of those signs are present, the situation may seem so trivial that the patient does not seek health care. Many patients develop purplish skin lesions known as Kaposi's sarcoma. Kaposi's sarcoma is a cancerous lesion that was quite rare until HIV appeared (Figure 10-9). As the disease progresses, many patients develop life-threatening opportunistic infections such as *P. jiroveci* pneumonia. Secondary infections caused by *M. tuberculosis* may also be present. As AIDS progresses, it involves the central nervous system; dementia, psychosis, encephalopathy, and peripheral neurologic disorders may develop.

Close monitoring of AIDS-related parameters helps physicians monitor, stage, and manage the disease. Routine testing of the following laboratory parameters is recommended:

- ***CD4 count.*** The CD4 cells are also called T-helper cells. Examination of CD4 counts gives an indication of how well the immune system is functioning. HIV infects CD4 cells and uses the cellular machinery to replicate the virus. A normal CD4 count is 500 to 1,500 cells per milliliter of blood. Generally speaking, a falling CD4 count in a patient with HIV infection indicates disease progression. When the count is very low, the risk of opportunistic infections increases.
- ***Viral load.*** The viral load is the number of copies of the HIV virus in the patient's blood. A high viral load (>10,000 copies) indicates that the virus is reproducing

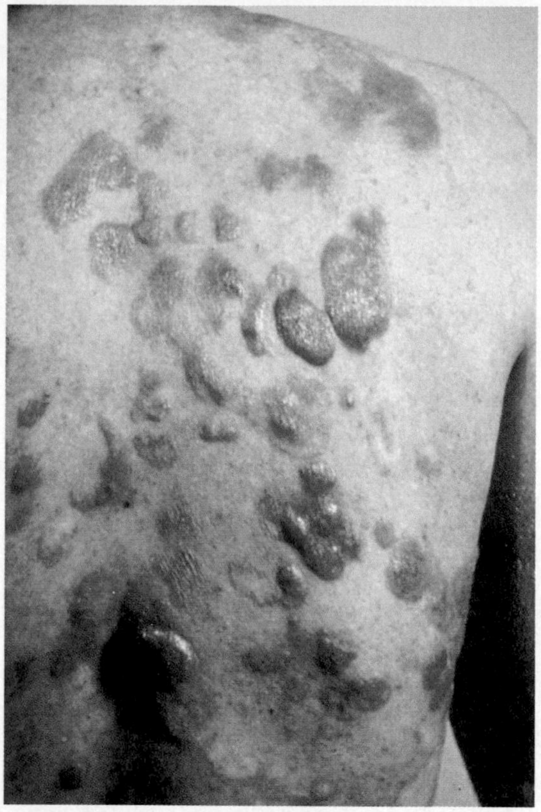

FIGURE 10-9 AIDS patient with Kaposi's sarcoma.
(National Cancer Institute)

and the disease is progressing. A low viral load (200–500 copies) means that HIV may not be actively reproducing and the disease may progress more slowly. In patients with known HIV infection, the inability to detect a viral load does not imply a cure—only that the load is beneath the sensitivity of the test to detect it.

POSTEXPOSURE PROPHYLAXIS There is no cure or vaccine for AIDS. After an exposure to a confirmed HIV-positive source patient, the health care worker should immediately seek evaluation and possible initiation of treatment by an occupational medicine or infectious disease physician. Current CDC recommendations include prompt initiation of postexposure therapy (within hours of the exposure).[4] The basic regimen typically includes antiretroviral drugs and is based on the risk of the exposure and the toxicity of the drugs. Early aggressive treatment may decrease the viral load and alter the set point. Counseling by the infectious disease control officer (IDCO) or a trained occupational infectious disease specialist must supplement the postexposure evaluation as part of the agency's exposure control plan. EMS personnel should not attempt to determine their own risk and need for postexposure prophylaxis. Health care workers have significantly underestimated their own risk and need for medical intervention regarding other infections, and the element of denial in HIV increases that tendency.

SUMMARY OF HIV HIV-positive patients generally do not present to EMS in life-threatening situations; however, they pose substantial psychosocial challenges. Despite changes in societal attitudes and increased tolerance of differences, HIV-positive individuals are often marginalized and shunned. Their subsequent feeling of social isolation is often worsened by depression. In spite of this, these patients are usually forthcoming about their infection status when dealing with health care workers. Although a paramedic generally has little to offer in terms of treatment, it is vitally important that care be compassionate, understanding, and nonjudgmental. Take appropriate precautions to prevent disease transmission, but if you truly understand the risk as it applies to you as a health care worker, it should be no barrier to your providing professional and emotionally supportive care, including a caring touch. In the EMS environment, physical isolation of the HIV-positive patient is unjustified.

Hepatitis

Hepatitis is an inflammation of the liver caused by viruses, bacteria, fungi, parasites, excessive alcohol consumption, or medications. Viruses are by far the most common cause of hepatitis. The clinical signs and symptoms of hepatitis secondary to viral infection are the same regardless of the type of virus. Initially they include headache, fever, weakness, joint pain, anorexia, nausea and vomiting, and, in some cases, right upper quadrant abdominal pain. As the disease progresses, the patient may become jaundiced, with fever often resolving at the onset of jaundice. This stage is sometimes marked by darkened urine and the development of clay-colored stools. The various types of hepatitis are transmitted in specific ways. Hepatitis A, B, C, D, and E represent the greatest potential for communicable disease. Paramedics who practice Standard Precautions against bloodborne and fecal–oral transmission will drastically reduce their risk of contracting hepatitis through occupational exposure (Table 10-3).[5]

HEPATITIS A Hepatitis A (infectious or viral hepatitis) is transmitted by the fecal–oral route. The causative agent, hepatitis A virus, is usually found in the stool of infected persons, who may not exercise suitable personal hygiene. After these individuals handle food or contact another individual even as casually as shaking hands, the virus can then be transmitted via contaminated hands, food, water, ice, and eating utensils. Furthermore, the virus can exist on unwashed hands for as long as 4 hours. Many hepatitis A infections are asymptomatic. They do not present with obvious signs like jaundice and are recognizable only by liver function studies. This is especially true of children, who represent most cases of infection and often transmit the virus to others by close social contact. Sexual contact can also spread the virus. Transmission by needle-stick injury is unlikely and has not been reported.

Table 10-3 Comparisons of Viral Hepatitis Infections

Disease	Virus	Incubation Period (Average)	Spread	Chronicity	Vaccine
Hepatitis A	HAV	15–30 days (30 days)	Fecal/oral	No	Yes
Hepatitis B	HBV	45–160 days (120 days)	Blood/body fluids	Yes	Yes
Hepatitis C	HCV	2–25 weeks (7–9 weeks)	Blood/body fluids	Yes	No
Hepatitis D	HDV	2–8 weeks	Blood/body fluids	Yes	HBV vaccine
Hepatitis E	HEV	2–9 weeks (40 days)	Fecal/oral	No	No

Diaper changing, especially in child care centers with an infected child, is known to increase risk. Travelers to areas with poor sanitary conditions are also at risk. Two doses of inactivated hepatitis A vaccine provide effective active immunization. A combination vaccine against hepatitis A and B is available for children. Health care workers serving on disaster medical teams to Africa, the Middle East, Central and South America, and Asia should be immunized. Immunization is not generally recommended for health care workers in the United States but may be advised in some areas where hepatitis A prevalence is unusually high. Passive preexposure immunization with immune globulin (gamma globulin) is therefore falling out of favor, but immunization may be used after exposure in selected incidents.

The hepatitis A virus's incubation period averages from three to five weeks, with the greatest probability of transmission in the latter half of that period. Afflicted individuals are most infectious during the first week of symptoms. The disease follows a mild course, is rarely serious, and lasts from two to six weeks. Fortunately, the incidence of hepatitis A infection has decreased significantly following the introduction of the vaccine.

HEPATITIS B The hepatitis B (serum hepatitis) virus is transmitted through direct contact with contaminated body fluids (blood, semen, vaginal fluids, and saliva) and therefore represents a substantial risk to EMS providers. Hepatitis B is much more contagious than HIV. The potential for transmitting hepatitis B following exposure to infected blood ranges from 1.9 to 40 percent and by needle stick from 5 to 35 percent. The incidence of antibodies to hepatitis B in health care workers has been reported to be two to four times greater than in the community at large. Health care workers infected by hepatitis B can develop acute hepatitis, cirrhosis, and liver cancer. From 5 to 10 percent of infected health care workers may become asymptomatic chronic carriers and pose an infection risk to family and other intimate contacts. The effectiveness of the three series of immunizations has been reported to be close to 90 percent in adults and higher in children, but low rates of health care worker compliance with immunization are distressingly common. No clearly identifiable populations are at risk except for individuals who are exposed to high-risk body fluids in the course of their employment.

In the general populace, sexual transmission of hepatitis B is common—but declining. This is due to the fact that most individuals who now become sexually active have been vaccinated for hepatitis B as a part of their childhood vaccines. Transmission has also been known to occur with transfusion, dialysis, needle and syringe sharing in IV drug use, tattooing, acupuncture, and communally used razors and toothbrushes. The virus is stable on surfaces with dried, visible blood for more than seven days. Infection of toddlers from household contacts with family member carriers has been reported. Transmission by insect vectors or the fecal–oral route has not been reported.

Serum markers that reflect amounts of antigen or antibody from surface or core molecules of the virus reliably reflect active infection, communicability, the window phase of infection, and peak virus replication levels. A detailed discussion of the clinical significance of these markers and how they guide therapy is beyond the scope of this text.

Hepatitis B vaccination is generally required before employment as a health care provider. This has significantly reduced occupational exposure to hepatitis B for health care workers—including those in EMS. Hepatitis B vaccines are safe and effective. The immunization regimen is a series of three intramuscular injections. Following the initial dose, booster doses are administered at one and six months. After the immunization regimen, antibody assays are obtained to confirm active immunity. Children are now routinely immunized against hepatitis B.

An additional booster may be necessary if the individual does not develop adequate antibody levels. The duration of protection is thought to be five years, perhaps longer. The vaccine is safe in pregnancy. Its side effects include local redness, occasional low-grade fever, rash, nausea, joint pain, or mild fatigue.

Hepatitis B's incubation period lasts from 8 to 24 weeks. Joint pain and rash are more common with hepatitis B infection than with other types of hepatitis, but 60 to 80 percent of hepatitis B infections are asymptomatic. The incidence of hepatitis B began to decline in the late 1980s with the introduction of an effective vaccine. The incidence was further reduced following universal vaccination of infants in 1991.

HEPATITIS C The prevalence of hepatitis C virus (HCV) in the United States is believed to be 1.6 percent in the adult population. The virus is transmitted primarily by IV drug abuse and sexual contact. Sexual contact, however, does not appear to transmit hepatitis C as effectively as it does hepatitis B. After 1989, effective blood donor screening for hepatitis C practically eliminated the risk of transfusion-associated infection.

Hepatitis C is a chronic condition in about 85 percent of infected people. Because of its chronic nature and its ability to cause active disease years later, it poses a great international public health problem. Antibodies can be produced against hepatitis C and provide the laboratory method for determining infection. However, the antibodies are not effective in eliminating the virus, and their presence does not indicate immunity. The ineffectiveness of antibodies is attributed to the virus's high mutation rate. Consequently, the cellular immune response, which results in the immune system's killing infected cells, is very aggressive and is believed, ironically, to cause most of the associated liver injury.

Hepatitis C infection—formerly called non-A, non-B hepatitis—often causes liver fibrosis which progresses over decades to cirrhosis and is estimated to develop in about 20 percent of infected individuals. This progression is known to be accelerated in persons older than 50 at the time of initial infection, in those consuming more than 50 g of alcohol per day, and in men. Cirrhosis has also been known to occur in those who have not consumed alcohol, however, and can worsen to end-stage liver disease with jaundice, ascites, and esophageal varices.

No effective vaccination for hepatitis C exists. Treatment with alpha interferon has had limited success, with about 15 to 20 percent of patients responding positively, as defined by the liver enzymes' return to normal levels. Several antiviral drugs—including ledipasvir, paritaprevir, ombitasvir, and dasabuvir—are being used in the treatment of hepatitis C, but the results have been mixed. Another drug, ribavirin (an antiviral), administered orally, is known to potentiate interferon's immune system effects, and researchers are now focusing their efforts on improving the results of combination therapy with ribavirin and alpha interferon.

HEPATITIS D The hepatitis D virus (HDV), formerly called delta hepatitis, depends on a surface antigen of the hepatitis B virus (HBV) to produce its structural protein shell. Thus, HDV infection seems to exist only with a coexisting HBV infection. Immunization against HBV therefore confers immunity to HDV. When a patient who has HBV infection with liver disease develops an overlying HDV infection, mortality rates are very high.

Parenteral HDV transmission occurs similarly to HBV in western Europe and North America. Fortunately, cases in health care workers are extremely rare. Frequent epidemics of nonparenteral transmission occur in central Africa, the Middle East, and the Mediterranean countries. HDV's incubation period has not been determined. No vaccine exists for hepatitis D.

HEPATITIS E Hepatitis E (HEV) is transmitted like hepatitis A virus (HAV), through the fecal–oral route, and seems to be associated with contaminated drinking water more commonly than HAV is. It occurs primarily in young adults, with highest rates in pregnant women. First described in India, outbreaks have occurred in Russia, Nepal, Southeast Asia, the Middle East, Pakistan, and China. Only six cases were reported in the United States from 1989 to 1992, most likely because of more sanitary sources of drinking water. It does not lead to chronic infection.

Tuberculosis

Tuberculosis (TB) is the most common preventable adult infectious disease in the world. Bacteria known collectively as the Mycobacterium tuberculosis complex, which includes *M. tuberculosis*, *M. bovis*, and *M. africanum*, cause TB. Other bacteria in the *Mycobacterium* family can cause tuberculosis, particularly in immunocompromised patients. These other types of *Mycobacterium* are referred to as atypicals. TB primarily affects the respiratory system, including a highly contagious form in the larynx. When untreated or undertreated, it may spread to other organ systems, causing extrapulmonary TB and other complications. The disease appeared about 7,000 years ago and peaked in the 18th century. The number of new cases in the United States has increased steadily since 1985, in large part because of TB in AIDS patients and in recently arrived immigrants from countries where the disease is prevalent. More recently, there has been an overall decline in TB cases in the United States.[6]

The development of multiple drug resistant tuberculosis (MDR-TB) has been known since the late 1940s. Drug resistance occurs when drug-resistant bacteria outgrow drug-susceptible bacteria. These bacteria acquire resistance because of either patient noncompliance with therapy or inadequate treatment regimens. Drug resistance occurs early in therapy, especially when only one drug is used. For this reason, most current CDC recommendations for the initiation of therapy in the United States involve several options for treatment, each calling for multiple medications, including isoniazid (INH), rifampin, pyrazinamide, ethambutol, and streptomycin, among others.

M. tuberculosis is most commonly transmitted through airborne respiratory droplets but may also be contracted by direct inoculation through mucous membranes and broken skin or by drinking contaminated milk. Animal reservoirs for the bacteria include cattle, swine, badgers, and primates. Coughing and other expiratory actions (sneezing, speaking, singing) create bacteria-containing droplets from 5 to 10 microns in size, which susceptible individuals inhale into the alveoli.

The risk of transmitting tuberculosis is not as high as that for measles. Although the average case infects only about a third of close contacts, prolonged exposure to a person with active TB is always listed as a risk factor. Communicability varies from case to case. Although a single occupational exposure to a patient with active TB is highly unlikely to transmit the disease to a paramedic, Standard Precautions against TB should still be employed.

SKIN TESTING The commonly used purified protein derivative (PPD) skin test effectively identifies candidates for prophylactic drug therapy (to prevent active TB) in large groups of health care workers. It has limited value in guiding individual therapy in those with active TB because a positive PPD indicates previous infection but does not distinguish active from dormant disease. Another health care worker experienced in interpreting the results should read the skin test, rather than the worker tested, because health care workers are known to underinterpret positive results. In addition, the skin test must be interpreted on the basis of the disease's prevalence in the community. A negative test does not rule out active disease, particularly in immunosuppressed individuals or in those who were infected so recently that their immune systems have not yet had time to mount the cellular mediated response that causes a positive PPD.

Most EMS agencies require skin testing at least annually. This may be sufficient, but again, decisions about the frequency of testing should be based on the disease's prevalence in the community. For individuals who have not been previously skin tested or who have no documentation of a negative PPD in the last 12 months, two-step testing may be reasonable. In these individuals, an initial negative test may be due to weak reactivity to the PPD. A second skin test is administered from one to three weeks later. A positive reaction to the second test probably represents a boosted reaction, which means that the individual has been previously infected, and should be evaluated for possible prophylaxis. If the second test is negative, that individual is classified as uninfected. A positive reaction to any subsequent test would represent a new infection by *M. tuberculosis*.

PATHOGENESIS TB's incubation period is 4 to 12 weeks. In most people with subclinical infections, immediate disease (primary TB) does not develop because of a cell-mediated immune response. Development of disease normally occurs 6 to 12 months after infection. Susceptibility to primary infection is increased in people who are malnourished and those whose immune systems are suppressed, such as the elderly, HIV patients, and people taking immunosuppressant drugs, such as transplant recipients. Children less than three years of age are at risk because of underdeveloped immune systems, with older children identified at lowest risk. As expected, the aged are at high risk, and the reactivation of latent infections in this age group implies that the immune system has difficulty dealing with the complex nature of the *M. tuberculosis* infection. Once the bacteria enter the lungs, alveolar macrophages attack them and attempt to "wall them off" (forming granulomas) in a localized immune response. For this reason, most TB infections do not produce disease. Healed sites leave lesions of calcified areas known as Ghon foci. When Ghon foci combine with lymph nodes, they form a Ghon complex, which creates small, sharply defined shadows on a chest X-ray.

If the macrophages cannot destroy them, the bacteria lie dormant within the macrophages and are then distributed to other sites within the body. They remain dormant until some event, usually a depression of the immune system, triggers their reactivation into secondary TB. The sites of reactivation are greatest in areas of the lung with the highest oxygen tension, the apices or upper lobes. Reactivation in extrapulmonary sites such as lymph nodes, pleura, and pericardium are much more common in HIV-infected persons. In AIDS patients, the disease may spread to the thoracic and lumbar spine, destroying intervertebral disks and adjacent vertebral bodies. TB is also known to lead to subacute meningitis and granulomas in the brain.

CLINICAL PRESENTATION The signs and symptoms of active TB can be very nonspecific and can be manifestations of other clinical conditions. However, a typical list would include chills, fever, fatigue, productive or nonproductive chronic cough, and weight loss. Many patients report night sweats, leaving their bed linens drenched with perspiration. Hemoptysis (expectorating blood) is very suggestive of active TB. Reactivation of dormant TB manifests as signs and symptoms specific to the organ systems involved.

EMS RESPONSE Your acceptance of responsibility for protecting yourself from *M. tuberculosis* is the most important step in preventing disease transmission. A proactive, high-index-of-suspicion-driven response is essential. The factors that increase a paramedic's risk of transmission are close and sometimes prolonged contact with the patient. Care and transport are provided in a very small, often ineffectively ventilated space, and the patient may affect various expiratory actions while in contact with EMS personnel. Placing a mask over the patient, when it does not create undue anxiety or dyspnea, effectively decreases the number of expectorated droplet nuclei. Also, nebulized medications may be administered more safely with a nebulization mask. Use appropriate respiratory precautions while performing CPR and intubation.

You should don a protective **respirator** on contact with a patient you suspect may have TB. Your knowledge of the prevalence of TB and the most susceptible populations in your jurisdiction should reinforce your index of suspicion. The most current NIOSH/OSHA standards for protecting health care workers from TB call for N95 masks, which are designed to prevent contaminated air from reaching the health care workers wearing them (Figure 10-10a). The more cumbersome negative-pressure respirators and powered air-purifying respirators (PAPRs) (Figure 10-10b) are no longer required in routine TB exposure except when high-risk procedures such as bronchoscopy or autopsy are conducted, when respiratory protection exceeding the CDC standard performance criteria may be needed. These respirators (negative-pressure and PAPRs) are more expensive, bulky, and sometimes difficult to breathe through.[7]

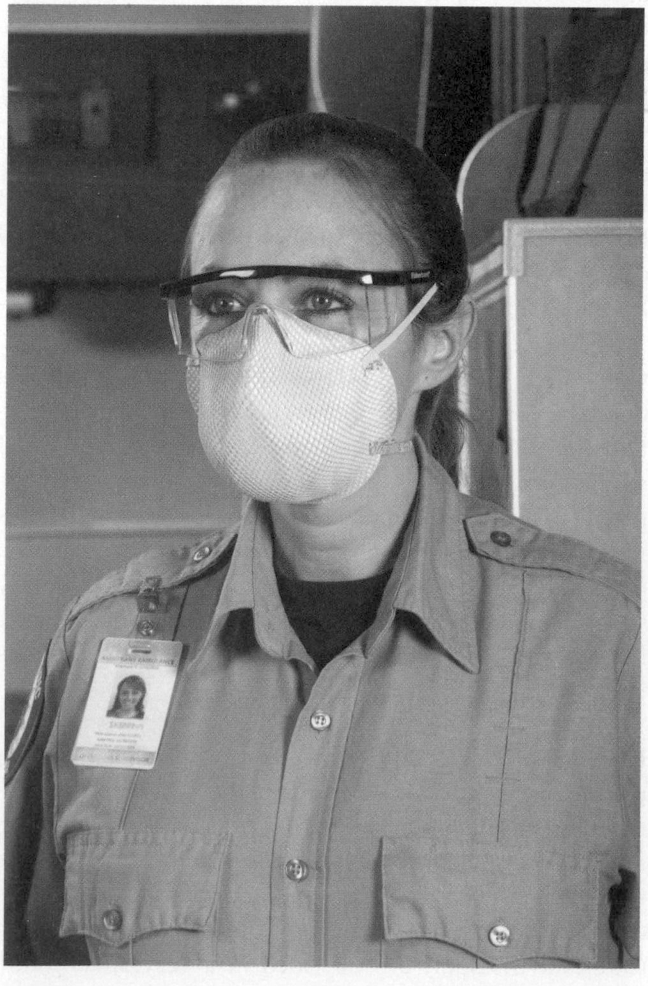

FIGURE 10-10a NIOSH/OSHA standards call for N95 masks when caring for patients with tuberculosis.

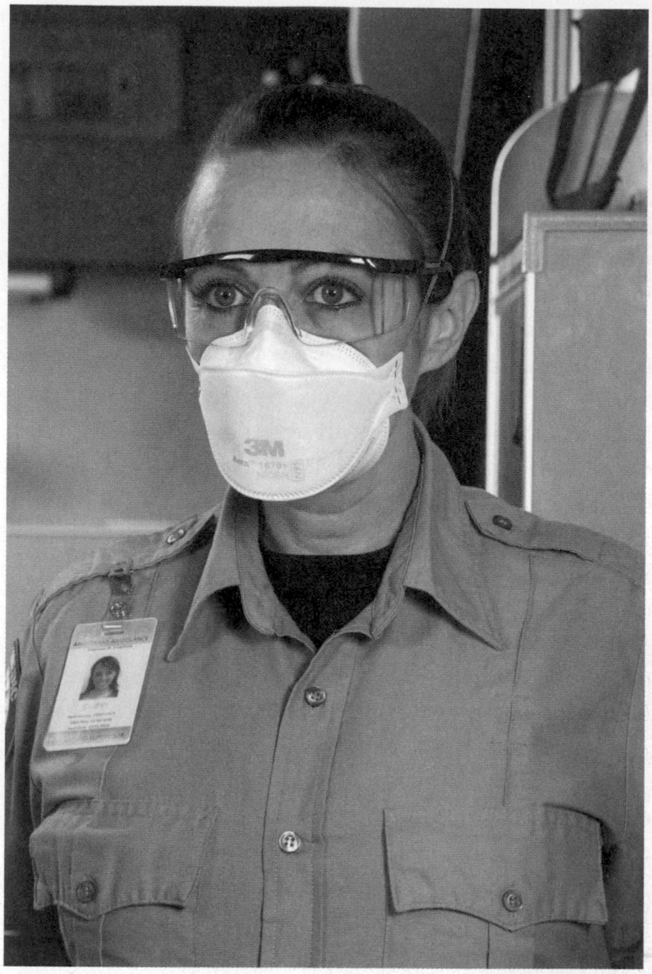

FIGURE 10-10b EMS agencies may opt to use high-efficiency respiratory protection for select cases.

Masks, as opposed to respirators, work primarily as barriers against larger particles and are not certified to prevent contaminated air from reaching the paramedic. However, they effectively prevent the transmission of many airborne pathogens, especially when both provider and patient wear them. They also provide a more comfortable and cost-effective alternative to the routine use of respirators. The extensive terminology and guidelines relative to the design, construction, and classification of various respirators is beyond the scope of this text. EMS agencies and their IDCOs are responsible for educating their personnel in the proper use and application of respirators and for ensuring proper fit and easy access. According to the NIOSH classification, N series respirators provide protection against non–oil-based aerosols, including the droplet nuclei from TB patients. These N type respirators must filter 95 percent of particles that are no larger than 0.3 microns in diameter; hence the designation N95. This is a very safe standard since the diameter of TB aerosol droplets ranges from 5 to 10 microns. Health care workers' noncompliance causes most respirator failures.

Ventilation systems currently being marketed in selected ambulances claim to effectively recycle and filter enough air to ensure the expulsion of infected droplet nuclei. Such ventilation systems should include HEPA filtration in addition to recycling the patient compartment air volume according to OSHA standards. Do not open patient compartment windows to increase ventilation and dilute the concentration of droplet nuclei. The moving ambulance may create a Bernoulli effect that draws engine exhaust, including carbon monoxide, into the patient compartment.

POSTEXPOSURE IDENTIFICATION AND MANAGEMENT Early identification of exposure and drug prophylaxis, if deemed necessary, are the keys to effectively preventing active TB in health care workers. An occupational medicine physician should assess TB skin test results and determine the appropriateness of chest X-rays, sputum cultures, and a myriad of other diagnostic procedures to confirm infection or the presence of frank disease. The polymerase chain reaction (PCR) test, which eliminates the need to wait for cultures and provides a diagnosis in 6 hours, may soon become the gold standard for identifying the presence of *M. tuberculosis.*

Pneumonia

Patients with difficulty breathing often confront paramedics with the enigma of differentiating pneumonia from mild exacerbations of congestive heart failure and its more severe form, acute pulmonary edema. The mistaken assumption that a patient has CHF may lead to aggressive treatment that reduces the patient's respiratory drive, dries protective mucus secretions, and contributes to hypotension.

Pneumonia, an acute lung inflammation, is not a single disease but a family of diseases that result from respiratory infection by viruses, bacteria, or fungi. The infectious agent most often associated with pneumonia, and against which the pneumococcal vaccine is targeted, is *Streptococcus pneumoniae,* Gram-positive spheres found in pairs or chains. Other microorganisms known to cause pneumonia are *Mycoplasma pneumoniae* (primary atypical pneumonia), *H. influenzae, Klebsiella pneumoniae, M. catarrhalis, Legionella, S. aureus* in nosocomial infections, and *P. jiroveci.* These agents are also known to cause meningitis, ear infections, and pharyngitis. In addition to droplet nuclei, the infectious agents are also spread by direct contact and through linens soiled with respiratory secretions.

Those at highest risk for pneumonia are the immunocompromised; patients with sickle cell disease, transplanted organs, cardiovascular disease, diabetes mellitus, kidney disease, multiple myeloma, lymphoma, Hodgkin's disease, or prolonged automatic ventilator use (vent-acquired pneumonia); those without a functioning spleen; and the elderly, particularly those in common residential situations. Low–birth-weight neonates and malnourished infants are very susceptible. In otherwise healthy individuals, susceptibility is increased by a previous respiratory infection like influenza, exposure to inhaled toxins, chronic lung disease, and aspiration (post-alcohol ingestion, near drowning, ingested toxins, or gastric distention from BVM ventilation). When patients contract infectious agents of pneumonia outside a hospital or other health care institution, they are referred to as cases of community-acquired pneumonia.

HISTORY AND ASSESSMENT Always consider the possibility of community-acquired pneumonia. In geriatric communities where residents live in their own home but may share common social facilities, ask if neighbors recently have been diagnosed with pneumonia or other respiratory infections. Signs and symptoms in previously healthy individuals include an acute onset of chills, high-grade fever, dyspnea, pleuritic chest pain worsened by deep inspiration, and cough, which may be productive with phlegm of various colors. The absence of fever does not rule out pneumonia. Breath sounds may include adventitious lung sounds (crackles, wheezes) and signs of consolidation. When purulent fluids accumulate in many lobes of the lung because of inflammation, alveoli collapse and their acoustic properties change to those of solid tissue; hence the name *consolidation.* Consolidation causes the expiratory sounds in the peripheral lung fields to develop the same duration as inspiration and to be just as loud (Figure 10-11). Assessment with pulse oximetry may be useful. In geriatric patients, the only presenting sign may be an altered mental status; fever is often absent, and headache, aches and pains, nausea, diarrhea, and nonproductive cough, if present, do not allow you to rule out pneumonia. In children, fever, tachypnea, and retractions are ominous signs but are not specific to pneumonia; this triad of signs, however, reliably indicates respiratory distress secondary to an infectious process in pediatric patients.

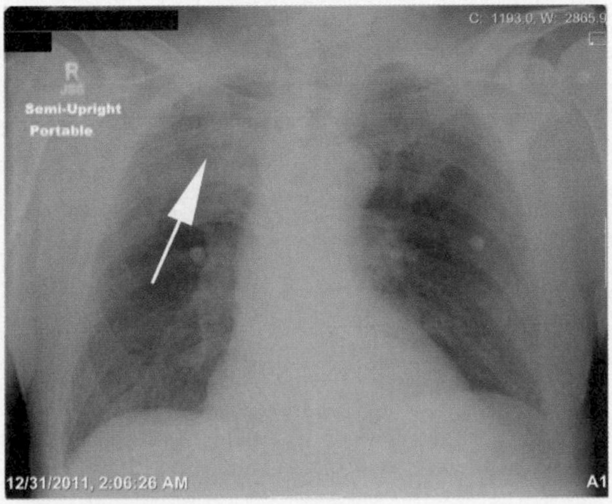

FIGURE 10-11 Pneumonia in the right lung.

(© Dr. Bryan E. Bledsoe)

PATIENT MANAGEMENT AND PPE Management of the pneumonia patient aims at supporting adequate ventilation and oxygenation. Supplemental oxygen should be administered to correct hypoxia. Also, in some patients with pneumonia, CPAP has proven to be of benefit in increasing oxygenation and ventilation. Always consider TB a possibility in any patient with pneumonia and place a mask either on yourself or on your patient.

IMMUNIZATION AND POSTEXPOSURE MANAGEMENT An effective vaccination exists against most serotypes of *S. pneumoniae* known to cause disease. It is highly recommended for children 2 years old and younger, for adults over 65, and for those without a spleen. Routine vaccination of EMS workers is not necessary. In health care settings, workers who routinely treat elderly, immunocompromised, or other at-risk patients may be required to be immunized because they pose the risk of patient transmission. Because EMS workers are predominantly healthy, exposure to a single patient with pneumonia generally will not result in infection or disease. A number of antimicrobial agents are effective against the infectious agents known to cause pneumonia. However, multidrug-resistant strains have been reported.

Severe Acute Respiratory Syndrome

As noted in the "Pulmonology" chapter, **severe acute respiratory syndrome (SARS)** is a viral respiratory illness that first appeared in southern China in 2002 and became a global threat in 2003 by spreading internationally. In that outbreak, 8,098 people worldwide were affected, of whom 774 died. Toronto, Ontario, was particularly affected, placing a significant stress on the Toronto EMS system. Four paramedics contracted the disease, reportedly before mandatory PPE measures were undertaken (Figure 10-12). SARS is considered to be an ongoing threat because of its highly infectious nature.

PATHOPHYSIOLOGY The virus that causes SARS, unrecognized before its 2002 appearance, is called SARS-associated coronavirus (SARS-CoV). Coronaviruses play a major role in upper respiratory infections and the common cold. SARS-CoV apparently may survive in the environment for several days and is spread by close person-to-person contact via respiratory droplets when an infected person coughs or sneezes. SARS-CoV can also be contracted by touching a contaminated object.

The incubation period is generally 2 to 7 days but in some cases has been as long as 10 to 14 days. A person with SARS is considered to be contagious as long as he has symptoms. There have been no reported cases of disease transmission before the source patient develops symptoms. Persons with documented SARS should be quarantined to their home for at least 10 days after the fever has abated and symptoms cleared.

Description:	An outbreak in 2002 caused concern about global spread. There has not been a SARS outbreak since 2004, but the severity of the disease warrants ongoing preparedness.
Transmission:	Respiratory, airborne, direct contact
Signs and Symptoms:	Fever and pneumonia
Prevention:	Standard Precautions, including face mask
Treatment:	Use respiratory droplet precautions when dealing with suspected cases. Treat hypoxia and respiratory distress IV fluids for dehydration.

FIGURE 10-12 Severe acute respiratory syndrome (SARS) is a viral respiratory illness that first appeared in China in November 2002.

ASSESSMENT If a SARS outbreak has been identified, all personnel should use appropriate PPE on every call or as directed by local health authorities. If a case is encountered in a non–SARS-epidemic area that has SARS-like symptoms, all involved should immediately don appropriate PPE.

As with any respiratory illness, first address signs of severe respiratory distress: altered mental status, one-to-two-word speech dyspnea, cough, cyanosis, and hypoxia. Patients with underlying respiratory disease (asthma, emphysema, chronic bronchitis) and those with chronic illnesses are at increased risk.

Signs and symptoms associated with SARS include sore throat, rhinorrhea (runny nose), chills, rigors (sudden paroxysmal chills), myalgias (muscle aches), headache, and diarrhea. This can progress to cough, sputum production, respiratory distress, and eventual respiratory failure.

MANAGEMENT Any patient suspected of having SARS should be treated as a patient with suspected pneumonia or other respiratory illness. Place the patient in a comfortable position and administer oxygen to correct hypoxia. Use pulse oximetry to assess the patient's oxygenation requirements. Provide ventilatory assistance and, if necessary, consider placement of an advanced airway device such as an endotracheal tube. Establish IV access and administer fluids if the patient is dehydrated. If the patient is wheezing, consider administering a nebulized bronchodilator. Notify the receiving hospital if you suspect SARS so that it can take appropriate protective measures.[8]

Middle East Respiratory Syndrome

An emerging infection, similar to SARS, is **Middle East respiratory syndrome (MERS).** It was first identified in Saudi Arabia and Jordan in 2012 and has subsequently spread to several other countries, including the United States. It is caused by the Middle East respiratory syndrome coronavirus (MERS-CoV), which is similar to the SARS virus. It primarily affects the respiratory system, has a fatality rate that ranges from 30 to 40 percent, and has affected persons from 1 to 99 years of age. The incubation period is usually 5 to 6 days but can range from 2 days to 2 weeks. The clinical findings include fever, cough, and shortness of breath. Some patients report gastrointestinal symptoms such as nausea, vomiting, and diarrhea. Most related deaths are caused by pneumonia and acute renal failure; most people who died from the disease had associated comorbidities. Cases reported in the United States have almost always been linked to travel to, or residence in, affected countries in the Middle East.

Ebola Virus Disease

Ebola virus disease (EVD) appeared in the United States in 2014 when a resident of Liberia in Western Africa flew to Dallas, Texas. Five days after arriving in Dallas, he began to develop the initial symptoms of EVD (fever, abdominal pain) and went to a local hospital for treatment, but he was subsequently diagnosed with sinusitis and discharged home on antibiotics. His symptoms worsened and the Dallas Fire Rescue EMS service was summoned. He was evaluated by paramedics and transported by ambulance to the same hospital where he was treated previously. He was admitted to the hospital and was later found to have EVD. He eventually died, and a member of the nursing staff who cared for him developed the infection. The paramedics and other health care workers were placed in isolation. This case, though tragic, pointed out deficiencies in the U.S. EMS and health care system when highly infectious diseases occurred. This led to numerous studies and recommendations from the CDC for highly infectious diseases such as EVD.

PATHOPHYSIOLOGY EVD, formerly called Ebola hemorrhagic fever (EHF), is a disease of humans and other primates that is caused by the virus *Ebolavirus*, of which there are four types (Figure 10-13). EVD is transmitted between people via direct contact through broken skin and mucous membranes of blood or other body fluids of a person who is infected with the virus. These body fluids include saliva, mucus, vomit, feces, sweat, tears, urine, semen, and breast milk. EVD can also be found in fruit bats and in other primates such as gorillas, monkeys, and chimpanzees. It was initially discovered in 1976 along the Bowl River in the Congo. It is now located primarily in West Africa.

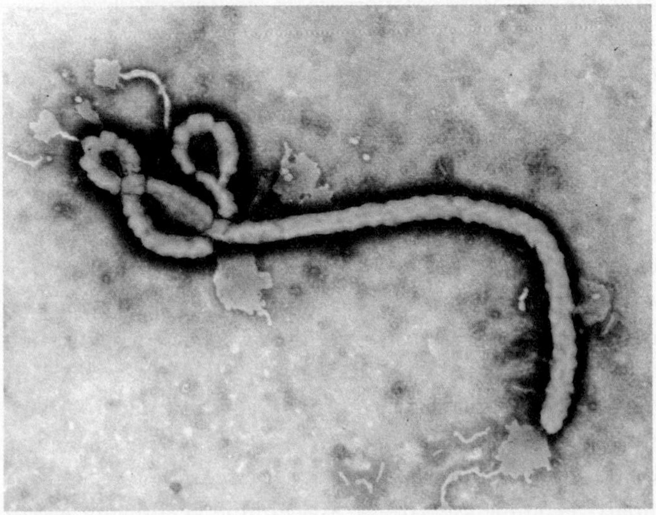

FIGURE 10-13 Ebola virus disease (EVD).

(Centers for Disease Control and Prevention)

ASSESSMENT The signs and symptoms of EVD vary somewhat, depending the stage of infection, and include:

- Fever
- Severe headache
- Loss of appetite
- Joint and muscle pain
- Weakness
- Fatigue
- Vomiting
- Diarrhea
- Abdominal pain
- Unexplained hemorrhage (bleeding or bruising)

Symptoms can appear anytime from two days to three weeks following exposure to EVD However, the average onset is about eight to ten days.

Any patient with signs and symptoms suggestive of EVD should be approached with extreme caution. The primary assessment should be conducted at least 3 feet from the patient. Once a patient has been suspected of having EVD, he is considered a "patient under investigation" until proven otherwise. Protection from EVD includes strategies and PPE significantly beyond what is usually used in prehospital care. These were detailed earlier in the chapter under "Enhanced Precautions," but additional information is available from the CDC and from the World Health Organization (WHO). Every EMS system, regardless of size or volume, should have operational and medical protocols and the necessary PPE available in case a suspected EVD patient is encountered.

MANAGEMENT Recovery from EVD depends on several factors, including the quality of supportive care that incorporates hydration, maintenance of oxygen saturation and blood pressure, and the treatment of concomitant infections. In addition, the condition of the patient's immune system is a factor in recovery from EVD. People who ultimately recover from EVD develop antibodies that appear to provide protection from the disease for at least 10 years.

Zika Virus

Zika virus disease (ZVD) is caused by the Zika virus. It was first identified in Africa and appeared in the Western

Hemisphere in Brazil and has spread to equatorial regions of the Americas, including many Caribbean islands. It is primarily spread through mosquito bites—specifically from the *Aedes* species of mosquitoes. There is evidence that the virus can be spread from mother to fetus during pregnancy. There is also some evidence that it can be contracted through sexual contact. The signs and symptoms of ZVD include fever, rash, joint pain, headache, and conjunctivitis (red eyes). The illness is mild and usually lasts several days to a week. Many persons (80 percent) who contract the disease remain asymptomatic. Deaths are rare, and no specific treatment is available. Maternal–fetal transmission of the disease has been associated with some birth defects (e.g., microcephaly) and fetal deaths. There has been a reported association between ZVD and Guillain-Barré syndrome.

Chikungunya Virus

Chikungunya virus disease is caused by the Chikungunya virus and is spread by the *Aedes* species of mosquitoes. It has occurred in outbreaks in numerous countries, including the Americas and the Caribbean islands. Symptoms usually begin 3 to 7 days after being bitten by an infected mosquito. The most common signs and symptoms of Chikungunya virus infection are fever and joint pain. In addition, many may suffer headaches, muscle pain, joint swelling, and/or rash. It is more severe in newborns and older adults, as well as those who have hypertension, diabetes, or heart disease. There is no specific treatment and most patients recover uneventfully.

Chickenpox (Varicella)

Chickenpox is caused by the varicella zoster virus (VZV). The varicella zoster virus is in the herpesvirus family. Although chickenpox (**varicella**) in pediatric patients is considered a self-limited disease that rarely causes severe complications, it is much more lethal in adults. It results in fewer than 100 deaths per year in the United States, but whereas adults represent only 2 percent of the morbidity, they account for 50 percent of the mortality. Thus, health care workers who have not been immunized against VZV nor been exposed to it as children must increase their awareness of this infection and its consequences. It is estimated that 10 percent of adults have not contracted VZV during childhood. VZV is also the infectious agent of shingles (herpes zoster), a painful condition that causes skin lesions along the course of peripheral nerves and dermatome bands. Approximately 15 percent of patients with chickenpox will eventually develop shingles.

CLINICAL PRESENTATION Chickenpox usually occurs in clusters during winter and spring and presents with respiratory symptoms, malaise, and low-grade fever, followed by a rash that starts on the face and trunk and progresses to the rest of the body, including mucous membranes. The rash may be the first sign of illness, and infected persons may have anywhere from a few to 500 lesions. It is more profuse on the trunk, with less distribution to the extremities and scalp. The fluid-filled vesicles that form the rash soon rupture, forming small ulcers that eventually scab over within one week, at which point the patient is no longer contagious (Figure 10-14). Transmission occurs through inhalation of airborne droplets and direct contact with weeping lesions and tainted linen. The incubation period is from 10 to 21 days.

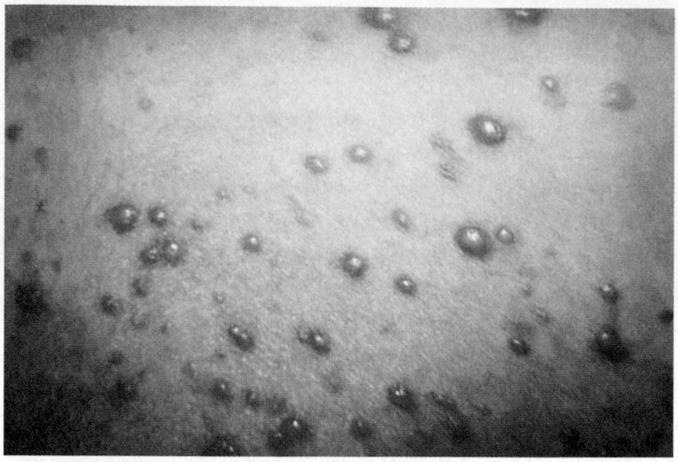

FIGURE 10-14 Varicella (chickenpox).
(Centers for Disease Control and Prevention/Joe Miller)

In adults, varicella's most common complication is a VZV pneumonia. A large percentage of adult deaths from VZV occur in immunocompromised patients. The most alarming aspect of adult epidemiology, however, is a significant death rate in previously healthy patients. Therefore, it is important for unexposed or unvaccinated paramedics to be immunized.

ASSESSING IMMUNITY Most people develop immunity for life after recovery from childhood chickenpox infections. Thus, a history of chickenpox is considered adequate evidence of immunity. An available blood test can determine immunity in those who are unsure about their history or who have not had chickenpox.

IMMUNIZATION A chickenpox vaccine, Varivax, has been licensed in the United States since 1995, and the CDC's Advisory Committee on Immunization Practices (ACIP) now recommends that all states require children entering child care facilities and elementary school to be vaccinated or have some other evidence of immunity. Such evidence would include a primary care provider's diagnosis of chickenpox, a reliable history of the disease, or a blood test confirming immunity. Vaccination is also routinely recommended for all susceptible health care workers. ACIP has also strengthened its recommendations for all other susceptible persons 13 years old or younger to include any adolescents living in the same household with younger children.

The vaccine is administered as one subcutaneous dose in children under age 12 and as two doses in susceptible adolescents and adults. Among vaccinated people 13 years or older, 78 percent developed protective antibodies, with 99 percent seroconverting after the second dose. Health care workers who receive the vaccination should have their antibody level checked six weeks after the second vaccination.

Patients with active TB, malignant conditions, or those being treated with immunosuppressants should not receive the varicella vaccine. Its use in those taking steroids depends on a variety of factors beyond the scope of this discussion. Few adverse effects have been reported through the CDC's Vaccine Adverse Events Reporting System (VAERS). The most frequent was rash, with some cases of herpes zoster. No incidents of chickenpox have been reported. Although a few serious adverse effects were reported, no cause-and-effect relationship was clearly established with the vaccination. The vaccine manufacturer discourages taking aspirin within six weeks after receiving the vaccination.

EMS RESPONSE AND POSTEXPOSURE Observe Standard Precautions and place masks on patients. If a patient has only chickenpox, he should remain at home until the lesions are crusted and dry. If a susceptible paramedic is exposed to chickenpox, postexposure vaccination may be warranted. Recent data indicate that if used within three days, and possibly up to five days, Varivax may be effective in preventing chickenpox or lessening its severity. Varicella zoster immune globulin (VZIG) is an alternative postexposure prophylaxis. Unlike Varivax, it provides passive immunity, and the most current recommendation for its use is in immunocompromised patients. The use of acyclovir, which inhibits replication of the virus, within 24 hours of the onset of rash may decrease the disease's severity in adults and adolescents.

Meningitis

Meningitis is an inflammation of the meninges (the membranes protecting the brain and spinal cord) and cerebrospinal fluid, caused by bacterial and viral infections. Meningococcal meningitis (spinal meningitis), caused by *Neisseria meningitidis,* is the disease variant of greatest concern to EMS responders.

Other agents are, or have been, known to cause meningitis. *Streptococcus pneumoniae,* the primary infectious agent of concern in pneumonia, is the second most common cause of pneumonia in adults and the most common cause of otitis media in children. Vaccines have proven very effective, especially in children. *Haemophilus influenzae* type B, a Gram-negative rod, was once the leading cause of meningitis in children age 6 months to 3 years. However, with the implementation of effective childhood vaccination against *H. influenzae* since 1981, *N. meningitidis* has become the bacterium most commonly implicated in serious meningitis cases. Viruses and other microorganisms are known to cause meningitis, with similar disease profiles. Enteroviruses are implicated in 90 percent of patients with viral (aseptic) meningitis. In healthy individuals, viral meningitis is a self-limited disease that lasts about seven to ten days.

TRANSMISSION FACTORS *N. meningitidis* asymptomatically colonizes the upper respiratory tract of healthy individuals and is then transmitted by respiratory droplets. Up to 35 percent of the general population may be infected with the bacterium, which is prevented from gaining access to the CSF by the epithelial lining of the pharynx. Almost every human has probably been a carrier at some point in his life. Conversion from carrier to clinical disease is rare in developed countries and occurs in clusters in developing nations. The disease appears to peak in midwinter months with low temperature and humidity. This has been validated by observations of epidemic seasonal variations in the "meningitis belt" of sub-Saharan Africa. Epidemiologists have hypothesized that this pattern may represent a herd immunity, in which host resistance factors may be more a function of the population's general immunity than of the immunity of individuals within that population. One theory that could explain the phenomenon of herd immunity holds that another species within the genus *Neisseria* may be "mistaken" for *N. meningitidis* (a cross reaction), resulting in effective antibody production against the pathogen. Meningococcal meningitis occurs more commonly in some areas of the United States, and the world, for reasons not yet understood. Other factors that have been implicated in transmission of *N. meningitidis* include contacting oral secretions of the index case (kissing, sharing food or drink), crowding, close contact, smoking, and lower socioeconomic status. For the EMS responder, contact with secretions during mouth-to-mask ventilation, intubation, or suctioning would increase the probability of transmission.

CLINICAL PRESENTATION The incubation period most commonly ranges from two to four days but may last as long as ten days. As with most bacterial infections, signs and symptoms develop rapidly within a few hours or one to two days of exposure and include fever, chills, headache, nuchal rigidity with flexion, arthralgia, lethargy, malaise, altered mental status, vomiting, and seizures. An upper respiratory or ear infection may precede the disease. A characteristic rash may appear and develop into hemorrhagic spots, or petechiae. Roughly 10 percent of patients may develop septic shock. Acute adrenal insufficiency, disseminated intravascular coagulation (DIC), and coma are other consequences. Death can ensue in 6 to 8 hours.

Newborns and infants may seem slow or inactive, vomit, appear irritable, or feed poorly. Fever in newborns should be evaluated with a high index of suspicion for meningococcemia. Rarely, bulging of an open anterior fontanel is seen. In older children, assessment techniques that stretch the inflamed meninges and cause pain may reveal positive Brudzinski's and Kernig's signs. **Brudzinski's sign** is a physical exam finding suggestive of meningitis. As a result of irritation of the meninges, flexion of the neck causes flexion of the hips and knees. To test for Brudzinski's sign, have the patient lie supine without a pillow. Flex the neck while observing the hips and knees. Flexion of the hips or knees when the neck is flexed is considered a positive Brudzinski's sign. **Kernig's sign** is likewise suggestive of meningitis. To elicit Kernig's sign, have the patient sit or lie and flex the hips. With the hips flexed, attempt to extend (straighten) the knee. Inability to fully extend the knee is due to meningeal irritation and is considered a positive Kernig's sign. Maternal antibodies protect newborns from meningitis and other infections until up to 6 months of age (slightly longer in breast-fed children). Infants from 6 months to 2 years of age are especially susceptible to meningitis because they no longer have circulating maternal antibodies and their immune systems are immature and incompetent.

IMMUNIZATION *N. meningitidis* has several serotypes (A, B, C, X, Y, Z, 29-E, W-135), with B and C causing most disease outbreaks in the United States. The A serotype is the most common cause of epidemics in Africa and Asia. An effective vaccine has been developed against the A, C, Y, and W-135 serotypes. Attempts to develop one against the B serotype have so far resulted in weak immune responses. The meningococcal vaccine is not currently recommended for routine immunization of health care workers. Travelers to endemic areas and children younger than 2 years old who are asplenic (without a spleen) or have a certain deficiency in their complement system are candidates for vaccination.

EMS RESPONSE AND POSTEXPOSURE Observing Standard Precautions and using masks on yourself and/or your patients with suspected meningococcal meningitis will adequately protect you against all the infectious agents of meningitis. Postexposure prophylaxis with rifampin, ciprofloxacin (Cipro), or ceftriaxone (Rocephin) is the primary means of preventing meningococcal disease in patients with significant exposures. Prophylaxis should be started within 24 hours after exposure because the rate of effective transmission in close contacts (EMS responders) with the index-case patient has been estimated to be 500 to 800 times that of the general population. Initiation of chemoprophylaxis 14 days or more after the onset of illness in the index case is of limited or no value. All postexposure medications are easily complied with and have few side effects.

Other Job-Related Airborne Diseases

Influenza and colds, rubella, measles, mumps, and respiratory syncytial virus (RSV) are viral infections that may be contracted in the EMS environment. Pertussis, a highly contagious bacterial disease, also poses a risk. These diseases are transmitted by direct inhalation of infected droplets or through exposed mucosal surfaces. Handling contaminated surfaces or objects and subsequently introducing the virus by scratching, wiping, or other activities with unwashed hands (autoinoculation) is another route of transmission. Masks and ventilation are recommended for measles. Precautions against autoinoculation with RSV infections, influenza, and colds include masks, more practically placed on patients, and possibly gloves, gowns, and goggles. Avoid touching your face and areas of broken skin while in contact with the patient. Effective, vigorous hand washing with soap and warm water after patient contact is the most important personal precaution against disease transmission.

INFLUENZA AND THE COMMON COLD **Influenza** is caused by viruses designated types A, B, and C. Within these types are various subtypes that mutate so often that they are identified on the basis of where they were isolated, the culture number, and year of isolation—for instance, A/Japan/305/57. Two glycoproteins, hemagglutinin and neuraminidase, on the outer membrane of an influenza virus determine its virulence. The letters H and N, which denote these two glycoproteins, are often seen in parentheses along with a number, as in A (H1N1). This method of classification helps epidemiologists to more specifically identify a flu virus, as it is based on the immune responses to hemagglutinin and neuraminidase.[9]

Influenza is a leading cause of respiratory disease worldwide, and various strains cause epidemics, mainly during the winter months. It is easily transmittable in crowded spaces such as public transportation vehicles, and can be spread by direct contact. The virus can persist on environmental surfaces for hours, especially in low humidity and cold temperatures. Thus, it has a high potential for transmission by autoinoculation. It is much more serious than the common cold and has caused worldwide epidemics with high mortality rates. The last great epidemic was in 1918, and the CDC and the World Health Organization (WHO) closely monitor worldwide disease outbreaks.

CONTENT REVIEW

- Other Job-Related Airborne Diseases
  - Influenza and the common cold
  - Measles
  - Mumps
  - Rubella
  - Respiratory syncytial virus
  - Pertussis

Influenza is characterized by the sudden onset of fever, chills, malaise, muscle aches, nasal discharge, and cough. The disease is more serious in the very young, the very old, and those with underlying disease. Its incubation period is from one to three days. Fever generally lasts three to five days. Signs include mild sore throat, nonproductive cough, and nasal discharge. The cough may be severe and of long duration. Secondary infections may occur as the virus damages respiratory epithelial cells, thereby decreasing resistance to other, primarily bacterial, disorders. Severe cases may result in pneumonia, hemorrhagic bronchitis, and death. The uncomplicated disease usually lasts two to seven days and full recovery is the norm.

Management is primarily supportive. Fever may increase body temperature to as high as 105°F. Begin cooling measures for patients with temperatures of 104°F or greater. Increased body temperature may lead to significant insensible fluid loss and dehydration. Determine hydration status early and begin fluid replacement, if indicated.

Everyone is susceptible to influenza. Although infection confers resistance after recovery, the influenza viruses mutate so rapidly that protection is effective only against the particular strain or variant from which the person has just recovered. An immunization is available and is recommended for the elderly, those who live or work in correctional institutions, and military recruits. Patients should be immunized between early September and mid-November for maximum effectiveness. The CDC recommends vaccination for EMS personnel to reduce transmission of influenza to patients and to decrease worker absenteeism. EMS responders who are diabetics, especially those requiring frequent medical follow-up, are strongly urged to be immunized. Three antiviral drugs, amantadine (Symmetrel), oseltamivir (Tamiflu), and rimantadine (Flumadine), are available for the prevention and treatment of influenza; however, they work only against the type A influenza virus. They are as effective as vaccines when used preventively, and they shorten the illness's duration when used as a treatment. A new agent, zanamavir (Relenza), which is effective against type B, was recently released. However, its use is limited because only 35 percent of influenza cases are type B and because it must be delivered by aerosol nebulizer.

The common cold, or viral rhinitis, is caused by the rhinoviruses, of which there are more than 200 serotypes. Its incidence in the United States rises in fall, winter, and spring, is highest in children younger than 5 years of age, and declines in older adults, displaced by more serious diseases. Transmission is by direct contact, airborne droplets, or, more importantly, by hands and linen soiled with discharges from infected individuals. The incubation period ranges from 12 hours to 5 days and averages 48 hours. The disease's course is mild, often without fever and generally without muscle aching. Aside from severity, it is often difficult to differentiate from influenza. Mortality has not been reported, but a cold may lead to more serious complications such as otitis media and sinusitis.

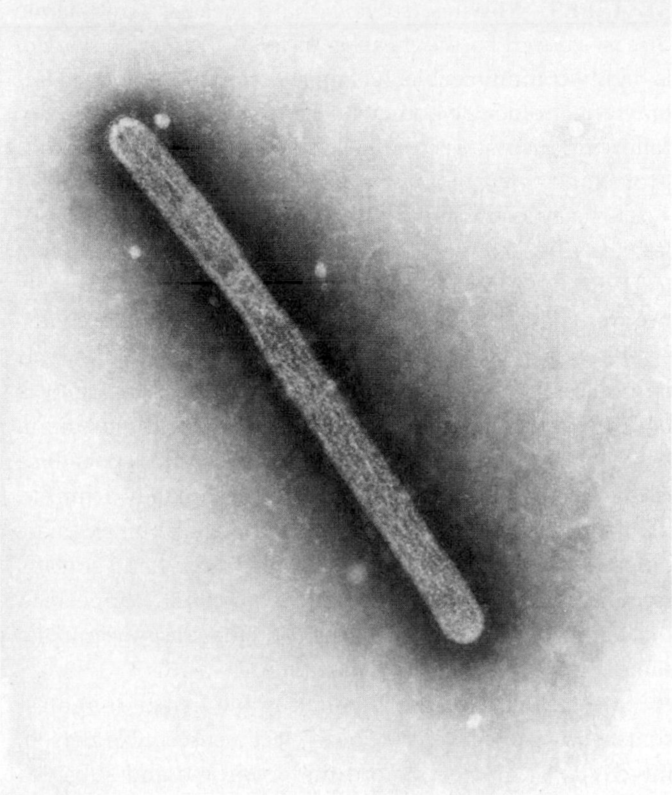

FIGURE 10-15 H5N1 influenza virus responsible for avian influenza ("bird flu").

(Centers for Disease Control and Prevention/Cynthia Goldsmith; Jackie Katz)

AVIAN INFLUENZA Influenza viruses are common in birds. Most avian influenza viruses do not infect humans except in cases of prolonged contact. However, some avian viruses can mutate or merge with a human influenza virus to form a virus that can infect humans. This was the case with the three largest influenza pandemics of the past 100 years. Not long ago, a particularly infectious form of avian influenza virus (H5N1) was identified in Asia (Figure 10-15). There were cases in which the virus infected humans—often causing death. Most of the human infections were in those who worked with poultry or lived around domestic birds. The H5N1 virus has been colloquially called the "bird flu" and is particularly pathogenic. It tends to affect younger people and has a high mortality rate. The H5N1 virus is a particular risk because it may "jump species." This means that the virus may mutate or merge with another human influenza virus, resulting in a highly pathogenic human influenza virus. If this were to occur, a worldwide pandemic might result with thousands (if not millions) of deaths. There is a vaccine available.

The reported symptoms of avian influenza in humans have ranged from typical influenza-like symptoms (e.g., fever, cough, sore throat, and muscle aches) to eye infections (conjunctivitis), pneumonia, acute respiratory distress, viral pneumonia, and other severe and life-threatening complications.

MEASLES **Measles** (rubeola, hard measles), a systemic disease caused by the measles virus of the genus *Morbilli,* is highly communicable. It is most common in children but may affect older persons who have not had it. Immunity following disease is usually lifelong. Maternal antibodies protect neonates for about four to five months after birth.

Measles is transmitted by inhalation of infective droplets and direct contact. The incubation period ranges from 7 to 14 days, averaging 10 days. The infected person presents prodromally like a severe cold, with fever, conjunctivitis, swelling of the eyelids, photophobia, malaise, cough, and nasopharyngeal congestion. The fever increases, rising to as high as 104°F to 106°F, when the rash reaches its maximum. A day or two before the rash develops, Koplik's spots (bluish-white specks with a red halo approximately 1 mm in diameter) appear on the oral mucosa. The red, bumpy (maculopapular) rash normally lasts about six days and spreads from head to feet by the third day. At that point, it appears to thicken on the head and shoulders and then disappear in the same direction as its progression (Figure 10-16).

Measles is so highly communicable that the slightest contact with an active case may infect a susceptible person. Infectivity is greatest before the prodrome and subsides about four days after the rash appears or as it fades. Everyone should be immunized. Immunization is 99 percent effective in children, for whom vaccination is mandatory because there is no specific treatment. However, despite an effective vaccine, there has been an increase in the occurrence of measles in the United States largely due to the so-called anti-vaccine movement, whereby some parents have chosen not to immunize their children. Unimmunized or previously unexposed paramedics should mask their measles patients and be vigilant about handling linens and touching their face during and after the call. Postexposure hand washing is critical.

In otherwise healthy children or adults, uncomplicated measles has a low mortality rate. Potential complications include bacterial pneumonia, eye damage, and myocarditis. The most life-threatening sequela is encephalitis in children and adolescents, which causes gradual decreases in mental capacity and muscle coordination.[10]

MUMPS The **mumps** virus, a member of the genus *Paramyxovirus,* is transmitted through respiratory droplets and direct contact with the saliva of infected patients. It is characterized by painful enlargement of the salivary glands. Most cases occur in the 5- to 15-year age group. After a 12- to 25-day incubation period, mumps presents as a feverish cold that is soon followed by swelling and stiffening of the parotid salivary gland in front of the ear. The condition is often found bilaterally. The patient may also experience earache and difficulty chewing and swallowing. In most cases, the submaxillary and sublingual glands are very tender to palpation (Figure 10-17). Most cases resolve spontaneously within one week without intervention.

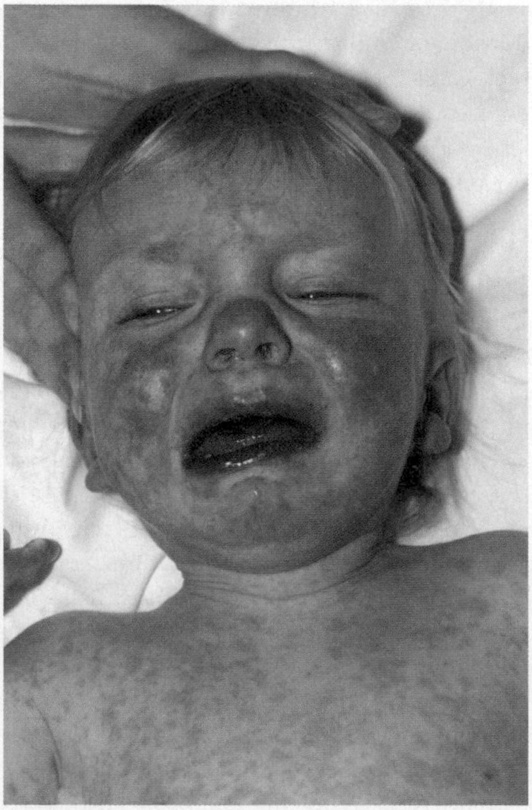

FIGURE 10-16 Measles (rubeola).

(DR M.A. Ansary/Science Source)

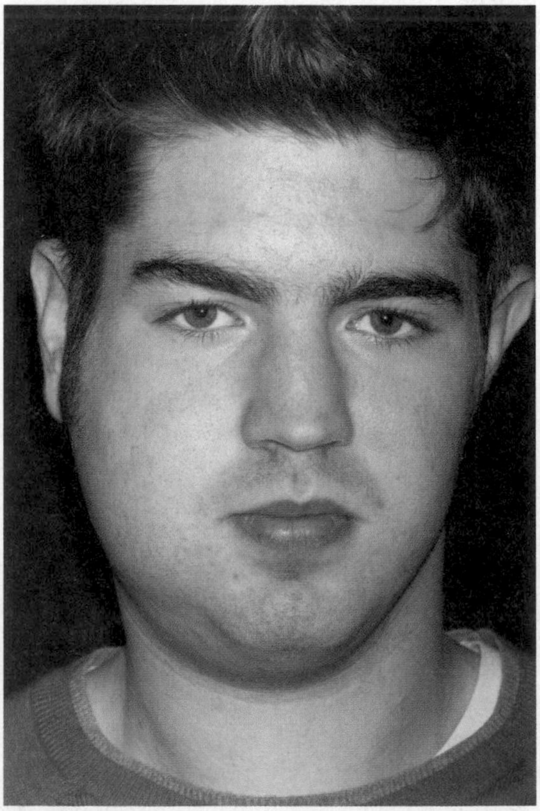

FIGURE 10-17 Mumps.

(Dr. P. Marazzi/Science Source)

Mumps occurs in epidemics, with danger of transmission beginning one week before the infected person feels sick and lasting about two weeks. Lifelong immunity is generally conferred after infection, even in the absence of disease (subclinical infection).

Mumps is generally benign and self-limiting; however, complications may occur. In postpubescent patients, inflammation of the testicles (orchitis), breasts (mastitis), or ovaries (oophoritis) may occur, but is of short duration and of no serious consequence. Meningoencephalitis is fairly common but resolves without residual neurologic sequelae.

A mumps live-virus vaccine is available and should be administered with measles and rubella vaccines to all children over 1 year of age. Mumps is not easily transmitted, and with Standard Precautions the risk of contracting the disease is minimal. For the benefit of their patients, EMS workers should not work without an established mumps/measles/rubella (MMR) immunity.[11]

RUBELLA **Rubella (German measles)** is a systemic viral disease caused by the rubella virus, of the genus *Rubivirus*, transmitted by inhalation of infective droplets. Generally milder than measles, it is characterized by sore throat and low-grade fever, accompanied by a fine pink rash on the face, trunk, and extremities that lasts about three days (Figure 10-18). The incubation period is 12 to 19 days, with natural infection conferring lifelong immunity, as does immunization. Transfer of maternal antibodies does not confer lifelong immunity but does protect the neonate. There is no specific treatment for rubella. The more serious complications that occur in measles do not occur in rubella, but young females sometimes develop a short course of arthritis.

Rubella is devastating to a developing fetus. Mothers infected during the first trimester are at risk for abnormal fetal development, with offspring often developing congenital rubella syndrome and shedding large quantities of virus in their secretions. An infant acquiring this infection *in utero* is likely to be developmentally delayed and suffer eye inflammation, deafness, and congenital heart defects. All women, therefore, should be immunized against rubella before becoming pregnant.

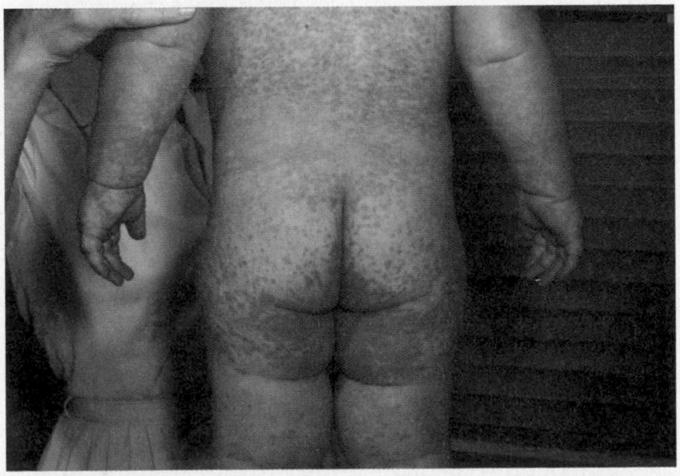

FIGURE 10-18 Typical rash of German measles (rubella).

(Centers for Disease Control and Prevention)

Vaccines for measles, mumps, and rubella are commonly combined in an MMR vaccination, which can be given safely with the varicella vaccine. Immunization is 98 to 99 percent effective but is not recommended for pregnant women because of a theoretical possibility of birth defects. Health care workers have been identified as the source in numerous outbreaks. For this reason, and for their own protection, all EMS providers should be required to receive the MMR vaccination before they are allowed to work. Immunizations, along with placing a mask on the patient, are an effective method of preventing these diseases.[12]

RESPIRATORY SYNCYTIAL VIRUS **Respiratory syncytial virus (RSV)** is a common cause of pneumonia and bronchiolitis in infants and young children. In this age group, RSV may be fatal. In older children and adults RSV is less common, and its symptoms are generally milder. RSV is often associated with outbreaks of lower respiratory infections from November to April. If a patient with pneumonia or bronchitis simultaneously contracts this virus, the disease becomes more severe. RSV commonly begins as an upper respiratory infection, and is often misdiagnosed as a simple cold. Children with RSV infection will initially develop a runny nose and nasal congestion. Later, this will spread to lower airway involvement, evidenced by wheezing, tachypnea, and signs of respiratory distress. It is a common infection that can be diagnosed by a rapid assay using nasal washings. In winter months, wheezing in children under 1 year of age should be presumed to be due to RSV until proven otherwise. High-risk children (those with congenital heart conditions, prematurity, or cancers, for instance) can be treated with the antiviral agent ribavirin (Virazole). However, this treatment is quite expensive and poses a significant risk to unborn babies of pregnant health care workers. Postexposure prophylaxis with RespiGam (RSV immune globulin) is also an option.[13]

PERTUSSIS The word *pertussis* means "violent cough." **Pertussis** (whooping cough) is caused by the bacterium *Bordetella pertussis*, affecting the oropharynx in three clinical phases after an incubation period of from 6 to 20 days. The *catarrhal phase*, characterized by symptoms similar to those of the common cold, lasts from one to two weeks. The *paroxysmal phase*, during which the fever subsides, can last a month or longer. The patient develops a mild cough that quickly becomes severe and violent. Rapid consecutive coughs are followed by a

CONTENT REVIEW

➤ Phases of Pertussis
- Catarrhal
- Paroxysmal
- Convalescent

deep, high-pitched inspiration. (This characteristic "whoop" often is not present in infants and adults.) The cough often produces large amounts of thick mucus, and vomiting may also occur. Sustained coughing may lead to increased intracranial pressure and intracerebral hemorrhage. Continually high intrapulmonary pressure and vigorous chest movement may cause pneumothorax. During the *convalescent phase*, the frequency and severity of coughing attacks decrease, and the patient is not contagious.

The widespread vaccination of children in a combination diphtheria-tetanus-pertussis (DTP) vaccine caused a dramatic decrease in the incidence of pertussis until the early 1980s. Over the past 20 years, however, its incidence has steadily grown, with the greatest increase in persons aged 5 years or older. This has occurred in spite of unprecedented pertussis vaccination coverage. One factor in the increase may be a waning effectiveness of the vaccine among adolescents and adults vaccinated during childhood. Although the disease is likely to confer immunity against pertussis, the duration of that immunity is unknown. Previously immunized and exposed adolescents and adults therefore may be at risk of infection. Thus, booster doses are recommended. For patients with pertussis, EMS is most likely to be requested during the paroxysmal phase, when the primary treatment will be calming and oxygenating the patient. Anticipate the needs to intubate patients with respiratory failure and to perform chest decompression for those whose coughing paroxysms might have caused a pneumothorax. During the response, remember that pertussis is highly contagious. Fortunately, the communicable period is thought to be greatest before the paroxysmal phase. Transmission occurs via respiratory secretions or in an aerosolized form. Mask the patient and observe Standard Precautions, including postexposure handwashing.

Everyone is susceptible to *B. pertussis* infection. Routine immunization of EMS workers against pertussis is not yet recommended. Evaluation of pertussis vaccination is ongoing, however, and considering the unknown duration of immunity with past immunization or exposure, adolescent and adult immunization may be recommended in the future. Erythromycin (and other macrolide antibiotics) is known to decrease the period of communicability, but can reduce symptoms only if administered before the onset of violent coughing.[14]

Viral Diseases Transmitted by Contact

Mononucleosis and herpes simplex type 1 infections pose little risk to EMS providers who observe Standard Precautions and wash their hands after patient contact. Because these diseases cause relatively minor symptoms, patients may not even be aware of their infection status. The public is highly aware of these two diseases, however, so as health care providers, paramedics should be familiar with them.

CONTENT REVIEW

- Viral Diseases Transmitted by Contact
  - Mononucleosis
  - Herpes simplex virus type 1

MONONUCLEOSIS **Mononucleosis** is caused by the Epstein-Barr virus (EBV). It affects the oropharynx, tonsils, and the reticuloendothelial system (the phagocytes). A four- to six-week incubation period precedes the development of symptoms, which characteristically begin with fatigue. Fever, severe sore throat, oral discharges, and enlarged, tender lymph nodes generally follow several days to weeks later. Splenomegaly (enlargement of the spleen) is present in approximately one-half of patients. The disease is common; more than 95 percent of the general population has antibodies to the virus. One-half of all children will have contracted it before the age of 5 years. Infection by EBV generally confers immunity for life.

Mononucleosis is most commonly transmitted through oropharyngeal contact involving the exchange of saliva between an uninfected person and one who has the disease but who is asymptomatic. Kissing is implicated in adolescents and adults, and transmission from caregivers to young children is common. Blood transfusions can be a mode of transmission, but few cases of disease are attributed to it. Active disease is most common in those between 15 and 25 years of age. The risk of contracting the disease without close facial contact is minimal. Symptoms generally dissipate within a few weeks, but full recuperation may take several months. There is no specific treatment for mononucleosis, and immunization is unavailable. Corticosteroids are occasionally administered to help minimize tonsillar swelling. Nonsteroidal anti-inflammatory drugs (NSAIDs) may provide symptomatic relief.[15]

HERPES SIMPLEX VIRUS TYPE 1 There are two types of **herpes simplex virus**, herpes simplex virus type 1 (HSV-1) and herpes simplex virus type 2 (HSV-2) (Figure 10-19). HSV-2 will be discussed in the section on sexually transmitted diseases. HSV-1 is transmitted in the saliva of carriers and commonly infects the oropharynx, face, lips, skin, fingers, and toes. Everyone is susceptible. Infections of health care workers' hands and fingers can result in herpetic whitlow, weeping inflammations at the distal fingers and toes. The incubation period following exposure ranges from 2 to 12 days. In the oral cavity, fluid-filled vesicles develop into cold sores or fever blisters that soon deteriorate into small ulcers. Fever, malaise, and dehydration may accompany these primary lesions. The lesions usually disappear in two to three weeks. They may recur spontaneously, especially following periods of stress or other illness. Recurrent HSV labialis (lip lesions) may cause problems for many years in some adults.

Although recognized primarily for causing skin and mucous membrane disorders, HSV-1 can cause meningoencephalitis in newborns and aseptic meningitis in adults.

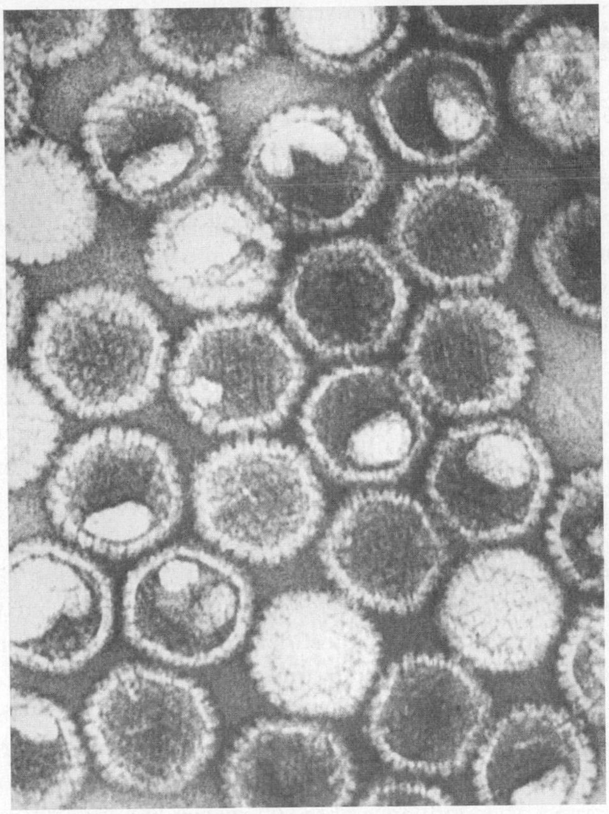

FIGURE 10-19 Herpes virus, the causative agent of herpes infections. *(Centers for Disease Control and Prevention/Dr. Fred Murphy; Sylvia Whitfield)*

A high index of suspicion for HSV-1 in these situations may result in timely treatment with antiviral agents such as acyclovir, which is somewhat effective against HSV-1.

Standard Precautions—primarily gloves—are absolutely essential, especially if an intimate contact or family member of the EMS worker is afflicted. Breaks in the skin place everyone at greater risk, and may not be visible to the naked eye. Treatment with acyclovir (Zovirax) provides relief when used topically or orally. Immunization is not available.

Other Infectious Conditions of the Respiratory System

The majority of profiles in this section discuss pathological conditions of the airway caused by a variety of infectious agents. They are not diseases, per se. The "Pediatrics" chapter discusses croup and epiglottitis in greater detail. Hantavirus is included here, although its sites of pathology extend beyond the airways.

CONTENT REVIEW

- Other Infectious Respiratory Conditions
  - Epiglottitis
  - Croup
  - Pharyngitis
  - Sinusitis
  - Hantavirus

Epiglottitis

Epiglottitis is an inflammation of the epiglottis and may also involve the areas just above and below it. In children it is a true emergency, usually caused by *H. influenzae*, with an abrupt onset over several hours and without any immediate history of upper respiratory disease. Patients present with one or more of the "four Ds": dysphonia, drooling, dysphagia, or distress. Epiglottitis can also occur in teenagers and adults. In the older age groups, stridor, sore throat, fever, and drooling usually develop over days, not hours. Because of natural immunity from the initial infection, epiglottitis is not known to reoccur in any age group. Increased immunization against *H. influenzae* has reduced the incidence of epiglottitis caused by this bacterium. However, *S. pneumoniae* and *S. aureus* have been implicated as causative agents of epiglottitis.

Croup

Croup (laryngotracheobronchitis) is a common cause of acute upper airway obstruction in children. A viral illness characterized by inspiratory and expiratory stridor and a seal-bark-like cough, it is most common in children under the age of 3 years. Although generally not life threatening, croup may create panic in parents and children alike. Viruses implicated in croup include the parainfluenza viruses, rhinoviruses, and RSV. Croup is often preceded by an upper respiratory infection. The child commonly awakens during the night with acute respiratory distress, tachypnea, and retractions. Seasonal outbreaks of this disease are common. Total airway obstruction is rare.[16]

Pharyngitis

Pharyngitis is a common infection of the pharynx and tonsils. It may be caused by a virus or bacteria and is characterized by a sudden onset of sore throat and fever. The tonsils and palate become red and swollen, and the cervical lymph nodes enlarge. Headache, neck pain, nausea, and vomiting may also be present. Most cases occur in late winter and early spring. Although this disease may occur in any age group, most cases are seen in 5- to 11-year-olds.

Group A streptococcus (strep throat) causes a particularly serious pharyngitis that, if left untreated, can progress to rheumatic fever in certain cases. There are several subtypes of group A streptococcus. One strain causes rheumatic fever. Another strain is responsible for scarlet fever (scarletina). Patients infected with this bacterium may present with a scarlet-colored rash. Because strep throat is very contagious, wear a mask when assessing and managing these patients. Although laboratory tests can easily determine which cases of pharyngitis are caused by strep, it is virtually impossible to tell clinically. Assume that all cases of pharyngitis are serious and contagious until proven otherwise. Antibiotics (penicillin, amoxicillin, erythromycin, azithromycin) effectively treat strep throat.

Sinusitis

Sinusitis is an inflammation of the paranasal (ethmoid, frontal, maxillary, or sphenoid) sinuses. It occurs when mucus and pus cannot drain and become trapped in the sinus. Sinusitis is usually preceded by a viral upper respiratory infection or exposure to allergens, either of which may cause nasal congestion and blocked sinus passages. Postnasal drip may develop and nasal drainage may be blood tinged and purulent. As fluids collect in the sinus, a sensation of pressure or fullness generally develops. If left untreated, the condition may become painful, and the infection can cause an abscess or spread into the cranium and attack the brain. Discomfort often worsens when the patient bends forward or when pressure is applied over the affected sinus. Sinusitis is occasionally a causative factor of meningitis. Management includes corticosteroids, decongestants, and supportive care. Apply a heat pack directly over the affected sinus to help relieve pain and facilitate drainage.

Hantavirus

Hantavirus is a family of viruses carried by rodents such as the deer mouse. Other known carriers are the rice and cotton rats in the southeastern United States and the white-footed mouse of the northeastern states. The common house mouse is not known to carry the virus. Most cases of hantavirus infection have occurred in the southwestern United States, particularly in the Four Corners region. Transmission is primarily by inhalation of aerosols created by stirring up the dried urine, saliva, and fecal droppings of these rodents. Contamination of food and autoinoculation after handling objects tainted by rodent droppings may also cause transmission. Direct bites are possible routes, but are thought to be rare. Person-to-person transmission is not possible.

The virus causes hantavirus pulmonary syndrome (HPS), to which anyone is susceptible. The initial symptoms are fatigue, fever, and muscle aches, especially of large muscle groups. Headaches, nausea, vomiting, diarrhea, and abdominal pain are also common. Earache, sore throat, and rash are uncommon. Approximately four to ten days later, symptoms of pulmonary edema occur. Patients with fatal infections appear to have severe myocardial depression, which can progress to sinus bradycardia and subsequent electromechanical dissociation, ventricular tachycardia, or fibrillation. Hemodynamic compromise occurs a median of five days after symptoms' onset—usually dramatically within the first day of hospitalization. The only specific treatment is intensive supportive care, and no immunization is available.

EMS responders who find themselves in dusty, unoccupied buildings for extended times should wear face masks to prevent inhaling aerosolized rodent droppings.[17]

GI System Infections

CONTENT REVIEW

- GI System Infections
  - Gastroenteritis
  - Food poisoning

You may, on occasion, respond to scenes with single or multiple cases of foodborne illness. Although you cannot determine the causative agent outside the hospital, you must have a basic knowledge of the infectious process and guidelines for assessment, management, and safe handling of these patients. Many EMS personnel are being recruited and volunteering for domestic and international disaster medical teams. In these situations, when the sanitation infrastructure (water treatment and distribution, sewer, animal control, and so forth) is disrupted, GI system infections increase significantly.

Gastroenteritis

Gastroenteritis is a gastrointestinal disorder manifested by nausea, vomiting, gastrointestinal cramping or discomfort, anorexia, and diarrhea. In more advanced cases, which are rare, it can cause lassitude and shock. It is a common disease that many of us in developed countries have experienced. The reference to "stomach flu" in these situations is incorrect, as an influenza of the GI system has not yet been identified. What this distressing and uncomfortable condition usually represents, at least in developed countries, is a viral gastroenteritis. The causative agents may be viruses (norovirus, rotavirus, and others), bacteria (*E. coli*, *K. pneumoniae*, *C. jejuni*, *E. aerogenes*, *V. cholerae*, *Shigella*, and *Salmonella*), and parasites (*G. lamblia*, *C. parvum*, *C. cayetensis*). Gastroenteritis is highly contagious via the fecal–oral route, including the ingestion of contaminated food and water. It is especially contagious during natural disasters in epidemic proportions. International travelers into endemic areas are very susceptible, whereas native populations are generally resistant.

In otherwise healthy persons, gastroenteritis is generally self-limiting and benign; however, in the very young, the very old, or those with preexisting disease, it can be serious and often fatal. Prolonged vomiting and/or diarrhea may result in dehydration and electrolyte disturbances. Patients generally experience painful and severe abdominal cramping, and some develop hypovolemic shock. Always consider dehydration in any patient who presents with signs of gastroenteritis. If a patient has vomited many times or is actively vomiting, has multiple medical problems, is debilitated, or is at risk by virtue of age and general health, start an IV with isotonic saline. Pay careful attention to hydration status. If the patient is in shock, the management objectives are no different than for hemorrhagic shock. If the patient is not in shock, the judicious use of fluids is warranted. A good rule of thumb is to replace fluids at approximately the rate they are lost. The World Health Organization and other international disaster response agencies have found oral rehydration very effective in treating fluid loss, even with cholera. Do not feel compelled to pour in IV fluids. If prolonged vomiting or retching is present, administer an antiemetic such as ondansetron (Zofran). Remember that vehicle movements often aggravate symptoms and increase the probability of vomiting.

With isolated cases of gastroenteritis, compliance with Standard Precautions and postexposure hand washing are critical to avoiding infection. In times of disaster, EMS responders must be more focused on environmental health and sanitation issues: preparing food, identifying clean sources of water, using mosquito netting while sleeping, and general sanitation. Eat only hot foods and drink hot beverages that have been brisk-boiled. Be careful to avoid personal habits that facilitate fecal–oral transmission. Prevention is important because even though antimicrobials may be available to treat isolated cases, resources for treating gastroenteritis during disasters or in developing countries may be limited. In those situations, many people receive symptomatic treatment.

Food Poisoning

Food poisoning is a nonspecific term often applied to gastroenteritis. Food poisoning occurs suddenly and is caused by eating. Diarrhea, vomiting, and gastrointestinal discomfort characterize its more benign presentation. Most cases are caused by bacteria and their toxic products. In the majority of cases, only the GI system is affected, but other systems may be affected in some cases, as with botulism or *Escherichia coli* O157:H7, causing debilitating illness or death. *Clostridium botulinum* produces a very potent neurotoxin that causes flaccid paralysis by blocking the release of acetylcholine at motor end plates and preganglionic autonomic synapses.

E. coli O157:H7, transmitted by the ingestion of uncooked or undercooked ground beef, often causes severe bloody diarrhea and abdominal cramps; sometimes the infection causes nonbloody diarrhea or no symptoms. Drinking unpasteurized milk and swimming in or drinking sewage-contaminated water can also cause infection. Little or no fever is usually present, and the illness resolves in five to ten days. In some persons, particularly children under 5 years of age and the elderly, the infection can cause a complication called hemolytic uremic syndrome, in which the red blood cells are destroyed and the kidneys fail. About 2 to 7 percent of infections lead to this complication. In the United States, hemolytic uremic syndrome is the principal cause of acute kidney failure in children, and *E. coli* O157:H7 causes most cases of hemolytic uremic syndrome.

Other bacteria implicated in food poisoning include *Campylobacter, Salmonella, Shigella,* and *Vibrio cholerae.* Microorganisms may be transmitted in other meats that are insufficiently cooked. *Salmonella* is commonly transmitted through incompletely cooked poultry. It may also be spread through contaminated cookware and utensils used in preparation of poultry. Hepatitis A and norovirus are known to have been ingested in undercooked seafood. Bacterial gastrointestinal infections tend to be much more severe than viral gastrointestinal infections. With bacterial infections, the patient will appear more toxic. There is often a history of bloody, foul-smelling diarrhea (especially with shigellosis). The presence of leukocytes in a fecal smear is suggestive of bacterial disease. Ultimately, stool cultures are required to confirm a bacterial cause of gastroenteritis.

Initiate standard advanced life support (ALS) protocols, including assessment of airway and ventilatory status, oxygenation, initiation of an IV, and cardiac monitoring. Fluid resuscitation with isotonic crystalloids is often required. It is not uncommon for an adult with severe gastroenteritis to require 2 to 3 liters of fluid. In patients with significant vomiting or diarrhea, also consider antiemetics. Constant reassessment of ventilatory status is essential because the neurotoxin in *C. botulinum* ingestion may cause respiratory arrest. Observing Standard Precautions should protect against foodborne transmission of infectious agents. No immunization against these agents or their toxins exists.

Prevention efforts are the primary means of reducing foodborne illness. Advances in technology may provide better alternatives for food supply surveillance, an aspect of foodborne disease prevention that could be improved. Lawrence Berkeley National Laboratory has developed plastic strips that turn from blue to red in the presence of toxic strains of *E. coli.* This technology's basis could become a prototype for other simple reagent strips that can detect foodborne pathogens.

Nervous System Infections

Encephalitis, rabies, tetanus, and Lyme disease all have significant effects on the nervous system. These infectious conditions or diseases do not necessarily pose occupational risks to EMS providers. They are well known to the general public, however, and are often associated with recreational activities in which EMS responders participate.

Encephalitis

Encephalitis is an inflammation caused by infection of the brain and its structures, usually by viruses such as equine viruses, arboviruses, the rubella virus, or the mumps virus. These viral infections usually result in one of the following:

- They cause no pathology until they are transported to cerebral neurons, which they invade, and then replicate (the rabies and arthropod-borne viruses, for instance), or

CONTENT REVIEW

➤ Nervous System Infections
- Encephalitis
- Rabies
- Tetanus
- Lyme disease

- They first injure nonnervous tissues and then, rarely, invade the cerebral neurons (for example, herpes simplex 1 and varicella zoster virus).

Bacteria, fungi, or parasites may also cause encephalitis, but the viruses are the predominant infectious agents.

The clinical presentation of encephalitis is similar to that of meningitis, as they often coexist. Signs and symptoms include decreased level of consciousness, fever, headache, drowsiness, coma, tremors, and a stiff neck and back. Seizures may occur in patients of any age but are most common in infants. Characteristic neurologic signs include uncoordinated and involuntary movements; weakness of the arms, legs, or other portions of the body; or unusual sensitivity of the skin to various types of stimuli.

Treatment is difficult, even when the virus is known. Despite the severity of illness, many patients suffer no long-term neurologic deficits; however, as many as 50 percent of children younger than 1 year of age may suffer irreversible brain damage after contracting Eastern or Western equine encephalitis, diseases of horses and mules transmitted to humans by mosquitoes.

Rabies

Rabies is transmitted by the rabies virus, a member of the Rhabdovirus family and *Lyssavirus* genus, which affects the nervous system. It exists in two epidemiological forms: *urban,* propagated chiefly through unimmunized domestic dogs and cats, and *sylvatic,* propagated by skunks, foxes, raccoons, mongooses, coyotes, wolves, and bats. Humans are especially susceptible when bitten by infected animals. The virus is transmitted in the saliva of infected mammals by bites, an opening in the skin, or direct contact with a mucous membrane. It passes along motor and sensory fibers to the spinal ganglia corresponding to the site of invasion, and then to the brain, creating an *encephalomyelitis* that is almost always fatal. Although rare, transmission is also known to occur by inhalation of aerosolized virus, through nasal nerve fibers and mucosa, along the olfactory nerve, and then to the brain. Mammals are highly susceptible to infection. Transmission is known to be affected by the severity of the wound, abundance of the nerve supply close to the wound, the distance to the CNS, the amount and strain of virus, protective clothing, and other undetermined factors. The highly variable incubation period is usually from three to eight weeks but can be as short as nine days (rare) or as long as ten years. It is believed to be dependent on the bite site, with bites to the head and neck generally followed by shorter incubation periods.

Rabies is characterized by a nonspecific *prodrome* (symptoms that precede the appearance of a disease) of malaise, headache, fever, chills, sore throat, myalgias, anorexia, nausea, vomiting, and diarrhea. The prodrome typically lasts from one to four days. The next phase, the *encephalitic phase,* begins with periods of excessive motor activity, excitation, and agitation. This is soon followed by confusion, hallucinations, combativeness, bizarre aberrations of thought, muscle twitches and tetany, and seizures. Soon, focal paralysis appears. When left untreated, it can cause death within two to six days. Attempts to drink water may produce laryngospasm, causing the characteristic profuse drooling commonly known as hydrophobia (fear of water).

Rabies in the United States has become more prevalent in the wild (more than 90 percent of cases occur in wildlife). The number of rabies-related human deaths in the United States has declined from more than 100 annually at the turn of the 20th century to one or two per year in the modern era. Modern-day prophylaxis has proven nearly 100 percent successful. In Africa, Asia, and Latin America, dogs remain the major source. Although human rabies is rare in the United States, 16,000 to 39,000 people receive postexposure prophylaxis each year. This is not a matter of paranoia. The CDC estimates that up to one-third of persons who have contracted rabies cannot accurately relate a history of having been bitten by an animal. Thus, epidemiologists now believe that the inhalation route, once thought to be theoretical, may be more common than previously believed. Human-to-human transmission of rabies is not known to occur; however, paramedics should take Standard Precautions to protect themselves from contact with infectious saliva. The use of masks in environments where a patient has been exposed may be prudent, judging from the recent epidemiological evidence in the United States with bats.

When caring for a bite patient, first inspect the site of the wound for a bite pattern and the presence of saliva. Then rinse the wound with copious amounts of normal saline to remove saliva and blood. Do not bandage or dress the wound, but allow it to drain freely during transport. Irrigation en route from a 10- or 15-drop/mL IV administration set may be beneficial. If the patient refuses transport to the emergency department, inform him of the consequences of the bite and the importance of medical follow-up. If time and circumstances permit, ensure that the suspect animal has been secured and contained for transport to the hospital or animal control shelter for subsequent postmortem examination of cerebral tissue.

If you are bitten or exposed to an animal you believe is rabid, take the following measures:

1. Vigorously wash the wound with soap and warm water.
2. Debride and irrigate the wound, and allow it to drain freely on the way to the emergency department.
3. Discuss postexposure prophylaxis with the physician. Consultation with public health officials may be

necessary. Unless you have an actual bite from an animal whose behavior is consistent with rabies infection, exposure is a medical urgency, not emergency.

4. Consider the need for tetanus and other antibiotic therapy as the attending physician deems appropriate.

The strategy for postexposure prophylaxis is determined by the animal's status. It generally includes both passive and active immunity. For people who have never been vaccinated against rabies previously, postexposure anti-rabies vaccination should always include administration of both passive antibody (human rabies immune globulin [HRIG]) and the vaccine for both bite and nonbite exposures, regardless of the interval between exposure and initiation of treatment. People who have previously been vaccinated or are receiving preexposure vaccination for rabies should receive only vaccine. The first dose of the four-dose course should be administered as soon as possible after exposure. Additional doses should be administered on days 3, 7, and 14 after the first vaccination.[18]

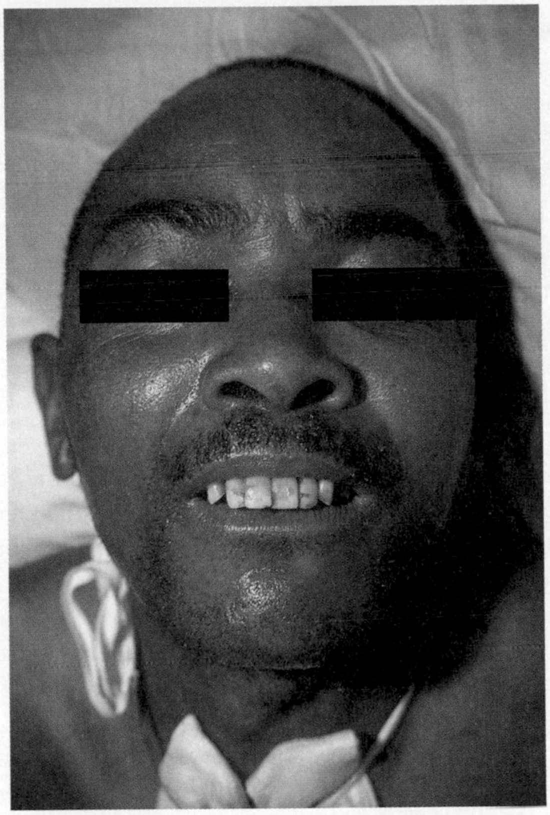

FIGURE 10-20 Tetanus.
(Centers for Disease Control and Prevention/Dr. Thomas F. Sellers/Emory University)

Tetanus

Tetanus is an acute bacterial infection of the central nervous system. It presents with musculoskeletal signs and symptoms caused by tetanospasmin, an exotoxin of the *Clostridium tetani* bacillus. *C. tetani* is present as extremely durable spores in the soil, street dust, and feces and is in the same genus as *C. perfringens,* the causative organism of gas gangrene. Because *Clostridium* species favor an anaerobic environment, the bacteria are particularly suited to colonizing dead or necrotic tissue. Infection has been contracted through wounds considered too minor to warrant medical attention, and through burns. Although puncture wounds are classically associated with *C. tetani* infection, deep lacerations can also be suitable environments. Transmission can even occur by injection of contaminated drugs and surgical procedures, leading to the conclusion that *C. tetani* spores are found everywhere (Figure 10-20). The incubation period is variable (usually from 3 to 21 days, sometimes from 1 day to several months) and depends on the wound's severity and location. Generally, a shorter incubation period leads to a more severe illness. The mortality rate increases in direct proportion to age. The general population is susceptible, but incidence is highest in agricultural areas where unimmunized people are in frequent contact with animal feces. The disease is rare in the United States, with fewer than 100 cases reported each year.

Localized tetanus symptoms include rigidity of muscles in close proximity to the injury site. Subsequent generalized symptoms may include pain and stiffness in the jaw muscles and may progress to cause muscle spasm and rigidity of the entire body. Respiratory arrest may result. In children, abdominal rigidity may be the first sign. Rigidity occurs after the toxin is taken up at the myoneural junction and transported to the CNS. The toxin then acts on inhibitory neurons, which normally suppress unnecessary efferent impulses and muscle movements. The reduction in inhibitory action results in the muscles' receiving more nervous impulses and tetany. Sometimes a sardonic grin, *risus sardonicus,* accompanies the lockjaw and conjures memories of the Cheshire Cat in *Alice in Wonderland.*

EMS responders will rarely encounter this disease, much less recognize its signs and symptoms until they are advanced to the point of tetany. A possible EMS scenario would be the transfer of a patient from a rural community hospital to an urban medical center for intensive care. Standard Precautions should provide adequate protection. Masks probably are not necessary unless the infectious agent is unknown. Respiratory arrest is a possibility, so you should consider wearing masks while performing endotracheal intubation. If you incur a wound in the course of treating a patient, wash the wound thoroughly or, if warranted, have it inspected and debrided in the emergency department. Wounds that are cared for within 6 hours pose a lower risk for growth of anaerobic microorganisms. Consideration should be given to postexposure prophylaxis with tetanus immune globulin

CONTENT REVIEW

➤ Stages of Lyme Disease
- Early localized
- Early disseminated
- Late

(TIG), diphtheria-tetanus toxoid (Td), or diphtheria-tetanus-pertussis (DTP).

Immunizations, which generally begin in childhood as DTP vaccinations, include boosters before entering elementary school and every ten years thereafter. A booster administered every ten years is believed to confer effective active immunity. Previous documented infection is not known to confer lifelong immunity.[19]

Lyme Disease

Lyme disease is a recurrent inflammatory disorder accompanied by skin lesions, polyarthritis, and involvement of the heart and nervous system. Caused by the tick-borne spirochete *Borrelia burgdorferi,* similar in shape to the causative organism of syphilis, it is the most commonly reported vector-borne disease in the United States. The tick that carries Lyme disease is common in the Northeast, the Upper Midwest, and along the Pacific Coast. Deer and mice are both reservoirs of the tick, and the disease is common in people living and engaging in recreation near wooded areas with high deer populations. Most infections occur in spring and summer, when tick exposure is most likely. Everyone is susceptible, and natural infection does not appear to confer immunity. The incubation period ranges from 3 to 21 days.

Lyme disease progresses in three stages:

- ***Early localized stage***—A painless, flat, red lesion appears at the bite site. In some patients, a ringlike rash, *erythema migrans (EM),* develops and spreads outward. The outer border remains bright red, with the center becoming clear, blue, or even necrotic. The rash—often called a "bull's eye" rash—usually disappears in time, whether treated or not (Figure 10-21). At this stage, patients also may complain of headache, malaise, and muscle aches. Although uncommon, the patient's neck may be stiff.
- ***Early disseminated stage***—The spirochete spreads to the skin, nervous system, heart, and joints. More EM lesions develop. CNS sequelae include meningitis, seventh-cranial-nerve Bell's palsy, and peripheral neuropathy. Cardiac abnormalities include conduction defects and myopathy. Arthritis and myalgia are common months after infection. Approximately 8 percent of patients will have some cardiac involvement. The most common manifestations are varying degrees of atrioventricular block (first degree, Wenckebach, and complete heart block). Less commonly, myocarditis and left ventricular dysfunction are seen. Cardiac involvement typically lasts only a few weeks, but can recur.

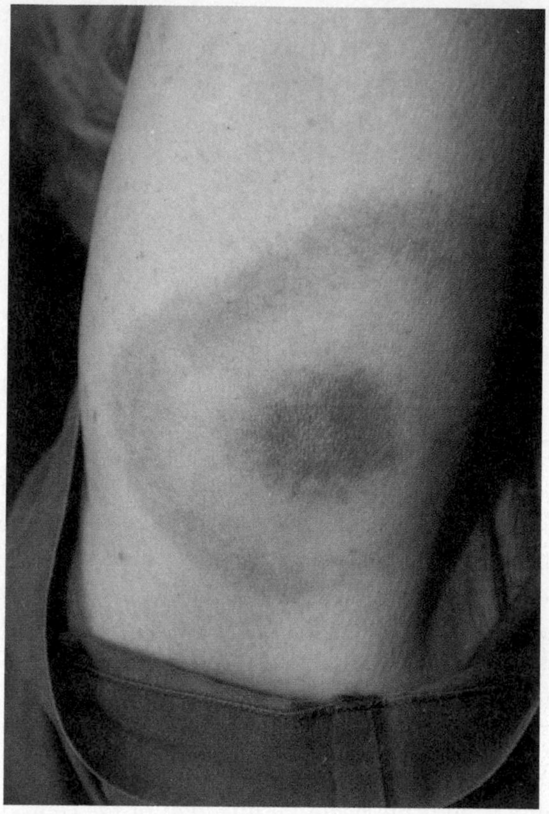

FIGURE 10-21 Characteristic target rash of Lyme disease.
(Centers for Disease Control and Prevention/James Gathany)

- ***Late stage (persistent infection)***—The late stage can occur months or years after the initial exposure. Although the incidence of cardiac problems is lower, it involves the same neurologic complications as the second stage, as well as encephalopathy with cognitive deficits, depression, and sleep disorders. Monoarthritis of large joints and more than one joint concurrently (polyarthritis) is common.

Development of erythema migrans, the bull's eye rash, usually 3 to 30 days after tick exposure, is presumptive for the diagnosis.

The EMS response to Lyme disease will probably be to treat its clinical consequences, especially those of the disseminated and late stages. ALS treatment is directed toward those consequences, not the infection. Adhere to Standard Precautions. After responding to calls in heavily wooded areas infested by ticks, always check both your and the patient's clothing, shoes, socks, and body for ticks. Spray the ambulance compartment with an insecticide

CONTENT REVIEW

➤ Sexually Transmitted Diseases
- Gonorrhea
- Syphilis
- Genital warts
- Herpes simplex type 2
- Chlamydia
- Trichomoniasis
- Chancroid

effective against arthropods. Available antibiotic therapies are effective for the stages of the disease progression. The vaccine for Lyme disease is no longer available.[20]

Sexually Transmitted Diseases

Infectious diseases transmitted through sexual contact are known as **sexually transmitted diseases, or STDs**. They represent some of the most prevalent communicable diseases. A variety of bacterial (gonorrhea, syphilis, chancroid, chlamydia), viral (HIV, herpes), and parasitic (*Pediculosis, Trichomonas*) infections are spread by this route. Other illnesses that are generally not considered STDs, including hepatitis A, B, C, D, salmonella, and shigella, may also be transmitted through sexual contact. STDs affect the genital organs, often resulting in pathology to reproductive structures. Although EMS responders do not treat these diseases, other emergency health care personnel commonly know the information in the following profiles. Your knowledge of these diseases will put you on a "level playing field" with those other health care workers and bolster your credibility. When you treat or transport patients with STDs, observe Standard Precautions, avoid contact with lesions and exudates, and wash your hands vigorously after exposure.

Gonorrhea

Gonorrhea, caused by *Neisseria gonorrhoeae,* a Gram-negative bacterium, is one of the most commonly diagnosed communicable diseases in the United States. More than 1 million cases are treated annually. Everyone is susceptible to infection, and although antibodies develop after exposure and confer immunity, they do so only for the specific serotype that caused the infection. Thus, persons contracting gonorrhea would not be immune to penicillinase-producing *N. gonorrhoeae* (PPNG), a strain of *N. gonorrhoeae* known by military personnel during the Vietnam War as "black clap." Most commonly seen in males in their early 20s, gonorrhea is transmitted by direct contact with exudates of mucous membranes, primarily from direct sexual contact. In men, the disease presents as painful urination and a purulent urethral discharge (Figure 10-22). Untreated, it can lead to epididymitis, prostatitis, and urethral strictures. The majority of women contracting the disease have no pain and minimal discharge. In some cases, symptoms include urinary frequency, vaginal discharge, fever, and abdominal pain. Pelvic inflammatory disease (PID) often results after menstruation when bacteria spread from the cervix to the upper genital tract. Affected women are at increased risk for sterility, ectopic pregnancy, abscesses within reproductive structures, and peritonitis.

Gonorrhea may occasionally become systemic, causing sepsis or meningitis. Septic arthritis may result, presenting with fever, pain, swelling, and limited range of motion in one or two joints, sometimes leading to progressive deterioration. In the United States, single dosing is often effective in treating localized gonorrhea (genitourinary only). Treating systemic gonorrhea often involves additional chemotherapy. When gonorrhea infection coexists with chlamydial infections (as is estimated to occur in about 50 percent of gonorrhea patients), two-drug therapy is routinely advised. No immunization is available.

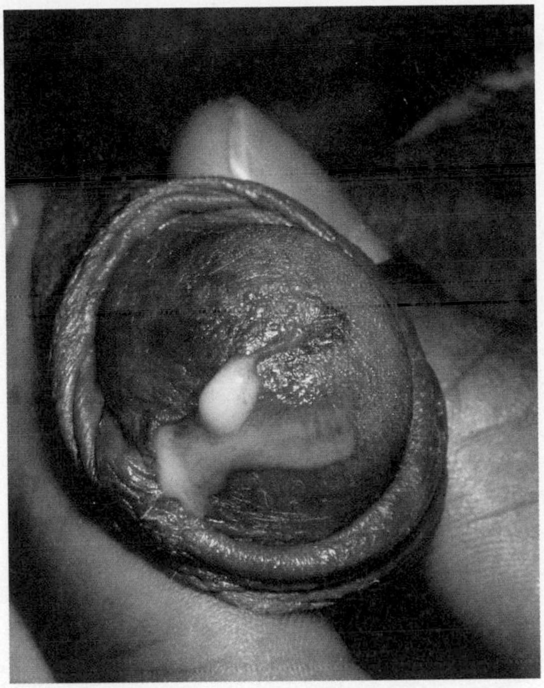

FIGURE 10-22 Penile discharge due to gonorrhea.
(Centers for Disease Control and Prevention)

Syphilis

Syphilis is a disease caused by the spirochete *Treponema pallidum.* It is transmitted by direct contact with exudates from other syphilitic lesions of skin and mucous membranes, semen, blood, saliva, and vaginal discharges. It is therefore most commonly contracted through sexual intercourse but also may be transmitted by kissing or close contact with an open lesion. An estimated 30 percent of exposures result in infection. In congenital syphilis, infants contract the disease before birth from an infected mother. Everyone is susceptible to infection. Although the risk of transmission by blood transfusion or needle-stick injury is low, health care workers have been infected after physical examination involving manual contact with a lesion. A gradual immunity does develop after infection, but aggressive antimicrobial therapy may interfere with this natural antibody formation, especially during the primary and secondary stages.

CONTENT REVIEW

➤ Stages of Syphilis
- Primary
- Secondary
- Latent
- Tertiary

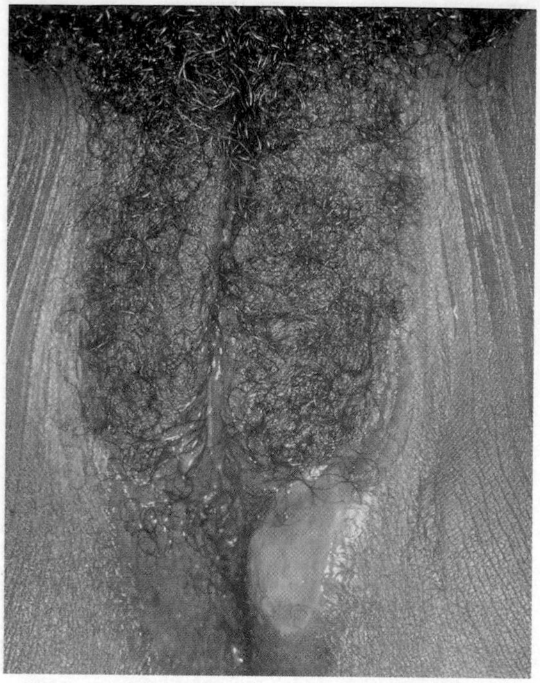

FIGURE 10-23 Syphilis chancre on female labia.
(Armed Forces Institute of Pathology)

Syphilis is characterized by lesions that may involve virtually any organ or tissue. It usually has cutaneous manifestations with frequent relapses, and it may remain latent for years. The incubation period is three weeks. Syphilis may occur in four stages, depending on how early and aggressively treatment is initiated:

- *Primary syphilis (first stage)* presents as a painless lesion, or chancre. In heterosexual men, the chancre is usually on the penis. In homosexual men, the chancre is often found on the anal canal, rectum, tongue, lips, or other point of entry (Figure 10-23). The chancre typically occurs three to six weeks after exposure. Nontender enlargement of regional lymph nodes may also occur.
- *Secondary syphilis (second stage)*, or the bacteremic stage, begins five to six weeks after the chancre has healed. It is characterized by a maculopapular skin rash (small, red, flat lesions) on the palms and soles, condyloma latum (painless, wartlike lesions on warm, moist skin areas that are very infectious), and cutaneous infection in areas of hair growth causing loss of hair and/or eyebrows. These skin signs last for about six weeks. CNS disease (syphilitic meningitis) and arthritis may occur, as can infections of the eyes and kidneys.
- *Latent syphilis (third stage)*, a period when symptoms improve or disappear completely, may last from months to many years. Twenty-five percent of cases may relapse with secondary stage symptoms; however, relapses usually do not occur after four years. Thirty-three percent of cases will progress to tertiary syphilis, and the rest will remain asymptomatic.
- *Tertiary syphilis (fourth stage)* is the stage of syphilis that justifies its reputation as a "great imitator." Lesions with sharp borders, called *gummas*, may appear on skin and bones, causing a deep, gnawing pain. Cardiovascular syphilis may appear, usually ten years after the primary infection, resulting in aortic aneurysms that antibiotic therapy does not reverse. Neurosyphilis is diagnosed when there are neurologic signs in seropositive patients. Meningitis may result, with possible spinal cord disease causing loss of reflexes and reduced sensation of pain and temperature. The spirochetes can also invade the cerebral vessels, causing a stroke. A progressive dementia can also occur during this stage.

EMS responders may treat a variety of clinical complications of syphilis, often without being aware of infection as the primary etiology. ALS is directed toward treating the clinical presentation, which may include seizures, an acute onset of dementia, signs of a stroke, aortic aneurysm, or acute myocardial infarction. Avoid frequent contact with lesions on any part of the patient's body, and pay attention to hand washing technique after patient contact, as *T. pallidum* is easily killed by heat, soap, and water.

For presumptive screening after exposure, rapid plasmin reagin (RPR) and venereal disease research labs (VDRL) tests are available. Because RPR or VDRL have fairly high rates of false positive reactions, however, more specific tests should always follow. Treatment of primary syphilis is benzathine penicillin, with erythromycin and doxycycline (Vibramycin) as alternatives for patients allergic to penicillin. No immunization is available.

Genital Warts

Genital warts (condyloma acuminatum) are caused by the human papillomavirus (HPV), a DNA virus. To date, research has identified 70 HPV types, with most known to cause specific clinical manifestations. Some of the types known to cause genital warts are associated with cervical cancer. Genital warts are contagious and easily spread. In men, they generally appear as cauliflower-like, fleshy growths on the penis, anus, and mucosa of the anal canal. In women, they usually appear on the labial surfaces (Figure 10-24). Genital warts are sometimes difficult to distinguish from the condyloma latum seen in the secondary stage of syphilis. HPV has been implicated as a causative factor of cervical cancer in women. A vaccine is now available for HPV and primarily serves as a cervical cancer prevention agent.

Herpes Simplex Virus Type 2

HSV-2 causes 70 to 90 percent of all genital herpes cases. Transmission is usually by sexual contact. Everyone is susceptible, but adolescents and young adults are most commonly afflicted. Neonates are often infected during passage through the birth canal. The prevalence of HSV-2

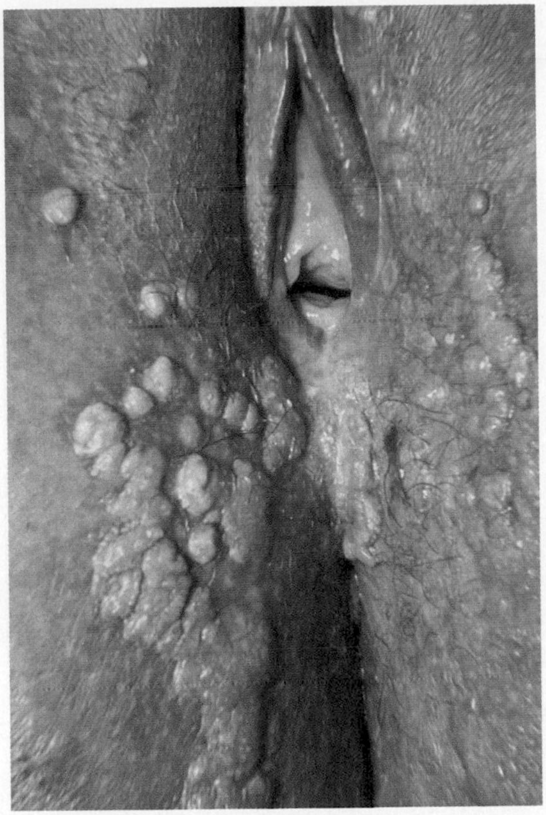

FIGURE 10-24 Genital warts (condyloma) on female labial surfaces caused by human papillomavirus.

(Centers for Disease Control and Prevention/Joyce Ayers)

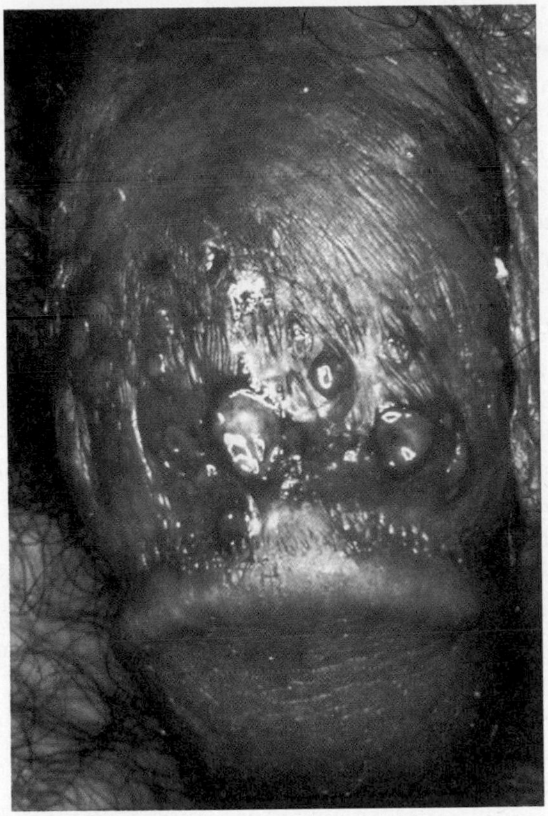

FIGURE 10-25 Genital herpes.

(Centers for Disease Control and Prevention/Dr. N. J. Flumara; Dr. Gavin Hart)

antibody, which does not confer immunity, is greater in lower socioeconomic groups and persons with multiple sex partners. The disease presents as vesicular lesions on the penis, anus, rectum, and mouth of a man, depending on sexual activity. Women are sometimes asymptomatic, but can display lesions of the vagina, vulva, perineum, rectum, mouth, and cervix. Recurrent infections in women are often found on the vulva, buttocks, legs, and the perineum. Patients may present with fever and enlarged lymph nodes during the initial infection. Lesions may last up to several weeks before eventually crusting over and healing (Figure 10-25). The most serious consequence of HSV-2 infection is that painful lesions may recur periodically during the patient's lifetime, significantly diminishing quality of life. Recent evidence suggests that symptomatic treatment with the antiviral agent acyclovir orally, intravenously, or topically may decrease the incidence of recurrences and lessen the severity of their symptoms. Other treatment alternatives include cryotherapy (freezing and removal) with liquid nitrogen, electrical cauterization, and interferon. Immunization is not currently available.

Chlamydia

Chlamydia is a genus of intracellular parasites most like Gram-negative bacteria. Once thought to be viruses, the chlamydiae are now known to have an inner and outer membrane, to contain both DNA and RNA, and to be susceptible to numerous antibiotics. However, they lack peptidoglycan, a net of polysaccharides found in all true bacterial walls.

From the standpoint of STDs, *Chlamydia trachomatis* is the most clinically significant species, affecting the genital area, eyes, and respiratory system. Everyone is susceptible, and up to 25 percent of men may be carriers. *C. trachomatis* is responsible for roughly 50 percent of all cases of nongonococcal urethritis (NGU) in men, with dysuria and penile discharge common. It is transmitted by sexual activity and by hand-to-hand transfer of eye secretions, causing conjunctivitis. Internationally, this is the leading cause of preventable blindness. Because children are the major reservoir and the common use of infected linen can transmit chlamydia, child care center and school workers should exercise caution in handling blankets, sheets, and towels.

The symptoms are similar to those of gonorrhea but less severe, often making the clinical differentiation difficult. In addition, the progression of disease in women is identical, with both causing a mucopurulent discharge that often accompanies cervicitis. Some women may have retrograde infections of the reproductive tract, causing pelvic inflammatory disease. Sterility may result. Newborns may be infected during passage through an infected birth canal, resulting in infant pneumonia or blindness.

No immunization is available, but *C. trachomatis* infection responds to a variety of antimicrobial agents such as tetracycline, doxycycline (Vibramycin), erythromycin (PCE), and orally administered azithromycin (Zithromax). Natural infection is not known to confer immunity.

Another species of Chlamydia, *C. pneumoniae,* has been found in atherosclerotic lesions of patients who have died of myocardial infarction. This has led to speculation about the relationship between *C. pneumoniae* infection and atherosclerosis as an inflammatory process.

Trichomoniasis

Trichomonas vaginalis, a protozoan parasite, is a common cause of vaginitis. In women, the symptoms of **trichomoniasis** include a greenish-yellow vaginal discharge, irritation of the perineum and thighs, and dysuria. This disease is frequently present with gonorrhea. Men are generally asymptomatic carriers of the disease. When present, symptoms include dysuria, urethral discharge, and discomfort in the perineum. The infection is currently treated with metronidazole (Flagyl).

Chancroid

Chancroid is a highly contagious ulcer caused by *Haemophilus ducreyi,* a Gram-negative bacterium. It is more frequently diagnosed in men, particularly those who have sex with prostitutes. Uncircumcised men are at higher risk. It is spread by direct contact, mostly sexual, with open lesions and pus. Autoinoculation has occurred in infected persons. Its incubation period is typically 3 to 5 days, but may be as long as 14 days.

The disease begins with a painful, inflamed pustule or ulcer that may appear on the penis, anus, urethra, or vulva (Figure 10-26). It spreads easily to other sites, such as breasts, fingers, and thighs. Lymph nodes may become swollen and tender, and fever may be present. Chancroid ulcer is linked with increased risk of HIV infection. Chancroid lesions in children beyond the neonatal period should alert EMS responders to the possibility of reportable child sexual abuse.

Health care workers have contracted the disease by contacting patients' ulcers. Immunization is not available, and infection does not appear to confer immunity. Several effective antimicrobials (for example, erythromycin) are available.

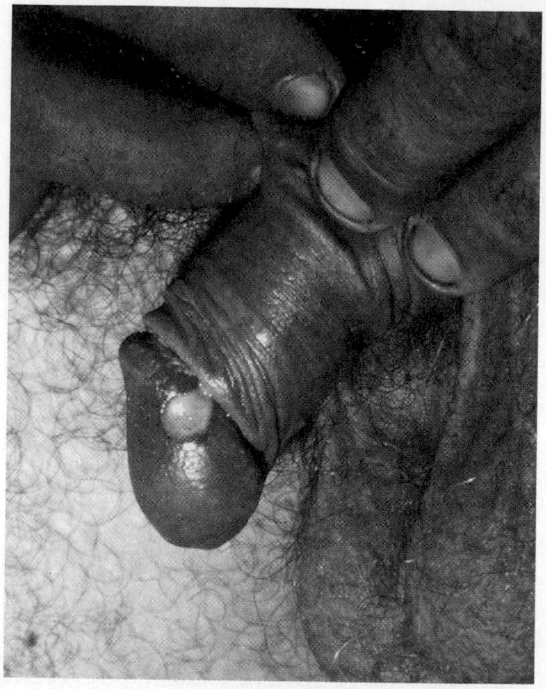

FIGURE 10-26 Chancroid.

(Centers for Disease Control and Prevention/Joe Miller)

Diseases of the Skin

EMS responders' interactions with patients or the general public may expose them to contagious skin infections such as impetigo or the ectoparasites lice and scabies. Because the public frequently attempts to consult paramedics about general topics in personal and community health, your knowledge of ectoparasites may enable you to provide education and customer service. As always, use Standard Precautions and effective postexposure handwashing.

CONTENT REVIEW

- Diseases of the Skin
  - Impetigo
  - Lice
  - Scabies

Impetigo

Impetigo is a very contagious infection of the skin caused by staphylococci or streptococci. The disease begins as a single vesicle that ruptures and forms a thick, honey-colored crust with a yellowish-red center. Lesions most commonly occur on the extremities and joints. Although few patients call an ambulance for this condition, it often appears on patients who seek EMS for other reasons. EMS responders who develop impetigo should not report for work until cleared by their physician. It is easily transmitted by direct skin-to-skin contact, so Standard Precautions should provide ample protection.

Lice

Lice (pediculosis) is a parasitic **infestation** of the skin of the scalp, trunk, or pubic area. Lice infest hosts rather than infect them because they do not break the skin. The three different varieties of infestations are *Pediculus humanus var. capitis* (head lice), *Pediculus humanus var. corporis* (body lice), and *Pthirus pubis* (pubic lice, or crabs). Historically, head lice have been involved in outbreaks of typhus, trench fever in World War I, and relapsing fever. Head and body lice appear similar, both being 3 to 4 mm long. Head lice are transmitted by sharing of combs or hats and are fairly common among young school-age children, regardless of socioeconomic status. Outbreaks in child care centers and schools are common. Head lice are easily diagnosed by the presence of small, white, oval-shaped eggs (nits) attached to the hair shafts. Nits can be seen with the naked eye but are more easily found with a magnifying glass. Lice themselves are rarely seen. They tend to leave febrile hosts, so high environmental temperatures and crowding favor transmission. Lice have a three-stage life cycle of eggs, nymphs, and adults. Eggs hatch in 7 to 10 days but cannot hatch below 72°F. The nymph stage lasts about 7 to 13 days, again depending on temperature, with a total egg-to-egg cycle of 3 weeks.

Anyone can be infested, and repeated infestations may cause an allergic response. Infestation often occurs on eyebrows and eyelashes, hair, mustaches, and beards. Symptoms are generally limited to severe itching. Body lice often infest clothing along seams close to skin surfaces and attach to the skin only to feed. They can be vectors of bacteria. Red macules, papules, and urticaria commonly appear on the shoulders, buttocks, and abdomen. Pubic lice infest through sexual contact by attaching to hair in the genital and anal regions, but can also infest facial hair.

Any EMS responder exposed to a patient with lice may be treated with one of several nonprescription agents. Pyrethrin preparations, such as RID, are commonly used, but require two applications one week apart because they do not kill eggs. Permethrin agents, such as Nix or Elimite, theoretically require only a single application because they kill adults and eggs. Lindane 1% shampoo (Kwell) may be used, but it is available only by prescription and is more toxic than the other treatments. Eliminating the eggs by combing the hair is essential. Nits are more easily removed (nit picking) after soaking combs in a white vinegar solution or using a commercial preparation such as the Step 2 Nit Removal System. Separately bagging linen in an occupational setting is unnecessary. At home, however, isolating infested linen and clothing is advisable to avoid exposing uninfested laundry for extended periods. Lice are not known to jump great distances, as fleas do, so spraying the ambulance's interior close to the cot and the area by the patient's head with an insecticide, preferably one containing permethrin, should be sufficient after a call. Clean and wipe all sprayed areas to remove insecticide residues.

Scabies

Scabies is caused by infestation of a mite (*Sarcoptes scabiei*) that is barely visible without magnification. Exposure to the mite is through close personal contact, from hand holding to sexual relations. The mite can remain viable on clothing or in bedding for up to 48 hours.

Upon attaching to a new host, the female tunnels into the skin within 2.5 minutes and lays up to three eggs a day along the "burrow" in the epidermis. The larvae hatch shortly thereafter, leading to full-grown adults 10 to 20 days later. The adults remain near hair follicles and forage for nourishment with their jaws and the claws of their forelegs.

The primary symptom is intense itching (hence the name "seven-year itch"), usually at night. It generally occurs from two to six weeks after infestation. The irritation results from sensitization to the mite and its droppings. Inflammatory lesions appear as fine, wavy, dark lines, usually not more than 1 cm long. In males, they most commonly occur on the webs of the fingers, wrists, elbows, armpits, belt line, thighs, and external genitalia. In females, they most often involve the areolae and nipples, abdomen, and lower portions of the buttocks. In infants, the head, neck, palms, and soles are frequently involved. Older children exhibit patterns similar to adults. Complications are generally due to infections of lesions that are broken by scratching.

Although everyone is susceptible to infection, immunocompromised patients sometimes develop Norwegian scabies, a more severe form of scabies. Persons with previous exposure appear to have fewer mites on subsequent exposures and develop symptoms much sooner (in from one to four days), suggesting an amnestic (remembered) immune system response. Outbreaks of scabies resistant to lindane (Kwell) have been reported in several nursing homes across the country.

Scabies remains communicable until all mites and eggs are destroyed. Because of the long incubation period, all household members and/or close contacts of infested EMS responders should be treated simultaneously. Although some experts recommend that clothing and uniforms worn within two days of treatment, along with towels and bed linen, should be washed in hot water or dry cleaned, this necessity is questionable for most infestations. It is essential, however, for articles contacting patients with Norwegian scabies. Bag and remove all linens from the ambulance immediately after you deliver the patient. To prevent spread of the mite, clean the stretcher and patient compartment as recommended for lice. Remove and decontaminate any clothing that may have contacted the patient.

The scabicides of choice are permethrin cream (Elimite) or lindane (Kwell), which is applied to the skin from the neck down, left on for 8 to 14 hours, and then washed off. This should be repeated within one week. If permethrin is ineffective, 10% crotamiton (Eurax) and ivermectin (Stromectol) are also available.

Bedbugs

There has been a recent increase in the occurrence of bedbug infestations and resultant bedbug bites. Bedbugs (*Cimex lectularius*) are small, flat, parasitic insects that feed solely on the blood of people and animals while they sleep. Bedbugs are reddish-brown in color, are wingless, range from 1 to 7 mm in size (roughly the size of Lincoln's head on a penny), and can live several months without a blood meal. Bedbugs are found throughout the globe. At one time, they were limited primarily to developing countries. Now they have spread into many other parts of the world, including the United States. Bedbugs have been found in five-star hotels and resorts and are not necessarily related to the cleanliness of the facility. They primarily infest regions around or near the areas where people sleep. These areas include apartments, shelters, rooming houses, hotels, cruise ships, buses, trains, and dorm rooms. They hide during the day in places such as seams of mattresses. They have been shown to be able to travel more than 100 feet in a night but tend to live within 8 feet of where people sleep. Although bedbugs generally do not transmit disease, they can be an annoyance because they can cause itching and loss of sleep. Bedbugs affect different people differently and responses can range from an absence of any physical signs of the bite to a small bite mark to a serious allergic reaction.

Nosocomial Infections

Hospitalized patients, especially those with compromised immune function, often acquire new infectious diseases. Especially virulent strains of microorganisms may cause these **nosocomial** (hospital-acquired) diseases. Bacteria that resist antibiotics are of particular concern. Recently, vancomycin-resistant enterococcus (VRE) and methicillin-resistant *Staphylococcus aureus* (MRSA) have become especially alarming. Both these organisms can cause severe host damage, and both are difficult to treat. They rapidly colonize patients in whom broad-spectrum antibiotics have eliminated normal flora. Hospitalized patients may also contract resistant strains of tuberculosis that spread easily from patient to patient if protective clothing and handwashing precautions are not strictly observed.

Patient Education

In spite of increased emphasis in public education and extensive media attention in recent years, a lack of understanding of infectious diseases remains widespread among the public. The one exception may be HIV, owing to its extensive and relatively objective media exposure. Media coverage of other infectious diseases such as hantavirus, Ebola, "flesh-eating bacteria," and others has been so sensational that it has accomplished little from an educational perspective and, in some cases, has spread misinformation and created undue fear.

As with more publicized topics in emergency medicine, such as trauma and substance abuse, prevention is without question the most effective intervention in preventing transmission of infectious diseases. The key to effective prevention is education; however, because these diseases are less "glamorous" than other illnesses, attracting public attention is difficult, and influencing behavior poses a formidable challenge. Paramedics have an opportunity to assume a leadership role in this area. EMS personnel are often active in public and community education and are ideally positioned to influence the public's behavior. CPR and first-aid classes offer a platform to also introduce and discuss issues related to disease transmission. Leading by example is extremely important. Paramedics, especially those working in rural and suburban areas, reflect the general community. They are in close contact with the people they serve and are well respected in their communities. Taking an active part in public disease-prevention education will be among your most important roles as a paramedic.

Many of the diseases covered in this chapter are not emergencies and may not require emergency treatment. As prehospital emergency medicine evolves from vocation to profession, however, it will require more education and greater knowledge in these areas. Infectious diseases' serious personal and public health implications require you to be knowledgeable in this area and take the lead in educating others.

Preventing Disease Transmission

Preventing or limiting exposure to infectious or communicable diseases cannot be overemphasized. Although some infectious diseases are relatively minor with no long-term effects, others can be very serious and even life threatening. As a paramedic, you must be extremely vigilant during patient contact and take every step possible to ensure your health and safety. Personal accountability is important.

Do not go to work if you:

- Have diarrhea.
- Have a draining wound or any type of wet lesions. Allow them to dry and crust over before returning to work.
- Are jaundiced.
- Have mononucleosis.
- Have been exposed to lice or scabies and have not yet been treated.
- Have strep throat and have not been taking antibiotics for at least 24 hours.
- Have a cold.

Keep the following immunizations current: MMR, hepatitis A (if deemed appropriate in your jurisdiction), hepatitis B, DPT, polio, chickenpox, influenza (seasonal), and rabies (if appropriate).

Always approach the scene cautiously, with a high index of suspicion. On arrival, control the scene to decrease the likelihood of body fluid exposure for everyone present. Use Standard Precautions. If there is the remotest possibility of splashing or aerosolization of body fluids, wear protective eyewear or a mask with face shield. If large volumes of blood or other fluids may result from the response, don a gown. When contacting a patient who has or may have active TB, wear the appropriate N95 masks.

Patients who have coughs, fever, headache, general weakness, recent weight loss, or nuchal rigidity or are taking certain medications may raise your awareness of the potential for contracting an infectious agent. With experience, you will develop your intuition and associate certain symptoms with infectious patients you have treated. Bolster your experience by increasing your knowledge, particularly your clinical acumen in recognizing the immunocompromised patient.

After a call, wash your hands first. Decontaminate and disinfect your equipment and the interior of the ambulance. Using commercially available disinfectants that certify bactericidal activity against *M. tuberculosis* should provide ample disinfection of those infectious agents that pose your greatest occupational risk. Remember that HIV is a fragile virus that any vigorous application of soap and water will kill. Use high-level disinfection on airway equipment. If the patient or the situation surrounding the response presents the possibility of lice, scabies, or ticks, spray the gurney and interior of the ambulance with the appropriate insecticide and wipe or mop up any residue. Ensure that linens will not be taken home. If practical, do not wear uniforms home. To discourage that practice, some EMS agencies consider uniforms as PPE. Report any infectious exposure to the IDCO, human resources director, or appropriate designated official.

The topics mandated by OSHA/NIOSH for compliance with published standards and guidelines (i.e., bloodborne pathogens and TB) reflect the paramedic's minimum needed knowledge of infectious diseases. Proactive EMS agencies offer their personnel continuing education in infectious diseases that have high incidence or prevalence in the communities they serve. Continuing education sessions should include identification of causative agents, modes of transmission, epidemiological patterns within the community, signs and symptoms, methods to avoid infection, and special postexposure considerations, including postexposure prophylaxis, if appropriate.

To maintain a perspective on personal risk, always consider the interaction of three major factors: infectious agent, host, and environment. Are you aware of the infectious agent's virulence? Do you have some idea of the dose of the organism involved? For example, was a large volume of body fluid involved? How healthy are you? Do you have any chronic medical conditions or take any medications that would classify you as immunocompromised? What was the nature of the exposure? Is it significantly high? The probability of risk is sometimes just a measure of exposure. Not all infectious diseases are communicable. If they are communicable, they may not necessarily pose a high probability of developing disease. The risk and potential for HIV transmission to health care workers may be high, for example, but the probability of transmission, which averages approximately 0.3 percent, is very low.

As you are promoted within your organization, your first additional responsibility may be as a preceptor for a new paramedic or student. You therefore assume responsibility for his well-being. Are you familiar with your local protocols and procedures for reporting and recording an exposure? Can you adequately document the circumstances surrounding the exposure to facilitate review by the IDCO, physician, or agency administrator? If you cannot, what kind of a role model are you for that new employee or student?

Paramedics cannot allow their personal prejudices to interfere with providing optimum care for their patients. Patients should not be treated differently because they have an infectious disease that might reflect on their ethnicity, culture, sexual preference, or social status. You should not avoid certain procedures because you find a disease process or its consequences personally repulsive. It is sometimes helpful to think about doing things *for* patients, as opposed to doing things *to* them.

Paramedics work in a profession fraught with uncertainty. They make clinical decisions based on limited data. They rarely deal with infectious disease emergencies but must be constantly and consistently vigilant to protect themselves, their patients, and other responders. The exposures are often unknown and involve intangible infectious agents. Thus, Standard Precautions, which are EMS practice standards, are predicated on the possibility that all body fluids, in any situation, are infectious. Adhering to those standards will markedly decrease your risk of occupational infection.

Sepsis/Systemic Inflammatory Response Syndrome (SIRS)

Sepsis is the tenth most common cause of death in the world and the most common cause of death in debilitated patients in hospital intensive care units. Sepsis, sometimes called **septicemia**, is a life-threatening medical condition caused by a whole-body inflammatory state called **systemic inflammatory response syndrome (SIRS)**. It occurs in response to a known or suspected infection (usually bacterial). The original site of infection can be anywhere in the body, and the infection usually spreads to the vascular system or other sterile areas. Common sites of SIRS origin include the gastrointestinal system (peritonitis, pancreatitis), the genitourinary system (pyelonephritis, UTI), the neurologic system (meningitis), the hepatobiliary system (liver, gallbladder), the respiratory system (pneumonia), or the skin (cellulitis). Sepsis can also result from medical interventions and devices, including IV lines, surgical wounds and drains, decubitus ulcers, urinary catheters, and others.

Those most at risk of developing sepsis are:

- People with immunosuppression (e.g., from AIDS, chemotherapy, steroids)
- Patients who are hospitalized (e.g., with surgery, pneumonia)
- People with preexisting infections or medical conditions (e.g., diabetes, pancreatitis)
- People with severe trauma (e.g., burns, polytrauma)
- People with a genetic tendency for sepsis
- The very old or very young

Sepsis

The diagnosis of sepsis is made when the patient has an infection (documented or suspected) and at least two of the following signs and symptoms (Figure 10-27):

- Heart rate >90 beats per minute
- Abnormal body temperature (>100.4°F [>38°C] or <96.8°F [<36°C])
- Tachypnea (>20 breaths per minute or a $PaCO_2$ <32 mmHg)
- Abnormal white blood cell count (<4,000 or >12,000 cells/microliter) on a complete blood count (CBC)

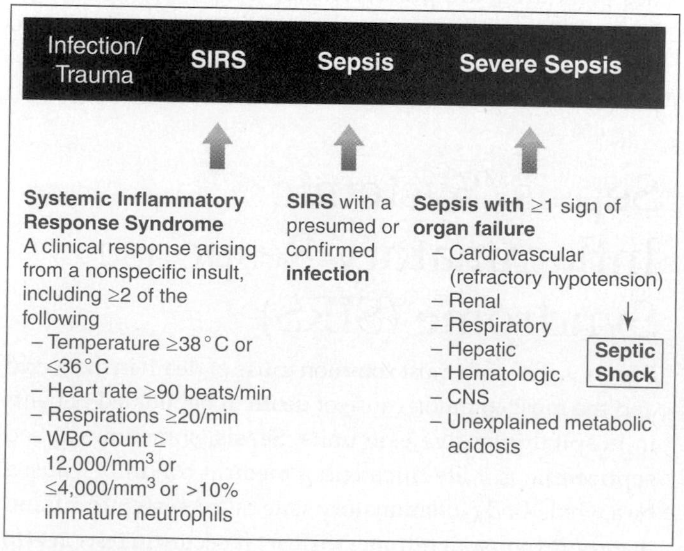

FIGURE 10-27 The spectrum of sepsis.

Severe Sepsis

Severe sepsis includes the presence of sepsis (as defined in the previous section) and evidence of hypoperfusion:

- Mottled skin
- Delayed capillary refill (>3 seconds)
- Decreased urine output (<0.5 mL/kg/hr)
- Lactate >1 mmol/L
- Altered mental status
- Abnormal findings in electroencephalogram (EEG)
- Platelet count <100,000 cells/mL
- Disseminated intravascular coagulation (DIC)
- Acute lung injury or acute respiratory distress syndrome (ARDS)
- Cardiac dysfunction, shown on echocardiography or direct measurement of cardiac output

Septic Shock

Septic shock is defined as severe sepsis associated with one or both of the following conditions:

- Mean systemic blood pressure below 60 mmHg (or less than 80 mmHg if the patient has known hypertension).
- The maintenance of mean arterial pressure above 60 mmHg (or greater than 80 mmHg, if there is prior history of hypertension) requires vasopressor therapy.[21]

Management

Early recognition and aggressive treatment for sepsis is necessary for the best outcome. The early signs and symptoms of sepsis/SIRS can be subtle. Many septic patients are initially cared for by EMS. Hospitals and physicians have developed specific treatment strategies for sepsis, referred to as early goal-directed therapy (EGDT) (Figure 10-28).[22] This includes:

- Supplemental oxygen (if the patient is hypoxic) with or without intubation and mechanical ventilation
- Fluid resuscitation
- Maintenance of systolic blood pressure >90 mmHg with vasopressors
- Administration of broad-spectrum antibiotics

Components of EGDT that can be started in the prehospital setting include oxygenation (if the patient is hypoxic), ventilation, fluid resuscitation, and pressor support.[23] In rural areas, consideration should be given to developing protocols for early empiric broad-spectrum antibiotic therapy. In addition, the availability of point-of-care lactate testing in the field may allow better diagnostic accuracy (lactate is the anion of lactic acid). Always remember: Sepsis kills, and prompt intervention is required.

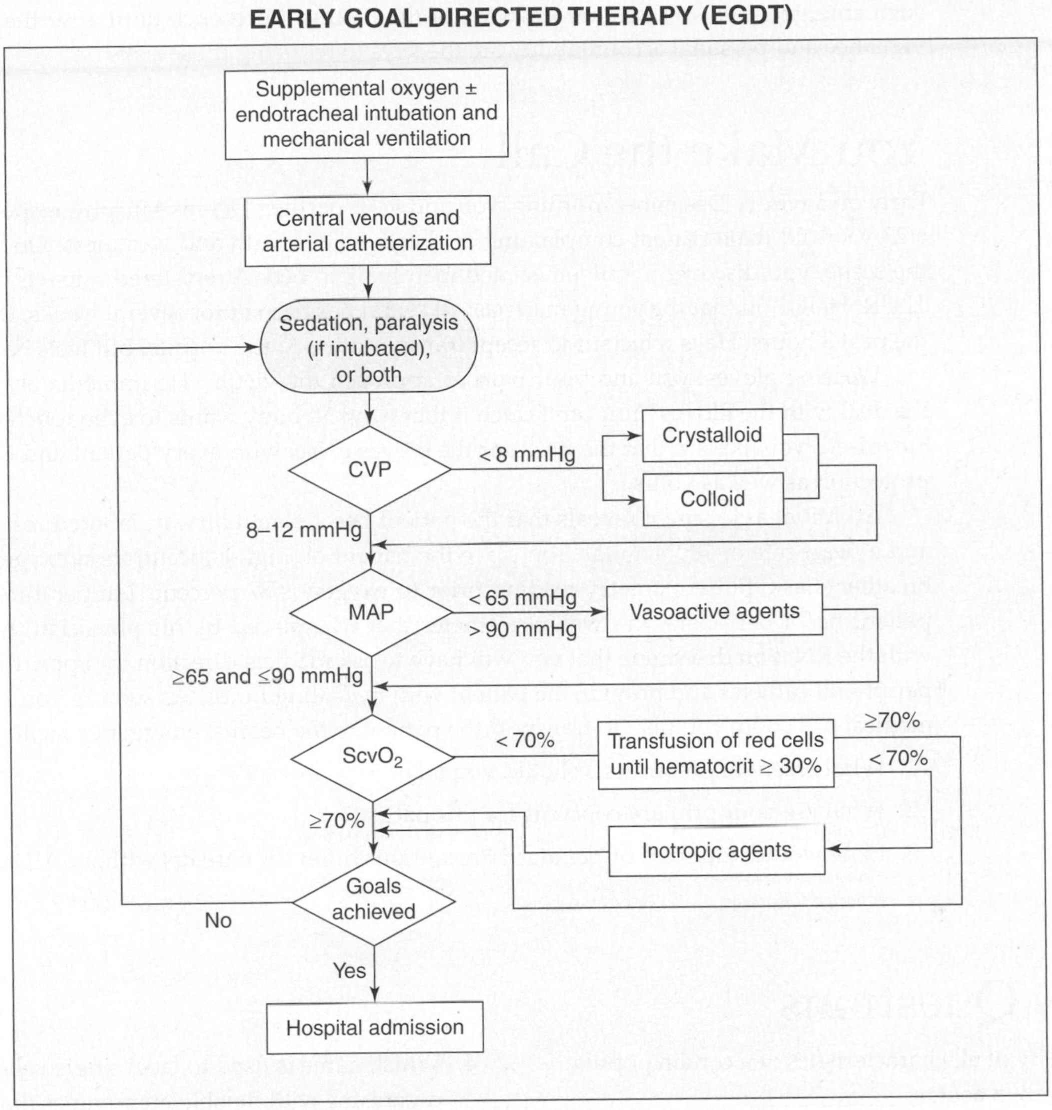

FIGURE 10-28 Overview of early goal-directed therapy (EGDT) sepsis treatment.

Summary

Over the past 30 years, medical science has made tremendous progress in diagnosing and treating infectious diseases. New vaccines and antibiotics are continually being developed. Advances in laboratory technology, notably the polymerase chain reaction (PCR), have made the presence and identification of microorganisms easier, quicker, and more accurate. Despite these tremendous advances, many infectious diseases cannot be treated effectively. Specific treatments for most viral diseases remain elusive, and each year countless people die from AIDS, hepatitis, pneumonia, sexually transmitted diseases, and other infectious diseases.

EMS can have a significant impact on the incidence of infectious disease if providers remain knowledgeable, are leaders in public education, and are consistently alert in protecting themselves and their patients. The title of the International Association of Fire Fighters (IAFF) hepatitis B curriculum, *The Silent War,* provides a metaphor for the dilemma of infectious diseases in EMS: EMS personnel deal with few infectious disease emergencies; however, when we do respond to such emergencies, we often are unaware of the disease's presence until after the call. Constant vigilance and personal accountability are the keys to reducing those risks.

You Make the Call

Early on a wintry December morning, you and your partner, Dennis Murphy, respond to a call for a 27-year-old male patient complaining of shortness of breath and weakness. On your arrival at the scene, you discover a frail, emaciated man lying in bed. A registered nurse is caring for him. The RN tells you that the young man has AIDS and has been ill for several weeks, worsening over the past 3 hours. He is reluctant to accept transportation to the hospital but feels he has no choice.

Wearing gloves, you and your partner approach the victim. He immediately says, "What's the deal with the gloves? You can't catch it that way! Nobody wants to even touch me anymore!" Surprised, you explain that the need for the gloves exists with every patient and that it is for his protection as well as yours.

An initial assessment reveals that the patient has a patent airway, labored respirations of 22, and a heart rate of 100/regular. You place the patient on high-concentration oxygen via a nonrebreather mask. Pulse oximetry reading prior to oxygen is 87 percent. Temperature is 101°F. The patient has a peripheral in-dwelling catheter that was placed by his physician. As you consult with the RN, you determine that you will have to ask medical direction for approval to access the peripheral catheter and provide the patient with hydrating fluids. As soon as you have contacted medical direction, you plan to transport the patient to the nearest emergency facility.

1. What essential precautions should you take?
2. What are your primary concerns for this patient?
3. How would your care or Standard Precautions differ for patients without AIDS?

See Suggested Responses at the back of this book.

Review Questions

1. The totality of all characteristics of a certain population is known as its ____________
   a. boundary.
   b. workplace.
   c. parameters.
   d. demographics.
2. Which organization monitors national disease data and freely disseminates this information to all health care providers?
   a. AHA
   b. CDC
   c. OSHA
   d. HHHS
3. The infectious agent of toxic shock syndrome, *S. aureus*, releases a(n) ____________, as does anthrax, which can be delivered as a biological weapon of mass destruction.
   a. protein
   b. exotoxin
   c. endotoxin
   d. polysaccharide
4. Which name is used to label single-celled parasitic organisms with flexible membranes that have the ability to move?
   a. Fungi
   b. Pinworms
   c. Protozoa
   d. Parasites
5. Factors that affect the likelihood that an exposed individual will become infected and then actually develop disease include which of the following?
   a. Virulence
   b. Correct mode of entry
   c. Number of organisms
   d. All of the above
6. The ____________ is an essential organ in the lymphatic system that is located in the left upper abdominal quadrant.
   a. liver
   b. spleen
   c. pancreas
   d. gallbladder

7. All of the following fluid types pose a high risk for effective transmission of HIV to health care workers *except* ______________
   a. semen.
   b. blood.
   c. saliva.
   d. vaginal secretions.
8. Which virus is transmitted through direct contact with contaminated body fluids (blood, semen, vaginal fluids, and saliva) and therefore represents a substantial risk to EMS providers?
   a. Hepatitis A
   b. Hepatitis B
   c. Hepatitis C
   d. Hepatitis E
9. What is the most common preventable adult infectious disease in the world?
   a. TB
   b. AIDS
   c. Pneumonia
   d. Hepatitis B
10. Which viral illness is characterized by inspiratory and expiratory stridor and a seal-bark-like cough, and is most common in children under the age of 3 years?
    a. Sinusitis
    b. Pharyngitis
    c. Epiglottitis
    d. Laryngotracheobronchitis

See Answers to Review Questions at the back of this book.

References

1. Centers for Disease Control and Prevention (CDC). "HIV Surveillance—United States 1981–2008." *MMWR* 60 (2011): 689–699.
2. Kuhn, L., C. Reitz, and E. J. Abrams. "Breastfeeding and AIDS in the Developing World." *Curr Opin Pediatr* 21 (2009): 83–93.
3. CDC. "Diagnosis of HIV Infection and AIDS in the United States and Dependent Areas, 2009." (Available at http://www.cdc.gov/hiv/surveillance/resources/reports/2009report/.)
4. CDC. "Updated U.S. Public Health Service Guidelines for the Management of Occupational Exposure to HIV and Recommendations for Postexposure Prophylaxis." *MMWR* (2005): 541–617.
5. CDC. "Viral Hepatitis." (Available at http://www.cdc.gov/hepatitis/.)
6. CDC. "Decrease in Reported Tuberculosis Cases–United States, 2009." *MMWR* 59 (2010): 289–294.
7. CDC/NIOSH. "TB Respiratory Protection Program in Health Care Facilities Administrator's Guide." (Available at http://www.cdc.gov/niosh/docs/99-143/.)
8. Vijayanand, P., E. Wilkins, and M. Woodhead. "Severe Acute Respiratory Syndrome (SARS): A Review." *Clin Med* 4(2) (2004): 152–160.
9. Kasowski, E. J., R. J. Garten, and C. B. Bridges. "Influenza Pandemic Epidemiologic and Virologic Diversity: Reminding Ourselves of the Possibilities." *Clin Infect Dis* 52 (2011): Supplement.
10. Gershon, A. A. "Measles Virus (Rubeola)," in Mandell G. L., J. E. Bennett, and R. Dolin, eds. *Principles and Practice of Infectious Diseases*. 7th ed., ch. 160. Philadelphia: Elsevier Churchill Livingstone, 2009.
11. Dayan, G. H., M. P. Quinisk, A. A. Parker, et al. "Recent Resurgence in Mumps in the United States." *NEJM* 358 (2008): 1580–1589.
12. Weisberg, S. S. "Vaccine Preventable Diseases: Current Perspectives in Historical Context." *Dis Mon* 53 (2007): 467–528.
13. "Respiratory Syncytial Virus," in Mandell, G. L., J. E. Bennett, and R. Dolin, eds. *Principles and Practice of Infectious Diseases*. 7th ed., ch. 158. Philadelphia: Elsevier Churchill Livingstone, 2009.
14. Hewlett, E. L. and K. M. Edwards. "Clinical Practice. Pertussis—Not Just for Kids." *NEJM* 352 (2005): 1215–1222.
15. Luzuriaga, K. and J. L. Sullivan. "Infectious Mononucleosis." *NEJM* 27 (2010): 1993–2000.
16. Sobol, S. E. and S. Zapata. "Epiglottitis and Croup." *Otolarynol Clin North Am* 41 (2008): 551–556.
17. Bell, M. "Viral Hemorrhagic Fevers," in Goldman, L. and D. Ausiello, eds. *Cecil Medicine*. 23rd ed., ch. 404. Philadelphia: Saunders Elsevier, 2007.
18. Rupprecht, C. E., D. Briggs, C. M. Brown, et al. "Centers for Disease Control and Prevention (CDC). Use of a Reduced (4-Dose) Vaccine Schedule for Postexposure Prophylaxis to Prevent Human Rabies: Recommendations of the Advisory Committee on Immunization Practices." *MMWR Recomm Rep* 59(RR-2) (Mar 19, 2010): 1–9. Erratum in: *MMWR Recomm Rep* 59(16) (Apr 30, 2010): 493.
19. Reddy, P. and T. P. Bleck. "*Clostridium tetani* (Tetanus)," in Mandell G. L., J. E. Bennett, and R. Dolin, eds. *Mandell, Douglas, and Bennett's Principles and Practice of Infectious Diseases*. 7th ed., ch. 244. Orlando, FL: Saunders Elsevier, 2009.
20. Clark, R. P. and L. T. Hu. "Prevention of Lyme Disease and Other Tick-Borne Infections." *Infect Dis Clin North Am* 22 (2008): 381–396.
21. Levy, M. M., M. P. Fink, J. C. Marshall, et al. "2001 SCCM/ESICM/ACCP/ATS/SIS International Sepsis Definitions Conference." *Crit Care Med* 31 (2003): 1250–1256.
22. Rivers, E., B. Nguyen, S. Havstad, et al. "Early Goal-Directed Therapy in the Treatment of Severe Sepsis and Septic Shock." *N Engl J Med* 345 (2001): 1368–1377.
23. Wang, H. E., M. D. Weaver, N. I. Shapiro, and D. M. Yealy. "Opportunities for Emergency Medical Services Care of Sepsis." *Resuscitation* 81 (2010): 193–197.

Further Reading

Heyman, D. L., ed. *Control of Communicable Diseases Manual*. 20th ed. Washington, DC: American Public Health Association, 2014.

Chapter 11
Psychiatric and Behavioral Disorders

Bryan Bledsoe, DO, FACEP, FAAEM, EMT-P

STANDARD
Medicine (Psychiatric)

COMPETENCY
Integrates assessment findings with principles of epidemiology and pathophysiology to formulate a field impression and implement a comprehensive treatment/disposition plan for a patient with a medical complaint.

Learning Objectives

Terminal Performance Objective: After reading this chapter, you should be able to integrate patient assessment findings, patient history, and knowledge of anatomy, physiology, pathophysiology, and basic and advanced life support interventions to recognize and manage patients with psychiatric and behavioral disorders.

Enabling Objectives: To accomplish the terminal performance objective, you should be able to:

1. Define key terms introduced in this chapter.
2. Discuss the biological, psychosocial, and sociocultural influences on psychiatric and behavioral disorders.
3. Adapt the scene size-up, primary assessment, history, secondary assessment, and use of monitoring technology to arrive at a field impression and differentials for behavioral emergencies.
4. Discuss the pathophysiology and assessment findings that would be present in a patient experiencing specific psychiatric disorders in the prehospital environment.
5. Describe the epidemiology and risk factors for suicide.
6. Use a process of clinical reasoning to guide and interpret the patient assessment findings and develop a treatment plan for patients displaying a behavioral emergency in the prehospital environment.
7. Describe special considerations for assessment and management of psychiatric and behavioral disorders in geriatric and pediatric populations.
8. Explain the characteristics and management of excited delirium syndrome.

9. Describe special considerations in the assessment and management of TASERed patients.
10. Describe the indications, procedures, precautions, and necessary documentation associated with the use of physical and chemical restraint to manage violent patients.
11. Given a variety of scenarios, discuss the integration of assessment and management guidelines as they relate to behavioral, suicidal, and violent patient emergencies.

KEY TERMS

affect, p. 448
anger, p. 452
anorexia nervosa, p. 455
anxiety, p. 451
anxiety disorder, p. 451
behavior, p. 446
behavioral emergency, p. 446
bereavement, p. 452
biological/organic , p. 446
bipolar disorder, p. 453
bulimia nervosa, p. 455
catatonia, p. 451
confusion, p. 448
delirium, p. 450
delusions, p. 450
dementia, p. 450
depersonalization, p. 454
depression, p. 452
dissociative disorder, p. 454
dissociative identity disorder, p. 454
excited delirium syndrome, p. 457
factitious disorder, p. 454
fear, p. 448
flat affect, p. 451
fugue state, p. 454
hallucinations, p. 450
impulse control disorder, p. 456
manic, p. 453
mental status, p. 448
mental status examination (MSE), p. 449
mood disorder, p. 452
panic attack, p. 451
personality disorder, p. 455
phobia, p. 452
positional asphyxia, p. 462
post-traumatic stress disorder (PTSD), p. 452
posture, p. 448
psychogenic amnesia, p. 454
psychosis, p. 456
psychosocial, p. 447
schizophrenia, p. 450
sociocultural, p. 447
somatoform disorder, p. 454

Case Study

On a hot August night, paramedic ambulance crew Kelly Underwood and Charles Bear have been dispatched to a possible psychiatric emergency at a local supermarket. They carefully approach the scene and observe a man standing in front of the store with his back to them. The manager approaches the ambulance and tells Kelly and Charles that the man came to the store and announced that the produce was poisonous. The manager also warns them that the man's behavior is somewhat bizarre. The man turns and begins shouting loudly, "Don't come in here! They're selling poison. They're trying to kill us all!" Charles radios for police assistance. He and Kelly remain in the ambulance and observe the patient until police arrive.

When the police arrive, Kelly quickly briefs them on the situation and the patient's status. The officers recognize the man as a psychiatric patient with whom they have recently had contact at a local motel. The man begins yelling and says he is working for the government. He yells at the top of his voice, "We'll close this place down!" The police ask Kelly and Charles to prepare the stretcher and restraints as a precaution. As the police approach the man, he calls them "poisoners." His agitation continues to escalate despite the efforts of the crew and officers to calm him. It becomes obvious that restraint is needed. The officers make the initial approach and control the patient's arms. Kelly is able to safely control the man's legs while Charles moves the stretcher into place. After placing the patient supine on the stretcher, they restrain his arms and legs using wide roller bandages. Kelly performs an assessment to rule out medical or traumatic causes of the patient's altered mental status. She monitors the man carefully en route to the emergency department. From there the patient is eventually transferred to the psychiatric center.

Introduction

Many of the topics you have studied up to this point have had objective diagnostic criteria. For example, you know that a tachycardia is a heart rate of more than 100 beats per minute, and a bradycardia is a rate of less than 60. Behavioral and psychiatric emergencies, however, are not so clear cut. Nonetheless, they include patient presentations that require a complete patient history, physical exam, and a skilled approach to the situation.

Another significant difference between behavioral and psychiatric conditions and other types of medical emergencies is that most of your assessment and care will depend on your people skills. You can evaluate a bradycardia with a cardiac monitor and treat it with atropine or a pacing unit. You provide psychological care for the cardiac patient to reduce anxiety and offer emotional support. You evaluate the psychiatric patient, on the other hand, by observing his behavior, by gathering information from his family and bystanders, and by interviewing him. Your care, which includes support, calming reassurance, and occasionally restraint, requires interpersonal skills more than diagnostic equipment.

Behavioral Emergencies

Behavior is a person's observable conduct and activity. A **behavioral emergency** is a situation in which a patient's behavior becomes so unusual, bizarre, threatening, or dangerous that it alarms the patient or another person, such as a family member or bystander, and requires the intervention of emergency service and/or mental health personnel.

Notice that the definition of behavioral emergency does not use the word *abnormal*. Saying that a behavioral emergency involves "abnormal behavior" would be easy, but the differentiation between normal and abnormal is largely subjective. What is "normal" varies based on culture, ethnic group, socioeconomic class, and personal interpretation and opinion. What one person considers normal, another might consider highly abnormal. Generally, however, normal behavior can be defined as behavior that is readily acceptable in a society.

Objective factors that may indicate a behavioral or psychological condition include actions or situations that:

- Interfere with core life functions (eating, sleeping, ability to maintain housing, interpersonal or sexual relations)
- Pose a threat to the life or well-being of the patient or others
- Significantly deviate from society's expectations or norms

We discuss specific diseases and conditions later in the chapter.

Pathophysiology of Psychiatric Disorders

The National Institutes of Health (NIH) estimates that up to 20 percent of the population has some type of mental health problem and that as many as one person in seven will actually require treatment for an emotional disturbance. These problems may be severely disabling and require inpatient care, or the patient may quietly tolerate them with no outward symptoms. That all people with psychiatric conditions exhibit bizarre or unusual behavior is a misconception. The small percentage of patients with psychiatric disorders who publicly exhibit bizarre behavior tend to create this misconception among lay people. In reality, most patients who suffer from disorders such as anxiety, depression, eating disorders, or mild personality disorders function normally on a daily basis, going unnoticed in society. Nonetheless, according to the Centers for Disease Control and Prevention (CDC), behavioral and psychiatric disorders incapacitate more people than all other health problems combined. Most patients with mental illness are cared for in outpatient settings such as public mental health centers. Only those with severe psychiatric illnesses remain institutionalized. Because of this, EMS providers are increasingly being called to care for patients with behavioral complaints. A common reason for EMS intervention in psychiatric illness is patients' failure to take their psychiatric medications. When mental health patients such as schizophrenics begin to deteriorate and develop bizarre behavior, more often than not they have not been adhering to their psychiatric medication regimen.

Another common misconception is that all mental patients are unstable and dangerous and that their conditions are incurable. This is simply not true. Research in psychiatry, like other areas in medicine, has made great strides in determining causes and treatments for many psychiatric conditions. Suffering from a mental disorder is not reason for embarrassment or shame, although society often stigmatizes these patients unfairly. The general causes of behavioral emergencies are biological (or organic), psychosocial, and sociocultural. Each of these three possible causes should guide your questioning during the patient interview. Keep in mind, however, that a patient's condition may result from more than one pathological process.

Biological

CONTENT REVIEW

➤ General Causes of Behavioral Emergencies
- Biological (organic)
- Psychosocial (personal)
- Social (situational)

For many years, medical practitioners have used the terms **biological** and **organic** interchangeably when discussing certain types of psychiatric disorders whose causes are physical rather than purely psychological. They result from disease processes such as infections and tumors or from structural changes in the brain such as those brought on by the abuse of alcohol or drugs (including over-the-counter and prescription medications). It could be argued, however, that even purely psychological conditions originate in the brain and, for that very reason, they are organic. Indeed, many psychiatric conditions do originate from alterations in brain chemistry.

Behavioral emergencies frequently involve biological conditions. Never assume that a patient with an altered mental status or unusual behavior is suffering from a purely psychological condition or disease until you have completely ruled out medical conditions and substance abuse.

Psychosocial

Psychosocial (personal) conditions are related to a patient's personality style, dynamics of unresolved conflict, or crisis management methods. These disorders are not attributable to substance abuse or medical conditions.

Environment plays a large part in psychosocial development. Traumatic childhood incidents may affect a person throughout life. Parents or other persons in positions of authority can have a tremendous impact on a child's development. Dysfunctional families, abusive parents, alcohol or drug abuse by parents, or neglect can cause behavioral problems from childhood through adulthood. Such conditions—in addition to, or in combination with, genetic predisposition and brain chemistry—form the basis for psychosocial conditions.

Patho Pearls

Medical Causes for Behavioral Emergencies. Although you may encounter a patient with a bona fide psychiatric problem, it is important to keep in mind that drug and alcohol use cause a significant number of aberrant and violent behavior problems. Whenever you encounter a violent patient or a patient with apparent acute psychosis, first try to identify a medical or toxicologic cause of the behavior. Many medical conditions, such as diabetes mellitus, can cause behavioral changes, as can trauma. Likewise, many medications and recreational drugs can cause behavior that is similar to that caused by mental illness. Always consider the possibility of drugs, alcohol, or an underlying medical condition or trauma in a patient with a behavioral emergency.

Sociocultural

Sociocultural (situational) causes of behavioral disorders are related to the patient's actions and interactions within society and to factors such as socioeconomic status, social habits, social skills, and values. These problems are usually attributable to events that change the patient's social space (relationships, support systems), social isolation, or otherwise have an impact on socialization.

Some events in the lives of children and adults that may cause a profound psychological change are rape, assault, witnessing the victimization of another, death of a loved one, and acts of violence such as war or riots. Events that occur over time may also have an impact on the individual. These include the loss of a job, economic problems such as poverty, and ongoing prejudice or discrimination. Sometimes, simply doing anything outside the norms of society can lead to stress and psychological changes.

Assessment of Behavioral Emergency Patients

The assessment and care of behavioral emergency patients is similar to that for other medical conditions. The order of assessment (scene size-up, primary assessment, focused history and physical examination) remains unchanged. Potential medical conditions that mimic behavioral emergencies require you to perform a thorough medical assessment.

Among the differences between your assessment and care of a patient with a medical condition and one with a behavioral emergency is that, as already noted, you actually begin your care at the same time you begin your assessment by developing a rapport with the patient. Interpersonal skills are important for all patients, but perhaps never more than for one who is experiencing a behavioral emergency. Additionally, the focused history and physical exam for a behavioral emergency includes a mental status examination.

Scene Size-Up

As with any call, determining scene safety is of the utmost importance. Approach the scene carefully. If a patient is experiencing a behavioral emergency that is significant enough to warrant EMS, it is most likely significant enough to have law enforcement authorities respond. Most patients experiencing behavioral emergencies or crises will not attack you; however, those who are behaving unusually, experiencing hallucinations or delusions, or are under the effect of a substance may become violent. Approach every patient cautiously to protect yourself and your crew from injury (Figure 11-1).

The scene size-up also includes making observations that relate to patient care. Look for evidence of substance use or abuse, for therapeutic medications that may indicate an underlying medical condition (or abuse of that medication), and for signs of violence or destruction of property. Examine the general environmental

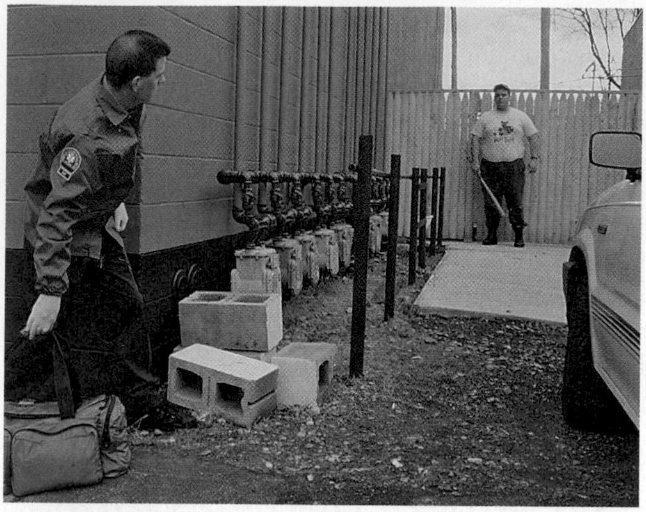

FIGURE 11-1 Approach every patient cautiously. If you determine a potential for violence, request police assistance.

condition and, when possible, observe the patient from a distance to note any visible behavior patterns or violent behavior.

Primary Assessment

Because many behavioral emergencies are caused by or concurrent with medical conditions, you should be acutely suspicious of life-threatening emergencies. As with any other injury or condition, assess the ABCs and intervene when necessary. Continue to observe the patient for any clues to his underlying condition. Be cautious of any overt behavior such as **posture** or hand gestures. Note any emotional response such as rage, **fear**, anxiety, **confusion**, or anger. Early in the evaluation try to determine the patient's **mental status**, the state of his cerebral functioning. Continue assessing mental status throughout the patient encounter by evaluating his awareness, orientation, cognitive abilities, and **affect** (visible indicators of mood).

Control the scene as soon as possible. Remove anyone who agitates the patient or adds confusion to the scene. Generally, a limited number of people around the patient is best. At times, performing an effective assessment and care may necessitate totally clearing a room or moving the patient to a quiet area. Finally, observe the patient's affect in greater detail. To avoid being grabbed or struck by the patient, stay alert for signs of aggression.

Secondary Assessment

Your examination of a patient experiencing a behavioral emergency is largely conversational. This makes your interpersonal technique very important. Just as starting an IV with poor technique most likely will not establish a patent IV line, interviewing with poor interpersonal skills most likely will not obtain significant information. Remove the patient from the crisis area and limit interruptions. Focus your questioning and assessment on the immediate problem and follow these guidelines:

- ***Listen.*** Ask open-ended questions (those that require more than a yes or no response). These will encourage your patient to respond in detail and share important information. Listen to the answer. Pay attention. No one likes being ignored. When you need information from a patient, listen.
- ***Spend time.*** Rushing the patient's answers, cutting him off, or appearing hurried will cause him to "shut down" and stop answering questions.
- ***Be assured.*** Communicate self-confidence, honesty, and professionalism.
- ***Do not threaten.*** Avoid rapid or sudden movements or questions that the patient might interpret as threats. Approach him slowly and confidently.
- ***Do not fear silence.*** Silence can be appropriate. Encourage the patient to tell his story, but do not be forceful or antagonizing.
- ***Place yourself at the patient's level.*** Standing over the patient may be intimidating. Unless you are intentionally attempting to gain a position of authority, crouch, kneel, or sit near the patient. Do not position yourself where you cannot respond appropriately to danger or attack.
- ***Keep a safe and proper distance.*** The surest way to make a behavioral emergency patient violent is to invade his "personal space" (Figure 11-2). This is an area within an approximately 3-foot radius around every person; encroaching on it causes anxiety. If appropriate, however, you may touch the patient's

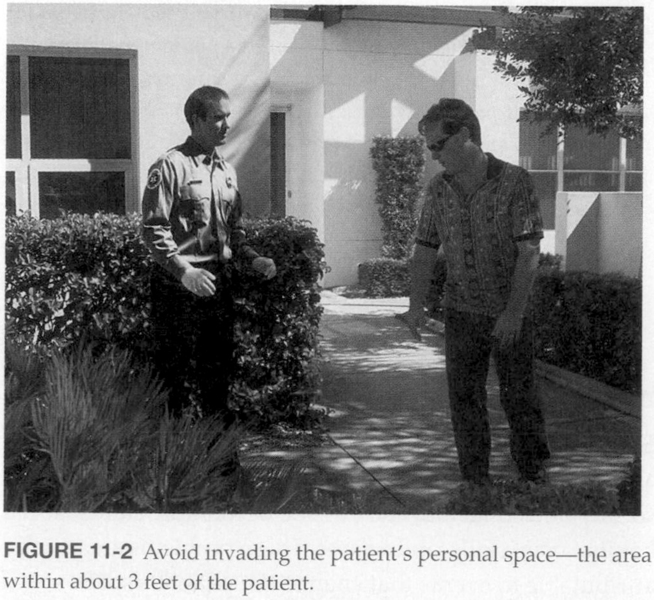

FIGURE 11-2 Avoid invading the patient's personal space—the area within about 3 feet of the patient.

shoulder or use another consoling touch when he allows.

- *Appear comfortable.* Do not appear uncomfortable—even if you are. Talking to patients about suicide, self-mutilation, or other psychological conditions is difficult. If the patient sees that you are uncomfortable, however, he is unlikely to open up to you. Would you expect a patient to tell you his reasons for attempting suicide when you appear uncomfortable even saying the word? To help, use terms the patient has used. If he says he wanted to "end it all," begin with that. Caregivers sometimes hesitate to use the word *suicide* because it might give the patient ideas of suicide. If you are there to care for a suicidal or potentially suicidal patient, however, he has already had those thoughts.
- *Avoid appearing judgmental.* Patients who are experiencing behavioral emergencies may feel strong emotions toward their caregivers. The patient should believe that you are interested in his condition and welfare. Be supportive and empathetic, and avoid judgments, pity, anger, or any other emotions that may damage your relationship with the patient.
- *Never lie to the patient.* Honesty is the best policy. Do not reinforce false beliefs or hallucinations or mislead the patient in any way.

Mental Status Examination

As part of the focused history and physical examination for behavioral emergencies, do not overlook any physical or medical complaint. In addition to the medical evaluation, which is covered in depth throughout this and the other volumes of this program, your examination of the patient with psychiatric or behavioral disorders should include a psychological evaluation, also known as a **mental status examination (MSE)** . The components of the MSE include:

- *General appearance.* The patient's appearance can provide important information when looking at his "big picture." Observe hygiene, clothing, and overall appearance.
- *Behavioral observations.* Observe verbal or nonverbal behavior, strange or threatening appearance, or facial expressions. Note tone of voice, rate, volume, and quality.
- *Orientation.* Does the patient know who he is and who others are? Is he oriented to current events? Can he concentrate on simple questions and answer them?
- *Memory.* Is the patient's memory intact for recent and long-term events?
- *Sensorium.* Is the patient focused? Paying attention? What is his level of awareness?
- *Perceptual processes.* Are the patient's thought patterns ordered? Does he appear to have any hallucinations, delusions, or phobias?
- *Mood and affect.* Observe for indicators of the patient's mood. Is it appropriate? What is his prevailing emotion? Depression, elation, anxiety, or agitation? Other?
- *Intelligence.* Evaluate the patient's speech. What is his level of vocabulary? His ability to formulate an idea?
- *Thought processes.* What is the patient's apparent form of thought? Are his thoughts logical and coherent?
- *Insight.* Does the patient have insight into his own problem? Does he recognize that a problem exists? Does he deny or blame others for his problem?
- *Judgment.* Does the patient base his life decisions on sound, reasonable judgments? Does he approach problems thoughtfully, carefully, and rationally?
- *Psychomotor.* Does the patient exhibit an unusual posture or is he making unusual movements? Patients with hallucinations may react to them. For example, a patient who believes he is covered with insects may be picking at his skin to remove the "bugs."

Psychiatric Medications

Many patients who suffer from psychiatric or behavioral disorders are under the care of a mental health professional and may be taking prescription medications. During the interview and history-taking process, determine whether the patient is taking medications and, if so, what type. The patient's use of such medications can provide clues to his underlying condition. Additionally, if a patient is not taking a medication as directed, his condition may deteriorate. Some schizophrenic patients may receive periodic injections of extremely long-acting antipsychotics (for example, haloperidol decanoate) because of poor compliance. They will often carry an identification card or may report that they "go to the clinic every three weeks for a shot." Types of psychiatric medications are discussed in the chapter "Emergency Pharmacology."

Specific Psychiatric Disorders

Almost all psychiatric disorders have two diagnostic elements: symptoms of the disease or disorder and indications that the disease or disorder has impaired major life functions, resulting in loss of relationships, a job, or housing, or in another significant social problem. To define specific conditions, mental health professionals use the *Diagnostic and*

Statistical Manual of Mental Disorders, Fifth Edition (DSM-5). Published by the American Psychiatric Association (APA), the DSM-5 details diagnostic criteria for all currently defined psychiatric disorders, which are grouped according to the patient's signs and symptoms. The recognized types of behavioral and psychiatric disorders include:

- Cognitive disorders
- Schizophrenia
- Anxiety disorders
- Mood disorders
- Substance-related disorders
- Somatoform disorders
- Factitious disorders
- Dissociative disorders
- Eating disorders
- Personality disorders
- Impulse control disorders

The following summaries of these illnesses' major criteria do not imply that you should diagnose behavioral disorders. Even for skilled psychologists and psychiatrists, diagnosis is complicated by the considerable overlap in symptoms from one disease to another. A patient may actually fit into several categories. You should use the information here only as a guide to better understand the science of psychiatry and the criteria applied to patients with behavioral emergencies. Knowledge of these terms and conditions will also allow you to communicate better with psychiatric care providers.

Cognitive Disorders

Psychiatric disorders with organic causes, such as brain injury or disease, are known as *cognitive disorders*. This family of disorders includes conditions caused by metabolic disease, infections, neoplasm, endocrine disease, degenerative neurologic disease, and cardiovascular disease. They might also be caused by physical or chemical injuries due to trauma, drug abuse, or reactions to prescribed drugs. The specific brain pathology will differ based on the type of disease. Two types of cognitive disorders are delirium and dementia.

DELIRIUM **Delirium** is characterized by a relatively rapid onset of widespread disorganized thought. These patients suffer from inattention, memory impairment, disorientation, and a general clouding of consciousness. In some cases, individuals may experience vivid visual hallucinations. Delirium is characterized by a fairly acute onset (hours or days) and may be reversible. Delirium may be due to a medical condition, substance intoxication, substance withdrawal, or multiple etiologies. Confusion is a hallmark of delirium.

CONTENT REVIEW

➤ Cognitive Disorders
- Delirium
- Dementia

DEMENTIA **Dementia** may be due to several medical problems. Included among the more common causes of dementia are Alzheimer's disease (both early and late onset), vascular problems, AIDS, head trauma, Parkinson's disease, and substance abuse. Regardless of its cause, dementia involves memory impairment, cognitive disturbance, and pervasive impairment of abstract thinking and judgment. Unlike delirium, dementia usually develops over months and, in many cases, is irreversible.

Dementia involves cognitive deficits manifested by both memory impairment (diminished ability to learn new information or to recall previously learned information) and one or more of the following cognitive disturbances:

- *Aphasia*—impaired ability to communicate.
- *Apraxia*—impaired ability to carry out motor activities despite intact sensory function.
- *Agnosia*—failure to recognize objects or stimuli despite intact sensory function.
- ***Disturbance in executive functioning***—impaired ability to plan, organize, or sequence.

These conditions must significantly impair social or occupational functioning and represent a significant decline from a previous level of functioning. Your approach to patients with either of these conditions should be supportive. Assess and manage any medical complaints or conditions and transport to an appropriate medical facility.

Schizophrenia

Schizophrenia is a common mental health problem, affecting an estimated 1 percent of the U.S. population. Its hallmark is a significant change in behavior and a loss of contact with reality. Signs and symptoms often include hallucinations, delusions, and depression. The schizophrenic patient may live in his "own world" and be preoccupied with inner fantasies. Although several biological and psychosocial theories attempt to explain the condition and its manifestations, its definitive cause is unknown.

The symptoms of schizophrenia include:

- **Delusions**—Fixed, false beliefs that are not widely held within the context of the individual's cultural or religious group
- **Hallucinations**—Sensory perceptions with no basis in reality; often auditory ("hearing voices")
- ***Disorganized speech***—Frequent derailment or incoherence

CONTENT REVIEW

➤ Major Types of Schizophrenia
- Paranoid
- Disorganized
- Catatonic
- Undifferentiated

- **Catatonia**—Grossly disorganized behavior
- **Flat affect** Reduced or absent emotional expressiveness

A diagnosis of schizophrenia requires that two or more symptoms must each be present for a significant portion of each month over the course of six months. The symptoms must cause a social or occupational dysfunction (decline in social relations or work from the predisease state). Most schizophrenics are diagnosed in early adulthood.

The DSM-5 defines several major types of schizophrenia:

- *Paranoid*—the patient is preoccupied with a feeling of persecution and may suffer delusions or auditory hallucinations.
- *Disorganized*—the patient often displays disorganized behavior, dress, or speech.
- *Catatonic*—the patient exhibits catatonic rigidity, immobility, stupor, or peculiar voluntary movements. Catatonic schizophrenia is exceedingly rare.
- *Undifferentiated*—the patient does not readily fit into one of the categories above.

Your approach to the schizophrenic patient should be supportive and nonjudgmental. Do not reinforce the patient's hallucinations, but understand that he considers them real. Speak openly and honestly with him. Be encouraging, yet realistic. Remain alert for aggressive behavior, and restrain the patient if he becomes violent or presents a danger to you, to himself, or to others.

Anxiety and Related Disorders

The group of illnesses known as **anxiety disorders** is characterized by dominating apprehension and fear. These disorders affect approximately 2 to 4 percent of the population. Broadly defined, **anxiety** is a state of uneasiness, discomfort, apprehension, and restlessness. More specifically, anxiety disorders fall into three categories: panic disorder, phobia, and post-traumatic stress disorder.

CONTENT REVIEW

➤ Anxiety-Related Disorders
- Panic attack
- Phobia
- Post-traumatic stress syndrome

PANIC ATTACK The DSM-5 does not list **panic attacks** in themselves as a disease. Characterized by recurrent, extreme periods of anxiety resulting in great emotional distress, they are symptoms of disease and are included among the criteria for other disorders (panic disorder, agoraphobia). Panic attacks differ from generalized feelings of anxiety in their acute nature. They are usually unprovoked, peaking within 10 minutes of their onset and dissipating in less than 1 hour.

The presentation of panic and anxiety may resemble a cardiac or respiratory condition. This presents a dilemma for EMS personnel. Ruling out those conditions is difficult in the prehospital setting; psychiatrists usually diagnose anxiety or panic disorders by excluding known medical conditions. Keys to identifying panic or anxiety in the field are the patient's having a history of the condition and being outside the expected age range for certain cardiac or respiratory illnesses. This, of course, is not to say that young people cannot have myocardial infarction. Many symptoms of panic resemble those of hyperventilation, and some do appear to be correlated, such as the paresthesia from panic being due largely to hyperventilation.

The diagnostic criteria for a panic attack require a discrete period of intense fear or discomfort, during which four or more of the following symptoms develop abruptly and reach a peak within 10 minutes:

- Palpitations, pounding heart, or accelerated heart rate
- Sweating
- Trembling or shaking
- Sensations of shortness of breath or smothering
- Feeling of choking
- Chest pain or discomfort
- Nausea or abdominal distress
- Feeling dizzy, unsteady, lightheaded, or faint
- Derealization (feelings of unreality) or depersonalization (being detached from oneself)
- Fear of losing control or going crazy
- Fear of dying
- Paresthesia (numbness or tingling sensations)
- Chills or hot flashes

Management for anxiety disorders is generally simple and supportive. Show empathy. Assess any medical complaints and manage them appropriately. If the patient experiences hyperventilation, calm and reassure him to help decrease his respiratory rate to normal. Patients with severe or incapacitating symptoms may benefit from the administration of a sedative. Benzodiazepines, such as diazepam (Valium) and lorazepam (Ativan), can be administered in the prehospital setting. In addition, antihistamines, such as hydroxyzine (Vistaril) and diphenhydramine (Benadryl), have sedative effects and are useful in treating patients with significant anxiety. Consult medical direction in accordance with local protocol and transport to an appropriate medical facility.

PHOBIAS Everyone has some source of fear or anxiety that they consciously avoid. When this fear becomes excessive and interferes with functioning, it is termed a **phobia**. A phobia—generally considered an intense, irrational fear—may be due to animals, the sight of blood (or injection or injury), situational factors (elevators, enclosed spaces), or environmental conditions (heights or water). Exposure to the situation or item will induce anxiety or a panic attack. Some patients experience extreme phobias that prevent or limit their normal daily activities. For example, a patient suffering from agoraphobia (fear of crowds) may confine himself to his home and avoid ever venturing outdoors. In most patients, however, the phobia is less severe; the patient realizes that his fear is unreasonable, and the anxiety dissipates.

Management for a patient with a phobia is supportive. Understand that the patient's fear is very real. Do not force him to do anything that he opposes. Manage any underlying problems and transport for evaluation.

POST-TRAUMATIC STRESS DISORDER EMS providers often are particularly interested in **post-traumatic stress disorder (PTSD)** because their responsibilities may make them susceptible to it. Originally recognized on the battlefields of war, post-traumatic stress disorder (PTSD) is a reaction to an extreme, usually life-threatening stressor such as a natural disaster, victimization (rape, for instance), or other emotionally taxing situation. It is characterized by a desire to avoid similar situations, recurrent intrusive thoughts, depression, sleep disturbances, nightmares, and persistent symptoms of increased arousal. The patient may feel guilty for having survived the incident, and substance abuse may frequently complicate his condition.

Treat any PTSD patient with respect, empathy, and support, and transport the patient to an appropriate facility for evaluation.

Mood Disorders

The DSM-5 defines mood as "a pervasive and sustained emotion that colors a person's perception of the world." Common examples of mood alterations include depression, elation, **anger**, and anxiety. The main **mood disorders** are depression and bipolar disorder.

DEPRESSION **Depression** is characterized by a profound sadness or feeling of melancholy. It is common in everyday life and is to be expected following the breakup of a relationship or the loss of a loved one. Most of us have experienced some sort of depression, at least in its mildest form. It is one of the most prevalent psychiatric conditions, affecting from 10 to 15 percent of the population. When depression becomes prolonged or severe, however, it is diagnosed as a *major depressive episode.*

CONTENT REVIEW

- Mood Disorders
  - Depression
  - Bipolar disorder

The symptoms of major depressive disorder include:

- Depressed mood most of the day, nearly every day, as indicated by subjective report or observation by others
- Markedly diminished interest in pleasure in all, or almost all, activities most of the day nearly every day
- Significant weight loss (without dieting) or weight gain—a 5 percent change in body weight is considered significant
- Insomnia or hypersomnia nearly every day
- Psychomotor agitation or retardation every day (observable by others, not just the subjective feeling of the patient)
- Feelings of worthlessness or excessive inappropriate guilt (may be delusional) nearly every day
- Diminished ability to think or concentrate, or indecisiveness nearly every day
- Recurrent thoughts of death (not just fear of dying), recurrent suicidal ideation without a specific plan, or a suicide attempt or a specific plan for committing suicide (Depression greatly increases the risk of suicide.)

The diagnostic criteria for major depressive disorder require that five or more of the symptoms have been present during the same two-week period and represent a change from previous functioning; at least one of the symptoms must be either a depressed mood or loss of interest in pleasure. The condition must cause clinically significant distress or impairment in social, occupational, or other important functions. Further, it must not meet the criteria for a mixed episode (mixtures of mania and depression); it must not be due to the direct physiologic effects of a substance such as drug abuse or a medication, or to a general medical condition such as hypothyroidism; finally, it must not be better accounted for by **bereavement**. The acronym *In SAD CAGES* provides a screening mnemonic for major depression.

- **I**nterest
- **S**leep
- **A**ppetite
- **D**epressed mood
- **C**oncentration
- **A**ctivity
- **G**uilt
- **E**nergy
- **S**uicide

Depression may occur as an isolated condition, but it is often accompanied by other disorders such as substance abuse, anxiety disorders, and schizophrenia. Depression can also affect a patient without meeting all the identified clinical criteria. It can affect different people in different ways and is often atypical. Bereavement is one of the situations in which depression is expected. If the depression lasts longer than two months or is accompanied by suicidal ideation or marked functional impairment, however, it could be classified as a major depressive episode. Depression is more prevalent in females and is spread evenly throughout the life span.

BIPOLAR DISORDER **Bipolar disorder** is characterized by one or more **manic** episodes (periods of elation), with or without subsequent or alternating periods of depression. In the past, the term *manic-depressive* was used to describe this condition. Bipolar disorder is not particularly common, affecting approximately less than 1 percent of the population.

Manic-depressive episodes are not the "Jekyll and Hyde" transformations that television and the movies often portray. However, they often begin suddenly and escalate rapidly over a few days. In contrast to major depressive disorders, bipolar disorders usually develop in adolescence or early adulthood and occur as often in males as in females. Some patients with major depressive episodes will eventually develop a bipolar disorder and experience manic episodes. Commonly, patients have several depressive episodes before having a manic episode.

The diagnostic criteria for a manic episode require a distinct period of abnormally and persistently elevated, expansive, or irritable mood lasting for at least one week (or for any duration when hospitalization is necessary). Three or more (four or more if the mood is only irritable) of the following symptoms must have been present to a certain degree and must have persisted during that time:

- Inflated self-esteem or grandiosity
- Decreased need for sleep
- More talkative than usual or pressure to keep talking
- Flight of ideas or subjective experience that thoughts are racing
- Distractibility
- Increase in goal-directed activity (socially, at work or school, or sexually) or psychomotor agitation
- Excessive involvement in pleasurable activities that have a high potential for painful consequences (buying sprees, sexual indiscretions, foolish business investments)
- Delusional thoughts (grandiose ideas or unrealistic plans)

The symptoms must not meet the criteria for a mixed episode. The mood disturbance must be severe enough to markedly impair occupational or social functioning, to require hospitalizing the patient to prevent harm to him or others, or present with psychotic features. As with depression, the symptoms must not be due to the direct physiologic effects of a substance or a general medical condition. Patients with bipolar illness are often prescribed medications for treatment. These may include lithium, selected anticonvulsants, antidepressants, antipsychotics, and/or benzodiazepines.

Management of these patients includes maintaining a calm, protective environment. Avoid confronting the manic patient. Never leave a depressed or suicidal patient alone. Assess and manage any other coexisting medical problems, and transport to an appropriate medical facility. Bipolar patients in an extreme manic phase may be overtly psychotic. In these cases, medication with an antipsychotic medication such as haloperidol may be indicated. Always contact medical direction for treatment options.

Substance-Related Disorders

Substance abuse is a common disorder. Many patients you will encounter in EMS will be under the influence of one or many substances (Figure 11-3). Any patient exhibiting symptoms of a psychiatric or behavioral disorder should be screened for substance use and/or abuse. Substance abuse patients may present as being depressed, psychotic, or delirious, and their signs and symptoms may mimic those of many behavioral disorders. The DSM-5 lists substance abuse as a psychiatric disorder; you should consider it a serious condition. Any mood-altering chemical has the potential for abuse. Alcohol is a common part of our culture, but can be abused. The user of a substance may be intoxicated from the effects of the

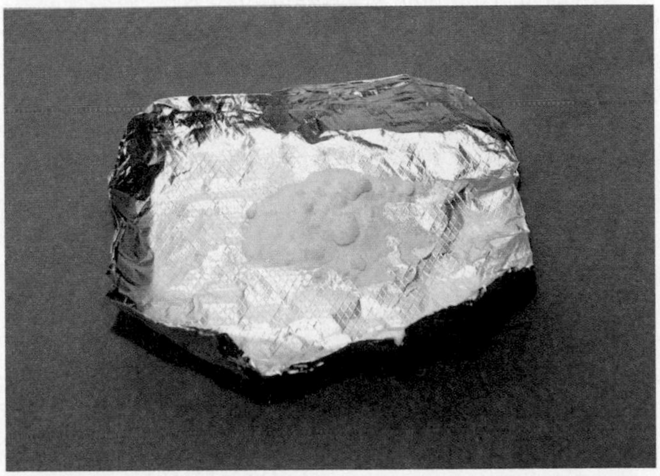

FIGURE 11-3 Crystal meth (powder amphetamine) is an intensely addictive drug that has a stimulant effect on the user's central nervous system. Created in underground labs across the country and around the world, its ingredients are easily found in most households and over-the-counter products.

(U.S. Drug Enforcement Administration)

chemical or may be ill from addiction or withdrawal of the chemical. Intoxication, in and of itself, may cause behavioral problems.

Repetitive use of a mood-altering chemical may lead to dependence or addiction. Dependence on a substance is characterized by repeated use of the substance. Dependence may be psychological, physical, or both. Psychological dependence is marked by a compelling desire to use the substance, inability to reduce or stop use, and repeated efforts to quit. Physical dependence is characterized by the need for increased amounts of the chemical to obtain the desired effect. Also, the presence of withdrawal symptoms when the substance is reduced or stopped is characteristic of physical dependence. All drugs have the potential to cause psychological dependence; many have the potential to cause physical dependence as well.

Somatoform Disorders

Somatoform disorders are characterized by physical symptoms that have no apparent physiologic cause. They are believed to be attributable to psychological factors. People who suffer from somatoform disorders believe their symptoms are serious and real. The major types of somatoform disorder are:

- ***Somatization disorder***—the patient is preoccupied with physical symptoms.
- ***Conversion disorder***—the patient sustains a loss of function, usually involving the nervous system (for instance, blindness or paralysis), unexplained by any medical illness.
- ***Hypochondriasis***—exaggerated interpretation of physical symptoms as a serious illness.
- ***Body dysmorphic disorder***—the patient believes he has a defect in physical appearance.
- ***Pain disorder***—the patient suffers from pain, usually severe, that is unexplained by a physical ailment.

Somatoform disorders are often difficult to identify and diagnose. They can mimic and be confused with various bona fide physical conditions. Never attribute physical symptoms to a behavioral disorder until medical conditions have been ruled out.

CONTENT REVIEW

- ➤ Somatoform Disorders
  - Somatization disorder
  - Conversion disorder
  - Hypochondriasis
  - Body dysmorphic disorder
  - Pain disorder

Factitious Disorders

Factitious disorders are sometimes confused with somatoform disorders. They are characterized by the following three criteria:

- An intentional production of physical or psychological signs or symptoms.
- Motivation for the behavior is to assume the "sick role."
- External incentives for the behavior (e.g., economic gain, avoiding work, avoiding police) are absent.

Although patients suffering from factitious disorders essentially feign their illnesses, that does not preclude the possibility of true physical or psychological symptoms. The disorder is apparently more common in males than in females. In severe cases, patients will go to great length to obtain medical or psychological treatment. Patients with factitious disorders often will voluntarily produce symptoms and will present with a very plausible history. They often have an extensive knowledge of medical terminology and can be very demanding and disruptive. In severe cases (Munchausen syndrome), patients will undergo multiple surgical operations and other painful procedures.

Dissociative Disorders

Dissociative disorders occur as a response to significant, usually multiple or ongoing, life-threatening traumatic experiences. The person unconsciously disassociates, or separates themselves, from the trauma as a way of coping. Dissociation is a disruption of identity, memory, emotions, perceptions, and even behavior (Potter & Moller, 2020). Dissociative disorders include dissociative identity disorder, dissociative amnesia, and depersonalization/derealization disorder.

PSYCHOGENIC AMNESIA Whereas amnesia is a partial or total *inability* to recall or identify past events, **psychogenic amnesia** is a *failure* to recall. The "forgotten" material is present but "hidden" beneath the level of consciousness.

FUGUE STATE An amnesic individual may withdraw even further by retreating in what is known as a **fugue state**. A patient in a fugue state actually flees as a defense mechanism and may travel hundreds of miles from home.

DISSOCIATIVE IDENTITY DISORDER **Dissociative identity disorder** occurs when an individual develops one or more separate identities as a way of coping with traumatic memories, usually of horrific and ongoing abuse.

CONTENT REVIEW

- ➤ Dissociative Disorders
  - Psychogenic amnesia
  - Fugue state
  - Dissociative Identity Disorder
  - Depersonalization

DEPERSONALIZATION **Depersonalization** is a relatively more frequent dissociative disorder

CONTENT REVIEW

- Eating Disorders
  - Anorexia nervosa
  - Bulimia nervosa

that occurs predominantly in young adults. Patients experience a loss of the sense of one's self. Such individuals suddenly feel "different"—that they are someone else or that their body has taken on a different form. The disorder is often precipitated by acute stress.

Eating Disorders

The two classifications of eating disorders are anorexia nervosa and bulimia nervosa. Both generally occur between adolescence and the age of 25. The condition afflicts women more than men at a rate of 20:1.

ANOREXIA NERVOSA Anorexia is the loss of appetite. **Anorexia nervosa** is a disorder marked by excessive fasting. Individuals with this disorder have an intense fear of obesity and often complain of being fat even though their body weight is low. They suffer from weight loss (25 percent of body weight or more), refusal to maintain body weight, and often a cessation of menstruation from severe malnutrition.

BULIMIA NERVOSA Recurrent episodes of seemingly uncontrollable binge eating with compensatory self-induced vomiting or diarrhea, excessive exercise, or dieting and with a full awareness of the behavior's abnormality characterize **bulimia nervosa**. Individuals often display personality traits of perfectionism, low self-esteem, and social withdrawal.

The weight loss and body changes experienced by anorexic and bulimic patients can lead to serious physical problems. Starvation and attempts to purge can have drastic consequences, such as anemia, dehydration, vitamin deficiencies, hypoglycemia, and cardiovascular problems. In addition to psychological support, prehospital care is likely to include treatment for dehydration and physical problems. Both disorders have a high potential morbidity and mortality.

Personality Disorders

Most adults' personalities are attuned to social demands. Some individuals, however, often seem ill equipped to function adequately in society. These people might be suffering from a **personality disorder**. Stemming largely from immature and distorted personality development, these personality, or character, disorders result in persistently maladaptive ways of perceiving, thinking, and relating to the world.

The broad category of personality disorder includes problems that vary greatly in form and severity. Although others might describe them as "eccentric" or "troublesome," some patients with personality disorders function adequately. In extreme cases, patients act out against or attempt to manipulate society.

Personality Disorder Clusters

The DSM-5 groups similar personality disorders into three broad types: cluster A, cluster B, and cluster C. The disorders in each cluster have similar features.

CLUSTER A Individuals in cluster A often act odd or eccentric. Their unusual behavior can take drastically different forms. This cluster includes the following:

- ***Paranoid personality disorder***—pattern of distrust and suspiciousness
- ***Schizoid personality disorder***—pattern of detachment from social relationships
- ***Schizotypal personality disorder***—pattern of acute discomfort in close relationships, cognitive distortions, and eccentric behavior

CLUSTER B Individuals in cluster B often appear dramatic, emotional, or fearful. This cluster includes the following:

- ***Antisocial personality disorder***—pattern of disregard for the rights of others
- ***Borderline personality disorder***—pattern of instability in interpersonal relationships, self-image, and impulsivity
- ***Histrionic personality disorder***—pattern of excessive emotions and attention seeking
- ***Narcissistic personality disorder***—pattern of grandiosity, need for admiration, and lack of empathy

CLUSTER C Individuals in cluster C often appear anxious or fearful. This cluster includes the following:

- ***Avoidant personality disorder***—pattern of social inhibition, feelings of inadequacy, and hypersensitivity to criticism
- ***Dependent personality disorder***—pattern of submissive and clinging behavior related to an excessive need to be cared for
- ***Obsessive-compulsive disorder***—pattern of preoccupation with orderliness, perfectionism, and control

CONTENT REVIEW

- Personality Disorder Clusters
  - Cluster A personality disorders
    - Paranoid
    - Schizoid
    - Schizotypal
  - Cluster B personality disorders
    - Antisocial
    - Borderline
    - Histrionic
    - Narcissistic
  - Cluster C personality disorders
    - Avoidant
    - Dependent
    - Obsessive-compulsive

Diagnosing a personality disorder requires evaluating the individual's long-term functioning and behavior. In many cases, the individual suffers from multiple disorders. A complete interview, history, and assessment will assist you in determining your approach. Your prehospital care will vary based on the patient's chief complaint and overall presentation.

Impulse Control Disorders

Related to the personality disorders are the **impulse control disorders**. Recurrent impulses and the patient's failure to control them characterize these disorders. Examples of impulse control disorders include:

- ***Kleptomania***—a recurrent failure to resist impulses to steal objects not for immediate use or for their monetary value
- ***Pyromania***—a recurrent failure to resist impulses to set fires
- ***Pathological gambling***—a chronic and progressive preoccupation with gambling and the urge to gamble
- ***Trichotillomania***—a recurrent impulse to pull out one's own hair
- ***Intermittent explosive disorder***—recurrent and paroxysmal episodes of significant loss of control of aggressive responses

Disorders of impulse control may be harmful to the patient and others. Before committing the act, the patient will have an increasing sense of tension. After the act, he will either have pleasure gratification or release.

Suicide

Suicide, simply stated, occurs when a person intentionally takes his own life. Suicide is alarmingly common. It is the ninth leading cause of death overall, and it is the third leading cause in the 15- to 24-year age group. Suicide rates have risen dramatically in the younger age groups and have also increased significantly in the elderly population. Women attempt suicide more than men, but men—especially those over 55 years of age—are more likely to succeed. Statistically, suicide successes and methods vary widely by race, sex, and culture. The most common methods of suicide (2014) are:

1. Bullet wound (60 percent)
2. Poisoning/overdose (18 percent)
3. Strangulation/suffocation (15 percent)
4. Cutting (1 percent)
5. Other, or unspecified (6 percent)

Assessing Potentially Suicidal Patients

In cases of attempted suicide, many focus on whether the patient really wanted to kill himself. Indeed, this question will be at the heart of the patient's future psychiatric care, and information from the paramedic will be crucial to making that determination. However, never lose sight of patient care while probing the psychological nature of attempted suicide.

Perform an appropriate focused history and physical exam concurrently with providing sound psychological care. Mental health professionals are rarely on the scene. It is up to you to document observations at the scene, especially any detailed suicide plans, any suicide notes, and any statements of the patient and bystanders. This information may not be available after the event when the patient receives psychiatric screening at the hospital. Such care and observations at the scene, combined with detailed documentation, are critical to the patient's long-term psychological care.

Risk Factors for Suicide

The risk factors for suicide are numerous. When assessing a patient who has indicated suicidal intentions, screen for any of these risk factors:

- Previous attempts (Eighty percent of persons who successfully commit suicide have made a previous attempt.)
- Depression (Suicide is 500 times more common among patients who are severely depressed than those who are not.)
- Age (Incidence is high between the ages of 15 and 24 years and over the age of 40.)
- Alcohol or drug abuse
- Divorce or widowhood (The rate is five times higher than among other groups.)
- Giving away personal belongings, especially cherished possessions
- Living alone or in increased isolation
- The presence of **psychosis** with depression (for example, suicidal or destructive thoughts or hallucinations about killing or death)
- Homosexuality (especially homosexuals who are depressed, aging, alcoholic, or HIV infected)
- Major separation trauma (mate, loved one, job, money)
- Major physical stresses (surgery, childbirth, sleep deprivation)
- Loss of independence (disabling illness)
- Lack of goals and plans for the future
- Suicide of same-sexed parent or other family member

- Expression of a plan for committing suicide
- Possession of the mechanism for suicide (gun, pills, rope)

Patients who have attempted suicide must be evaluated in a hospital or psychiatric facility. Many people assume that "they were just looking for attention." Applied to the wrong patient, that conjecture may contribute to his death.

Age-Related Conditions

Some behavioral disorders are particularly common among patients at the ends of the age spectrum—the young and the elderly. Your awareness of age-related conditions will help you to assess and interact with these patients.

Crisis in the Geriatric Patient

Common physical problems among the elderly include dementia, chronic illness, and diminished eyesight and hearing. The elderly also experience depression that is often mistaken for dementia. When confronted with an elderly person in a crisis, take the following steps:

- Assess the patient's ability to communicate.
- Provide continual reassurance.
- Compensate for the patient's loss of sight and hearing with reassuring physical contact.
- Treat the patient with respect. Call the patient by name and title, such as "Mrs. Jones." Avoid such terms as "dear," "honey," and "babe."
- Avoid administering medication.
- Describe what you are going to do before you do it.
- Take your time. Do not convey the impression that you are in a hurry.
- Allow family members and friends to remain with the patient, if possible.

Crisis in the Pediatric Patient

Behavioral emergencies are not limited to adults. Children also have behavioral crises. Although the child's developmental stage will affect his behavior, these general guidelines will assist you when confronting an emotionally distraught or disruptive child.

- Avoid separating a young child from his parent.
- Attempt to prevent the child from seeing things that will increase his distress.
- Make all explanations brief and simple, and repeat them often.
- Be calm and speak slowly.
- Identify yourself by giving both your name and your function.
- Be truthful with the child. Telling the truth will develop trust.
- Encourage the child to help with his care.
- Reassure the child by carrying out all interventions gently.
- Do not discourage the child from crying or showing emotion.
- If you must be separated from the child, introduce the person who will assume responsibility for his care.
- Allow the child to keep a favorite blanket or toy.
- Do not leave the child alone, even for a short period.

Always be mindful of every young or elderly patient's uniqueness. Treat him equally and fairly, as you would any other patient.

Excited Delirium Syndrome

Excited delirium syndrome, also called *agitated delirium*, appears to be a factor in sudden death associated with restraint situations. Excited delirium is both a mental state and physiologic arousal that appears to result from increased dopamine levels in the brain. Excited delirium can be caused by drug intoxication (including alcohol), psychiatric illness, or a combination of both. Cocaine and other stimulants are well-known causes of drug-induced excited delirium. Often, however, an exact cause cannot be determined.[1]

Differentiating someone in excited delirium from someone who is simply violent is often difficult. People suffering from excited delirium may have:

- An abnormal tolerance of pain (100%)
- Tachypnea (100%)
- Sweating (95%)
- Agitation (95%)
- Skin that feels hot to touch (95%)
- Noncompliance toward police (90%)
- Lack of tiring (90%)
- Unusual strength (90%)
- Inappropriate clothing (70%)

It may become apparent that a patient is suffering from excited delirium only when he suddenly collapses. Beware of the patient who becomes suddenly tranquil after frenzied activity. This is often followed by cardiac collapse and death.[2,3]

Many deaths from excited delirium cannot be prevented. However, excited delirium must always be suspected when a patient is restrained. Paramedics should have a low threshold for using chemical restraint in the patient with possible excited delirium. Allowing the patient to struggle against restraints is a risk factor for sudden death.

Management of Behavioral Emergencies

Patients who are experiencing behavioral emergencies require both medical and psychological care. In general, take the following measures when you treat a patient who is experiencing a behavioral emergency:

1. Ensure scene safety and use Standard Precautions.
2. Provide a supportive and calm environment.
3. Treat any existing medical conditions.
4. Do not allow the suicidal patient to be alone.
5. Do not confront or argue with the patient.
6. Provide realistic reassurance.
7. Respond to the patient in a direct, simple manner.
8. Transport to an appropriate receiving facility.

Remember to treat the whole patient. Never overlook any serious, or potentially serious medical complaints while focusing on the psychiatric assessment.

TASERed Patients

In the course of your duties as a paramedic, you may be called on to examine a patient who has been restrained with a TASER device. A TASER is a nonlethal (sometimes called less-lethal) weapon used by law enforcement officers to subdue subjects. It uses an electrical current to disrupt voluntary control of the skeletal muscles and cause pain. The term TASER is an acronym for "Thomas A. Swift's Electric Rifle." Tom Swift, the character in many juvenile science fiction books, was the childhood hero of the inventor of the device. TASERs are highly effective and can decrease the use of lethal force by law enforcement officers. They also decrease the injury rate in both officers and subjects/prisoners. Although these weapons are considered less lethal, they can cause injury. Fortunately, most of these injuries are minor. However, it has become common practice for law enforcement to ask EMS personnel to evaluate subjects/prisoners who have been tased before they go to jail or after they have arrived at jail.

The TASER fires two small dart-like electrodes that make contact with the skin. These darts are powered by compressed nitrogen gas. Each dart is connected to the weapon by a small wire. Once in place, an electrical current is sent through the wires and into the subject. This usually results in incapacitation of the subject and/or pain. Generally speaking, the darts will work virtually anywhere on the body and do not need to penetrate or contact the skin to function properly. The benefit of the TASER is that it is immediately effective. It works as soon as the darts come into contact with the suspect. Typically, the electrical pulse lasts for 5 seconds. In some instances, it is necessary to repeat the electrical pulse to subdue some subjects.

Injuries from a TASER are generally classified as direct or secondary. Direct injuries generally result from the impact of the probe. The probes are propelled by nitrogen gas and can travel 20 to 25 feet (less in the civilian model). They can damage sensitive structures such as the eyes, face, and genitalia. Secondary injuries can result from the muscle contraction that occurs with the electrical pulse. They can also occur from resultant blunt trauma when the patient falls as a result of the muscle contraction. There is a danger of igniting combustible gases, if present. There have been some concerns expressed about the cardiorespiratory effects of the electrical pulse on certain subjects. However, research has failed to document or reproduce changes in electrolyte distribution, respiratory inhibition, or the development of cardiac arrhythmias. Although the device uses high voltage, the wattage is actually very low. The energy delivered with a TASER pulse is approximately 0.36 joules. This is considerably less than the amount of energy necessary to affect the heart.

As a paramedic, you may be summoned to evaluate a patient who has been subdued with a TASER. In many instances, the TASER darts may still be in place. First, before you approach any patient who has been subdued by a TASER or other less lethal weapon, you should ensure that the scene is safe. Most patients who have been subdued by these devices will have no injury. In most instances, they can be observed for approximately 15 minutes and then allowed to go with law enforcement if no further problems occur. Patients should have the following findings before being released to law enforcement:

- Glasgow Coma Scale score of 15
- Heart rate <110 per minute
- Respiratory rate >12 per minute
- Normal SpO_2 (>94 percent)
- Systolic blood pressure >100 mmHg
- The dart must not have penetrated the eye, face, neck, breast (females), axilla, or genitalia.
- The patient has no other acute medical condition including trauma, hypoglycemia, and/or acute psychiatric disturbances such as excited delirium syndrome.

If the subject meets the criteria above, the TASER darts can be removed. The procedure is as follows:

1. Ensure that the TASER is no longer active and has been secured.
2. Use scissors to cut the wire at the base of each dart, thus disconnecting it from the device.
3. While wearing gloves, grasp the cylinder of the TASER dart between your thumb and index finger and remove the dart with a quick, firm hold directed perpendicular to

the skin surface. Dispose of the dart in a sharps container, being careful not to sustain an injury with the device.

4. Clean each dart wound with an appropriate antiseptic solution.
5. Cover each dart wound with a bandage or other sterile dressing. The bandage or dressing can be removed in 24 to 48 hours if there are no problems.
6. Offer the patient transport to the hospital, if necessary. Document your findings and obtain appropriate releases. Encourage the subject/patient to seek follow-up care if he develops signs of infection around one or both of the punctures. These signs include fever, increasing pain, erythema, warmth, swelling, and/or purulent drainage.

Your local protocols may vary somewhat. Always follow local protocols in this regard. If you encounter any other issues, such as arrhythmias or other abnormalities, treat the patient accordingly. When in doubt, err on the side of safety and transport the patient to the emergency department for subsequent evaluation. Remember, patients with excited delirium syndrome are at high risk for sudden death. These patients should be treated aggressively and transported emergently to a hospital.

Medical Care

Patients who are experiencing apparent behavioral emergencies often have concurrent medical conditions—some of which may be responsible for the behavioral problem. Current literature indicates that medical conditions and/or substance abuse cause a much higher proportion of behavioral emergencies than previously believed. Medical care may include treatment for overdose, lacerations, toxic inhalation, hypoxia, or metabolic conditions. Many patients with chronic psychiatric conditions take medications for their illnesses; when abused, those medications have extremely toxic side effects. (Refer to the chapter "Emergency Pharmacology.") Additionally, these patients often live in conditions ranging from substandard housing to the street. This existence may predispose them to other medical problems such as exposure, infections, and untreated illnesses.

Psychological Care

Patients who present with an apparent behavioral emergency also require psychological care. The time you spend developing a rapport with the patient—before, during, and after assessment—is actually a part of the care you provide. In effect, when you begin an assessment you are also beginning your care, and you will continue to perform psychological assessment and care concurrently with medical assessment and care. Be calm and reassuring while you interview your patient.

Because much of your care will be aimed at the psychological problem, you should steer your conversation and actions in that direction. Visualize your patients on a continuum ranging from agitated and out of control to introverted and depressed (Figure 11-4). As a paramedic, you will need to defuse the agitated patient and attempt to communicate with the withdrawn patient. These situations especially will require the interviewing skills you learned earlier in this chapter.

As you approach the patient, introduce yourself and state that you want to help, as this might not be intuitively

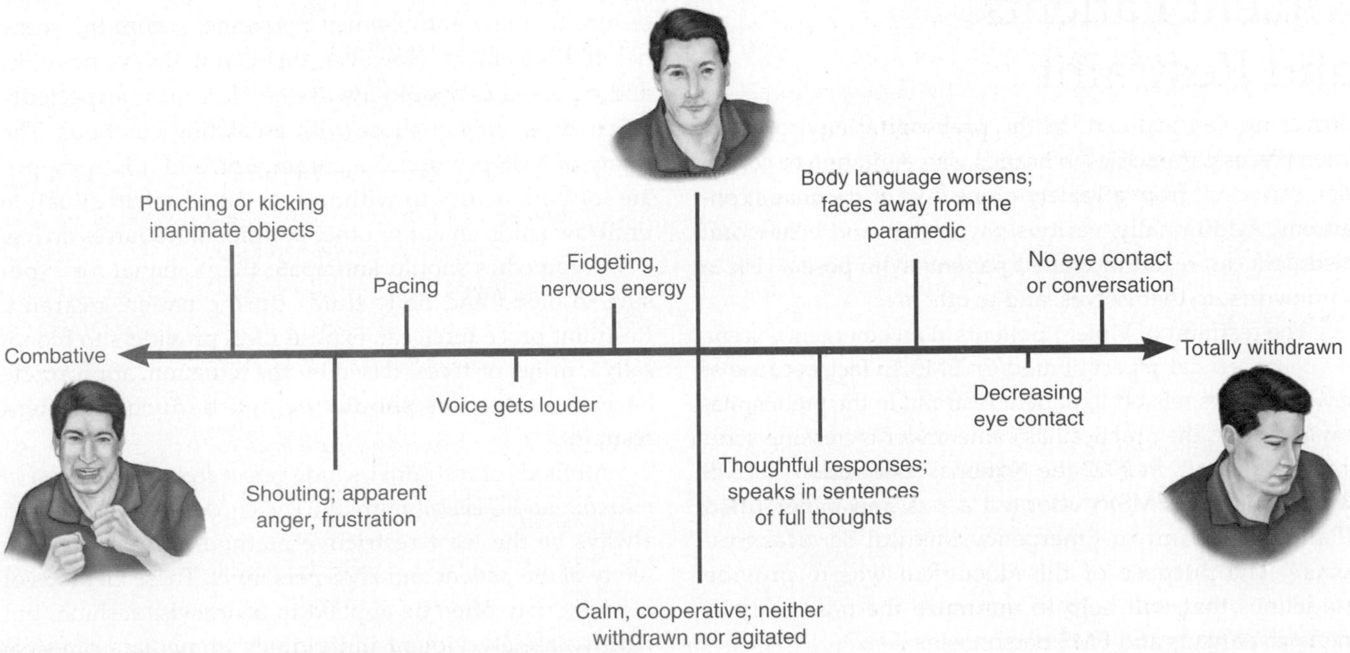

FIGURE 11-4 Continuum of patient responses during behavioral emergency. Whether dealing with an agitated or a withdrawn patient, you will use your interpersonal skills to bring him to the calm, cooperative state in the middle of the continuum.

clear to a person with distorted perceptions. As you begin to converse, note how the patient reacts to you. Generally, if he responds appropriately to your actions, you should continue what you are doing. If the patient becomes more agitated or further withdrawn, rethink. Perhaps you are getting too close, talking too fast, or addressing difficult topics too early. Be sure your exit path is not blocked.

Your approach to these patients requires excellent people skills—especially listening and observing. If you do not use these skills or if you rush or seem disinterested, your care will likely fail. Therapeutic communication, as this interaction has been called, is an art. "Talking down" the behavioral emergency patient requires effort and skill. Some patients, however, will not react favorably even to the best people skills. Extremely withdrawn patients or those with severe psychotic symptoms may never fully respond during the time you spend with them out of the hospital. These patients still deserve quality care and compassion, even when they are uncommunicative or restrained.

Just as we must observe the patient, the patient observes us. Patients may actually be able to "read" us as accurately (or more accurately) than we read them. Perform your assessment and care confidently and competently. If patients sense uneasiness or indecision, they are more likely to act out. Never play along with a patient's hallucinations or delusions. It may seem to be the easiest route, but ultimately it may be harmful. Often the patient will recognize that you are patronizing him. Or the patient may talk of hallucinations or appear delusional, but not fully believe what he says. If you play along, you will lose credibility.

Violent Patients and Restraint

Providing medical care in the prehospital environment often places paramedics in harm's way. Agitation or confusion can result from a variety of medical or traumatic conditions. Additionally, various psychiatric and behavioral disorders can result in violent patients who pose a risk to paramedics, to themselves, and to others.

The restraint of violent patients at an emergency scene is a controversial aspect of modern EMS. In fact, because of several deaths related to patient restraint in the prehospital environment, the practice has come under increasing scrutiny. As a result, in 2002 the National Association of EMS Physicians (NAEMSP) adopted a position paper titled "Patient Restraint in Emergency Medical Services Systems." The purpose of this document was to provide guidelines that will help to minimize the possibility of injury to patients and EMS personnel.

It is important to remember that many medical and trauma conditions can result in agitation and combativeness. Because of this, paramedics must be knowledgeable about these conditions and their appropriate treatment. All EMS systems should have protocols in place for the restraint and management of agitated and combative patients.

Legal Considerations

Medical–Legal Issues in Patient Restraint. EMS systems and medical directors must be aware of the laws of their state. Local legislation related to an individual's rights, the processes for involuntarily restraining or holding patients with mental health disorders, an individual's right to refuse treatment, and other related legal issues must be considered when developing a patient restraint protocol. In general, legislation attempts to ensure the safety of individuals who are an immediate threat to themselves or others. It may be necessary to involve law enforcement or a mental health official to restrain a competent individual against his will.

When possible, EMS systems should ensure that patients are accompanied by personnel of the same gender as the patient during treatment and transportation. This is of particular importance when pharmacological agents are used for chemical restraint.

The application of physical and chemical restraints to a patient must be performed with the understanding that overstepping the boundaries of proper restraint may be perceived as battery, assault, or false imprisonment. Restraint of an individual may even lead to serious allegations of civil rights violations. For these reasons, the EMS service should always review patient restraint policies with appropriate legal counsel.

Methods of Restraint

If a patient is known to be violent, EMS personnel should ensure that law enforcement personnel secure the scene before EMS enters. However, this is not always possible, and paramedics should always be alert for unexpectedly agitated patients or those with escalating emotions. The safety of EMS personnel is paramount, and it is appropriate for paramedics to withdraw from a violent situation until law enforcement or other additional resources arrive.

Paramedics should anticipate the potential for exposure to blood and body fluids during patient restraint. Restraint procedures can expose EMS providers to blood, saliva, urine, or feces. Based on the situation, appropriate barrier protection should be worn during patient restraint.[4]

Methods of restraint include *verbal deescalation, physical restraint,* and *chemical restraint*. The chosen method should always be the least restrictive method that ensures the safety of the patient and EMS personnel. These methods of restraint may often be applied in a stepwise fashion, but with extremely violent individuals immediate physical restraint may be indicated to ensure the safety of the patient, EMS personnel, and bystanders.

Verbal Deescalation

The application of verbal techniques to calm the patient is usually the first method paramedics should employ. This method is safest because it does not require any physical contact with the patient. The conversation must be honest and straightforward, with a friendly tone. Avoid direct eye contact and encroachment on the patient's "personal space," which may create added stress and anxiety. Always attempt to have equally open escape routes for both paramedics and the patient should it become necessary. Always assess the patient for suicidal and/or homicidal ideation. Verbal intervention sometimes defuses the situation or at least prevents further escalation and may avert the need for further restraint tactics.

Physical Restraint

When physically restraining a patient, paramedics must make every effort to avoid injuring the patient. Patient restraint policies must, therefore, recommend restraint devices that are associated with the least chance of inflicting injury. Physical restraint is accomplished with materials and techniques that will restrict the movement of a person who is considered to be a danger to himself or others. Examples include both soft restraints (sheets, wristlets, and chest Posey) and hard restraints (plastic ties, handcuffs, and leathers).

In general, EMS personnel should avoid using hard restraints. If an EMS system chooses to use hard restraints, all personnel should be trained to proficiency in their use, and the patient's extremities should be evaluated frequently for injury or possible neurovascular compromise.

Ideally, a minimum of five people should be present to safely apply physical restraint to a violent patient, which allows for control of the head and each limb. This requirement may be difficult for some EMS systems to accomplish because of limits on the number of available personnel. At the least, however, four rescuers should work together to accomplish restraint (Procedure 11-1). Before beginning physical restraint, there should be a plan and a team leader who will direct the restraining process.

Procedure 11-1 Restraining a Patient

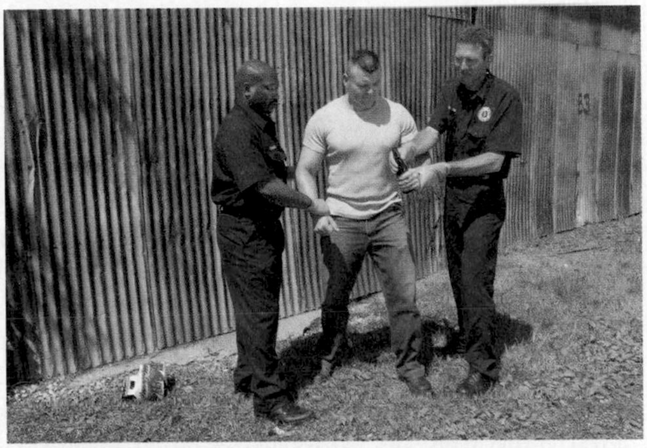

11-1a Two rescuers should be present.

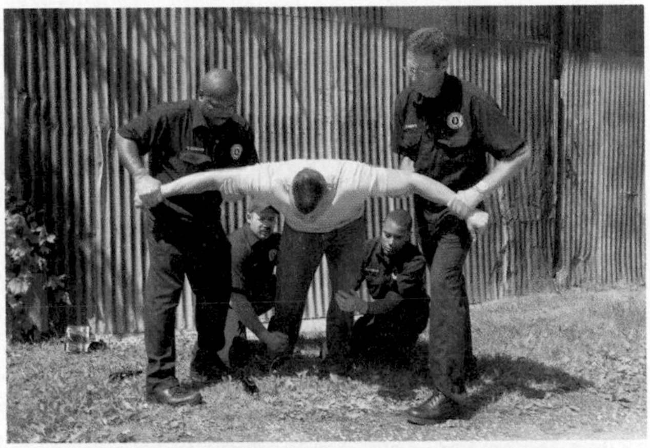

11-1b Plan the maneuver.

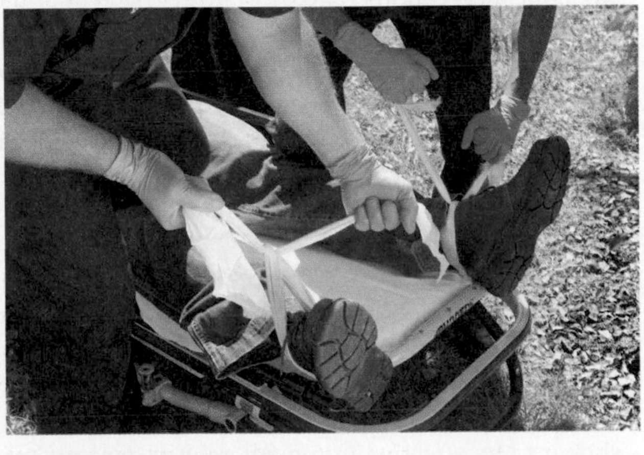

11-1c Place the patient supine.

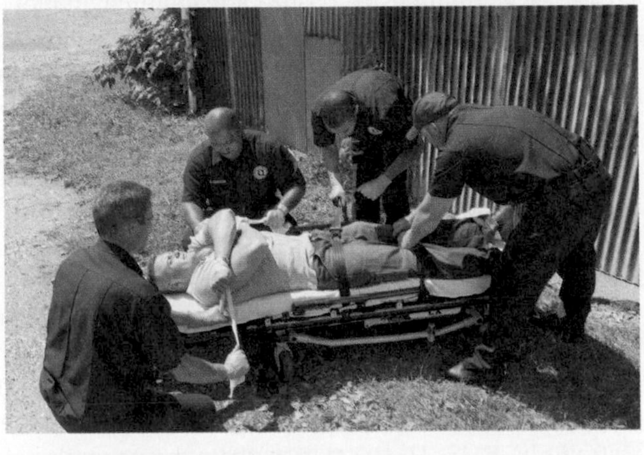

11-1d One method is to pull arms across the patient's chest and tie on opposite sides of the stretcher frame.

Four-point restraints (restraining both arms and both legs) are preferred over two-point restraints. It is often helpful to tether the hips, thighs, and chest. Tethering the thighs just above or below the knees is often more effective in preventing kicking than restraint of the ankles.

Contrary to the methods recommended in the U.S. DOT National Standard Curriculum for EMT-Paramedics, patients should *not* be transported while restrained in a prone position. Restraint in a prone position has been associated with **positional asphyxia**. In addition, nothing should be placed over the face, head, or neck of the patient. A surgical mask placed loosely on the patient may prevent spitting. A hard cervical collar may limit the mobility of the patient's neck and may decrease the range of head motion necessary for the patient to attempt to bite.

While gaining initial control of the patient, it may be acceptable to restrain him in a prone position *temporarily*—or to sandwich the patient with mattresses or backboards *temporarily*—but *personnel must be extremely vigilant for respiratory compromise*. Gaining initial control of the patient in the prone position limits the patient's visual awareness of the environment and decreases the range of motion of the extremities. As soon as the team has control of the patient's movement, however, the team must work to move the patient into a supine four-point restrained position.

A patient should *never* be hobbled or "hog-tied" with the arms and legs tied together behind the back. During transport, a patient should *never* be restrained to a stretcher in the prone position or sandwiched between backboards or mattresses.

Once the patient has been restrained, he should never be left unattended. If a patient vomits, it will be necessary to immediately position him and possibly to suction him to protect the airway. Also, paramedics should perform and document frequent neurovascular assessments of the restrained extremities to ensure adequate circulation. A patient who has undergone physical restraint should not be allowed to continue to struggle against the restraints (see the Chemical Restraint section). Struggling against restraints may lead to severe acidosis and fatal arrhythmia. In general, for the safety of the patient and EMS personnel, physical restraints applied in the field should not be removed until the patient is reevaluated on arrival at the receiving hospital.

Weapons used by law enforcement officers—including, but not limited to, pepper spray, mace defensive spray, stun guns, air TASERs, stun batons, and telescoping steel batons—are *not* appropriate choices for patient restraint by EMS. They can exacerbate the patient's agitation and increase the risk of injury or death. Although appropriately trained law enforcement officers may use these weapons, their use should be excluded from routine EMS protocols.

Chemical Restraint

Chemical restraint is defined as the administration of specific pharmacological agents to decrease agitation and increase the cooperation of patients who require medical care and transportation. EMS systems may use a variety of agents for chemical restraint of the agitated or combative patient. The goal is to subdue excessive agitation and struggling against physical restraints. Ideally, this pharmacological sedation will change the patient's behavior without reaching the point of amnesia or altering the patient's level of consciousness.

Butyrophenones (haloperidol, droperidol) and/or benzodiazepines (diazepam, midazolam, lorazepam) are the medications most commonly used for chemical restraint in emergency departments and in prehospital care. Other historical but less advisable medications include the barbiturates (Pentothal), opioids (morphine), and phenothiazines (chlorpromazine).

Chemical restraint protocols often include a butyrophenone, a benzodiazepine, or a combination of both. Diazepam (Valium), lorazepam (Ativan), and midazolam (Versed) are the benzodiazepines that are most commonly used for patient restraint. Droperidol (Inapsine) and haloperidol (Haldol) are the butyrophenones that are commonly used. All five of these medications can be given intramuscularly or intravenously. Ketamine is being used with increasing frequency in the prehospital management of excited delirium and in situations where chemical restraint is deemed necessary. It is typically effective and has a good safety profile. It is sometimes used in conjunction with benzodiazepines. As with any medications that can alter mental status, the patient's vital signs and respiratory status must be constantly monitored when using ketamine or any of the sedative/hypnotic medications.

Although several limited prehospital studies support the effectiveness of droperidol in decreasing the agitation of combative patients in the prehospital setting, the FDA has issued a warning of possible arrhythmias associated with droperidol administration. Droperidol has been associated with problems in patients who have a prolonged QT interval on their ECG. Because of this, many experts recommend obtaining a 12-lead ECG on patients prior to administering droperidol. This is not always practical in agitated or combative patients, however, and this makes droperidol a less desirable agent for chemical restraint. Haloperidol and the benzodiazepines have been shown to be effective in the emergency department setting, and they are probably also effective in the prehospital environment.

Ketamine is being used with increasing frequency for patient restraint in the prehospital setting. It is relatively safe and highly effective—particularly in patients with excited delirium. Ketamine is a dissociative agent and can be administered intramuscularly and intravenously. It is sometimes used in conjunction with benzodiazepines (e.g., lorazepam, diazepam, midazolam).

Neuromuscular-blocking medications that are used with endotracheal intubation are never indicated to paralyze a patient solely for the purpose of restraining violent behavior. Only patients who have coexisting medical conditions—for example, severe head injury or respiratory failure—may benefit from paralysis and intubation. In all cases, the decision to paralyze a patient should be based on medical indications beyond violent or combative behavior.

When considering the use of chemical restraint, paramedics must weigh the risks of the patient struggling while physically restrained against the side-effect profile of the medications being considered for sedation of the agitated patient. At present, there is no consensus on the best medication or dosage for chemical restraint, and these decisions are best deferred to the individual EMS system and its medical director.

Summary

Calls involving psychiatric and behavioral emergencies will challenge your skills and at times your patience as a paramedic. Differentiating physiologic and psychological conditions will try your diagnostic skills, and developing the interview abilities that form the basis of psychiatric assessment and care will test your people skills. Ultimately, you will be called on to help patients in a time of great need—the time of crisis. Once you determine that the patient is experiencing a purely behavioral emergency, your compassion and communication skills, rather than medications and procedures, will benefit him most.

Emergency medical services providers routinely encounter patients who are violent or combative as a result of behavioral illness, a medical condition, or trauma. Verbal, physical, and chemical restraint techniques provide effective ways of restraining patients who are a threat to themselves or others or who require medical assessment and treatment for a condition associated with combative or agitated behavior. Life-threatening adverse events have occurred in restrained individuals, but adherence to the principles of restraint presented in this chapter will minimize the occurrence of such adverse events. EMS personnel and their medical directors should ensure that their systems are prepared to treat violent or combative patients responsibly by providing appropriate training, policies, and protocols to deal with these situations.

Situations involving crisis can drain your emotions. Observing a suicide or attempted suicide or struggling with or restraining a patient can take its toll. Take care of yourself before, during, and after these calls.

You Make the Call

You are called for a behavioral emergency in an office-building parking lot on a cold February day. You arrive to find the police watching over a man in a car. They tell you he is a psychiatric patient who has crashed his car into several others in the parking lot. The crashes were low speed and you do not suspect spinal injuries. Your primary assessment is unremarkable. The patient responds verbally but is not alert. He is talking about "the coming of the Lord." He is nonviolent and does not resist your assessment. He has no obvious injuries. Religious literature and several Bibles are scattered about the car. You note the patient is wearing only a shirt in below-zero temperatures and is sweating profusely.

1. What do you suspect this patient's problem is? What are the possibilities?
2. Is the sweating significant? The religious literature? The car crashes?
3. Should this patient be treated as a psychiatric emergency?

See Suggested Responses at the back of this book.

Review Questions

1. ____________ is defined as a person's observable conduct and activity.
   a. Affect
   b. Conduct
   c. Behavior
   d. Personality
2. The general causes of behavioral emergencies are ____________
   a. social.
   b. biological.
   c. psychosocial.
   d. all of the above.
3. ____________ causes of behavioral disorders are related to the patient's actions and interactions within society.
   a. Organic
   b. Personal
   c. Sociocultural
   d. Psychosocial
4. Visible indicators of mood describe a person's ____________
   a. fear.
   b. affect.
   c. posture.
   d. behavior.
5. Encroachment on an area within an approximately 3-foot radius around every person causes anxiety. This area is known as one's ____________
   a. comfort zone.
   b. safety zone.
   c. personal space.
   d. private space.
6. Observing hygiene and clothing describes which component of the MSE?
   a. Orientation
   b. General appearance
   c. Perceptual processes
   d. Thought processes
7. Published by the American Psychiatric Association (APA), which work details diagnostic criteria for all currently defined psychiatric disorders, which are grouped according to the patient's signs and symptoms?
   a. PDR
   b. CDC
   c. Cecil's *Textbook of Medicine*
   d. DSM-5
8. Psychiatric disorders with organic causes such as brain injury or disease are known as what type of disorders?
   a. Mood
   b. Cognitive
   c. Anxiety
   d. Dissociative
9. Failure to recognize objects or stimuli despite intact sensory function describes ____________
   a. agnosia.
   b. aphasia.
   c. apraxia.
   d. dysphagia.
10. Feeling detached from oneself defines ____________
    a. fugue state.
    b. psychogenic amnesia.
    c. depersonalization.
    d. dissociative identity disorder.

See Answers to Review Questions at the back of this book.

References

1. Vilke, G. M., M. L. Debard, T. C. Chan, et al. "Excited Delirium Syndrome (ExDS): Defining Based on a Review of the Literature." *J Emerg Med* (2011).
2. Otahbachi, M., C. Cevik, S. Bagdure, and K. Nugent. "Excited Delirium, Restraints, and Unexpected Death: A Review of Pathogenesis." *Am J Forensic Med Pathol* 31 (2010): 107-112.
3. Stratton, S. J., C. Rogers, K. Brickett, et al. "Factors Associated with Sudden Death of Individuals Requiring Restraint for Excited Delirium." *Am J Emerg Med* 19 (2001): 187–191.
4. National Association of EMS Physicians. "Patient Restraint in Emergency Medical Services Systems." *Prehospital Emergency Care* 6(3) (2002): 340–345.

Further Reading

American Psychiatric Association. *Diagnostic and Statistical Manual of Mental Disorders*, 5th ed. Washington, DC: American Psychiatric Press, 2013.

Marcus, E. *Why Suicide?* San Francisco: Harper Collins, 1996.

Soreff, S. M. and R. T. Cadigan. *EMS Street Strategies*. Albany, NY: Delmar Learning, 2004.

Chapter 12

Diseases of the Eyes, Ears, Nose, and Throat

Bryan Bledsoe, DO, FACEP, FAAEM, EMT-P

STANDARD

Medicine (Diseases of the Eyes, Ears, Nose, and Throat)

COMPETENCY

Integrates assessment findings with principles of epidemiology and pathophysiology to formulate a field impression and implement a comprehensive treatment/disposition plan for a patient with a medical complaint.

Learning Objectives

Terminal Performance Objective: After reading this chapter, you should be able to integrate patient assessment findings, patient history, and knowledge of anatomy, physiology, pathophysiology, and basic and advanced life support interventions to recognize and manage patients with disorders of the eyes, ears, nose, and throat.

Enabling Objectives: To accomplish the terminal performance objective, you should be able to:

1. Define key terms introduced in this chapter.
2. Review the anatomy and physiology of the eyes, ears, nose, and throat structures.
3. Adapt the scene size-up, primary and secondary assessment, medical history, and use of monitoring technology to arrive at a field impression for eyes, ears, nose, and throat emergencies.
4. Discuss the pathophysiology and assessment findings that would be present in a patient experiencing specific eyes, ears, nose, and throat emergencies in the prehospital environment.
5. Use a process of clinical reasoning to guide and interpret the patient assessment findings and develop a treatment plan for patients with eyes, ears, nose, and throat emergencies.
6. Given a variety of scenarios, discuss the integration of assessment and management guidelines as they relate to emergencies of the eyes, ears, nose, and throat.

KEY TERMS

aqueous humor, p. 467
cataract, p. 471
cerumen, p. 472
chalazion, p. 468
endolymph, p. 473
hyphema, p. 470
Kiesselbach's plexus, p. 475
Ludwig's angina, p. 481
orbital septum, p. 470
photopigments, p. 468
pterygium, p. 469
sebum, p. 467
sty, p. 468
vitreous humor, p. 467

Case Study

MedicWest Ambulance paramedics are dispatched to an "unknown emergency" in a relatively decaying part of town. Because of the unknown nature of the emergency, Metro police officers are dispatched as well. On arrival at the ramshackle house, paramedics and police officers find a large quantity of blood throughout the living room. A trail of blood leads to the bathroom, where an elderly man is seated on a closed toilet, holding his nose, constantly spitting blood out of his mouth. It is difficult to get information from the patient, but the paramedics learn that his nose started bleeding approximately 12 hours earlier. Initially, the bleeding was limited to a small trickle. However it has become progressively worse, despite the measures the man has employed to stop the bleeding.

The paramedics move the patient back to the living room, where the lighting is better and where there is more room to complete the necessary assessment and treatment. Because there appears to be no evidence of foul play, police officers clear the scene. The paramedics complete the primary assessment and find no threat to the airway, breathing, or circulation. They then turn their attention to the secondary assessment.

The patient reports that he is usually cared for at the Veterans Administration clinic and is currently on multiple medications, including Coumadin for an irregular heartbeat. The patient states that he missed his last few appointments at the clinic but has continued to take his medications as prescribed. He said that the nosebleed started spontaneously early in the morning and has continued through the course of the day. He has tried tissues, Vaseline, and other strategies to stop the bleeding—all to no avail. Initially, he reported that the bleeding was primarily out of the anterior portion of the nose. Now, much of it appears to be posterior. He complains of facial and abdominal pain, as well as nausea. He is weak and pale.

The paramedics inspect the nasopharynx and oropharynx and cannot readily identify the source of bleeding because of the sheer volume of blood present and the multiple clots. They place a nasal clamp on the nose and apply a cold pack. The patient's vital signs are stable, with the exception of a tachycardia of 108 beats per minute.

The paramedics place the patient in a semi-Fowler's position and start a saline lock. They administer 4 mg of ondansetron and 50 mcg of fentanyl. They place a commercial nose clip onto the nose and transport the patient to University Medical Center. The trip to the hospital is uneventful.

Examination by the emergency physician reveals multiple bleeding sites. Laboratory studies obtained in the emergency department reveal the patient's prothrombin time, as measured by the INR (International Normalized Ratio), is six times normal. Based on this, an ear, nose, and throat (ENT) physician is consulted, and the patient is admitted to the hospital.

The patient receives vitamin K to reverse the effects of the Coumadin, as well as fresh frozen plasma. Although he is anemic, he does not require transfusion. The emergency physician placed nasal packing that controlled the bleeding. The ear, nose, and throat physician evaluates the patient and determines that no further care is warranted. Following discharge, the patient is referred back to the Veterans Administration clinic for social care and monitoring of his prothrombin levels and Coumadin dose.

Introduction

The head and neck contain many of the body's essential sensory organs and other important structures. Numerous medical conditions and injuries can affect the head and neck and associated structures. This is particularly true in the case of the pediatric patient. Many of these conditions do not readily fit into the chapters previously presented in this text. They are discussed here in detail to assist prehospital practitioners in caring for patients with these conditions. Trauma of the head and neck is discussed in detail in the chapter "Head, Neck, and Spinal

Trauma." This chapter addresses nontraumatic conditions of the head and neck.

The numerous important structures contained in the head and neck include the eyes, ears, nose, throat, and associated structures. The following sections contain brief reviews of the anatomy and physiology of these important structures.

Eyes

The eyes are the organs of sight. They gather light and focus the light onto various receptors in the back of the eye that, in turn, produce an image that is interpreted by the brain. This allows us to see and function in the environment in which we live.

Anatomy of the Eye

The anatomy of the eye can be divided into the external anatomy and the internal anatomy.

External Anatomy of the Eye

The eyes are well protected by a group of bones that form the *ocular orbit*. The orbit is padded with subcutaneous tissue that cushions and protects the eye from injury. Movement of the eyes is controlled by six *extraocular muscles* that allow us to look in various directions. Two movable folds of skin, the *eyelids*, protect the eyes from the environment. The *eyelashes* function as sensors to cause rapid closure of the eyelids when a foreign substance approaches the eyes. Several accessory glands secrete an oily substance called **sebum** onto the eyelids to keep them soft and pliable.

A membrane called the *conjunctiva* covers and protects the exposed surface of the eye. Each eye has a lacrimal apparatus that manufactures and stores tears. The tears are manufactured in the *lacrimal glands* and then spread across the eye laterally to medially, where they then drain through the *lacrimal ducts* into the nose (Figure 12-1).

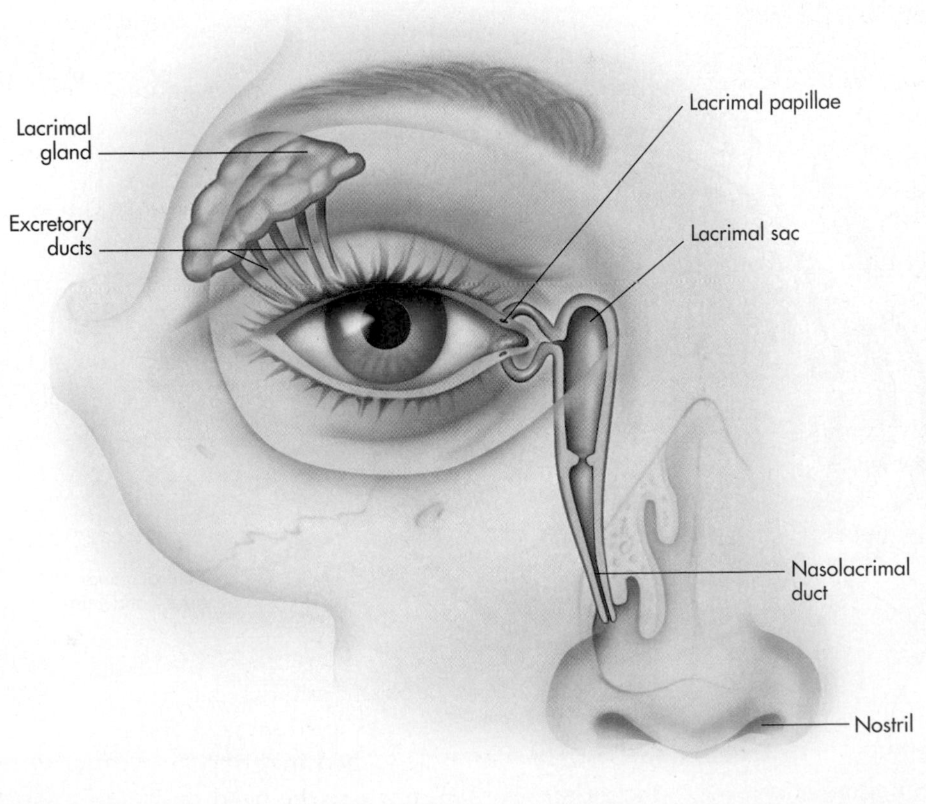

FIGURE 12-1 External anatomy of the eye.

Internal Anatomy of the Eye

The globe of the eye contains two distinct fluid-filled cavities. *The posterior cavity*, the portion of the eye behind the lens, contains the **vitreous humor**. The vitreous humor is a clear, jellylike fluid that fills the entire vitreous cavity. The *anterior cavity*, the portion of the eye in front of the lens, contains the **aqueous humor**. The aqueous humor is a waterlike fluid that surrounds the iris, pupil, and lens. The anterior cavity is divided into the *anterior chamber* and the *posterior chamber*. Both chambers are filled with aqueous humor.

The eye comprises three layers. The innermost layer is the *retina*. The middle layer is the *choroid*. The outermost layer is the *sclera*.

The sclera is a tough, fibrous, protective tissue. It is also referred to as the "white of the eye." The anterior, transparent portion of the sclera is the *cornea*. The cornea allows light to pass into the eye and onto the retina. The cornea is curved, which allows it to focus the incoming image onto the curved surface of the retina.

The *choroid* is a highly vascular tissue that provides essential nutrients to the tissues of the eye. The choroid contains both the iris and the pupil. The *iris* is the colored portion of the eye and controls the size of the *pupil*. It is a sphincter that can contract or relax, thereby changing the diameter of the pupillary opening. Immediately behind the pupil is the *lens*. The lens is the structure that focuses the incoming light images onto the retina. Specialized muscles called *ciliary muscles* surround the lens. The ciliary muscles can change the shape of the lens to precisely focus the incoming image.

The retina contains the nerve endings that receive and interpret the incoming image. The retina also contains two types of light-sensing receptors called rods and cones. The *rods* are effective in dim light and do not perceive color. The *cones* are more effective in bright light and do perceive color. These *photoreceptors* contain **photopigments** that undergo a chemical change when contacted by light. This chemical change sends impulses to the optic nerve and on to the brain, where the image is eventually interpreted (Figure 12-2).

Medical Conditions of the Eye

Most eye emergencies that paramedics will be called on to treat are traumatic. However, there are a few medical conditions of the eye that you may encounter in the course of your work that are nontraumatic.[1] These include the following:

- ***Sty (external hordeolum).*** A **sty** (alternative spelling: *stye*), also referred to as an *external hordeolum*, is an infection of the eyelid that results from blockage of the oil glands associated with an eyelash. It is typically located at the lash line and has the appearance of a small pustule or lump. The lump can point externally or internally. There is often associated swelling of the lid. The sty typically resolves when the gland blockage is relieved. This can be facilitated by the use of warm soaks. Occasionally, topical antibiotics are needed.
- ***Chalazion (internal hordeolum).*** A **chalazion**, also referred to as an *internal hordeolum*, is inflammation or infection that results from blockage of one of the *meibomian glands* in the tarsal plate of the eyelid. The meibomian glands produce the fluid that lubricates the eyelids. Approximately 50 to 100 of these glands are located near the eyelashes. Typically, a chalazion is seen as a red, tender lump in the eyelid or eyelid margin. The treatment is similar to that for a sty and sometimes requires antibiotics.
- ***Conjunctivitis.*** Conjunctivitis is an infection or inflammation of the conjunctiva. There are three major causes of conjunctivitis:
  - ***Bacterial conjunctivitis.*** Bacterial conjunctivitis is an infection and inflammation of the conjunctiva of the eye caused by infectious bacteria. It is often associated with a purulent drainage and erythema. The infection and inflammation are limited to the conjunctiva. The cornea is clear. Bacterial conjunctivitis is often called "pinkeye." The eye is usually red and itching and producing more

CONTENT REVIEW

➤ Medical Conditions of the Eye
- Sty
- Chalazion (internal hordeolum)
- Conjunctivitis
- Pterygium
- Iritis (uveitis)
- Herpes simplex virus (HSV) keratitis
- Herpes zoster ophthalmicus
- Corneal ulcers
- Cellulitis
- Atraumatic hyphema
- Glaucoma
- Cataract
- Optic neuritis
- Papilledema
- Central retinal artery occlusion
- Central retinal vein occlusion
- Retinal detachment

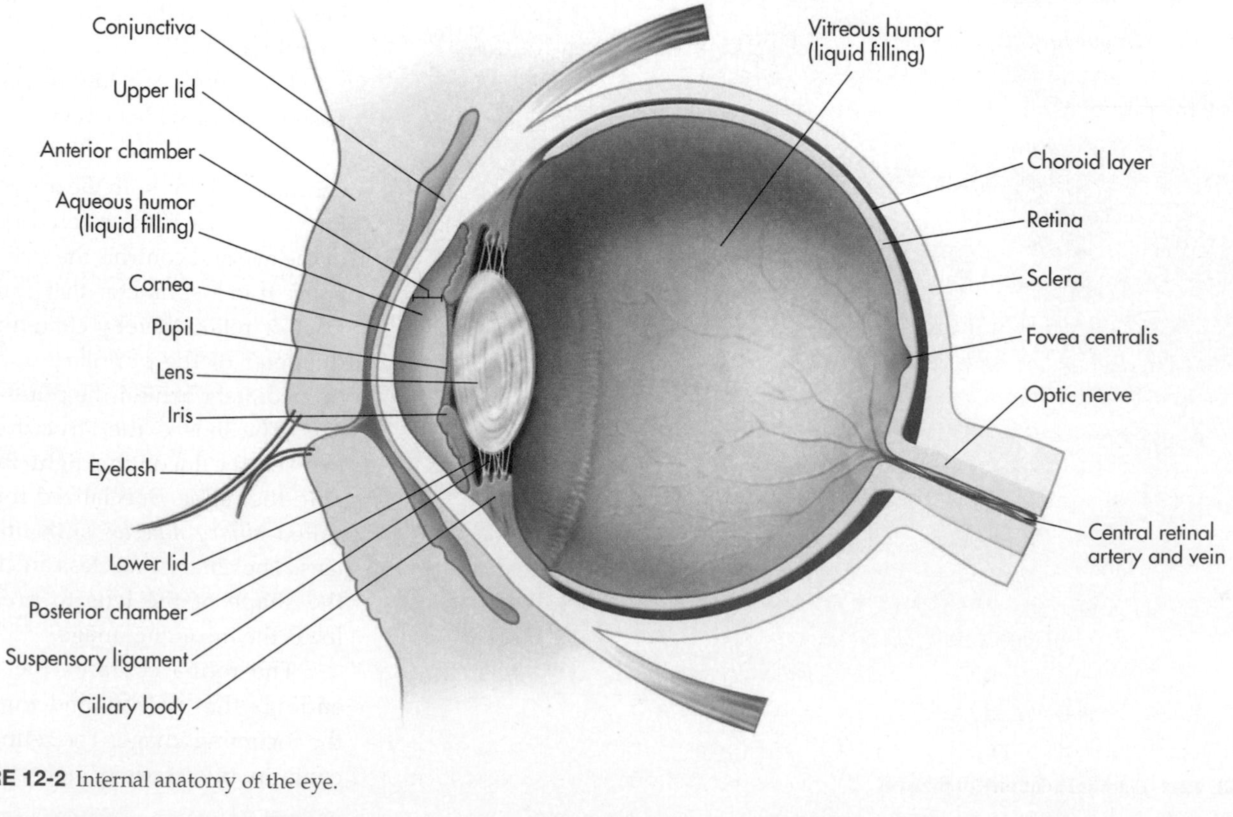

FIGURE 12-2 Internal anatomy of the eye.

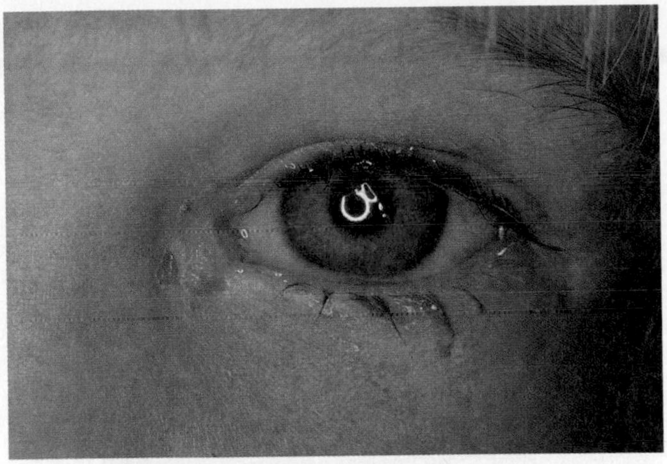

FIGURE 12-3 Conjunctivitis.

(© Dorling Kindersley)

tears than usual (Figure 12-3). There may be some sensitivity to light. Bacterial conjunctivitis is less common than viral conjunctivitis but can spread rapidly between individuals. It is commonly passed from eye, to hand, to eye. Topical antibiotics are usually indicated for bacterial conjunctivitis. Preventive measures include hand washing and similar hygienic techniques.

- ***Viral conjunctivitis.*** Viral conjunctivitis is similar to bacterial conjunctivitis except that the cause is viral. It is more common than bacterial conjunctivitis, but follows a similar course. It often occurs in schools and day care centers. Treatment is symptomatic. Antibiotics are generally not indicated.
- ***Allergic conjunctivitis.*** Allergic conjunctivitis is a common condition related to exposure to pollen and other antigens to which the patient is allergic. Typically, allergic conjunctivitis is characterized by redness, watery discharge, itching, and swelling. It tends to be seasonal, depending on the specific pollen or pollens to which the patient is allergic. Treatment is primarily oral and topical ocular antihistamines.

- ***Pterygium.*** A **pterygium** is a conjunctival condition characterized by a raised, wedge-shaped growth of the conjunctiva. It is noncancerous and is readily visible over the white sclera. It can sometimes extend over the cornea and invade the visual axis of the eye. Although the cause of a pterygium is unknown, it is more common in people who have increased outdoor exposure to sun, wind, and dust. It is more common in southern climates and is rare in children. Generally, no treatment is indicated other than protective strategies such as goggles and sunglasses.
- ***Iritis.*** Iritis, also called *uveitis*, is a swelling and irritation of the middle layer of the eye. The *uvea* consists of the iris, *ciliary body*, and choroid. Uveitis is most often seen in patients with autoimmune diseases such as rheumatoid arthritis or ankylosing spondylitis. Uveitis is also seen in other conditions, including AIDS, ulcerative colitis, and certain infections. Uveitis is usually classified as *anterior uveitis* or *posterior uveitis*. Anterior uveitis generally involves inflammation of the front part of the eye. This is typically called *iritis*. Posterior uveitis affects the back part of the choroid, and is also called *choroiditis*. Uveitis can affect one or both of the eyes. Signs and symptoms include blurred vision, eye pain, erythema, photosensitivity, and occasionally the appearance of floaters in the eye. Treatment usually includes protection from light, analgesia, and corticosteroid eye drops.
- ***Herpes simplex virus (HSV) keratitis.*** Herpes simplex virus (HSV) keratitis is an infection and inflammation of the cornea that results from the herpes simplex virus. The herpes simplex virus is the same virus that causes fever blisters and mouth ulcers. HSV keratitis is primarily a disease of adults and typically occurs many years after the initial infection. HSV keratitis is the most frequent cause of corneal blindness in the United States and is a common reason for corneal transplantation. The signs and symptoms of HSV keratitis include pain, photophobia, blurry vision, tearing, and erythema. Initially, close examination of the cornea reveals raised clear vesicles similar to cutaneous herpes lesions. Eventually, these will coalesce into a spiderlike pattern that will ultimately form a corneal ulcer.
- ***Herpes zoster ophthalmicus.*** Herpes zoster ophthalmicus is a condition in which herpes zoster (shingles) affects the eye. In herpes zoster, the varicella (chickenpox) virus is reactivated, spreads along a nerve root, and inflames and infects the tissues supplied by the nerve root. In the case of herpes zoster ophthalmicus, the virus spreads along the first division of the trigeminal nerve. The viral particles take approximately three to four days to reach the nerve endings. Ultimately, damage can result to the eye itself. Typically, there will be an ulcer or similar lesion on the cornea.
- ***Corneal ulcers.*** There are numerous causes of nontraumatic corneal ulcers. Most nontraumatic ulcers are due to infection of the cornea by an infectious agent that breaks through the epithelial border of the cornea. These can be serious and sight-threatening infections. Typically, the patient has a painful red eye, tearing, and photophobia. It is important to determine the likely cause of the infection. Viral infections are treated differently from bacterial infections. Treatment typically includes topical antibiotics and analgesia. Prompt evaluation by an ophthalmologist is essential.
- ***Cellulitis.*** The soft tissues surrounding the eye can become infected, resulting in cellulitis. It can be both

sight-threatening and life-threatening. Cellulitis around the eye is typically classified as periorbital or orbital.[2]

- ***Periorbital cellulitis.*** Periorbital cellulitis, also called *preseptal cellulitis,* is a cellulitis that has not breached the **orbital septum**. The orbital septum, also called the *palpebral ligament,* is a membranous structure that separates the anterior aspect of the eye from the posterior aspect of the eye. Typically, the condition is characterized by edematous, erythematous, and warm eyelids and surrounding tissues. The eye itself is not involved. The infection is usually bacterial and is a particular risk for children under the age of 5 years in whom the infection can rapidly expand to the postseptal region. Patients typically complain of pain, conjunctivitis, blurred vision, and increased tear production. Swelling of the eyelids is common—often to the point at which the patient cannot open his eyes. Treatment generally involves potent antibiotics and hospital admission (Figure 12-4).
- ***Orbital cellulitis.*** Orbital cellulitis, also called *postseptal cellulitis,* is a serious infection that has involved the structures behind the orbital septum. It is often a complication of periorbital cellulitis and sinus infections. Orbital cellulitis is somewhat more common in winter months. The patient often presents with fever, headache, eyelid edema, a runny nose, and generalized malaise. On physical exam, there is often protrusion of the eye (*proptosis*) and inability to move the eye because of the effect of the infection and swelling on the extraocular muscles. There is often pain with attempted eye movement, decreased vision, and inflammation of the conjunctiva. Orbital cellulitis requires hospitalization, potent antibiotics, and, often, surgical drainage. It is a true emergency.

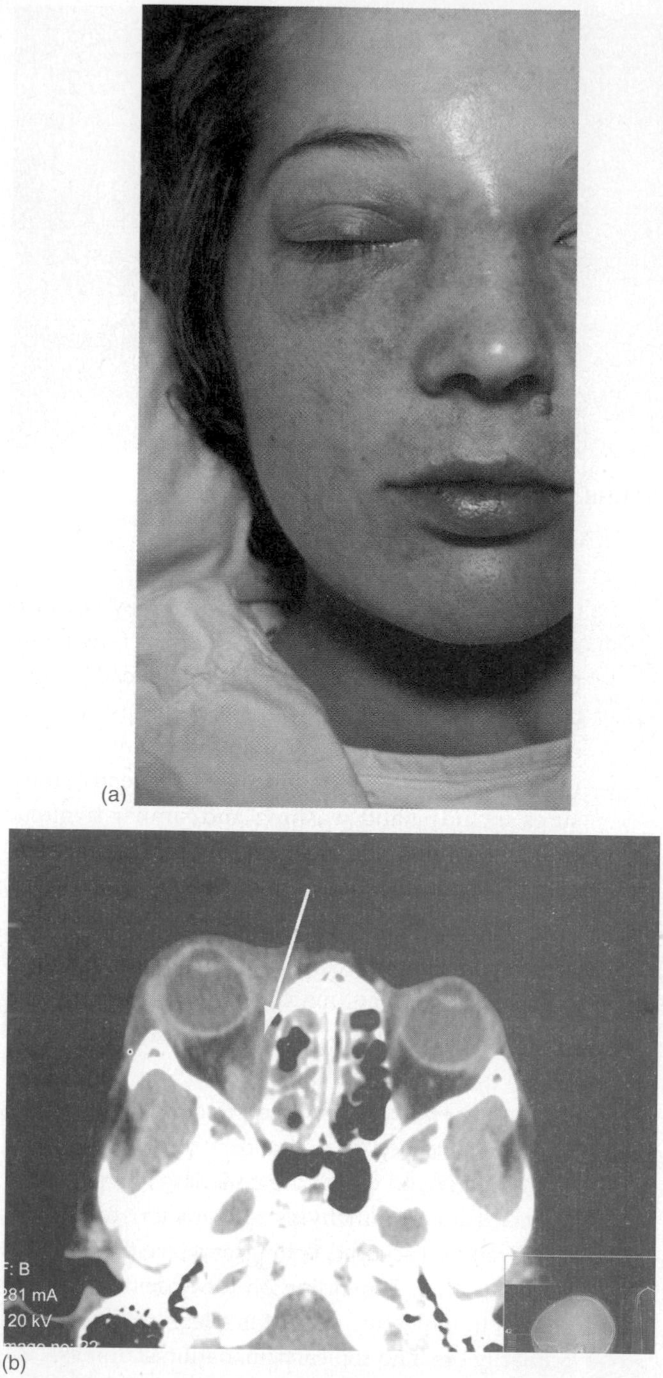

(a) (b)

FIGURE 12-4 Periorbital cellulitis.

(Photo a: Centers for Disease Control and Prevention; Photo b: Dr. Bryan E. Bledsoe)

- ***Atraumatic hyphema.*** A **hyphema** is a collection of blood in the anterior chamber of the eye. In most instances, a hyphema is the result of trauma. However, there are a few nontraumatic conditions that can cause a hyphema. The most common of these is sickle cell disease. It can also be seen with diabetes and with certain tumors of the eye. Close examination of the anterior chamber of the eye will reveal the presence of blood. This may be difficult to see if the blood has layered out in the bottom portion of the chamber. In some cases, blood can fill the entire anterior chamber, resulting in what is referred to as an "eightball hyphema." A hyphema can be a sight-threatening condition, and prompt evaluation by an ophthalmologist is usually indicated.
- ***Glaucoma.*** Glaucoma is a group of eye conditions that can be sight threatening. Glaucoma is characterized by an increase in the pressure within the eye (*intraocular pressure [IOP]*). This increased pressure can ultimately damage the optic nerve. Glaucoma is the second most common cause of blindness in the United States. There are two major classes of glaucoma: *open-angle (chronic) glaucoma* and *angle-closure (acute) glaucoma.*[3]

  Glaucoma results from the blockage of the flow of aqueous humor from the anterior chamber. This increases the IOP in the anterior chamber. Angle-closure glaucoma occurs when the outflow of aqueous humor is suddenly blocked. This causes a rapid and severe increase in the IOP. This is characterized by pain in the eye. Open-angle glaucoma is the most common type of glaucoma encountered. Although the cause is unknown, the IOP increases slowly over time. This subsequently places pressure on the optic nerve and the retina that can lead to blindness. Open-angle glaucoma tends to run in families and is more prevalent in people of African descent.

The signs and symptoms of glaucoma vary based on the type of disease. With open-angle glaucoma, most patients have no symptoms until they begin to lose vision. With angle-closure glaucoma, the patient will suddenly develop severe pain in the affected eye. This is often accompanied by a decreased or cloudy vision in the affected eye. There is often associated nausea and vomiting. The patient will often report rainbow- or halo-like effects around lights. The eye will often be red and appear swollen. If touched, the globe will appear tenser when compared to the opposite eye.

- In acute angle-closure glaucoma, the goal of treatment is to reduce the IOP. This may be done with medications or surgery. In the prehospital setting, emphasis should be on identifying glaucoma as a possible cause and treating the associated symptoms, including pain as well as nausea and vomiting.
- ***Cataract.*** A **cataract** is a clouding of the lens of the eye. It is associated with aging and results from a breakdown of proteins within the lens. Risk factors for cataract development include diabetes, eye injury, radiation exposure, smoking, and exposure to ultraviolet light (sunlight). Patients with a cataract will complain of decreased vision that they may describe as being cloudy or fuzzy, light sensitivity, diplopia, loss of color intensity, and seeing halos around lights. Treatment is usually prevention and surgical removal (Figure 12-5).

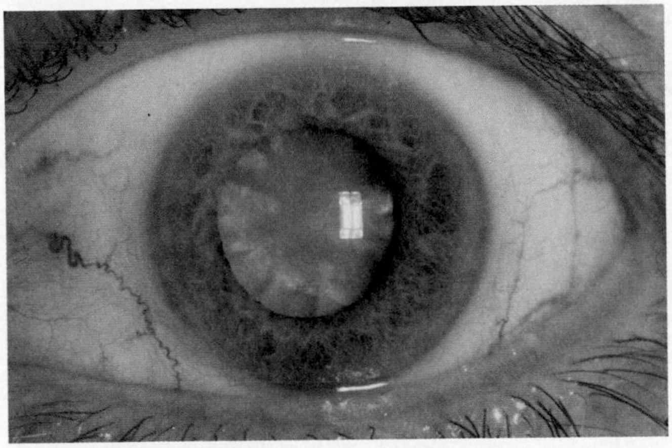

FIGURE 12-5 Cataract.

(National Eye Institute, National Institutes of Health)

- ***Optic neuritis.*** Optic neuritis is an inflammation of the optic nerve. It typically occurs as a result of autoimmune disease (e.g., systemic lupus erythematosus) but is also seen with infections, drug toxicity, and multiple sclerosis. The patient will typically develop loss of vision in a single eye—generally over the course of an hour or so. The patient may also exhibit loss of color vision, changes in the pupillary reaction to light, and pain with eye movement. In many cases, vision returns to normal within two to three weeks without treatment. In some cases, corticosteroids are used. Ophthalmological evaluation is essential.
- ***Papilledema.*** Papilledema is not a condition per se but a swelling of the optic disk secondary to increased intracranial pressure. The optic disk is the region of the retina where fibers of the optic nerve enter the eye. It is a small, circular structure and contains no rods or cones. The finding of papilledema requires examination with an ophthalmoscope. There are numerous causes of papilledema, including trauma, infections within the brain (e.g., encephalitis), stroke, tumors, and hydrocephalus. The presence of papilledema is a worrisome finding and requires additional evaluation if the cause is unknown.
- ***Central retinal artery occlusion.*** Central retinal artery occlusion is a blockage of one of the small arteries that supply the retina. The blockage typically results from a thrombus or atherosclerotic plaque. The carotid arteries are the most common source of clots in central retinal artery occlusion. Central retinal artery occlusion is more common in diabetics, patients with arrhythmias (e.g., atrial fibrillation), those with valvular heart disease, and intravenous drug abusers. The symptoms of central retinal artery occlusion typically involve all or part of one eye and appear to last from a few seconds to minutes. In some cases, it can be permanent. Several treatments are used, including fibrinolytics as well as massaging the eye. In many cases, the blockage is permanent.[4]
- ***Central retinal vein occlusion.*** Central retinal vein occlusion is a blockage of the small veins that drain the retina. It is most commonly caused by atherosclerosis or a thrombus. Central retinal vein occlusion is more common in diabetics, patients with hypertension, patients with atherosclerosis, and those with other eye conditions such as glaucoma. The symptoms of central retinal vein occlusion typically include sudden blurring or vision loss in all or part of one eye. Most patients regain vision without treatment, although it rarely returns to normal.
- ***Retinal detachment.*** A retinal detachment is a separation of the retina from the supporting structures. While

many cases of retinal detachment result from unknown causes, it can be seen in trauma, diabetes, and similar disorders. The patient will typically complain of bright flashes of light that are most evident in the peripheral vision. They will also report blurred vision and the presence of "floaters" in the eye. There may be a shadow or blindness in part of the visual field of the affected eye. Retinal detachment is typically treated surgically.[5]

Patho Pearls

Diabetes mellitus commonly affects the eyes. The most common eye-related complication of diabetes mellitus is *diabetic retinopathy,* which affects up to 80 percent of diabetics who have had the disease for more than ten years. Hyperglycemia causes damage and death of certain cells and structures, including small blood vessels, within the retina. As the disease progresses, new small blood vessels develop and proliferate (prolific diabetic retinopathy). The new vessels can bleed (ocular hemorrhage) and cloud the retina, affecting vision. The signs and symptoms of diabetic retinopathy include blurred vision, floaters (spots before the eyes from hemorrhagic flecks), shadows or missing areas of vision, and problems with night vision. Treatment is directed at glycemic control and avoidance of contributing habits (e.g., smoking). Occasionally, medications are used to try to limit angiogenesis (blood vessel development).

Ears

The ear is the organ of sound. It gathers sound waves from the environment and processes these for interpretation by the brain. In addition to gathering sounds, the ears play an important role in balance and equilibrium. There are numerous conditions, both medical and traumatic, that can affect the ear. Traumatic conditions of the ear are discussed in the "Head, Neck, and Spinal Trauma" chapter. This chapter details nontraumatic disorders of the ear and associated structures.

Anatomy of the Ear

The ears are located on the lateral aspects of the head. Most of the structure of the ear is well protected by the bones of the skull. Anatomically, the ear comprises three regions: the external ear, the middle ear, and the inner ear.

The External Ear

The external ear is the part of the ear that we can readily see on physical examination. The major portion of the external ear is called the *pinna* or *auricle*. The pinna collects sound waves and directs them into the *external auditory canal* through the *external auditory meatus to* contact the *tympanic membrane*. The external auditory canal extends to the tympanic membrane. The canal contains a protective substance called **cerumen** (earwax) that is secreted by specialized glands within the canal (Figure 12-6).

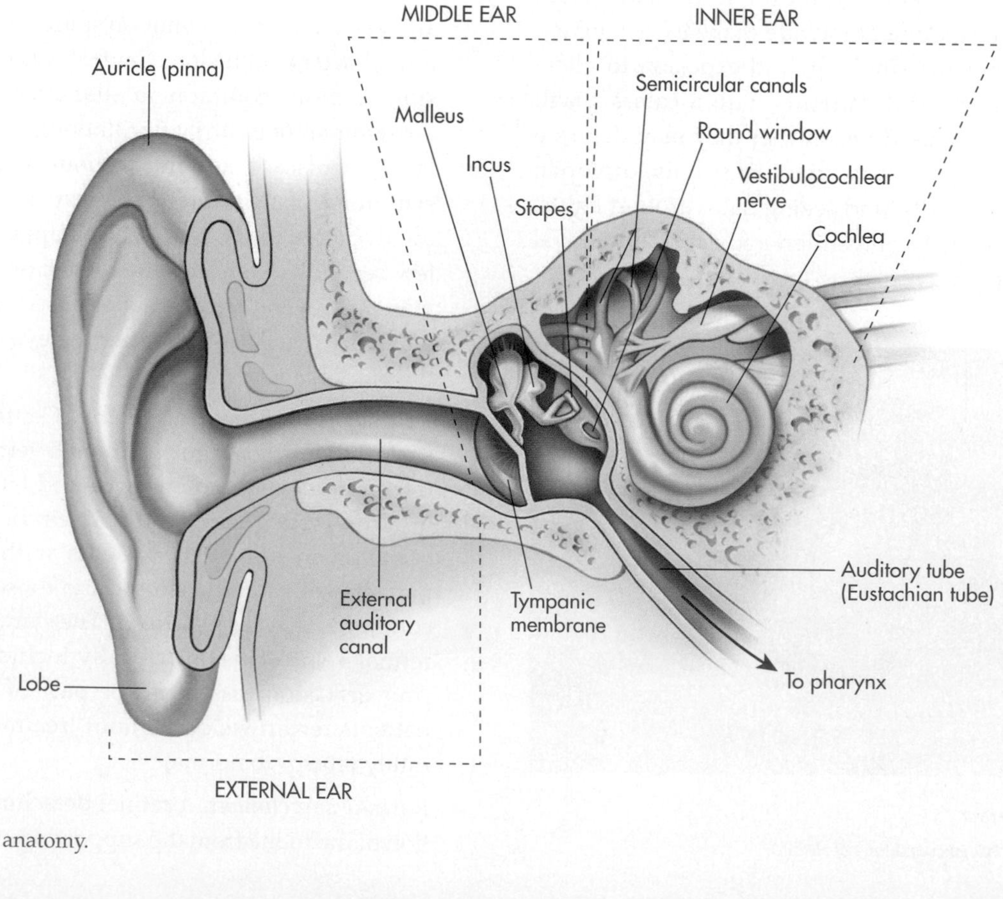

FIGURE 12-6 Ear anatomy.

The Middle Ear

The middle ear is the portion of the ear that contains the *auditory ossicles*. The auditory ossicles are three small bones that are joined together and function to amplify sound waves received by the tympanic membrane. These three bones, called the *malleus*, *incus*, and *stapes*, are well protected within the *tympanic cavity*. The middle ear is connected to the pharynx by the *Eustachian (auditory) tube*. This connection to the pharynx enables equalization of pressure between the middle ear and the environment.

The Inner Ear

The inner ear is separated from the middle ear by the *oval window*. Hearing and *equilibrium* are provided by specialized receptors within the inner ear. These receptors are well protected by the *bony labyrinth*. The bony labyrinth is surrounded by a collection of tubes and chambers called the *membranous labyrinth*. The membranous labyrinth is filled with a fluid called **endolymph**. The bony labyrinth can generally be divided into three parts:

- ***Vestibule.*** The vestibule contains membranous sacs that sense gravity and linear acceleration.
- ***Semicircular canals.*** The semicircular canals contain sensory structures that detect rotation of the head. The vestibule and semicircular canals are often called, collectively, the *vestibular complex*.
- ***Cochlea.*** The cochlea is a spiral-shaped structure that contains the *cochlear duct* of the membranous labyrinth. Receptors within the cochlea provide our sense of hearing (Figure 12-7).

Medical Conditions of the Ear

Although the ear is vulnerable to trauma, there are multiple medical conditions that also can affect the ear. These include the following:

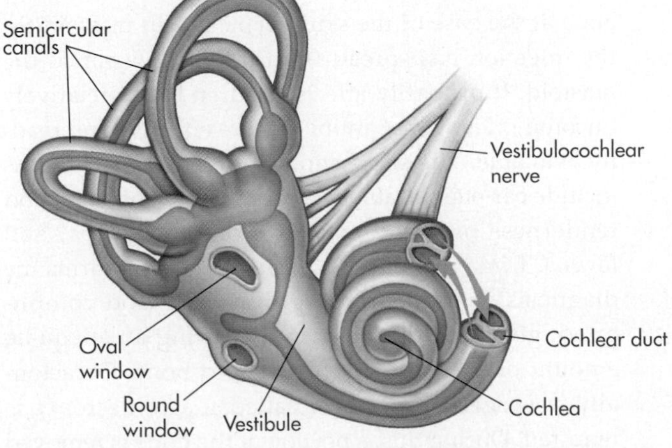

FIGURE 12-7 Internal ear anatomy.

CONTENT REVIEW

➤ Medical Conditions of the Ear
- Foreign body
- Impacted cerumen
- Infections
- Perforated tympanic membrane
- Mastoiditis
- Labyrinthitis
- Ménière's disease

- ***Foreign body.*** A foreign body in the external auditory canal is not uncommon. It is particularly common in children—especially toddlers. Any object small enough to fit into the external auditory canal is suspect. The vast majority of foreign bodies in the ear are placed there voluntarily. However, insects can also crawl into the ear—especially when the patient is asleep.

  Although foreign bodies rarely are a medical emergency, they can be quite painful and disturbing to the patient. Typically, patients will complain of ear pain. They are occasionally nauseated. Bleeding is common. If the foreign body is an insect, the patient may feel the insect moving or buzzing within the canal. In many instances, the foreign body can be removed with gentle suction or small forceps. Metallic objects can be removed with a small magnet. Alternatively, the external auditory canal can be gently irrigated with warm water.

  An insect within the ear can cause trauma and infection. The insect can be difficult to remove, because it moves and is easily broken up by forceps and other surgical instruments. A simple solution is to fill the external auditory canal with mineral oil. This will suffocate the insect, allowing easier removal with forceps.
- ***Impacted cerumen.*** Cerumen protects the ear by trapping dust. However, excess cerumen can block the external auditory canal and interfere with hearing. This is a common condition in some individuals. The symptoms of cerumen impaction include earache, a sensation of ear plugging, tinnitus, and a partial hearing loss. Examination with an otoscope reveals a cerumen plug occluding the canal. The plug can be removed with various agents including mineral oil, baby oil, commercial drops, detergents, and hydrogen peroxide.
- ***Infections.*** Infections of the ear are common. In fact, ear infections are one of the most common conditions for which people, particularly children, receive health care. Ear infections are typically divided into two classes: external ear infections (*otitis externa*) and middle ear infections (*otitis media*):
  - ***Otitis externa.*** Otitis externa, also called *swimmer's ear*, is an inflammation, irritation, or infection of the outer ear and/or the external auditory canal. It is a common condition and can result from infection, allergic reactions, and chronic skin conditions. Signs and symptoms of otitis externa include ear pain, drainage, itching of the ear or ear canal, and hearing

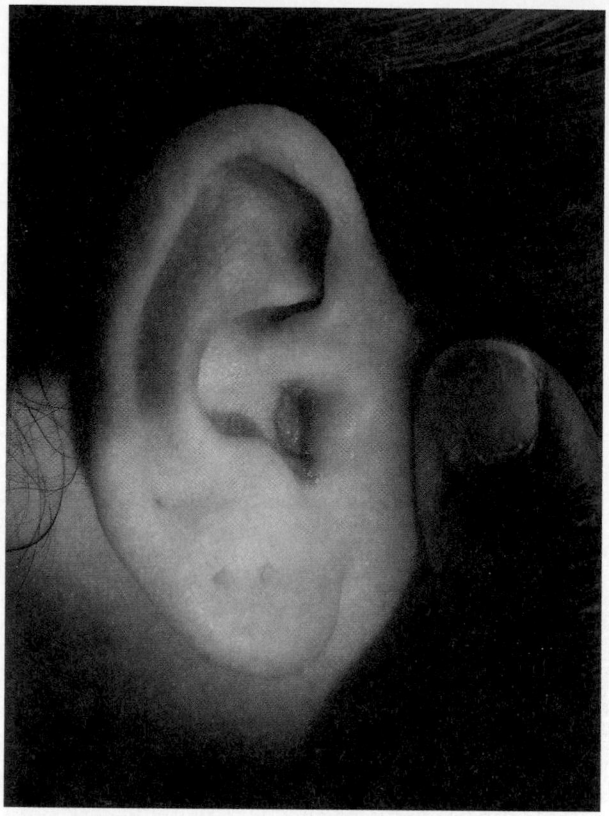

FIGURE 12-8 Otitis externa.

(Reproduced with permission from Otolaryngology Houston, www.ghorayeb.com)

loss. Examination of the external auditory canal will typically reveal erythema and swelling. Movement of the pinna often causes pain (Figure 12-8). Treatment typically involves analgesia and topical otic antibiotics and anti-inflammatory drugs.

A serious form of otitis externa is *malignant otitis externa*. Malignant otitis externa is an infection of the external ear that has spread to the bones and cartilage at the base of the skull. It is an uncommon complication of otitis externa and is typically caused by difficult-to-treat bacterial infections. Patients who are diabetic, who are immunosuppressed, or who are receiving chemotherapy are at increased risk. The signs and symptoms of malignant otitis externa include the signs and symptoms of regular otitis externa (earache, ear pain, drainage) as well as fever, difficulty swallowing, loss of voice, and facial weakness. Treatment generally involves hospitalization and appropriate antibiotic therapy.[6]

- ***Otitis media.*** Otitis media is a common condition, particularly in children. Blockage of the Eustachian tube is often the cause, as blockage of the tube can increase fluid pressure within the middle ear. This can result in a bacterial or viral infection. Ear infections are common in children because their Eustachian tubes are more easily blocked than those of adults. Anything that causes blockage of the Eustachian tube can cause otitis media, including allergies, upper respiratory infections, excessive mucus and saliva during teething, and irritants. The signs and symptoms of otitis media include earache, fullness or pressure, general malaise, hearing loss, and fever. In children, pulling at the ear may be noted. Vomiting and diarrhea are common. On physical exam, the tympanic membrane will appear red and distended.

  Although it was once common practice to treat all middle ear infections with antibiotics, it is now known that most ear infections, particularly in children, clear without antibiotic therapy. Middle ear infections are generally classified as acute or chronic. These conditions are treated somewhat differently. A chronic middle ear infection is one that persists or recurs and places the individual at risk of permanent ear damage. In addition to antibiotics, chronic middle ear infections may require the placement of tympanostomy tubes to decompress the middle ear.

- ***Perforated tympanic membrane.*** The tympanic membrane is a delicate structure that separates the external ear from the middle ear. The membrane is easily perforated or ruptured by trauma (including changes in pressure—barotrauma), by foreign objects in the ear, and by infection. The patient typically complains of decreased hearing, earache, drainage of blood or pus from the ear, and noise or buzzing in the ear. Symptoms often begin acutely (or the patient notes an acute change in the condition). Physical examination of the membrane with an otoscope will reveal a perforation or damage to the structure. In most instances, the perforation will heal. Treatment primarily involves analgesia and strategies to prevent infection. Protecting the ear and using topical antibiotics is the primary therapy (Figure 12-9).

- ***Mastoiditis.*** Mastoiditis is an infection of the mastoid bone at the base of the skull. Typically, in mastoiditis, the infection has spread from the middle ear to the mastoid. It primarily affects children but is relatively uncommon now that antibiotics are effective and readily available. The signs and symptoms of mastoiditis include ear pain, drainage, hearing loss, erythema and tenderness over the mastoid bone, headache, and fever. CT imaging of the mastoid usually confirms the diagnosis. Treatment is typically long and complicated, given the difficulty in delivering an adequate amount of antibiotic to the mastoid bone. Occasionally, a surgical procedure called mastoidectomy is required. During this, a portion of the bone is removed and the infection drained.

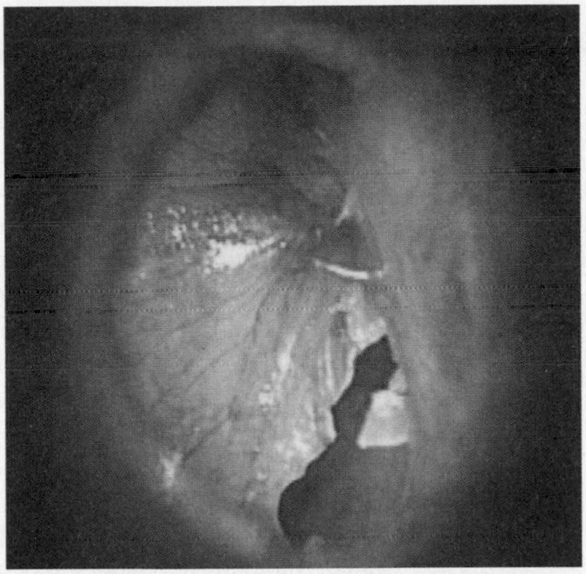

FIGURE 12-9 Perforated tympanic membrane.

(Reproduced with permission from Otolaryngology Houston, www.ghorayeb.com)

- ***Labyrinthitis.*** Labyrinthitis is a swelling and irritation of the inner ear. It tends to occur following a middle ear infection or upper respiratory infection. It can also occur with allergies and with use of certain medications. Inflammation of the inner ear can affect normal functioning, causing vertigo, involuntary eye movements (nystagmus), dizziness, loss of balance, nausea and vomiting, hearing loss, and tinnitus. Treatment is primarily symptomatic and includes the use of antiemetic medications and/or benzodiazepines. Nausea and vomiting are common complaints and can be treated with antiemetic medications such as ondansetron.
- ***Ménière's disease.*** Ménière's disease is a disease of the inner ear that affects balance and hearing. It occurs when the labyrinths within the inner ear become swollen. Although the cause of Ménière's disease is unknown, it may be related to middle ear infections and prior head injury. The signs and symptoms of Ménière's disease often begin acutely and include severe vertigo and dizziness, severe nausea and vomiting, and hearing loss. Typically, the hearing loss is unilateral. Symptoms are usually worsened by sudden movement and can last from minutes to hours. There is no known cure for Ménière's disease. However, symptoms can be attenuated through the use of a low-salt diet, diuretic medications, and preventive strategies such as avoiding sudden movement, bright lights, and similar factors that can provoke an attack. In the prehospital setting, treatment of nausea and vomiting with an antiemetic such as ondansetron or a similar medication may be beneficial.[7]

Assessment Pearls

What is the difference between dizziness and vertigo? Many people think they are synonymous, but the words are not actually interchangeable. *Dizziness*, also called light-headedness, is a nonspecific term often used to indicate true vertigo, imbalance, or a form of near syncope. *True vertigo* is a more specific condition. It is an illusion of rotary motion caused by differences in nervous signals between the right and left *vestibular nuclei*. The brain interprets these as rotary motion (e.g., "the room is spinning"). It is usually worsened by head movement and is almost always temporary. The diagnosis of general dizziness or of true vertigo can usually be made based on the history and physical examination. Treatment depends on the underlying cause and is usually symptomatic.

Nose

The nose is the organ of smell. It also has other important functions, including filtering, warming, and humidifying incoming air. There are several nontraumatic conditions of the nose that you may encounter in the prehospital setting. These are detailed next. Traumatic nasal conditions are discussed in the chapter "Head, Neck, and Spinal Trauma."

Anatomy and Physiology of the Nose

As just stated, the nose (referred to anatomically as the *nasal cavity*) has numerous functions. From the standpoint of sensory function, the nose is the organ of smell. The sense of smell originates from receptors in the olfactory region of the upper part of the nasal cavity. The nerves that arise from the olfactory receptors are a part of the first cranial nerve (the olfactory nerve) and enter the brain through the cribriform plate. When the brain processes the incoming signals, we smell. The senses of smell and taste are closely related. The warming, cleansing, and humidification of air are also important functions of the nose.

The structures of the nose are highly vascular. A specific area, called **Kiesselbach's plexus**, is a network of four arteries located in the anteroinferior region of the nasal septum. It is the region where approximately 90 percent of nosebleeds occur (Figure 12-10).

In addition to the nose, the sinuses can give rise to certain nontraumatic conditions. There are four sinuses (air-filled cavities separated from the nasal cavity by a mucous membrane): the *maxillary sinuses*, *the frontal sinuses*, the *ethmoid sinuses*, and the *sphenoid sinuses* (Figure 12-11).

CONTENT REVIEW

- Medical Conditions of the Nose
  - Epistaxis
  - Foreign body
  - Rhinitis
  - Sinusitis

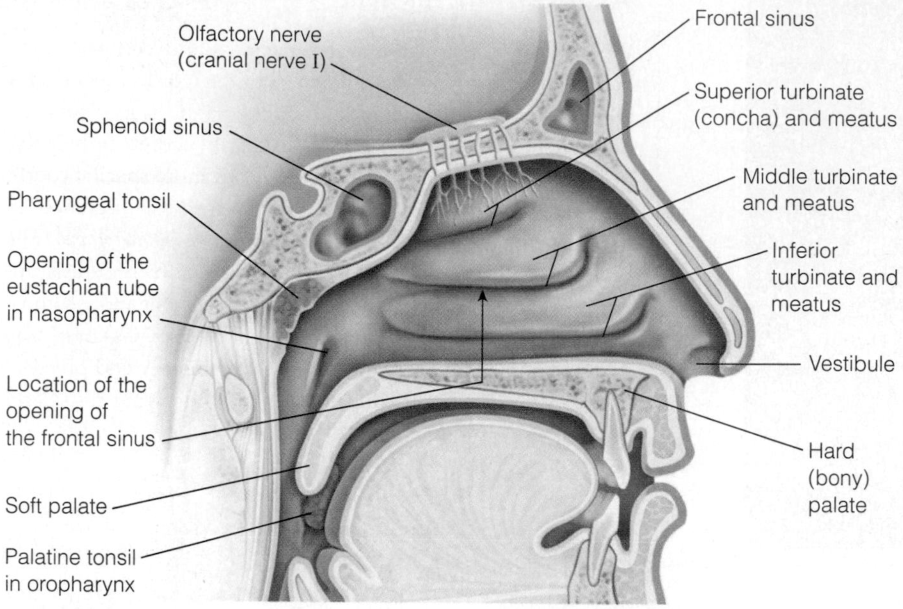

FIGURE 12-10 Nasal anatomy.

Medical Conditions of the Nose

Although the nose is vulnerable to trauma, there are also several nontraumatic (medical) conditions related to the nose and sinuses. These include:

- ***Epistaxis.*** Epistaxis is a nosebleed. Nosebleeds are quite common, with most occurring secondary to minor irritations or upper respiratory infections. Bleeding usually occurs when the nasal mucosa becomes eroded and the underlying blood vessels are exposed. These subsequently rupture, leading to bleeding. Fortunately, most nosebleeds are not life threatening. Epistaxis is typically divided into two categories: anterior bleeds and posterior bleeds. The vast majorities of nosebleeds are anterior bleeds and arise from Kiesselbach's plexus, as described earlier. Posterior bleeds arise from blood vessels further back in the nasal cavity. Posterior bleeds tend to be arterial in origin and tend to be more profuse than anterior bleeds.

  Nosebleeds can arise from such conditions as low humidity, topical medications (e.g., cocaine), structural abnormalities (e.g., deviated septum), inflammation, tumors, blood coagulation disorders, and hypertension. In some instances, the cause of epistaxis is not readily evident. The signs and symptoms of epistaxis are easy to detect. Often, the bleeding is painless. With anterior bleeds, blood flow drains through the nares. Posterior bleeds, which are more often associated with hypertension, tend to drain into the nasopharynx and into the mouth (where much of the blood is swallowed) (Figure 12-12). Nausea and vomiting are more common with posterior bleeds.

  Treatment of nosebleeds is based on the location of the bleed and the cause. In many instances, bleeding stops with simple pressure. In other instances, medications and devices are needed to control the source of the bleeding. Cauterization of the bleeding site can sometimes be accomplished if the site is readily identified. Prehospital treatment of epistaxis includes strategies to stop bleeding such as simply pinching the nose. In some EMS systems, paramedics may insert catheters or nasal tampons to control bleeding. Pain can be present and should be treated with analgesics. With posterior bleeds, nausea and vomiting are often present and should be treated with antiemetics.

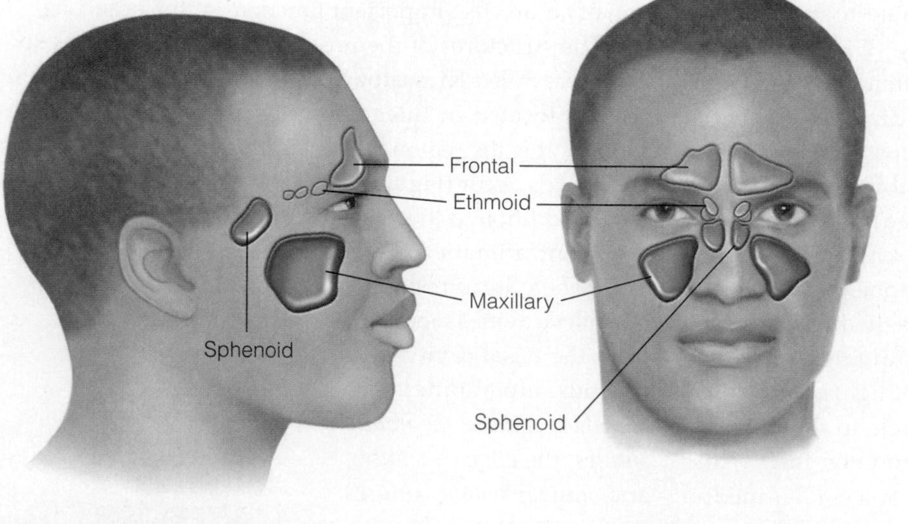

FIGURE 12-11 Sinus anatomy.

- ***Foreign body.*** Nasal foreign bodies are common—especially in pediatric patients. Anything small enough to be placed in the nares and into the nose is a potential nasal foreign body. Common items include pieces of toys, beads, small rocks, and similar items, including food items. In many instances, the patient will be asymptomatic. There may be whistling with respiration. In others, there may be pain and even infection. The primary treatment is removal of the foreign body. There are several methods to achieve this. However, in very young children, the procedure can be somewhat difficult. Repeated

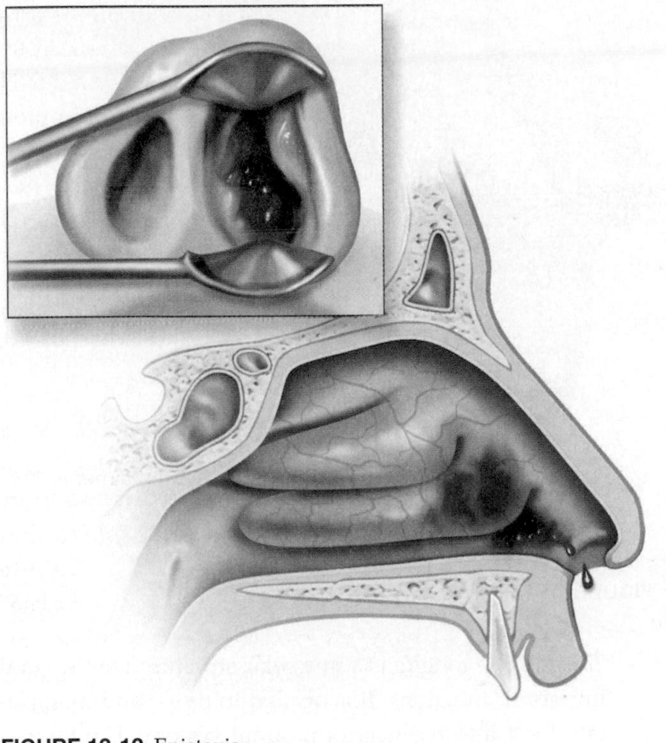

FIGURE 12-12 Epistaxis.

attempts at foreign body removal can cause additional trauma.[8]

- *Rhinitis.* Rhinitis is an inflammation of the nose. It is most commonly associated with an upper respiratory infection but also occurs with allergies and similar conditions (Figure 12-13). It can occur in both adults and children. It is significantly more common in infants, who are obligate nasal breathers. The treatment of rhinitis depends on the cause. In infants, rhinitis is usually treated with humidification of air, saline nose drops, and bulb suctioning. Nasal decongestants are not recommended for children because of well-documented complications. In adults, decongestants can help decrease the swelling of the nasal mucosa and improve airflow and congestion. With allergic rhinitis, antihistamines and nasal corticosteroids are the preferred treatments.
- *Sinusitis.* Sinusitis is an infection or inflammation of the sinuses. It can result from several causes, including infections (both bacterial and viral) as well as allergies and similar conditions. Sinus infections often occur secondarily to upper respiratory infections. The signs and symptoms of sinusitis include facial pressure, headache, sore throat, posterior nasal drip, cough (often worse at night, when secretions drain), bad breath, loss of smell, malaise, and occasionally fever. On physical exam, there is usually tenderness to percussion over the frontal or maxillary sinus. The pharynx is often injected (that is, red or erythematous) with posterior drainage noted. There may be swelling of the anterior cervical lymph nodes. The treatment of sinusitis is based on the cause. Bacterial sinusitis is often treated with antibiotics and decongestants in adults. Allergic and viral sinusitis is treated symptomatically. Antihistamines, decongestants, and corticosteroids are sometimes used (Figure 12-14).

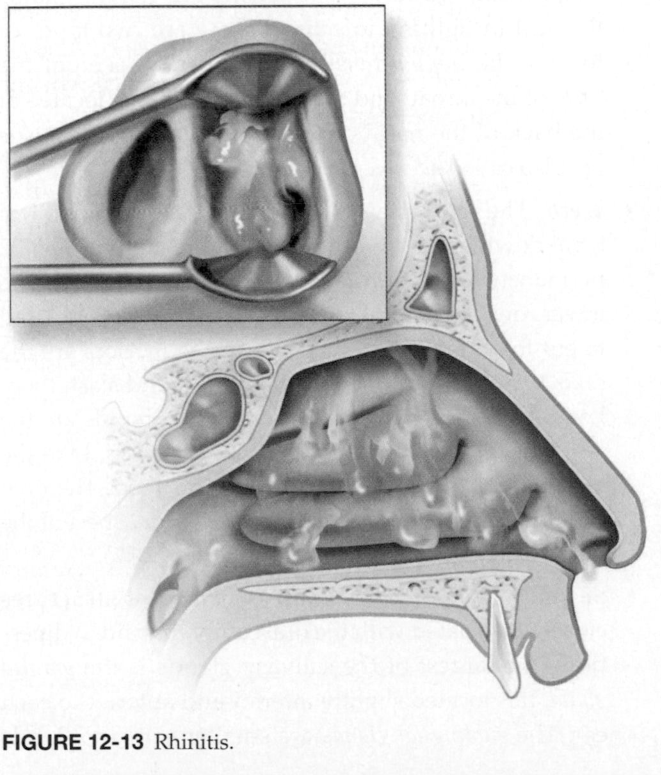

FIGURE 12-13 Rhinitis.

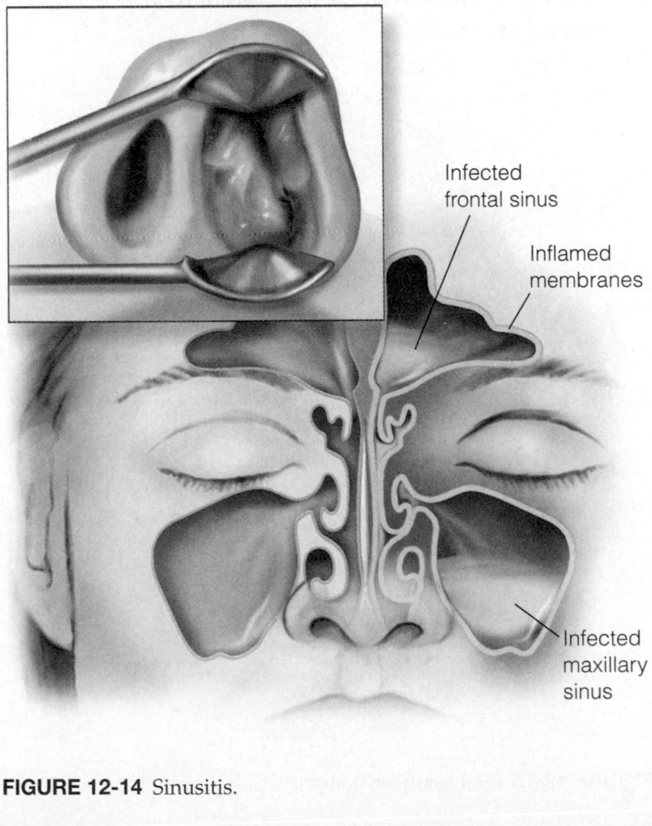

FIGURE 12-14 Sinusitis.

Throat

The mouth and throat are the route of entry into the gastrointestinal system. They are also an important part of the route of entry to the respiratory system. Disorders of the throat and mouth are common conditions. In many instances, these infections are not limited to the anatomic structures of the mouth and throat, but also involve adjoining structures such as the nose and lower airway. There are many nontraumatic medical conditions of the throat and mouth that will be detailed next. Traumatic conditions of the throat and mouth are detailed in the "Head, Neck, and Spinal Trauma" chapter.

Anatomy and Physiology of the Mouth and Throat

The mouth is the opening to the oral cavity and is the entrance to the gastrointestinal tract. These structures also serve as a conduit for the respiratory gases entering and leaving the respiratory system. The oral cavity senses and analyzes substances before swallowing, mechanically processes food, and enhances digestion through the introduction of lubrication and digestive enzymes. The many structures within the oral cavity (Figure 12-15) include:

- ***Labia (lips).*** The lips are the structures that protect the mouth from the environment. They are contiguous with the cheeks that make up the lateral walls of the oral cavity. Within the oral cavity, the cheeks are covered by the buccal mucosa as a protective layer.
- ***Palate.*** The palate is the upper portion (roof) of the oral cavity. It is divided into the hard palate and the soft palate.

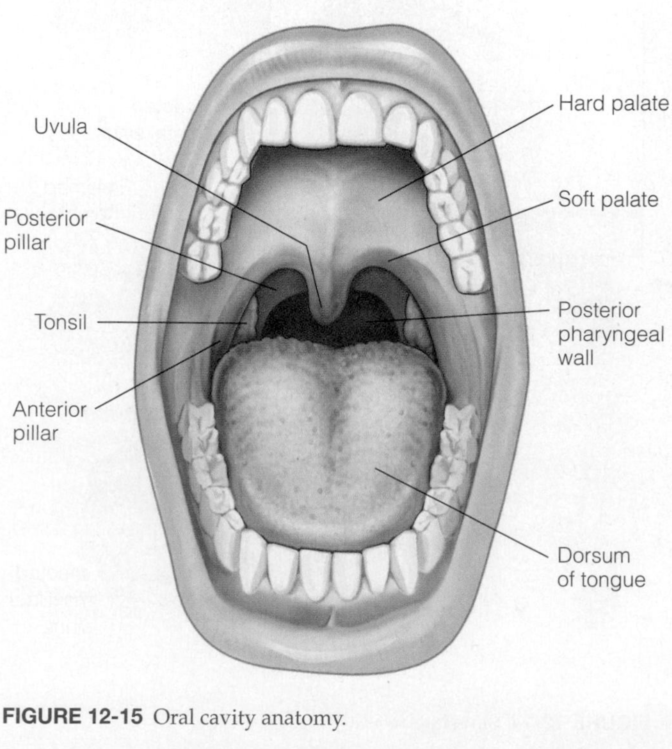

FIGURE 12-15 Oral cavity anatomy.

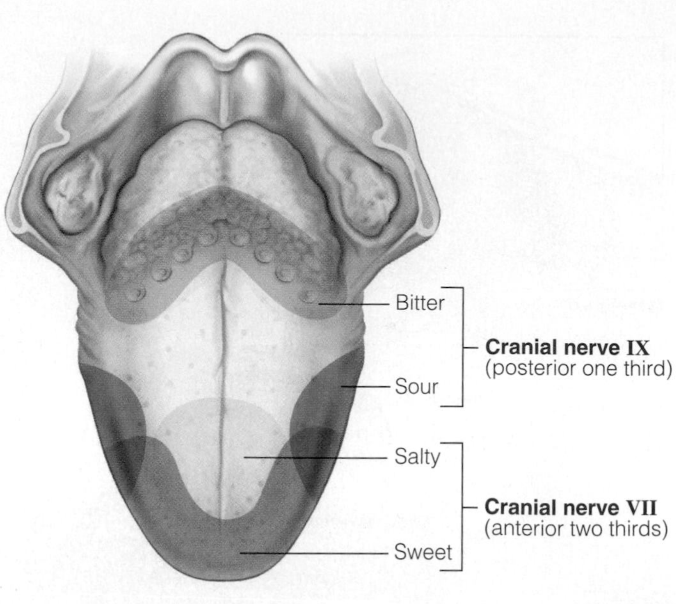

FIGURE 12-16 The tongue.

- ***Tongue.*** The tongue is a muscular structure with several important functions. It is needed to move and manipulate food into the gastrointestinal system. The tongue contains sensory structures (taste buds) that allow us to taste and identify substances in the mouth (Figure 12-16).
- ***Pharynx.*** The posterior aspect of the oral cavity is the pharynx, which is bounded by the posterior pharyngeal wall and associated structures.
- ***Uvula.*** The uvula is a singular structure hanging from the posterior aspect of the mouth. It helps to block food and other substances from entering the nose during swallowing.
- ***Tonsils and adenoids.*** The tonsils are lymph glands that aid in fighting infection. There are two types of tonsils: the *lingual tonsils* (which can be seen at the back of the throat) and the *pharyngeal tonsils* (located at the back of the nasal cavity). The pharyngeal tonsils are also called *adenoids*.
- ***Teeth.*** The teeth play a major role in the mechanical breakdown of food for digestion. There are typically 32 permanent teeth, with 16 in the upper row and 16 in the lower row. The central teeth, called the *incisors*, are used to cut food. Immediately lateral to the incisors are the *canine* or *cuspid* teeth, which hold, tear, and slash food. Lateral and somewhat posterior to the cuspids are the *bicuspids*, which are also called the *premolars*. Like the bicuspids, the premolars primarily tear food. The final type of teeth are the *molars*, at the posterior aspect of the dental ridges, which grind food (Figure 12-17).
- ***Salivary glands.*** The *salivary glands* are structures closely associated with the oral cavity that aid in digestion. The largest of the salivary glands is the *parotid gland*. It is located slightly inferior and anterior to each ear. The *sublingual glands* are smaller salivary glands

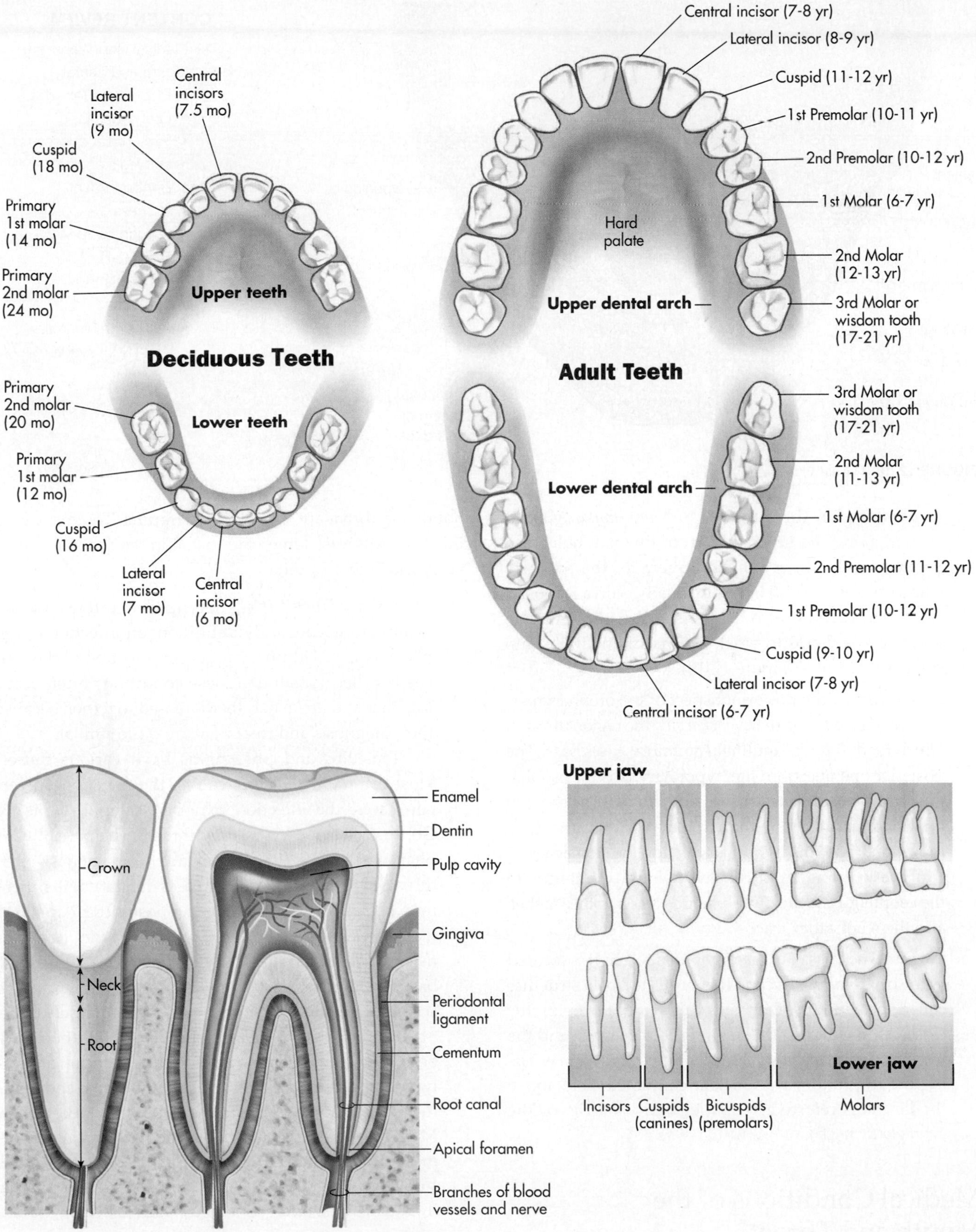

FIGURE 12-17 The teeth.

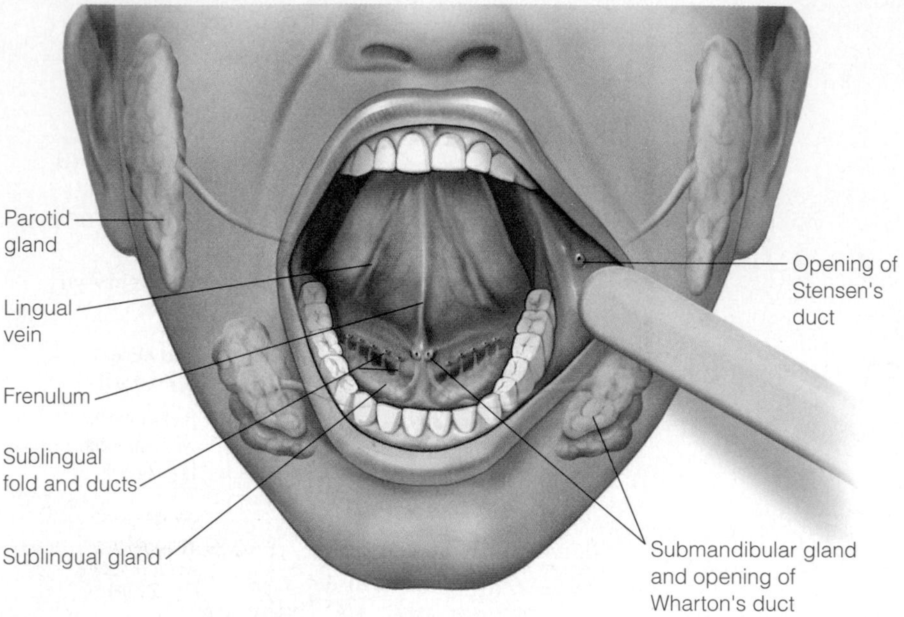

FIGURE 12-18 The salivary glands and ducts.

CONTENT REVIEW

➤ Medical Conditions of the Mouth and Throat
- Pharyngitis/tonsillitis
- Oral candidiasis
- Peritonsillar abscess
- Ludwig's angina
- Dentalgia/dental abscess
- Foreign body
- Epiglottitis
- Laryngitis
- Tracheitis
- Temporomandibular joint (TMJ) syndrome

located under the tongue. *Submandibular glands*, located along the inner surface of the mandible, also participate in digestion. On average, the salivary glands secrete 1 to 1.5 L of saliva daily. Saliva is mostly water. However, it also contains a digestive enzyme, amylase, that helps to break down carbohydrates into smaller molecules (Figure 12-18).

- ***Esophagus.*** At the posterior aspect of the oropharynx is an area referred to as the *hypopharynx*, the region through which food, liquids, and the respiratory gases pass. The posterior opening from the hypopharynx is the esophagus, which is the route for food and liquids. The esophagus is a muscular tube that systematically contracts to move food from the hypopharynx into the stomach.

  The opening from the hypopharynx, anterior to the esophagus, is the glottis, which leads to the trachea and the respiratory tract.

- ***Larynx.*** The larynx is the organ of speech. It is located at the origin of the *trachea*. It is protected by a structure called the *epiglottis*. During swallowing, the epiglottis closes off the glottis, the opening to the larynx and the trachea, to prevent food, liquids, and saliva from entering the respiratory tract. The area immediately above the larynx is referred to as the *laryngopharynx* or the *supraglottic region*.

Medical Conditions of the Mouth and Throat

Medical conditions of the mouth and throat are common. A number of these are infectious in origin and were discussed in the "Infectious Diseases and Sepsis" chapter. Some of this material is reviewed briefly in the next section. Certainly, the mouth and throat are vulnerable to trauma. Traumatic conditions are discussed in greater detail in the chapter "Head, Neck, and Spinal Trauma."

- ***Pharyngitis/Tonsillitis.*** Pharyngitis and tonsillitis are common infections. By definition, an infection of the pharynx is called pharyngitis; an infection of the tonsils is called tonsillitis. These conditions often occur together and are generally discussed together, because their diagnosis and treatment are quite similar.

  Tonsillitis and pharyngitis have various causes. Most commonly, a virus causes the infection. In certain cases, the infection may be bacterial—typically Group A streptococcus (strep throat). The patient with pharyngitis/tonsillitis will exhibit a red and swollen throat (Figure 12-19). In some cases of pharyngitis, there may be an exudate (pus) on the posterior pharyngeal wall or tonsils. This finding, called *exudative pharyngitis* or *exudative tonsillitis*, tends to be associated with a bacterial infection such as strep. However, it can also be seen in some viral infections, such as mononucleosis.

  In many cases of pharyngitis/tonsillitis, there may be enlargement and tenderness of the anterior cervical lymph nodes. Headache, neck pain, nausea, and vomiting may also be present. The patient is often febrile. Most cases occur in late winter and early spring. Treatment of pharyngitis/tonsillitis is based on the cause. Viral infections often resolve with only symptomatic treatment. Bacterial infections, such as strep throat, may require antibiotics.

- ***Oral candidiasis.*** Oral candidiasis, commonly called *thrush*, is a fungal (yeast) infection of the mouth. The most common causative agent is the fungus *Candida albicans*. Oral candidiasis is most common in infants,

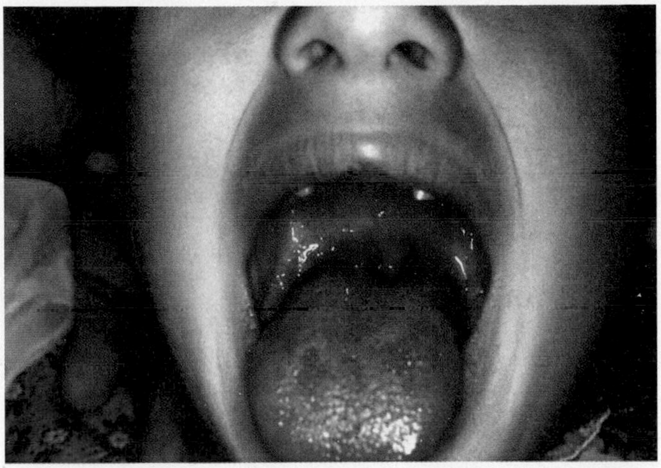

FIGURE 12-19 Tonsillitis.

(Centers for Disease Control and Prevention)

diabetics with poor glucose control, and AIDS patients, and is a side effect to taking antibiotics. *Candida albicans* is normally present in the flora of the mouth. However, bacteria, also present in the normal mouth flora, keep the quantity of the fungus present at an acceptable level. However, during disease states and with use of antibiotics, bacteria are reduced and the yeast grows as an opportunistic infection.

On physical examination the patient typically exhibits a white- or cream-colored deposit on mucous membranes. The oral mucosa may be erythematous and swollen. In babies, there may be poor feeding and irritability. In adults, the most common complaint is pain or difficulty swallowing. Treatment includes removing the offending agent, correcting risk factors, and the use of antifungal agents.

- ***Peritonsillar abscess.*** A peritonsillar abscess is a collection of infected material (pus) in the area around the tonsils. In most cases, it is a complication of tonsillitis and is usually caused by group A beta-hemolytic streptococcus. Peritonsillar abscess is usually a disease of older children, adolescents, and young adults. It has become less common with the use of antibiotics to treat tonsillitis. Generally, peritonsillar abscess is unilateral although it can be bilateral. The infection may spread over the roof of the mouth (palate), and to the neck and chest, including the lungs. Swollen tissues may block the airway, which is a life-threatening medical emergency. In some cases, the abscess can break open (rupture) into the throat, infecting or further blocking the airway.

  The signs and symptoms of peritonsillar abscess include:

  - Chills
  - Difficulty opening the mouth (or pain with opening the mouth)
  - Difficulty swallowing (dysphagia)
  - Drooling or inability to swallow saliva
  - Facial swelling
  - Fever
  - Headache
  - Muffled voice
  - Sore throat (may be severe and is usually on one side)
  - Tender glands of the jaw and throat

  Treatment is drainage of the abscess and antibiotics. Prehospital treatment should ensure airway protection and treatment of hypoxia. If the patient is having trouble swallowing secretions, allow him to self-suction his mouth with a Yankauer suction tip. Pain and nausea are common, and analgesics and antiemetics may be indicated.[9]

- ***Ludwig's Angina.*** **Ludwig's angina** is a type of oral bacterial cellulitis, or inflammation, that involves the floor of the mouth under the tongue. It often occurs after an infection of the roots of the teeth (dental abscess) or a mouth injury. It is uncommon in children. Ludwig's angina develops quickly, and swelling of the tissues occurs quickly and occludes the airway. It can be life threatening.

  The symptoms of Ludwig's angina include:

  - Breathing difficulty
  - Confusion or other mental changes
  - Fever
  - Neck pain
  - Neck swelling
  - Redness of the neck
  - Weakness, fatigue, excess tiredness
  - Difficulty swallowing
  - Drooling
  - Earache
  - Speech that is unusual and sounds like the person has a "hot potato" in the mouth

  Examination of the neck and head typically shows erythema and swelling of the upper neck and under the chin. The swelling may reach across the floor of the mouth. The tongue may be swollen or out of place.

  The primary prehospital concern is protection of the airway. In severe cases, a surgical airway (e.g., cricothyrotomy) may be required. Hospital care generally includes parenteral antibiotics. Surgery is sometimes required. Ludwig's angina can be life threatening. However, it can be cured with proper protection of the airways and appropriate antibiotics.[10]

- ***Dentalgia and dental abscess.*** Dental problems are a common reason for people to seek emergency care. Dental injury, infection, and abscess can lead to pain, fever, and similar complaints. The teeth, if properly cared for, will last a lifetime. However, without dental care, cavities and infections will ultimately damage and destroy the teeth. Most issues related to dental pain (with the exception of trauma) are a direct result of lack of preventive dental care and restorative care. Most dental emergencies are not life threatening.

  Dental pain, called *dentalgia*, occurs when the exterior of the tooth is broken down, allowing the sensitive interior structures, including the nerve, to be exposed. In the case of infection, the development of closed-space infections, called abscesses, is common and can cause pain. Abscesses are usually seen at the gum line. Although nontraumatic dental problems are troublesome, they are rarely an emergency. Emergency care includes the alleviation of pain, treatment of infection (if present), and appropriate dental care.

- ***Foreign body.*** Foreign bodies can lodge in the mouth or throat, sometimes creating an emergency situation. The oral cavity is large enough that few foreign bodies become stuck in this region. However, some foreign objects can lodge in the hypopharynx and obstruct the airway. It is not uncommon for patients to seek emergency care for swallowed foreign bodies or foreign bodies that become lodged or stuck in the mouth and throat.

  Three groups are at increased risk for such gastrointestinal foreign bodies: children, psychiatric patients and prisoners, and patients who do not have their natural teeth. Most foreign bodies seen in children are objects they simply picked up and placed into their mouth. In adults, the foreign bodies are more likely animal bones, especially fish bones, and food boluses. In addition, toothpicks, dentures, and similar items can become stuck or lodged in the mouth or throat. In psychiatric patients, virtually anything can become a foreign body.

  The patient with a potential oral or swallowed foreign body will complain of an inability to swallow or a foreign-body sensation. Prehospital treatment is always aimed at ensuring a proper airway, making the patient comfortable, and transporting him to a facility where the foreign body can be removed. If it is uncertain that a foreign body is present, examination of the oropharynx and hypopharynx with a laryngoscope or a video laryngoscope may help identify the source of the problem.

- ***Epiglottitis.*** Epiglottitis is an inflammation or infection of the epiglottis and can be a life-threatening emergency. The infection or inflammation can cause swelling of the epiglottis, thus potentially causing obstruction of the proximal airway. Fortunately, the condition is now relatively uncommon because of immunizations and antibiotics. The signs and symptoms of epiglottitis include fever and a sore throat. The patient may have drooling from inability to swallow saliva, stridor, hoarseness, difficulty breathing, and even cyanosis. Treatment includes protection of the airway and administration of appropriate antibiotics and other therapies. The treatment of epiglottitis is discussed in greater detail in the chapters "Pulmonology" and "Pediatrics."[11]

- ***Laryngitis.*** Laryngitis is a swelling and inflammation of the larynx. It is most commonly caused by a viral infection or draining from an upper airway/sinus infection. However, there are other causes, including allergies, bacterial infections, injury, chemical exposures, gastroesophageal reflux disease (GERD), and pneumonia. Signs and symptoms of laryngitis include fever, hoarseness, and loss of voice. Because laryngitis is primarily viral, symptomatic treatment is all that is required. If there is a concern about the airway, consideration should be given to more serious conditions such as croup or epiglottitis.

- ***Tracheitis.*** Tracheitis is an inflammation or infection of the trachea. It is similar to laryngitis except that it involves lower airway structures. Unlike laryngitis, tracheitis is usually a bacterial infection and is limited to the trachea below the level of the larynx. The signs and symptoms of tracheitis include a deep cough (similar to that seen in croup), dyspnea, fever, and stridor. In some cases, the patient may be hypoxic. The primary concern in the prehospital setting is prevention of airway obstruction and ventilation of the patient. This can be achieved through the use of mechanical airways and ventilation.

- ***Temporomandibular joint (TMJ) syndrome.*** Temporomandibular joint (TMJ) disorders result from problems with the joint between the temporal bone and the mandible (jaw). There are various causes of TMJ disorders, including malocclusion of the teeth. It can also result from orthodontic appliances and other factors. The signs and symptoms of TMJ disorders include difficulty in biting or chewing, pain with biting or chewing, and a clicking or popping of the TMJ joint when the patient closes or opens his mouth. In addition, patients with TMJ disorders often have dull facial pain, earache, jaw pain, or headache. The treatment depends on the underlying cause.

Summary

There will be instances during your career as a paramedic when you encounter a patient with a nontraumatic condition involving the ears, eyes, nose, mouth, throat, and/or associated structures. Some of these conditions may be life threatening. Others may not. However, prehospital treatment priorities remain the same. These include protection of the airway, ventilation (if required), and circulation. Once these have been established, paramedics should try to identify the cause of the problem and begin appropriate treatment. In many instances, treatment of the conditions discussed in this chapter is symptomatic. Pain should be treated with the appropriate analgesic. Nausea and vomiting should be treated with an appropriate antiemetic. Other issues should be treated as directed by local protocols. Regardless, many nontraumatic conditions involving the ears, eyes, nose, mouth, and throat can be true emergencies. Prompt recognition and treatment are essential.

You Make the Call

You are called to examine a 46-year-old man who states that he has "something stuck in my throat." He was eating dinner with some business associates and, while talking and eating, he quickly inhaled an unknown food particle. You take note of two empty martini glasses, without the olives, on the table near the patient. The patient keeps pointing to the back of his throat saying, "Look. Can't you see it? It's right there. I can feel it."

You complete your primary assessment and take the patient to the back of the ambulance, where it is more private and where you have medical equipment immediately available. The patient is seated on the squad bench, and you carefully look at the oropharynx and posterior pharynx with a bright light. You don't identify any particular foreign body. You then take a sterile tongue depressor and look a little deeper into the oropharynx. The patient keeps saying, "Surely you have to see it. It's right there. I can feel it." Despite a detailed exam, you cannot identify any foreign body.

1. At this point, what is your primary concern regarding this patient?
2. What alternative methods are available to evaluate this patient?
3. What should you do if you cannot visualize a foreign body or an injury secondary to the foreign body?

See Suggested Responses at the back of this book.

Review Questions

1. ___________ is a conjunctival condition characterized by raised, wedge-shaped growth on the conjunctiva. It is noncancerous and is readily visible over the white sclera and can sometimes extend over the cornea and invade the visual axis of the eye.
   a. Sty
   b. Chalazion
   c. Conjunctivitis
   d. Pterygium
2. Movements of the eyes are controlled by six ________ muscles, allowing us to look in various directions.
   a. sensory
   b. extraocular
   c. intraocular
   d. orbital
3. What is the name of the clear jellylike fluid that is contained in the posterior cavity of the eye?
   a. squamous humor
   b. aqueous humor
   c. vitreous humor
   d. synovial humor
4. Which condition is characterized by an increase of pressure in the eye?
   a. Hyphema
   b. Orbital cellulitis
   c. Uveitis
   d. Glaucoma

5. The ______________ collects sound waves and directs them into the external auditory canal.
   a. pinna
   b. external auditory meatus
   c. tympanic membrane
   d. malleus

6. What is the name of the spiral-shaped structure that contains the cochlear duct of the membranous labyrinth?
   a. cochlea
   b. stapes
   c. vestibule
   d. semicircular canal

7. What condition may exist if the patient is complaining of symptoms that include earache, fever, malaise, and partial hearing loss?
   a. Otitis externa
   b. Otitis media
   c. Cerumen impaction
   d. Mastoiditis

8. Which disease of the inner ear affects balance and hearing and occurs when the labyrinths within the inner ear become swollen?
   a. Otic disease
   b. Labyrinthitis
   c. Vertigo
   d. Ménière's disease

9. Which gland is the largest of the salivary glands?
   a. Parotid
   b. Salivary
   c. Sublingual
   d. Submandibular

10. Which fungal infection of the mouth is common in infants, diabetics with poor glucose control, and AIDS patients, and is a common side effect of taking antibiotics?
    a. Candida albicans
    b. Candidicans oral
    c. Oral candidiasis
    d. Peritonsillar abscess

See Answers to Review Questions at the back of this book.

References

1. Bledsoe, B. E. and B. Ho. "Sight-Threatening Eye Injuries: Prehospital Management of Ophthalmological Emergencies." *JEMS* 29 (2004): 94–106.
2. Hauser, A. and S. Fogarasi. "Periorbital and Orbital Cellulitis." *Pediatr Rev* 31 (2010): 242–249.
3. Dargin, J. M. and R. A. Lowenstein. "The Painful Eye." *Emerg Med Clin North Am* 26 (2008): 199–216.
4. Haymore, J. G. and L. J. Mejico. "Retinal Vascular Occlusion Syndromes." *Int Ophthalmol Clin* 49 (2008): 63–79.
5. Vortmann, M. and J. I. Schneider. "Acute Monocular Visual Loss." *Emerg Med Clin North Am* 26 (2008): 76–96.
6. Carfrae, M. J. and B. W. Kesser. "Malignant Otitis Externa." *Otolaryngol Clin North Am* 41 (2008): 537–549.
7. Kutz, J. W., Jr. "The Dizzy Patient." *Med Clin North Am* 94 (2010): 989–1002.
8. Heim, S. W. and K. L. Maughan. "Foreign Bodies in the Ear, Nose, and Throat." *Am Fam Physician* 76 (2007): 1185–1189.
9. Galioto, N. J. "Peritonsilar Abscess." *Am Fam Physician* 77 (2008): 199–202.
10. Saifeldeen, K. and R. Evans. "Ludwig's Angina." *Emerg Med J* 21 (2004): 242–243.
11. Nentwich, L. and A. S. Urich. "High-Risk Chief Complaints II: Disorders of the Head and Neck." *Emerg Med Clin North Am* 27 (2009): 713–746.

Further Reading

Koop, K. and L. Stack,. *The Atlas of Emergency Medicine.* 4th ed. Columbus, OH: McGraw-Hill, 2016.

Roberts, J. R. and J. R. Hedges. *Clinical Procedures in Emergency Medicine.* 6th ed. St. Louis: Saunders, 2013.

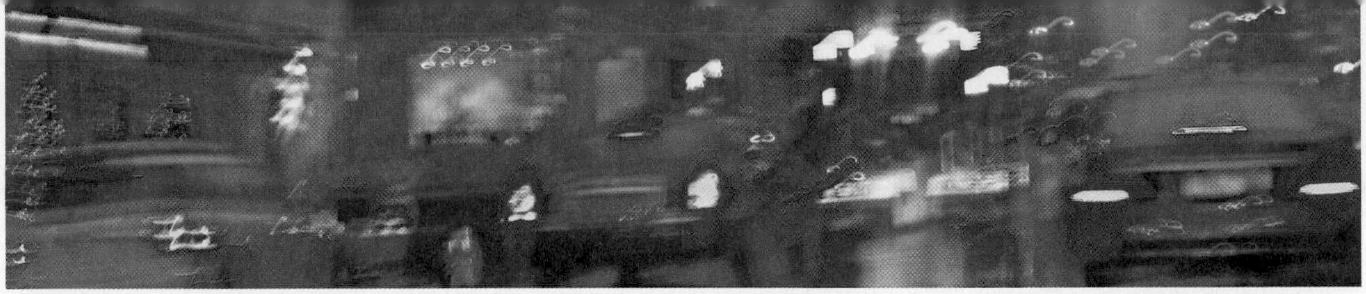

Chapter 13

Nontraumatic Musculoskeletal Disorders

Bryan Bledsoe, DO, FACEP, FAAEM, EMT-P

STANDARD

Medicine (Nontraumatic Musculoskeletal Disorders)

COMPETENCY

Integrates assessment findings with principles of epidemiology and pathophysiology to formulate a field impression and implement a comprehensive treatment/disposition plan for a patient with a medical complaint.

Learning Objectives

Terminal Performance Objective: After reading this chapter, you should be able to integrate patient assessment findings, patient history, and knowledge of anatomy, physiology, pathophysiology, and basic and advanced life support interventions to recognize and manage patients with nontraumatic musculoskeletal disorders.

Enabling Objectives: To accomplish the terminal performance objective, you should be able to:

1. Define key terms introduced in this chapter.
2. Review the anatomy and physiology of the musculoskeletal system.
3. Adapt the scene size-up, primary and secondary assessment, medical history, and use of monitoring technology to arrive at a field impression for nontraumatic musculoskeletal disorders.
4. Discuss the pathophysiology and assessment findings that would be present in a patient experiencing specific nontraumatic musculoskeletal disorders in the prehospital environment.
5. Use a process of clinical reasoning to guide and interpret the patient assessment findings and develop a treatment plan for patients displaying nontraumatic musculoskeletal disorders.
6. Given a variety of scenarios, discuss the integration of assessment and management guidelines as they relate to nontraumatic musculoskeletal disorder emergencies.

KEY TERMS

ankylosing spondylitis, p. 494
carpal tunnel syndrome (CTS), p. 492
cellulitis, p. 496
chronic pain syndrome (CPS), p. 498
epicondylitis, p. 492
fasciitis, p. 496
fibromyalgia, p. 499
gangrene, p. 496
gout, p. 495
necrotizing fasciitis (NF), p. 496
Osgood-Schlatter disease, p. 499
osteoarthritis (OA), p. 493
osteomyelitis, p. 497
osteoporosis, p. 493
reflex sympathetic dystrophy (RSD), p. 499
repetitive-motion disorders, p. 491
rheumatoid arthritis (RA), p. 494
septic arthritis, p. 497
systemic lupus erythematosus (SLE), p. 495
tendonitis, p. 492
tenosynovitis, p. 492

Case Study

On a busy Saturday morning in early summer, Watkins Hollow Volunteer Ambulance Corps is called to the local hardware store for an injured person. EMT Chris Kelly and paramedic Larry Johnson respond the short distance from the ambulance station to the store. On arrival, store employees escort the crew to the home and garden center where a man has fallen on a wet floor. As Larry turns the corner, he recognizes the man as a distant relative. He approaches him and says, "Bill, what on earth happened to you?" The patient states that he reached up for a bottle of plant food and slipped on the floor and struck his head. He sustained a laceration to the right temporal region. He thinks he was "knocked out for a second." There was a moderate amount of bleeding, but a store employee controlled it with a towel until the ambulance arrived. Bill says that he has a headache and that his neck is very sore. He denies other injury.

Everybody in town knows Bill Landers. He has been active in local politics and community events. He is also well recognized because he has severe ankylosing spondylitis. His disease is fairly advanced for a man in his 50s. He walks, always stooped, looking at the floor. He will look up to people, as best he can, through his glasses, without being able to raise his head. Bill has had ankylosing spondylitis as long as Larry can remember, but he has not let the disease slow his active and interesting life.

The paramedics remove the towel and inspect the wound. It is an approximately 5 cm linear laceration to the right side of his head. It will require sutures or staples. They place a dressing and bandage before turning their attention to preparing Bill for transport. The crew knows that Bill's ankylosing spondylitis has made his spinal column rigid and permanently curved. Because he has so much neck pain, they're assuming he has a potential fracture or injury to the spine. The crew is able to place a rigid cervical collar, but they know that Bill will not be able to lie flat and be placed on the long spine board. In anticipation of transport, Chris retrieves several blankets and towels from the ambulance. The crew members carefully move Bill to the ambulance stretcher and fill the void areas behind his neck and back with the towels to maintain his neck and back in a neutral position. Because of the excessive pain Bill is feeling, Larry places a saline lock and administers 50 mcg of fentanyl. This provides significant pain relief, and they move Bill to the ambulance for transport to the hospital.

The transport is uneventful, and the crew delivers Bill to the emergency department in improved condition. At the hospital, CT imaging of Bill's head, neck, and thoracic spine reveals no fractures, and the emergency department staff repairs the laceration with staples. Bill remains in the emergency department for several hours and is later discharged home in good condition.

Introduction

From the standpoint of emergency services, most musculoskeletal complaints are related to recent trauma. However, there are numerous nontraumatic conditions that involve the musculoskeletal system. Although these conditions are generally chronic, during acute exacerbations the patient may summon EMS for emergency medical care.

Many nontraumatic (medical) musculoskeletal disorders are inflammatory or autoimmune in nature. Rheumatologists—physicians who specialize in the treatment of nontraumatic conditions that affect the muscles, joints, and bones—often care for these patients. Physiatrists—physicians who specialize in physical medicine and rehabilitation—also manage many medical conditions of the musculoskeletal system.

In this chapter, we detail several conditions of the musculoskeletal system that are nontraumatic. Even though these do not commonly prompt calls to EMS, from time to time during your career you will probably be called on to treat a patient who has one of these conditions.

Anatomy and Physiology Review

The musculoskeletal system, as its name indicates, is made up of the muscular system and the skeletal system. It provides the body with form, support, stability, and the ability to move about the environment. The skeletal system consists of the body's bones, joints, ligaments, and associated connective tissues. The muscular system consists of the muscles, tendons, and associated connective tissues. Nontraumatic medical conditions can affect any of these structures. Other body systems, such as the nervous system, also play a major role in nontraumatic medical conditions.

Skeletal System

The human skeleton, the framework of the body, consists of approximately 206 bones. These are typically classified based on their shape:

- Long bones
- Short bones
- Flat bones
- Irregular bones

The long bones are generally found in the extremities, whereas the short bones are found in the wrists and ankles. The flat bones form the skull, ribs, and sternum. Irregular bones are typically found in joints and in the spine (see Figures 13-1 and 13-2).

Bones are joined together by ligaments to form the *joints*. The joints allow us to move. Joints are grouped into six classes:

- ***Gliding joints.*** Gliding joints contain flat, plate-like surfaces that glide back and forth (although usually very slightly), allowing movement in various planes. The wrists and ankles are examples of gliding joints.
- ***Hinge joints.*** Hinge joints, which permit angular movement in a single plane, include the elbows and knees.
- ***Saddle joints.*** Saddle joints contain articular faces that fit together like a rider on a saddle. This allows angular movement but restricts rotation. The joint of the base of the thumb, the carpometacarpal joint, is an example of a saddle joint.
- ***Pivot joints.*** Pivot joints are found between the atlas (C-1) and axis (C-2) in the cervical spine. This joint allows only rotation. A similar pivot joint is found in the forearm, allowing pronation and supination of the wrist.
- ***Ellipsoidal joints.*** Ellipsoidal joints allow movement in two planes. An ellipsoidal joint connects the radius with the proximal carpal bones of the wrist, and the phalanges to the metatarsal bones in the foot.

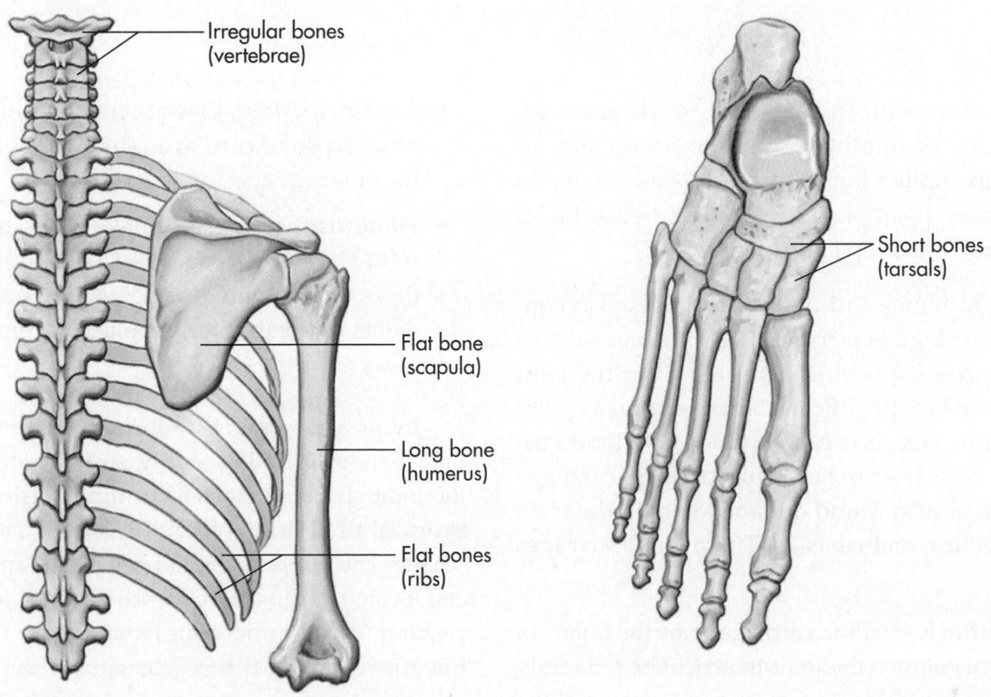

FIGURE 13-1 Bone shapes.

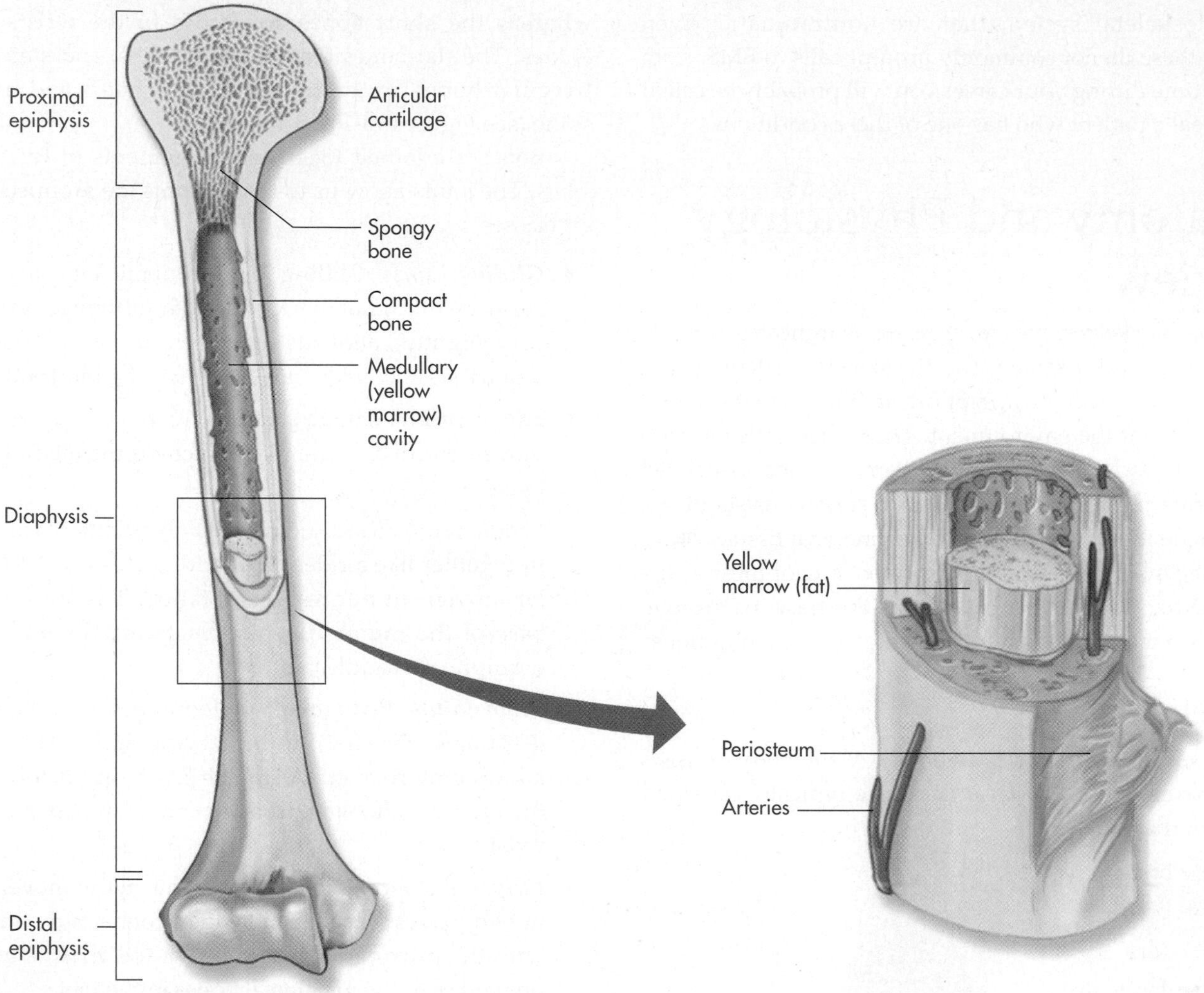

FIGURE 13-2 Basic bone anatomy.

- ***Ball-and-socket joint.*** In a ball-and-socket joint, the rounded head of one bone fits into a cup-shaped depression in another bone. This allows movement in multiple planes. Examples of the ball-and-socket joint are the shoulder and hip joints (Figure 13-3).

In addition to bones and ligaments, joints also contain *cartilage*. Cartilage is a form of flexible connective tissue that provides support and structure for the joint and provides a cushioning effect. Cartilage is an avascular tissue, meaning that it is not supplied by blood vessels. Instead, it receives nutrients through the cartilage matrix. Cartilage is also found outside joints in the ears, nose, larynx, trachea, and rib cage. There are three types of cartilage:

- ***Hyaline cartilage.*** Hyaline cartilage lines the bones in the joints. This allows the joint to articulate smoothly and reduces friction. Most of the cartilage found in the body is hyaline cartilage.
- ***Elastic cartilage.*** Elastic cartilage is more flexible than other types of cartilage. This is the cartilage found in the outer ear and in the larynx.
- ***Fibrocartilage.*** Fibrocartilage is the strongest and most rigid type of cartilage. It makes up the intervertebral disks of the spine. It also connects tendons and ligaments to bones. Fibrocartilage is found in high-stress areas.

Joints also contain a lubricant, referred to as *synovial fluid*. Synovial fluid is an oily, straw-colored fluid that fills the joint space and serves to reduce friction in the joint. Synovial fluid is also found in tendon sheaths and in the bursae. The bursae are fluid-filled sacs and synovial pockets, located throughout the musculoskeletal system, that cushion tendons and bones and reduce friction, allowing free movement. All these structures can become sites of inflammation in nontraumatic musculoskeletal disorders (Figure 13-4).

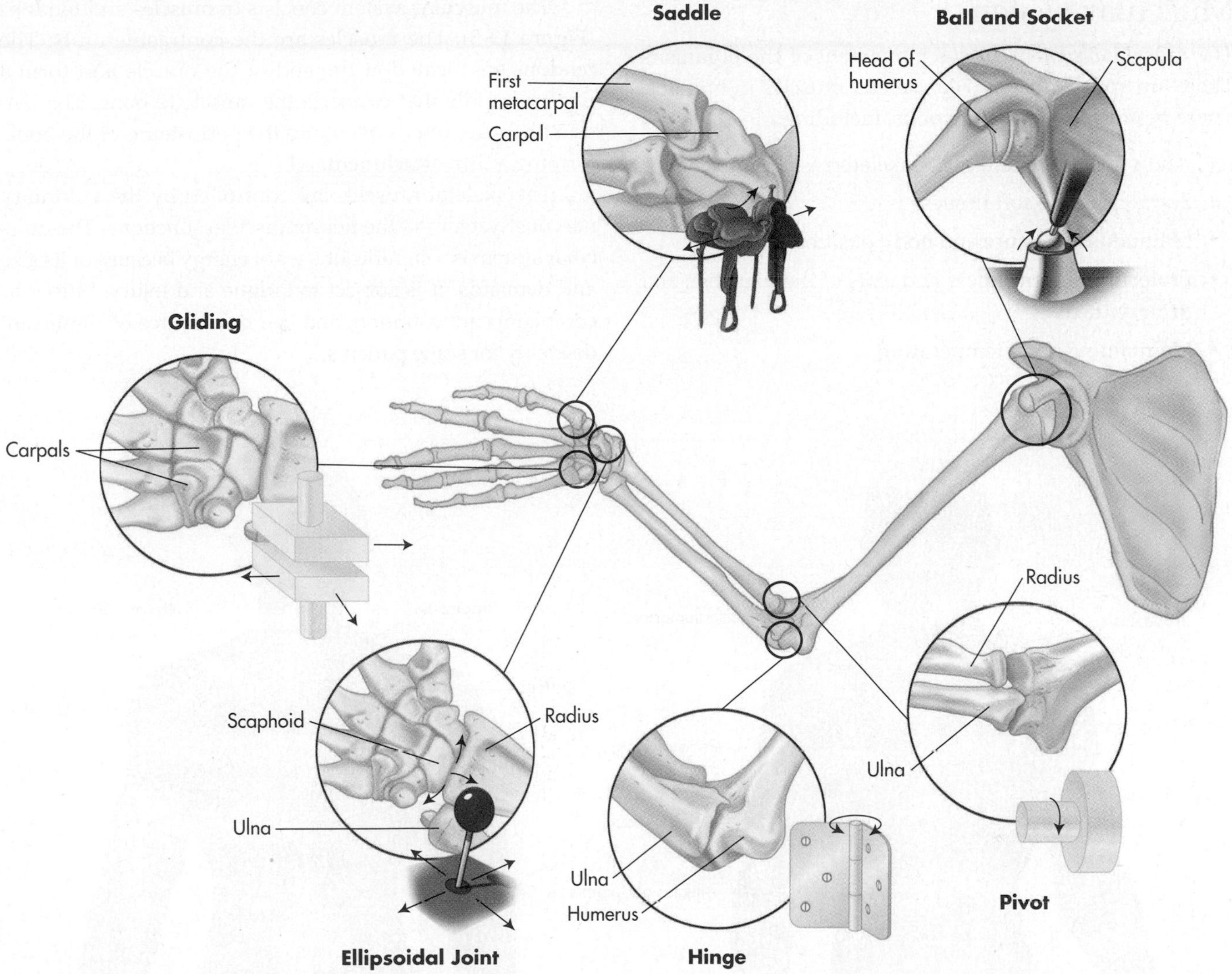

FIGURE 13-3 Types of joints.

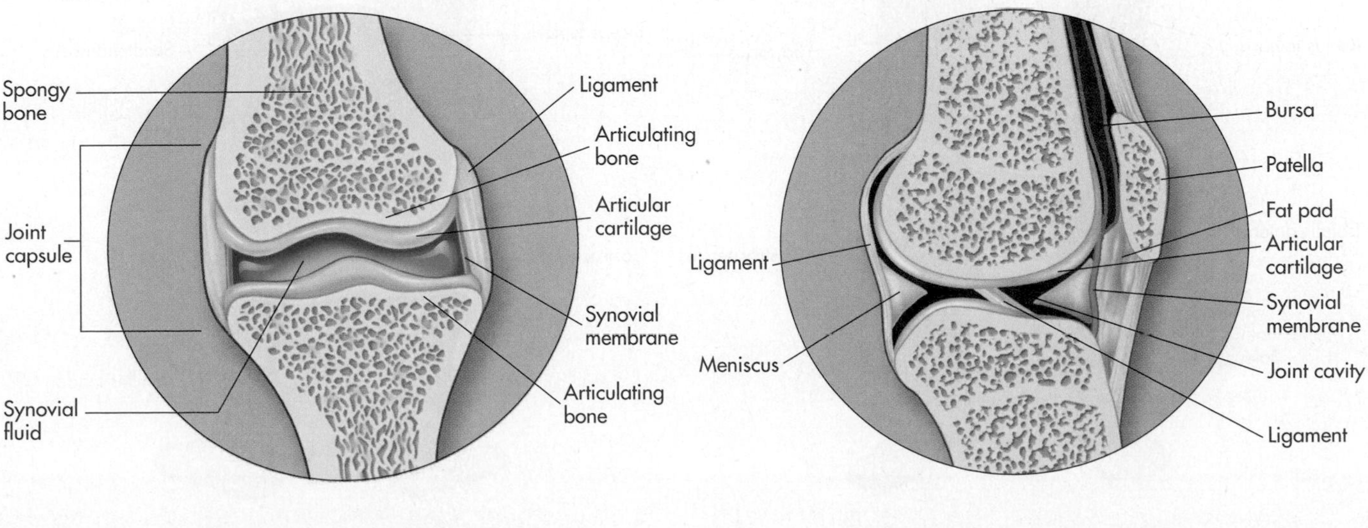

FIGURE 13-4 Articular cartilage and synovial joint.

Muscular System

The muscular system allows movement of the organism. There are approximately 700 skeletal muscles in humans. These perform multiple functions, including:

- Allowing movement of the skeleton
- Supporting the soft tissues
- Maintaining posture and body position
- Protecting the entrances and exits of the digestive and urinary tracts
- Maintaining body temperature

The muscular system consists of muscles and tendons (Figure 13-5). The muscles are the contractile units. The tendons are located at the end of the muscle and form a fibrous bundle that connects the muscle to bone. The tendon fibers are interwoven into the periosteum of the bone, forming a firm attachment.

The skeletal muscles are controlled by the voluntary nervous system via the neuromuscular junctions. The muscular system is a significant user of energy because of its size and demands. It is subject to fatigue and injury. Muscular complaints are common, and can be a source of significant disability for some patients.

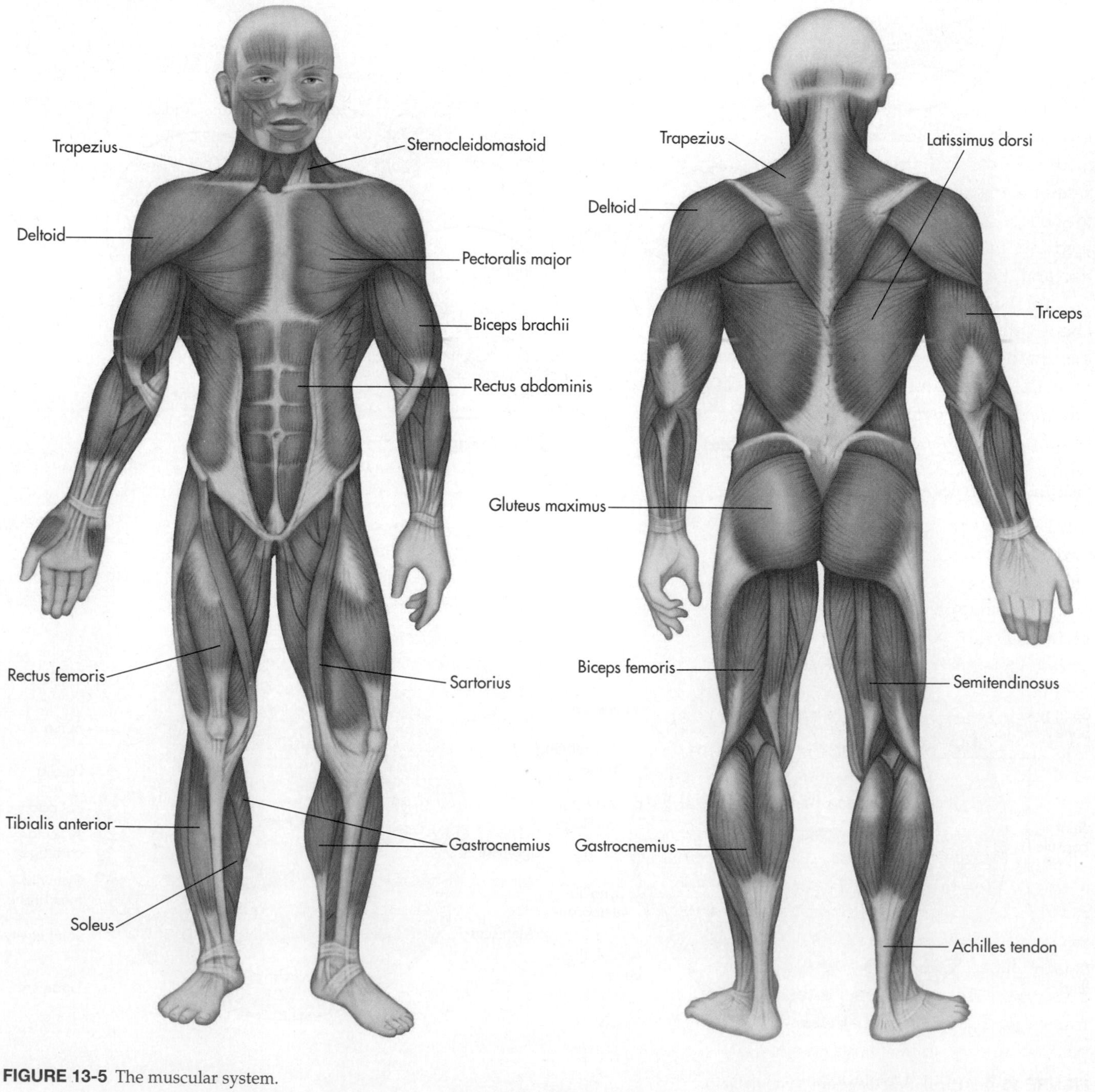

FIGURE 13-5 The muscular system.

Assessment and Findings

Most patients with nontraumatic musculoskeletal disorders will present with pain or tenderness. The physical examination findings you encounter will be as varied as the patients. As already stated, patients will often complain of pain and tenderness that is much worse than usual or typical for the condition. They may complain of associated swelling or other abnormality. In some cases, specifically with the inflammatory disorders, there will be some loss of movement of the affected joints and associated structures. This can be due to pain or due to abnormalities in the structure of the joint itself. With some of these conditions, the neurologic and vascular systems may be affected as well. As many of these diseases progress, deformity, either temporary or permanent, can occur.

Your assessment of the patient with a nontraumatic musculoskeletal disorder will employ the same techniques and strategies as for a patient with any other complaint. This includes the primary assessment and ensuring the adequacy of the airway, breathing, and circulation. The secondary assessment should include a fairly focused and detailed history of the illness. It is often helpful to review the patient's medications for additional information regarding the condition and the level of pain the patient is suffering.

You should pay particular attention to the body region about which the patient is complaining. If your patient has joint pain, examine the joint for tenderness, swelling, erythema, and restriction in the range of motion. For muscle disorders, look for restrictions in the range of motion, as well as for particular tender points and muscle spasm. For patients who are complaining of back pain, a more detailed exam is necessary to exclude conditions that require emergency treatment, such as *cauda equina* syndrome. The examination of the patient with back pain should include examination of the affected area and a neurologic exam including deep tendon reflexes (knee and ankle) as well as the search for sensory or motor deficits. Look particularly for signs of urinary or fecal incontinence as well as saddle anesthesia (numbness in the crotch and perineum). Many patients with chronic back pain have discogenic disease and will present with radicular symptoms (e.g., sciatica). These should be noted and considered as you formulate a treatment plan.

For the most part, treatment of these conditions is supportive and symptomatic. Pain management can be provided with opiate analgesics as well as with nonsteroidal anti-inflammatory drugs. In some cases, nonpharmacological treatments, such as splinting, application of cold or heat packs, and similar strategies, may be beneficial. In certain conditions, such as ankylosing spondylitis, the patient may present a challenge in terms of packaging and preparing for transport. Because many of these conditions include chronic pain, some patients will have an overlay of depression, anxiety, or both. Communication, empathy, and quality care will help to alleviate some of this. In many cases, the complaints related to these conditions may seem trivial. However, the patient knows his body and his disease and may summon EMS during a severe exacerbation of the illness.

Nontraumatic Musculoskeletal Conditions

There are numerous causes of nontraumatic (medical) musculoskeletal conditions that you may encounter during the course of your work as a paramedic. Some of these conditions are common; others are rare. In actuality, the cause of many of these conditions is traumatic in nature, including overuse and repetitive-motion injuries. Others are inflammatory or autoimmune conditions, including such diseases as rheumatoid arthritis and ankylosing spondylitis. Still others are due to degenerative changes within the musculoskeletal system that occur with aging, including osteoarthritis and osteoporosis.

The following sections detail the more common types of nontraumatic musculoskeletal disorders you may encounter in the prehospital setting.

Overuse/Repetitive-Motion Disorders

Repetitive motions such as repeatedly lifting a patient or using a computer keyboard can, over time, injure or inflame the tissues and structures that are being used. Technically speaking, overuse and **repetitive-motion disorders** are a form of trauma. However, because they tend to be chronic, they are often considered medical conditions.[1] Despite the clinical similarities between overuse/repetitive-motion injuries and other types of musculoskeletal trauma, the pathophysiology is somewhat different. Whereas most injuries result from a single recognizable event, overuse and repetitive-motion disorders occur from repetitive events that ultimately lead to signs and symptoms that are similar to those associated with acute trauma.

Repetitive-motion injuries are quite common and are due to microscopic tears of the affected tendons or muscles. However, unlike what occurs with acute trauma, the body is unable to repair the affected tissues because of continued use. Most repetitive-motion disorders are related to a vocation or

CONTENT REVIEW

- Nontraumatic Musculoskeletal Conditions
  - Overuse/repetitive-motion disorders
  - Degenerative conditions
  - Inflammatory conditions
  - Infectious conditions
  - Neoplastic processes
  - Chronic pain syndrome

avocation, and the patient often must or will continue to use the affected body part. In addition to repetitive movements, causes of repetitive-motion disorders include trauma, crystal deposits within the joint (e.g., gout), friction, and as a result of systemic diseases. Most patients with repetitive-motion disorders will complain of pain or tenderness in the affected area. Range of motion may be restricted because of swelling and/or pain. Examples of repetitive-motion injuries include tendonitis, bursitis, myalgias, carpal tunnel syndrome, and similar conditions.

- *Tendonitis.* **Tendonitis** (alternative spelling: *tendinitis*) is an inflammation of the tendon. The most common sites of tendonitis are the elbow, the biceps muscle, and the shoulder. Depending on the patient's activities, other tendons may be involved. Tendonitis is somewhat more common in males and generally occurs where the tendon inserts to the bone. Examples of tendonitis include:
  - *Tennis elbow.* Tennis elbow, also called lateral **epicondylitis**, is an inflammation of the common extensor tendon on the lateral aspect of the elbow. It is common in people who play racquet sports that involve repetitive twisting of the wrists. Tennis elbow causes worsening elbow pain that often radiates to the forearm. There is often a weakening of the grasp in the affected hand.
  - *Golfer's elbow.* Golfer's elbow, also called medial epicondylitis, is similar to tennis elbow except that it involves the common tendonous sheath that inserts into the medial epicondyle. This tenderness is felt during activities such as swinging a golf club or throwing a baseball.
- *Tenosynovitis.* A condition similar to tendonitis is **tenosynovitis**, which is an inflammation of the lining of the sheath (synovium) that surrounds the tendon. The signs and symptoms are identical to those of tendonitis.
- *Bursitis.* Bursitis is inflammation of the bursae. The bursae are small synovial sacs that are located along tendons at points where friction can develop. They serve to lubricate the area between the tendon and the associated bone. There are more than 150 bursae located throughout the body. The most common locations for bursitis include the elbow, knee, and hip (trochanteric bursae). Bursitis can be traumatic (as occurs with repetitive-motion injuries), infectious, or secondary to gout (Figure 13-6).
- *Myalgias.* The term *myalgia* means muscle pain. It is not a condition as much as it is a symptom of other disease processes. Chronic myalgia is a painful condition of various causes. In many instances, it results from repetitive injuries such as lifting, moving, or turning. Any muscle that is overused or repetitively used is at risk for developing myalgia.

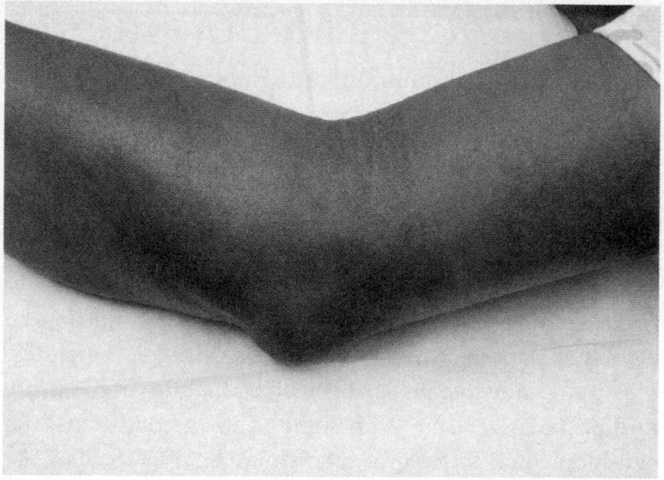

FIGURE 13-6 Olecranon bursitis.

(American Society for Surgery of the Hand; www.aash.org)

- *Carpal tunnel syndrome.* **Carpal tunnel syndrome (CTS)** is a condition caused by pressure on the median nerve in the wrist. There are numerous causes of CTS, but repetitive motion is the most common cause. The signs and symptoms of CTS include tingling, numbness, weakness, or pain that is felt in the fingers and hand. Sometimes the pain extends up into the distal forearm. The repetitive motion that originally led to the condition typically exacerbates the pain. The median nerve enters the hand through the wrist via a structure called the carpal tunnel. Repetitive motions, such as the use of tools, the use of a computer keyboard, and similar movements, can place pressure on the carpal tunnel, thus impinging the median nerve. CTS is a common cause of work-related disability (Figure 13-7).

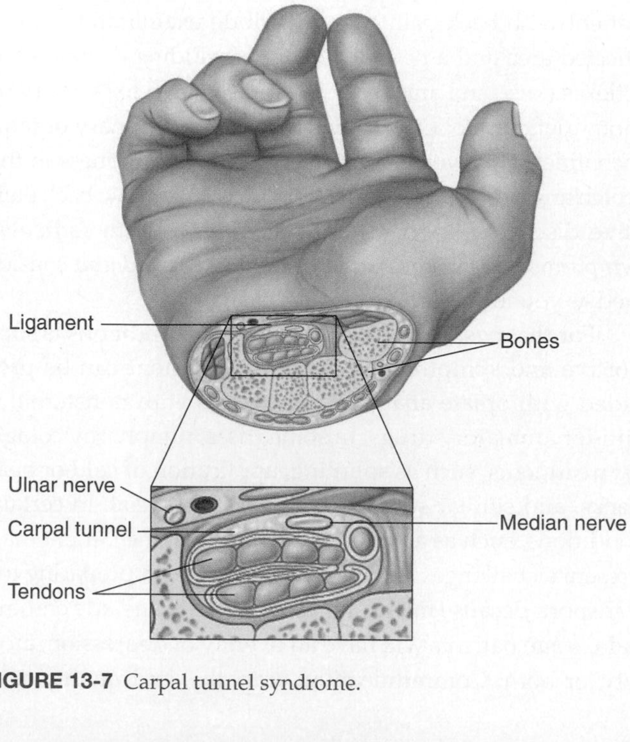

FIGURE 13-7 Carpal tunnel syndrome.

Degenerative Conditions

A degenerative condition or disorder is one that results from a disturbance in normal functioning of the affected tissues or organ system. In some cases, the degeneration is due to age and simple wear and tear. Although degenerative conditions can affect virtually any body system, this discussion is limited to those that affect the musculoskeletal system. Some of the most common degenerative musculoskeletal conditions are osteoarthritis, osteoporosis, and degenerative disk disease.

Osteoarthritis

Osteoarthritis (OA), also called *degenerative joint disease*, is a common condition caused by wear and tear on the joints. Although the precise cause of OA may not be known, it is certainly associated with aging. Virtually every person will have some signs and symptoms of OA by the age of 70. However, it can occur in younger individuals, particularly women, who are in their fifth or sixth decades of life. OA tends to run in families. It is exacerbated by obesity, which places particular stresses on the weight-bearing joints, especially the hips, knees, ankles, and feet. OA can also result from medical disorders such as hemophilia, avascular necrosis (interruption of blood supply to the joint), and other arthritic disorders, including gout and rheumatoid arthritis.

The signs and symptoms of OA include pain and stiffness that are present primarily on arising in the morning. This usually improves with movement and the activities of daily living. However, OA often becomes worse over time. In some patients, there may be swelling or crackling (crepitation) in the joint. There may also be limited range of motion. You may note tenderness in the joint when the joint is touched or compressed. Routine movement and activities are often painful (Figure 13-8).

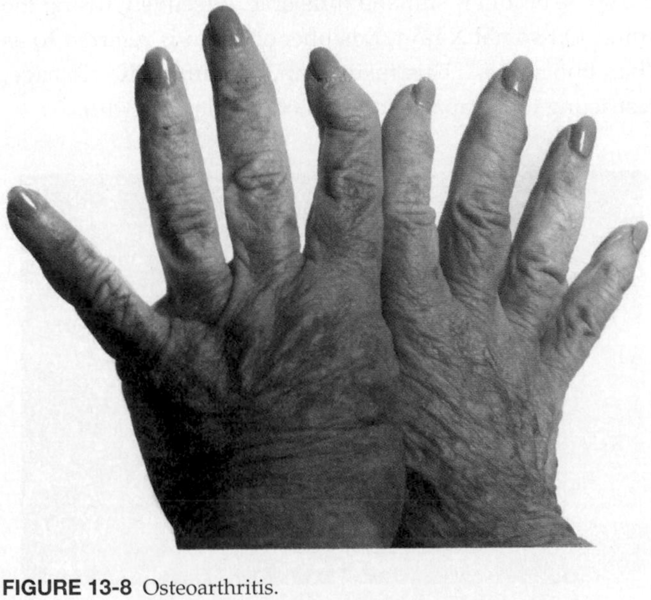

FIGURE 13-8 Osteoarthritis.

(Laurin Rinder/Fotolia)

OA is a chronic condition but will improve with medications such as nonsteroidal anti-inflammatory drugs and with physical therapy modalities including exercise, weight loss, and similar strategies.

Osteoporosis

Osteoporosis is the most common form of bone disease. It is a thinning of bone tissue and loss of bone density (from mineral loss) that occurs over time. It is estimated that approximately 1 in 5 American women over the age of 50 have some degree of osteoporosis. Osteoporosis occurs when the body fails to produce enough new bone to replace bone that is being resorbed or used. The minerals calcium and phosphate are the two major substances essential for normal bone formation. The primary cause of osteoporosis is the loss of estrogen effect in women as they enter menopause. It also occurs following a drop in testosterone levels in men. Women over the age of 50 and men over the age of 70 are at increased risk for developing osteoporosis. Others at risk include those who have chronic arthritis such as rheumatoid arthritis, patients taking corticosteroids, those with hyperparathyroidism, people with vitamin D deficiency, or those who are bedridden. It is also somewhat more common in women who drink a large amount of alcohol, who smoke, or who have a family history of osteoporosis.

Osteoporosis is generally asymptomatic until late in the disease process. Later, as the condition progresses, the patient may develop bone pain, tenderness, or even a fracture with little or no trauma. In addition, as the vertebral bodies collapse and compress from osteoporosis, the patient may lose body height—often as much as 6 inches over time. Patients with osteoporosis also are more prone to having low back pain and neck pain. Women, particularly, tend to develop increased kyphosis of the spine that is sometimes referred to as a "dowager's hump." From an emergency standpoint, osteoporosis can be a contributing factor to several conditions—especially trauma.

The treatment of osteoporosis includes pain control, medications and therapies to reduce bone loss and promote bone development, and preventive strategies to minimize falls and other injuries. Calcium replacement, hormonal therapy, and other strategies are often used. Exercise plays an important role in prevention. As with many chronic conditions, prevention is the best treatment.

Degenerative Disk Disease

Degenerative disk disease is one of the most common causes of low back pain. It is actually not a disease per se, but often is a result of normal age-related changes in the spinal disks.

Each of the vertebral bodies of the spine is separated and cushioned by a cartilaginous disk. These disks function essentially as shock absorbers for the spine. They allow for relatively painless movement of the spine. There are 23 disks in the spine. Each disk consists of two basic structures: the *nucleus pulposus* and the *annulus fibrosus*. The outer portion of the disk is the annulus fibrosus, a tough circular structure that gives the disk its shape. The inner aspect of the disk is the nucleus pulposus, which contains a network of fibers in a jellylike substance. This is the region of the disk that acts as a shock absorber.

During youth, roughly 80 percent of the disk is composed of water. However, as we age, the disks slowly dehydrate and become stiff. When this occurs, the disk functions less effectively as a shock absorber. In addition, the outer layer will crack, allowing the jellylike material to be forced out through the cracks, causing the disk to bulge or rupture. When this occurs, the herniated portion of the disk can place pressure on the adjoining spinal nerves, causing pain and weakness. Because the disk is primarily cartilage, it does not have a blood supply and is thus inefficient in repairing itself. Thus, discogenic back problems become worse as we age.

The most common symptom of degenerative disk disease is back or neck pain. However, this can vary significantly among individuals. Some people will have no pain, whereas others with the same degree of degenerative disk disease will have debilitating pain. The pain is often worsened with movement. Other spinal conditions, including osteoarthritis of the spinal facet joints and narrowing of the spinal canal, called spinal stenosis, can worsen the signs and symptoms of degenerative disease.

Inflammatory Conditions

Inflammatory joint diseases are a group of rheumatologic conditions that result from inflammation within the joint. Inflammatory joint diseases are typically characterized by pain, stiffness, erythema, warmth, and swelling of the joint. The presence of increased fluid within the joint, called an *effusion*, is also common. In some cases, the inflammation can be so severe that range of motion of the joint is lost. There are several inflammatory musculoskeletal disorders. These include rheumatoid arthritis, ankylosing spondylitis, gout, and others.

Rheumatoid Arthritis

Rheumatoid arthritis (RA) is a chronic disease that leads to inflammation and injury to the joints and the surrounding tissues. Although the specific cause of RA is unknown, it is considered to be an autoimmune disease. Normally, the body's immune system is able to discern self from nonself. However, with certain autoimmune conditions such as RA, the immune system confuses healthy tissue with a foreign substance. This results in the immune system actually attacking normal body structures. In the case of RA, the immune system attacks the synovium and surrounding tissues, causing inflammation and subsequent damage. RA is common and can occur at any age—including childhood. Women are more often affected than men. RA usually affects joints on both sides of the body. The joints of the wrists, fingers, knees, ankles, and feet are the most commonly affected.

The signs and symptoms of RA are subtle initially and include fatigue, low-grade fever, malaise, and weakness. Eventually the joint will become painful and swollen, with prolonged morning stiffness. The joints will become swollen to an extent that they lose range of motion. In severe and/or untreated cases, RA can cause significant damage to the joints, with subsequent deformity—a condition called "burned out" RA (Figure 13-9). RA often adversely affects other body systems. These include the kidneys, the eyes, and other structures.

RA is a chronic condition that cannot be cured but can be treated with medications. Surgery can be used to restore damaged joints to a fairly normal level of function. Many of the medications used to treat RA can be quite toxic. Physical therapy modalities have been found to be beneficial in patients with various stages of RA. From an EMS standpoint, the most common complaint related to RA would most likely be pain or general malaise.

Ankylosing Spondylitis

Ankylosing spondylitis (AS) is a form of inflammatory arthritis that primarily affects the spine. It is estimated that approximately 500,000 people in the United States have the condition. AS primarily causes inflammation of the joints between the vertebrae of the spine and the sacroiliac joints in the pelvis. It can also cause inflammation and pain in other parts of the body. As the condition worsens and the inflammation persists, new bone forms as a part of the healing process. The bone may grow from the edge of the vertebra across the disk space between two vertebrae, resulting in a bony bridge. This may occur throughout the spine, so the spine becomes stiff and inflexible, effectively fusing the spine. On spinal X-rays, this phenomenon is referred to as "bamboo spine." This fusion can also affect the rib cage, restricting lung capacity and function (Figure 13-10).

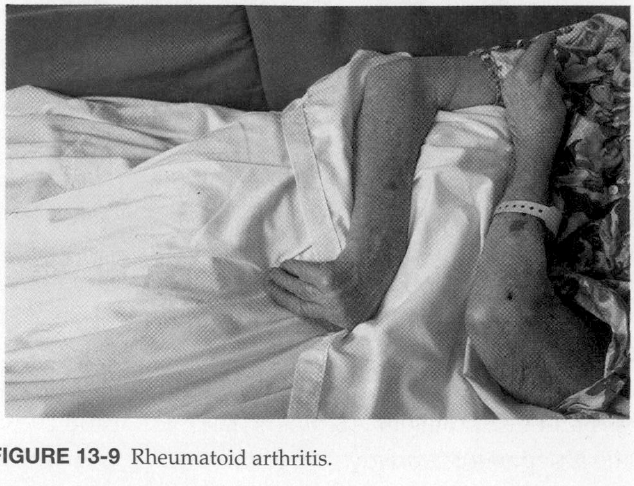

FIGURE 13-9 Rheumatoid arthritis.

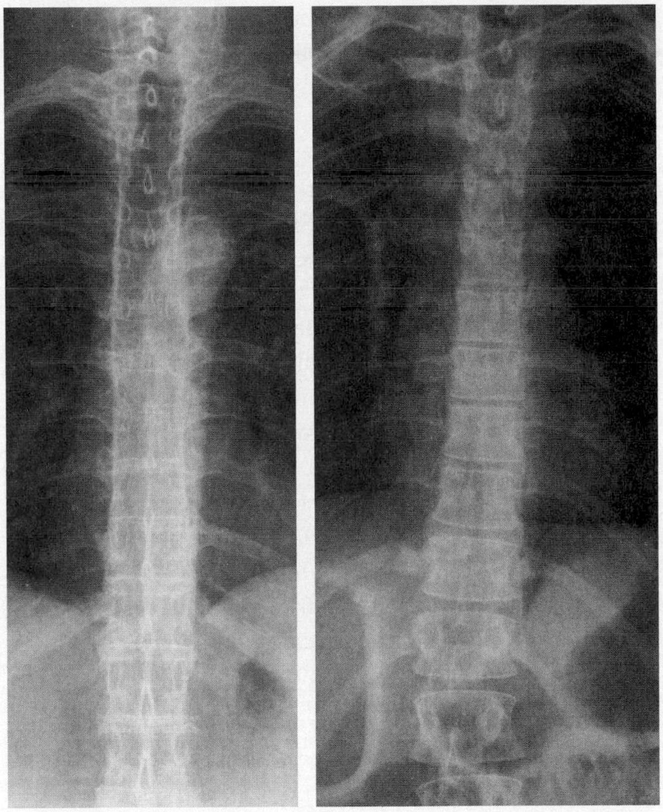

FIGURE 13-10 Ankylosing spondylitis causes inflammation and fusion of the joints of the spine, causing "bamboo spine." The spinal X-ray on the left shows the characteristic "bamboo spine" changes when compared to a normal spinal X-ray on the right.

(Both photos: © Spondylitis Association of America)

As the disease progresses, the spine becomes fused into a single unit incapable of flexion, extension, or lateral movement. Usually the fusion progresses with the spine assuming a flexed position and the patient forced to walk bent over.

EMS providers called to care for a victim of AS must remember that their patient's spine is inflexible and cannot be moved. Furthermore, the fused spine can be extremely fragile and subject to fracture with resultant spinal cord injury.[2] Numerous EMS techniques must be modified to accommodate patients with AS. These include airway management techniques, splinting techniques, and transport considerations.[3] Because most AS patients have chronic spinal flexion, it is important to adequately pad underneath the patient's head, neck, and upper back with sheets or pillows.

Likewise, airway management techniques must be applied without extending the neck. Airway devices that do not require visualization (e.g., extraglottic airways) should be considered instead of endotracheal intubation, with cricothyrotomy used as a last resort. Although patients with AS are not commonly encountered, improper EMS care of them can be devastating. Learn to identify the signs and symptoms of AS and be careful to protect the patient's spine accordingly.

Systemic Lupus Erythematosus

Systemic lupus erythematosus (SLE) is a chronic autoimmune disease that can affect the skin, joints, kidneys, and other organs. As with rheumatoid arthritis, in SLE the immune system fails in the ability to recognize self versus nonself. Thus, the overreactive immune system attacks otherwise healthy cells and tissues, causing chronic inflammation. As with rheumatoid arthritis, the underlying cause of SLE is unknown. It has been associated with certain medications and tends to run in families. It is more common in women than in men and can occur at any age.

The signs and symptoms of SLE vary significantly. Generally speaking, patients with SLE will have joint pain and swelling. Some will develop a full-blown arthritis. The fingers, wrists, and knees are the joints most commonly affected by SLE. Other signs and symptoms of SLE include chest pain (often pleuritic), fatigue, fever, malaise, skin rash, and swollen lymph nodes. Later, as the disease progresses, the patient can develop more severe complications, such as renal failure. SLE can be diagnosed with laboratory testing and physical exam.

As with RA, SLE is a chronic disease and treatment is aimed at mitigating symptoms and stopping disease progression. In many instances, corticosteroids are required to suppress the overactive immune response. As with RA, most SLE patients who summon EMS will primarily be complaining of pain and similar problems. Treatment is symptomatic.

Gout

Gout is a form of inflammatory arthritis that occurs when uric acid accumulates in the joints. Uric acid is a normal byproduct of the body's breakdown of purine. With gout, patients have an abnormal elevation of the amount of uric acid in the body. This can cause accumulation of uric acid crystals in the joints, causing what is called gouty arthritis. Not every patient with an elevated uric acid will develop gout. Although the exact cause of gout is unknown, it does tend to occur in families and affects men more often than women. It can be worsened by certain medications, such as diuretics. The signs and symptoms of acute gouty arthritis include severe pain, swelling, and erythema of the affected joint. Often, gout affects the joint between the foot and the great toe (first metatarsal joint) (Figure 13-11). The pain can be so severe that even the presence of a sheet resting on the joint is unbearable. Some patients will also have fever during gouty attacks. Diagnosis is confirmed by analysis of the synovial fluid demonstrating the presence of uric acid crystals. Treatment includes medications for pain, inflammation, and the use of a medication (e.g., allopurinol) to lower uric acid levels in the blood. Dietary restrictions will also help in keeping uric acid levels at a minimum.

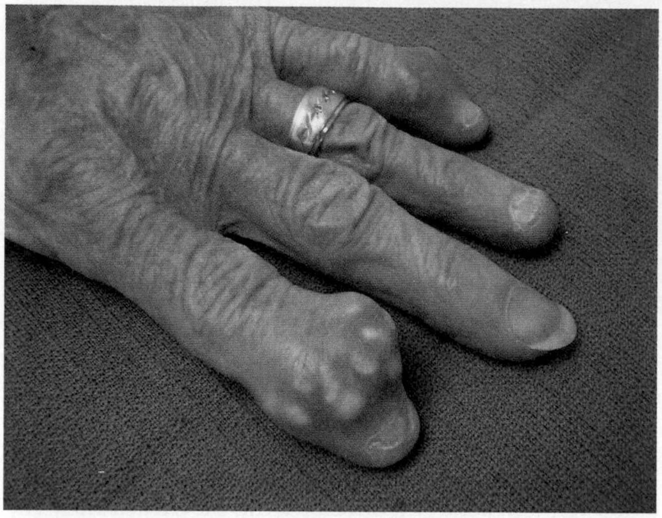

FIGURE 13-11 Gout.

(American Society for Surgery of the Hand)

Infectious Conditions

As with other body tissues, the tissues of the muscular and skeletal systems (and surrounding structures) are vulnerable to infection by various pathogens—primarily bacteria. Soft-tissue infections are fairly common, but infections of the bones and joints are less so. Because bone and joint infections tend to involve deeper structures, infection is relatively uncommon—but also more difficult to treat.

Soft Tissue Infections

Soft tissue infections are infections that involve the skin, the underlying tissues, and the fascia, as well as tendons and even muscle. The following are different types of soft tissue infections that may be encountered in prehospital care:

- ***Cellulitis.*** **Cellulitis** is an infection of the skin and often involves the associated soft tissues. Most cases of cellulitis are mild and heal with appropriate treatment, including antibiotics. However, in certain cases, the infection can involve deeper tissues and become more serious. Patients who have coexisting medical conditions, such as diabetes mellitus, are at increased risk of complications from cellulitis and soft tissue infections. The signs and symptoms of cellulitis include swelling and tenderness of the affected area. There may also be erythema and even exudate (pus). In many cases, a prior injury or skin break led to the infection. The treatment of cellulitis includes antibiotics and pain medication. In certain cases, surgical drainage and expiration may be required.
- ***Fasciitis.*** **Fasciitis** is an inflammation and infection of the fascia. The fascia is a layer of fibrous connective tissue found throughout the body. It surrounds muscles, muscle groups, blood vessels, nerves, and similar structures. The fascia may be superficial or deep. Once an infection reaches the fascia, it can disseminate along the various fascial planes to adjoining structures, causing significant infection.

  In some cases, fasciitis can become life threatening. This is most evident in the condition called **necrotizing fasciitis (NF)** —also called *flesh-eating disease*. NF is a bacterial infection that can rapidly destroy the skin, muscles, and surrounding tissues and is often due to multiple bacteria. These bacteria release toxins that cause widespread tissue damage. In many cases, the bacteria are resistant to commonly used, even potent, antibiotics, including methicillin. It is most common in patients who have preexisting chronic disease or malignancies, or those who are immunosuppressed. Typically, the infection begins at a single site and spreads rapidly through the fascial planes. Patients who develop NF are critically ill, and the mortality rate is very high. Treatment usually involves surgery, parenteral antibiotics, and other therapies.[4]
- ***Tenosynovitis.*** Tenosynovitis was discussed earlier under repetitive-motion disorders. The term *tenosynovitis* refers to inflammation of the fibrous sheath that surrounds the tendon. Such inflammation can also result from infection. When infection enters the tendon sheath, it can spread readily to adjoining tissues. Tenosynovitis is often seen following wounds to the hand, including animal and human bites. In many instances, infectious tenosynovitis can be a threat to the affected body appendage (usually the hand). It is treated with parenteral antibiotics and, in some instances, surgical drainage.
- ***Gangrene.*** Soft tissue infections can lead to gangrene. **Gangrene** is the death of tissue in the affected part of the body. It usually occurs when the blood supply in the affected tissue is interrupted. This occurs following a significant injury and in patients with peripheral vascular disease or diabetes, those who are immunosuppressed, or following surgical procedures.

  The signs and symptoms of gangrene depend on the location and the cause. Often, there is no pain. Typically, there is a discoloration of the skin that is usually blue or black. Gangrene of tissues below the skin often presents as a red or bronze appearance. There is often a foul-smelling discharge, as well as loss of sensation in the affected area. In most cases, gangrene requires surgery to remove the dead tissue and/or to restore blood supply. Antibiotics are sometimes of benefit. In many instances, amputation remains the only alternative (Figure 13-12).
- ***The Diabetic Foot.*** A common soft tissue condition is the diabetic foot. The feet, and, to a lesser degree, the hands, are affected by the complications of poorly controlled

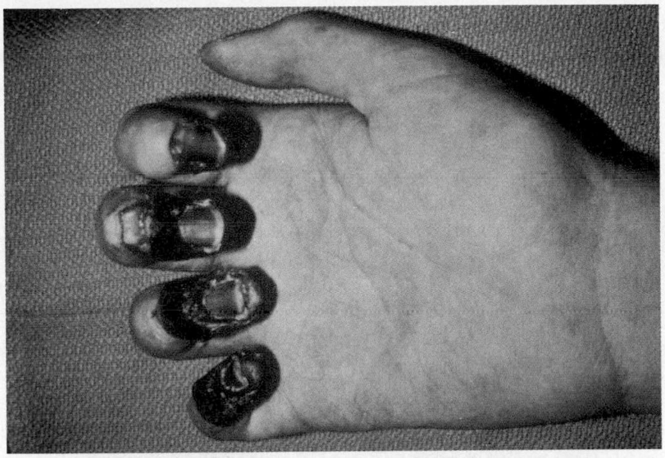

FIGURE 13-12 Gangrene.
(Centers for Disease Control and Prevention)

diabetes mellitus. Diabetes adversely affects peripheral blood vessels and nerves. This can result in decreased blood supply in the foot, as well as decreased sensation. Later, a minor injury, such as a laceration or skin ulcer, may go unrecognized. This can lead to development of a serious foot infection that often spreads to bone, causing osteomyelitis. The effects of diabetes on the peripheral blood vessels and the resultant decrease in blood supply worsen this condition.

Another complication of diabetes that affects the foot is called *neuropathic arthropathy* or *Charcot joint disease*. It is a progressive degeneration of the weight-bearing joints, particularly in the foot. It is characterized by bone destruction and deformity. This actually worsens the possibility of subsequent ulceration and can lead to amputation of the affected extremity or death. Typically, the patient with neuropathic arthropathy will have erythema, edema, and warmth in the affected joint or joints. Ulcers may or may not be present. It is often difficult to determine whether a patient with a Charcot joint actually has concomitant osteomyelitis. Treatment is based on the findings and generally involves preventive care and bracing.[5]

Bone and Joint Infections

An infection of the bone is referred to as osteomyelitis. Joints can also become infected—a condition called septic arthritis.

Osteomyelitis

Osteomyelitis is an infection of the bone. It can be either acute or chronic, based on the duration of the infection. The most common cause of osteomyelitis is a bacterial infection. In some cases, the cause of the infection may be fungal. Generally, osteomyelitis results from a spread of infection from the skin, muscles, and/or tendons to the affected bone. Osteomyelitis is most commonly seen following chronic wounds or with a chronic skin ulcer, such as is seen in patients with diabetes or with decubitus ulcers (bedsores). It is also seen following trauma. In some cases, osteomyelitis results from an infection that is in another part of the body but has spread to the bone via the bloodstream. Patients at risk for developing osteomyelitis are diabetics, patients on chronic hemodialysis, intravenous drug users, patients with peripheral vascular disease, and those who have sustained recent trauma. In addition, people who have undergone a splenectomy are at increased risk of developing osteomyelitis, because they are vulnerable to bacteria that are encapsulated (surrounded by an envelope). Many of the bacteria that cause osteomyelitis are caused by encapsulated bacteria species. The spleen plays a major role in the immune system's response to these bacterial types.

The signs and symptoms of osteomyelitis can vary based on the patient's underlying condition. For example, diabetics will have little, if any, pain. Other patients will have bone pain, fever, malaise, and localized erythema and warmth overlying the infection. Other symptoms include chills, diaphoresis, and swelling. The diagnosis of osteomyelitis is made based on diagnostic imaging and laboratory analysis. Treatment primarily involves the administration of appropriate antibiotics, often over a long interval. Surgical drainage and resection of the affected bone is sometimes necessary.

Septic Joints

A *septic joint*, also called **septic arthritis**, is an infection of a joint by various microorganisms, primarily bacteria but possibly, to a lesser degree, viruses and fungi. Surgical procedures and the presence of a prosthetic joint place the patient at increased risk for developing a septic joint. Approximately 20,000 cases of septic arthritis occur each year. Septic arthritis due to bacterial infection is typically divided into two categories: gonococcal and nongonococcal arthritis. Monarticular (single joint) septic arthritis, particularly in younger sexually active individuals, is often due to infection by *Neisseria gonorrhoeae*. Nongonococcal causes are generally due to bacteria of the streptococcal species. As with osteomyelitis, the infection spreads to the joint through direct contact with the skin, as occurs during a surgical procedure or joint injection or aspiration. It can also occur from spread via the bloodstream.

Those at risk for septic arthritis include patients with prosthetic joints, those with a bacterial infection elsewhere in the body, and those who are taking immunosuppressant drugs or have AIDS. In addition, those who have sustained recent joint trauma, who are IV drug abusers, and who have had a recent surgical procedure (e.g., arthroscopy) are at increased risk. Septic joints can also occur in children—particularly children under the age of 3. In this age group, the hip is the most commonly affected joint.

The most common presenting complaint with septic arthritis is joint pain. This is often accompanied by an inability to move the joint, as well as joint swelling, redness, and a low-grade fever. The diagnosis is made by diagnostic imaging and by withdrawing fluid from the joint and performing laboratory analyses. Treatment generally involves antibiotics, although surgical drainage and irrigation may be required. If a joint prosthesis is in place, it may be necessary to remove and replace the prosthesis.

Neoplastic Processes

A *neoplasm* is an abnormal growth of body tissue and is often called a *tumor*. Tumors can arise from bone and muscle tissue. A primary musculoskeletal tumor is one that arises from muscle, bone, or one of the associated tissues (e.g., synovium). A secondary musculoskeletal tumor is one that spreads to the muscle or bone from another site or tissue type (e.g., breast cancer, prostate cancer).

Bone tumors can be benign or malignant (cancerous). The most common benign bone tumors are the osteochondromas. Most malignant bone tumors are sarcomas. Sarcomas arise from bone, cartilage, muscle, fat, and similar tissues. Malignant bone tumors include:

- Chondrosarcoma (arises from cartilage)
- Ewing's sarcoma (round cell tumor)
- Osteosarcoma (arises from bone)
- Fibrosarcoma (arises from fibrous tissue)

Malignant tumors that arise from muscle and the associated connective tissues include:

- Rhabdomyosarcoma (arises from skeletal muscle)
- Synovial sarcoma (arises from the synovium)
- Liposarcoma (arises from fatty tissue)

In most instances, patients will know that they have a musculoskeletal tumor. In others, the diagnosis may not yet have been made. Pain, swelling, and deformity are common complaints with these conditions (Figure 13-13). Fractures secondary to the tumor, referred to as *pathological fractures*, can also result. In patients with a known diagnosis of a musculoskeletal tumor, an acute onset of pain or inability to use the affected part may be related to a pathological fracture.

In the prehospital setting, treatment of musculoskeletal tumors and pathological fractures is symptomatic. Patients in pain should be provided adequate analgesia. If a fracture is suspected, standard treatment, including splinting and local measures, is also indicated.

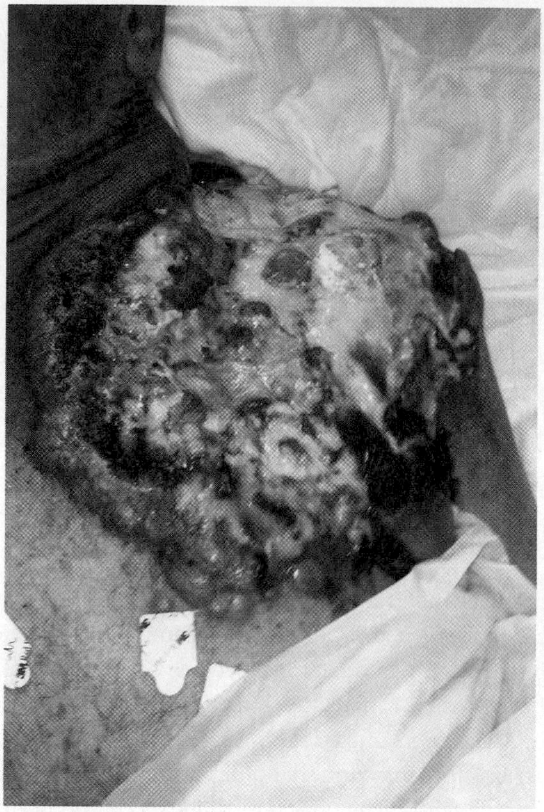

FIGURE 13-13 Untreated sarcoma of the left shoulder.
(© Dr. Bryan E. Bledsoe)

Chronic Pain Syndrome

Pain is the most common reason people seek medical care. In some individuals, pain will persist longer than typically seen in others who have the same condition. This is referred to as **chronic pain syndrome (CPS)**. CPS is a poorly defined condition, but generally includes ongoing pain that lasts anywhere in excess of three to six months. It typically includes multiple symptoms and complaints and has multiple causes, although these causes are complex and poorly understood. Chronic pain is somewhat more common in women. There are often associated psychological syndromes including depression, anxiety, and hypochondriasis. CPS is often characterized by the presence of the six D's:

- Dramatization of complaints
- Drug misuse
- Dysfunction/disuse
- Dependency
- Depression
- Disability

Regardless of the cause, the chief complaint is pain.

The patient with CPS will often present with nonspecific musculoskeletal pain. However, even chronic pain can be due to other causes and must be investigated. It is important to determine the location of the pain, any exacerbating or alleviating factors, the quality of the pain, and the overall intensity and severity of the pain using a pain-scoring system.

It is not uncommon for patients with CPS to call EMS when the pain becomes unbearable. Often, there is an event that leads to exacerbation of the pain. From a pathophysiologic standpoint, chronic pain is somewhat different from acute pain in origin. Some treatments, including short-acting opiates, can actually worsen CPS. Whereas acute treatment of CPS is similar to acute treatment of other painful conditions, long-term treatment of CPS involves other medications, including antidepressants and similar agents.[6]

Fibromyalgia (Central Sensitivity Syndrome)

Fibromyalgia is a somewhat enigmatic condition characterized by widespread pain in the muscles and soft tissues throughout the body. It is more common in young or middle-aged women than in other groups. The exact cause of fibromyalgia is unknown. However, more recent research into the possible causes of fibromyalgia has led to its reclassification as *central sensitivity syndrome (CSS)*. The signs and symptoms of fibromyalgia include pain in the muscles and soft tissues of the neck and back. A unique finding in fibromyalgia is the presence of tender spots that are referred to as trigger points. Fibromyalgia is associated with chronic fatigue, as well as difficulty in sleeping. In some patients, associated symptoms include headaches, difficulty concentrating, morning stiffness, and irritable bowel syndrome. Because fibromyalgia is a chronic pain syndrome, many patients have an overlay of anxiety and depression that can worsen the condition. The diagnosis is based on the physical examination and tenderness in at least 11 of the 18 predefined tender points. There are various treatment strategies, including regular exercise and stress management. Any associated depression is treated as well.[7]

Reflex Sympathetic Dystrophy

Reflex sympathetic dystrophy (RSD) is a chronic pain condition characterized by diffuse pain, swelling, and limitation of movement that follows an injury to an arm or leg. The symptoms are significantly out of proportion to the severity of the injury and may continue long after the injury is healed. The signs and symptoms of RSD typically include pain, swelling, and vasomotor dysfunction. RSD is often considered a type of *complex regional pain syndrome (CRPS)*. The exact pathogenesis of RSD is unknown. Typically, following an injury, the patient will have persistent pain and subsequently develop an abnormal sympathetic reflex. This results in vasoconstriction in the affected joint that can cause ischemia and escalating pain. Typically, on physical exam, the patient with RSD will have a swollen, painful, stiff, and poorly functioning extremity. There are two major approaches to treatment of RSD. The first includes blockade of the portion of the sympathetic nervous system supplying the affected extremity. In addition, corticosteroids and medications that block the sympathetic nervous system can be used. In severe cases, surgical removal of parts of the sympathetic nervous system may be necessary.[8]

Pediatric Conditions

Although most nontraumatic musculoskeletal disorders occur in adults, some such conditions occur in children. For example, *juvenile rheumatoid arthritis* is a debilitating condition of children. There are other nontraumatic musculoskeletal disorders that can affect children. Among these are Osgood-Schlatter disease and slipped capital femoral epiphysis.

- ***Osgood-Schlatter disease.*** **Osgood-Schlatter disease** is a painful swelling of the anterior tibial tubercle (often involving both legs). This is the bump on the upper tibia just below the knee. It is primarily a disease of children and is thought to be caused by repetitive injuries to the area before growth is complete. The primary symptom of Osgood-Schlatter disease is painful swelling over the shin. There is often associated knee and leg pain made worse with jumping, running, or climbing stairs. Physical examination often reveals tenderness over the affected area. Treatment primarily involves rest, ice, and other local measures. Nonsteroidal anti-inflammatory medications are often used.
- ***Slipped capital femoral epiphysis.*** A slipped capital femoral epiphysis is a separation of the ball of the hip joint from the femur. It occurs in children at the growth plate (epiphysis) in the proximal femur. It may affect one or both hips. The condition is somewhat more common in boys ages 11 to 15 who are somewhat obese or growing rapidly. The signs and symptoms of slipped capital femoral epiphysis include a limp, difficulty walking, hip or knee pain, hip stiffness, and restricted range of motion. Diagnosis is generally made by X-ray and physical exam. Treatment involves surgery to stabilize the bone using pins. It is not uncommon to treat both hips, despite the fact that only one is initially involved.

Summary

Most musculoskeletal problems you will encounter as a paramedic will be traumatic in origin. However, there are some nontraumatic conditions that can become emergent. Although these are primarily chronic, they are often characterized by acute exacerbations that may warrant prehospital care. Because these conditions are chronic, most emergency care is symptomatic. In most cases, the patient's primary complaint will be pain. Pain should be treated appropriately using the medications recommended for the condition and by local EMS protocols. It is important to remember that measures such as rest, ice, compression, heat, and elevation can be beneficial. In chronic pain conditions, there is often a significant overlay of anxiety and depression that contributes to the pain. Chronic pain patients can often be difficult to deal with and can require greater-than-expected doses of medications to alleviate pain. The role of the paramedic is to address the immediate problem and provide needed treatment—even if only symptomatic and supportive care.

You Make the Call

It has been a quiet day. You're preparing to watch the NBA playoffs when the dispatcher notifies you of a "medical emergency" at 2011 West Pecan Street. You and your partner immediately recognize the address as that of one of your regular patients. The patient, Wendy Rush, has chronic pain and frequently summons EMS for transportation to the local emergency department. As you think back, you realize that you transported Wendy just last week.

You and your partner depart the station and take the regular route to Wendy's house. As usual, her daughter meets you at the door and leads you through clutter to a back bedroom, where Wendy is in bed. There are multiple medication containers on the nightstand. Today, Wendy is complaining of severe abdominal pain. Your partner looks at you and says, "I'll get the stretcher and we'll take her to the ED." Softly, so Wendy and her daughter don't hear it, he adds, "We'll be back at the station before the first quarter is finished." You smile, but your instincts and experience warn you that something is different today. You tell your partner, "Wait. Let's take a closer look."

You and your partner complete a fairly comprehensive examination. The findings on this occasion are certainly different from those Wendy usually exhibits. She is tachycardic, slightly diaphoretic, and is having nausea and vomiting. Examination of her abdomen reveals diffuse tenderness and decreased bowel sounds. There appears to be some degree of rebound tenderness.

Based on your findings, you place an IV catheter and begin fluid administration. Because you know that Wendy has a high tolerance to pain medications, you administer 10 mg of morphine intravenously, as well as 4 mg of ondansetron. Then you move her to the ambulance and complete an uneventful transport to the hospital.

On arrival at the emergency department, the triage nurse takes a quick look at Wendy, rolls her eyes, and says, "Take her to the hallway." This is a nurse who is familiar with Wendy's frequent visits. Now, however, you pull her aside and explain that something is different today. You suggest that Wendy be placed into a regular treatment bed.

Later, you learn that your instincts were correct. Wendy had acute appendicitis and underwent a laparoscopic appendectomy.

1. What mistakes could have been made in the care of Wendy Rush?
2. When responding to a patient like Wendy with whom you are very familiar, what kind of shortcuts should you take with your assessment?

See Suggested Responses at the back of this book.

Review Questions

1. All of the following are examples of repetitive-motion injury *except* ____________
   a. tennis elbow.
   b. tenosynovitis.
   c. carpal tunnel syndrome.
   d. osteoarthritis.

2. The most common form of bone disease is ________
   a. osteoporosis.
   b. osteomyelitis.
   c. rheumatoid arthritis.
   d. osteoarthritis.

3. __________ is a chronic disease that leads to inflammation and injury to the joints and the surrounding tissues. It is also considered an autoimmune disease.
   a. Septic arthritis
   b. Degenerative joint disease
   c. Rheumatoid arthritis
   d. Ankylosing spondylitis

4. What is a form of inflammatory arthritis that occurs when uric acid accumulates in the joints?
   a. Osteoarthritis
   b. Rheumatoid arthritis
   c. Systemic lupus erythematosus
   d. Gout

5. ____________ is an inflammation or infection of the fibrous sheath that surrounds the tendon. It is often seen following wounds to the hand, including animal and human bites.
   a. Gangrene
   b. Tenosynovitis
   c. Arthropathy
   d. Fasciitis

6. What is the name of an infection that invades the bone and often arises from a bacterial cause?
   a. Osteomyelitis
   b. Gout
   c. Septic arthritis
   d. Neoplastic infection

7. Your patient is complaining of pain in the muscles and soft tissues of the neck and back, chronic fatigue, and difficulty sleeping. What could be the cause?
   a. Chronic pain syndrome
   b. Muscle strain
   c. Fibromyalgia
   d. Rheumatoid arthritis

8. Osgood-Schlatter disease is a painful swelling of which body region in children?
   a. Medial humeral epicondyle
   b. Femoral synovial bursae
   c. Anterior tibial tubercle
   d. Carpal tunnel sheath

9. A separation of the ball of the hip joint from the femur, commonly occurring in children, is known as ____________
   a. childhood rheumatoid arthritis.
   b. slipped capital femoral epiphysis.
   c. degenerative disc disease.
   d. pediatric ischial osteoporosis.

10. All of the following are malignant bone tumors except ____________
    a. chondrosarcoma.
    b. osteosarcoma.
    c. rhabdomyosarcoma.
    d. fibrosarcoma.

11. In the prehospital environment, the primary treatment strategies for most nontraumatic musculoskeletal disorders include all of the following *except* ________
    a. IV therapy with a large-bore catheter.
    b. opiate analgesics for pain relief.
    c. placing the patient in a position of comfort.
    d. providing emotional support.

See Answers to Review Questions at the back of this book.

References

1. Szabo, R. M. and K. J. King. "Repetitive Stress Injury: Diagnosis or Self-Fulfilling Prophecy?" *J Bone Joint Surg Am* 82 (2000): 1314–1322.
2. Carnell, J., J. Fahimi, and C. P. Wills. "Cervical Spine Fracture in Ankylosing Spondylitis." *West J Emerg Med* 10 (2009): 267.
3. Nee, P. A., J. Benger, and R. M. Walls. "Airway Management." *J Emerg Med* 25 (2008): 98–102.
4. Usatine, R. P. and N. Sandy. "Dermatologic Emergencies." *Am Fam Physician* 82 (2010): 773–780.

5. Anderson, C. A. and T. S. Roukis. "The Diabetic Foot." *Surg Clin North Am* 87 (2007): 1149–1177.
6. Baker, K. "Chronic Pain Syndromes in the Emergency Department: Identifying Guidelines for Management." *Emerg Med Australas* 17 (2005): 65–72.
7. Smith, H. S. and R. L. Barkin. "Fibromyalgia Syndrome: A Discussion of the Syndrome and Pharmacotherapy." *Am J Ther* 17 (2010): 418–439.
8. Hsu, E. S. "Practical Management of Complex Regional Pain Syndrome." *Am J Ther* 16 (2009): 147–154.

Further Reading

Koop, K., and L. Stack. *The Atlas of Emergency Medicine*. 4th ed. Columbus, OH: McGraw-Hill, 2016.

Roberts, J. R. and J. R. Hedges. *Clinical Procedures in Emergency Medicine*. 6th ed. St. Louis, MO: Saunders, 2013.

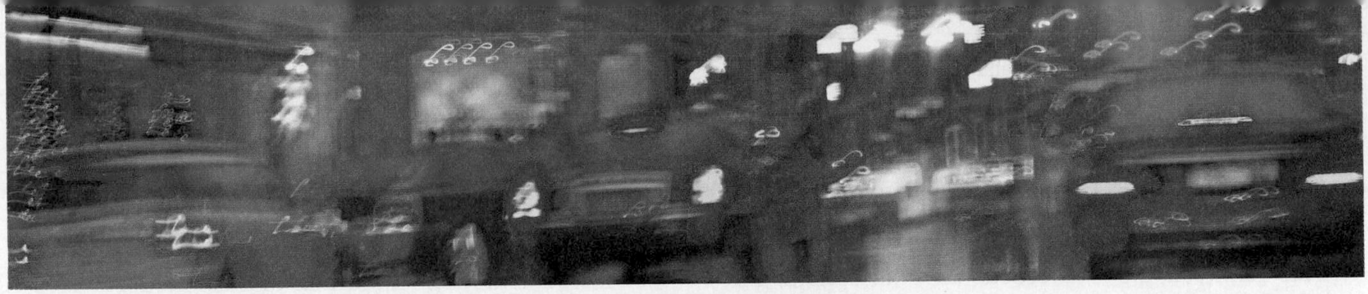

Precautions on Bloodborne Pathogens and Infectious Diseases

Prehospital emergency personnel, like all health care workers, are at risk for exposure to bloodborne pathogens and infectious diseases. In emergency situations it is often difficult to take or enforce proper infection control measures. However, as a paramedic, you must recognize your high-risk status. Study the following information on infection control carefully.

Infection control is designed to protect emergency personnel, their families, and their patients from unnecessary exposure to communicable diseases. Laws, regulations, and standards regarding infection control include:

- *Centers for Disease Control and Prevention (CDC) Guidelines.* The CDC has published extensive guidelines on infection control. Proper equipment and techniques that should be used by emergency response personnel to prevent or minimize risk of exposure are defined.
- *The Ryan White Act.* The Ryan White Act of 1990 allows emergency personnel to find out if they were exposed to an infectious disease while rendering patient care. Employers are required to name a "designated officer" to coordinate communications with the treating hospital.
- *Americans with Disabilities Act.* This act prohibits discrimination against individuals with disabilities, including those with contagious diseases. It guarantees equal employment opportunities and job protection if the infected individual can perform essential job functions and does not pose a threat to the safety and health of patients and coworkers.
- *Occupational Safety and Health Administration (OSHA) Regulations.* OSHA has enacted a regulation entitled Occupational Exposure to Bloodborne Pathogens that classifies emergency response personnel as being at the greatest risk of occupational exposure to communicable diseases. This regulation requires employers to provide hepatitis B (HBV) vaccinations free of charge, maintain a written exposure control plan, and provide personal protective equipment. These requirements primarily apply to private employers. Applicability to local and state governmental employees varies by locality. Many states have developed their own OSHA plans.
- *National Fire Protection Association (NFPA) Guidelines.* This is a national organization that has established specific guidelines and requirements regarding infection control for emergency response agencies, particularly fire departments and EMS services.

Standard Precautions and Personal Protective Equipment

Emergency response personnel should practice Standard Precautions by which ALL body substances are considered to be potentially infectious. To practice Standard Precautions, all emergency personnel should utilize personal protective equipment (PPE). Appropriate PPE should be available on every emergency vehicle. The minimum recommended PPE includes the following:

- *Gloves.* Disposable gloves should be donned by all emergency response personnel BEFORE initiating any emergency care. When an emergency incident involves more than one patient, you should attempt to change gloves between patients. When gloves have been contaminated, they should be removed as soon as possible. To properly remove contaminated gloves, grasp one glove approximately 1 inch from the wrist. Without touching the inside of the glove, pull the glove halfway off and stop. With that half-gloved hand, pull the glove on the opposite hand completely off. Place the removed glove in the palm of the other glove, with the inside of the removed glove exposed. Pull the second glove completely off with the ungloved hand, only touching the inside of the glove. Always wash hands after gloves are removed, even when the gloves appear intact.

- *Masks and Protective Eyewear.* Masks and protective eyewear should be present on all emergency vehicles and used in accordance with the level of exposure encountered. Masks and protective eyewear should be worn together whenever blood spatter is likely to occur, such as during arterial bleeding, childbirth, endotracheal intubation, invasive procedures, oral suctioning, and cleanup of equipment that requires heavy scrubbing or brushing. Both you and the patient should wear masks whenever the potential for airborne transmission of disease exists.
- *HEPA and N-95 Respirators.* Due to the resurgence of tuberculosis (TB), prehospital personnel should protect themselves from TB infection through use of an N-95 or a high-efficiency particulate air (HEPA) respirator, as approved by the National Institute of Occupational Safety and Health (NIOSH). It should fit snugly and be capable of filtering out the tuberculosis bacillus. An N-95 or HEPA respirator should be worn when caring for patients with confirmed or suspected TB. This is especially true when performing "high-hazard" procedures such as administration of nebulized medications, endotracheal intubation, or suctioning on such a patient.
- *Gowns.* Gowns protect clothing from blood splashes. If large splashes of blood are expected, such as with childbirth, wear impervious gowns.
- *Resuscitation Equipment.* Disposable resuscitation equipment should be the primary means of artificial ventilation in emergency care. Such items should be used once, then disposed of.

Remember, the proper use of personal protective equipment ensures effective infection control and minimizes risk. Use ALL protective equipment recommended for any particular situation to ensure maximum protection.

Consider ALL body substances potentially infectious and ALWAYS practice Standard Precautions.

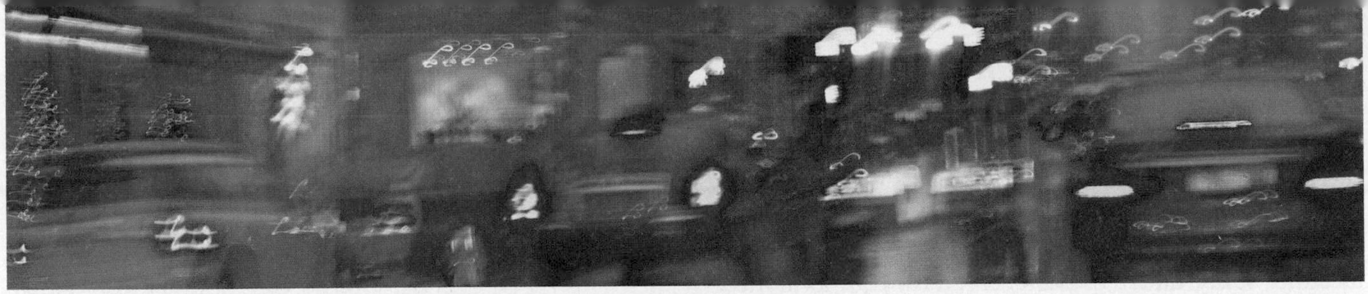

Suggested Responses to "You Make the Call"

The following are suggested responses to the "You Make the Call" scenarios presented in each chapter of Volume 3, Medicine. Each represents an acceptable response to the scenario but should not be interpreted as the only correct response.

Chapter 1—Pulmonology

1. *What pathophysiologic abnormality of the respiratory system do you suspect?*

This patient clearly has a severe disruption in diffusion of oxygen into his blood. The fever and cough in this patient will lead you to suspect pneumonia or support a possible diagnosis of ARDS. This patient is a very high priority due to the cyanosis and especially his altered mental status. The fact that the patient's mental status is altered lets you know that there is significant decompensation. Without rapid interventions, this patient is likely to progress to respiratory and cardiac arrest.

2. *How would you initially manage this patient?*

Your initial focus should be on high-concentration oxygen and assisting his ventilations with either a BVM or CPAP. Due to his long history of COPD, we want to avoid intubation unless absolutely necessary. (Intubation should be used cautiously in COPD patients. They have a tendancy to be very difficult to wean from assisted ventilations and extubation.) CPAP could prevent the necessity of an endotracheal tube as well as reverse the patient's hypoxia. Listening to lung sounds will help you determine the need for bronchodilators along with corticosteroid treatments. An IV line should be established, but not before taking care of controlling the respiratory distress. The cardiac monitor should be placed and obtain a 12-lead ECG at the first available moment. This is more of a precautionary measure just to rule out additional issues.

3. *Why is the finding of a cough and fever significant in this patient?*

Upper respiratory tract infection and pneumonia are common in patients with underlying lung disorders because their normal defenses, including mucous production and cilia action, are limited. These conditions also worsen underlying diseases such as COPD and pneumonia.

Chapter 2—Cardiology

1. *What is your assessment of the patient's condition?*

This patient is presenting with classic signs and symptoms of a myocardial infarction. Additionally, he has ST segment elevation in two or more contiguous leads; therefore, he is having a STEMI event. The elevation is seen in the "Inferior" leads with reciprocal changes in the lateral leads (serving to reinforce the diagnosis of an "Inferior MI").

2. *What prehospital care should be provided?*

This patient should be loaded and transport begun as soon as possible. Transport should be directed to the closest appropriate facility, preferably one with a designated cardiac care team and percutaneous coronary intervention (PCI) lab. Since the elevation is in his inferior leads, a right-sided assessment should be accomplished by moving the patient's V4 (at a minimum, if time allows, an entire right-sided ECG could be completed) to its mirror side on the right and looking for right-sided involvement. If the patient is not having right-sided involvement, then treatment can begin with nitrates. If right ventricular involvement is suspected, nitrates should not be used as the right ventricular involvement can cause a significant reduction in preload. Thus, administration of nitrates would cause a significant drop in pressure. This can be avoided by preparing the patient with fluid boluses before beginning the nitrate treatment.

Your first treatment for this patient would be supplemental oxygen followed by administration of ASA and nitroglycerin (see above regarding nitrate use with right ventricular infarct). Also note: Nitroglycerin can be given as either spray, tablet, or paste, based on your local medical direction. Subsequent 12-lead ECGs should be performed every 5–10 minutes, and transport should be emergent.

3. *What additional orders or directives could you expect to receive from Medical Direction?*

Ideally, your EMS system will have early STEMI activation (from the field), making it very possible to bypass the emergency room and move straight into the cardiac catheterization lab. Other options could include the use of fibrinolytics if your service has long transport times and carries them.

You should continue to monitor this patient for abnormal rhythms and be prepared to progress into a cardiac arrest scenario if necessary. Remember that time is of the essence with this patient, so your IV should be established en route to the hospital if at all possible. If your local protocols allow, you may begin a second IV line or lock for the receiving facility. Ultimately, you should do everything you can possibly do to decrease the time to definitive treatment for this patient.

Chapter 3—Neurology

1. *Based on the clinical symptoms present, what might be wrong with this patient?*

Based on the clinical symptoms that you were presented with initially, this patient appears to have been suffering from a stroke.

2. *What would account for the quickly dissipating symptoms?*

The fact that the symptoms have subsided makes it clear that this patient is most likely suffering from a transient ischemic attack (TIA). The symptoms subsided once the brain began to receive oxygen again. This could have been helped by the oxygen therapy that you started or it could have subsided itself.

3. *What is the priority in managing this patient's care?*

Whether she is having a stroke or a TIA, this patient should be treated as if she is having a stroke and transported to the closest appropriate stroke facilty.

4. *What are the appropriate steps in caring for this patient?*

Your treatment should include a full neurologic assessment, pulse-oximetry, glucometer reading, and vital signs. Additionally, you should perform a Cincinnati or Los Angeles Prehospital Stroke Screen. Continue to monitor the patient throughout transport for any additional changes and note all trends.

Chapter 4—Endocrinology

1. *What is your first priority?*

This patient is presenting with myriad signs and symptoms. First and foremost, make sure her airway is patent and her breathing is adequate.

2. *What additional intervention is needed?*

Adding supplemental oxygen should be accomplished early on in the treatment if the patient is hypoxic. Listen to the patient's lung sounds to determine if there is a possible bronchoconstriction or other airway narrowing causing the shortness of breath. If her lungs present with wheezes, you may begin treating the patient with a beta agonist such as albuterol. Began an IV for possible administration of additional medications as necessary. Due to the patient's low blood sugar and complaint of weakness, administration of dextrose to improve the level of glucose is acceptable. Monitor the patient for improvements with treatments and document all vital signs including lung sounds before and after any treatment. The patient should be transported to the hospital via EMS to allow you the opportunity to provide necessary monitoring and treatment.

3. *What do you suspect is the likely cause of her signs and symptoms?*

Most likely, this patient is suffering from hypoglycemia secondary to the decreased intake and vomiting. Another situation to note is that this patient has stopped taking her prednisone four days ago. It is imperative to note when a patient is not taking medications as ordered, because many of these medications have to be stopped gradually to avoid serious side effects. Additionally, the fact that the patient has been taking antibiotics could also have added to her current condition. It is possible that the antibiotics could have had an effect on the medications that the patient was taking, thereby making them less or more effective than normal.

4. *Should you transport this patient to the hospital or could her husband take her in their private vehicle?*

This is a life-threatening emergency. Under no circumstances should she be allowed to go by car.

Chapter 5—Immunology

1. *What is the most likely explanation of the patient's emergency?*

This patient is clearly having a hypersensitive reaction to the toxin from the fish.

2. *How would you treat this patient?*

As with all of your patients, the primary concern is with the patient's airway and breathing status. One of you should begin quickly applying oxygen while the other begins to remove the patient's shoe to expose the injury.

Treat the local injury for bleeding and apply heat if your protocols will allow. Heat in marine animal stings tends to break down the toxins and reduce the pain associated with it. The local injury is NOT your top priority as it will not result in immediate danger. Assessment of the patient's airway status for progression of the reaction should be done quickly while an IV is established. The patient should be treated with epinephrine. (Depending on the vitals, if the blood pressure is low the patient should receive IV epinephrine in a 1:10,000 solution. If he is normotensive, then IM epinephrine would be effective.) Additionally, the patient may receive steroids via IV, and, if necessary, additional epinephrine can be administered either via IV or IV infusion.

3. *Should the local marine institute be advised of a potentially toxic strain of hardhead catfish?*

In this patient, the local catfish sting resulted in normal reactions. However, the extensive general reaction was abnormal and most likely a hypersensitivity of this patient—not necessarily something that would require notification of the local marine institute. However, it is always a good idea to pass the information along to the receiving facility and the marine institute so they may watch for additional patients/victims with the same situations.

Chapter 6—Gastroenterology

1. *What are your first steps in caring for this patient?*

Unfortunately, this is a common location for EMS to work. You will respond to more than your share of calls in bathrooms. Since this patient has just passed out in front of you, the first step for this patient is to get him supine on the floor. Quickly assess his airway and pulses to determine his circulatory status. Provide oxygenation, if hypoxic, and ventilatory support as necessary. Quickly obtain a set of vital signs and begin to prepare to move the patient to the ambulance for transport.

2. *What are possible causes for the patient's condition? and 3. What information would you attempt to ascertain from the patient's wife?*

Try to obtain a history and determine any previous medical conditions such as GI history including hemorrhoids and ulcers. Additionally, you would want to determine if the patient has been complaining of any pain or discomfort prior to the event, anything that may help you clue in to the cause. Once the patient is in the ambulance, an IV should be started en route to the hospital and fluid therapy given to maintain a blood pressure of 90 mmHg systolic.

4. *What physical clues might you identify in this situation?*

Removing him from the toilet will quickly give you an impression of what is in the toilet. Do you see bloody stools? Dark black stools or bright red blood? Additionally, the odor of a GI bleed is very unique and can be identified from the door once you have been exposed to it for the first time. The possible causes for the patient's condition are most likely either a GI bleed or potentially a vagal response due to the patient straining. A physical assessment should concentrate on the patient's abdomen and include palpation of the abdomen, looking for any rigid areas, masses, and, specifically, pulsating masses that would indicate a potential abdominal aortic aneurysm. Transport should be rapid to the closest appropriate facility with the ability to assess and potentially treat with surgery.

Chapter 7—Urology and Nephrology

1. *What is your first management priority?*

Your first management priority of this patient is to build a rapport with him in an effort to convince him to allow you to treat him.

2. *What risk factors, if any, might the patient have for a renal complication to his conditions? Which renal complication, if any?*

It is apparent that the patient is dehydrated, at a minimum, and potentially in early stages of renal failure as indicated by his decreased urinary output.

3. *Should you agree to the neighbor's driving the patient to the hospital after he finishes dressing? If no, why not?*

It is important that you try to convince the patient to allow you to take him to the hospital and begin treatment as soon as possible. He appears to be confused, potentially from increased ammonia levels in his blood from a decrease in his renal function. It is important for you to help the patient be comfortable with your assessment and treatment and allow your transport. Initial treatment should begin with oxygen therapy and then establishing an IV and adjusting the flow to provide him with the necessary fluids he needs. Transporting him to the hospital and providing the receiving facility with all of your observations, as well as the neighbor's observations, will help the treating team and physician make decisions on what additional treatments and assessment/tests they should obtain.

Chapter 8—Toxicology and Substance Abuse

1. *What class of toxin are you dealing with?*

You are dealing with a pesticide poisoning; these poisonings fall into the category of organophosphates.

2. *What toxidrome (including signs and symptoms) will you expect to find when you make a further assessment of the patient?*

With organophosphates you are dealing with a cholinergic toxidrome. The best way to remember the accompanying symptoms with a cholinergic toxidrome is the acronym SLUDGE. You can suspect this patient to present with excessive Salivation, Lacrimation (tearing), Urination, Defecation, GI distress, and Emesis.

3. *What are your priorities in managing this patient?*

Your number-one priority is to get the patient removed from the garage and decontaminate him by removing his clothing and washing him down with copious amounts of water. (The solution to pollution is dilution!) The problem that you are faced with here is that the patient is in the garage, which is obviously an unsafe environment for you to enter. You need the support of the Fire Department hazmat team. If they have not been notified and requested, now is the time to do so. At this point you really have only two choices. (1) Yell to the patient (or use your PA speaker on your siren) and see if he can follow commands. If the patient can understand you and follow your commands, have him remove himself (self-rescue) from the environment and walk/crawl out to a safe environment and remove his clothes (his clothes will be contaminated with the poison as well, so removal of his clothes will effectively remove greater than 75 percent of the toxins) BEFORE you make contact with him. If the patient is unable to self-rescue, you are forced to wait for trained hazmat technicians to arrive and remove the patient. (This is a very difficult situation for you to be in, but your safety and the safety of those around you are always your number-one priority.)

Once the patient has been removed from the environment and has been properly decontaminated, your number-one priority is to assess, monitor, and ensure a patent airway. With the potential of copious amounts of salivation and vomiting, a secure airway is paramount. Be prepared to provide ventilations if ventilatory support is necessary. Try to identify the specific poison that was being used; if this is a place of business, there should be an MSDS sheet on the poison. Rapid transport should begin as quickly as possible. Establish IV access.

4. *Beyond standard supportive measures, what other intervention will help treat this patient?*

This patient would benefit from treatment with a Mark I kit, or specifically atropine and pralidoxime chloride (2-PAM). If a Mark I kit is not available, you can begin treatment with atropine. Initially, doses of 2–5 mg are common. Your local protocols and/or medical direction will aid you in dosing of atropine. Treatment is normally continued with atropine until the symptoms subside or the patient begins to show signs and symptoms of atropine toxicity.

Chapter 9—Hematology

1. *What hemostatic responses will seek to control this blood loss?*

At the initial time of injury, the body will vasoconstrict to attempt to reduce the bleeding. Additionally, platelets will begin rushing to the site of injury to form a plug followed by a fibrin mesh to help the blood to coagulate. In this particular situation, the problem with this occuring naturally is the pressure and amount of blood rushing through the site. The blood is flushing the platelet plug and fibrin mesh away faster than it can build to reduce the flow.

2. *Why are the heart rate and respiratory rate elevated?*

The patient's heart and respiratory rate are increased due to a number of factors. First, the release of adrenaline from the initial injury naturally will cause the increase in heart rate. Additionally, as he begins to compensate for the blood loss his body will release additional catecholamines that will cause both vasoconstriction and increased heart rate.

3. *What will the body do to replace red blood cells?*

His body should begin to note the decrease in blood, which will then cause him to produce more erythropoietin, which in turn will stimulate the production of blood cells.

4. *What body mechanisms will fight off an infection?*

To fight the infectious process, the patient's white blood cells begin to respond to the infection by chemotaxis to the infection site. At the site, macrophages may begin destroying the invaders through phagocytosis while lymphocytes begin stimulating the immune responses that will help rid the body of the infection-causing agent.

Chapter 10—Infectious Diseases and Sepsis

1. *What essential precautions should you take?*

AIDS is a bloodborne pathogen that is only found in the blood or body fluids. Precautions you take for this patient should not be any different than you should take for all patients. By wearing gloves, you are not only protecting yourself, but you are actually protecting the patient from you and any bacteria that you may be carrying that could be detrimental to the patient.

2. *What are your primary concerns for this patient?*

Your primary concerns for this patient are to monitor his airway and provide oxygenation if he is hypoxic. Your general care for this patient will be predominately supportive in nature.

3. *How would your care or Standard Precautions differ for patients without AIDS?*

All patients deserve the same treatment whether they are suffering from HIV, Hep. B, the common cold, or trauma. To that end, Standard Precautions are used for all patients. Wearing gloves on all patients is a practice that should be adhered to for all EMS providers.

Chapter 11—Psychiatric and Behavioral Disorders

1. *What do you suspect this patient's problem is? What are the possibilities?*

The most detrimental mistake any medic can make is to get tunnel vision and forget his basics. Anytime you are presented with a patient with a possible "behavioral emergency" you should treat it as an "altered level of consciousness." All patients deserve the best treatment you can provide them and that begins with a proper, unbiased assessment. Unfortunately for some patients, they are first met by people who assume the problem is psychiatric and begin treating it as that, only to find that the underlying problem was medically induced. For this patient, your primary concerns about airway and breathing have been addressed. Therefore, move on to assessing his glucose. He is presenting as someone with an altered LOC that could possibly be brought on by a bout of hypoglycemia.

2. *Is the sweating significant? The religious literature? The car crashes?*

The fact that he is diaphoretic (sweating) helps to point you in that direction, but it could also be pointing you toward other medications/drugs that could alter his LOC.

3. *Should this patient be treated as a psychiatric emergency?*

The patient's diagnosis can be blurred by the fact that he is acting as a religous fanatic and his car is strewn with religious literature, but the fact that he has been crashing into vehicles at low speeds does not fit the mold. Therefore, it is imperative to do additional assessments and evaluations to rule out an underlying medical condition. At all costs, you want to protect the patient and yourselves from (additional) injury. Make sure you follow local protocols if the patient condition changes and he becomes violent, thereby requiring more aggressive therapy and even restraints.

Chapter 12—Diseases of the Eyes, Ears, Nose, and Throat

1. *At this point, what is your primary concern regarding this patient?*

This scenario is very real and not that uncommon. As with all situations, your primary concern for this patient is to make sure he has a patent airway and is breathing adequately. In this case, the patient does not appear to be in any distress and does not seem to be having any airway issues currently. Even though you are not able to visualize the object in the patient's oropharynx, you should assume the patient does have something lodged just out of sight. Since the patient can feel what you may not be able to see, this patient should be treated as if there is an object present.

2. *What alternative methods are available to evaluate this patient?*

Additional evaluation strategies would include listening to the patient's lung sounds and even listening to the air movement over the trachea. Additionally, more advanced procedures for assessing his airway would include X-ray studies and laryngoscopy/bronchoscopy.

3. *What should you do if you cannot visualize a foreign body or an injury secondary to the foreign body?*

All of these procedures would require a physician and specialized equipment. Therefore, if you are unable to visualize and remove an object and the patient is unable to clear it with coughing or drinking water, transport to the hospital would be in order. In this case, transport with EMS would be advisable because the object could potentially dislodge and create an airway emergency. It would be important for the patient to be with EMS in the event of such an emergency.

Chapter 13—Nontraumatic Musculoskeletal Disorders

1. *What mistakes could have been made in the care of Wendy Rush?*

It is easy to assume that chronic patients will only suffer chronic conditions. In this situation, the patient has a chronic condition that was not related to the acute complaint. Because of preexisting bias, it is easy to overlook the acute problems and assume that any current complaints are chronic. A critical mistake can be made if you allow yourself to become complacent. Especially in situations where paramedics work long shifts with high call volumes, these biases begin to crop up more regularly. Luckily for Wendy, you noticed the abnormality and investigated it further.

2. *When responding to a patient like Wendy with whom you are very familiar, what kind of shortcuts should you take with your assessment?*

There is a tendency to take "shortcuts" in your assessment of selected patients—especially those whom you know or who have chronic conditions. This failure to perform a systematic and detailed assessment could have led to a delay in the diagnosis of appendicitis. The same attitude and shortcuts could have occurred in the emergency department with similar delays. However, when the nurse began to discount the patient's condition, your patient advocacy made her rethink her decision, saving precious time and potentially even Wendy's life—all by simply letting the receiving nurse know that you felt there was more to this than her normal complaints.

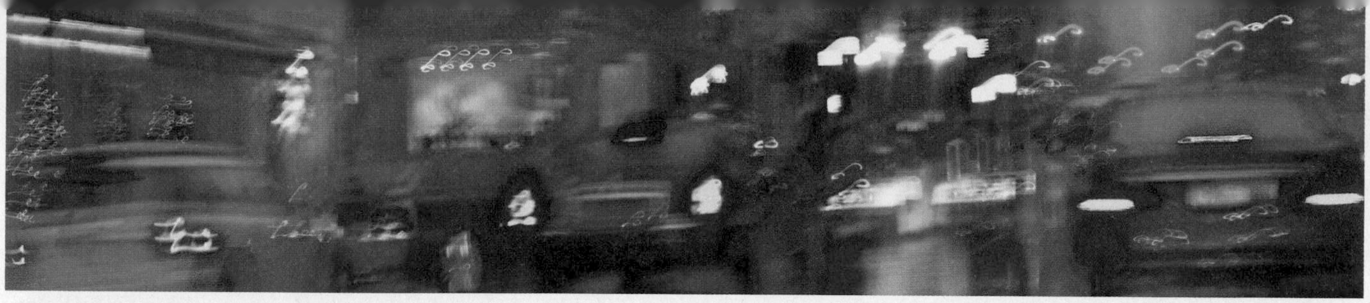

Answers to Review Questions

Below are the answers to the Review Questions presented in each chapter of Volume 3.

Chapter 1—Pulmonology

1. a
2. d
3. c
4. c
5. a
6. c
7. d
8. c
9. b
10. d
11. d
12. b
13. c
14. c
15. c
16. b
17. b
18. c

Chapter 2—Cardiology

1. b
2. c
3. b
4. b
5. c
6. b
7. a
8. a
9. a
10. c
11. c
12. d
13. a
14. c
15. b
16. d
17. c
18. a
19. a
20. d

Chapter 3—Neurology

1. c
2. a
3. a
4. b
5. b
6. b
7. d
8. a
9. b
10. b
11. c
12. a
13. b
14. c
15. a
16. c
17. b
18. d
19. a
20. b

Chapter 4—Endocrinology

1. b
2. c
3. d
4. a
5. b
6. d
7. d
8. c
9. a
10. c

Chapter 5—Immunology

1. a
2. b
3. b
4. a
5. c
6. d
7. d
8. d
9. b
10. d

Chapter 6—Gastroenterology

1. a
2. b
3. c
4. d
5. b
6. c
7. b
8. c
9. b
10. d

Chapter 7—Urology and Nephrology

1. a
2. c
3. b
4. d

5. b
6. c
7. d
8. d
9. c
10. d
11. a

Chapter 8—Toxicology and Substance Abuse

1. b
2. c
3. b
4. b
5. c
6. a
7. b
8. b
9. b
10. d
11. d

Chapter 9—Hematology

1. d
2. a
3. b
4. c
5. c
6. b
7. c
8. a
9. d
10. b
11. a

Chapter 10—Infectious Diseases and Sepsis

1. d
2. b
3. b
4. c
5. d
6. b
7. c
8. b
9. a
10. d

Chapter 11—Psychiatric and Behavioral Disorders

1. c
2. d
3. c
4. b
5. c
6. b
7. d
8. b
9. a
10. c

Chapter 12—Diseases of the Eyes, Ears, Nose, and Throat

1. d
2. b
3. c
4. d
5. a
6. a
7. b
8. d
9. a
10. c

Chapter 13—Nontraumatic Musculoskeletal Disorders

1. d
2. a
3. c
4. d
5. b
6. a
7. c
8. c
9. b
10. c
11. a

Glossary

2,3-biphosphoglycerate (2,3-BPG) chemical in the red blood cells that affects hemoglobin's affinity for oxygen.

abdominal aortic aneurysm dilation of the abdominal aorta that generally occurs below the renal arteries and above the bifurcation of the common iliac arteries.

aberrant conduction conduction of the electrical impulse through the heart's conductive system in an abnormal fashion.

absence seizure type of generalized seizure with sudden onset, characterized by a brief loss of awareness and rapid recovery.

absolute refractory period the period of the cardiac cycle when stimulation will not produce any depolarization whatsoever.

acid a substance that liberates hydrogen ions (H^+) when in solution.

acquired immunity immunity that develops over time and results from exposure to an antigen.

action potential the stimulation of myocardial cells, as evidenced by a change in the membrane electrical charge, that subsequently spreads across the myocardium.

activated charcoal a powder, usually premixed with water, that will adsorb (bind) some poisons and help prevent them from being absorbed by the body.

active immunity acquired immunity that occurs following exposure to an antigen and results in the production of antibodies specific for the antigen; protection against disease developed after birth as a result of a direct exposure to the disease.

active transport movement of a molecule through a cell membrane from a region of lower concentration to one of higher concentration; movement requires energy consumption within the cell.

acute arterial occlusion the sudden occlusion of arterial blood flow.

acute coronary syndrome (ACS) a spectrum of coronary artery disease processes from myocardial ischemia and myocardial injury to myocardial infarction that includes the clinical entities of stable and unstable angina and acute myocardial infarction.

acute gastroenteritis sudden onset of inflammation of the stomach and intestines.

acute kidney injury (AKI) the sudden onset of severely decreased urine production; also called *acute renal failure (ARF).*

acute pulmonary embolism blockage that occurs when a blood clot or other particle lodges in a pulmonary artery.

acute renal failure (ARF) *see* **acute kidney disease (AKI).**

acute respiratory distress syndrome (ARDS) form of pulmonary edema that is caused by fluid accumulation in the interstitial space within the lungs.

acute tubular necrosis a particular syndrome characterized by the sudden death of tubular cells.

addiction compulsive and overwhelming dependence on a drug; an addiction may be physiologic dependence, a psychological dependence, or both.

Addison's disease endocrine disorder characterized by adrenocortical insufficiency. Symptoms may include weakness, fatigue, weight loss, and hyperpigmentation of skin and mucous membranes.

Addisonian crisis form of shock associated with adrenocortical insufficiency and characterized by profound hypotension and electrolyte imbalances.

adhesion union of normally separate tissue surfaces by a fibrous band of new tissue.

affect visible indicators of mood.

afferent carrying impulses toward the central nervous system. Sensory nerves are afferent nerves.

afterload the resistance against which the heart must pump.

airborne transmitted through the air by droplets or particles.

alkali a substance that liberates hydroxyl ions (OH^-) when in solution; a strong base.

allergen a substance capable of inducing allergy of specific hypersensitivity. Allergens may be protein or nonprotein, although most are proteins.

allergic reaction an exaggerated response by the immune system to a foreign substance.

allergy a hypersensitive state acquired through exposure to a particular allergen.

Alzheimer's disease a degenerative brain disorder; the most common cause of dementia in the elderly.

amyotrophic lateral sclerosis (ALS) progressive degeneration of specific nerve cells that control voluntary movement characterized by weakness, loss of motor control, difficulty speaking, and cramping. Also called *Lou Gehrig's disease.*

anabolism the constructive or "building up" phase of metabolism.

anaphylaxis an unusual or exaggerated allergic reaction to a foreign protein or other substance. Anaphylaxis means the opposite of phylaxis, or protection.

anastomosis communication between two or more vessels.

anemia an inadequate number of red blood cells or inadequate hemoglobin within the red blood cells.

aneurysm dilation of a blood vessel.

anger hostility or rage to compensate for an underlying feeling of anxiety.

angina pectoris chest pain that results when the heart's oxygen requirements exceed oxygen supply available from blood.

angioneurotic edema marked edema of the skin that usually involves the head, neck, face, and upper airway; a common manifestation of severe allergic reactions and anaphylaxis.

ankylosing spondylitis a form of inflammatory arthritis that primarily affects the spine.

anorexia nervosa psychological disorder characterized by voluntary refusal to eat.

antibody protein that is produced in response to and that attacks a disease antigen.

antidiuresis formation and passage of a concentrated urine, preserving blood volume.

antidote a substance that will neutralize a specific toxin or counteract its effect on the body.

antigen surface protein on most viruses and bacteria that identifies them as self or nonself; any substance that is capable, under appropriate conditions, of inducing a specific immune response.

anuria no elimination of urine.

anxiety disorder condition characterized by dominating apprehension and fear.

anxiety state of uneasiness, discomfort, apprehension, and restlessness.

apnea absence of breathing.

apneustic respiration breathing characterized by a prolonged inspiration unrelieved by expiration attempts, seen in patients with damage to the upper part of the pons.

appendicitis inflammation of the vermiform appendix at the juncture of the large and small intestines.

aqueous humor a waterlike fluid that surrounds the iris, pupil, and lens of the eye.

arachnoid membrane middle layer of the meninges.

arrhythmia any deviation from the normal electrical rhythm of the heart. Also called *dysrhythmia.*

arteriosclerosis a thickening, loss of elasticity, and hardening of the walls of the arteries from calcium deposits.

artifact deflection on the ECG produced by factors other than the heart's electrical activity.

ascending loop of Henle the part of the tubule beyond the descending loop of Henle.

asphyxia a decrease in the amount of oxygen and an increase in the amount of carbon dioxide as a result of some interference with respiration.

ataxic respiration poor respirations due to CNS damage, causing ineffective thoracic muscular coordination.

atherosclerosis a progressive, degenerative disease of the midsize and large arteries.

augmented leads another term for unipolar limb leads, reflecting the fact that the ground lead is disconnected, which increases the amplitude of deflection on the ECG tracing.

aura a subjective sensation that may precede a seizure.

autoimmune disease condition in which the body makes antibodies against its own tissues.

autoimmunity the body's formation of antibodies against itself.

automaticity pacemaker cells' capability of self-depolarization.

autonomic nervous system part of the nervous system controlling involuntary bodily functions. It is divided into the sympathetic and the parasympathetic systems.

B lymphocytes cells that attack invaders in humoral immune responses.

bacteria microscopic single-celled organisms that range in length from 1 to 20 micrometers.

bactericidal capable of killing bacteria.

bacteriostatic capable of inhibiting bacterial growth or reproduction.

basophil type of white blood cell that participates in allergic responses.

behavior a person's observable conduct and activity.

behavioral emergency situation in which a patient's behavior becomes so unusual that it alarms the patient or another person and requires intervention.

Bell's palsy one-sided facial paralysis with an unknown cause characterized by the inability to close the eye, pain, tearing of the eyes, drooling, hypersensitivity to sound, and impairment of taste.

benign prostatic hypertrophy a noncancerous enlargement of the prostate associated with aging.

bereavement death of a loved one.

biological/organic related to disease processes or structural changes.

bipolar disorder condition characterized by one or more manic episodes, with or without periods of depression.

bipolar leads electrocardiogram leads applied to the arms and legs that contain two electrodes of opposite (positive and negative) polarity; leads I, II, and III, also called *limb leads*.

bloodborne transmitted by contact with blood or body fluids.

Bohr effect phenomenon in which a decrease in PCO_2 acidity causes an increase in the quantity of oxygen that binds with the hemoglobin and, conversely, an increase in PCO_2 acidity causes the hemoglobin to give up a greater quantity of oxygen.

bowel obstruction blockage of the hollow space within the intestines. An obstructed bowel segment can be catastrophic if not rapidly diagnosed and treated.

Bowman's capsule the hollow, cup-shaped first part of the nephron tubule.

bradycardia a heart rate less than 60 beats per minute.

bradypnea slow respiration.

brain abscess a collection of pus localized in an area of the brain.

brainstem part of the brain connecting the cerebral hemispheres with the spinal cord. It consists of the mesencephalon (midbrain), pons, and medulla oblongata.

Brudzinki's sign physical exam finding in which flexion of the neck causes flexion of the hips and knees.

bruit the sound of turbulent blood flow through a vessel; usually associated with atherosclerotic disease.

bulimia nervosa recurrent episodes of binge eating.

bundle branch block a kind of interventricular heart block in which conduction through either the right or left bundle branch is blocked or delayed.

bundle of Kent an accessory AV conduction pathway that is thought to be responsible for the ECG findings of preexcitation syndrome.

carbaminohemoglobin hemoglobin with carbon dioxide bound.

carboxyhemoglobin hemoglobin with carbon monoxide bound.

cardiac arrest the absence of ventricular contraction.

cardiac cycle the period of time from the end of one cardiac contraction to the end of the next.

cardiac output the amount of blood pumped by the heart in 1 minute.

cardiac tamponade accumulation of excess fluid inside the pericardium.

cardiogenic shock the inability of the heart to meet the metabolic needs of the body, resulting in inadequate tissue perfusion.

cardiovascular disease (CVD) disease affecting the heart, peripheral blood vessels, or both.

cardiovascular system the heart and the blood vessels.

carina the point at which the trachea bifurcates into the right and left mainstem bronchi.

carpal tunnel syndrome a condition caused by pressure on the median nerve in the wrist, with repetitive motion being the primary cause.

catabolism the "breaking down" phase of metabolism.

cataract a clouding of the lens of the eye.

catatonia condition characterized by immobility and stupor, often a sign of schizophrenia.

***cauda equina* syndrome** condition caused by significant narrowing of the spinal canal that compresses the nerve roots below the level of the spinal cord, causing back pain, leg pain, numbness in the groin or perineal region, and bowel and bladder disturbances, as well as diminished reflexes, muscle weakness, and loss of sensation in the lower extremities.

cell-mediated immunity generalized, temporary defense against any invader.

cellular immunity immunity resulting from a direct attack of a foreign substance by specialized cells of the immune system.

cellulitis an infection of the skin that often involves the associated soft tissues.

central nervous system (CNS) the brain and the spinal cord.

central neurogenic hyperventilation hyperventilation caused by a lesion in the central nervous system, often characterized by rapid, deep, noisy respirations.

central pain syndrome condition resulting from damage or injury to the brain, brainstem, or spinal cord characterized by intense, steady pain described as burning, aching, tingling, or a "pins and needles" sensation.

cerebellum portion of the brain located dorsally to the pons and medulla oblongata. It plays an important role in the fine motor movement, posture, equilibrium, and muscle tone.

cerebrospinal fluid watery, clear fluid that acts as a cushion, protecting the brain and spinal cord from physical impact. The cerebrospinal fluid also serves as an accessory circulatory system for the central nervous system.

cerebrum largest part of the brain, consisting of two hemispheres. The cerebrum is the seat of consciousness and the center of the higher mental functions such as memory, learning, reasoning, judgment, intelligence, and the emotions.

cerumen earwax; a protective substance secreted by glands within the ear canal.

chalazion an inflammation or infection resulting from blockage of a gland of the eyelid.

chancroid highly contagious sexually transmitted ulcer.

chemotaxis the movement of white blood cells in response to chemical signals.

Cheyne-Stokes respirations a breathing pattern characterized by a period of apnea lasting 10 to 60 seconds, followed by gradually increasing depth and frequency of respirations.

chickenpox *see* varicella.

Chikungunya virus disease a disease caused by the Chikungunya virus and spread by the *Aedes* species of mosquitoes.

chlamydia group of intracellular parasites that cause sexually transmitted diseases.

cholecystitis inflammation of the gallbladder.

chronic ambulatory peritoneal dialysis (CAPD) a dialysis procedure that relies on the patient's peritoneal membrane as the semipermeable membrane. Dialysate is introduced into the abdomen via a closed system that allows the patient to be ambulatory during dialysis. Also called just *peritoneal dialysis*.

chronic gastroenteritis nonacute inflammation of the gastrointestinal mucosa.

chronic kidney disease (CKD) permanently inadequate renal function due to nephron loss; also called *chronic renal failure (CRF)*.

chronic obstructive pulmonary disease (COPD) a disease characterized by a decreased ability of the lungs to perform the function of ventilation.

chronic pain syndrome pain that persists longer than that typically seen in others who have the same condition.

chronic renal failure (CRF) *see* **chronic kidney disease (CKD).**

chronotropy pertaining to heart rate.

circumcision the surgical removal of the foreskin of the penis.

cirrhosis degenerative disease of the liver.

claudication severe pain in the calf muscle due to inadequate blood supply. It typically occurs with exertion and subsides with rest.

clonic phase phase of a seizure characterized by alternating contraction and relaxation of muscles.

colic acute pain associated with cramping or spasms in the abdominal organs.

collecting duct the larger structure beyond the distal tubule into which urine drips.

coma a state of unconsciousness from which the patient cannot be aroused.

communicable period time when a host can transmit an infectious agent to someone else.

communicable capable of being transmitted to another host.

community-acquired infection an infection occurring in a nonhospitalized patient who is not undergoing regular medical procedures, including the use of instruments such as catheters.

compensatory pause the pause following an ectopic beat when the SA node is unaffected and the cadence of the heart is uninterrupted.

complex partial seizure type of partial seizure usually originating in the temporal lobe characterized by an aura and focal findings such as alterations in mental status or mood.

conductivity ability of the cells to propagate the electrical impulse from one cell to another.

confusion state of being unclear or unable to make a decision easily.

congestive heart failure (CHF) condition in which the heart's reduced stroke volume causes an overload of fluid in the body's other tissues.

contamination presence of an agent only on the surface of the host without penetrating it.

contractility ability of muscle cells to contract, or shorten.

cor pulmonale hypertrophy of the right ventricle resulting from disorders of the lung.

coronary artery disease (CAD) a type of CVD; the single largest killer of Americans.

corrected QT (QTc) The QT interval divided by the square root of the RR interval.

cortex the outer tissue of an organ such as the kidney.

coupling interval distance between the preceding beat and the PVC.

cranial nerves twelve pairs of nerves that extend from the lower surface of the brain.

creatinine a waste product caused by metabolism within muscle cells.

crepitus crackling sounds.

Creutzfeldt-Jakob disease (CJD) a rare form of brain damage that leads to a rapid decrease in mental function and movement characterized by dementia, ataxia, hallucinations, jerking, and general decline.

Crohn's disease idiopathic inflammatory bowel disorder associated with the small intestine.

croup viral illness characterized by inspiratory and expiratory stridor and a seal bark-like cough.

Cullen's sign ecchymosis in the periumbilical area.

current of injury (injury current) the flow of current between the pathologically depolarized area of myocardial injury and the normally depolarized areas of the myocardium.

Cushing's disease pathological condition (a form of Cushing's syndrome) caused by a tumor of the pituitary (adenoma) that causes excess production of adrenocorticotropic hormone (ACTH) that, in turn, elevates cortisol production from the adrenal glands, causing excess cortisol in the blood.

Cushing's syndrome pathological condition resulting from excess adrenocortical hormones. Symptoms may include changed body habitus, hypertension, and vulnerability to infection.

Cushing's triad a collective change in vital signs (increased blood pressure, decreased pulse rate, and irregular respirations) associated with increasing intracranial pressure.

cyanosis bluish discoloration of the skin due to an increase in reduced hemoglobin in the blood. The condition is directly related to poor ventilation.

cyclical vomiting syndrome (CVS) a disorder of unknown cause characterized by repeated, sudden episodes of severe nausea, vomiting, and physical exhaustion,

cystic medial necrosis a death or degeneration of a part of an artery wall.

cystitis infection of the bladder.

decerebrate posturing sustained contraction of extensor muscles of the extremities resulting from a lesion in the brainstem. The patient presents with stiff and extended extremities and retracted head.

decontaminate to destroy or remove pathogens.

decontamination the process of minimizing toxicity by reducing the amount of toxin absorbed into the body.

decorticate posturing characteristic posture associated with a lesion at or above the upper brainstem. The patient presents with the arms flexed, fists clenched, and legs extended.

deep venous thrombosis a blood clot in a vein.

defibrillation the process of passing an electrical current through a fibrillating heart to depolarize a critical mass of myocardial cells. This allows them to repolarize uniformly, resulting in an organized rhythm.

degenerative neurologic disorders a collection of diseases that selectively affect one or more functional systems of the central nervous system.

delayed hypersensitivity a hypersensitivity that develops after the elapse of some time following reexposure to an antigen. Delayed hypersensitivity reactions are usually less severe than immediate reactions.

delirium tremens (DTs) disorder found in habitual and excessive users of alcoholic beverages after cessation of drinking for 48 to 72 hours. Patients experience visual, tactile, and auditory disturbances. Death may result in severe cases.

delirium condition characterized by relatively rapid onset of widespread disorganized thought.

delusions fixed, false beliefs not widely held within the individual's cultural or religious group.

dementia condition involving gradual development of memory impairment and cognitive disturbance.

denervated lacking nervous system connections, as in a transplanted heart.

deoxyhemoglobin hemoglobin without oxygen.

depersonalization feeling detached from oneself.

depolarization a reversal of charges at a cell membrane so that the inside of the cell becomes positive in relation to the outside; the opposite of the cell's resting state, in which the inside of the cell is negative in relation to the outside. *See also* repolarization.

depression profound sadness or feeling of melancholy.

dermatome area of the skin innervated by spinal nerves.

descending loop of Henle the part of the tubule beyond the proximal tubule.

diabetes insipidus excessive urine production caused by inadequate production of antidiuretic hormone.

diabetes mellitus disorder of inadequate insulin activity, due either to inadequate production of insulin or to decreased responsiveness of body cells to insulin.

diabetic ketoacidosis complication of type 1 diabetes due to decreased insulin intake. Marked by high blood glucose, metabolic acidosis, and, in advanced stages, coma. Ketoacidosis is often called *diabetic coma.*

dialysate the solution used in dialysis that is hypoosmolar to many of the wastes and key electrolytes in blood.

diaphoresis sweatiness.

diastole the period of time when the myocardium is relaxed and cardiac filling and coronary perfusion occur.

diencephalon portion of the brain lying beneath the cerebrum and above the brainstem. It contains the thalamus, hypothalamus, and limbic system.

diffusion the movement of molecules through a membrane from an area of greater concentration to an area of lesser concentration.

disease period the duration from the onset of signs and symptoms of disease until the resolution of symptoms or death.

disinfection process that destroys certain forms of microorganisms, but not all.

dissecting aortic aneurysm aneurysm caused when blood gets between and separates the layers of the aortic wall.

disseminated intravascular coagulation (DIC) a disorder of coagulation caused by systemic activation of the coagulation cascade.

dissociative disorder condition in which the individual avoids stress by separating from his core personality.

distal tubule the part of the tubule beyond the ascending loop of Henle.

diuresis formation and passage of a large amount of dilute urine, decreasing blood volume.

diverticula small outpouchings in the mucosal lining of the intestinal tract.

diverticulitis inflammation of diverticula.

diverticulosis presence of diverticula, with or without associated bleeding.

downtime duration from the beginning of the cardiac arrest until effective CPR is established.

dromotropic pertaining to the speed of impulse transmission.

drug overdose poisoning from a pharmacological substance in excess of that usually prescribed or that the body can tolerate.

dura mater tough outermost layer of the meninges.

dyspnea difficult or labored breathing; a sensation of "shortness of breath."

dysrhythmia abnormal rhythm; see *arrhythmia*.

dystonias a group of disorders characterized by muscle contractions that cause twisting and repetitive movements, abnormal postures, or freezing in the middle of an action.

early repolarization ST-segment elevation without underlying disease.

Ebola virus disease (EVD) disease of humans and other primates caued by the virus *Ebolavirus* and transmitted between people by direct contact.

ectopic beat cardiac depolarization resulting from depolarization of ectopic focus.

ectopic focus nonpacemaker heart cell that automatically depolarizes; plural ectopic foci.

efferent carrying impulses away from the brain or spinal cord to the periphery. Motor nerves are efferent nerves.

Einthoven's triangle the triangle around the heart formed by the bipolar limb leads.

ejection fraction ratio of blood pumped from the ventricle to the amount remaining at the end of diastole.

electrocardiogram (ECG) the graphic recording of the heart's electrical activity. It may be displayed either on paper or on an oscilloscope. Also abbreviated *EKG*.

encephalitis acute infection of the brain, usually caused by a virus.

endocrine gland gland that secretes chemical substances directly into the blood; also called a *ductless gland*.

endolymph fluid that fills the membranous labyrinth of the inner ear.

endotoxin toxic products released when bacteria die and decompose.

end-stage kidney disease (ESKD) *see* end-stage renal failure (ESRF).

end-stage renal failure (ESRF) an extreme failure of kidney function due to nephron loss; also called *end-stage kidney disease (ESKD)*.

enterotoxin an exotoxin that produces gastrointestinal symptoms and diseases such as food poisoning.

epicondylitis inflammation of an epicondyle (a prominence on the distal part of a long bone to which muscles and ligaments attach). *Lateral epicondylitis* is often called *tennis elbow*.

epididymis a saclike duct adjacent to a testis that stores sperm cells.

epiglottitis infection and inflammation of the epiglottis.

erythrocyte red blood cell.

erythropoiesis the process of producing red blood cells.

erythropoietin a hormone produced by kidney cells that stimulates maturation of red blood cells.

esophageal varix swollen vein of the esophagus.

excitability ability of the cells to respond to an electrical stimulus.

excited delirium syndrome a mental state and a state of physiologic arousal that appears to result from increased dopamine levels in the brain. It can be caused by drug intoxication (including alcohol) or psychiatric illness or a combination of both. Also called *agitated delirium*.

exocrine gland gland that secretes chemical substances to nearby tissues through a duct; also called a *ducted gland*.

exotoxin a soluble poisonous substance secreted during growth of a bacterium.

facilitated diffusion a form of molecular diffusion in which a molecule-specific carrier in a cell membrane speeds the molecule's movement from a region of higher concentration to one of lower concentration.

factitious disorder condition in which the patient feigns illness to assume the sick role.

fasciitis infection of the fascia (a layer of fibrous connective tissue that surrounds muscles, blood vessels, nerves, and similar structures throughout the body). *See also* necrotizing fasciitis.

fear feeling of alarm and discontentment in the expectation of danger.

fecal–oral route transmission of organisms picked up from the gastrointestinal tract (e.g., feces) into the mouth.

fibrinolysis the process through which plasmin dismantles a blood clot.

fibromyalgia a condition characterized by widespread pain in the muscles and soft tissues throughout the body. Also called *central sensitivity syndrome (CSS)*.

filtrate the fluid produced in Bowman's capsule by filtration of blood.

flail chest one or more ribs fractured in two or more places, creating an unattached rib segment.

flanks the part of the back below the ribs and above the hip bones.

flat affect appearance of being disinterested, often lacking facial expression.

food poisoning nonspecific term often applied to gastroenteritis that occurs suddenly and that is caused by the ingestion of food containing preformed toxins.

free radicals molecules, atoms, or ions with an odd number of electrons (unpaired electrons) that can be formed through interaction with oxygen and can cause damage to body cells. Also called *reactive oxygen species*.

fugue state condition in which an amnesiac patient physically flees.

fungus plantlike microorganism; plural *fungi*.

gangrene death of body tissue.

gastric lavage removing an ingested poison by repeatedly filling and emptying the stomach with water or saline via a gastric tube; also known as "pumping the stomach."

gastroenteritis generalized disorder involving nausea, vomiting, gastrointestinal cramping or discomfort, and diarrhea.

generalized seizures seizures that begin as an electrical discharge in a small area of the brain but spread to involve the entire cerebral cortex, causing widespread malfunction.

genital warts warts occurring in the genital area caused by the human papillomavirus (HPV).

genitourinary system the male organ system that includes reproductive and urinary structures.

German measles *see* rubella.

Glasgow Coma Scale (GCS) tool used in evaluating and quantifying the degree of coma by determining the best motor, verbal, and eye-opening response to standardized stimuli.

glomerular filtration rate (GFR) the volume per day at which blood is filtered through capillaries of the glomerulus.

glomerular filtration the removal of water and other elements from blood in the nephron tubule.

glomerulus a tuft of capillaries from which blood is filtered into a nephron.

gluconeogenesis conversion of protein and fat to form glucose.

glucose intolerance the body cells' inability to take up glucose from the bloodstream.

glycogenolysis the breakdown of glycogen to glucose, primarily by liver cells.

glycosuria glucose in urine, which occurs when blood glucose levels exceed the kidney's ability to reabsorb glucose.

gonorrhea sexually transmitted disease caused by a Gram-negative bacterium.

gout a form of inflammatory arthritis that occurs when uric acid accumulates in the joints.

Gram stain method of differentiating types of bacteria according to their reaction to a chemical stain process.

Graves' disease endocrine disorder characterized by excess thyroid hormones, resulting in body changes associated with increased metabolism; primary cause of thyrotoxicosis.

Grey Turner's sign ecchymosis in the flank.

Guillain-Barré syndrome a condition caused when the immune system attacks the peripheral nerves, leading to nerve inflammation that causes muscle weakness that can worsen to paralysis.

hallucinations sensory perceptions with no basis in reality.

hantavirus family of viruses that are carried by the deer mouse and transmitted by ticks and other arthropods.

heart failure clinical syndrome in which the heart's mechanical performance is compromised so that cardiac output cannot meet the body's needs.

hematemesis bloody vomitus.

hematochezia bright red blood in the stool.

hematocrit the packed cell volume of red blood cells per unit of blood.

hematology the study of blood and the blood-forming organs.

hematopoiesis the process through which pluripotent stem cells differentiate into various types of blood cells.

hemodialysis a dialysis procedure relying on vascular access to the blood and on an artificial membrane.

hemoglobin oxygen-bearing molecule in the red blood cells. It is made up of an iron-rich red pigment called heme and a protein called globin.

hemolysis destruction of red blood cells.

hemophilia a blood disorder in which one of the proteins necessary for blood clotting is missing or defective.

hemoptysis expectoration of blood from the respiratory tree.

hemorrhoid small mass of swollen veins in the anus or rectum.

hemostasis the combined three mechanisms that work to prevent or control blood loss.

hemothorax a collection of blood in the pleural space.

hepatitis inflammation of the liver characterized by diffuse or patchy tissue necrosis.

hepatitis injury with inflammation or infection of the liver cells.

hernia protrusion of an organ through its protective sheath.

herpes simplex virus organism that causes infections characterized by fluid-filled vesicles, usually in the oral cavity or on the genitals.

hilum the notched part of the kidney where the ureter and other structures join kidney tissue.

histamine a product of mast cells and basophils that causes vasodilation, capillary permeability, bronchoconstriction, and contraction of the gut.

homeostasis the natural tendency of the body to keep the internal environment and metabolism steady and normal.

hookworm parasite that attaches to the host's intestinal lining.

hormone chemical substance released by a gland that controls or affects processes in other glands or body systems.

human immunodeficiency virus (HIV) organism responsible for acquired immunodeficiency syndrome (AIDS).

humoral immunity specialized, permanent defense against a particular foreign antigen resulting from attack of an invading substance by antibodies.

Huntington's disease a disease caused by a genetic defect and characterized by rigidity, slow movements, tremor, behavioral changes, unusual movements, and dementia.

Hymenoptera any of an order of highly specialized insects such as bees and wasps.

hyperglycemia excessive blood glucose.

hyperglycemic hyperosmolar nonketotic (HHNK) coma *see* **hyperosmolar hyperglycemic state (HHS).**

hyperosmolar hyperglycemic state (HHS) complication of type 2 diabetes due to inadequate insulin activity. Marked by high blood glucose, marked dehydration, and decreased mental function. Often mistaken for ketoacidosis. Also called *hyperglycemic hyperosmolar nonketotic (HHNK) coma.*

hyperosmolar having a concentration in one substance greater than that of a second solution.

hyperoxia higher than normal levels of oxygen.

hypersensitivity an unexpected and exaggerated reaction to a particular antigen. It is used synonymously with the term *allergy*.

hypertensive emergency an acute elevation of blood pressure that requires the blood pressure to be lowered within 1 hour; characterized by end-organ changes such as hypertensive encephalopathy, renal failure, or blindness.

hypertensive encephalopathy a cerebral disorder of hypertension indicated by severe headache, nausea, vomiting, and altered mental status. Neurologic symptoms may include blindness, muscle twitches, inability to speak, weakness, and paralysis.

hyperthyroidism excessive secretion of thyroid hormones, resulting in an increased metabolic rate.

hypertrophy stretching; enlargement without any additional cells.

hyphema a collection of blood in the anterior chamber of the eye.

hypoglycemia deficiency of blood glucose. Sometimes called *insulin shock*.

hypoglycemic seizure seizure that occurs when brain cells are not functioning normally due to low blood glucose.

hypoosmolar having a concentration in one substance lower than that of a second solution.

hypothyroidism inadequate secretion of thyroid hormones, resulting in a decreased metabolic rate.

hypoxia state in which insufficient oxygen is available to meet the oxygen requirements of the cells.

immediate hypersensitivity a hypersensitivity that develops swiftly following reexposure to an antigen. Immediate hypersensitivity reactions are usually more severe than delayed reactions. The swiftest and most severe of such reactions is anaphylaxis.

immune response complex of events within the body that works toward the destruction or inactivation of pathogens, abnormal cells, or foreign molecules.

immune system the body's mechanism for defending against foreign invaders.

immunoglobulin (Ig) alternative term for *antibody*.

impetigo infection of the skin caused by staphylococci or streptococci.

impulse control disorder condition characterized by the patient's failure to control recurrent impulses.

incubation period time between a host's exposure to an infectious agent and the appearance of symptoms.

indeterminate axis a calculated axis of the heart's electrical energy from –90° to –180°. (Indeterminate axis is often considered to be extreme right axis deviation.)

index case the individual who first introduces an infectious agent to a population.

induced active immunity immunity achieved through vaccination given to generate an immune response that results in the development of antibodies specific for the injected antigen; also called artificially acquired immunity.

induced therapeutic hypothermia (ITH) the practice of cooling survivors of cardiac arrest in the immediate post-resuscitation period.

infarction area of dead tissue caused by lack of blood.

infection presence of an agent within the host, without necessarily causing disease.

infectious disease illness caused by infestation of the body by biological organisms.

infestation presence of parasites that do not break the host's skin.

inflammatory process a nonspecific defense mechanism that wards off damage from microorganisms or trauma.

influenza disease caused by a group of viruses.

ingestion entry of a substance into the body through the gastrointestinal tract.

inhalation entry of a substance into the body through the respiratory tract.

injection entry of a substance into the body through a break in the skin.

injury current *see* current of injury.

inotropy pertaining to cardiac contractile force.

intercalated disks specialized bands of tissue inserted between myocardial cells that increase the rate in which the action potential is spread from cell to cell.

interpolated beat a PVC that falls between two sinus beats without effectively interrupting this rhythm.

interstitial nephritis an inflammation within the tissue surrounding the nephrons.

intrarenal abscess abscess that forms within the renal parenchyma.

intussusception condition that occurs when part of an intestine slips into the part just distal to itself.

irritable bowel syndrome (IBS) a gastrointestinal system disorder characterized by symptoms that include abodominal pain, cramping, increased gas, altered bowel habits, food intolerance, and bloating; also called *spastic colon.*

isosthenuria the inability to concentrate or dilute urine relative to the osmolarity of blood.

Kernig's sign inability to fully extend the knees with hips flexed.

ketone bodies compounds produced during the catabolism of fatty acids, including acetoacetic acid, β-hydroxybutyric acid, and acetone.

ketosis the presence of significant quantities of ketone bodies in the blood.

kidney an organ that produces urine and performs other functions related to the urinary system.

Kiesselbach's plexus a region in the anteroinferior part of the nasal septum where four arteries form a network, or vascular plexus, that is the site of most nosebleeds.

Korsakoff's psychosis psychosis characterized by disorientation, muttering delirium, insomnia, delusions, and hallucinations. Symptoms include painful extremities, bilateral wrist drop (rarely), bilateral foot drop (frequently), and pain on pressure over the long nerves.

Kussmaul's respirations rapid deep respirations caused by severe metabolic and CNS problems.

latent period time when a host cannot transmit an infectious agent to someone else.

left axis deviation a calculated axis of the heart's electrical energy that equals or exceeds –30° (or in a simplified formula, from 0° to –90°).

leukemia a cancer of the hematopoietic cells.

leukocyte white blood cell.

leukocytosis too many white blood cells.

leukopenia too few white blood cells.

leukopoiesis the process through which stem cells differentiate into the white blood cells' immature forms.

lice parasitic infestation of the skin of the scalp, trunk, or pubic area.

ligament of Treitz ligament that supports the duodenojejunal junction.

limb leads *see* augmented leads; bipolar leads; unipolar leads.

lower gastrointestinal bleeding bleeding in the gastrointestinal tract distal to the ligament of Treitz.

Ludwig's angina a type of oral bacterial cellulitis, or inflammation, that involves the floor of the mouth under the tongue.

Lyme disease recurrent inflammatory disorder caused by a tick-borne spirochete.

lymph overflow circulatory fluid in spaces between tissues.

lymphatic system secondary circulatory system that collects overflow fluid from the tissue spaces and filters it before returning it to the circulatory system.

lymphocyte cell that attacks invader in immune response.

lymphoma a cancer of the lymphatic system.

macrophage after neutrophils, the most common phagocytic white blood cell.

major basic protein (MBP) a larvacidal peptide.

Mallory-Weiss syndrome esophageal laceration, usually secondary to vomiting, with resultant bleeding.

manic characterized by excessive excitement or activity (mania).

mask a device for protecting the face.

mast cell specialized cell of the immune system that contains chemicals that assist in the immune response.

McBurney's point common site of pain from appendicitis, 1 to 2 inches above the anterior iliac crest in a direct line with the umbilicus.

measles highly contagious, acute viral disease characterized by a reddish rash that appears on the fourth or fifth day of illness.

medulla oblongata lower portion of the brainstem, connecting the pons and the spinal cord. It contains major centers for control of respiratory, cardiac, and vasomotor activity.

medulla the inner tissue of an organ such as the kidney.

melena dark, tarry, foul-smelling stool indicating the presence of partially digested blood.

meninges membranes covering and protecting the brain and spinal cord. They consist of the pia mater, arachnoid membrane, and dura mater.

meningitis inflammation of the meninges, usually caused by an infection.

mental status examination (MSE) a structured exam designed to quickly evaluate a patient's level of mental functioning.

mental status the state of the patient's cerebral functioning.

mesencephalon portion of the brain connecting the pons and cerebellum with the cerebral hemispheres; also called the midbrain. It controls motor coordination and eye movement.

mesenteric ischemia occlusion or narrowing of one of the mesenteric arteries, causing a reduction in oxygen and nutrients to the portion of the intestine that is normally supplied by the artery, leading, if untreated, to tissue death and infection.

metabolism the sum of cellular processes that produce the energy and molecules needed for growth and repair.

microangiopathy a disease affecting the smallest blood vessels.

Middle East respiratory syndrome (MERS) viral respiratory infection caused by the Middle East respiratory syndrome coronavirus (MERS-CoV).

mononucleosis acute disease caused by the Epstein-Barr virus.

mood disorder pervasive and sustained emotion that colors a person's perception of the world.

multiple myeloma a cancerous disorder of plasma cells.

multiple personality disorder manifestation of two or more complete systems of personality.

multiple sclerosis disease that involves inflammation of certain nerve cells followed by demyelination, or the destruction of the myelin sheath, which is the fatty insulation surrounding nerve fibers.

mumps acute viral disease characterized by painful enlargement of the salivary glands.

Murphy's sign pain caused when an inflamed gallbladder is palpated by pressing under the right costal margin.

muscular dystrophy a group of genetic diseases characterized by progressive muscle weakness and degeneration of the skeletal or voluntary muscle fibers.

myocardial infarction (MI) death and subsequent necrosis of the heart muscle caused by inadequate blood supply; also acute myocardial infarction (AMI).

myocardial injury injury to the myocardium (heart muscle), typically following myocardial ischemia that results from loss of blood and oxygen supply to the tissue. The injured myocardium tends to be partially or completely depolarized.

myocardial ischemia deprivation of oxygen and other nutrients to the myocardium (heart muscle), typically causing abnormalities in repolarization.

myoclonus temporary, involuntary twitching or spasm of a muscle or group of muscles.

myoglobin an iron-containing protein found in muscle fibers that is similar to hemoglobin but has a much higher affinity for oxygen and provides oxygen to the muscle cells during periods of extreme demand.

myxedema coma life-threatening condition associated with advanced myxedema, with profound hypothermia, bradycardia, and electrolyte imbalance.

myxedema condition that reflects long-term exposure to inadequate levels of thyroid hormones with resultant changes in body structure and function.

nasal flaring excessive widening of the nares with respiration.

natural immunity genetically predetermined immunity that is present at birth; also called *innate immunity*.

naturally acquired immunity immunity that begins to develop after birth and is continually enhanced by exposure to new pathogens and antigens throughout life.

necrotizing fasciitis a life-threatening bacterial infection that can rapidly destroy skin, muscles, and surrounding tissues. Also called *flesh-eating disease. See also* fasciitis.

neoplasm literally meaning "new form"; a new or abnormal formation; a tumor.

nephrology the medical specialty dealing with the kidneys.

nephron a microscopic structure within the kidney that produces urine.

neuron nerve cell; the fundamental component of the nervous system.

neurotransmitter a substance that is released from the axon terminal of a presynaptic neuron on excitation and that travels across the synaptic cleft to either excite or inhibit the target cell. Examples include acetylcholine, norepinephrine, and dopamine.

neutropenia a reduced number of neutrophils.

neutrophil the most common phagocytic white blood cell.

noncompensatory pause pause following an ectopic beat where the SA node is depolarized and the underlying cadence of the heart is interrupted.

non–ST segment elevation myocardial infarction (NSTEMI) *see* subendocardial infarction.

normal flora organisms that live inside our bodies without ordinarily causing disease.

normal sinus rhythm the normal heart rhythm.

normoxia normal levels of oxygen.

nosocomial infection an infection acquired in a medical setting.

nosocomial acquired while in the hospital.

obligate intracellular parasite organism that can grow and reproduce only within a host cell.

oliguria decreased urine elimination to 400–500 mL or less per day.

opportunistic pathogen ordinarily nonharmful bacterium that causes disease only under unusual circumstances.

orbital septum a membranous structure that separates the anterior aspect of the eye from the posterior aspect of the eye. Also called the *palpebral ligament*.

organophosphates phosphorus-containing organic chemicals.

orthopnea difficulty breathing while lying supine.

Osgood-Schlatter disease a painful swelling of the anterior tibial tubercle (bump on the upper tibia just below the knee), often involving both legs.

osmolarity the measure of a substance's concentration in water.

osmosis the diffusion pattern of water in which molecules move to equalize concentrations on both sides of a membrane.

osmotic diuresis greatly increased urination and dehydration that results when high levels of glucose cannot be reabsorbed into the blood from the kidney tubules and the osmotic pressure of the glucose in the tubules also prevents water reabsorption.

osteoarthritis (OA) degradation of the joints. Also called *degenerative joint disease.*

osteomyelitis an infection of the bone.

osteoporosis thinning of bone tissue and loss of bone density from mineral loss that occurs over time.

oxidative stress damage to body cells and tissues caused by the presence of free radicals, which may form when molecules, atoms, or ions interact with oxygen.

oxyhemoglobin hemoglobin with oxygen bound.

pallor paleness.

pancolitis ulcerative colitis that affects the entire colon.

pancreatitis inflammation of the pancreas.

panic attack extreme period of anxiety resulting in great emotional distress.

papilla the tip of a pyramid; it juts into the hollow space of the kidney.

parasite organism that lives in or on another organism from which it derives nutriment.

parasympathetic nervous system division of the autonomic nervous system that is responsible for controlling vegetative functions. Parasympathetic nervous system actions include decreased heart rate and constriction of the bronchioles and pupils. Its actions are mediated by the neurotransmitter acetylcholine.

Parkinson's disease chronic and progressive motor system disorder characterized by tremor, rigidity, bradykinesia, and postural instability.

paroxysmal nocturnal dyspnea (PND) a sudden episode of difficult breathing that occurs after lying down; most commonly caused by left-heart failure.

partial seizures seizures that remain confined to a limited portion of the brain, causing localized malfunction. Partial seizures may spread and become generalized.

passive immunity acquired immunity that results from administration of antibodies either from the mother to the infant across the placental barrier (natural passive immunity) or through vaccination (induced passive immunity).

pathogen a disease-producing agent or invading substance.

penis the male organ of copulation.

peptic ulcer erosion caused by gastric acid.

perfusion the circulation of blood through the capillaries.

perinephric abscess a pocket of infection in the layer of fat surrounding the kidney.

peripheral arterial atherosclerotic disease a progressive degenerative disease of the midsize and large arteries.

peripheral nervous system (PNS) part of the nervous system that extends throughout the body and is composed of the cranial nerves arising from the brain and the peripheral nerves arising from the spinal cord. Its subdivisions are the somatic and the autonomic nervous systems.

peripheral neuropathy any malfunction or damage of the peripheral nerves. Results may include muscle weakness, loss of sensation, impaired reflexes, and internal organ malfunctions.

peritoneal dialysis *see* chronic ambulatory peritoneal dialysis (CAPD).

peritonitis inflammation of the peritoneum, which lines the abdominal cavity.

personality disorder condition that results in persistently maladaptive behavior.

pertussis disease characterized by severe, violent coughing.

pH abbreviation for potential of hydrogen. A measure of relative acidity or alkalinity. Because the pH scale is inverse to the concentration of acidic hydrogen ions, the lower the pH, the greater the acidity and the higher the pH, the greater the alkalinity. A normal pH range for humans is 7.35 to 7.45.

phagocytosis process in which white blood cells engulf and destroy an invader.

pharyngitis infection of the pharynx and tonsils.

phobia excessive fear that interferes with functioning.

photopigments material located in the cones of the retina of the eye that undergoes a chemical change when contacted by light, sending impulses to the optic nerve and the brain.

pia mater delicate innermost layer of the meninges.

Pick's disease a rare, permanent form of dementia similar to Alzheimer's disease but affecting only certain areas of the brain; characterized by incorrect behavior in social settings and difficulty with decision making, complex tasks, and language.

pinworm parasite that is 3–10 mm long and lives in the distal colon.

plasma thick, pale yellow fluid that makes up the liquid part of the blood.

pleuritic sharp or tearing, as a description of pain.

pluripotent stem cell a cell from which the various types of blood cells can form.

pneumonia acute infection of the lung, including alveolar spaces and interstitial tissue.

pneumothorax a collection of air in the pleural space, causing a loss of the negative pressure that binds the lung to the chest wall. In an *open pneumothorax*, air enters the pleural space through an injury to the chest wall. In a *closed pneumothorax*, air enters the pleural space through an opening in the pleura that covers the lung. A *tension pneumothorax* develops when air in the pleural space cannot escape, causing a buildup of pressure and collapse of the lung.

Poiseuille's law a law of physiology stating that blood flow through a vessel is directly proportional to the radius of the vessel to the fourth power.

poliomyelitis (polio) infectious, inflammatory viral disease of the central nervous system that sometimes results in permanent paralysis.

polycythemia an excess of red blood cells.

pons process of tissue connecting the medulla oblongata and cerebellum with upper portions of the brain.

portal pertaining to the flow of blood into the liver.

positional asphyxia death from positioning that prevents sufficient intake of oxygen.

positive end-expiratory pressure (PEEP) a method of holding the alveoli open by increasing expiratory pressure. Some bag-valve units used in EMS have PEEP attachments. Also, EMS personnel sometimes transport patients who are on ventilators with PEEP attachments.

postrenal ARF acute renal failure (ARF) caused by obstruction distal to the kidney.

post-traumatic stress disorder (PTSD) reaction to an extreme stressor.

posture position, attitude, or bearing of the body.

PPD purified protein derivative, the substance used in a test for tuberculosis.

precordial (chest) leads electrocardiogram leads applied to the chest in a pattern that permits a view of the horizontal plane of the heart; leads V_1, V_2, V_3, V_4, V_5, and V_6.

preload the pressure within the ventricles at the end of diastole; commonly called the end-diastolic volume.

prerenal ARF acute renal failure (ARF) caused by decreased blood perfusion of the kidneys.

preventive strategy a management plan to minimize further damage to vital tissues.

priapism a painful, prolonged erection of the penis.

primary response initial, generalized response to an antigen.

Prinzmetal's angina variant of angina pectoris caused by vasospasm of the coronary arteries, not blockage per se; also called vasospastic angina or atypical angina.

prions particles of protein, folded in such a way that protease enzymes cannot act on them.

proctitis ulcerative colitis limited to the rectum.

prolonged QT interval QT interval greater than 0.44 sec.

prostate gland a gland that surrounds the male bladder neck and the first portion of the urethra; it produces fluid that mixes with sperm to make semen.

prostatitis infection and inflammation of the prostate gland.

protozoa single-celled parasitic organisms with flexible membranes and the ability to move.

proximal tubule the part of the tubule beyond Bowman's capsule.

psychogenic amnesia failure to recall, as opposed to inability to recall.

psychosis extreme response to stress characterized by impaired ability to deal with reality.

psychosocial related to a patient's personality style, dynamics of unresolved conflict, or crisis management methods.

pterygium a raised, wedge-shaped growth of the conjunctiva of the eye.

pulmonary embolism (PE) blood clot in one of the pulmonary arteries.

pyelonephritis an infection and inflammation of the kidney.

pyramids the visible tissue structures within the medulla of the kidney.

QRS axis reduction of all the heart's electrical forces to a single vector represented by an arrow moving in a single plane.

QT interval period from the beginning of the QRS to the end of the T wave.

rabies viral disorder that affects the nervous system.

reabsorption the movement of a substance from a nephron tubule back into the blood.

reactive oxygen species *see* free radicals.

reciprocal a mirror image seen typically on the opposite wall of the injured area.

reduced nephron mass the decrease in number of functional nephrons that causes chronic renal failure.

reduced renal mass the decrease in kidney size associated with chronic renal failure.

referred pain pain felt in a location other than that of its origin.

reflex sympathetic dystrophy (RSD) a chronic pain condition characterized by diffuse pain, swelling, and limitation of movement that follows an arm or leg injury.

refractory period the period of time when myocardial cells have not yet completely repolarized and cannot be stimulated again.

relative refractory period the period of the cardiac cycle when a sufficiently strong stimulus may produce depolarization.

renal ARF acute renal failure (ARF) caused by pathology within the kidney tissue itself.

renal calculi kidney stones.

renal dialysis artificial replacement of some critical kidney functions.

renal pelvis the hollow space of the kidney that junctions with a ureter.

renal pertaining to the kidneys.

renin an enzyme produced by kidney cells that plays a key role in controlling arterial blood pressure.

repetitive-motion disorders injury or inflammation of tissues caused by repeated motions.

repolarization return of a muscle cell to its preexcitation resting state in which the inside of the cell is negative in relation to the outside. *See also* depolarization.

reservoir any living creature or environment (water, soil, etc.) that can harbor an infectious agent.

resistance a host's ability to fight off infection.

respiration the exchange of gases between a living organism and its environment.

respirator an apparatus worn that cleanses or qualifies the air.

respiratory syncytial virus (RSV) common cause of pneumonia and bronchiolitis in children.

resting potential the normal electrical state of cardiac cells.

resuscitation provision of efforts to return a spontaneous pulse and breathing.

reticular activating system the system responsible for consciousness. A series of nervous tissues keeping the human system in a state of consciousness.

reticuloendothelial system (RES) the cells involved in the immune response.

return of spontaneous circulation (ROSC) resuscitation resulting in the patient's having a spontaneous pulse.

rheumatoid arthritis (RA) a chronic disease that leads to inflammation and injury to the joints and the surrounding tissues.

rhythm strip electrocardiogram printout.

right axis deviation a calculated axis of the heart's electrical energy that equals or exceeds +105° (or, in a simplified formula, from +90° to +180°).

rubella (German measles) systemic viral disease characterized by a fine pink rash that appears on the face, trunk, and extremities and fades quickly.

Ryan White Act federal law that outlines the rights and responsibilities of agencies and health care workers when an infectious disease exposure occurs.

scabies skin disease caused by mite infestation and characterized by intense itching.

schizophrenia common disorder involving significant change in behavior, often including hallucinations, delusions, and depression.

scrotum a muscular sac outside the abdominal cavity that contains the testes, epididymis, and vas deferens.

sebum an oily substance secreted onto the eyelids that keeps the lids soft and pliable.

secondary response response by the immune system that takes place if the body is exposed to the same antigen again; in secondary response, antibodies specific for the offending antigen are released.

secretion the movement of a substance from the blood into a nephron tubule.

seizure a temporary alteration in behavior due to the massive electrical discharge of one or more groups of neurons in the brain. Seizures can be clinically classified as generalized or partial.

semen male reproductive fluid.

sensitization initial exposure of a person to an antigen that results in an immune response.

sepsis a life-threatening medical condition caused by a whole-body inflammatory state called systemic inflammatory response syndrome (SIRS). Sepsis is also sometimes called *septicemia*.

septic arthritis infection of a joint, usually by bacteria but sometimes by viruses or fungi. Also called *septic joint*.

septicemia *see* sepsis.

sequestration the trapping of red blood cells by an organ such as the spleen.

seroconversion creation of antibodies after exposure to a disease.

severe acute respiratory syndrome (SARS) a highly infectious viral respiratory illness that first appeared in southern China in 2002.

sexually transmitted disease (STD) illness most commonly transmitted through sexual contact.

sickle cell disease an inherited disorder of red blood cell production, so named because the red blood cells become sickle shaped when oxygen levels are low. Also called *sickle cell anemia*.

simple diffusion the random motion of molecules from an area of high concentration to an area of lower concentration.

simple partial seizure type of partial seizure that involves local motor, sensory, or autonomic dysfunction of one area of the body. There is no loss of consciousness.

sinusitis inflammation of the paranasal sinuses.

slow-reacting substance of anaphylaxis (SRS-A) substance released from basophils and mast cells that causes spasm of the bronchiole smooth muscle, resulting in an asthma-like attack and occasionally asphyxia.

sociocultural related to the patient's actions and interactions within society.

somatic nervous system part of the nervous system controlling voluntary bodily functions.

somatic pain sharp, localized pain that originates in walls of the body such as skeletal muscles.

somatoform disorder condition characterized by physical symptoms that have no apparent physiologic cause and are attributable to psychological factors.

sperm cell male reproductive cell.

spina bifida (SB) a neural defect that results from the failure of one or more of the fetal vertebrae to close properly during the first month of pregnancy.

spontaneous pneumothorax a pneumothorax (collection of air in the pleural space) that occurs spontaneously, in the absence of blunt or penetrating trauma.

Starling's law of the heart law of physiology stating that the more the myocardium is stretched, up to a certain amount, the more forceful the subsequent contraction will be.

status epilepticus series of two or more generalized motor seizures without any intervening periods of consciousness.

sterilization process that destroys all microorganisms.

stroke volume the amount of blood ejected by the heart in one cardiac contraction.

stroke neurologic deficit caused by either ischemic or hemorrhagic lesions to a portion of the brain, resulting in damage or destruction of brain tissue. Previously called a *cerebrovascular accident*.

ST-segment elevation myocardial infarction (STEMI) *see* transmural infarction.

sty an infection of the eyelid caused by blockage of the oil glands associated with an eyelash. Alternative spelling: *stye.* Also called an *external hordeolum*.

subcutaneous emphysema presence of air in the subcutaneous tissue.

subendocardial infarction myocardial infarction that affects only the deeper levels of the myocardium; also called non–Q-wave infarction because it typically does not result in a significant Q wave in the affected lead. Commonly referred to as a *non-ST-segment elevation myocardial infarction (NSTEMI).*

substance abuse use of a pharmacological substance for purposes other than medically defined reasons.

sudden death death within 1 hour after the onset of symptoms.

surface absorption entry of a substance into the body directly through the skin or mucous membrane.

surfactant a compound secreted by the lungs that contributes to the elastic properties of the pulmonary tissues.

survival continuing to live under conditions in which death would be the expected outcome.

sympathetic nervous system division of the autonomic nervous system that prepares the body for stressful situations. Sympathetic nervous system actions include increased heart rate and dilation of the bronchioles and pupils. Its actions are mediated by the neurotransmitters epinephrine and norepinephrine.

synchronized cardioversion the passage of an electric current through the heart during a specific part of the cardiac cycle to terminate certain kinds of dysrhythmias.

syncope transient loss of consciousness due to inadequate flow of blood to the brain with rapid recovery of consciousness on becoming supine; fainting.

syncytium group of cardiac muscle cells that function physiologically as a unit.

syphilis bloodborne sexually transmitted disease caused by the spirochete *Treponema pallidum*.

systemic inflammatory response syndrome (SIRS) a whole-body inflammatory state. *See also* sepsis.

systemic lupus erythematosus (SLE) a chronic autoimmune disease that can affect the skin, joints, kidneys, and other organs.

systole the period of the cardiac cycle when the myocardium is contracting.

T lymphocytes cells that attack invaders in cell-mediated immune responses.

tachycardia a rapid heart rate greater than 100 beats per minute.

tachypnea rapid respiration.

tactile fremitus vibratory tremors felt through the chest by palpation.

tendinitis *see* tendonitis.

tendonitis an inflammation of a tendon. Alternative spelling: *tendinitis*.

tenosynovitis an inflammation of the lining of the sheath (synovium) that surrounds a tendon.

testes male sex organs.

testicular torsion twisting of the spermatic cord, resulting in blockage of the blood supply to the testicle and surrounding structures within the scrotum.

tetanus acute bacterial infection of the central nervous system.

therapeutic index the maximum tolerated dose divided by the minimum curative dose of a drug; the range between curative and toxic dosages; also called *therapeutic window*.

thrombocyte blood platelet.

thrombocytopenia an abnormal decrease in the number of platelets.

thrombocytosis an abnormal increase in the number of platelets.

thrombosis clot formation, which is extremely dangerous when it occurs in coronary arteries or cerebral vasculature.

thyrotoxic crisis toxic condition characterized by hyperthermia, tachycardia, nervous symptoms, and rapid metabolism; also known as *thyroid storm*.

thyrotoxicosis condition that reflects prolonged exposure to excess thyroid hormones with resultant changes in body structure and function.

tolerance the need to progressively increase the dose of a drug to reproduce the effect originally achieved by smaller doses.

tonic phase phase of a seizure characterized by tension or contraction of muscles.

tonic–clonic seizure type of generalized seizure characterized by rapid loss of consciousness and motor coordination, muscle spasms, and jerking motions.

total downtime duration from the beginning of the arrest until the patient's delivery to the emergency department.

toxicology study of the detection, chemistry, pharmacological actions, and antidotes of toxic substances.

toxidrome a toxic syndrome; a group of typical signs and symptoms consistently associated with exposure to a particular type of toxin.

toxin any poisonous chemical secreted by bacteria or released following destruction of the bacteria; any chemical (drug, poison, or other) that causes adverse effects on an organism that is exposed to it.

tracheal deviation any position of the trachea other than midline.

tracheal tugging retraction of the tissues of the neck due to airway obstruction or dyspnea.

transient ischemic attack (TIA) temporary interruption of blood supply to the brain.

transmural infarction myocardial infarction that affects the full thickness of the myocardium and almost always results in a pathological Q wave in the affected leads. Commonly referred to as an *ST-segment elevation myocardial infarction (STEMI).*

trichinosis disease resulting from an infestation of *Trichinella spiralis*.

trichomoniasis sexually transmitted disease caused by the protozoan *Trichomonas vaginalis*.

tuberculosis (TB) disease caused by a bacterium known as *Mycobacterium tuberculosis* that primarily affects the respiratory system.

ulcerative colitis an inflammatory bowel disorder of unknown origin. If spread throughout the colon, it is called *pancolitis;* if confined to the rectum, it is called *proctitis*.

unipolar leads electrocardiogram leads applied to the arms and legs, consisting of one polarized (positive) electrode and a nonpolarized reference point that is created by the ECG machine combining two additional electrodes; also called augmented limb leads; leads aVR, aVL, and aVF.

upper gastrointestinal bleeding bleeding within the gastrointestinal tract proximal to the ligament of Treitz.

urea waste derived from ammonia produced through protein metabolism.

uremia the syndrome of signs and symptoms associated with chronic renal failure.

ureter a duct that carries urine from the kidney to the urinary bladder.

urethra the duct that carries urine from the bladder out of the body; in men, it also carries reproductive fluid (semen) to the outside of the body.

urethritis an infection and inflammation of the urethra.

urinary bladder the muscular organ that stores urine before its elimination from the body.

urinary stasis a condition in which the bladder empties incompletely during urination.

urinary system the group of organs that produces urine, maintaining fluid and electrolyte balance for the body.

urinary tract infection (UTI) an infection, usually bacterial, at any site in the urinary tract.

urine the fluid made by the kidney and eliminated from the body.

urology the surgical specialty dealing with the urinary/genitourinary system.

urticaria the raised areas, or wheals, that occur on the skin, associated with vasodilation due to histamine release; commonly called "hives."

varicella viral disease characterized by a rash of fluid-filled vesicles that rupture, forming small ulcers that eventually scab; commonly called *chickenpox*.

varicose veins dilated superficial veins, usually in the lower extremity.

vas deferens the duct that carries sperm cells from the epididymis to the urethra.

vasculitis inflammation of blood vessels.

vector a force that has both magnitude and direction.

ventilation the mechanical process of moving air in and out of the lungs.

virulence an organism's strength or ability to infect or overcome the body's defenses.

virus disease-causing organism that can be seen only with an electron microscope.

visceral pain dull, poorly localized pain that originates in the walls of hollow organs such as the ureter or bladder.

vitreous humor clear, jellylike fluid that fills the vitreous cavity of the eye.

volvulus twisting of the intestine on itself.

von Willebrand's disease condition in which the vWF component of factor VIII is deficient.

Wernicke's syndrome condition characterized by loss of memory and disorientation, associated with chronic alcohol intake and a diet deficient in thiamine.

whole bowel irrigation administration of polyethylene glycol continuously at 1–2 L/hour through a nasogastric tube until the effluent is clear or objects are recovered.

window phase time between exposure to a disease and seroconversion.

withdrawal referring to alcohol or drug withdrawal in which the patient's body reacts severely when deprived of the abused substance.

Zika virus disease (ZVD) a disease caused by the Zika virus and spread by the *Aedes* species of mosquitoes.

Zollinger-Ellison syndrome condition that causes the stomach to secrete excessive amounts of hydrochloric acid and pepsin.

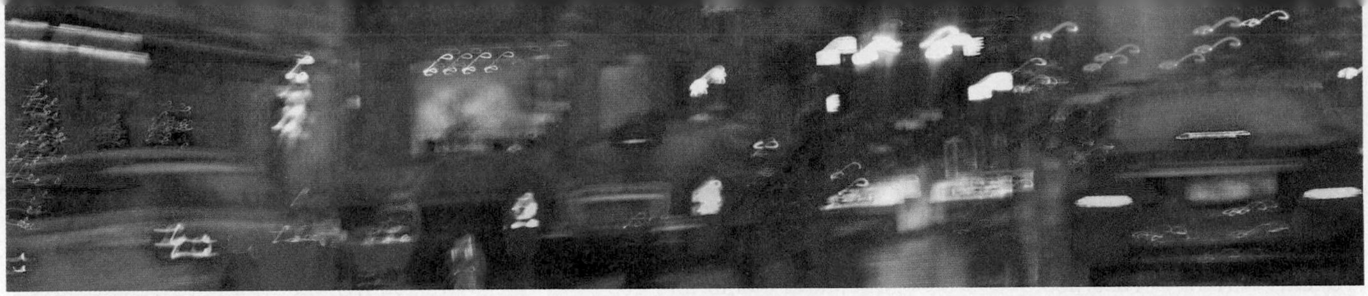

Index

A

Abdomen, examination of, 310
Abdominal aorta, 55
Abdominal aortic aneurysm, 154
Aberrant conduction, 108
Absence seizure, 221
Absolute refractory period, 72
Accelerated idioventricular rhythm, 97–98, 99
Accelerated junctional rhythm, 96, 97
Acetaminophen toxicity, 349
Acids, 344
Acini, 244
Acquired immunity, 264
Acquired immunodeficiency syndrome (AIDS), 410–412
Action potential, 63, 65
Activated charcoal, 330
Active immunity, 264, 401
Active transport, 305
Acute arterial occlusion, 155
Acute coronary syndrome (ACS)
- defined, 131
- evolution of, 166–167
- pathophysiology, 131

Acute gastroenteritis, 283–284
Acute kidney injury (AKI). *See also* Renal and urologic emergencies
- assessment, 313–314
- causes of, 312
- defined, 311
- management, 314
- pathophysiology, 312–313
- postrenal, 313
- prerenal, 312
- renal, 312

Acute myocardial infarction
- anterior infarct, 170, 173–175
- anterolateral infarct, 170–171
- high lateral infarct, 171
- inferior infarct, 171, 172
- inferolateral infarct, 171
- lateral infarct, 171
- localization grid, 169
- localization of, 167–176
- location table, 170
- true posterior infarct, 171–176

Acute pulmonary embolism, 155
Acute respiratory distress syndrome (ARDS)
- assessment, 27
- causes of, 26
- defined, 26
- end-stage, 29
- initiation of, 28
- management, 27
- pathophysiology, 27

Acute tubular necrosis, 312
Acute ulcerative colitis, 288
Addiction, 359
Addisonian crisis, 258
Addison's disease, 257
Adenosine, 120
Adhesions, 292
Adrenal cortex, 245
Adrenal glands
- defined, 245
- disorders of, 257–258
- hormones, 245–246

Adrenal insufficiency, 258
Adrenal medulla, 245
Affect, 448
Afferent fibers, 203
Africanized honeybees (AHBs), 353–354
Afterload, 58
Agonal rhythm, 103, 105
AIDS (acquired immunodeficiency syndrome), 410–412
Airborne route, 397
Airway
- anaphylaxis and, 270
- asthmatic, 33
- in primary assessment, 16
- resistance, 9

AKI. *See* Acute kidney injury
Alcohol abuse
- alcohol withdrawal syndrome, 363–364
- consequences of chronic ingestion, 363–364
- general alcoholic profile, 363
- overview, 362
- physiologic effects, 362–363
- prehospital management, 361
- signs and symptoms of, 361

Alcoholism, 214, 363
Aldosterone, 246
Alkalis, 344
Allergens, 265
Allergic conjunctivitis, 469
Allergic reactions. *See also* Anaphylaxis
- assessment findings in, 271
- defined, 263
- introduction, 263
- management, 269, 271–272
- pathophysiology, 263–266
- patient education, 272
- signs and symptoms of, 271

Allergies
- cardiovascular patient, 113
- clinical presentation of, 268
- defined, 264
- delayed hypersensitivity, 265
- immediate hypersensitivity, 265–266

Alteplase (tPA), 122
Altered mental status, 213–214
Alveolar collapse, 29
Alveolar dead space, 10
Alveoli, 6–7
Alzheimer's disease, 228
Amiodarone, 120
Amphetamines/stimulants, 360, 361

Amyotrophic lateral sclerosis (ALS), 230
Anabolism, 248
Anaphylaxis
- agents that may cause, 263
- airway protection, 270
- assessment findings in, 266–268
- clinical presentation of, 268
- defined, 263
- management, 268–271
- medication administration, 270–271
- occurrence of, 266
- pathophysiology, 267
- patient education, 272
- psychological support, 271
- signs and symptoms of, 271
- slow-reactive substance of (SRS-A), 266

Anastomoses, 56
Anatomical dead space, 10
Androgenic hormones, 246
Anemias, 383–384
Aneurysm, 154–155
Anger, 452
Angina pectoris
- defined, 131–132
- field assessment, 132–133
- management, 133

Angioneurotic edema, 266
Angiotensin-converting enzyme (ACE), 247
Angiotensinogen, 247
Ankylosing spondylitis (AS), 494–495
Anorexia nervosa, 455
ANP (atrial natriuretic peptide), 62
Anterior infarct, 170, 173–175
Anterior pituitary, 243–244
Anterolateral infarct, 170–171
Antiarrhythmics, 120
Antibodies, 263, 399
Antidepressant overdose
- management, 348
- newer, 347–348
- serotonin syndrome, 347–348
- signs and symptoms, 347
- tricyclic antidepressants, 346

Antidiuresis, 305–306
Antidotes, 330–331
Antigens, 263, 377, 399
Antihistamines, 270–271
Antisocial personality disorder, 455
Antivenin, 357
Anuria, 311
Anxiety disorders, 451–452
Apnea, 13
Apneustic respiration, 14, 209
Appendicitis, 293–294
Aqueous humor, 467
Arachnoid membrane, 200
ARDS. *See* Acute respiratory distress syndrome
Arrhythmias
- accelerated idioventricular rhythm, 97–98, 99
- accelerated junctional rhythm, 96, 97
- artificial pacemaker rhythm, 105–108
- asystole, 103–105
- atria origination, 82–88
- atrial fibrillation, 87–88
- atrial flutter, 86–87
- atrioventricular blocks, 89–93
- AV junction (AV blocks) origination, 88–93
- classification of, 76
- from conduction disorders, 108–109
- defined, 75
- first-degree AV block, 89, 90
- junctional bradycardia, 95–96
- junctional escape complexes and rhythms, 94–95
- multifocal tachycardia (MAT), 83
- paroxysmal supraventricular tachycardia (PSVT), 84–85
- preexcitation syndromes and, 109
- premature atrial contractions (PACs), 83–84
- premature junctional contractions (PJCs), 94
- premature ventricular contractions, 98–101
- pulseless electrical activity (PEA), 108
- SA node origination, 76–82
- sick sinus syndrome, 80–82
- sinus arrest, 78–79
- sinus arrhythmia, 78
- sinus block, 79–80
- sinus bradycardia, 76–77
- sinus pause, 80
- sinus tachycardia, 77–78
- by site of origin, 76
- supraventricular tachycardia, 86
- third-degree AV block, 92–93
- 2:1 AV block, 92
- type I second-degree AV block, 89–91
- type II second-degree AV block, 91
- ventricles origination, 96–105
- ventricular conduction disturbances and, 108–109
- ventricular escape complexes and rhythms, 97, 98
- ventricular fibrillation, 102–103
- ventricular tachycardia, 101–102
- wandering atrial pacemaker, 82

Arterial system, 57
Arteries, 57
Arterioles, 57
Arteriosclerosis, 154
Artifacts. *See* Electrocardiogram
Artificial pacemaker rhythm
- description, 105–106
- magnet use, 107–108
- management considerations, 107
- pacemaker problems and, 106–107

AS (ankylosing spondylitis), 494–495
Ascending aorta, 55
Ascending loop of Henle, 304
Asphyxia, 16
Aspirin, 122
Assessment
- acute kidney injury (AKI), 313–314
- acute respiratory distress syndrome (ARDS), 27
- adrenal insufficiency, 258
- allergic reactions, 271
- altered mental status, 213–214
- anaphylaxis, 266–268
- angina pectoris, 132–133
- asthma, 33–34
- back pain, 232–233
- carbon monoxide inhalation, 42
- cardiac arrest, 152
- cardiac tamponade, 143–145
- cardiogenic shock, 147
- cardiovascular patient, 111–116
- central nervous system dysfunction, 45
- chronic bronchitis, 32
- chronic kidney disease (CKD), 315–316
- degenerative neurologic disorders, 230–231
- diabetic ketoacidosis, 252
- dysfunction of spinal cord, nerves, or respiratory muscles, 45–46
- Ebola virus disease (EVD), 419
- emphysema, 31
- gastrointestinal emergencies, 278–280
- general treatment, 280

Graves' disease, 256
headache, 224
heart failure, 140–142
hematopoietic disorders, 379–382
hyperadrenalism, 258
hyperosmolar hyperglycemic state (HHS), 254
hypertensive emergencies, 145–146
hyperventilation syndrome, 45
hypoglycemia (insulin shock), 255
hypothyroidism, 256–257
infectious disease patients, 408–409
ingested toxins, 331
inhaled toxins, 332
lung cancer, 40–41
myocardial infarction (MI), 135–136
myxedema, 256–257
neoplasm, 227–228
neurologic patient, 207–213
nontraumatic musculoskeletal disorders, 491
pneumonia, 38, 417
pulmonary embolism, 43
renal and urologic emergencies, 308–311
renal calculi, 319–320
respiratory system, 14
right ventricular infarctions, 176
seizures, 221–222
severe acute respiratory syndrome (SARS), 39, 418
spontaneous pneumothorax, 44
stroke, 216–217
surface-absorbed toxins, 333
syncope, 223
thyrotoxic crisis (thyroid storm), 256
toxic inhalation, 41
toxicologic emergencies, 329
upper airway obstruction, 25–26
upper respiratory infections (URIs), 37
urinary tract infection (UTI), 321–322
vascular disorders, 156
"weak and dizzy," 226

Asthma
airway, 33
assessment, 33–34
in children, 36
defined, 32
management, 34–36
nebulized medication administration, 35–36
occurrence of, 27
pathophysiology, 32–33
peak expiratory flow rate (PEFR) and, 34
phases, 34
presenting symptoms, 33
respiratory rate and, 34
status asthmaticus, 36

Asystole, 103–105
Ataxic (Biot's) respirations, 14, 209
Atherosclerosis, 154
Atherosclerotic heart disease (ASHD), 133
Atraumatic hyphema, 470
Atria, 53
Atrial contraction, 70
Atrial enlargement, 182, 185
Atrial excitation, 70, 71
Atrial fibrillation, 87–88
Atrial flutter, 86–87
Atrial natriuretic hormone (ANH), 247
Atrial natriuretic peptide (ANP), 62
Atrial syncytium, 63
Atrioventricular (AV) blocks
classification of, 89
conduction abnormalities, 177
defined, 89
first-degree AV block, 89, 90, 177
third-degree AV block, 92–93, 177
2:1 AV block, 92
type I second-degree AV block, 89–91, 177
type II second-degree AV block, 91, 177

Atrioventricular (AV) bundle, 63
Atrioventricular valves, 53
Atropine sulfate, 120
Augmented leads, 68
Aura, 220
Auscultation
cardiovascular patient, 115–116
chest, 19

Autoimmune disease, 375
Autoimmunity, 400
Automaticity, 64
Autonomic nervous system. *See also* Nervous system
defined, 197
disorders, 207
hypothalamus and, 240
parasympathetic nervous system, 198, 204–205
sympathetic nervous system, 198, 204

AV junction
arrhythmias sustained or originating in, 82–88, 93–96
impulse delay at, 71
problems in, 88
transitional fibers, 88

AV node
arrhythmias origination in, 93
organization of, 88–89

Avian influenza, 423
Avoidant personality disorder, 455
AVPU method, 207
Axis deviation, 162–164

B

B lymphocytes, 400
Back pain
assessment, 232–233
causes of, 231–232
low, 231
management, 233
overview, 231

Bacteria, 395–396
Bacterial conjunctivitis, 468–469
Bactericidal, 396
Bacteriostatic, 396
Ball-and-socket joint, 488
Barbiturates, 360, 361
Basophils, 265, 374
Bedbugs, 437–438
Behavior, 446
Behavioral emergency patients. *See also* Psychiatric disorders
assessment, 447–449
defined, 446
management of, 458–460
medical care, 459
mental status examination, 449
primary assessment, 448
psychiatric medications, 449
psychological care, 459–460
scene size-up, 447–448
secondary assessment, 448–449
TASERed, 458–459
violent, and restraints, 460–463

Bell's palsy, 225
Benign prostatic hypertrophy, 303
Benign tumors, 226–227
Benzodiazepines, 360, 362
Bereavement, 452
Beta blocker poisoning treatment algorithm, 344
Beta-agonists, 271
Biological (organic) disorders, 446–447

Bipolar leads, 67, 158–159
2,3-bisphosphoglycerate (2,3-BPG), 372
Bites and stings
- Africanized honeybees, 353–354
- black widow spider bites, 354–355
- brown recluse spider bites, 354
- insect stings, 353
- scorpion stings, 355–356
- snakebites, 356–358

Black widow spider bites, 354–355
Blood. *See also* Hematopoietic disorders
- components of, 370–376
- hemostasis, 376–377
- plasma, 370–371
- platelets, 375–376
- red blood cells, 371–373
- white blood cells, 373–375

Blood delivery, stress response factors affecting, 60
Blood flow, heart, 54–55, 56
Blood glucose
- determination, 253–254
- meter, 212
- regulation, 248–249

Blood transfusion
- fluid added by, 379
- reactions, 379
- types of, 378
- universal donors, 378

Bloodborne diseases, 397
BNP (brain natriuretic peptide), 62
Body dysmorphic disorder, 454
Bohr effect, 12, 372
Bone
- anatomy, 488
- infections, 497
- joints, 487–489
- shapes, 487
- tumors, 498

Borderline personality disorder, 455
Bowel obstruction, 292–293
Bowman's capsule, 304
Bradycardia, 74
Brain
- areas of specialization, 202
- division of, 200–202
- external anatomy, 201
- illustrated, 201
- inferior view, 203
- vascular supply, 202

Brain abscess, 228
Brain natriuretic peptide (BNP), 62, 247
Brainstem, 200
Breath sounds, 115
Breathing
- abnormal sounds, 19
- normal sounds, 19
- in primary assessment, 16

Bronchi, 5–6
Bronchial vessels, 7
Bronchospasm, 9
Brown recluse spider bites, 354
Brudzinski's sign, 422
Brugada syndrome, 151
Bruits, 85
Bulimia nervosa, 455
Bundle branch blocks
- conduction abnormalities, 178–182, 183–184
- defined, 108
- left anterior hemiblock, 181–182
- left bundle branch block, 179–181, 183
- left posterior hemiblock, 181
- right bundle branch block, 179, 184

Bundle of His, 64
Bundle of Kent, 109
Bursitis, 492

C

CAD (coronary artery disease), 52
Calcium channel blocker poisoning treatment algorithm, 343
Cancer, lung, 40–41
CAPD (chronic ambulatory peritoneal dialysis), 317
Capillaries, 57
Capnograms, 22, 23–24
Capnography, 22–24, 212
Capnometry, 22
Carbaminohemoglobin, 12
Carbon monoxide
- defined, 333
- detection, 338
- pathophysiology, 335–337
- sources of, 333–335

Carbon monoxide inhalation
- assessment, 42
- management, 42–43
- overview, 41–42
- pathophysiology, 42
- poisoning inhalation, 42

Carbon monoxide poisoning
- acute, 337
- chronic, 337
- cyanide poisoning and, 342
- diagnosis, 340
- hyperbaric oxygen (HBO) therapy, 335, 341
- management, 338–341
- signs and symptoms of, 337
- treatment, 340–341
- treatment algorithm, 340

Carboxyhemoglobin, 42, 335
Carboxyhemoglobinemia, 335
Cardiac action potential, 63, 65
Cardiac arrest
- causes of, 149
- circulatory phase, 149–150
- defined, 149
- electrical phase, 149
- field assessment, 152
- field termination of resuscitation, 153–154
- management, 152–153
- metabolic phase, 150–151
- pathophysiology, 149–151
- three-phase model, 150
- treatment of, 104
- unusual causes, 151–152
- withholding of resuscitation, 153

Cardiac conductive system
- automaticity, 64
- conductivity, 64
- contractility, 64
- excitability, 63
- illustrated, 66
- overview, 63
- rate of self-excitation, 65
- review, 157

Cardiac cycle
- defined, 57–60
- diastole, 57
- illustrated, 59
- systole, 57–58

Cardiac depolarization, 63
Cardiac enzymes, 138
Cardiac function, role of electrolytes, 62
Cardiac medication overdose, 343–344
Cardiac output, 58
Cardiac polarization, 66
Cardiac tamponade, 143–145
Cardinal positions of gaze, 209
Cardiogenic pulmonary edema, 28
Cardiogenic shock, 147–149
Cardiology, 49–194

Cardiovascular anatomy
heart, 53–56
overview, 53
peripheral circulation, 57
Cardiovascular disease (CVD), 52–53
Cardiovascular emergencies
acute arterial occlusion, 155
acute coronary syndrome (ACS), 131, 166–167
acute pulmonary embolism, 155
advanced life support, 117
aneurysm, 154–155
angina pectoris, 131–133
atherosclerosis, 154
basic life support, 117
cardiac arrest, 149–154
cardiac tamponade, 143–145
cardiogenic shock, 147–149
carotid sinus massage, 128–130
defibrillation, 122–125
ECG monitoring in the field, 117–119
heart failure, 139–143
hypertensive, 145–147
management of, 117–130
myocardial infarction (MI), 133–139
noncritical peripheral vascular conditions, 155–156
peripheral vascular, 154–156
pharmacological management, 120–122
precordial thump, 119–120
specific, managing, 130–156
support and communication, 130
synchronized cardioversion, 125, 126
transcutaneous cardiac pacing (TCP), 125–128
vagal maneuvers, 119
vasculitis, 155
Cardiovascular patient
allergies, 113
assessment, 111–116
assessment overview, 111
auscultation, 115–116
chest pain, 112
common symptoms, 112–113
cough, 112
dyspnea, 112
emergency management, 117–130
events preceding incident, 114
history, 111–114
inspection, 114–115
last oral intake, 114
medications, 113–114
palpation, 116
past medical history, 114
physical examination, 114–116
primary assessment, 111
scene size-up, 111
Cardiovascular system, 53
Carina, 5
Carotid artery bruit, 116
Carotid sinus massage, 128–130
Carpal tunnel syndrome (CTS), 492
Carpopedal spasm, 19
Catabolism, 248
Cataract, 471
Catatonia, 451
Cauda equina syndrome, 232
Caustic substances, 344–345
Cell-mediated immunity, 400
Cellular immunity, 263
Cellulitis, 469, 496
Central nervous system (CNS). *See also* Nervous system
brain, 200–203
defined, 197
disorders, 206
dysfunction, 45
neurons, 198
protective structures, 198–200
respiratory patterns with dysfunction, 209
spinal cord, 203, 204
Central neurogenic hyperventilation, 14, 209
Central pain syndrome, 230
Central retinal artery occlusion, 471
Central retinal vein occlusion, 471
Central sensitivity syndrome (CSS), 498
Cerebellum, 200–202
Cerebral cortex, 200
Cerebral homeostasis, 206
Cerebrospinal fluid, 10, 200
Cerebrum, 200
Chalazion, 468
Chamber enlargement
atrial, 182, 185
types of, 182
ventricular, 182, 186
Chemical restraint, 462–463
Chemotaxis, 373
Chest pain
in cardiovascular patient, 112
causes of, 130–131
pleuritic, 38
Cheyne-Stokes respirations, 13, 209
CHF (congestive heart failure), 140, 141–142
Chickenpox (varicella), 420–421
Chikungunya virus disease, 420
Children. *See* Pediatric patients
Cholecystitis, 294–295
Chronic alcoholism, 214
Chronic ambulatory peritoneal dialysis (CAPD), 317
Chronic bronchitis, 31–32
Chronic gastroenteritis, 285
Chronic kidney disease (CKD). *See also* Renal and urologic emergencies
assessment, 315–316
causes of, 314
common elements of, 316
defined, 314
intermediate management, 316
long-term management, 316–318
management, 316–318
pathophysiology, 314–315
peritoneal dialysis, 317
renal dialysis, 316–318
Chronic obstructive pulmonary disease (COPD)
defined, 3
occurrence of, 27
regulation of ventilation and, 10–11
Chronic pain syndrome (CPS), 498–499
Chronic renal failure (CRF). *See* Chronic kidney disease (CKD)
Chronotropy, 61
Ciguatera (bony fish) poisoning, 351, 359
Cincinnati Prehospital Stroke Scale (CPSS), 217, 219
Circumcision, 307
Cirrhosis, 283, 297
CKD. *See* Chronic kidney disease
Claudication, 154
Clonic phase, 220
Clostridium botulinum, 351
Clotting abnormalities, 386–388
CNS. *See* Central nervous system
Cocaine, 360, 361
Cognitive disorders, 450
Cognitive systems
alteration in, 205–206
autonomic nervous system disorders, 207

Cognitive systems (*continued*)
central nervous system disorders, 206
cerebral homeostasis, 206
peripheral nervous system disorders, 206
Colic, 288
Collateral circulation, 56
Collecting duct, 304
Color, patient, 15
Colorimetric devices, 22–23
Coma, 206
Commotio cordis, 152
Communicable diseases, 398
Communicable period, 399
Community-acquired infections, 321
Compensatory pause, 94
Complement system, 400
Complete block, 92–93
Complex partial seizures, 221
Complex regional pain syndrome (CRPS), 498
Conduction abnormalities
AV blocks, 177
bundle branch blocks, 178–182, 183–184
chamber enlargement, 182–186
Conductivity, 64
Confusion, 448
Congenital adrenal hyperplasia (CAH), 258
Congestive heart failure (CHF), 140, 141–142
Conjunctivitis, 468
Contaminated food, 351–352
Contamination, 398
Continuous positive airway pressure (CPAP)
in acute respiratory distress syndrome (ARDS), 27
in cardiovascular emergencies, 142–143
defined, 142
device, 142
indications for, 143
procedure illustration, 144
steps for, 143
Contractility, 64
Conversion disorder, 454
CO-oximetry, 212, 338, 339
COPD. *See* Chronic obstructive pulmonary disease
Copperhead, 356
Cor pulmonale, 30
Coral snake bites, 357, 358
Corneal ulcers, 469
Coronary arteries, 55–56
Coronary artery bypass grafting (CABG), 137
Coronary artery disease (CAD), 52
Coronary veins, 56
Corpus callosum, 200
Correct QT (QTc), 72
Corticosteroids, 271
Cortisol, 245
Cottonmouth, 356
Coupling interval, 100
CPAP. *See* Continuous positive airway pressure
Crackles, 19
Cranial nerves
defined, 203–204
disorders, 225–226
illustrated, 205
status, 211
Creatine kinase (CK), 138
Creatine phosphokinase (CPK), 138
Creatinine, 306
Crepitus, 18
Creutzfeldt-Jakob disease (CJD), 228–229
Crohn's disease, 289–290
Croup, 427
CTS (carpal tunnel syndrome), 492
C-type natriuretic peptide (CNP), 62
Cullen's sign, 280
Current of injury, 164
Cushing's disease, 257
Cushing's syndrome, 257
Cushing's triad, 212
CVD (cardiovascular disease), 52–53
CVS (cyclical vomiting syndrome), 286–287
Cyanide
antidote kit, 342
as cellular toxin, 341–342
defined, 341
exposure management, 342–343
signs and symptoms of exposure, 342
Cyanosis, 15
Cyclical vomiting syndrome (CVS), 286–287
Cystic medial necrosis, 154
Cystitis, 321
Cytochrome, 335

D

Decerebrate posturing, 210
Decontamination, 329–330, 407
Decorticate posturing, 210
Deep venous thrombosis, 155
Defibrillation
defined, 122
procedure illustration, 123–124
steps, 123–125
success factors, 123
Defibrillators, 122–123
Degenerative conditions, 493–494
Degenerative disk disease, 493–494
Degenerative neurologic disorders
Alzheimer's disease, 228
amyotrophic lateral sclerosis (ALS), 230
assessment, 230–231
central pain syndrome, 230
Creutzfeldt-Jakob disease (CJD), 228–229
defined, 228
dystonias, 229
Guillain-Barré syndrome, 229
Huntington's disease, 228
management, 231
multiple sclerosis (MS), 229
muscular dystrophy (MD), 229
myoclonus, 230
Parkinson's disease, 229–230
Pick's disease, 228
poliomyelitis (polio), 230
spina bifida, 230
types of, 228–231
Dehydration, in infectious disease patients, 409
Delayed hypersensitivity, 265
Delirium, 450
Delirium tremens (DTs), 363
Delusions, 450
Demargination, 373
Dementia, 450
Denervated, transplanted heart, 62
Dentalgia and dental abscess, 481
Deoxyhemoglobin, 11
Dependent personality disorder, 455
Depersonalization, 454–455
Depression, 452–453
Dermatomes, 203, 204
Descending loop of Henle, 304
Diabetes insipidus, 243
Diabetes mellitus
blood glucose regulation and, 248–249
defined, 247
glucose metabolism and, 248

overview, 247
type 1, 249
type 2, 250
Diabetic emergencies, 247–255
Diabetic foot, 496–497
Diabetic ketoacidosis
assessment and management, 252
defined, 250
pathophysiology, 250–252
signs and symptoms, 252
Diagnostic and Statistical Manual of Mental Disorders, Fifth Edition (DSM-5), 449–450
Diagnostic testing, respiratory patient, 20–24
Dialysate, 317
Diaphoresis, 15
Diaphragm, 7, 13
Diastole, 57
Diazepam/lorazepam, 122
Diencephalon, 200
Diffusion, 11, 14
Disease period, 399
Disinfection, 407–408
Disk injury, 232
Dissecting aortic aneurysms, 154–155
Disseminated intravascular coagulation (DIC), 388
Dissociative disorders, 454–455
Distal tubule, 304
Diuresis, 249, 305
Diverticula, 290
Diverticulitis, 290–291
Diverticulosis, 290
Dobutamine, 121
Dopamine, 121
Downtime, 152
Dromotropy, 61–62
Drug overdose, 360
Dura mater, 200
Dyspnea, 16
Dysrhythmia, 75
Dystonias, 229

E

E. coli, 351
Early goal-directed therapy (EGDT), 440, 441
Early repolarization, 177, 178
Ears
anatomy of, 472–473
external ear, 472
foreign body, 473
illustrated, 472
impacted cerumen, 473
infections, 473
inner ear, 473
labyrinthitis, 475
mastoiditis, 474
medical conditions of, 473–475
Ménière's disease, 475
middle ear, 473
otitis externa, 473–474
otitis media, 474
overview, 472
perforated tympanic membrane, 474, 475
Eating disorders, 455
Ebola virus disease (EVD), 419
ECG. *See* Electrocardiogram
ECG leads. *See also* 12-lead ECG
axes, 160
bipolar, 67, 158–159
defined, 67
illustrated, 160
limb, 67, 158–161
precordial, 68, 161, 162
types of, 67, 158
unipolar (augmented), 68, 159–161
Ecstasy, 360
Ectopic (abnormal beats), 75
Ectopic foci, 75
Ectopic tachycardia, 82
Efferent fibers, 203
18-lead ECGs, 176–177
Einthoven's triangle, 67, 161
Ejection fraction, 58
EKG. *See* Electrocardiogram (ECG)
Elastic cartilage, 488
Electrocardiogram (ECG). *See also* ECG leads
artifacts, 67
changes from electrolyte abnormalities and hypothermia, 109–111
defined, 66
graph paper, 68
illustrated, 73
lead groupings overview, 73
lead systems and heart surfaces, 73
monitoring in the field, 117–119
P wave, 69
PR interval (PRI), 71
prehospital monitoring, 187–190
QRS complex, 69
QRS interval, 71
recording, 68, 157–158
relationship to electrical vents in heart, 68–73
routine monitoring, 67–68
ST segment, 71, 73
T wave, 69
U wave, 71
Electrocardiograph waves, 159
Electrocardiographic monitoring, 65–75
Electrolytes
in cardiac function, 62
tubular handling of, 305–306
Electrophysiology, 62–65
Ellipsoidal joints, 487, 489
Embolic strokes, 215–216
Emphysema
assessment, 31
defined, 30
management, 31
pathophysiology, 30–31
EMS response and postexposure, 422
Encephalitis, 429–430
Endocardium, 53
Endocrine disorders and emergencies
adrenal glands, 257–258
adrenal insufficiency, 258
diabetes mellitus, 247–250
diabetic emergencies, 247–255
diabetic ketoacidosis, 250–252
Graves' disease, 255–256
hyperadrenalism, 257–258
hyperosmolar hyperglycemic state (HHS), 252–254
hypoglycemia (insulin shock), 254–255
hypothyroidism and myxedema, 256–257
pancreas, 247–255
thyroid gland, 255–257
thyrotoxic crisis (thyroid storm), 256
Endocrine glands. *See also specific glands*
defined, 239
illustrated, 240
table of, 241–242
Endocrine system
adrenal glands, 245–246
anatomy and physiology of, 239–247
gonads, 246
hypothalamus, 240
introduction to, 239
pancreas, 244–245
parathyroid gland, 244
pineal gland, 246

Endocrine system (*continued*)
pituitary gland, 243–244
thymus gland, 244
thyroid gland, 244
Endocrinology, 237–260
Endolymph, 473
Endotoxins, 395–396
End-stage kidney disease (ESKD), 314
End-stage renal failure (ESRF), 314
End-tidal CO2 (ETCO2), 22, 23, 24
Enterotoxins, 351
Eosinophils, 374
Epicondylitis, 492
Epididymis, 307
Epigastrium, 115, 116
Epiglottitis, 427, 482
Epinephrine, 121, 245, 270
Epistaxis, 476
Erythrocyte, 371
Erythropoiesis, 372
Erythropoietin, 247, 306, 370
Esophageal varices, 282–283
Esophagus, 480
Estrogen, 246
EVD (Ebola virus disease), 419
Excitability, 63
Excited delirium syndrome, 457
Exocrine glands, 239
Exotoxins, 351, 395
Expiration, 8–9
Expiratory reserve volume, 9
Eyes
anatomy of, 467–468
atraumatic hyphema, 470
cataract, 471
cellulitis, 469
central retinal artery occlusion, 471
central retinal vein occlusion, 471
chalazion, 468
conjunctivitis, 468
corneal ulcers, 469
external anatomy of, 467
glaucoma, 470–471
herpes simplex virus keratitis, 469
herpes zoster ophthalmicus, 469
internal anatomy of, 467–468
iritis, 469
medical conditions of, 468–472
optic neuritis, 471
orbital cellulitis, 470
papilledema, 471
periorbital cellulitis, 470
pterygium, 469
retinal detachment, 471–472
sty, 468

F

Factitious disorders, 454
Fasciitis, 496
Fear, 448
Fecal-oral route, 397
Fentanyl, 121–122
Fibrinogen, 376
Fibrinolysis, 136, 377
Fibrinolytic agents, 122
Fibrocartilage, 488
Fibromyalgia, 499
15-lead ECGs, 176–177
Filtrate, 304
First-degree AV block, 89, 90, 177
Flail chest, 13
Flanks, 303
Flat affect, 451
Food contamination, 351–352
Food poisoning, 429
Forced expiratory volume (FEV), 10
Foreign body
ears, 473
mouth and throat, 481
nose, 476–477
Free radicals, 25
Fugue state, 454
Functional residual capacity, 9
Fungi, 396
Furosemide, 122

G

Gallbladder, 294
Gallstones, 295
Gangrene, 496
Gastric lavage, 330
Gastrin, 247
Gastroenteritis, 428–429
Gastroenterology, 275–299
Gastrointestinal emergencies
accessory organ diseases, 293–297
acute gastroenteritis, 283–284
appendicitis, 293–294
assessment, 278–280
bowel obstruction, 292–293
cholecystitis, 294–295
chronic gastroenteritis, 285
Crohn's disease, 289–290
cyclical vomiting syndrome (CVS), 286–287
diverticulitis, 290–291
esophageal varices, 282–283
hemorrhoids, 291
hepatitis, 296–297
introduction, 277
irritable bowel syndrome (IBS), 291
lower gastrointestinal bleeding, 287–288
lower gastrointestinal diseases, 287–293
mesenteric ischemia, 293
OPQRST-ASPN history, 279
pancreatitis, 295–296
pathophysiology, 277–278
peptic ulcers, 285–286
primary assessment, 278–279
rectal foreign body, 291–292
scene size-up, 278–279
secondary assessment, 279–280
specific illnesses, 280–297
treatment, 280
ulcerative colitis, 288–289
upper gastrointestinal diseases, 281–287
upper GI bleeding, 281–282
Gastrointestinal tract, 281
GCS (Glasgow Coma Scale), 211–212
Generalized seizures, 220–221
Genitourinary system
anatomy of, 307
defined, 302
hematopoietic problems and, 382
Geriatric patients
crisis in, 457
neurologic assessment, 212–213
German measles, 425
Glasgow Coma Scale (GCS), 211–212
Glaucoma, 470–471
Gliding joints, 487, 489
Glomerular filtration, 304
Glomerular filtration rate (GFR), 304
Glomerulus, 304
Glottic opening, 5
Glucagon, 245
Glucocorticoids, 245–246
Gluconeogenesis, 245
Glucose intolerance, 315
Glucose metabolism, 248
Glycogen, 245
Glycogenolysis, 245
Glycosuria, 249
Golfer's elbow, 492
Gonads, 246
Gout, 495–496
Gram stain, 395
Granulocytes, 373–374

Graves' disease, 255–256
Grey Turner's sign, 280
Guillain-Barré syndrome, 229

H

Haldane effect, 12
Hallucinations, 450
Hallucinogens, 360, 362
Hantavirus, 428
HCM (hypertrophic cardiomyopathy), 151–152
Headache
  assessment, 224
  management, 225
  organic, 224
  pain, 224
  statistics, 223–224
  tension, 224
  vascular, 224
  worrisome signs and symptoms, 224
Heart
  anatomy of, 53–56
  blood flow, 54–55, 56
  cardiac cycle, 57–60
  cardiac output, 58
  chambers, 53, 54
  coronary circulation, 55–56
  electrophysiology, 62–65
  as endocrine organ, 62
  location within chest, 53
  nervous control of, 61–62
  tissue layers, 53, 54
  transplanted, 62
  valves, 53–54, 55
Heart failure. *See also* Cardiovascular emergencies
  congestive (CHF), 140, 141–142
  CPAP, 142–143
  defined, 139
  field assessment, 140–142
  left ventricular failure, 139, 140
  management, 142
  right ventricular failure, 139–140, 141
  types and etiologies, 139–140
Heart rate calculator rulers, 74
Heart sounds, 115–116
Heavy metal toxicity, 350–351
Hemarthrosis, 387
Hematemesis, 282
Hematochezia, 284
Hematologic crisis, 384
Hematology, 368–390
Hematopoiesis, 370
Hematopoietic disorders
  anemias, 383–384
  assessment, 379–382
  cardiorespiratory effects, 382
  as chronic conditions, 379
  disseminated intravascular coagulation (DIC), 388
  gastrointestinal effects, 381
  genitourinary effects, 382
  hemophilia, 387
  introduction to, 369–370
  leukemias, 386
  leukocytosis, 385–386
  leukopenia, 385
  lymphatic effects, 381
  lymphomas, 386
  management of, 382–383
  multiple myeloma, 388
  musculoskeletal effects, 382
  physical examination, 380–382
  polycythemia, 383, 385
  primary assessment, 379–380
  scene size-up, 379
  secondary assessment, 380–382
  sickle cell disease, 384–385
  skin and, 381
  thrombocytopenia, 387
  thrombocytosis, 387
  von Willebrand's disease, 388
Hemiblocks, 181–182
Hemodialysis, 317
Hemoglobin, 11, 371, 372–373
Hemoglobin oxygen saturation, 20
Hemolysis, 372
Hemolytic anemias, 383
Hemolytic disease, 378
Hemophilia, 387
Hemoptysis, 16
Hemorrhoids, 291
Hemostasis, 376–377
Hemothorax, 13
Hepatitis
  defined, 296, 412
  hepatitis A, 297, 412–413
  hepatitis B, 297, 413–414
  hepatitis C, 297, 414
  hepatitis D, 297, 414
  hepatitis E, 297, 414
  infections comparison, 413
Hering-Breuer reflex, 10
Hermorrhagic strokes, 216
Hernias, 292
Herpes simplex virus, 426–427
Herpes simplex virus keratitis, 469
Herpes zoster ophthalmicus, 469
HHS. *See* Hyperosmolar hyperglycemic state
High lateral infarct, 171
Hilum, 303
Hinge joints, 487, 489
Histamine, 266
History
  cardiovascular patients, 111–114
  gastrointestinal patients, 279–280
  hematopoietic disorders and, 380
  infectious disease patients, 409
  ingested toxins and, 331
  neurologic patients, 208
  pneumonia patients, 417
  renal and urologic patients, 308
  respiratory patients, 16–17
HIV. *See* Human immunodeficiency virus (HIV)
Homeostasis, 239
Hookworms, 397
Hormones
  adrenal, 245–246
  androgenic, 246
  anterior pituitary, 243
  defined, 239
  ovaries, 246
  pancreas, 245
  parathyroid glands, 244
  pineal gland, 246
  posterior pituitary, 243
  regulation of, 242
  table of, 241–242
  testes, 246
  thymus gland, 244
  thyroid gland, 244
  tubular handling of water and electrolytes, 305
Human chorionic gonadotropin (hCG), 246–247
Human immunodeficiency virus (HIV)
  clinical presentation, 411–412
  defined, 410
  overview, 410
  pathogenesis, 410–411
  postexposure prophylaxis, 412
  risk to general public, 411
  risk to health care workers, 411
  summary of, 412
Humoral immunity, 263, 400
Huntington's disease, 228
Hyaline cartilage, 488
Hydrocarbons, 345
Hydrofluoric acid, 345

Hymenoptera, 263, 328, 353
Hyperadrenalism, 257–258
Hyperbaric oxygen (HBO) therapy, 335, 341
Hypercalcemia, 110
Hyperglycemia, 248–249
Hyperkalemia, 109–110, 313
Hyperosmolar hyperglycemic state (HHS)
  assessment and management, 254
  defined, 252
  pathophysiology, 252–254
  signs and symptoms, 254
Hyperosmolar solution, 305
Hyperoxia, 25
Hypersensitivity
  defined, 264
  delayed, 265
  immediate, 265–266
Hypertensive emergencies. *See also* Cardiovascular emergencies
  conditions, 146
  defined, 145
  field assessment, 145–146
  management, 146–147
Hypertensive encephalopathy, 145
Hyperthyroidism, 255
Hypertrophic cardiomyopathy (HCM), 151–152
Hypertrophy, 182
Hyperventilation syndrome, 44–45
Hyphema, 470
Hypocalcemia, 110
Hypochondriasis, 454
Hypoglycemia, 248, 254–255
Hypoglycemic seizure, 255
Hypokalemia, 109
Hypo-osmolar solution, 305
Hypotension, 409
Hypothalamus, 200, 240
Hypothyroidism, 255, 256–257
Hypoxia, 14, 25

I

IBS (irritable bowel syndrome), 291
Immediate hypersensitivity, 265–266
Immune response, 263, 375
Immune system
  defined, 263, 399
  disease and, 399–400
Immunity
  active, 401
  autoimmunity, 400
  cell-mediated, 400
  humoral, 263, 400
  individual host, 401
  passive, 401
  white blood cells (WBCs) and, 375
Immunoglobulins (Igs), 263, 400
Immunology, 261–274
Impacted cerumen, 473
Impetigo, 436
Impulse control disorders, 456
Impulse formation mechanism, 75–76
Incubation period, 399
Indeterminate axis, 162
Index case, 394
Induced active immunity, 264
Induced therapeutic hypothermia (ITH), 152–153
Infarction, 292
Infection, 398
Infectious crisis, 384
Infectious disease patients
  assessment, 408–409
  assessment precautions, 404–405
  contact with, 403–406
  management precautions, 405–406
  past medical history, 409
  physical examination, 409
  prehospital care considerations, 406
Infectious diseases
  airborne, 397
  avian influenza, 423
  bedbugs, 437–438
  bloodborne diseases, 397
  body's defenses against, 399–401
  chancroid, 436
  chickenpox (varicella), 420–421
  Chikungunya virus disease, 420
  chlamydia, 435–436
  communicable period, 399
  confidentiality of exposure records, 408
  contraction, transmission and stages of, 397–399
  croup, 427
  decontamination methods and procedures, 407–408
  defined, 393
  disease period, 399
  Ebola virus disease (EVD), 419
  encephalitis, 429–430
  enhanced precautions, 404–406
  epiglottitis, 427
  exposures, 408
  fecal-oral route, 397
  food poisoning, 429
  gastroenteritis, 428–429
  genital warts, 434
  GI system, 428–429
  gonorrhea, 433
  hantavirus, 428
  hepatitis, 412–414
  herpes simplex virus, 426–427
  herpes simplex virus type 2, 434–435
  human immunodeficiency virus (HIV)/AIDS, 410–412
  of immediate concern to EMS providers, 410–427
  impetigo, 436
  incubation period, 399
  infection and development of, 398–399
  influenza, 422–423
  interruption of transmission, 402
  introduction to, 393
  latent period, 399
  lice, 436–437
  Lyme disease, 432–433
  measles, 424
  meningitis, 421–422
  microorganisms, 395–397
  Middle East respiratory syndrome (MERS), 418–419
  modes of transmission, 398
  mononucleosis, 426
  mumps, 424–425
  nervous system, 429–433
  nosocomial, 438
  patient contact, 403–406
  patient education, 438
  pertussis, 425–426
  pharyngitis, 427
  pneumonia, 417–418
  postexposure, 408
  in prehospital care, 401–408
  preparation for response, 401–402
  process phases, 399
  rabies, 430–431
  recovery, 406–407
  reporting, 394, 408
  respiratory syncytial virus (RSV), 425
  response, 402–403
  rubella (German measles), 425
  scabies, 437
  severe acute respiratory syndrome (SARS), 418
  sexually transmitted, 433–436
  sinusitis, 428
  skin, 436–437

standard precautions, 403–404
syphilis, 433–434
tetanus, 431–432
transmission prevention, 438–439
trichomoniasis, 436
tuberculosis (TB), 414–417
viral, transmitted by contact, 426–427
window phase, 399
Zika virus disease (ZVD), 419–420
Inferior infarct, 171, 172
Inferior mesenteric artery (IMA), 293
Inferior vena cava, 54–55
Inferolateral infarct, 171
Infestations, 436
Inflammatory joint conditions
ankylosing spondylitis (AS), 494–495
defined, 494
gout, 495–496
rheumatoid arthritis (RA), 494
systemic lupus erythematosus (SLE), 495
Inflammatory process, 375
Influenza, 422–423
Infranodal block, 91
Ingested toxins, 331–332. *See also specific toxins*
Ingestion, 328
Inhalation, 328
Inhaled toxins, 332–333. *See also specific toxins*
Injected toxins
bites and stings, 353–358
ciguatera poisoning, 358
general principles of management, 352–353
marine animal injection, 358
snakebites, 358
Injection, 328
Injury current, 164
Inotropy, 61
Insect stings, 353
Inspection
cardiovascular patient, 114–115
respiratory patient, 18
Inspiration, 8–9
Inspiratory capacity, 9
Inspiratory reserve volume, 9
Insulin, 245, 249
Insulin-dependent diabetes mellitus (IDDM), 249
Interbrain, 200
Intercalated disks, 62
Intercostal muscles, 7, 8
Internodal atrial pathways, 64
Interpolated beat, 99
Interstitial nephritis, 312
Interventricular septum, 53
Intracerebral hemorrhage, 216
Intracranial pressure
increased, 214
shock vital signs comparison, 212
Intrarenal abscesses, 321
Intussusception, 292
Iritis, 469
Iron overdose, 351
Irritable bowel syndrome (IBS), 291
Islets of Langerhans, 244
Isosthenuria, 315
ITH (induced therapeutic hypothermia), 152–153

J

Joints
ball-and-socket, 488, 489
ellipsoidal, 487, 489
gliding, 487, 489
hinge, 487, 489
illustrated, 489
inflammatory conditions, 494–496
pivot, 487, 489
saddle, 487, 489
septic, 497–498
types of, 487–488, 489
Jugular vein distension, 17
Junctional bradycardia, 95–96
Junctional escape complexes and rhythms, 94–95
Juvenile rheumatoid arthritis, 498

K

Kernig's sign, 422
Ketamine, 463
Ketone bodies, 248
Ketosis, 248
Kidney stones. *See* Renal calculi
Kidneys
control of arterial blood pressure, 306
control of erythrocyte development, 306
cross section, 303
defined, 303
gross and microscopic anatomy, 303–304
nephron physiology, 304–305
physiology, 304–306
tubular handling of glucose and urea, 306
tubular handling of water and electrolytes, 305–306
Kiesselbach's plexus, 5, 475
Korsakoff's psychosis, 214
Kussmaul's respirations, 13, 209, 252

L

Labyrinthitis, 475
Lactic dehydrogenase (LDH), 138
Laryngitis, 482
Larynx, 5, 480
Latent period, 399
Lateral infarct, 171
Lead and mercury toxicity, 351
Left anterior hemiblock, 181–182
Left axis deviation, 162, 163
Left bundle branch block, 179–181, 183
Left posterior hemiblock, 181
Left ventricular failure, 139, 140
Leukemias, 386
Leukocytes, 373, 399
Leukocytosis, 385–386
Leukopenia, 385
Leukopoiesis, 373
Lice, 436–437
Lidocaine, 120
Ligament of Treitz, 281
Limb leads, 67
Limbic system, 200
Lithium toxicity, 348
Liver, 382
Liver cirrhosis, 297
Lloyd's sign, 322
Long QT syndrome (LQTS), 151
Los Angeles Prehospital Stroke Screen (LAPSS), 217, 218
Low back pain, 231
Lower airway anatomy, 5–7
Lower gastrointestinal bleeding, 287–288
Lower gastrointestinal diseases, 287–293
Ludwig's angina, 481
Lung cancer, 40–41
Lung compliance, 9
Lungs
capacities, 9
characteristics of, 7
defined, 7
diffusion, 11
perfusion, 11
ventilation, 7–11
volumes, 9–10

Lyme disease, 432–433
Lymph, 400
Lymphatic system, 400–401
Lymphocytes, 374, 400
Lymphomas, 386

M

Macrophages, 400
Major basic protein (MBP), 374
Major depressive disorder, 452
Malignant tumors, 226, 227
Mallory-Weiss syndrome, 281
Manic episodes, 453
Marijuana, 361
Marine animal injection, 358
Masks, 416
Mast cells, 265
Mastoiditis, 474
MAT (multifocal tachycardia), 83
MBP (major basic protein), 374
McBurney's point, 294
MDMA, 360
Measles, 424
Medical conditions, 480–482
Medications. *See also specific medications*
  anaphylaxis, 270–271
  antiarrhythmics, 120
  cardiovascular emergencies, 120–122
  cardiovascular patient, 113–114
  fibrinolytic agents, 122
  myocardial ischemia, 121–122
  nebulized, administration of, 35–36
  psychiatric, 449
  vasopressor agents, 120–121
Medulla, 10, 303
Medulla oblongata, 200
Melatonin, 246
Melena, 282
Ménière's disease, 475
Meninges, 200, 201
Meningitis
  clinical presentation, 421–422
  defined, 421
  immunization, 422
  signs and symptoms of, 224
  transmission factors, 421
Mental status
  defined, 448
  examination, 449
  in respiratory assessment, 15
MERS (Middle East respiratory syndrome), 39–40, 418–419
Mesencephalon, 200
Mesenteric ischemia, 293
Metabolism, 239
Metals overdose, 350–351
Methemoglobin, 336
Methemoglobinemia, 342
Methylene chloride, 335
Microangiopathy, 312
Microorganisms
  bacteria, 395–396
  fungi, 396
  hookworms, 397
  pinworms, 397
  prions, 396
  protozoa, 396–397
  trichinosis, 397
  viruses, 395–396
Middle East respiratory syndrome (MERS), 39–40, 418–419
Mineralocorticoids, 246
Minute respiration volume, 10
Mitral valve, 53
Monoamine oxidase inhibitors (MAOIs) overdose, 346–347
Monocytes, 374
Mononeuropathy, 206
Mononucleosis, 426
Mood disorders, 452–453
Morphine sulfate, 121–122
Motor system status, 211
Mouth and throat
  anatomy of, 478–480
  dentalgia and dental abscess, 481
  epiglottitis, 482
  esophagus, 480
  foreign body, 481
  laryngitis, 482
  larynx, 480
  Ludwig's angina, 481
  medical conditions of, 480–482
  oral candidiasis, 480–481
  oral cavity anatomy, 478
  overview, 478
  peritonsillar abscess, 481
  pharyngitis/tonsillitis, 480, 481
  pharynx, 478
  salivary glands and ducts, 478–480
  teeth, 478, 479
  temporomandibular joint (TMJ) syndrome, 482
  tongue, 478
  tonsils and adenoids, 478
  tracheitis, 482
  uvula, 478
Multifocal tachycardia (MAT), 83
Multiple drug resistant TB (MDR-TB), 414
Multiple myeloma, 388
Multiple organ dysfunction syndrome (MODS), 336
Multiple personality disorder, 454
Multiple sclerosis (MS), 229
Mumps, 424–425
Murphy's sign, 295
Muscular dystrophy (MD), 229
Muscular system, 490
Musculoskeletal system. *See also* Nontraumatic musculoskeletal disorders
  anatomy and physiology of, 487–490
  muscular system, 490
  skeletal system, 487–489
Mushrooms, poisonous, 352
Myalgias, 492
Myocardial infarction (MI). *See also* Cardiovascular emergencies
  acute, localization of, 167–176
  defined, 133
  field assessment, 135–136
  in-hospital management, 139
  illustrated, 134
  localization grid, 169
  management, 137–139
  prehospital management, 137–139
  reperfusion therapies, 136–137
  subendocardial infarction, 166
  tissue damage, 134
  transmural infarction, 166
  types of, 134
Myocardial injury, 164
Myocardial ischemia
  defined, 164
  drugs used for, 121–122
Myocardium, 53
Myoclonus, 230
Myoglobin, 138, 149, 335
Myxedema, 255, 256–257
Myxedema coma, 256

N

Narcissistic personality disorder, 455
Narcotics/opiates, 360, 361
Nasal anatomy, 476
Nasal cavity, 4–5
Nasal flaring, 16
Natural immunity, 264
Naturally acquired immunity, 264

Nebulized medication administration, 35–36
Necrotizing fasciitis (NF), 496
Neoplasms
assessment, 227–228
benign tumors, 226–227
bone, 498
brain, locations and manifestations, 227
defined, 226, 498
malignant tumors, 226, 227
management, 228
Neoplastic processes, 498
Nephrology, 302
Nephrons, 303, 304
Nervous control of the heart, 61–62
Nervous system
anatomy and physiology, 197–205
central nervous system (CNS), 197, 198–203
in hematopoietic evaluation, 380–381
infections, 429–433
introduction, 197
overview illustration, 197
pathophysiology, 205–207
peripheral nervous system (PNS), 197–198, 203–205
Nervous system emergencies
airway and breathing, 213
altered mental status, 213–214
back pain and nontraumatic spinal disorders, 231
brain abscess, 228
circulatory support, 213
cranial nerve disorders, 225–226
degenerative neurologic disorders and dementia, 228–231
headache, 223–225
neoplasms, 226–228
pharmacological interventions, 213
psychological support, 213
seizures, 220–223
steps for reducing symptoms, 213
stroke, 214–220
syncope, 223
transport considerations, 213
"weak and dizzy," 226
Neurologic patient
assessment, 207–213
assessment tools, 212
cardiovascular status, 210
cranial nerves status, 211
eyes, 208–209
face, 208
geriatric considerations, 212–213
Glasgow Coma Scale (GCS), 211–212
history, 208
mental status assessment, 211–212
motor system status, 211
nervous system status, 210–211
nose/mouth, 209
ongoing assessment, 213
physical examination, 208–212
primary assessment, 207–208
respiratory status, 209–210
scene size-up, 207–208
secondary assessment, 208–213
sensorimotor evaluation, 210
vital signs, 212
Neurology, 195–236
Neuromuscular-blocking medications, 463
Neurons, 198
Neurotransmitters, 198
Neutropenia, 374
Neutrophils, 374, 399–400
NF (necrotizing fasciitis), 496
Nitric oxide (NO), 336
Nitroglycerin, 121
Nitrous oxide, 121
Noncompensatory pause, 83
Non-insulin-dependent diabetes mellitus (NIDDM), 250
Nonsteroidal anti-inflammatory drugs (NSAIDs) overdose, 349–350
Non-ST-segment elevation myocardial infarction (NSTEMI), 134, 168
Nontraumatic musculoskeletal disorders. *See also* Musculoskeletal system
ankylosing spondylitis (AS), 494–495
assessment, 491
bone and joint infections, 497
bursitis, 492
carpal tunnel syndrome (CTS), 492
cellulitis, 496
chronic pain syndrome (CPS), 498–499
conditions, 491–499
degenerative conditions, 493–494
degenerative disk disease, 493–494
diabetic foot, 496–497
fasciitis, 496
fibromyalgia, 499
findings, 491
gangrene, 496
golfer's elbow, 492
gout, 495–496
infectious conditions, 496–498
inflammatory conditions, 494–496
introduction to, 486–487
myalgias, 492
neoplastic processes, 498
Osgood-Schlatter disease, 499
osteoarthritis (OA), 493
osteomyelitis, 497
osteoporosis, 493
pediatric conditions, 499
reflex sympathetic dystrophy (RDS), 499
repetitive-motion disorders, 491–492
rheumatoid arthritis (RA), 494
septic joints, 497–498
slipped capital femoral epiphysis, 499
soft tissue infections, 496–497
systemic lupus erythematosus (SLE), 495
tendonitis, 492
tennis elbow, 492
tenosynovitis, 492, 496
Nontraumatic spinal disorders, 231–233. *See also* Back pain
Norepinephrine, 121, 245
Normal 12-lead ECG, 164, 165
Normal flora, 395
Normal sinus rhythm, 75
Normoxia, 25
Nose
anatomy and physiology of, 475–476
epistaxis, 476
foreign body, 476–477
medical conditions of, 476–477
nasal anatomy, 476
rhinitis, 477
sinus anatomy, 476
sinusitis, 477
Nosocomial infections, 321, 438
NSTEMI (non-ST-segment elevation myocardial infarction), 134, 168

O

OA (osteoarthritis), 493
Obligate intracellular parasites, 396
Obsessive-compulsive disorder, 455
Obstructive lung disease, 28–30. *See also* Asthma; Chronic bronchitis; Chronic obstructive pulmonary disease (COPD); Emphysema

Occlusive strokes, 215
Oliguria, 311
Oncotic pressure, 371
Ondansetron, 122
Opportunistic pathogens, 395
OPQRST questions, 16, 309
Optic neuritis, 471
Oral candidiasis, 480–481
Oral cavity anatomy, 478
Orbital cellulitis, 470
Orbital septum, 470
Organic headaches, 224
Organophosphates, 328
Orthopnea, 16
Osgood-Schlatter disease, 499
Osmolarity, 305
Osmosis, 304–305
Osmotic diuresis, 249, 306
Osmotic pull, 371
Osteoarthritis (OA), 493
Osteomyelitis, 497
Osteoporosis, 493
Otitis externa, 473–474
Otitis media, 474
Ovaries, 246
Oxidative stress, 25
Oxygen
  for anaphylaxis, 270
  content, 21
  dissociation curve, 11
  for myocardial ischemia, 121
Oxygenation, 25
Oxyhemoglobin, 11, 335

P

P wave
  analysis, 74
  asystole, 106
  defined, 69
$PaCO_2$, 22
PACs (premature atrial contractions), 83–84
Pain
  referred, 278, 308
  renal and urologic patients, 308
  somatic, 278
  visceral, 277, 308
Pain disorder, 454
Pallor, 15
Palpation
  cardiovascular patient, 116
  chest, 18
Pancolitis, 288
Pancreas
  anatomy of, 296
  defined, 244
  disorders of, 247–255
  hormones, 244
  internal anatomy of, 244
Pancreatitis, 295–296
Panic attack, 451
Papilla, 303
Papilledema, 471
Paralytic shellfish poisoning, 351
Paranasal sinuses, 4
Paranoid personality disorder, 455
Parasites, 397
Parasympathetic nervous system, 198, 204–205
Parathyroid glands, 244
Parietal pleura, 7
Parkinson's disease, 229–230
Paroxysmal nocturnal dyspnea (PND), 16, 141
Paroxysmal supraventricular tachycardia (PSVT), 84–85
Partial seizures, 220, 221
Passive immunity, 264, 401
Past medical history
  cardiovascular patients, 114
  infectious disease patients, 409
Pathogens, 263, 395
Pathological fractures, 498
Patient education
  allergic reactions, 272
  anaphylaxis, 272
  infectious diseases, 438
PEA (pulseless electrical activity), 108
Peak expiratory flow rate (PEFR), 34
Peak flow, 21–22
Pediatric patients
  asthma in, 36
  crisis in, 457
  nontraumatic musculoskeletal disorders in, 499
PEEP (positive end-expiratory pressure), 27
Penis, 307
Peptic ulcers, 285–286
Percussion, chest, 18–19
Percutaneous coronary intervention, 136–137
Perforated tympanic membrane, 474, 475
Perfusion, 11, 14
Pericardium, 53
Perinephric abscesses, 321
Periorbital cellulitis, 470
Peripheral arterial atherosclerotic disease, 155
Peripheral circulation, 57
Peripheral nervous system (PNS). *See also* Nervous system
  autonomic nervous system, 197–198, 204–205
  cranial nerves, 203–204, 205
  defined, 197
  disorders, 206
  nerve categories, 204
  somatic nervous system, 197
  subdivisions, 197–198
Peripheral neuropathy, 206
Peritoneal dialysis, 318
Peritonitis, 277–278
Peritonsillar abscess, 481
Personality disorder clusters, 455–456
Personality disorders, 455
Pertussis, 425–426
PETCO2, 22
pH, arterial PCO2 and, 10
Phagocytosis, 373, 400
Pharmacological interventions
  cardiovascular emergencies, 120–122
  nervous system emergencies, 213
  renal and urologic patients, 311
Pharyngitis, 427, 480, 481
Pharynx, 5, 478
Phobias, 452
Photopigments, 468
Physical examination
  cardiovascular patients, 114–116
  gastrointestinal patients, 280
  hematopoietic disorders and, 380–382
  infectious disease patients, 409
  ingested toxins and, 331
  neurologic patients, 208–212
  renal and urologic patients, 310–311
  respiratory patient, 17–19
Physical restraint, 461–462
Pia mater, 200
Pick's disease, 228
Pineal gland, 246
Pinworms, 397
Pit viper bites, 356–358
Pituitary gland, 243–244
Pivot joints, 487, 489
PJCs (premature junctional contractions), 94
Plants, poisonous, 352

Plasma, 370–371
Platelets
  activation of, 375–376
  defined, 375
  diseases of, 386–388
Pleura, 7
Pleural friction rub, 19
Pleuritic chest pain, 38
Pluripotent stem cells, 370
PND (paroxysmal nocturnal dyspnea), 16, 141
Pneumonia
  assessment, 38, 417
  defined, 37, 417
  history, 417
  immunization and postexposure management, 418
  management, 38–39
  pathophysiology, 38
  patient management and PPE, 418
  risk of, 37
  types of, 38
Pneumothorax, 13
PNS. *See* Peripheral nervous system
Poiseuille's law, 57
Poisonous plants and mushrooms, 352
Poliomyelitis (polio), 230
Polycythemia, 30, 383, 385
Polyneuropathy, 206
Polypeptide cells, 245
Pons, 200
Portal pressure, 282
Position, patient, 15
Positional asphyxia, 462
Positive end-expiratory pressure (PEEP), 27
Posterior pituitary, 243
Postrenal AKI, 313
Post-traumatic stress disorder (PTSD), 452
Posture, 448
PPD, 402, 415
PR interval (PRI)
  analysis, 75
  defined, 71
Precordial leads, 67, 161, 162
Precordial thump, 119–120
Preexcitation syndromes, 109
Pregnancy-induced hypertension, 145
Prehospital 12-lead ECG monitoring, 187–190
Preload, 58
Premature atrial contractions (PACs), 83–84
Premature junctional contractions (PJCs), 94
Premature ventricular contractions (PVCs). *See also* Arrhythmias
  clinical significance, 101
  coupling interval, 100
  description, 98–99
  etiologies, 100–101
  illustrated, 99
  interpolated beat, 99
  multifocal, 100
  patterns of group beating, 100
  treatment, 101
  unifocal, 100
Prerenal AKI, 312
Preventative strategies, 303
Priapism, 320
Primary assessment
  behavioral emergency patient, 448
  cardiovascular patient, 111
  gastrointestinal patient, 278–279
  hematopoietic disorders, 379–380
  neurologic patient, 207–208
  renal and urologic patient, 308
  respiratory patient, 15–16
  toxicologic emergencies, 329
Primary response, 264
Prinzmetal's angina, 132
Prions, 396
Proctitis, 288
Progesterone, 246
Prolonged QT interval, 72
Prostate gland, 307
Prostatitis, 321
Prothrombin, 376
Protozoa, 396–397
Proximal tubule, 304
Pseudoseizures, 221
PSVT (paroxysmal supraventricular tachycardia), 84–85
Psychiatric disorders. *See also* Behavioral emergency patients
  age-related conditions, 457
  anorexia nervosa, 455
  antisocial personality disorder, 455
  anxiety disorders, 451–452
  avoidant personality disorder, 455
  biological (organic), 446–447
  bipolar disorder, 453
  body dysmorphic disorder, 454
  borderline personality disorder, 455
  bulimia nervosa, 455
  cognitive disorders, 450
  conversion disorder, 454
  delirium, 450
  dementia, 450
  dependent personality disorder, 455
  depersonalization, 454–455
  depression, 452–453
  diagnostic elements, 449–450
  dissociative disorders, 454–455
  eating disorders, 455
  excited delirium syndrome, 457
  factitious disorders, 454
  fugue state, 454
  hypochondriasis, 454
  impulse control disorders, 456
  mood disorders, 452–453
  multiple personality disorder, 454
  narcissistic personality disorder, 455
  obsessive-compulsive disorder, 455
  pain disorder, 454
  panic attack, 451
  paranoid personality disorder, 455
  pathophysiology, 446–447
  personality disorder clusters, 455–456
  personality disorders, 455
  phobias, 452
  post-traumatic stress disorder (PTSD), 452
  psychogenic amnesia, 454
  psychosocial, 447
  schizoid personality disorder, 455
  schizophrenia, 450–451
  schizotypal personality disorder, 455
  sociocultural, 447
  somatization disorder, 454
  somatoform disorders, 454
  substance-related disorders, 453–454
  suicide, 456–457
Psychiatric medications, 449
Psychogenic amnesia, 454
Psychosis, 456
Psychosocial conditions, 447
Pterygium, 469
PTSD (post-traumatic stress disorder), 452
Public health agencies, 394
Public health principles, 394
Pulmonary artery, 55
Pulmonary edema, 26–27, 28
Pulmonary embolism
  assessment, 43
  defined, 140
  management, 43–44

Pulmonary embolism (*continued*)
  overview, 43
  pathophysiology, 43
Pulmonary shunting, 14
Pulmonary veins, 55
Pulmonary vessels, 7
Pulmonology
  assessment, 14–24
  introduction to, 3
  pathophysiology, 12–14
  respiratory anatomy and physiology review, 3–12
  respiratory disease, 25–46
  respiratory disorder management, 24–25
Pulse, 116
Pulse oximetry, 20–21, 212
Pulseless electrical activity (PEA), 108
Pulsus paradoxus, 20
Purkinje system, 64–65
PVCs. *See* Premature ventricular contractions
Pyelonephritis, 321
Pyramids, 303

Q

QRS axis, 162
QRS complex
  analysis, 75
  defined, 69
QRS interval, 71
QT interval, 71, 72

R

RA (rheumatoid arthritis), 494
Rabies, 430–431
Rapid axis determination, 163
Rattlesnake, 356
RDS (reflex sympathetic dystrophy), 499
Reabsorption, 304
Reactive oxygen species (ROS), 25
Rectal foreign body, 291–292
Red blood cells (RBC)
  defined, 371
  diseases of, 383–385
  laboratory evaluation of, 372–373
  in oxygen transport, 371–372
  production, 372
Reduced nephron mass, 314–315
Reduced renal mass, 315
Reentry, 75–76
Referred pain, 278, 308
Reflex sympathetic dystrophy (RDS), 499
Refractory periods, 72, 73
Relative refractory period, 72
Renal, 302
Renal AKI, 312
Renal and urologic emergencies
  acute kidney injury (AKI), 311–314
  assessment, 308–311
  chronic kidney disease (CKD), 314–318
  management and treatment plans, 311
  pathophysiology, 308
  priapism, 320
  primary assessment, 308
  renal calculi, 318–320
  scene size-up, 308
  secondary assessment, 308–311
  testicular torsion, 320
  urinary tract infection (UTI), 320–322
Renal calculi
  assessment, 319–320
  defined, 303, 318
  management, 320
  pathophysiology, 319
  stone formation, 318–319
Renal dialysis, 316–318
Renal pelvis, 303
Renin, 306
Reperfusion, 133
Reperfusion therapies, 136–137
Repetitive-motion disorders, 491–492
Repolarization, 63
RES (reticuloendothelial system), 399
Reservoirs, 397
Residual volume, 9
Resistance, 399
Respirations
  abnormal patterns, 13–14
  apneustic, 14, 209
  ataxic (Biot's), 14, 209
  Cheyne-Stokes, 13, 209
  defined, 12
  Kussmaul's, 13, 209, 252
Respirators, 416
Respiratory disorders
  acute respiratory distress syndrome (ARDS), 26–27
  asthma, 32–36
  carbon monoxide inhalation, 41–43
  central nervous system dysfunction, 45
  chronic bronchitis, 31–32
  dysfunction of spinal cord, nerves, or respiratory muscles, 45–46
  emphysema, 30–31
  hyperventilation syndrome, 44–45
  lung cancer, 40–41
  management of, 24–25
  Middle East respiratory syndrome (MERS), 39–40
  obstructive lung disease, 27–30
  oxygenation, 25
  pneumonia, 37–39
  pulmonary embolism, 43–44
  severe acute respiratory syndrome (SARS), 39
  specific, 25–46
  spontaneous pneumothorax, 44
  toxic inhalation, 40–41
  types of, 27–28
  upper airway obstruction, 25–26
  upper respiratory infection, 36–37
Respiratory effort, 16
Respiratory muscles dysfunction, 45–46
Respiratory syncytial virus (RSV), 425
Respiratory system
  airway, in primary assessment, 16
  anatomy and physiology review, 3–12
  assessment, 14–24
  breathing, in primary assessment, 16
  diagnostic testing and, 20–24
  diseases, 25–46
  general impression, 15–16
  history and, 16–17
  introduction to, 3
  lower airway anatomy, 5–7
  management of disorders, 24–25
  pathophysiology, 12–14
  physical examination and, 17–19
  physiologic processes, 7–12
  primary assessment, 15–16
  scene size-up and, 14–15
  secondary assessment, 16–24
  upper airway anatomy, 3–5
  vital signs and, 20
Resting potential, 63
Restraint
  chemical, 462–463
  methods of, 460
  physical, 461–462
  verbal deescalation, 461
  violent patients and, 460–463
Resultant cardiac vector, 162

Resuscitation
ABCs, 152
defined, 152
field termination of, 153–154
withholding, 153
Reticular activating system (RAS), 202
Reticuloendothelial system (RES), 399
Retinal detachment, 471–472
Return of spontaneous circulation (ROSC), 152–153
Rheumatoid arthritis (RA), 494
Rhinitis, 477
Rhonchi, 19
Rhythm strips
defined, 66
interpretation of, 74–75
P wave analysis, 74
PR interval analysis, 75
QRS complex analysis, 75
rate analysis, 74
rhythm analysis, 74
Right axis deviation, 162, 163
Right bundle branch block, 179, 184
Right ventricular failure, 139–140, 141
Right ventricular infarctions, 176–177
Rohypnol, 360–362
ROSC (return of spontaneous circulation), 152–153
Routes of toxic exposure, 327–328
RR interval, 74
RSV (respiratory syncytial virus), 425
Ryan White Act, 408

S

SA node, arrhythmias originating in, 76–82
SAD CAGES mnemonic, 452
Saddle joints, 487, 489
Salicylate overdose, 349
Salivary glands and ducts, 478–480
Salmonella, 351
SAMPLE history, 16, 380
SARS (severe acute respiratory syndrome), 39
Scabies, 437
Scene size-up
behavioral emergency patient, 447–448
cardiovascular patient, 111
gastrointestinal patient, 278–279
hematopoietic disorders, 379
neurologic patient, 207–208
renal and urologic patient, 308
respiratory patient, 14–15
toxicologic emergencies, 329
Schizoid personality disorder, 455
Schizophrenia, 450–451
Schizotypal personality disorder, 455
Scombroid (histamine) poisoning, 351
Scorpion stings, 355–356
Scrotum, 307
Sebum, 467
Secondary assessment
behavioral emergency patient, 448–449
gastrointestinal patient, 279–280
hematopoietic disorders, 380–382
neurologic patient, 208–213
renal and urologic patient, 308–311
respiratory patient, 16–24
toxicologic emergencies, 329
Secondary response, 264
Second-degree Mobitz I block, 89–91
Second-degree Mobitz II block, 91
Secretin, 247
Secretion, 304
Sedatives, 362
Seizures
absence, 221
assessment, 221–222
complex partial, 221
defined, 220
generalized, 220–221
hypoglycemic, 255
management, 222
partial, 220, 221
patient protection, 222
simple partial, 221
status epilepticus, 222–223
tonic-clonic, 220
types of, 220–221
Selective serotonin reuptake inhibitor (SSRI) poisoning, 348
Semen, 307
Semilunar valves, 53
Sensitization, 264
Sensorimotor evaluation, 210
Sepsis
defined, 439
diagnosis, 440
early goal-directed therapy (EGDT), 441
management, 440
risk of developing, 440
severe, 440
spectrum of, 440
Septic joints, 497–498
Septic shock, 440
Septicemia, 439
Sequestration, 372
Seroconversion, 399
Serotonin syndrome, 347–348
Severe acute respiratory syndrome (SARS), 39, 418
Sexually transmitted diseases (STDs)
chancroid, 436
chlamydia, 435–436
defined, 433
genital warts, 434
gonorrhea, 433
herpes simplex virus type 2, 434–435
syphilis, 433–434
trichomoniasis, 436
Shigella, 351
Shock, 212
Sick sinus syndrome, 80–82
Sickle cell disease, 384–385
Simple diffusion, 304
Simple partial seizures, 221
Sinus anatomy, 476
Sinus arrest, 78–79
Sinus arrhythmia, 78
Sinus block, 79–80
Sinus bradycardia, 76–77
Sinus pause, 80
Sinus tachycardia, 77–78
Sinusitis, 428, 477
Six-second method, 74
Skeletal system, 487–489
Skin
cardiovascular patient, 115
diseases of, 436–437
hematopoietic problems and, 381
renal and urologic patients, 310
Skull, bones of, 199
SLE (systemic lupus erythematosus), 495
Slipped capital femoral epiphysis, 499
Slow-reactive substance of anaphylaxis (SRS-A), 266
Snakebites
antivenin, 357
coral snake bites, 358
overview, 356
pit viper bites, 356–358
Snoring, 19
Sociocultural conditions, 447
Sodium channels, 65
Soft tissue infections, 496–497

Somatic nervous system, 197
Somatic pain, 278
Somatization disorder, 454
Somatoform disorders, 454
Somatostatin, 245
Speaking ability, 15–16
Sperm cells, 307
Spina bifida, 230
Spinal cord
  characteristics of, 203
  dysfunction, 45–46
  illustrated, 203
  sectional view, 204
Spontaneous pneumothorax, 44
SRS-A (slow-reactive substance of anaphylaxis), 266
ST segment, 71, 73
Stable angina, 133
Standard precautions, infectious diseases, 403–404
Starling's law of the heart, 58
Status asthmaticus, 36
Status epilepticus, 222–223
STDs. *See* Sexually transmitted diseases (STDs)
STEMI. *See* ST-segment elevation myocardial infarction
Sterilization, 408
Stretch receptors, 10
Stridor, 19
Stroke
  arm drift and, 218
  assessment, 216–217
  causes of, 215
  defined, 214
  embolic, 215–216
  etiologies of, 215
  facial droop and, 217
  hermorrhagic, 216
  intracranial hemorrhage and, 214–220
  management, 219–220
  occlusive, 215
  prehospital scoring systems, 217–219
  signs and symptoms of, 216–217
  syndromes, 217
  thrombotic, 216
  TIAs and, 217–219
Stroke volume, 58
Structural lesions, 206
ST-segment elevation myocardial infarction (STEMI)
  defined, 134
  early repolarization versus, 177
  evolution of, 135
  illustrated, 167
Sty, 468
Subarachnoid hemorrhage, 216
Subcutaneous emphysema, 18
Subendocardial infarction, 134, 166
Substance abuse/overdose
  addiction, 359
  commonly abused drugs, 360, 361–362
  defined, 359
  drug overdose, 360
  drugs used for sexual purposes, 360–362
  tolerance, 359
  withdrawal, 359
Substance-related disorders, 453–454
Sudden death, 149
Suicidal patients, 331
Suicide, 456–457
Superior mesenteric artery (SMA), 293
Superior vena cava, 54
Supraventricular tachycardia, 86
Surface absorption, 328
Surface-absorbed toxins, 333. *See also specific toxins*
Surfactant, 6–7
Survival, 152
Sympathetic nervous system, 198, 204
Synapse, 198
Synchronized cardioversion, 125, 126
Syncope, 222, 223
Syncytium, 63
Synovial fluid, 488
Systemic inflammatory response syndrome (SIRS), 439–440
Systemic lupus erythematosus (SLE), 495
Systole, 57–58

T

T lymphocytes, 400
T wave, 69
Tachyarrhythmias, 75
Tachycardia, 16, 74
Tactile fremitus, 18
TASERed patients, 458–459
TB. *See* Tuberculosis
TCP. *See* Transcutaneous cardiac pacing
Teeth, 478, 479
Temporomandibular joint (TMJ) syndrome, 482
Tendonitis, 492
Tenecteplase, 122
Tennis elbow, 492
Tenosynovitis, 492, 496
Tension headaches, 224
Testes, 246, 307
Testicular torsion, 320
Testosterone, 246
Tetanus, 431–432
Thalamus, 200
Theophylline toxicity, 350
Third-degree AV block, 92–93, 177
Thoracic aorta, 55
Thorax, cardiovascular patient, 115, 116
Throat. *See* Mouth and throat
Thrombocytes, 375
Thrombocytopenia, 387
Thrombocytosis, 375, 387
Thrombosis, 377
Thrombotic strokes, 216
Thrombus, 133
Thymus gland, 244
Thyroid gland
  defined, 244
  disorders of, 255–257
  hormones, 244
Thyrotoxic crisis (thyroid storm), 256
Thyrotoxicosis, 255
TIAs (transient ischemic attacks), 217–219
Tidal volume, 9
Tissue plasminogen activator (tPA), 214
TMJ (temporomandibular joint) syndrome, 482
Tolerance, 359
Tongue, 478
Tonic phase, 220
Tonic-clonic seizure, 220
Tonsils and adenoids, 478
Torsades de pointes, 102, 103
Total downtime, 152
Total lung capacity, 9
Toxic inhalation, 41
Toxic-metabolic states, 206
Toxicologic emergencies
  antidotes, 330–331
  assessment, 329
  decontamination, 329–330
  epidemiology, 327
  ingested toxins, 331–332
  inhaled toxins, 332–333
  introduction to, 326–327
  poison control centers, 327
  as poisoning, 326

primary assessment, 329
routes of exposure, 327–328
scene size-up, 329
secondary assessment, 329
suicidal patients and, 331
surface-absorbed, 333
treatment, 329–331
Toxicology, 325–367
Toxidromes (toxic syndromes), 333, 334–335
Toxins
acetaminophen, 349
alcohol, 345
antidepressants, 347–348
carbon monoxide, 333–341
cardiac medications, 343–344
caustic substances, 344–345
contaminated food, 351–352
cyanide, 341–343
defined, 263, 326
hydrocarbons, 345
hydrofluoric acid, 345
ingested, 331–332
inhaled, 332–333
injected, 352–359
lead and mercury, 351
lithium, 348
MAO inhibitors, 346–347
metals, 350–351
nonsteroidal anti-inflammatory drugs (NSAIDs), 349–350
poisonous plants and mushrooms, 352
routes of exposure, 327–328
salicylates, 348–349
surface-absorbed, 333
theophylline, 350
tricyclic antidepressants, 346
Trachea, 5
Tracheal deviation, 18
Tracheal tugging, 16
Tracheitis, 482
Transcutaneous cardiac pacing (TCP)
defined, 125
procedure illustration, 127–128
steps, 125–128
Transient ischemic attacks (TIAs), 217–219
Transitional fibers, 88
Transmural infarction, 134
Transplanted heart, 62
Trichinosis, 397
Tricuspid valve, 53
Tricyclic antidepressants poisoning, 346
Trigeminal neuralgia, 225–226
Triplicate method, 74
Troponins, 138–139
True posterior infarct, 171–176
Tuberculosis (TB)
clinical presentation of, 415
defined, 414
EMS response, 415–417
multiple drug resistant (MDR-TB), 414
overview, 414–415
pathogenesis, 415
postexposure identification and management, 417
skin testing, 415
Turbinates, 4
12-lead ECG
acute coronary syndrome (ACS), 166–167
acute myocardial infarction, 167–176
angles, 161
axis deviation, 162–164
disease findings, 164–177
normal, 164, 165
prehospital monitoring, 187–190
right ventricular infarctions, 176–177
2:1 AV block, 92
Type 1 diabetes mellitus, 249
Type 2 diabetes mellitus, 250
Type I second-degree AV block, 89–91, 177
Type II second-degree AV block, 91, 177

U

U wave, 71
Ulcerative colitis, 288–289
Unipolar (augmented) leads, 68, 159–161
Universal donors, 378
Unstable angina, 133
Upper airway anatomy, 3–5
Upper airway obstruction
assessment, 25–26
conscious adult, 26
overview, 25
unconscious adult, 26
Upper gastrointestinal diseases, 281–287
Upper respiratory infections (URIs), 36–37
Urea, 302, 306
Uremia, 315
Ureter, 306
Urethra, 306–307
Urethritis, 321
Urinary bladder, 306
Urinary stasis, 320
Urinary system
anatomy and physiology of, 303–308
assessment, 308–311
defined, 302
introduction, 302–303
kidneys, 303–306
male genitourinary system, 307
management and treatment plans, 311
nontraumatic tissue problems, 308
pain types, 308
pathophysiology, 308
ureters, 306
urethra, 306–307
urinary bladder, 306
Urinary tract infection (UTI). *See also* Renal and urologic emergencies
assessment, 321–322
defined, 320
management, 322
pathophysiology, 321
stone formation and, 319
Urine, 302
Urology, 300–324
Urticaria, 268
Uvula, 478

V

Vagal maneuvers, 119
Valves, heart, 53–54, 55
Varicella, 420
Varicose veins, 156
Vas deferens, 307
Vascular headaches, 224
Vasculitis, 155
Vasoocclusive crisis, 384
Vasopressin, 121
Vasopressor agents, 120–121, 271
Vectors, 162, 163
Veins, 57
Venous system, 57
Ventilation
airway resistance and lung compliance, 9
defined, 7
disruption in, 13

Ventilation (*continued*)
inspiration and expiration, 8–9
lung volumes, 9–10
medulla control of, 10
regulation of, 10–11
Ventilation systems, 416–417
Ventricles
arrhythmias originating in, 96–105
electrical excitation of, 72
Ventricular conduction disturbances, 108–109
Ventricular enlargement, 182, 186
Ventricular escape complexes and rhythms, 97, 98
Ventricular fibrillation, 102–103
Ventricular repolarization, 72
Ventricular syncytium, 63
Ventricular tachycardia, 101–102
Venules, 57
Vertebral injury, 232
Vestibule, 5
Viral conjunctivitis, 469
Viral hepatitis, 297
Virulence, 398
Viruses, 395–396
Visceral pain, 277, 308
Visceral pleura, 7
Vital signs
comparison in shock and increased intracranial pressure, 212
neurologic patient, 212
renal and urologic patient, 311
respiratory patient, 20
Vitreous humor, 467
Volvulus, 292
von Willebrand's disease, 388

W

Wandering atrial pacemaker, 82
Waterhouse-Friderichsen syndrome (WFS), 258
"Weak and dizzy," 226
Wenckebach block, 89–91
Wernicke's syndrome, 214
Wheezing, 19
White blood cells (WBCs)
basophils, 374
defined, 373
diseases of, 385–386
eosinophils, 374
granulocytes, 373–374
illustrated, 373
lymphocytes, 374
monocytes, 374
neutrophils, 374
types of, 373
Whole bowel irrigation, 330
Window phase, 399
Withdrawal, 359
Wolff-Parkinson-White (WPW) syndrome, 109
Wright spirometer, 21

X

Xanthines, 350

Z

Zika virus disease (ZVD), 419–420
Zollinger-Ellison syndrome, 286